Connective Tissue

Histophysiology, Biochemistry, Molecular Biology

Connective Tissue

Histophysiology, Biochemistry, Molecular Biology

Nikolay Omelyanenko
Leonid Slutsky
Sergey Mironov, Editor

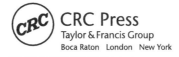

CRC Press
Taylor & Francis Group
Boca Raton   London   New York

CRC Press is an imprint of the
Taylor & Francis Group, an **Informa** business

CRC Press
Taylor & Francis Group
6000 Broken Sound Parkway NW, Suite 300
Boca Raton, FL 33487-2742

First issued in paperback 2016

© 2014 by Taylor & Francis Group, LLC
CRC Press is an imprint of Taylor & Francis Group, an Informa business

No claim to original U.S. Government works

Version Date: 20131114

ISBN 13: 978-1-138-03410-5 (pbk)
ISBN 13: 978-1-4822-0358-5 (hbk)

This book contains information obtained from authentic and highly regarded sources. Reasonable efforts have been made to publish reliable data and information, but the author and publisher cannot assume responsibility for the validity of all materials or the consequences of their use. The authors and publishers have attempted to trace the copyright holders of all material reproduced in this publication and apologize to copyright holders if permission to publish in this form has not been obtained. If any copyright material has not been acknowledged please write and let us know so we may rectify in any future reprint.

Except as permitted under U.S. Copyright Law, no part of this book may be reprinted, reproduced, transmitted, or utilized in any form by any electronic, mechanical, or other means, now known or hereafter invented, including photocopying, microfilming, and recording, or in any information storage or retrieval system, without written permission from the publishers.

For permission to photocopy or use material electronically from this work, please access www.copyright.com (http://www.copyright.com/) or contact the Copyright Clearance Center, Inc. (CCC), 222 Rosewood Drive, Danvers, MA 01923, 978-750-8400. CCC is a not-for-profit organization that provides licenses and registration for a variety of users. For organizations that have been granted a photocopy license by the CCC, a separate system of payment has been arranged.

Trademark Notice: Product or corporate names may be trademarks or registered trademarks, and are used only for identification and explanation without intent to infringe.

Visit the Taylor & Francis Web site at
http://www.taylorandfrancis.com

and the CRC Press Web site at
http://www.crcpress.com

CONTENTS

AUTHORS INFORMATION IX

INTRODUCTION XI

CHAPTER 1.
PECULIARITIES OF CONNECTIVE TISSUE
HISTOPHYSIOLOGY, BIOCHEMISTRY
AND MOLECULAR BIOLOGY

1.1. Definitions, organization principles,
and classification of connective tissue.........................2
1.2. Basic definitions, principles and emphasis
of modern biochemistry and molecular biology 4
1.3. General biochemical aspects of connective tissue.......8
1.4. Formation and histogenesis of connective tissue.......11
1.4.1. Embryology and histogenesis of connective tissue ...11
1.4.2. Molecular and biochemical regularities of initial
stages of connective tissue structures formation.......13

CHAPTER 2.
CELLULAR ELEMENTS OF CONNECTIVE TISSUE

2.1. Proper cells of connective tissue 18
2.2. Fibroblastic differon 19
2.2.1. Histophysiologic characteristics of fibroblastic
differon...19
2.2.2 Biochemical and molecular biological characteristics
offibroblastic differon 45
2.3. Adventitious cells...56
2.4. Adipose cells (lipocytes, adipocytes) 56
2.4.1. Histophysiologic characteristics of adipose cells........56
2.4.2. Biochemical and molecular biological characteristics
of adipose cells 64
2.5. Cells associated with connective tissue 68
2.5.1. Macrophages...68
2.5.2 Mast cells (tissue basophiles) (mc) 72
2.5.3. Plasma cells (plasmocytes) 76

CHAPTER 3.
EXTRACELLULAR MATRIX OF CONNECTIVE TISSUE.
HISTOPHYSIOLOGY, BIOCHEMISTRY AND MOLECULAR
BIOLOGY

3.1. Fibrous structures 80
3.1.1. Collagen fibrous structures.......................................80
3.1.1.1. Biochemistry of collagenous proteins. Collagen
classification. Collagen biosynthesis.........................80
3.1.1.2. Collagen fibrillogenesis and fiber formation 93
3.1.1.3. Composition of collagen fibrous structures.............95

3.1.2. Elastic fibrous structures..107
3.1.2.1. Biochemistry of fibrillin microfibrils 107
3.1.2.2. Elastin biochemistry 109
3.1.2.3. Formation of elastic fibers 112
3.1.2.4. Structure of elastic fibers 112
3.1.2.5. Organ peculiarities of elastic fiber structure..........118
3.2. Integrating buffer metabolic medium (ground
substance) of connective tissue extracellular
matrix 121
3.2.1. Biochemical characteristics of glycoconjugates
and their classification..121
3.2.1.1. Glycoproteins: structure and functions..................125
3.2.1.2. Proteoglycans: structures, properties
and biosynthesis 132
3.2.1.3. Structural organization of connective tissue
integrating buffer metabolic medium
(ground substance) 140
3.3. Basement membranes 144
3.3.1. Structure of basement membranes 144
3.3.2. Biochemistry of basement membranes 144
3.4. Interstitial (interfibrous and intercellular) space
of connective tissue..152
3.5. Structural peculiarities of connective tissue
various types and their organ specificity..................152
3.5.1. Morphological characteristics of connective
tissue of various types 152
3.5.2. Peculiarities of organ structure of fibrous
connective tissue..157
3.5.3. Biochemical and molecular biological
characteristics of fibrous dense connective
tissue 171
3.6. General regularities of molecular
and supramolecular organization of connective
tissue extracellular matrix. Molecular mechanisms
of cells and matrix interaction 177
3.6.1. Main general peculiarities of macromolecular
components of extracellular matrix 177
3.6.2. Interaction of extracellular matrix macromolecular
components and morphogenetic role of these
interactions 179
3.6.3. Proteins of cell (cytoplasmic) membrane.
Cells' interactions with extracellular matrix 181
3.7. Catabolism of macromolecular components
extracellular of the matrix 185
3.7.1. Metalloproteases (metalloproteinases) 185
3.7.2. Inhibitors of metalloproteases 189

CHAPTER 4.
REGULATION OF CONNECTIVE TISSUE
METABOLIC FUNCTIONS

4.1.   Systemic factors of regulation 192
4.2.   Local factors of regulation 193

CHAPTER 5.
BIOCHEMICAL AND MOLECULAR
MECHANISMS AND MANIFESTATIONS
OF CONNECTIVE TISSUE AGEING 199

CHAPTER 6.
BONE – AN ORGAN OF THE SUPPORT AND LOCOMOTOR
APPARATUS CONTAINING ALL TYPES OF CONNECTIVE
TISSUE

6.1.   Overview of bone structure and function 208
6.2.   General structural and functional characteristics
        of bone components 209

CHAPTER 7.
CARTILAGE – CARTILAGINOUS TISSUE: STRUCTURAL,
BIOCHEMICAL AND MOLECULAR BIOLOGICAL
CHARACTERISTICS

7.1.   Overview of structure and composition
        of cartilage tissue 246
7.2.   Hyaline cartilages – cartilage tissues 249
7.2.1. Hyaline articular cartilages 249
7.2.1.1. Cartilage cells differon 249
7.2.1.1.1. Morphology and histophysiology
        of chondroblast and chondrocyte 249
7.2.1.1.2. Biochemical and molecular biological
        characteristics of chondroblast and chondrocyte 265
7.2.1.2. Extracellular matrix 271
7.2.1.2.1. Fibrillar components of cartilaginous tissue 271
7.2.1.2.1.1. Biochemical characteristics 271
7.2.1.2.1.2. Morphologic characteristics 275
7.2.1.2.2. Structure of articular cartilage minerals 286
7.2.1.2.3. Organization of articular cartilage interstitial
        space 294
7.2.1.2.4. Glycoconjugates of cartilaginous tissue 294
7.2.1.2.4.1. Biochemical characteristics of glycoproteins
        and proteoglycans 294
7.2.1.2.4.2. Morphological characteristic of structured
        polysaccharide complexes 307
7.2.1.3. Cartilaginous tissue as an integrated system
        (structural functional unity of cells and matrix) 311

7.2.1.4. Metabolism of cartilaginous tissue 314
7.2.1.5. Regulation of cartilaginous tissue metabolic
        functions 317
7.2.1.5.1. Systemic factors of regulation 317
7.2.1.5.2. Local factors of regulation 320
7.2.1.6. Biomechanical (mechanochemical) aspects
        of articular cartilage 323
7.2.2. Hyaline non-articular cartilages – cartilaginous
        tissues 326
7.2.2.1. Morphologic characteristic 326
7.3.   Elastic cartilages – cartilaginous tissue 327
7.3.1. Morphologic characteristic 327
7.4.   Fibrous cartilages – cartilaginous tissue 334
7.4.1. Morphologic characteristic 334

CHAPTER 8.
BONE TISSUE: THE STRUCTURAL-FUNCTIONAL,
BIOCHEMICAL AND BIOMOLECULAR CHARACTERISTICS
OF ITS COMPONENTS

8.1.   General overview of bone tissue structure
        and composition 342
8.1.1. The structure of bone tissue 342
8.1.2. Chemical composition of bone tissue 343
8.2.   Differons of bone cells 346
8.2.1. Osteogenic cells (osteoblasts, osteocytes)
        and their progenitors 346
8.2.1.1. Morphology of preosteoblasts and osteoblasts 346
8.2.1.2. Molecular biological and biochemical
        characteristics of osteoblasts 354
8.2.1.3. Morphology of osteocytes 358
8.2.1.4. Biochemical and molecular biological
        characteristics of osteocytes 358
8.2.2. Osteoclasts. Osteoclastic resorption of bone
        tissue 361
8.2.2.1. Morphology of osteoclasts 361
8.2.2.2. Functions of osteoclasts and biochemical
        mechanisms of osteoclastic bone tissue
        resorption 362
8.3.   Extracellular matrix of bone tissue 370
8.3.1. Organic component of bone matrix 370
8.3.1.1. Biochemical characteristic of bone matrix
        organic component 370
8.3.1.1.1. Collagenous components of matrix. Fibrillin 370
8.3.1.1.2. Non-collagen components of bone matrix 371
8.3.1.1.3. Matrix non-specific components 374
8.3.1.2. Morphological characteristic of organic
        component of bone matrix 375
8.3.2. Mineral component of bone matrix 376

8.3.2.1. Chemical characteristic of mineral
component...376
8.3.2.2. Morphologic (structural) arrangement
of mineral component...............................386
8.3.2.3. Dynamics and biochemical mechanisms
of structuring (mineralization) bone minerals............387
8.3.2.4. Structuring of bone minerals in reparative
bone regeneration 400
8.3.2.5. Demineralization of bone matrix *in vitro*
and subsequent structuring (crystallization)
of bone minerals dissolved on its surface 405
8.3.2.6. Structure of coral skeleton 410
8.3.2.7. Structure of sea-shell mineral 410
8.3.2.8. Role of mineral component in bone
biomechanical properties 410
8.4.   Interstitial space of bone tissue...............................411
8.4.1. Morphologic characteristic of bone canals 411
8.4.2. Physico-chemical characteristics
of interstitial space of bone tissue..........................419
8.5.   Regulation mechanisms of bone tissue
metabolism and functions..421
8.5.1. Systemic factors and regulation mechanisms
(hormones, neuroendocrine factors, vitamins) 421
8.5.2. Local (short distance) regulation factors
of bone tissue metabolic functions 443
8.6.   Remodeling of bone tissue 450
8.6.1. Definition, classification, general characteristic........450
8.6.2. Molecular and biochemical mechanisms
of bone tissue remodeling 450
8.7.   Tooth connective tissue 457
8.7.1. Structural organization 457
8.7.1.1. Pulp 457
8.7.1.2. Dentin 457
8.7.1.3. Enamel 468

CHAPTER 9.
BIOCHEMICAL CHARACTERISTIC OF SYNOVIAL
MEMBRANE AND SYNOVIA

9.1. Synovial membrane..474
9.2. Synovia (synovial fluid)...476
9.2.1. General characteristics of synovia.
Protein components.....................................476
9.2.2. Synovia hyaluronan...480
9.2.3. Molecular mechanisms of synovia lubricating
function...482

CHAPTER 10.
MOLECULAR BIOLOGICAL AND BIOCHEMICAL
REGULARITIES OF CONNECTIVE TISSUE
STRUCTURES ONTOGENESIS

10.1. Molecular biological and biochemical mechanisms
of mesenchyme condensation. Regulation
systems of connective tissue structure
morphogenesis 486
10.2. Differentiation of connective tissue cells 500
10.2.1. Molecular biological and biochemical
mechanisms of fibroblast differentiation
and formation of fibrous (dense) connective
tissue structures 500
10.2.2. Molecular biological and biochemical
mechanisms of chondroblastic differentiation..........500
10.2.3. Molecular biological and biochemical
mechanisms of osteoblastic differentiation..............507
10.2.4. Molecular biological mechanisms
of osteoclastogenesis and its regulation..................518
10.3. Molecular biological and biochemical
regularities of skeleton formation and growth..........520
10.3.1. Molecular biological and biochemical
regularities of bone formation.................................520
10.3.1.1. Ossification types. Endochondral ossification 520
10.3.1.2. Molecular biological and biochemical
regularities of metaepiphyseal cartilage
function 521
10.3.1.3. Intramembraneous ossification 529
10.3.1.4. Type x collagen 533
10.4. Molecular biological and biochemical
mechanisms of joint formation 534
10.4.1. Mechanisms of joint formation............................534
10.4.2. Molecular factors of regulation of joint
formation..537

REFERENCES.. 541

LIST ABBREVIATIONS 595

INDEX 605

AUTHORS INFORMATION

Nikolay Petrovich OMELYANENKO

Doctor of Medicine, Professor, Member of the New York Academy of Sciences, Winner of the Prize of the Russian Federation Government, the Chief of the Laboratory of connective tissue of the Central Research Institute of Traumatology and Orthopedics of N.N. Priorov, the Department of Public Health of the Russian Federation. The scientific interests: structural and functional organization of bone, cartilaginous tissue and other connective tissue types in health, regeneration and pathology.

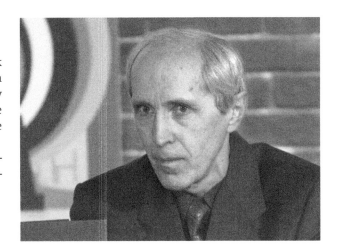

Leonid Ilyich SLUTSKY

Professor Emeritus, Doctor Habilitatus of Medicine. In 1960–1996–the Chief of the Laboratory of Biochemistry of the Riga Research Institute of Traumatology and Orthopedics (Latvia).
The main scientific interests: biochemistry of the connective tissue and skeleton.

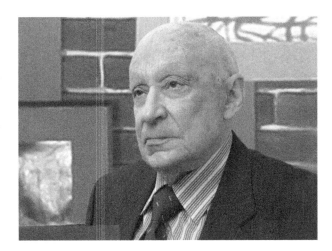

Sergey Pavlovich MIRONOV

Doctor of Medicine, Professor, Academician of the Russian Academy of Sciences and Russian Academy of Medical Sciences, Honoured Worker of Science of the Russian Federation, Winner of the State Prize and the Prize of the Russian Federation Government, the Head of the Central research institute of traumatology and orthopaedics of N.N. Priorov, the Department of Public Health of the Russian Federation.
Field of research: clinical and fundamental orthopedics and traumatology.

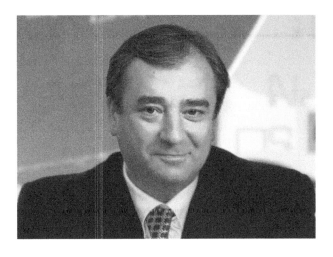

INTRODUCTION

One of the most important matter in a mammals' organism is connective tissue, which is the most complex structure and is responsible for numerous vital functions such as tissue-organ integration, metabolism, regulation, morphogenesis, homeostasis maintenance, biomechanical (support), protection, etc.

Connective tissue is the most prevalent tissue in the body, making up more than a half of human body weight and possessing a high functional activity, including metabolic and immunologic ones. The possibility to use the regeneration potential of the connective tissue as a basis for physiological renewal and reparation determines an effective healing of damaged tissues and organs in the body. Traumas, stress of various genesis, genetic factors, social problems, age, diet, ecology and other factors cause damage to the connective tissue structure and functions that, in turn, leads to numerous and frequently serious disorders with a long chronic course when the connective tissue and other tissues and organs depending on it are affected.

The basic knowledge of connective tissue in histophysiology, biochemistry and molecular biology is of both fundamental scientific interest, and applied relevance in clinical medicine. Its comprehensive study can promote mankind to new discoveries in the field of studying the body's internal processes.

The **first part** (chapters 1–5) of the monograph is devoted to the discussion of the patterns of structure, genesis and functions of cellular differons and the behaviour of connective tissue cells when cultured in an incubator integrated with an optical microscope, DIC-contrast and time-lapse imaging that are common to all types of connective tissue. The data on the multilevel (from the macro- to nanolevel) structural organization of extracellular matrix, the chemical nature of its macromolecular components and their metabolism, system and local regulation factors are presented.

The **second part** (chapters 6–10) contains an extensive review of the current data on biochemistry and molecular biology of skeletal connective tissue (bone and cartilaginous), their metabolism and regulation. It deals with a comprehensive analysis of the data in relation to molecular mechanisms of connective tissue ontogenesis, from the earliest stages of embryonic development and up to ageing. Essentially novel findings on the structural

dynamics of bone marrow stromal connective tissue cells when cultured are presented. These fundamental data are especially of immediate interest in relation to the vigorous development of cell-based technologies. The organization of interstitial channels in bone tissue is described in detail according to the morphological and physical and chemical data. The novel investigations results of a nanostructure of bone mineral, mineralized cartilage, teeth, recrystallized minerals (i.e. minerals derived from tissues and reconstituted as crystals) and in comparison with that of a coral and a seashell obtained with electron microscopy (SEM and TEM) are presented in the book. There are no analogues of these results in the worldwide science.

The monograph peculiarities are as follows:

— a logic combination of classic and modern complementary data on histophysiology, biochemistry and molecular biology of the connective tissue, as well as the results of the authors' original investigations of both known, and new, unpublished before;

— morphological illustrations (micrographs), represented in the monograph, are made by one of the monograph's authors–Omelyanenko;

— the majority of the presented authors' morphological data is gained while studying the human connective tissue;

— the monograph supplements, to a certain extent, to the existing guidelines on biochemistry.

On its content and novelty the book can be of interest, on the one hand, for fundamental researchers–histophysiologists, morphologists, pathologists, biochemists, specialists in molecular biology and embryology, on the other hand, for clinicians–rheumatologists, traumatic orthopedists, dental specialists, dermatologists, cosmeticians, ophthalmologists, gerontologists and many others.

The authors especially hope that the monograph will be useful to young researchers and will promote the further studying of various aspects of the connective tissue structure and functions.

Chapter 1

PECULIARITIES
OF CONNECTIVE
TISSUE
HISTOPHYSIOLOGY,
BIOCHEMISTRY
AND MOLECULAR
BIOLOGY

1.1. DEFINITIONS, ORGANIZATION PRINCIPLES AND CLASSIFICATION OF CONNECTIVE TISSUE

Connective tissue (CT) is a structural functional complex of specialized cells, which are derivatives of the mesenchyma, fibrous structures and the integrating buffer metabolic medium (ground substance) carrying out the integrating, regulatory, trophic, biomechanical, morphogenetic, plastic and protective functions in an organism.

The presence of an extracellular (intercellular) matrix (EM) in its structure is a distinct feature of the connective tissue. The EM considerably exceeds the mass of cell elements that produce it, carries out the basic functions of connective tissue, and serves as a medium for the existence of other cells, mesenchyma derivatives, as well as those involved in CT vital activities and in various metabolic processes.

The extracellular matrix, in turn, is a significantly complicated component of the connective tissue, comprising collagen and elastic type fibrous structures, which are surrounded by the integrating buffer metabolic medium (ground substance).

The specialized cellular elements of the connective tissue (the CT cells properly) are located between the fibrous structures and are surrounded by the integrating buffer metabolic medium. They produce and renew an intercellular matrix, thereby maintaining a quantitative proportion of its composition.

The specificity of connective tissues' organ structure is determined by a combination of qualitative and quantitative differences in the cell structure composition (the CT proper cells and the associated ones) and non-cellular components: the composition and structure of a fibrous framework, the proteoglycans' composition, the physical and chemical properties of the intercellular matrix, and the interstitial space volume.

The combination of these parameters is taken as a principle for the allocation of proper (fibrous) connective tissues, connective tissues with special properties, and skeletal tissues. It is necessary to emphasize that the convention of the proposed classification for fibrous structures is present in all types of connective tissue, but in the first of them, fibrous CT, there is much more of them than in the second group–CT with special properties. The group of skeletal CT is distinguished by the mineralization of all bone tissue and partially cartilaginous tissue. The latter is subdivided into three types of cartilaginous tissue (hyaline, elastic and fibrous) and three types of bone tissue (lamellar, rough-fibrous and reticular-fibrous).

In turn, fibrous structures' orientation and their volume ratio to interfibrous and intercellular spaces form the basis for the allocation of loose, dense regular (oriented) and dense irregular (non-oriented) connective tissues (the dermis, tendons, ligaments, aponeuroses and others). An analysis of the group of connective tissues with special properties has shown that reticular tissue, which belongs to this group, can undoubtedly be considered as loose irregular connective tissue as the reticular fibers are a type of the collagen fibers whose basis is composed of a type III collagenous protein. The jelly or mucous connective tissue normally encountered in the umbilical cord (Wharton's jelly) of the fetus should be referred to as embryonic tissues, along with the connective tissue of the provisory organs. Therefore, the group of CT with special properties is comprised of adipose connective tissue consisting of two types: white and brown.

Thus, three type of connective tissue will be subdivided as such:
1) fibrous connective tissue (loose, dense regular and dense irregular);
2) adipose connective tissue (white and brown); and
3) skeletal tissue (bone and cartilaginous).

If the existence of the organ-specific peculiarities of connective tissues is taken into consideration, it is pertinent to allocate *three groups of connective tissues*:
1) intraorgan (organ) connective tissue;
2) extraorgan (interorgan) connective tissue with a prominent trophic function; and
3) connective tissue of organs with a biomechanical function. The aforementioned information is combined and presented in *Fig.1.1*.

The intraorgan connective tissue forms intermediate layers between tissues of a different nature (epithelial, muscular, nervous), surrounds the blood vessels, and creates a microenvironment for organs' basic functional components. The extraorgan connective tissue (subcutaneous, retroperitoneal) fills in the spaces between organs. Structurally, it can be fibrous connective tissue (loose or dense) with greater or fewer adipocytes and fibers of different orientation. The vessels and nerves also pass therein.

The connective tissues of organs with a prominent biomechanical function include bones, cartilages, tendons, ligaments, teeth and the dermis. All of them are rich in fibers; these are mostly collagen fibers rather than elastic ones. The mineralization of the intercellular matrix occurs in a number of cases (i.e. for the teeth and bones). Given that, throughout life, the human body is constantly exposed to various damaging influences of a greater or lesser extent, resulting in the impairment of tissue structural organization of the supraphysiological limits (range), *reparative connective tissue*, which essentially differs from the unchanged (*physiologic*) CT, is always formed in the damaged area. These differences are associated with its formation under different biochemical and biomechanical conditions. In some topographical types, this connective tissue remains life-long in its specific kind, which is distinct from the unchanged connective tissue that induces its allocation as a separate type. In other topographical regions, the damaged connective tissue is restored or subsequently remodeled without subsequent visible morphological deviations.

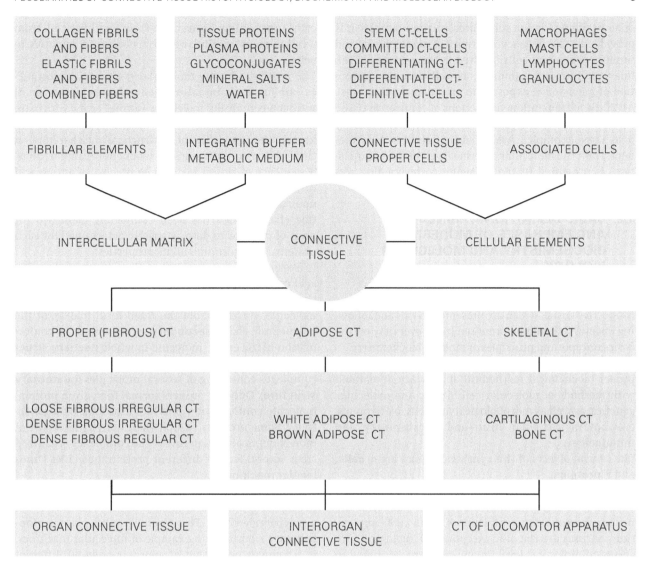

Fig.1.1
(according to Omelyanenko).

Evaluating the connective tissue in view of an organism's development, it is possible to determine:
1) the connective tissue of an embryo and its provisory organs;
2) the developing connective tissue of a fetus and in the early postnatal period; and
3) the connective tissue of an adult / mature organism. A considerable quantity of stem cells, glycoproteins and proteoglycans, the prominent asynchrony of development, and the high rates of differentiation in the provisory organs distinguish the connective tissue of an embryo and its provisory organs (the chorion and placenta, along with the umbilical cord, amnion, allantois).

The functions of connective tissues are manifold: integrating, trophic, regulatory, morphogenetic, biomechanical (supporting), plastic, protective and reparative. Being a uniform structural functional system, the connective tissue carries out an integrating function; hence it is named as such. It is this tissue that unites all the organism's organs and systems into an integral unit and maintains the particular, genetically determined spatial mutual relationships between them. The trophic function is associated with the nutrition regulation of tissue structures of the given region, and their participation in metabolism and homeostasis maintenance in the organism internal medium. Here the integrating buffer metabolic medium (ground substance) plays the leading role: the transport of water, salts, nutrients and waste products is carried out via it. The morphogenetic (structural educating) function manifests in the regulating influence of some connective tissue components on proliferation and the differentiation of cells of various tissues. The supporting, biomechanical function is one of the main functions. Collagen and elastic fibers form fibrous frameworks of all organs, determining their strength and elasticity (for example, tendons and ligaments). Connective tissues' plastic function is realized in their adaptation to changing living conditions, in regeneration, and in the restoration. The protective function consists of neutralizing foreign substances, microorganisms. It is provided by the phagocyte activity of macrophages and immunocompetent cells involved in the response of cellular and humoral immunity, as well as in the prevention of mechanical exposure to an organism (damages). All of the aforementioned functions of connective tissue are carried out by its structural components individually or as a tissue complex. A detailed analysis of each component, from the molecular to tissue levels of the organization, is presented in the following corresponding sections of the monograph.

1.2. BASIC DEFINITIONS, PRINCIPLES AND EMPHASES OF MODERN BIOCHEMISTRY AND MOLECULAR BIOLOGY

Data on the biochemistry of the locomotor apparatus connective tissue, which are presented in this and following chapters, should be premised by an overview on the basic concepts and principles of modern biochemistry. Modern biochemistry is a synthetic science based on the proper biochemical methodical approaches, integrated with methods of molecular cell biology and molecular genetics, as well as morphological methods, electron microscopy in particular, histo–and cytochemistry, and immunology.

The central objects of this synthetic science are *a)* **cells**, and *b)* **proteins**.

The significance of a cell as the central object of biochemistry is determined by the fact that the cell is the primary essential structural unit of life in all its implications; viruses are the only exception. All biological processes on molecular level, in any case, are attributed to the cell functions; all these processes are comprise the **metabolism**, and the basic part of metabolic reactions proceeds in cells. The cell produces (biosynthesis) the main substrate of life–proteins; this is a cell **anabolic** function. On the other hand, the cell also carries out degradation, the destruction of proteins; this is a cell **catabolic** function.

The proteins being the basic material from which both the cells and the **extracellular matrix** surrounding the cells are comprised determines their importance. According to some very approximate and probably a little exaggerated calculations, a human body contains about 400 000 various proteins. This number includes, first of all, **structural proteins** comprising the cells and the basic intracellular structures, and the extracellular matrix produced by cells. The basic active biochemical agents' functioning in the cells and tissues of living organisms are proteins. Firstly, these are the **enzymes** catalyzing almost all biochemical reactions both inside the cells and outside of them. (Some proteins combine both functions–being the structural components of living tissues while, at the same time, exhibiting enzymatic activity.) Secondly, these are extremely numerous **signaling molecules**, which transfer the information necessary for

cells' functioning: inside cells, from a cell to a cell, from a cell to an extracellular matrix,s and from a matrix to cells.

The proteins–highly molecular (polymeric) substances–are linear chains (also called **polypeptides**) of small nitrogen-containing molecules–amino acids, which are successively connected. 20 principal amino acids are known; they are different in structure and therefore, in their ability to enter various biochemical interactions. A sequence of amino acids (to be precise, of amino acid residues, as an amino acid molecule omits some atoms upon insertion into a polypeptide chain) in the polypeptide chain, which has been completely identified for most of proteins to date, is strictly determined for each protein and determines all its properties.

It is especially important that the sequence of amino acid residues (a protein **primary structure**) determines the 3D spatial structure (conformation) of a protein molecule, starting from the fixed local folding of the polypeptide chain (**secondary structure**) to the conformation of the entire molecule in whole (**tertiary structure**), and ending with the formation of **multimeric** complexes consisting of several molecules (**quaternary structure**). Only the proper (normal for a given protein) molecule conformation provides a protein biologic activity. Some proteins exhibit their activity as a part of more complicated structures–the complexes organized from several tens of different protein molecules (**"molecular machines"**).

The biosynthesis of proteins, which is carried out inside the cell, is considered as an assembly of amino acids into a polypeptide chain. This assembly takes place in **ribosomes**; a ribosome, an example of molecular machines, is a complex consisting of approximately 50 different proteins. The assembly has a matrix (template) character: it tales place on a **matrix**, where the **a matrix ribonucleic acid** (mRNA). Polymeric mRNA synthesized inside a cell nucleus by another protein molecular machine–**transcriptosome**–contains the information determining the sequence of amino acid residues in a protein, which is synthesized in the ribosome; this information is encoded in a **nucleotide** sequence forming mRNA. The process of polypeptide chain assembly is called a translation–a **translation** from the language whose letters (both in DNA and in RNA) are nucleotides into the language employing amino acids as letters.

The information contained in mRNA is operative, it is immediately used in protein biosynthesis. For its conservation from generation to generation, the cell has the essential additional material–**deoxyribonucleic acid** (DNA), which originated after ribonucleic acids in the course of evolution. DNA is located in a cell nucleus and is isolated by a nuclear membrane surrounding a nucleus. The information, necessary for the synthesis of each protein of an organism, is also encoded in DNA also as a particular nucleotide sequence; every sequence is a fragment of an extremely long–the longest of all molecules–DNA linear chain.

Such a fragment of a DNA molecule represents a **gene**, which contains the information essential for the correct and reproducible synthesis of a certain protein. The entire set of genes contained in a DNA molecule is united by the **genome** concept. A genome is different (individual) in different biological species, but it is identical in all cells of an organism of a given species without exception. Therefore, each particular cell possesses *all* genetic information, which is specific for the given organism. In other words, each cell is potentially capable of carrying out the synthesis of all proteins comprising it.

Multicellular organisms consist of many types of **differentiated** (specialized) cells, which perform different functions and form various tissues. The protein composition of different cells is not the same. Therefore, each cell type in the multicellular organism does not use all the information contained in DNA. Therefore, only some of genes, rather than all of them, is involved in the metabolic processes in a cell. It is the formation of a specific set of actively used genes (this formation is referred to as **differentiation**) that determines the biochemical peculiarities (peculiarities of a protein composition) and morphologic peculiarities of a cell, which are combined by the concept of a **phenotype**. Thus, the cell takes on the characteristics corresponding to its functions in an organism. These characteristics certainly are different in different types of cells. Moreover, they are not constant but change, depending upon the differentiation stage of a cell, the stage of an organism's development, and its physiologic or pathologic state. The cell phenotype is largely changeable.

While the stable genome is uniform for all the organism cells of a given biologic species, a **proteome** (the term has been proposed to designate the total set of the proteins in an organism) is a significantly more complicated concept. An organism's total proteome is *all* the proteins, which are present in its all cells and tissues during all stages of ontogenesis. This proteome is never manifested in full; it can be considered as a potential and actual biological activity express the certain dynamic proteome of each cell.

Here, we draw attention to one circumstance. The biological function or activity of a gene is often spoken about, although this language is not quite correct. The gene does not exhibit any activity or its own function. Its role is passive; it is only the carrier of the encoded information, which should be objectified in molecules of the corresponding protein. This objectification, which is carried out by molecular (protein) machines intended for it with the participation of some specialized regions, which do not contain the genetic information in a DNA, mRNA or other ribonucleic acid molecule, is called a gene **expression**. In other words, the activity of molecular machines employing the genetic information is referred to as the activity of a gene; we should speak of the activity of the gene expression rather than its activity. It is not the gene that "works" in a cell, but the protein it encodes; by entering biochemical interactions with other, primarily protein, components, it carries out the functions that inherent to it.

The term **expression** is quite often applied to proteins; in this meaning it is almost synonymous to **protein biosynthesis**. Quite often, a gene and the protein it encodes have the same name; therefore, **in bolde** are used in printed texts cross-out to indicate the names of genes for the purposes of their clarification.

The selectivity of gene expression is manifested in the very first stage of using the genetic information contained in DNA. Cell differentiation (when a cell takes on its phenotype) and its functional activity, as well as the expression intensity, depend on it. At this stage, which is ongoing in the cell nucleus and referred to as **transcription**, the information transfer–its "copying"–on mRNA synthesized in the nucleus occurs. This process involves numerous proteins forming the aforementioned transcriptosome and not only proteins exhibiting enzymatic activity, preparing DNA for the transcription's commencement and catalyzing the synthesis of high-molecular mRNA, but also the special proteins controlling the "switching in" of genes (this effect is known under the name of gene **induction**) and the intensity of their use. These latter proteins are known as **transcription factors**. Transcription factors, whose effect on the use of genetic information can be both positive (activating) and negative (inhibiting), play a decisive role in the formation of a cell phenotype during its differentiation (Tupler et al., 2001).

Transcription factors exert their influence on DNA under the control of intracellular biochemical regulation mechanisms, whose activity, in turn, is controlled by signals outcoming from the cell microenvironment and from the organism's regulating systems. In many cases, the transcription factors co-operate with other proteins, acting as cofactors in interaction with DNA. For example, by changing a cell's protein composition, the compliance of its functional properties with demands required by the development stage and an organism's physiological state is achieved. The role of transcription factors, just as the role of all other proteins, is demonstrated in two types of molecular-genetic experiments. In the first type of experiments, a so-called **null mutation** is artificially carried out–the gene encoding the studied factor is eliminated ("knocked out"), and the consequences of its absence in a cell are analyzed. In experiments of the second type, the consequences of an excess of the transcription factor, resulting from the introduction of an additional quantity of the corresponding gene into a cell, are analyzed.

The signals, which act on a cell from the outside, are molecules (it should be noted that the common term **signaling molecules** also refers to a great number of molecules functioning inside a cell), contacting with a cell. In their majority, these are molecules of a protein nature. But the cell is surrounded by a cell (cytoplasmic) membrane comprised of phospholipids and therefore, it is impenetrable for such molecules. Therefore, the molecules of a cell microenvironment, besides comparatively rare exceptions, can only transmit their signals inside a cell indirectly, by means of **receptors** of the cell (cytoplasmic) membrane. Membrane receptors are specific protein molecules embedded into the phospholipid membrane. The number of receptors of the same type on the surface of one cell ranges from several tens to several thousand; it changes depending on a cell's functional state. Each cell in a vertebrate's organism has receptors, capable of interacting with more than 100 types of signaling molecules. The receptor molecules have external (extracellular) and intracellular (cytoplasmic) regions (**domains**) connected with each other by a region, passing throughout the membrane. In some cases, the membrane receptors are complexes consisting of several different molecules.

Besides the receptor proteins, cytoplasmic membranes contain proteins and protein complexes, which form tunnels intended for the bilateral transport of water-soluble molecules, which are not soluble in lipids through the membrane–for example, of glucose entering the cells or urea excreted by the cells. These proteins of a cell membrane are classified as **transporters**.

As a rule, each of the numerous types of receptor proteins is strictly specialized and intended for interaction with particular **ligands**–this term covers any molecules interacting with receptors. Mostly each receptor binds a limited group of ligands related in structure and function or even binds selective only one ligand. In turn, each ligand can employ either one or several receptor or receptors close to each other in a structure in order to influence a cell.

The spatial structure (**conformation**) of a receptor's entire molecule and its cytoplasmic domain in particular changes with the interaction of a ligand and a receptor. In some cases, there are chemical alterations of this domain, for example, the phosphorylation of some amino acid residues. These changes result in the emergence of a complex, usually multiple-stage system of biochemical reactions in the cell. Various enzymes, predominantly **kinases**, are activated. The kinases are enzymes phosphorylating particular cytoplasmic proteins and thereby increasing their energy potential. The protein molecules activated in such a manner, take on the role of signals sequantially affecting each other. Eventually the signal enters a cell nucleus, where it reaches a transcription factor and converts its molecule into a state required for interaction with DNA. This entire system of intercellular reactions, started by the receptors, is considered as a **signaling pathway**; the signaling pathways vary for different receptors. But the total number of signaling pathways in a cell is small, and many pathways are employed by several receptors. In other cases, a receptor can transmit its signal along several pathways. It is conditionally considered that the signal is transferred downwards, and sometimes this process is compared to a cascade; the molecule giving the signal is referred to as upstream, while the one receiving the signal is downstream.

The terminology of the "cascade" is used to characterize the genes' **hierarchy**: a gene encoding the protein, upon which the induction of another gene depends, is referred to as an upstream gene in relation to the latter.

It is important to note that the expression of genes encoding receptor proteins follows the same regularities, which refer to all other proteins: it is activated and inhibited, depending on the cells' demands. The absence in a cell of the receptor, experimentally caused by the knockout of the gene encoding this receptor, excludes ligand exertion on the cells. On the contrary, an excess of receptor molecules enhances the ligand influence on a cell.

The number of proteins in an organism exceeds manifold the gene number in the genome: the human genome consists of approximately 22,000 genes. This is due to several reasons. **Post-translation modifications** are the common cause of the origin of several proteins encoded by the same gene. A post-translation modification is an alteration in a polypeptide chain that has already been assembled. These alterations can occur both inside a cell and in the extracellular matrix. Another reason is the rearrangement or exclusion of particular fragments of the same mRNA molecule (**exons**); the consequence of this phenomenon (**alternative splicing**) is theh generation of two protein molecules, which are close to each other but are still different from each other, so-called **isoforms**. In some cases, instead of using information of the entire gene, certain of its parts can be used (transcribed), resulting in the appearance of several different proteins. For example, the gene of lubricin, a protein involved in the formation of the lubrication properties of synovial fluid, is a fragment of a large gene, which encodes a growth factor of the megakaryocytes acting as a whole.

For all these reasons and even more important, owing to the reorganization of genes proceeding during the biological evolution, there appear whole **families** and even **superfamilies** (counting 100 and more members) of protein molecules, more or less close to each other in structure and having functions that are sometimes similar and sometimes opposite in action targeting. For example, extracellular signaling molecules combined under the name **transforming growth factors-beta** (TGF-β) are one of these superfamilies; wich includes also the family of bone morphogenetic proteins.

The cells produce not only proteins that the cell itself uses to build and renew its own structure and that carry out intracellular metabolic processes. Also, as already mentioned, the proteins form an **extracellular** matrix. The extracellular matrix is especially intensively developed in a number of connective tissue types; it plays the central role in functions of this tissue. The process of releasing proteins synthesized by a cell into the environment is called **secretion**, and these proteins, unlike those used by the cell, are referred to as **secreted**. Sometimes the expression of secreted proteins is also spoken about, implying in the term "expression" a wider sense as in this usage it includes both gene expression and protein biosynthesis, and the expression (secretion) of a finished (or nearly finished, distinctly formed) in an extracellular matrix) protein. The presence of a more or less extensive carbohydrate component, attached even inside a cell in the secreted protein molecules, is their essential feature. Such a "label" is a signal for a molecule's direction into the extracellular medium.

The molecular mass of proteins is very different, but in most cases it is high, which provides the basis for applying the term **macromolecule**. However, there is no generally accepted setting as to when this identity should be used. All proteins with a molecular mass exceeding 15kDa have a **domain** structure – they consist of several parts or regions (**domains**), which differ from each other in amino acid composition and accordingly in their spatial structural organization (conformation). We have already mentioned a protein domain structure, as exemplified by the proteins of membrane receptors; these proteins are distinctly divided into extracellular, transmembrane and cytoplasmic domains. The big protein molecules (macromolecules) quite often consist of many domains (more than 10), with each domain having its special function.

All representatives of the **collagenous** protein superfamily (29 types of collagens are presently known) are an illustrative example of the domain organization of the protein macromolecules of the extracellular matrix. In "classical" collagens, which form the matrix collagen fibrils and fibers, the macromolecule consists of three domains. The central domain, occupying almost all the molecule length, has a characteristic triple-helical structure and is distinguished by a peculiar amino acid composition. Relatively short domains with an absolutely different structure (**telopeptides**), participating in the formation of intra- and intermolecular cross-links between polypeptide chains, are located on both ends of this continuous domain, which determines the biomechanical properties of collagen fibers. The domain structure in so-called non-fibrillar collagens is more complicated: there are several triple helix domains, and they are connected by various non-spiralized ("non-collagen") domains, each of them performing a special function. In some collagens, these non-collagen domains form an appreciable part of a macromolecule.

The domain structure represents an almost universal structural pattern of the majority of extracellular matrix components. Thus, the same domains are part of absolutely different proteins. For example, domains that were primarily found in one of the proteins of the blood clotting system – the **von Willebrand factor** – are contained in approximately 500 matrix proteins and, moreover, in transmembrane receptors of the integrin class (Whittaker and Hynes, 2002). The complicated domain structure of protein macromolecules renders proteins classifications appreciably conditional.

In many cases, domains that are similar or close in amino acid composition are found in many proteins, often with a different biological role. These domains, common for several proteins, are referred to as **modules** – peculiar single-type building blocks, a certain set of which is used by cells in assembling polypeptide chains.

Along with the domains, the polypeptide chains of many proteins, including very different ones, have small regions with similar (uniform) amino acid sequences. These repeating amino acid sequences, repeating in several proteins, are called **motifs**. As it is the amino acid sequences (primary structure) that determine the spatial organization of polypeptide chains, the motifs manifest themselves at this structural level. Therefore, the concept of a motif is also used in referring to the structures of protein molecules. For example, there are single-type protrusions (**"zinc fingers"**) topped with the zinc atom in the conformation of a number of intracellular signaling protein molecules, regulating the expression of the gene interacting with DNA and mRNA (Ganss and Jheon, 2004).

The significant peculiarity of many structural extracellular proteins is the presence of specialized modules (domains) containing amino acid motifs within them, providing the proteins with adhesive properties ("stickiness"). A tripeptide RGD (arginine–glycine–asparagine) motif is the most common one among them. The adhesive motifs are of great importance for the matrix, assembling as a strong and stable construction.

The extracellular matrix is comprised not only of macromolecular structural protein components, which determine the matrix's biomechanical properties and provide for its supporting function. Numerous enzymes also act in the matrix; with their catalytic participation the final stages of the formation of structural macromolecules secreted by cells, the formation of more complicated **supramolecular** structures occur. Circulating in blood, the regulating factors of a systemic action – hormones – penetrate the cells via the matrix. Extremely numerous (estimated in hundreds) small (with a molecular mass of some tens of daltons) signaling protein molecules are also transferred from cell to a cell via the matrix; these signaling protein molecules are also referred to as **chemical mediators** and **short distance regulators** – growth factors, interleukins, cytokines and others.

The matrix is not a passive medium in relation to signaling molecules. The signaling molecules interact with the matrix's structural components; their activity as ligands to receptors of the cell cytoplasmic membrane largely depends on this interaction. Some cells secret special decoy receptors into the matrix, which are specially appropriated for binding an excess of the respective signaling molecules; in other words, to reduce the signal activity.

The signaling molecules in the matrix come into competitive interactions with specific molecules having an antagonist activity. For example, in comprising the growth factors, the **bone morphogenetic proteins** essential for regulating the morphogenesis of cartilaginous and bone tissues and many other processes, interact with a group of antagonistic proteins – *noggin, gremlin* and some others; the summary balance of these interactions determines the efficacy of bone morphogenetic proteins' influence on cells (Canalis et al.,2003).

The role of both intercellular and intracellular signaling molecules is extremely high in regulating the processes of cell **proliferation** and **differentiation**, especially in embryogenesis. These processes proceed in a strict conformity with the program of an organism's embryonic development. Herein, the transcription factors are used strictly coordinately for the time- and space-ordered induction of genes, the activity regulation (expression intensity) of genes, and their switching off in the transition of individual development to subsequent stages. The signaling molecules involved in these processes are sometimes referred to as **morphogens**.

The role of protein signaling molecules is not less significant in many physiological and pathological processes in the postnatal stages of ontogenesis, for example, during the life-long remodeling (reorganization) of bone tissue, and in the healing of wounds and fractures.

Proteins' **conservatism** is convincing evidence in favor of their fundamental role in biological processes. Conservatism consists of the fact that many protein macromolecules, despite their complexity, have retained the basic patterns of amino acid composition and structure, corresponding to their function, throughout the evolution. **Homologs** in lower invertebrates correspond to most proteins in higher vertebrates and human beings. Many homologs are found in a drosophila, for example, and therefore a lot of genes have names given to them when studying genetics of the drosophila–and even in unicellular organisms. These, phylogenetically old homologs have served as ancestors for proteins' modern families.

Certainly biochemistry cannot be restricted to only the biochemistry of proteins. Along with proteins, living organisms have numerous substances of a non-protein nature, which are also studied in biochemistry. During evolution, these substances have become essential for a great deal of metabolic processes and, therefore, for life as such. But the biosynthesis, transportation and metabolic use of all non-protein components of living tissues–nucleic acids, carbohydrates, lipids, hormones, vitamins, inorganic substances, as well as the accumulation (basically, in phosphorus compounds), transfer and use of energy–are carried out **only** with the mandatory participation of proteins, and enzymes in first place. At the same time, proteins themselves substantially carry out the regulation of biochemical reactions between proteins. Therefore, most proteins possess domains that provide "protein-protein" interactions.

Thus, it can be stated that, while all non-protein components are absolutely necessary for an organism, they have only a secondary, subordinated importance in relation to proteins. Therefore, **proteomics** have become one of the central trends in the development of modern biochemistry. This trend, by analogy with genomics, has completed the total characterization of the human genome and that of many other biological species. This, in general, challenges the full cataloguing of all proteins with the addition of their functional characteristics.

1.3. GENERAL BIOCHEMICAL ASPECTS OF CONNECTIVE TISSUE

The main peculiarity of connective tissue, which is common for all of its types, is the intensive development of the extracellular matrix.

Therefore, the main functional load for all specialized cells in connective tissue is the biosynthesis of macromolecular components of the extracellular matrix. Given that the matrix macromolecular composition of individual types of connective tissue is not the same due to their physiological role in an organism, the biochemical (biosynthetic) processes ongoing within the cells of these types are dissimilar. It is these processes that specify the **biochemical phenotype** of various connective tissue cells, i.e. the expression of a certain set of genes encoding the matrix protein components, which are typical for the given type of connective tissue. These components are considered as **phenotypic markers**, indicating the degree of cell maturation.

From a biochemical point of view, the extracellular matrix components can be subdivided into three main classes.

The first class comprises macromolecular **structural** components. They are cell-produced secreted macromolecules that comprise the matrix structures, as can be seen in a morphologic examination.

Structural macromolecules (almost all of them have a protein nature, the only significant exception being a highly polymeric polysaccharide hyaluronan) are characterized by stability and more or less evident insolubility.

The second class comprises **enzymes**, active protein macromolecules that are also secreted by cells. Some enzymes carry out biochemical reactions, anabolic in their essence, within the extracellular matrix, which are essential for the final formation of structural macromolecules; however, these reactions do not proceed within cells. Other enzymes catalyze the catabolic reactions also ongoing within the matrix.

The third class is represented by mobile, well-soluble **signaling** protein molecules (they can also be called informative) that transmit signals from cell to cell, and from cells to the matrix and visa versa. These molecules are small in comparison to the macromolecules of first two classes.

Apart from the components of these three classes, the connective tissue extracellular matrix contains other different molecules. First of all, blood plasma proteins should be mentioned: the albumin concentration in the matrix of most types of connective tissue is relatively high. The continuous motility of molecules, which are smaller than the proteins–metabolites takes place via the matrix. These molecules include glucose, amino acids, salts and others, directed towards the cells from the blood, and the metabolites eliminated from the cells. Systemic regulation factors such as hormones and vitamins are also directed towards the cells.

However, the components that play the determining role in the formation of the extracellular matrix structure are those constituting the first class of the three aforementioned classes. The same structural components, along with the enzymes and signaling molecules, facilitate the performance of all matrix main functions.

A morphologic examination carried out by means of light microscopy demonstrates that the connective tissue extracellular matrix consists of fibers and homogenous ground substance.

Collagen fibers that constitute aggregates of microscopic **collagen fibrils** consist of five members of the **collagenous proteins** (type I, II, III, V and XI collagens) superfamily. These collagenous proteins are recognized as fibrillar: their molecules' structure follows the generally accepted concept of **fibrillar** proteins as proteins, whose polypeptide chains are elongated, arranged in parallel to each other, and serve as a material for fibril formation.

Ultramicroscopic fibrils (protofibrils) formed by aggregating these collagens' macromolecules are further assembled in fibers.

Lately two more collagens (types XXIV and XXVII) have been identified, which are also referred to **fibrillar** collagens in accordance to the typical fibrillar structure of their macromolecules, which do not comprise collagen fibers (Wada et al., 2006). Therefore the collagens of large collagen fibers should be allocated into a special family, thereby designating them as **fiber-forming**.

Along with the fiber-forming (fibrillar) collagen family, the collagenous protein superfamily comprises other collagens, which all together are recognized as "non-fibrillar". It would be more correct to combine them in a large family of "collagenous proteins that do not form fibers". If considering the connective tissue extracellular matrix as a system consisting of two components – the fibers and ground substance as the matrix appears under a light microscope, then these collagens should have been referred to the ground substance although a lot of them form ultramicroscopic and sometimes are bound to fibers. With the advent of electron microscopy in biology, the allocation of the matrix into fibrous structures and the ground substance has actually become conditional.

If only collagen fibrils make up collagen fibers, then the composition (and therefore the structure) of the **elastic** fibers is more complicated. The elastic fibers originate by aggregating macromolecules of a globular elastomeric (providing the fibers with elasticity) protein **elastin** within a framework made by the microfibrils, which consist of other proteins, mainly **fibrillins** as well as related specific **glycoproteins**. Therefore, the ability to form fibers is intrinsic for elastin in interaction with other proteins, rather than for elastin itself. Consequently, elastin, whose polypeptide chains are elongated only in a stretched condition, can be considered as a fibrillar protein with particular exceptions.

Fibrillins are not only involved in the formation of elastic fibers. Fibrillin microfibrils are present in many tissues and organs, forming an independent system of connective tissue fibers exhibiting special functions. This is the third type of connective tissue fibrillar system after collagen and elastic fibers, which were revealed only during an electron-microscopic examination and can be called microfibrillar.

There is another local system of microfibril functions in the extracellular ground substance, especially during periods of tissue formation in embryogenesis or its regeneration, such as wound healing. This is a system of short-term fibrils, comprised of insoluble isoforms of a glycoprotein **fibronectin**, which are closely bond to the cells.

Table 1.1 summarizes the main characteristics of the biochemical nature of fibrous extracellular matrix structures, seen under a light microscope, and smaller extracellular matrix structures, including fibrillar ones, seen only under an electron microscope.

Thus, appearing structureless under a light microscope, the **ground (interfibrillar and intercellular) substance** of the extracellular matrix comprises the macromolecular components, which form functionally essential structures:

1) two systems of microfibrils –
a) fibrillin microfibrils containing, in addition to fibrillin, its related glycoproteins, and
b) microfibrils comprised of fibronectin around the cells under certain conditions;
2) various microfibrillar structures consisting of non-fibrillar collagens, which do not form "classical" fibrils and fibers.

The matrix ground substance, where all these structures are located, is comprised of an extremely large number of macromolecular components, which are **glycoconjugates** in their nature – proteins carrying various carbohydrate fragments attached to them. In accordance with the nature of these fragments, glycoconjugates are subdivided into two big classes – glycoproteins and proteoglycans.

Glycoprotein macromolecules contain a small amount of carbohydrates (not more than 10% of the molecular mass), which are attached to a polypeptide chain mostly as branched compounds of various monosaccharides.

The macromolecules of **proteoglycans** are glycoproteins that differ in that they contain peculiar linear (non-branched) polysaccharides – **glycosaminoglycans** – besides small branched, sometimes numerous carbohydrate fragments. Therefore, the proteoglycans are a special type of glycoproteins. Glycosaminoglycan chains can be of different length, and their number is different in different proteoglycans. In some cases, in so-called large proteoglycans, the total mass of glycosaminoglycans in a proteoglycan macromolecule was more than half of the macromolecule's total molecular mass.

It should be noted that, as a rule, fibers and fibril-forming proteins are also glycoproteins. The fact is that, as mentioned earlier, a carbohydrate fragment that is attached to a protein macromolecule in a cell (this attachment can occur during the assembly of a polypeptide

Table 1.1
Proteins of extracellular matrix fibrous structures

Proteins	Supramolecular	Peculiarities of Structures	Functions of Macromolecule
Large fiber-forming type I, II, III collagens	Collagen fibrils and fibers	Large central continuous triple helix domain	They are the main material for the formation of collagen fibrils and fibers
Minor fiber-forming type V and XI collagens	Embedded into the structure of large collagens	Large central continuous triple helix domain	They form a central core during the process of fiber formation
FACIT-collagens associated with collagen fibrils and fibers (types IX, XII, XIV, XVI, XIX, XX, XXI, XXII)	Unknown	Interrupted triple helix domain	Located on the surface of large collagen fibers, these collagens bind them to other matrix components
Fibrillar collagens forming collagen microfibrils (types VI, XXVIII, XXIX)	Rosary-like (resembling beads) microfibrils	Small triple helix domain	Bind cells to collagen fibers (?)
Fibrillar collagens that do not form fibers (types XXIV, XXVII)	Unknown	Large central continuous triple helix domain	Unknown
Elastin	Amorphous substance	Globular form of elastic fibers	Provides elastic fibers with elasticity
Fibrillins and the glycoproteins associated with them	Microfibrils	Rosary-like (resembling beads) long twisted macromolecules	Form a framework of elastic fibers where elastin macromolecules deposit
Fibrillins and the glycoproteins associated with them	Microfibrils forming a system of independent elastic-like fibers	Rosary-like (resembling beads) long twisted macromolecules	Provide little elasticity to connective tissue where they are located
Fibronectins	Microfibrillar network associated with cells and macromolecular components of ground substance	Macromolecules in the shape of an elongated letter V	Form a temporary dynamic microfibrillar construction in forming tissues that fixes cells and the macromolecular components of ground substance and directs their motility

Table 1.2
Characteristics of connective tissue extracellular matrix phases seen in light microscope

Fibrous Phase	Ground Substance
Collagenous proteins forming collagen fibers. Collagenous proteins associated with collagen fibrils (FACIT-collagens). Elastin and fibrillins with related glycoproteins comprising elastic fibers	Fibrillins and related glycoproteins comprising fibrillin microfibrils. Fibronectin(s) comprising fibronectin microfibrils. Collagens that do not form fibers (non-fibrillar), comprising various organized structures (collagen microfibrils, networks). Various glycoconjugates–proteoglycans and glycoproteins. Hyaluronan

chain or after the assembly has been completed), serves as a signal predetermining the macromolecule direction in the way of its secretion from a cell into the extracellular matrix. The presence of such a signal is obviously mandatory. Elastin is the exception; all other structural components of the matrix, including the collagenous proteins, are secreted by the cells with carbohydrate fragments. Upon entering the matrix, some proteins lose these fragments during the formation of supramolecular structures, but in most cases the carbohydrate fragments are retained and the secreted proteins retain a glycoprotein nature.

Moreover, the retained carbohydrate fragments of protein macromolecules in the matrix appear to be necessary for the protein's further functioning in the matrix. For example, the small carbohydrate fragments attached to collagen polypeptide chains are involved in the formation of intermolecular cross-links, which hold the macromolecules of fiber-forming collagens together, providing fibers' stability and strength. Therefore, collagenous proteins should be considered as glycoproteins.

It becomes evident that all potential classifications of extracellular matrix polymeric components cannot be regarded as strict by any single characteristic. For this reason, the division of these components in further chapters is based on various characteristics such as a macromolecule composition, a composition of supramolecular structures formed by macromolecules, localization in the matrix, and functions.

The biochemical characteristics of the extracellular matrix's two phases–the fibers and ground substance–is provided in *Table 1.2*.

1.4. FORMATION AND HISTOGENESIS OF CONNECTIVE TISSUE

1.4.1. Embryology and histogenesis of connective tissue

As the third germ layer, the mesoderm becomes differentiated in the second phase of gastrulation. The mesoderm axial parts differentiate in all vertebrates relatively early into dorsal, most massive regions–somites, which undergo progressive segmentation in the craniocaudal direction, and then differentiate into small intermediate regions–segment nephrotomes, which are also segmented, and ventral (lateral) regions–splanchnotoms, which remain non-segmented but are split into parietal and visceral layers. In a human embryo, mesoderm segmentation starts on the 20th–21st day of intrauterine development and continues in the 4th and 5th developmental weeks and is completed by the 35th day in the formation of 43–44 pairs of somites (Knorre, 1971). The differentiation of somites' material occurs in parallel to segmentation. Each somite, which is at first homologous and consists of epithelium-like organized columnar cells with nucleus localization at different levels, is then subdivided into the dorso-lateral region–a dermatome underlying the ectoderm and formed under its inducing exposure (Galera et al., 1996), the medio-ventral region–a sclerotome adjoining to the neural tube and the chorda, and the layer which is intermediate between them–a myotome. The dermatome and myotome protract into each other by their dorso-medial edges. The dermatome cells gradually take on a loose configuration, forming a mesenchyme from which a skin connective tissue base is further formed. In loosening, the sclerotome forms a skeletogenic mesenchyme, the cells of which migrate around the chorda and the neural tube, interact with them and then differentiate into a cartilaginous and bone tissue of an axial skeleton. In a culture on agar or on a Millipore filter, the sclerotome mesenchymal cells usually differ-

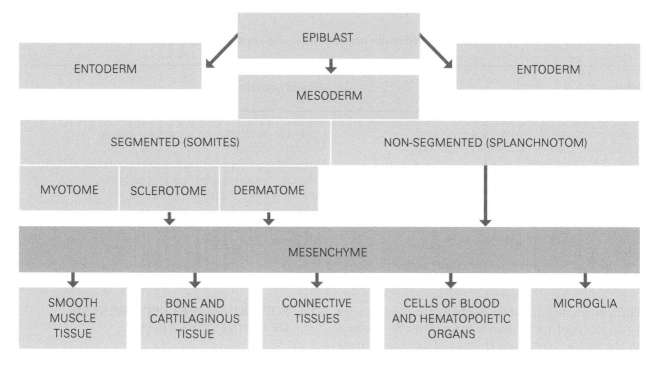

Fig.1.2 (according to Omelyanenko).

entiate into cartilage (Cheney & Lash, 1981). The chorda, neural tube, proteoglycans and collagens accelerate cartilage generation and enhance glycosaminoglycan synthesis. Removing an intercellular matrix from the chorda decreases its inductive ability (Kosher & Lash, 1975). Both the dermatome and the sclerotome are entirely spent in the formation of the mesenchyme, i.e. the mesenchyme originates due to the loosening of the somites' separate regions – the dermatomes and sclerotomes – and due to the migration of cells from the visceral and parietal layers of the splanchnotoms. The mesenchyme that migrated from the splanchnotoms forms most different tissue derivatives, being the source for hematopoietic differons and blood vessel cells, smooth muscle, and the connective tissue of many organs, involved in the formation of the skeleton's individual parts. The most specific characteristic of the histogenesis of most mesenchyme derivatives is the formation of a significant amount of an intercellular substance. The intercellular matrix is functionally leading in some organs or their parts (for example, in bone tissue), although genetically they are always CT-cell derivatives (Knorre, 1971).

In general, the mesenchyme is a complex of heterogeneous embryonic branched cells, which are loosely located and form a net-like (reticular) structure due to the interaction of cell processes. The mesenchyme fills in the gaps between the remaining, more compact anlages of other organs.

The mesenchyme sources and derivatives are summarized in *Fig.1.2.*

The initial stage of mesenchymal anlage differentiation involves the release of part of the cells from its general reticular organization, which takes on the properties of

wandering cells (Maximov, 1927). Another part intensifies the synthesis of intercellular matrix components, further differentiating in different ways. Thus, all types of connective tissue, i.e. hematopoietic, skeletal and so on, originate.

During its progressive growth and differentiation the mesenchyme is constantly changing, therefore in any stage of its development it is not similar to the previous stage especially if referring to the extracellular matrix. The adult connective tissue cannot be identified with any of these successive conditions. Mature connective tissue is a result of the continuous process of development. Therefore, the concept of "mesenchymal" should not be used to characterize any forms of mature connective tissue. The term "mesenchymal" can only indicate the origin of any cell type from a mesenchymal anlage (Eliseev,1961).

When the early tissue differentiation of some part of the mesenchyme occurs, then this anlage's part discontinues being a mesenchyme and becomes embryonic connective tissue.

In the embryonic histogenesis of connective tissue, the mesenchyme takes on the features of tissue structure earlier than those of the embryonic anlages of other tissues. This process occurs differently in different organs and systems and depends on their different physiologic significance in various stages of embryogenesis. Certain peculiarities have been found that make it possible to suggest that the connective tissue and the epithelium (or another tissue) located thereon comprise an integral complex, which starts to function only when the optimal correlative connections have been established. The connective tissue differentiates in provisory organs faster that in organ anlages due to the need to establish the connection between an embryo and a mother organism (for example, the placenta) and to ensure its development.

The chorion mesenchyme differentiates very early. As early as the first month of pregnancy, hyaluronic acid and chondroitin sulfates are detected in the villi, which are synthesized by the cells of a fibroblast type and aggregated in the ground substance. Their greatest quantity is present in the chorion villi during the second month of intrauterine development. In the beginning of the second month, collagen fibers are detected while they form in an embryo body later.

During the second month of development, the differentiation of the perimedullar, skeletogenic and skin mesenchyme, as well as the mesenchyme of the cardiac wall and large blood vessels, is the earliest to begin. This process vividly manifests in changes in the concentration of various polysaccharide compounds in the mesenchyme of the aforementioned organs. Following the development of these organs, the connective tissue of the lungs and digestive tube differentiates. Differentiation of the mesenchyme of human embryos in the 2nd developmental month (11–12 mm in length) starts with an increase in the glycogen amount and phosphatase activity. Hereafter, glycoproteins, RNA and protein aggregate in the sites of differentiation. The activity of SDH, LDH and leucine aminopeptidase increases in the cellular elements of the skin connective tissue in parallel to the intensity of fiber formation. The dependence of the dynamism of connective tissue metabolism on its localization in an organism is observed. Asynchronicity in connective tissue differentiation has been detected within the same organ (Afanasiev et al., 2001).

After birth, the development of the proper organ-specific structure of connective tissue occurs under the influence of genetic factors and the microenvironment. The organ specificity of the cellular elements is evident in their form (spindle-shaped, flattened, oval, ball-shaped and so on), which is optimally adapted to the function of a connective tissue or organ, in the interaction of cellular elements amongst each other (cell associations), and in the peculiarities of their internal structure (composition of organelles, a nucleus structure, the presence of enzymes and others).

1.4.2. Molecular and biochemical regularities of initial stages of connective tissue structures formation

The initial stages in the formation of connective tissue structures are associated with the function of **pluripotent stem cells** of the mesoderm directly originated from the epiblast totipotent cells. The pluripotency of these cells is the ability to differentiate into any cell of an organism (except for the germ cells) related to any of three germ layers–the ectoderm, endoderm and mesoderm. The pluripotent cells exhibit very high metabolic activity.

About 40 genes are found in human embryonic stem cells (hESC), the expression of which is intrinsic particularly for these cells. Among the proteins encoded by these genes in the earliest stage of embryogenesis, the key regulator of pluripotency is the transcription factor OCT4, localized in a cell nucleus, which is also called *Oct-3/4*. This protein, encoded by the gene *POU25F1* with a molecular mass of 38.5 kDa, consists of 360 amino acid residues.

OCT4 coordinates the expression of more than 1,000 genes, forming the most complex network of transcription factors that, all together, maintain the embryonic stem cells' pluripotency and ability to self-reproduce (proliferate); they also prevent the premature onset of differentiation. This network comprises a number of proteins of a cell nucleus, whose expression is directly influenced by OCT4. The influence of OCT4 is positive (stimulating) for some nuclear proteins, such as NANOG, SOX2, REX1, LEFTB, LEFTA/ EBAP, DPPA4, THY1, TDGF1). It is negative (inhibiting) for others (CDX2, EOMES, BMP4, TBX18, Brachyury, DKK1, RLX1, GATA6, ID2, DLX5). The effects caused by the OCT4-coordinated network of regulation factors include effects of an epigenetic character, such as chromatin remodeling and DNA modifications in stem cells, as well as their apoptosis (Babaie et al., 2007). Moreover, upon forming a complex with SOX2, OCT4 exerts an autoregulating effect on the activity of its own gene (*Oct3/4*) expression (Okumuro-Nakanishi et al., 2005).

A small signal protein CRIPTO (TDGF1), the glycoprotein LECT and the enzyme BUB1 with the activity of serin/ threonine protein kinase, which are secreted into the extracellular matrix, are also involved in maintaining the self-reproduction and pluripotency of hESC. These proteins activate the cell cycle, i.e. they facilitate the acceleration of cell proliferation (Li et al., 2006).

The micro-ribonucleic acids (microRNA) regulating gene functions also enable the maintenance of embryonic stem cells' pluripotency. The expression of a cluster (group) of micro RNA (miR-302b, miR302c, miR-367) by the stem cells is already seen in the first few days of embryogenesis (Hayer et al., 2008).

Apart from OCT4, the genes encoding transcription factors–SOX2, NANOG, zinc finger-containing proteins KLF2, KLF4, SALL4, the protein ESG1 and a number of other multifunctional proteins (c-Myc, Rex1, Foxd3, Gbx2, UTF1, Fgf4, Pem, Sall4, Zic3, Zfx) are of interest as markers of the embryonic stem cells (Yamanaka et al., 2008).

Embryonic pluripotent stem cells (hESC) differ from other cells by the significant peculiarities of the cytoplasmic membrane (plasmolemma) components. These peculiarities, which can be referred to specific markers, are glycolipid antigens SSEA3 and SSEA4 (molecules that consist of carbohydrates connected with the membrane's phospholipids), which are present on a membrane's outward surface, keratin sulfate proteoglycan antigens TRA-1–60, TRA-1–81, as well the protein antigens described as cell differentiation molecules (**CD**; some

CD are clusters of several molecules), CD9 and Thy1 (CD90) (Adewumi et al., 2007).

In the very early stage of vertebrates' embryonic development, as early as the stage of a **blastocyst** (in human it is the 5th day of embryogenesis) the stem cells start expressing numerous signaling molecules, particularly, some members of the transforming growth factor β (TGF-β) superfamily (Kitisin et al., 2007), the fibroblast growth factors family (Böttcher & Niehrs, 2005) and their receptors. For example, hESC express nodal and inhibin BC from the TGFβ superfamily, receptors ACVR1, ACVR2A, TGFBR1 and factors SMAD, comprising an intracellular signaling pathway of these molecules (Li et al., 2006). This and other signal pathways functioning at this stage (including the action of morphogens of the Wnt family) are also under the control of OCT4, acting in this direction by means of NANOG and SOX2 factors (Babaie et al., 2007).

In forming the **mesenchyme** from the mesoderm (segmented or non-segmented), alterations of the embryonic stem cells' phenotype occur. The main cell mass loses pluripotency; therefore the expression of factors maintaining the pluripotency decrease or discontinue therein. The ESC pluripotency changes to polypotency (or **multipotency**) in mesenchyme stem cells (MSC), which have a special proteome (Roche et al., 2006); multipotency is the ability to serve as a source for certain cell differons comprising the connective tissue system rather that all cell differons.

There is a point of view that multipotent mesenchymal stem cells are retained in an organism during its entire life, albeit in a very small quantity. They are mainly retained in the stroma of forming hematopoietic organs (in general, in the bone marrow stroma, where they account for 0.01–0.001% of the total cell number; therefore the acronym MSC can refer to multipotent stromal cells. At the same time, mesenchymal stem cells are retained in virtually all tissues and organs, where they predominantly have perivascular localization (Meirelles et al., 2006). With ageing, the number of MSC declines more and more and its ability to replicate and differentiate is reduced. Since the adult MSC (at present more than 200 cultured lines of these cells are known) are more available for investigation and clinical use than the cells of embryos, the general information on a phenotype of mesenchymal stem cells mainly refers to adult MSC.

In all varieties of phenotypes in different cultivated lines of MSC and changes of phenotypes depending on the degree of commitment (predestination of the way of the subsequent differentiation of multipotent progenitor cells), these phenotypes possess an essential general feature, which is a set of antigenic markers of a cytoplasmic membrane that differs from that of embryonic stem cells. The molecules of cell differentiation CD73 (ecto-5'-nucleotidase) and CD105 (endoglin) become the main markers of mesenchymal stem cells; CD90 (Thy-1) also retains its

Table 1.3*
Molecules, expressed by mesenchymal stem cells

Groups of Molecules	Molecules
Structural Macromolecules of the Extracellular Matrix	Type I, III, IV, V, VI and other collagens; hyaluronan, proteoglycans (versican, biglycan, decorin), fibronectins, laminins, perlecan, nidogen, syndecan
Adhesive Molecules	Integrins: $\alpha v\beta 3$, $\alpha v\beta 5$, integrin subunits: $\alpha 1$, $\alpha 2$, $\alpha 3$, $\alpha 4$, $\alpha 5$, αv, $\beta 1$, $\beta 3$, $\beta 4$; CAM-1, ICAM-2, VCAM1, ALCAM-1, LFA-3, L-selectin, endoglin, CD44
Cytokines/Growth Factors	Interleukins: 1α, 6, 7, 8, 11, 12, 14, 15, KIF, SCF, Flt-3 ligand, GM-CSF, G-CSF, M-CSF
Receptors of Cytokines/Growth Factors	L-1R, IL-3R, IL-4R, IL-6R, IL-7R, LIFR, SCFR, G-CSFR, IFNgR, TNFIR, TNFIIR, TGFβIR, TGFβIIR, bFGFR, PDGFR, EGFR

*Table comprises the data of Minguell et al., 2001.

significance (Roche et al., 2006). **SDF-1** (stromal cell-derived factor-1 or STRO-1) is considered as the most specific antigen; it is a small (its molecular mass is about 10 kDa) protein, secreted along with immunoglobulins CD106 (VCAM) and CD146 (MCAM), which actively enables cell growth and chemotaxis (Kortesidis et al., 2005).

Further, multipotency in most mesenchymal stem cells changes to **unipotency** – in retaining the ability for self-reproduction, they become progenitors of any connective tissue cell differon – osteoblastic, chondroblastic, adipocytic, as well as fibroblastic and myocytic (Suzdaltseva et al., 2007). Commitment of the progenitors – a choice of the way by which their differentiation would occur – is a complex process ongoing in the interaction of a number of regulating factors. In particular, they include the transcription factor Runx2, the zinc finger-containing transcription factor Osterix, the activating transcription factor 4 (ATF4), and the transcription modulator (co-activator) TAZ (Deng et al., 2008).

The development of the mesenchyme from the mesoderm involves the formation of a peculiar extracellular matrix by the multipotent cells; this matrix contains the main macromolecular components of the connective tissue matrix but differs from the matrix of connective tissue mature types due to some peculiarities. There is a high concentration of **hyaluronan**, which provides the matrix with viscosity, and the presence of **versican** as the main large proteoglycan produced by the fibroblasts, differentiating from MSC.

This matrix creates a microenvironment ("niche") providing the conditions necessary for the mesenchyme cells' functioning. These conditions include the inflow of signals maintaining the pluripotency of the retained embryonic stem cells (Lensch et al., 2006) and the mesenchymal progenitors, which restrain premature chondroblastic and osteoblastic differentiation (Chen et al., 2007).

The essential structural components of the extracellular mesenchymal matrix, as well as simultaneously expressed adhesive molecules, signaling molecules and the receptors of signaling molecules are listed in *Table 1.3*.

The presence of all essential components of basement membranes such as type IV collagens, laminins, perlecan and nidogen are noted in the table. The expression of these components, which will be covered in section 3.3.2, already starts in the mesoderm, where it is confirmed by the detection of the respective transport RNA, as well as direct immuno-histochemical findings (Gersdorf et al., 2006). These findings are evidence of the most important role of the basement membranes in all stages of morphogenetic processes, starting with the earliest ones.

Chapter 2

CELLULAR
ELEMENTS
OF CONNECTIVE
TISSUE

As has already been stated, all cellular elements of connective tissue (see section 1.4.1) are mesenchyme derivatives. Despite the structural and functional diversity of these cells, they can be divided into two major groups:

1) the proper cells of connective tissue, i.e. the synthesizing components of the intercellular matrix and constantly renewing it under physiological conditions and restoring it under reparative conditions; and

2) cells associated with connective tissue, for which the latter is a medium of their vital activities but are not directly involved in the formation of the intercellular (extracellular) matrix. In turn, every allocated group can be subdivided into several subgroups according to different features.

2.1. PROPER CELLS OF CONNECTIVE TISSUE

The proper cells of fibrous connective tissue (FCT) are cells that synthesize the molecular components of the intercellular matrix (fibrous proteins: collagens, elastin, fibrillin and others, adhesines, glycoconjugates), that secrete them into an extracellular space and are involved in establishing a supramolecular multilevel organization of supporting fibrous structures and a CT structured integrating buffer metabolic medium (ground substance), and that maintain their structural and functional physiologic state by means of its constant renewal both in physiologic state and under reparation and remodeling conditions due to synthesis and reabsorption. The proper FCT cells are involved in regulating the activity of cells of other tissue specificity, thereby affecting the homeostasis of other tissues.

Before characterizing the cells of a CT-differon*, it is necessary to distinguish two states of connective tissues as the physiologic and reparative. The first one can be conditionally divided into four types, including the states of development, stable maturation, functional remodeling and regression (ageing). The reparative state can also be subdivided into several stages, including formation, remodeling and post-reparation. All these states have their particular peculiarities in terms of CT-cell morphology and a qualitative ratio of their types. Therefore, when describing their structural and functional organization, the state of connective tissue in which the given cell is located shall be indicated.

The concept of "a cell differon" or a parent-progeny relationship (Klishov, 1984; Danilov, 2001) is successfully and widely applied to the structuring of tissue elements and the processes ongoing with them in modern biology. A differon is a special and temporary population of cells of the same differentiation line (histogenetic determination), which are at different levels of development, ranging from a stem to a definitive form.

The following cells should be referred to as part of the connective tissue differon:

1) stem polypotent CT-cells;
2) stem polypotent circulating (mobile) CT-cells;
3) organ-specific (committed) CT-cells- progenitors;
4) differentiating CT-cells;
5) mature (differentiated) CT-cells; and
6) definitive CT-cells.

A stem cell is any undifferentiated or poorly differentiated cell, which is capable of maintaining its own population by means of self-reproduction and originating at least one cellular differon.

Stem multipotent connective tissue (CT) cells are cellular elements, which are present in the connective tissue of different organs and are capable of self-reproduction and forming several differon types of CT-cells. A part of colony-forming units of fibroblast-like cells might be referred to these cells in bone marrow. These cells are isolated from the bone marrow using their ability to adhere to the bottom of a plastic or glass flask and generate colonies of fibroblast-like cells (Fridenstein & Lalykina, 1973). Upon increasing the cell number in a flask cultural medium, they can be repeatedly harvested (passage). Upon exposing these cells' culture by various factors, a targeted differentiation of the cultured cells can be induced into various CT-differons (Caplan, 2005). Obviously these cells' ability makes it possible to call the bone marrow-derived CT-cells multipotent. CT-cells derived from other organs' connective tissue exhibit the same polypotent properties. There exist different points of view on the identification of stem CT-cells in connective tissue of other types and topographies. The established opinion is that adventitial cells or pericytes comprise these cell groups (Caplan & Dennis, 2006).

Nondifferentiated multipotent circulating (mobile) CT-cells are a special population of blood-carried cells, called fibrocytes in the literature, which have a unique phenotype of a cell surface (type I collagen + / CD11b + / CD13 + / CD34 + /CD45RO + / MHC class II + / CD86 +) and prominent immuno-stimulating activity (stimulation of T-cells in an antigen-specific immunity) (Bucala et al., 1994; Chesney et al., 1997). These cells are likely to be derivatives of a stem polypotent fixed (resident) bone marrow CT-cell, i.e. they are common progenitor cells for several mesenchymal differons. The mobile fibrocytes comprise a small cell fraction (0.5–1%) amongst mononuclear cells (Bucala et al., 1994). In terms of their morphologic and phenotypic properties, these cells are similar to bone marrow CT-cells (possibly stem cells) isolated in the same way. But they differ from a fibroblast, monocyte/macrophage, T- and B-lymphocytes, dendritic cells or their progenitors, as well as epithelial and endothelial cells (Metz, 2003; Chesney et al., 1998). The circulating fibrocytes are found in unchanged connective tissue. The possibilities of the CT-cells' "operation reserve" replenishment in different types of intact connective tissue and the supply of a significant amount of reparative fibroblasts within the inflammatory foci by cells migrating from the peripheral blood are shown in publications authored by Khruschev (1976), Lange (1975), Sadykova (1974).

It is obvious that the differentiation of a circulating fibrocyte into a tissue-specific progenitor and then into a mature CT-cell is only possible under the influence of a respective tissue-specific microenvironment and at a particular time. This is confirmed by the fact that there was no spontaneous differentiation in the long-term culturing of fibrocytes isolated from the blood without special processing. The use of adipogenic induction has resulted in the origination of an adipocyte phenotype with the expression of the key adipogenic markers in the fibrocytes cultured. The fibrogenic multifunctional cytokine TGF-β1 causes the differentiation of these stem CT-progenitors into fibroblasts and their variety–α-SM actin-containing myofibroblasts (Chesney et al, 1998; Phillips et al., 2004; Chesney et al., 2000), and enhances the production of an intercellular matrix. By facilitating the differentiation of the myofibroblasts, TGF-β1 inhibits the fibrocyte differentiation into adipocytes (Abe et al., 2001).

According to Maximov (1927), wandering stem cells of the blood and connective tissue, which come close to the embryonic mesenchyme by their pluripotency, are retained in an adult organism.

Apart from the circulating fibrocytes enter tissue damage sites quickly, making it possible to assume that these cells play an important role in wound healing (Abe et al., 2001). The fibrocytes cultured *en vivo* can differentiate from a CD14+-enriched mononuclear cell population. This process requires contact with T-cells. The activated T-cells stimulate the early differentiation of the circulating fibrocyte into a fibroblast phenotype, which then migrate towards the wound area. Within a wound, these rapidly differentiating fibroblasts possibly interact with matured T-cells.

However, they achieve complete maturation and differentiation upon exposure by TGF-β1. The latter is an important fibrogenic and growth-regulating cytokine. It enhances the differentiation and functional activity of the cultured fibrocytes (Abe et al., 2001). The secondary lymphatic chemokine, the ligand CCR7 of a chemokine receptor, acts as a powerful stimulus of fibrocytes' chemotaxis *in vitro* and the movement of fibrocytes introduced towards the areas of damaged skin tissue *in vivo*.

The differentiated and cultured fibrocytes express a-SM actin and the contraction of collagen gels *in vitro*. This data provides an understanding of the process of fibrocyte differentiation in tissue reparation and significantly broadens their potential role in the wound-healing process (Abe et al., 2001).

Organ-specific (committed) CT-cells-progenitors are the cells that are the organ-specific "operation reserve" of connective tissue of a particular type, organ or specific affinity. In the physiologic state of the connective tissue, these cells obviously replenish the natural loss of differentiated adult CT-cells in their transformation to fibrocytes (tissue)–a definitive form.

2.2. FIBROBLASTIC DIFFERON

2.2.1. Histophysiologic characteristics of fibroblastic differon

The following cells should be referred as part of the fibroblastic differon:
1) stem polypotent CT-cells;
2) stem polypotent circulating (mobile) CT-cells;
3) committed organ-specific progenitor-CT-cells (prefibroblasts);
4) differentiating fibroblasts;
5) mature (differentiated) fibroblasts;
6) reparative fibroblasts;
7) myofibroblasts;
8) fibroclasts;
9) fibrocytes (tissue, definitive fibroblasts) (*Scheme 2.1*).

Organ-specific (committed) CT-cells-progenitors are the prefibroblasts that are the organ-specific "operation reserve" of fibrous connective tissue. Adventitious cells can presumably constitute such a reserve.

Differentiating fibroblasts are cells that are at different stages of differentiation into a mature fibroblast. Such single cells can be found extremely rarely in a physiologic stably mature or regressive state. They are more often found in a physiologic state of development or functional remodeling. Reparative connective tissue contains differentiating fibroblasts in the entire scale and significant number, especially at the stage of its formation. At the initial stages of differentiation, the fibroblasts have a round shape without projections. The cell size does not exceed 20–25 μm. The nucleus has a round or an oval shape and a small nucleolus. Chromatin is uniformly distributed. Incipient signs of euchromatin and heterochromatin generation are noted. A cytoplasm is basophilic and RNA-rich. Many free ribosomes are detected in the cytoplasm. The endoplasmic reticulum and mitochondria are underdeveloped. A lamellar complex is represented by aggregations of short tubules and vesicles. The fibroblasts exhibit a low level of synthesis and protein secretion at this stage of cytogenesis.

The fibroblasts are capable of proliferation at all stages of differentiation. As differentiation occurs in a fibroblast, its growth in size and development of all its organelles, including the cytoskeleton, is observed. This especially refers to a synthetic apparatus. The results of this development are provided in the following description of fibroblasts' differentiated forms in the physiologic and reparative states that connective tissue can be. It is supposed that there are two populations of fibroblasts, such as those that are short-lived (several weeks) and long-lived (several months) (Khruschov, 1976).

Mature differentiated organ-specific fibroblasts are cells that perform synthetic, regulating, resorbing and other functions to the extent necessary to maintain the physiologic state (homeostasis) of a connective tissue intercellular matrix, and its constant renewal or remodeling in accordance to the morpho-

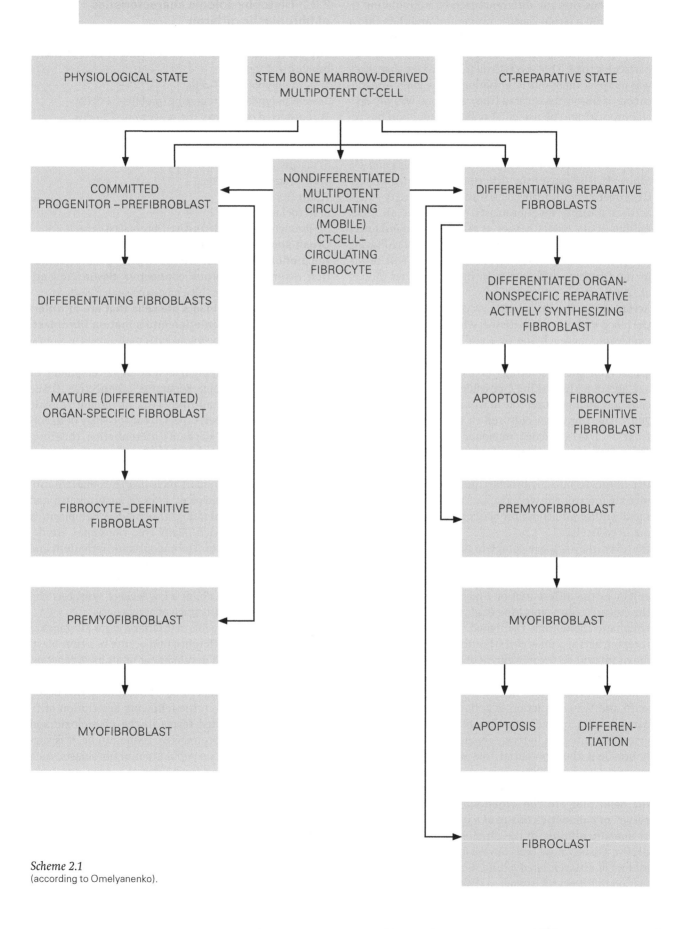

Scheme 2.1
(according to Omelyanenko).

functional specificity of a particular type of connective tissue or its topography. The fibroblasts are a complex, heterogeneous, and universal cell population, which plays an important role in development, morphogenesis and immune response. They exert a serious influence on the origin of many diseases, which are characterized by fibrosis, chronic inflammation and malignant alterations. The fibroblasts have mesenchymal CD-markers, which are intrinsic for them, and they have no CD-markers characteristic for other cell populations. Traditionally the fibroblasts are identified by the presence of vimentin fibers and the absence of cytokeratin fibers. These cells may have varied forms, including oval, polygonal, elongated or spindle-shaped, flattened, and branched. This polymorphism of the fibroblasts indicates their plasticity, i.e. the capability to change form depending on the functional state or particular conditions of their existence (to adapt). The cells can reach 40–50 µm in film-type specimens. A fibroblast surface exhibits a relatively prominent relief, formed by the folds of a cell membrane, secretory granules or crypts on a cell surface, which are formed by open secretory vacuoles (*Fig.2.1*). The number of folds on a fibroblast surface can increase under the impact of the epidermal growth factor (EFG). The folds can be considered as non-directional pseudopods or as a stage of macropinosome formation. Macropinosomes are large endocytic vesicles, which are formed as folds of a cell surface absorbing extracellular fluid.

Moreover, a cell membrane surface is an important receptor zone, which mediates the exposure of various regulating factors. There are receptor proteins on the cells' surface; these proteins are specific to the action of several types of regulating factors (growth factors, hormones and others). The fibroblasts' nuclei have a round or oval form with euchromatin and heterochromatin, 1–2 nucleoli. A nuclear membrane can have invaginations. A moderately developed granular endoplasmic reticulum (GER) contacts with a cytolemma in some regions. Its cisterns' length exceeds the width by several times. A lumen of the cisterns is diffusely filled with an amorphous or filamentous material of a medium electron density. The lamellar complex (Golgi apparatus) is generally represented by vesicles or saccules. The mitochondria are of different size and shape: round, elongated, branched, and the lysosomes are moderately developed (*Fig.2.1*). The cytoplasm is slightly basophilic and is characterized by a diplasmic vague division into an internal, denser part located at a nucleus–the endoplasm, and a peripheral, lighter one–the ectoplasm. The ratio of the endo- and ectoplasm depends on a cells' structural and functional state. The fibroblast cytoplasm contains a cytoskeleton or a fibroblast locomotive system. It is involved in performing all main cell functions. Most of the cells thread-like structures cross in the endoplasm, and all cell organelles are concentrated between them. Thread-like structures with a predominant orientation in different regions are located in the ectoplasm (*Fig.2.2*).

The cytoskeleton comprises five types of thread-like (microfibrillar) structures: **actin filaments, myosin filaments, microfilaments, intermediate filaments and microtubules**. The first three should be described in greater detail than the other cell organelles due to the fact that they are namely important for the fibroblasts. All these structures form a construction that, on the one hand, supports the cell shape, which is essential for the given moment, by adequately resisting external physical factors and, on the other hand, providing a dynamic change of this shape due to the cell's adaptation to the changing environment and spatial movements. Moreover, cytoskeleton elements regulate the shift of a hyaloplasm and provide cell organelles' movement within the cell.

The actin filaments (AF) in fibroblasts are linear helical structures, the subunits of which are oriented in the same direction, with a diameter of 8 nm. They are thinner and shorter than the microtubules. The AFs are composed by the globular molecules of the protein ε or γ-actin in the form of double-helical chain. Each actin subunit is one polypeptide consisting of 375 amino acid residues, to which an ATP molecule is bound. The actin molecules are subdivided into monomeric (globular) **G-actin** and polymerized or fibrillar **F-actin** (Fuller & Shield, 1998). There are five molecular actin isoforms, which have a similar amino acid sequence but differ from each other by the end regions of their molecules. The rate of actin polymerization and therefore, the activity of the structures bound to it, depend on the latter.

Actin filaments are assembled spontaneously and consist of actin subunits, connected as a trimer. Spontaneous polymerization starts with a late phase, when a core of new filaments is formed. Then the rapid polymerization follows, during which short filaments are elongated. One of the filament's ends (plus-end) is polymerized 10 times faster than the minus-end. In contrast to spontaneous polymerization, the elongation of present actin filaments occurs upon the subsequent attachment of actin separate molecules and, thus, is determined by the local concentration of free actin monomers. Various actin-binding proteins, such as **profilin**, **thymosine** and **spectrin**, regulate the actin properties and the amount of G-actin imbedded in a filament (Fuller & Shield, 1998). The actin filaments form a network or a peculiar framework (cortex) immediately beneath a plasmolemma, providing support for the cell membrane. The actin filaments form various types of aggregates by means of actin-coupling proteins. **Fimbrin** is a protein that binds actin filaments into parallel-arranged structures–bundles in a submembraneous cortex. α-actinin, which loosely binds actin and myosin filaments into temporary bundles, is involved in the formation of "stress fibers"; it is also involved in attaching the latter to the plasma membrane in **focal contacts**, which are sites where a cell is attached to an intercellular matrix. The continuous integration and disintegration of actin filaments make it possible for a submembraneous actin network to

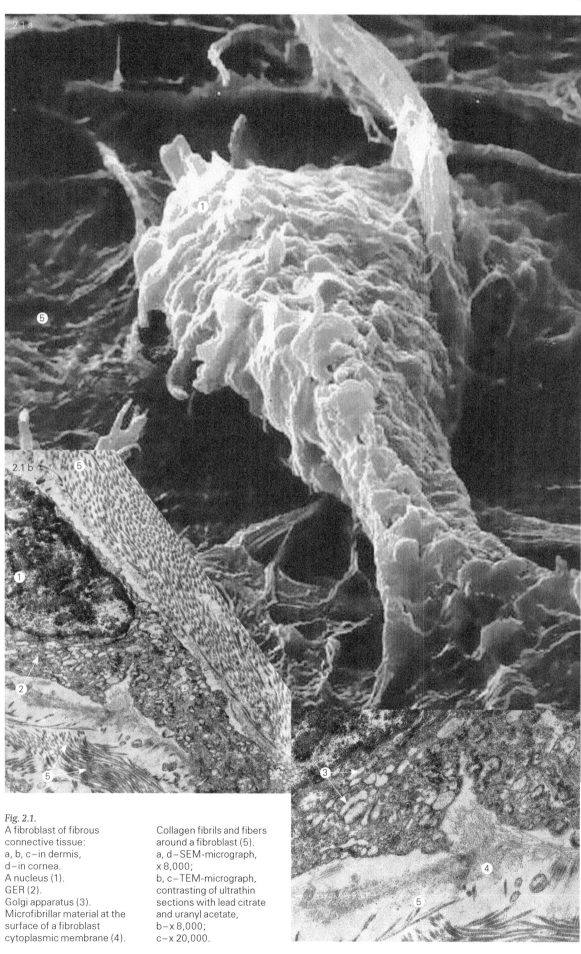

Fig. 2.1.
A fibroblast of fibrous
connective tissue:
a, b, c – in dermis,
d – in cornea.
A nucleus (1).
GER (2).
Golgi apparatus (3).
Microfibrillar material at the
surface of a fibroblast
cytoplasmic membrane (4).

Collagen fibrils and fibers
around a fibroblast (5).
a, d – SEM-micrograph,
x 8,000;
b, c – TEM-micrograph,
contrasting of ultrathin
sections with lead citrate
and uranyl acetate,
b – x 8,000;
c – x 20,000.

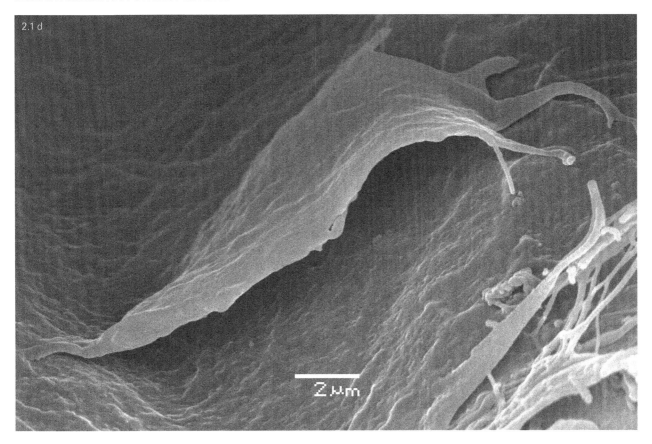

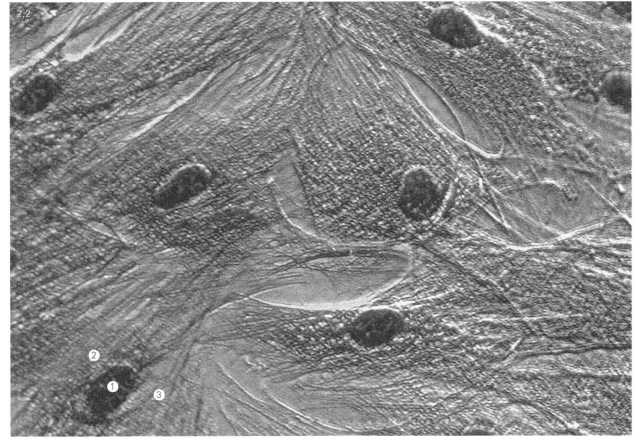

Fig. 2.2.
Skin fibroblasts in a culture.
A nucleus (1).

Endoplasm (2).
Thread-like (microfilaments)
structures in the ectoplasm (3).

LM-micrograph.
A light optic inverted
microscope Ti Nikon (Japan).

Staining with azure-eosin,
Hoffman modulation contrast.
x 400.

easily rearrange within the fibroblasts while moving and changing their form, as well as in endo-, pino- and exocytosis. Actin can become a transmembrane protein in plasmolemma specialized regions and adhesion contacts. The actin filaments are in a state of dynamic balance between the fibrillar (polymerized) F-actin and the monomeric (globular) G-actin, i.e. actin is constantly polymerized at the end of a motional edge where the actin filaments are attached to the plasma membrane and depolymerized from the inner side. Changes in cell form and motility are due to this constantly changing organization on the part of actin.

The **myosin filaments** in the fibroblasts are formed by molecules of the hexameric protein myosin and are unstable structures. Most of the molecules of non-muscle myosin—myosin II, minimyosin, the molecules which consist of two identical heavy chains, each 2,000 amino acids in length, and two light chains with 190 and 48 amino acids. The proteins with the light chains exhibit regions of calcium phosphorylation and binding. The heavy chains exhibit ATP activity and can bind to actin, temporarily forming a complex of actomyosin, i.e. **actomyosin microfilaments**.

The latter comprise the protein tropomyosin. The microfilaments are constantly present in a cell. Their supramolecular structure is formed in a fibroblast given the necessity of its movement from actin and myosin threads generally in the peripheral layer. The microfilament's thickness is 5–6 nm.

The organization of an actomyosin motor apparatus and its activity start with activation under the influence of a special Ca2+-dependent enzyme—the kinase of myosin light chains (KMLC), which transfers a phosphate residue from ATP onto myosin regular light chains. The phosphorylation of the myosin light chains KMLC activates myosin and disintegrates intramolecular bonds, leading to the straightening of myosin molecules and their spontaneous polymerization into active filaments, and the releasing of its heads, enabling them to bind actin and ATP and develop a pulling force (Shirinsky & Vorotnikova, 2005). At the same time, microfilaments are formed, consisting of actin threads and activated myosin filaments; during the interaction thereof, the transformation of a non-oriented actin network into bundles of actin-myosin filaments occurs. The strongest of these bundles are called fibrils of tension or stress-fibrils (fibers). They resemble fine microfibrils in their structure and functions. These fibers are bond to the plasma membrane at one end in special regions called focal contacts. In these regions, the cell cortex connects with components of the extracellular matrix by means of transmembrane binding proteins, by fibronectin, for example. The fibronectin receptor is a typical transmembrane binding protein comprised of two chains of glycoproteids from the integrin group. Its external part binds to fibronectin, while its internal (cytoplasmic) part is bond to the actin filaments in the stress-fibers. This connection is carried out by several proteins (for example, talin, vinculin and

others). The mechanical extension of a cell initiates the formation of stress-fibers, which disappear during mitosis when the cell becomes rounded and loses its connection with a substrate. In tissue fibroblasts, the stress fibers can contact and transfer a created effort to the surrounding extracellular matrix due to focal contacts. Thus, as a result, a temporary contracting apparatus is generated in a certain area of a non-muscle cell; this apparatus is inactivated and de-assembled by means of myosin dephosphorylation upon the completion of a movement. As in smooth muscles, an enzyme-antagonist of KMLC—**myosin light chain phosphatase**—is responsible for this. Such plasticity of non-muscle cells' locomotor system is obviously due to the necessity of their movements in different directions with a limited resource of contracting proteins (Shirinsky & Vorotnikova, 2005).

In a physiologic state, fibroblasts have insignificant mobility and low phagocytic activity. The fibroblasts' movement is made possible only upon their binding to the supporting fibrillar structures (fibrin, connective tissue fibers) by means of fibronectin—a glycoprotein, which is synthesized by fibroblasts and other proteins that provides adhesion of cells and non-cellular structures. During movements, the fibroblast is flattened; at the same time, its surface can increase manifold. During movement, the short-term stabilization of contracting filaments of the leading edge of the cytoplasm peripheral layer occurs, with the formation of a pseudopod cohering to a support point (in a tissue culture—to a solid wafer).

The **intermediate filaments** are comprised of polypeptides that are resistant to stretching and have a diameter of about 10 nm, which is between the diameter of the microfilaments and microtubules. Their main function is supportive. Upon being distributed throughout the cytoplasm, they form a network or a peculiar framework, which makes a cell resistant to mechanical stress on the one hand, and gives it elasticity on the other hand. The intermediate filaments of fibroblasts and other cells of mesenchymal origin are composed by vimentin with a molecular weight of 54 kDa. These proteins are long polypeptides, which form spiral dimmers by twisting with each other. Subsequent multilevel supramolecular lateral aggregation results in the formation of an intermediate filament.

The **microtubules** are present in all eukaryotic cells, including the fibroblasts. These are long thread-like structures with a thickness of 24 nm, extending throughout the entire cytoplasm. They are comprised of polymerized molecules of the protein tubulin and form a network that supports the structural organization and localization of some organelles, of the endoplasmic reticulum in particular. The microtubules are involved in cell division, intracellular transport, organelles' shift, and substance recirculation from the lamellar complex to the endoplasmic reticulum, as well as cell motility.

The cells can form thin, sharp projections or micropins. Lamellopodia and micropins are formed by means of rapid local polymerization on a plasma membrane, which projects frontwards or is squeezed out on a cell's moving edge. When the lamellopodia cannot attach to a substrate, a plasma membrane folding originates. In this case, the micropins and lamellopodia move backwards within a cell (Fuller & Shield, 1998).

Fibroblasts' activity involves the formation of the extracellular matrix: an integrating buffer metabolic medium and fibrous structures of connective tissue in a normal state, pathology and reparation (*Fig. 2.3*), i.e. the fibroblasts' main function is the construction and maintenance of specific architectonics and composition of the connective tissue intracellular matrix in an organ or a part thereof where a fibroblast is present. The fibroblasts synthesize and secret a number of humoral factors, thereby exerting a regulating influence on the growth, differentiation and functional activity of both their own population and macrophages, monocytes, lymphocytes, smooth muscle and epithelial cells. These cells can also be affected by components of the intracellular matrix produced by the fibroblasts, such as fibronectin, glycosaminoglycans, collagens of various types and so on.

At the same time, fibroblasts' activity is influenced by macrophages, monocytes, lymphocytes, smooth muscle and epithelial cells, tissue basophiles (mast cells) and others by means of different factors they secret into the intracellular space, such as lymphokines, monokines, fibrokines, labrokines and others. Apart from the specific mediators affecting the relevant receptors of cell membranes, there are non-specific ones such as prostaglandins, muramidase, fibronectin, and proteases. One of the systemic regulation factors of the fibroblast function is somatotropin, a hormone of the anterior pituitary. It stimulates the reproduction of connective tissue cells and the synthetic processes therein. In contrast, corticotrophin and glucocorticoids inhibit the proliferation and

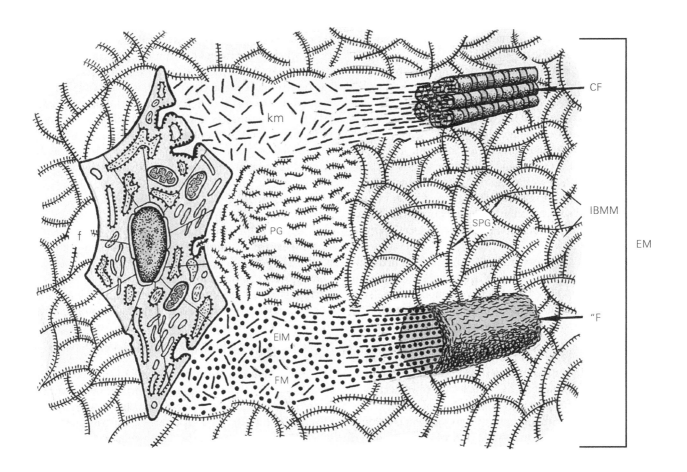

Fig. 2.3.
The organization image of a conditional structural functional unit of fibrous connective tissue. A fibroblast synthesizes and secrets molecules of collagen, elastin, fibrillin, proteoglycans (PG) and others into an extracellular space; the structural components of the extracellular matrix such as fibrous structures (collagen and elastic) and proteoglycans are formed from these molecules (according to Omelyanenko).

CF – collagen fiber
"F – elastic fiber
EM – extracellular matrix
F – fibroblast
CM – collagen molecules
EIM – elastin molecules

FM – fibrillin molecules
PG – proteoglycans
SPG – structured proteoglycans
IBMM – integrating buffer metabolic medium

cause the premature differentiation of fibroblasts, which is accompanied by disturbances in the synthesis of the intracellular matrix components.

The fibroblasts are significant for immunity. Being distributed throughout different tissues, they can be considered as "sentinel" cells that respond to warning signals and organize the tissue's response to infection or an injury. They synthesize many key mediators of inflammation, one of which is the *transcription factor RelB of the nuclear factor of the kB family (NF-kB).*

The fibroblasts lacking RelB produce a dysregulated response to stimuli, which leads to the large-scale overexpression of chemokines (Xia et al., 1997). Under natural conditions, the activated fibroblasts with a RelB deficiency are not capable to control the infiltration of the inflammatory cells, resulting in an intense increase of the granulocyte number within the tissue. The fibroblasts also play an important role in carcinogenesis. They are involved in the remodeling of the extracellular matrix in a tumor stroma and growth factors' secretion, thereby stimulating the growth of cancerous cells (Bhowmick et al., 2004, Silzle et al., 2004). Ageing fibroblasts are capable to stimulating the proliferation of malignant rather than normal epithelial cells (Krtolica et al., 2001).

Fibroblasts' activation is usually accompanied by the accumulation of glycogen and the increased activity of hydrolytic enzymes and the enzymes of glycolytic processes. The energy produced in glycogen metabolism is used for the synthesis of collagen polypeptides. The factors activating collagen biosynthesis are ions of iron, copper, chromium and ascorbic acid. The biosynthesis of RNA, collagen, elastin proteins and proteoglycans, which are essential for the formation of fibers and ground substance, is carried out rather intensively in mature fibroblasts, especially under conditions of reduced oxygen concentration.

The fibroblasts' phenotype significantly differs in different anatomical areas (regions) (Castor et al., 1962; Moulin et al., 1998; Lee & Eun, 1999; Chipev & Simon, 2002). These differences are called **topographic differentiation**. The latter is even maintained *in vitro* when the fibroblasts are isolated in a culture from the influence of other cell types. This suggests that the specificity of a topographic program implies a specific method of preserving a **position memory** (Chang et al., 2002). The fibroblasts are able to retain topographic differentiation *in vitro*. It is possible that cells' topographic differentiation is autonomous. The cells differ insofar as they can be considered as separate differentiated cell types. In using the expression profile of the whole genome, it has been shown that the topographic differences between fibroblasts are even more than the variability observed in the cultured cells derived from different individuals (Chang et al., 2002). Experimental data has shown that this position memory is based on the Hox-code. The Hox-genes encode the family of old transcription factors, which determine the orientation along the anterior-posterior and lateral axes in the process of development. Moreover, fibroblasts

derived from different regions differ in the expression of differentiation factors and transfer of signaling molecules. Therefore, a hypothesis has been proposed, whereby the fibroblasts serve as "traffic signs" that are conductors for other cell types in organogenesis (Chang вет al., 2002).

To date, the fibroblasts' phenotypes from a great number of topographic regions of a human adult have been studied and compared, including the skin (of the hands, abdomen, back, head, thigh, toes, the prepuce), the gingiva, oral mucous membrane, peritoneum, lungs and so on, as well as the embryonic lung and skin. More than 50 phenotypically different groups of fibroblasts have been detected (Witowski & Jörres, 2006; Chang, 2002; Sorrell & Caplan, 2004).

Their differences can manifest in the profiles and programs of genome expression, the degree of maturation, the ability to remodeling, migration behavior (Lepekhin et al., 2002), adhesive properties (Palaiologou et al., 2001), the expression of the extracellular matrix receptors (Palaiologou et al., 2001), the response to growth factors of the TGF-β 1 type (Lee & Eun, 1999) and the rate of division; the synthesis of the extracellular matrix components (various types and amount of glycosaminoglycans and collagens) and their aggregation and structuring; the intensity of contraction of a collagen gel fibrillar construction, the synthesis levels of metalloproteinase-2 (MMP-2) of the matrix and tissue inhibitors of metalloproteinases (TIMPs) (Stephens et al., 2001) and other factors. Based on the aforesaid, fibroblasts' phenotype differences can be divided and grouped as follows:
1) interindividual;
2) interorgan;
3) intraorgan (special-3D); and
4) ontogenetic (prenatal, postnatal).

The **fibrocytes (tissue)** are the definitive forms of fibroblasts. They have a spindle-like form, small processes, and a nucleus that occupies most of the cells. There is a narrow layer of the cytoplasm surrounding the nucleus. The cytoplasm contains few organelles, vacuoles, lipids and glycogen. The synthesis of collagen and other substances is sharply reduced in these cells; the capability to proliferate is also lost.

The **reparative fibroblasts**, as part of a fibroblastic differon, have possible common progenitors with "physiologic" fibroblasts. On the one hand, these are organ-specific (committed) CT-cells-progenitors–prefibroblasts, which are an organ-specific "operation" cell reserve of the fibrous connective tissue of the given region. On the other hand, as has already been mentioned (Chesney et al., 1998; Abe et al., 2001), these are the circulating (mobile) CT-cells, which have no commitment. It is these progenitors that form other reparative fibroblasts by means of their migration towards a damaged area through the differentiation process.

Differentiating reparative fibroblasts are cells at different stages of differentiation into mature, actively synthesizing reparative fibroblasts. By their structural organization, they are identical to differentiating fibroblasts of connective tissue, which is in a physiological state. However, their differentiation finishes by generating actively synthesizing organ-specific reparative fibroblasts.

Differentiated reparative fibroblasts are cells that actively synthesize components of the intercellular matrix and are involved in its formation under reparation conditions. This type of fibroblasts intensively produces the components of the connective tissue's intercellular matrix in reparative processes. The fibroblasts have a different form (round, spindle-shaped, pyriform, flattened) and from one to several processes, which are sometimes long. The surface relief is distinctly detected; it is formed by the folds in the form of scales and numerous short cylindrical processes (*Fig. 2.4 a, b, c, d*).

The reparative fibroblasts lie on the surface of previously formed collagen fibrils and fibers. Some cells are partially or entirely covered by fibrous structures (*Fig. 2.4 d*). The GER cisterns of these cells are abruptly dilated and filled in with a content of medium electron density. They occupy most of the cytoplasm (up to 90%). The lamellar complex is not prominent. It is significantly smaller than in the mature fibroblasts of connective tissue in a physiological state (*Fig. 2.5*). In some regions of the cytoplasm, the fusion of the GER cistern membrane with the cytolemma occurs, as well as the destruction of the latter, and release of the contents into the extracellular space.

A part of the cells can release synthesized products by means of the partial destruction of the cytolemma, i.e. there exists a holocrine type of secretion (Serov & Shekhter, 1981).

A peculiarity of fibroblasts' reparative activity is not only the high intensity of the synthesis of the extracellular matrix components, which is essential for the quick closure of a tissue defect but also the prevalence of type III collagen and the absence of the organ-specificity in a produced fibrous base of the organ damaged and therefore, the impossibility to form a developed part or an whole organ on this basis. Most of the reparative, actively synthesizing fibroblasts die by apoptosis upon completing the reparative process. Some fibroblasts become fibrocytes.

A myofibroblast is a fibroblast's specialized type with a well-developed contracting apparatus, which contains α-smooth muscle actin (α-SM actin) in its cytoskeleton, i.e. a structure that is characteristic for a smooth muscle cell and is involved in the contraction of the intercellular matrix.

Myofibroblasts were described for the first time in 1971 (Gabbiani et al., 1971). Since that time, their role has been intensively studied (Desmouliere, 1995; Desmouliere & Gabbiani, 1996; Powell et al., 1999; Moulin et al., 2000; Hinz et al, 2001).

Mature myofibroblasts express α-SM actin, an actin isoform that is present in smooth muscle cells in fine stress fibers and form large fibronexi (focal contacts) (Darby et al., 1990; Desmouliere & Gabbiani, 1996; Gabbiani,

1998, 2003; Tomasek et al., 2002). The myofibroblasts cause the compression of the extracellular matrix and are involved in regulating the proliferation and differentiation of epithelial, vascular and neurogenic cells (Saunders & D'Amore, 1992; Yamagish et al., 1993). The myofibroblasts are present in organs with a high ability to remodel, for example, in the kidneys, lungs and periodontal ligaments (Gabbiani, 1994, 1998; Desmouliere & Gabbiani, 1996; Lorena et al., 2002; Tomasek et al., 2002) or in the period of intensive remodeling, for example, during growth, development, inflammatory reactions and healing wound involution (Squier & Kremenak, 1980; Gabbiani, 1992). On the contrary, there are no fibroblasts in tissues with low remodeling activity, as in the normal dermis, for example (Squier & Kremenak, 1980; Cornelissen et al., 2000; Beurden et al., 2003). The myofibroblasts' contracting apparatus represents bundles of α-actin smooth muscle microfilaments and the contracting proteins bound to them, such as non-muscle myosin. It is supposed that this contracting apparatus is the main element generating a force, which causes intercellular matrix compression and therefore, local tissue deformation, for instance wound involution (Desmouliere, 1995), which has also been revealed in a fibroblast culture (Powell et al., 1999; Tomasek et al., 2002; Hinz & Gabbiani, 2003).

Actin-containing microfilaments end in specialized transmembrane adhesive complexes – focal contacts (fibronexi), through which cytoplasmic actin attaches to the extracellular fibronectin fibrils by means of integrins (Singer et al., 1984; Eyden, 1993; Powell et al., 1999). This provides a system of mechanotransduction, i.e. the transduction of a force generated by actomyosin microfilaments to the extracellular matrix (signaling from the inside out) (Tomasek et al., 2002). On the contrary, the extracellular signals can induce an intracellular response (signaling from the outside in) (Burridge & Chrzanowska-Wodnicka, 1996; Tomasek et al., 2002).

The bonds between the myofibroblasts are established by means of cohesion type desmosome-like and fissured contacts (nexi or gap-junctions). The myofibroblasts' nuclei have numerous crypts (Darby et al., 1990; Valentich et al., 1997; Powell et al., 1999). The aforementioned peculiarities are less prominent in ordinary fibroblasts (Eyden, 1993; Powel et al., 1999).

At present it is reasonable to subdivide the myofibroblasts into just two types (Hinz & Gabbiani, 2003). The first type – premyofibroblasts – is partially differentiated and only contains actin contracting microfilaments, but no α-SM actin. This cell type also produces extracellular fibronectin and has small, specialized transmembrane adhesive complexes – focal contacts (fibronexi) (Tomasek et al., 2002; Hinz & Gabbiani, 2003). The second type of myofibroblasts is characterized by a widespread network of actin contracting microfilaments, expresses α-SM actin and has large focal contacts and is supposed to be mature myofibroblasts (Tomasek et al., 2002; Hinz & Gabbiani, 2003).

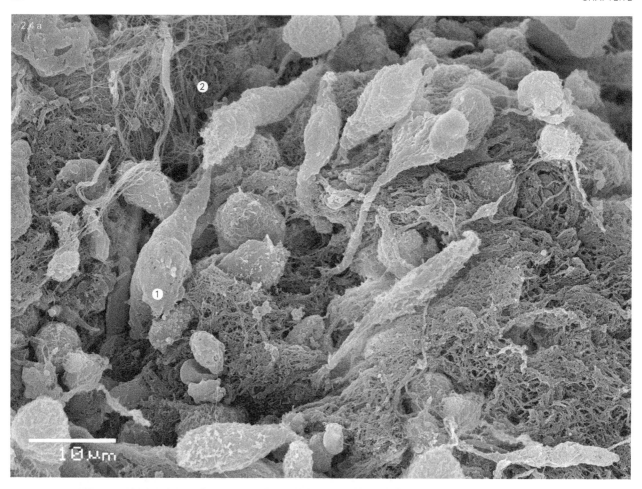

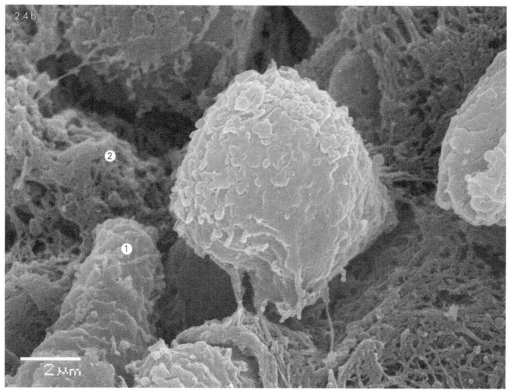

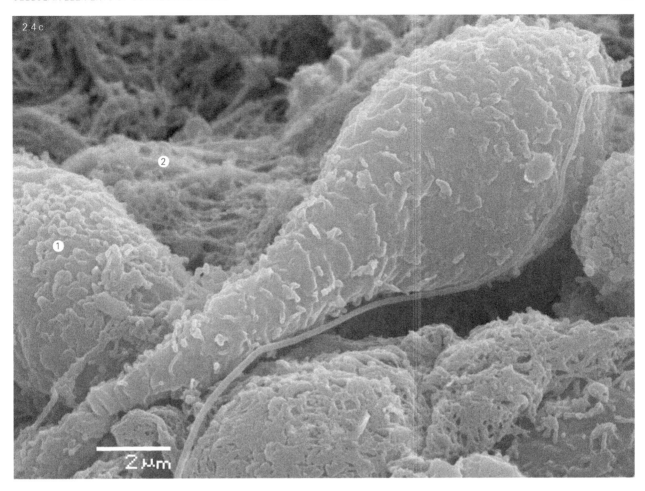

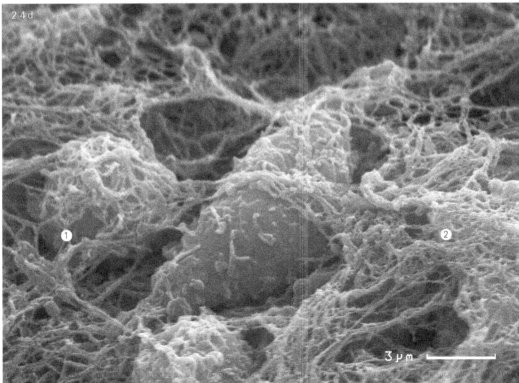

Fig. 2.4.
Reparative fibroblasts (1) in a healing skin wound.

Newly formed fibrous structures (2) of the extracellular matrix.

SEM-micrograph.
a–x 800;

b, d–x 6,000;
c–x 8,000.

The most common concept is that myofibroblasts originate from fibroblasts (Gabbiani et al., 1971, 1976; Gabbiani & Badonnel, 1976; Gokel & Hubner, 1977; Ariyan et al., 1978; Grinnell, 1994; Masur et al., 1996; Gabbiani, 2003). This process occurs in the following order. The fibroblasts migrating towards a remodeling or healing region primarily cause mechanical stress in the surrounding intracellular matrix containing fibrous structures (Tomasek et al., 2002), thereby stimulating the development of actin contracting microfilaments in other fibroblasts. The mechanical stress generated by the migrating fibroblasts promotes the assembly of stress fibers, which characterize premyofibroblasts (Tomasek et al., 2002; Hinz & Gabbiani, 2003). The increasing number of fibroblasts within the wound area secretes new collagen and fibronectin. The orientation of cells and fibers inside this matrix is parallel to a wound surface and goes along stress lines (Hinz et al., 2001). The fibroblasts exert little attractive forces on a newly formed matrix and strengthen the "cell–matrix" contacts, develop intracellular stress fibers and thus, become premyofibroblasts (Hinz & Gabbiani, 2003). The premyofibroblast phenotype is maintained by continuous interaction between the cell-generated stress and the substrate response, which is stable enough to counteract this force (Hinz & Gabbiani, 2003).

Thus, mechanical stress is the main factor enabling the differentiation of fibroblasts into premyofibroblasts. PDGF can also be involved in the process of this differentiation.

Such fibroblasts with a hypertrophic contracting apparatus can be referred to as premyofibroblasts, which generate contraction without α-SM actin expression. They are also capable of synthesizing and forming fibronectin and establishing small focal contacts (fibronexi). The premyofibroblasts can differentiate into mature myofibroblasts under the influence of such specific factors as TGF-β1, ED-A fibronectin (ED-A FN) and mechanical

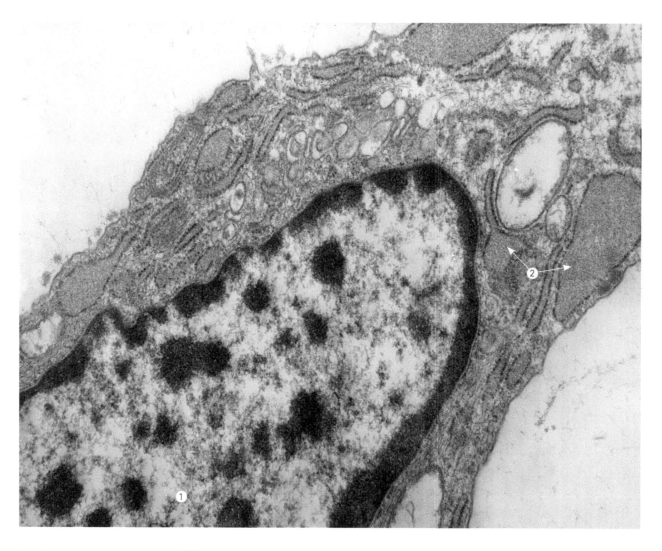

Fig. 2.5.
A reparative fibroblast fragment in a skin wound. A nucleus (1). Dilated GER cisterns, filled in with a secret (2).

TEM-micrograph. contrasting of ultrathin sections with lead citrate and uranyl acetate. x–30,000.

stress (Tomasek et al., 2002). Moreover, TGF-β1 is expressed by the fibroblasts (Varedi et al., 1997). Mature myofibroblasts express α-SM actin in fine contracting microfilaments and form large focal contacts. These differentiated myofibroblasts are present in later-contracting granulation tissue (Tomasek et al., 2002). A wound contraction is achieved by the simultaneous action of many myofibroblasts (Desmouliere & Gabbiani, 1996), is managed by numerous "cell–cell" and "matrix–cell" contacts, and is completed through the rearrangement or contraction of a network of collagen fibrils (Welch et al., 1990).

Mechanical stress, TGF-β1 and ED-A FN (a special type of fibronectin) are key factors in premyofibroblasts' differentiation into mature myofibroblasts (Tomasek, 2002; Gabbiani et al., 2003; Phan, 2003). TGF-β1 stimulates the expression of ED-A FN and α-SM actin, which enhances the assembly of stress fibers and focal contacts both *in vitro* and *in vivo* (Borsi et al., 1990; Desmouliere et al., 1993; Ronnov-Jessen & Petersen, 1993; Yokozeki et al., 1997; Vaughan et al., 2000).

The myofibroblasts preferably bind to ED-A FN via the integrins α9β1 and α4β1 (Liao et al., 2002; Muro et al., 2003). In the presence of ED-A FN and TGF-β1, the myofibroblast phenotype is lost with the disappearance of mechanical stress (Hinz et al., 2001). Thus, premyofibroblasts' differentiation into mature myofibroblasts is stimulated by the interaction of TGF-β1 and ED-A FN in the presence of mechanical stress (Serini et al., 1998; Vaughan et al., 2000).

There are also other factors that can contribute their share towards the differentiation of premyofibroblasts into mature myofibroblasts. The granulocyte and monocyte colony-stimulating factor (GM-CSF) appears to induce the synthesis of α-SM actin *in vivo* (Rubbia-Brandt et al., 1991; Feugate et al., 2001). Heparin induces α-SM actin *in vitro* (Desmouliere et al., 1992). The integrins are also involved in the premyofibroblasts' differentiation into mature myofibroblasts (Dugina et al., 2001). The expression of the receptor fibronectin α5β1 is simultaneously increased with the increase of α-SM actin in differentiating myofibroblasts (Masur et al., 1996, 1999). Large groups of this integrin are actually present in the focal contacts of mature myofibroblasts (Dugina et al., 1998, 2001; Masur et al., 1999).

At the same time, the binding of the αvβ1, αvβ3 and αvβ5 integrins to vitronectin inhibits the differentiation of mature myofibroblasts (Scaffid et al., 2001). Cytokines, which prevent myofibroblasts' differentiation, include interferon-γ (IFN-γ) (Hansson, et al., 1989), bFGF (Schmitt-Graff et al., 1994; Spyrou & Naylor, 2002) and prostaglandin E2 (PGE2) (Kolodsick et al., 2003). IFN-γ decreases the expression of α-SM actin both *in vitro* and *in vivo* (Pittet et al., 1994; Spyrou & Naylor, 2002). Further, IFN-γ reduces the contraction of collagen fibrils' network by means of dermal fibroblasts or the fibroblasts of the palate (Moulin et al., 1998; Yokozeki et al., 1999). bFGF also inhibits the myofibroblasts' differentiation *in vitro*

(Schmitt-Graff et al., 1994) and *in vivo* (Spyrou & Naylor, 2002; Kanda et al., 2003). Moreover, bFGF induces apoptosis of the myofibroblasts of the mucous membrane of a rat palate (Funato et al., 1997). Finally, PGE2 suppresses TGF-β1-induced expression of α-SM actin in primary embryonic and adult fibroblasts of the lung (Kolodsick et al., 2003).

Thus, mechanical stress is essential for the transformation of fibroblasts into premyofibroblasts. The interaction of mechanical stress, TGF-β1 and ED-A FN largely regulates the differentiation of premyofibroblasts into mature myofibroblasts (Tomasek et al., 2002).

Fibroclasts are specialized forms of the fibroblasts, the main function of which is resorption of a hypertrophic or reparative (primary) intercellular matrix with the help of a well-developed lysosomal apparatus. There are almost no fibroclasts in physiologically functioning connective tissue in a stable mature period. The resorbing function of a "worn-out" extracellular matrix is carried out by ordinary fibroblasts. The fibroclasts are the fibroblasts with a well-developed lysosomal apparatus, which enables the utilization (resorption) of the intracellular matrix, formed as a result of damaged tissue healing or hypertrophy and not complying with the surrounding tissues in terms of biomechanical characteristics. The fibroclasts correspond to the fibroblasts by morphology, but they contain numerous lysosomes, phagosomes and phagolysosomes in their cytoplasm, within which fragments of collagen fibrils are found.

The fibroblasts' phagocytic function differs from the corresponding functions of macrophages in that it is immune-independent due to the absence of receptors for immunoglobulins and a complement on its surface (Rabinovitch, 1995).

The fibroclasts mainly take on the components of the undestroyed intercellular matrix of connective tissue within the healing, hypertrophy or remodeling zone. The macrophages do not do this. They only absorb the partially destroyed intracellular matrix.

Fibroclasts, which are cells with higher phagocytic and hydrolytic activity involved in the resorption of an intercellular substance, are detected in connective tissue during the period of uterine involution after the termination of pregnancy. They combine in themselves the structural features of fibril-forming cells (developed GER, lamellar complex, mitochondria that are relatively large but few in number), as well as numerous lysosomes with hydrolytic enzymes specific for them. The proteolytic and glycolytic enzymes they secret outwards of the cell affect collagen fibers' cementing substance. Then collagenase breaks down a collagen molecule into two fragments, available for the action of nonspecific enzymes, which is followed by phagocytosis and the intracellular digestion of collagen by acidic cathepsins (Serov & Schekhter, 1981).

The term "fibroclast" is rarely used in the literature; however, much has been written about fibroblasts' phagocytic capabilities. Fibroclasts are known to mani-

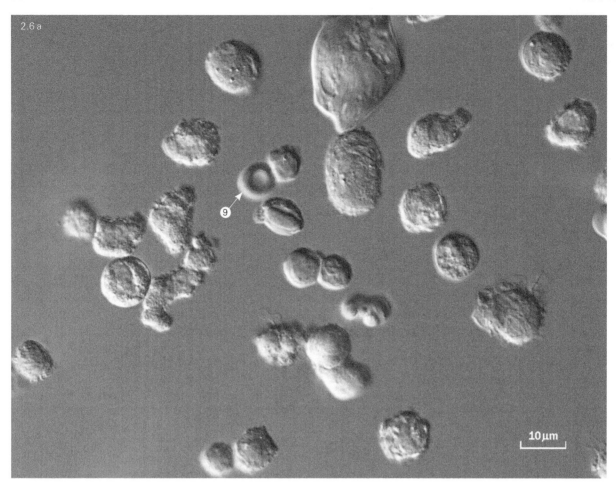

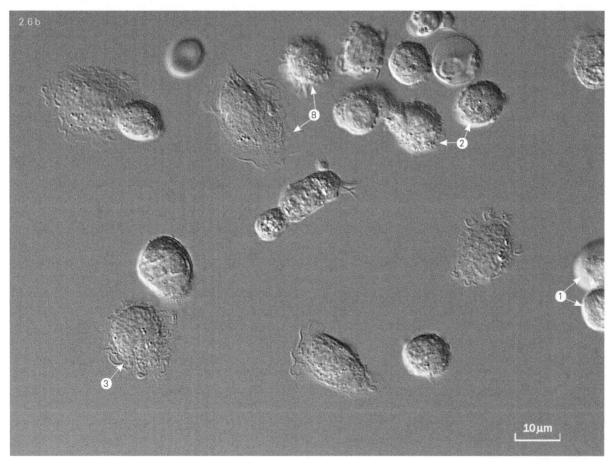

fest phagocytosis. The mechanisms they employ are similar to those used by macrophages to intake particles and weak neutrophiles; however, they are classified as "non-professional" phagocytes, as opposed to "professional" phagocytes – macrophages (Rabinovitch, 1995). Apoptotic neutrophiles are phagocyted by the fibroblasts (Hall et al., 1994). These mechanisms involve fibronectin, laminin-receptors or heparan sulfates, found in a cell. There are differences in capturing particles by macrophages and fibroblasts. Since there is a deficiency of Fc-receptors in fibroblasts, they are not capable of the phagocytosis of immunoglobulins and complementing them as effectively as the macrophages do (Rabinovitsch, 1995). *In vivo* investigations of fibroblastic phagocytosis have demonstrated the ultrastructural identification of absorbed collagen fibrils, which have been digested inside the fibroblasts. The ultrastructural mechanism of collagen intracellular lysis includes:
1) a cell's capturing of collagen fibrils' fragments (from 1–15) by the invagination of the cytolemma;

2) the formation of phagocytic vacuoles (phagosomes);
3) the fusion of phagosomes and primary lysomoses with the formation of secondary lysosomes (phagolysosomes); and
4) the gradual degradation of collagen fibrils – swelling, fragmentation, loss of cross striation and lysis.

Dense residual bodies of different types are retained in a site of phagolysosomes after collagen's complete destruction (Serov & Schekhter, 1981).

The investigation of fibroblasts under culturing conditions provides significant information on their structural organization, functions, and the peculiarities of their vital activities. The cells of a fibroblastic differon can be easily isolated to a sufficient extent from the human skin dermis by treating its bioptates with collagenase. In this case, the resulting suspension contains other cells (macrophages, plasma cells, mast cells, etc.), the environment of which contains connective tissue, and the cells of blood, epidermis and skin derivatives. These cells

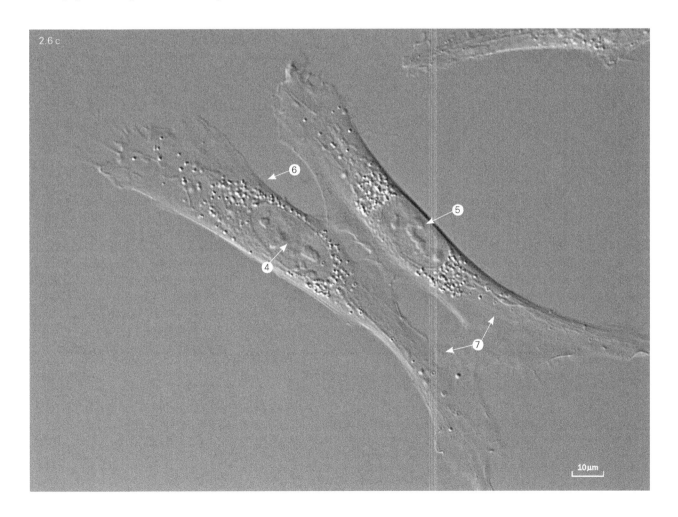

Fig. 2.6.
Human skin cells
in a cultural medium:
a – in a suspension
immediately after isolation;
b – after four hours
of culturing:

non attached (1),
attached (2),
attached-flattened (3);
c – fibroblasts spread on
a flask bottom.
A nucleus (4).
Nucleoli (5).

Endoplasm with
granules-organelles (6).
Ectoplasm (7).
Gel-like substance (8).
A red blood cell (9).
LM-micrograph.
A light optic inverted

microscope Ti Nikon (Japan)
integrated with an incubator.
Nomarsky (differential)
interference contrast (DIC),
x 900.

(apart from red blood cells) present in the suspension cannot be detected or differentiated (*Fig. 2.6 a*) although they differ noticeably from each other in form (round, circular-shaped, elongated-oval, irregular), and in size (2–4 µm, 5–7–10 µm, 10 × 20 µm, 20 × 45 µm in diameter). The surface of most cells has a prominent relief formed by round protrusions (peculiar folds) of a cytoplasmic membrane. These folds are formed as a result of changes in cells' natural tissue form when transferring them into a suspension in a cultural medium. The fold formation indicates cell membrane plasticity. The inner structure of the isolated cells, which is investigated by means of TEM, also significantly varies in different cells.

The cells are motile (possibly with the fluid flow), in contact with each other. Approximately 30 minutes after passage, i.e. the transfer into a cultural medium, the cells start attaching (not simultaneously) to the bottom of the cultural flask. After four hours of culturing, a significant part of the isolated cells have attached and flattened (*Fig. 2.6 b*). The cells' attachment occurs due to their secretion of a gel-like clear substance, possibly of a glycoconjugate nature, which "effuses" throughout the flask's bottom near the cell without losing contact with it and also without mixing with the cultural medium. The substance clings to the surface of the flask bottom and therefore, to the surface of the adjacent cell membrane. The borders of the produced secretion are clearly visible, which may be due to the varying light optical density of the secretion contact site and the cultural fluid surrounding it. A particular boundary structure – a membrane – seems to form in its place. In the literature, the feasibility of the formation of similar membranes along the contact border (separation) of solutions of two chemical compounds – proteins and polysaccharides – in the presence of calcium ions is known as an ionotropic effect (Thiale, 1967). The formed membrane limiting the gel can attach to the flask bottom on one side and to the cell membrane on the other side. The cell is likely to move along this gel intermediate layer or a "cushion" on the flask's bottom and can spread and also move. Part of the moving cells attaches along the entire surface towards the flask bottom by means of the secretion produced. Here in the area of the secretion's spread coverage somehow exceeds the equivalent diameter of the cell, which has already spread, extending beyond its borders (*Fig. 2.6 b*). Both the internal mechanism due to the polarization of actin filaments and the external mechanism, based on the capillary forces arising between the lower cell surface and its edge and the surface of the flask bottom covered by the gel produced, are involved in cells' spread and motility.

The produced secretion can shrink and form numerous folds, imitating cell processes around the attached cell, thereby substantiating the assumption of the presence of a coat or that a membrane arose on the border of its contact with the environment. Shrinking apparently results from the release of some water from the gel into the environment or inside the cell. Despite the attachment,

the cells move along the surface. Later they start to flatten out, thereby increasing the contact area with a flask bottom. The sizes of such flattened cells increase up to 20–40 µm and 15–30 µm.

Upon changing the cultural medium (24 hours after passage, i.e. at the beginning of culturing), single cells can detach in 1–2 hours and become suspended. The only cells remaining on the bottom of the flask are only attached flattened or partially spread. Such a phenomenon is apparently due to cells' response to a medium change in the form of some "contraction" and the due impairment of a gel-like substance structure, which binds the cells to the flask's bottom.

Cell attachment is a particular factor in the discriminating selection of connective tissue cells, which possess the ability to produce an adhesive substance in the form of a gel-like substance (secretion). In two days of culturing, there are cells at different stages of spreading on the flask bottom. Most of these cells have an elongated form. The lengthwise size (100–150 µm) several times exceeds the crosswise one (20–30 µm). The main part of organelles is located around the nucleus in the cell' central part, which is referred to as the endoplasm. Singular organelles and cytoskeleton threads are located in the ectoplasm – the cell peripheral part. Some organelles constantly move from the endoplasm into the ectoplasm and back (*Fig. 2.6 c*). Along the attached and flattened cells, there are microcells, whose primary size in a suspension was 2–4 µm in diameter; the length in flattened state was 20–30 µm, while it is 4–5 µm in the widest region.

The next stage in the cultured fibroblasts' vital activities is their division. Most of the attached and flattened cells – fibroblasts – have the potential to proliferate. It is owing to these cells that the cell culture grows and that a continuous monolayer is formed.

Only the spread cells divide. The whole division cycle is presented in detail by a series of successive micrographs of a single cell obtained using the technique of time-lapse photography. The flasks with cells cultured were placed in an incubator with an integrated inverted microscope (*Fig. 2.7*). The first stage, the preparation for division (*Fig. 2.7 a*), initially starts with a cell contraction in the width along its long axis. Its peripheral parts on the site of the spread ectoplasm contract and take the form of several thick long processes ranging from 2–5 (more often two with opposite poles) with a width of 5–10 µm

Fig. 2.7.
Structural dynamics of a skin (dermis) fibroblast division in a cultural medium in a cultural flask bottom.
a – a cell's preparation for division;
b – division proper;
c – division completion and spreading of daughter cells.

LM-micrograph.
A light optic inverted microscope Ti Nikon (Japan) integrated with an incubator. Nomarsky differential interference contrast (DIC), x 800.
Fragments of time-lapse photography

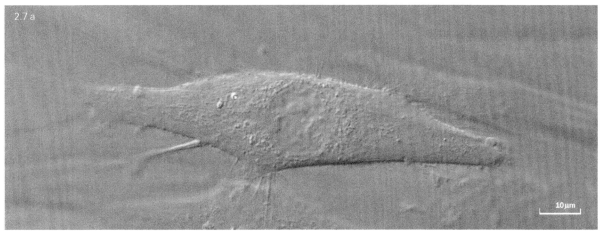

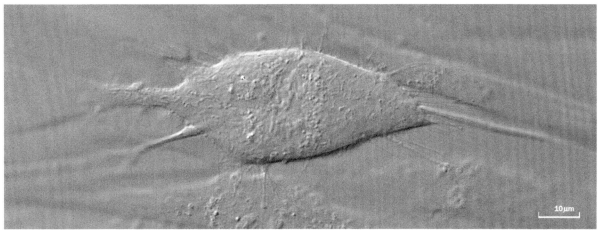

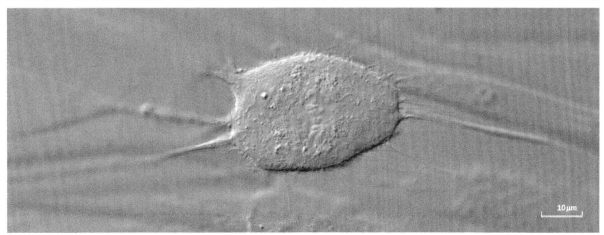

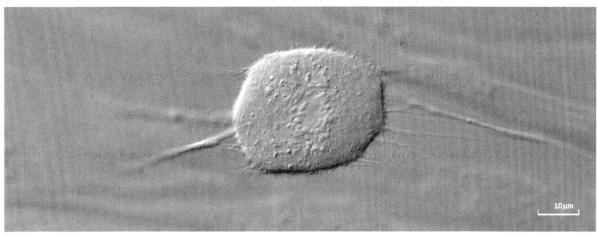

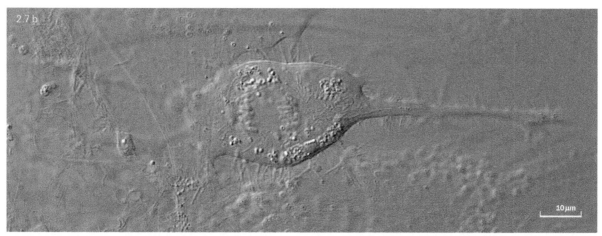

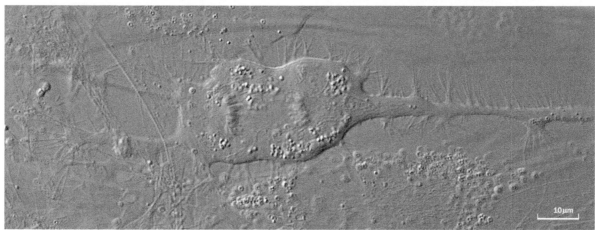

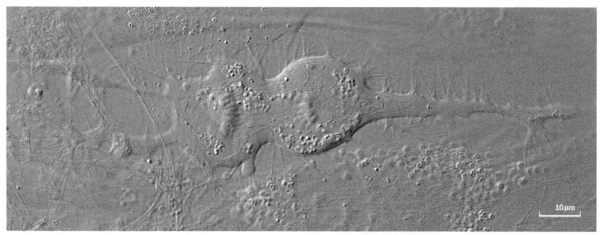

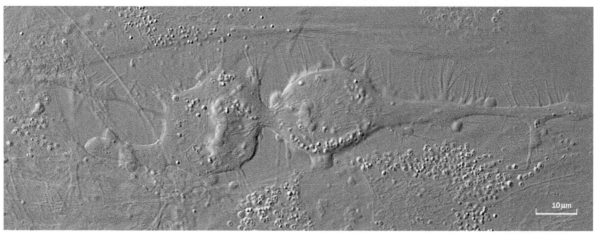

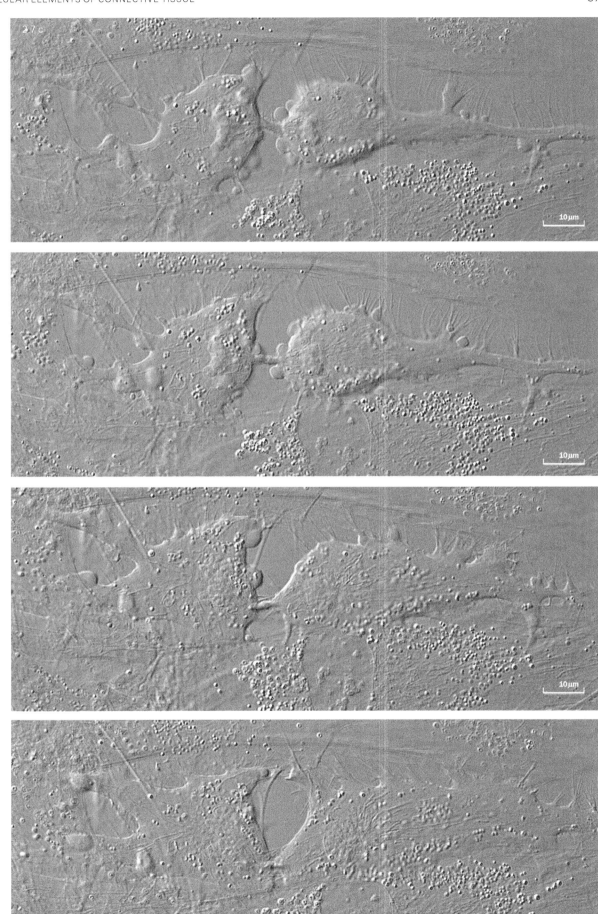

and a length of 20–50 µm. When the cell retains two processes with opposite poles, it becomes spindle-shaped. Fine threads in the form of rays perpendicularly branch from the processes. They might be residues of a gel substance, by means of which the cell attaches and fixes on the flask bottom. Later the processes contract in length approaching to the cell's central part. Their contraction can be uneven. One process (or processes) contracts quicker, while others do so more slowly. The aforementioned ray-like fine threads remain after the cell's contracted parts. The cell's central part also changes form. It becomes less spread and more prominent and circular. The radiating threads are left on the cells' sides. The cell rises more prominently over the flask bottom surface. The processes (more often two processes with opposite poles are left) become narrowed (2–3 µm) in width and shorter (10–30 µm). It should be noted that the processes are not drawn into the cell completely and are not detached from the flask's bottom, holding the cell in a certain position.

The aforementioned changes comprise the stage of mitosis–the prophase. Then the cell enters the next stage–the metaphase. It becomes circular-oval or ball-shaped and 20×30 µm in size, significantly rising over the flask bottom. The cell nucleus is not detected in such a state. Only granules-organelles in the cytoplasm and chromosomes along a cell's equatorial plane forming a metaphase plate or a mother star can be seen. Then the stage of division proper follows. A cell becomes oval-elongated and the chromosomes are pulled toward opposing poles (the stage–anaphase) (*Fig. 2.7 b*). Immediately after that, a division constriction appears on the cell's equator. The cell looks like a dumbbell. The constriction widens. The cell enters the telophase in such a manner, the significant event of which is cytokinesis (*Fig. 2.7 c*). Numerous protrusions of the cytoplasmic membrane, which can pull in and appear on other sites, arise on the two forming daughter cells. Their size ranges from 1–5 µm. The protrusion reaches its maximal size as the constriction deepens. Part of the cytoplasm with granules-organelles moves in the protrusions formed. In the period of generating protrusions, the future daughter cells take on an irregular bizarre form. This is a relatively short period of time, in which the cell's surface becomes relatively smooth and the cell starts to spread. In the division process, a fine cleavage furrow or a cell cytokinetic bridge resembling an umbilical cord is retained between future independent cells. Such a state is defined as incomplete cytokinesis as the communication between the daughter cells' cytoplasm is retained via the bridge (Danilov & Klishov, 1995). Later the protrusions are reduced in size and number. The daughter cells become more circular. Nuclear lines appear. The cells approach and come into close contact to one another. Then occurs the cells' slow elongation, and the process or processes by means of which cells are fixed to the flask bottom is maintained. Part of the cytoplasm migrates into them. If the process completely pulls in any daughter cell during con-

traction, a cytoplasmic membrane starts to protrude on the site of the former process in this cell, i.e. in an apical pole region, and part of the cytoplasm migrates into this protrusion. Before that, a cell produces a gel-like secretion, along which the protruding part of a cell spreads. The same mechanism that is observed in cell motility, flattening and spreading is reproduced. At first a gel is secreted, then a cell membrane protrusion is layered and the cytoplasm migrates into it and so on. The elongation of daughter cells continues and they start moving in opposite directions. Herein a disruption of the retained fine cell bridge occurs, i.e. cytokinesis is complete. The cells move apart. They can spread or become elongated and spindle-shaped. In the latter case, local protrusions appear and disappear quickly on the surface of spindle-shaped cells along their entire length. Irrespective of which cell starts spearing earlier, both cells spread eventually and continue dividing, albeit not simultaneously. As a rule, the first to start the following division is the daughter cell that has spread earlier. The division of the second cell can be delayed. The spread cells can take on various forms–elongated, multiangular, triangular. At the same time, the cells' form can constantly change. The adjacent cells contact with each other by their processes ("examine" or "inspect") or else temporarily overlap each other. The division rates of fixed and spread cells is not the same. Therefore, the rate of increasing cell clones also differs. This indicates the varying proliferative potencies of the cells, which depend on the degree of their development (differentiation) at the moment of their transfer into a culture, attachment and spreading. It is evident that a synthetic apparatus is to be formed in cells with a high proliferative potential to provide vital activities, to form a cell itself and its attachment to the bottom of a cultural flask by means of a gel-like secretion. At the same time, a highly differentiated or definite cell possesses less proliferative potencies. On the other hand, a relatively long stay in a cultural medium is required for a non-differentiated or poorly differentiated cell to form a synthetic apparatus, which is essential for the synthesis of a gel-like substance, by means of which the cell can attach to a cultural flask bottom and to cell proteins, which are essential for subsequent proliferation. After passage, most of skin-derived cells, which have attached to a flask bottom for 24 hours, start to divide. The continuous irregular proliferation of the cells results in uneven clone growth (i.e. monoclonal colonies) and the fusion of large clones with small ones

Fig. 2.8.
A monolayer of a skin fibroblast cell culture.
a – a disrupted monolayer;
b – a continuous (confluent) monolayer.
A nucleus (1).
Nucleoli (2).
Actin filaments in ectoplasm (3).
Granules-organelles in endoplasm (4).

An elongated microcell (7).
LM-micrograph.
A light optic inverted microscope Ti Nikon (Japan) integrated with an incubator. Nomarsky differential interference contrast (DIC), x 900.

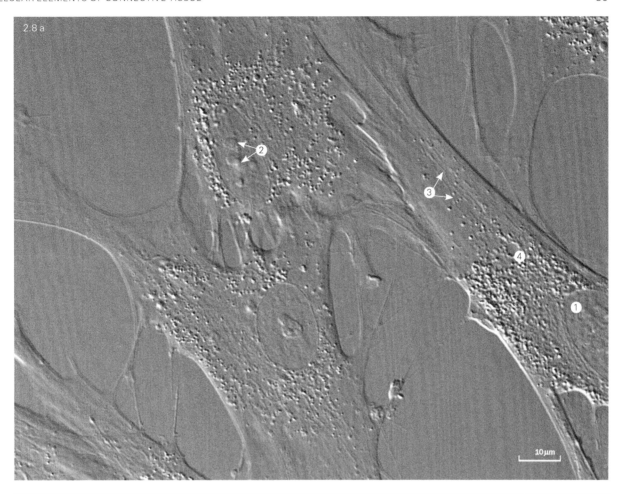

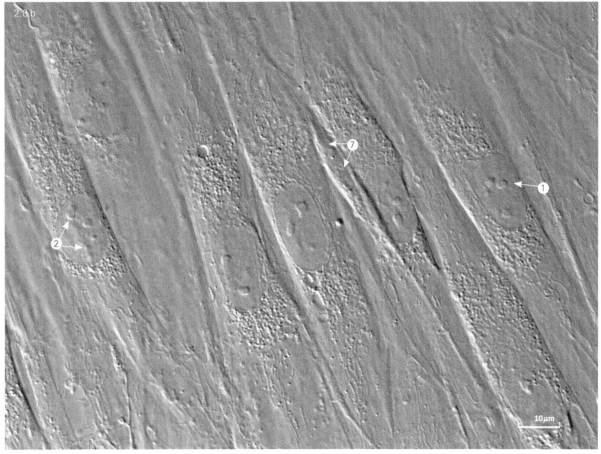

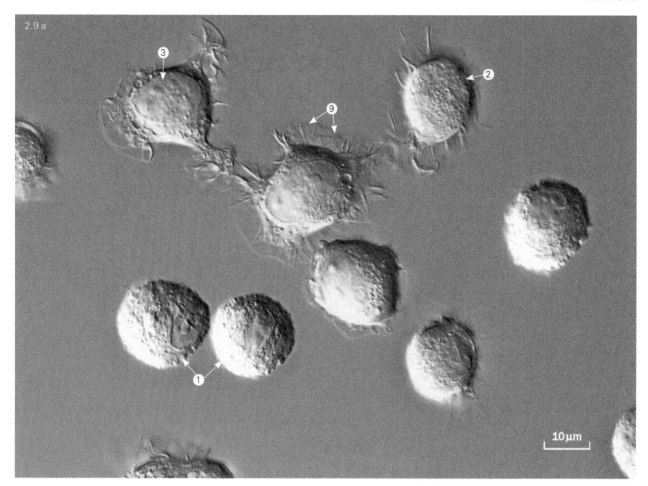

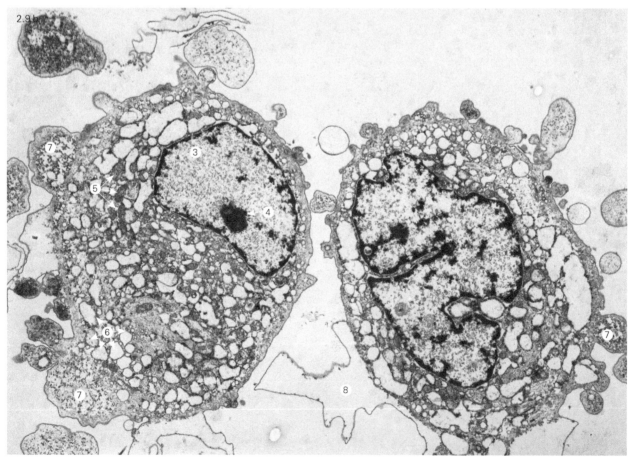

with the formation of polyclonal colonies, which represent a combination of several clones.

Due to proliferation, the cells gradually fill in the free space by limiting the range of their motion or movement therein and by affecting (changing) their form in spreading, i.e. the shape of newly formed cells and previously formed ones (*Fig. 2.8*). Thus, a continuous or confluent monolayer is formed, in which cells with a higher division rate will prevail. The interaction of cells with each other will lead to most of them becoming elongated and located in complexes, in which they are parallel or fan (radial) oriented. The thread-like and granular structures forming a cytoskeleton are visibly seen in the cells (*Fig. 2.8*). It seems that contact inhibition, delaying cell proliferation, manifests in the interaction involving the mutual pressure of the cells forming a continuous monolayer. The prevailing direction of cells' orientation is different in adjacent complexes. There are sites where the cells have a multiangular (non-elongated) form. The complexes of elongated cells surround aggregations of such cells. Among the aforementioned cells there are spindle-shaped small cells or microcells, 15–20 μm in size along the long axis and 3–5 μm along the cross axis. The division of such cells has not been observed.

Upon the continuous monolayer is fully formed, the culture of cells grown can be used for therapeutic purposes, exposed to cryoconservation for a long-term storage or passage in several flasks for subsequent culturing for the purpose of increasing a cell mass.

The structural dynamics of cultured cells of the first and subsequent passages differ from that of a zero (primary) passage (*Fig. 2.9*). Almost all cells of a continuous monolayer detached from a flask bottom and placed in a new cultural medium (i.e. being suspended) are ball-shaped with a diameter of 20–23 μm, i.e. they are more homogeneous and much bigger than the great mass of cells derived from a tissue and placed in a cultural medium. The prominent relief of a cell's surface is formed by circular protrusions of the cytoplasm or cytoplasmic membrane folds (*Fig. 2.9 a, b*). A peculiar "aureole" from the gel substances secreted by the cells is formed around the attached and flattened cells. The folds, which are possibly resulted from its osmotic dehydration, are also formed on a surface of this substance. An "aureole" accompanies

the spread cells (fibroblasts). The certain irrigation of a cytoplasm and a nucleus is general for all cells suspended. It manifests in a cytoplasm containing a considerable number of vacuoles of different size. The cytoplasm peripheral part near a cytoplasmic membrane looks structurally rarefied. In separate sites, the "lamination" or detaching of a cytoplasmic membrane from the cytoplasm structural part in the form of a protrusion, which does not contain any cell structural elements, is observed. Apart from vacuoles, there is a fine-granular material of moderate electron density in the cytoplasm's central part. Mitochondria and vacuoles of various size, with contents differing in density, have been detected. In such cells, the cell nucleus can be multilobed, which is formed due to invaginations of a nuclear membrane (*Fig. 2.9 b*). Euchromatin and heterochromatin are revealed in the nucleus. The rarefaction of a heterochromatin structure is also observed. The nucleus contains one or several nucleoli. Cytoplasm protrusions, folding of the cytoplasmic membrane and nucleus have obviously arisen due to the changing of the cell entire form as a result of the reduction of its volume after detaching from a surface of a flask bottom and the transition into a suspended state. In 15 minutes, the cells start fixing and spreading (*Fig. 2.10 a*). After four hours, almost every cell is attached. Most of the cells have a flattened form. Their spreading starts (*Fig. 2.10 b*). The time interval between the beginning of attachment and spreading of the first passage cultured cells is significantly less than that in a null passage. A layer (as an aureole) of a gel-like substance with the folds formed surrounds the cells in the periphery. The width of this layer significantly varies. Cell spreading is accompanied by the redistribution of the endoplasm's constituent elements (the cell organelles and intracellular matrix) adjusted for a cell becoming more flattened. The latter is associated with a flat surface of the supportive matrix (a cultural flask bottom), along which a cell membrane unfolds (unwraps) and possibly stretches out. The peripheral part of a flattened or spread cell referred to as the ectoplasm contains single organelles and the cytoskeleton elements in the form of actin threads (*Fig. 2.10 c*). The intracellular matrix or hyaloplasm prevails therein. As in the null passage, the spread cells start dividing by repeating the aforementioned proliferation cycle. The division onset of every cell depends on the progress of the preceding steps: attachment and spreading. Unlike the null passage, almost every subcultured cell divides in the first passage. Thereby a continuous monolayer, similar to that in the null passage, can be obtained in 2–3 days. This depends on the number of the cells cultured. The fibroblasts have the same locality and orientation therein as observed in the null passage (*Fig. 2.10 d*). Passaging leads to the elimination of a non-connective tissue differon form the cell culture, i.e. there are only fibroblasts free from other cells in the culture of the 3rd–4th passages.

The fibroblasts' structural dynamics during the second and following passages (including the division) are simi-

Fig. 2.9.
Human skin fibroblasts
in a cultural medium.
The first passage:
a – non-attached (1)
and attached (2) fibroblasts;
b – non-attached fibroblasts.
A nucleus (3).
Nucleoli (4).
Mitochondria (5).
Vacuoloo (6).
Protrusions of the cytoplasmic
membrane with cytoplasm (7).
Protrusions of the cytoplasmic
membrane with cleavage from
the cytoplasm structural
part (8).

Gel-like substance (9).
a – LM-micrograph.
A light optic inverted
microscope Ti Nikon (Japan)
integrated with an incubator.
Nomarsky (differential)
interference contrast (DIC),
x 900.
b – TEM-micrograph.
Contrasting of ultrathin sections
with lead citrate and uranyl
acetate.
b – x 5,000;
c – x 30,000; d – x 80,000.

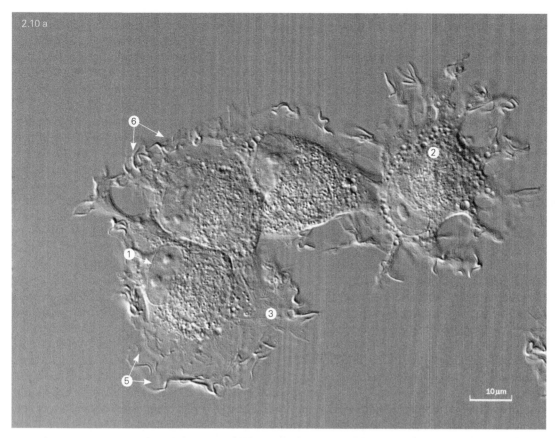

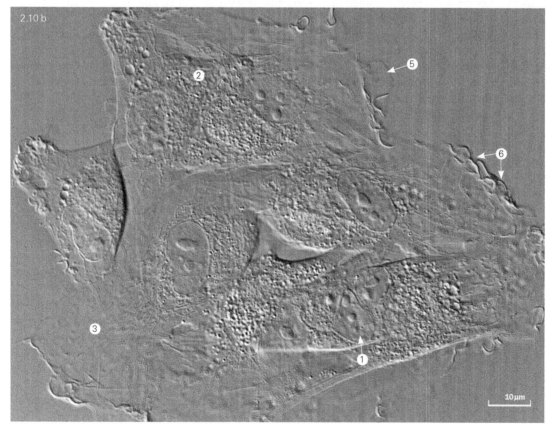

Fig. 2.10.
Human skin fibroblasts in a cultural medium.
The first passage:

a – attached and flattened fibroblasts;
b – flattened and partially spread fibroblasts;

c – spread fibroblasts in a discontinuous monolayer;
d – fibroblasts in a continuous monolayer.

A nucleus and nucleoli (1).
Granules-organelles in endoplasm (2).
Ectoplasm (3).

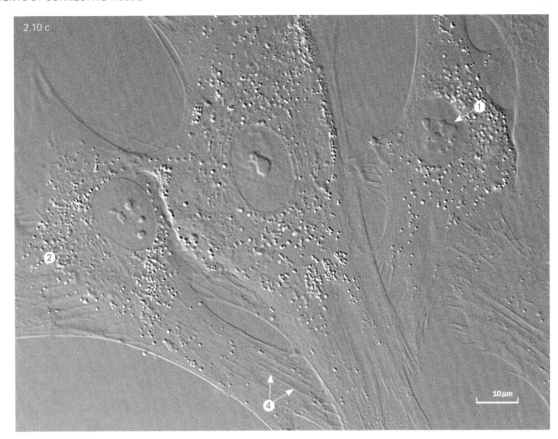

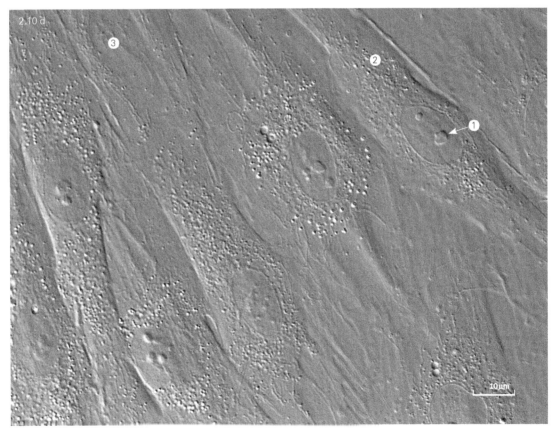

Microfilaments (actin threads) and microtubules of the cytoskeleton in ectoplasm (4). Gel-like substance (5). Folds of a gel-like substance (6). LM-micrograph. A light optic inverted microscope Ti Nikon (Japan) integrated with an incubator. Nomarsky differential interference contrast (DIC), x 800.

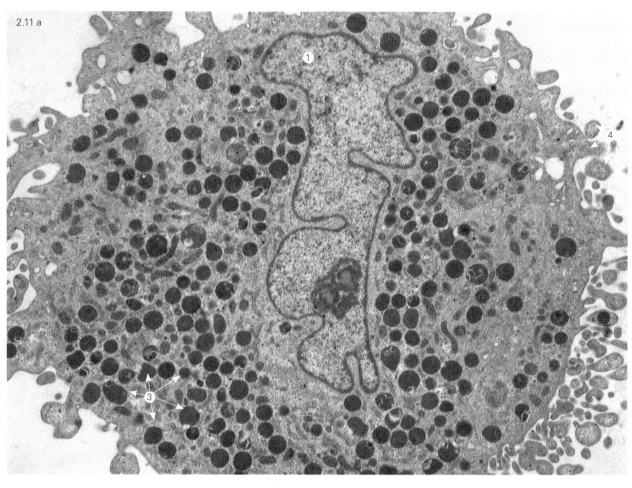

2.11 a

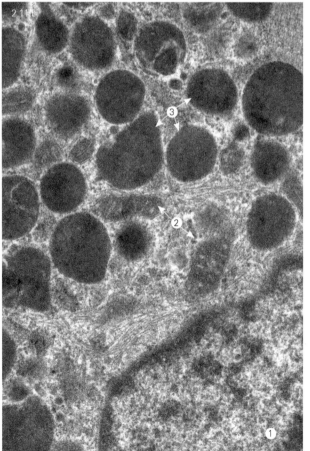

2.11 b

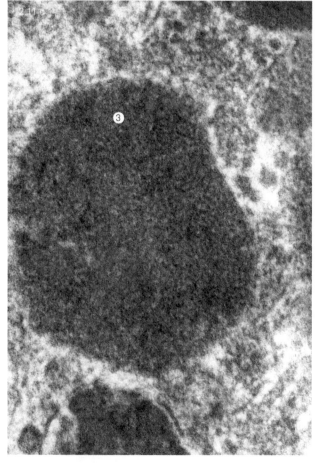

2.11 c

lar to that of the first passage. The generation and accumulation of a great number of fragments of microtubules, cytoskeleton microfibrillar and actin threads and electron dense bodies or aggregates with different electron density, which have diffuse or clear-cut outlines but are not surrounded by a membrane, are new (*Fig. 2.11 a, b, c*). Aggregates' size ranges from 0.2–1.0 µm in a diameter. They are discrete formations and consist of 10–20 nm electron dense granules. The aggregates seem to be formed from the fragments of the cytoskeleton elements in its depolarization, which is associated with cells' contraction in their detachment from a flask bottom. The cell cytoplasm is denser. These structures are more concentrated in the case of non-attached or just attached cells. The spread cells in a continuous monolayer also contain the aforementioned structures; however, there are noticeably fewer of them. This may be partially due to the larger area of the spread cells and the cytoskeleton restoration. A great number of vacuoles are located along the cytoplasmic membrane's inner surface. Some of them are open inside the environment. These vacuoles might carry out the function of exocytosis and endocytosis. Euchromatin and heterochromatin are revealed in the nucleus (*Fig. 2.11 d, e, f*). A newly synthesized intercellular matrix is located between the cells. In division, during the cells' contraction and their becoming circular, their cytoplasmic membranes do not form protrusions similar to those, which are formed in the cultured cells detached from a flask bottom (*Fig. 2.11 g*). Electron dense aggregates, approximately in equal numbers, are distributed between the daughter cells. In the metaphase stage, the chromosome structure is seen well in a metaphase plate (*Fig. 2.11 g*). There is no nuclear membrane. There are electron dense bodies-aggregates, single fragments of the rough endoplasmic reticulum, mitochondria, small vacuoles, and granular intracellular matrix in the cytoplasm. The cell exhibits single short fine processes.

The growth character and shape of the cells in a culture, to a large extent, depend on the properties of the material on which the cells grow, such as glass, plastic, or a collagen matrix (from a horse tendon or dematerialized bone matrix (DBM).

Upon being placed on a collagen matrix, the fibroblasts attach to fibrillar collagen structures and, for some time, they retain a round shape acquired in a cell suspension. Then the cells repeat all of the stages described above for fibroblasts placed on the bottom of glass or plastic flasks. Upon completing this process, they form a dense cell

layer. The fibroblasts attach to the collagen structures by their numerous processes rather than by their adjacent surface (apart from the glass flask or plastic bottom) (*Fig. 2.12 a*). The processes form a whole structural hierarchy. The processes of the first order branch directly from a cell body. Their thickness ranges from 1–10 µm. The processes of the second order branch from those of the first one and therefore have a smaller thickness (*Fig. 2.12 b*). There can also be processes of the third, fourth and other orders. The thickness, shape and extent of a process can vary. This obviously depends on the conditions of their existence.

2.2.2. Biochemical and molecular biological characteristics of fibroblastic differon

The concept of a fibroblastic differon has a complex "catch-all" character and the generalized term **fibroblast** does not convey the entire diversity of the cells comprising it (Chang et al., 2002). A fibroblastic differon is comprised of cells that have a formal resemblance but originate from the stem cells of different embryonic mesenchyme regions, including the hematopoietic mesenchyme (Ogawa et al., 2006). Moreover, the ectodermal genesis of a part of the fibroblasts, particularly the active fibroblasts involved in fibrous reactions resulting from the epithelial-mesenchymal transition, has recently been strongly confirmed (Wynn, 2008). This additionally increases the number of fibroblasts' differentiation ways. Such a variety of origin determines the generally recognized **phenotypic heterogeneity** of fibroblasts (Serov & Shekhter, 1981). This heterogeneity is manifested not only by the cells' morphological peculiarities and their behavior when cultured *in vitro* (Abercrombie, 1978), but also by the peculiarities of their functioning at the molecular level. Phenotypic heterogeneity is prominent in fibroblast populations in a different degree, depending on how their sources (progenitors) and differentiation ways differ. It also depends on the microenvironment influence, contacts with other cells, and interactions of regulatory factors. The fibroblast's state – whether it is resting or active – is of importance.

The fibroblasts' heterogeneity is so high that the **production program** of a **connective tissue extracellular matrix** can be considered as the only general phenotypic criterion that unifies all their populations (Robert, 1995). A fibroblast should be considered as a cell that synthesizes and secretes all main matrix protein components,

Fig. 2.11.
Human skin fibroblasts in a cultural medium.
The fourth passage:
a, b, c – non attached fibroblast in a cultural medium;
d, e, f – spread fibroblasts in a monolayer;
g – a fibroblast in a period of division at the stage of metaphase plate – a mother star.

A nucleus and nucleolus (1).
Mitochondria (2).
The cytoplasm contains circular electron dense bodies aggregates (3).
The protrusions of the cytoplasmic membrane (processes possibly) (4).
Microfilaments (actin threads) and microtubules of the cytoskeleton (5).

Chromosomes of the metaphase plate (6).
Vacuoles (7).
The granular intracellular matrix (8).
TEM-micrograph.
Contrasting of ultrathin sections with lead citrate and uranyl acetate.

a – x 6,000
b – x 40,000
c – x 80,000
d – x 10,000
e – x 20,000
f – x 40,000
g – x 6,000

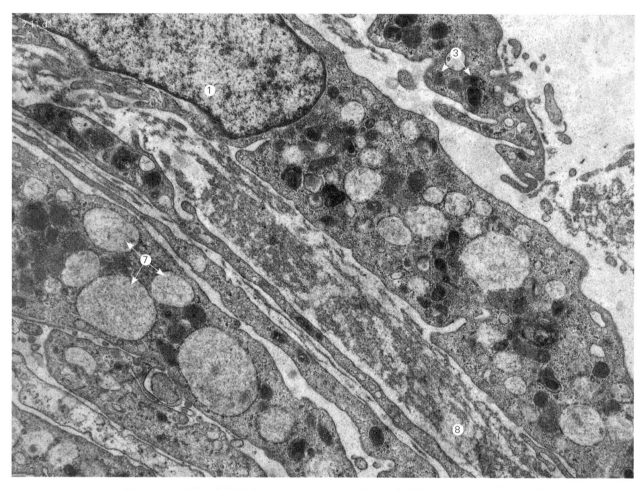

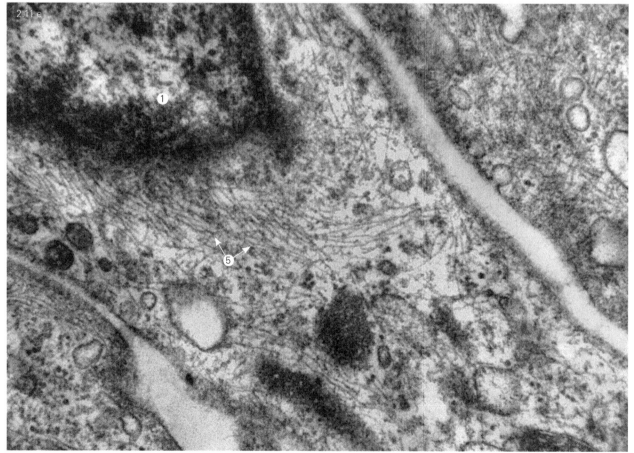

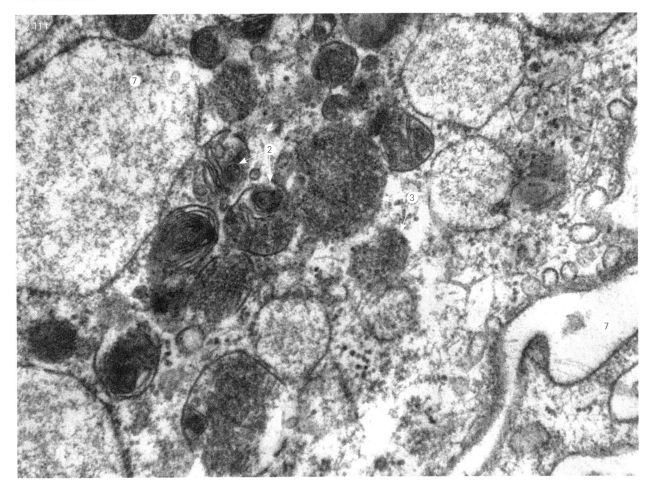

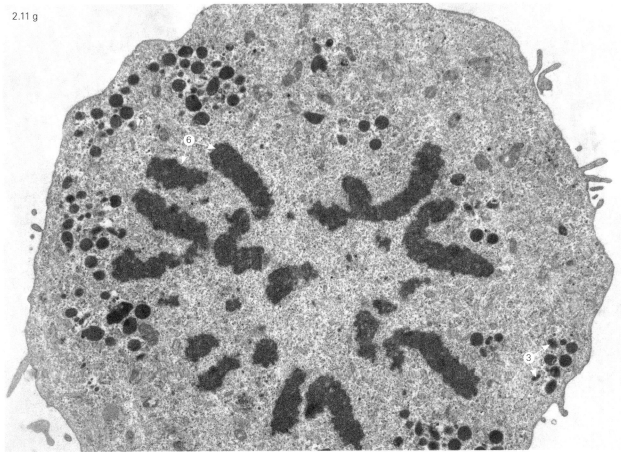

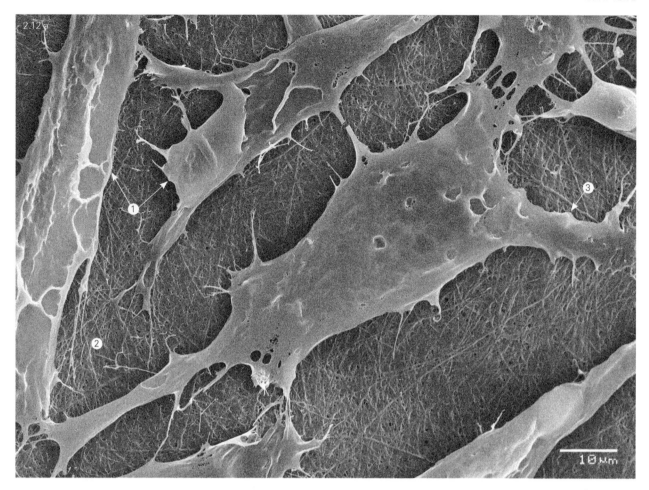

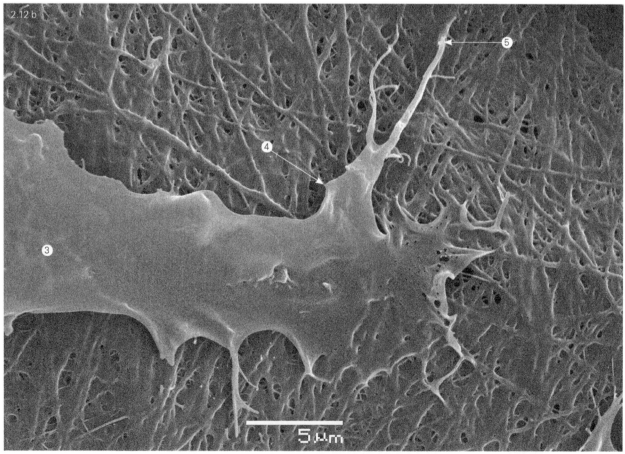

and primarily macromolecular structural components. The collagenous proteins, particularly fibrillar (fiber-forming) collagens, are most prominent among all these components. A fibroblast's biosynthetic "power" is extremely high: one differentiated cell in an active state is capable of producing 3.5 mln of collagen macromolecules per 24 hours (McAnulty, 2007). Along with collagens, the fibroblast produces other matrix fibrillar components (elastin, fibrillins) and structural protein components of the integrating buffer metabolic medium – glycoproteins and proteoglycans. Moreover, the fibroblasts produce and secrete the enzymes into the matrix, one part of which completes the post-translation processing of structural proteins and is involved in their integration into supramolecular structures, and the other part carries out the catabolic reactions necessary to maintain the matrix's dynamic balance.

The fibroblasts' phenotypic functional program, aimed at the construction of the connective tissue extracellular matrix, determines their main role in multicellular organisms. This role, referred to as "sculptural" (Doljanski, 2004), is manifested in morphogenetic processes and consists of providing organs, body individual parts and the body in whole with their **shape**.

The fibroblastic differon functional program, in its principal features, extends to differons of the specialized cells – chondroblast/chondrocyte in a cartilage, osteoblast/osteocyte in a bone, tenoblast/tenocyte in tendons and others, which perform the same function as the fibroblasts – namely, the formation of an extracellular matrix in various types of connective tissue. In this sense, a fibroblast is a **prototype** of the main class of different connective tissue cells that can be considered as modified or "sophisticated" fibroblasts, which differ from their prototype only by the selective activity of some genes' expression. This activity complies with the composition peculiarities of the matrix they synthesize. The set of collagens these cells synthesize and secrete is the selectivity most evident example; for example, a chondroblast produces type II, IX, XI collagens specific for a cartilaginous tissue.

As a prototype, a dermis fibroblast, which mainly produces fibril-forming type I collagen and, in embryonal and early postnatal periods, type III collagen, is recognized as a "classic" fibroblast. Serov & Shekhter (1981) proposed calling this fibroblast a collagenoblast, emphasizing that the main cell's biosynthetic load lies with collagen expression. The fibroblasts of loose connective tissue of various localization and those of visceral organs' connective tissue stroma and of dense fibrous connective tissue types, tendons and ligaments (tenoblasts), are similar to this fibroblast in terms of their phenotypic characteristics.

The biosynthesis mechanism and secretion ways of collagens by a fibroblast into the extracellular matrix will be the subject of section 3.1.1.1. A connection of procollagen polypeptide α-chains, assembled on the ribosomes into its macromolecules, and the macromolecules' movement via the lamella complex cisterns towards the cytoplasmic membrane occur with the involvement of accessory (accompanying) proteins – **chaperones**. A chaperone with a molecular mass of 47 kDa (**HSP47**, heat shock protein 47), also known as a collagen-binding protein or **colligin**, is especially important among them. HSP47 (as a member of the serpin family) exerts activity as a proteolytic enzyme inhibitor and is present in other cells, but its concentration is especially high in fibroblasts due to collagens' intensive synthesis; therefore, it is considered important as one of the relatively specific markers of the dermal fibroblast phenotype (Kuroda & Tajima, 2008).

Vimentin is considered to be a more specific marker of typical fibroblasts. It is a structural protein of the cytoskeleton's intermediate filaments, which promote the strengthening of the cytoskeleton's connection with hemidesmosomes (hemidesmosomes are a type of cell adhesive structures enabling the fibroblasts' interaction with the extracellular matrix). The fibroblasts contain this homodimeric phosphoprotein in a high amount relative to other cells, and mutations leading to switching off the vimentin gene are accompanied by serious impairments of fibroblasts' mechanic stability, mobility and contractility (Eckes et al., 1998). An increase in the intensity of cells' immunocytochemical staining of vimentin, coinciding with the beginning of type I collagen expression by the same cells, is considered as one of the main criteria of a epithelial-mesenchymal transition (EMT) (Kokkinos et al., 2007).

An intensified expression of the protein S100A4, which is also called a **fibroblast specific protein 1** (FSP1), by cells is another important marker of the phenomenon of epithelial-mesenchymal transition, which results in the formation of a significant part of fibroblasts (this will be discussed below) and therefore, as a fibroblast's marker (Teng et al., 2007). Blocking FSP1 expression by cultured epithelial cells delays their transition. Its expression is high in the fibroblasts of healing wounds and in fibroblasts involved in the fibrosis of parenchymal organs, for example, in the lungs (Lawson et al., 2005).

S100A4/FSP1, a small protein (with a molecular mass of 11.7 kDa) is a member of the large class of cytoplasmic S100-proteins of the calmodulin superfamily. The S100-proteins are involved in many intracellular processes (microtubules' dynamics, interaction of the cytoskeleton with the plasmolemma, calcium ions-mediated signals' transduction, cell cycle regulation and others). The functions of S100A4/FSP1 have not been exactly clarified. It is

Fig. 2.12.
Fibroblasts (1) of human skin on a collagen matrix (2) in a cultural medium. Fibroblast processes of the first order (3), the second order (4), the third order (5). SEM-micrograph.
a – x 3,000
b – x 10,000

supposed that this protein, whose molecule binds two calcium ions, relates to the maintenance of mesenchymal cells' shape and motility (Iwano et al., 2002).

All the aforementioned proteins play the role of fibroblastic markers in fibroblasts relating to reparative ones. The fibroblasts of these populations, which are involved in proliferative-reparative connective tissue reactions (e.g. wound healing, fibrosis of parenchymal organs, development of the malignant stroma), differ from mature organ-specific and tissue-specific resident (universal) fibroblasts by their increased activity. Fibroblasts generated as a result of epithelial-mesenchymal transition are in such an active state, as this transition occurs mainly when an abrupt increase in the fibroblasts' number is required. Therefore, the role of vimentin, S100A4/FSP1 and HSP47 as the markers of other less active fibroblast populations should be carefully evaluated.

This remark completely refers to the **fibroblast activation protein** α (FAPα). This integral transmembrane protein, passing throughout the cytoplasmic membrane (one-pass protein), is a proteolytic enzyme–serine protease dipeptidylpeptidase IV (its other name is seprase) (Wang et al., 2008). It contains 760 amino acid residues, has a glycoprotein nature and exerts gelatinase activity. FAPα is considered as a rather specific fibroblast marker, but again of fibroblasts that are in an active state. FAPα expression is especially evident in the fibroblasts of cancer tumor stroma and in sarcoma tumor cells (malignant transformed fibroblasts), making FAPα an important marker of the fibroblast state in oncological investigations (Henry et al., 2007). At the same time, seprase expression is detected in articular cartilage chondrocytes affected by anti-inflammatory stimuli, and this fact diminishes the FAPα specificity as a fibroblast marker (Milner et al., 2005).

The described molecular (cytochemical) markers, indicating the differences between the reparative (activated) and universal tissue fibroblasts, are only one possible manifestation of fibroblasts' heterogeneity.

Fibroblasts' heterogeneity is a large-scale concept, which is considered on two levels. At the first level, it comprises comparatively small functional (molecular biochemical) peculiarities of cells within separate genetically and morphologically homogenous cell populations, and, at the second level, significant morphological and molecular differences between the populations with different sources of their origin and their functions in an organism.

Heterogeneity at the first level–fibroblasts' intrapopulation heterogeneity–has been characterized in detail in cultured human dermis fibroblasts (Chang et al., 2002). When studying the expression of the whole set of genes comprising a genome of these cells, very significant differences of expression activity of the genes' entire sets have been established, depending on the skin anatomical area from which the fibroblasts were derived. Such transcription differences, called **topographic differentiation**, are detected in the sets of genes involved in the

synthesis of the extracellular matrix, lipids' metabolism, and the formation of signal pathways related to cell proliferation and migration.

Differences between the fibroblasts of the dermis reticular and superficial (papillary) layers have been found, where additional peculiarities distinguish the papillary fibroblasts located at a dermal-epidermal junction (**DEJ**) and fibroblasts associated with hair follicles. The differences manifest in a qualitative composition of the cell-synthesized extracellular matrix, i.e. in gene transcription. The papillary layer contains fibrill-associated FACIT XII and XVI type collagens, type IV collagen (in a basement membrane), type VI collagen in the DEJ (see section 3.1.1.1), tenascin-C (see section 3.2.1.1), and the large proteoglycan versican (see section 3.2.1.2), which are absent or present in a very small amount in the matrix reticular layer. As for the reticular layer, it contains FACIT type XIV collagen and tenascin-X, which are absent in the papillary layer. Versican is detected in the reticular layer only in connection with elastic fibers. These differences are partially intrinsic for the matrix produced *in vivo* by fibroblasts derived from various layers of the dermis (Sorrell & Caplan, 2004).

The differences between the subpopulations derived from a general population of dermis residential fibroblasts, which involve the expression of 337 genes, are collectively so significant that they justify the evaluation of these subpopulations as separate types of fibroblasts despite their morphologic similarity. This evaluation of dermal fibroblasts heterogeneity (position variability) is also confirmed by the fact that adult fibroblasts retain the local expression of so-called homeotic genes, which are specific for the embryonic period (see 1.4). These genes regulate the implementation of a general body pattern. Although the expression of many homeotic genes (for example, *DLX5, EYA2, LIMK1*), which is intrinsic for mesenchymal stem cells, discontinues upon their differentiation into fibroblasts (Brendel et al., 2005), the retaining activity of some of them (*HOXA5, HOXA11, HOXA13, HOXD8, TBX2, TBX15, EMX3, FOXF1, TRPS1*) is sufficient to provide fibroblasts with information on their locality. The differences between fibroblasts of the upper and lower body parts, the upper and lower extremities are most evident. All this implies that the phenotypic heterogeneity of the dermal fibroblasts' population is mainly due to genotypic peculiarities laid down in the earliest stages of differentiation rather than local peculiarities of the signals coming from the extracellular matrix (Rinn et al., 2006).

The range of genes' transcription activity is even wider upon comparing dermal and non-dermal (derived from the stroma of visceral organs and skeletal muscles' connective tissue) tissue fibroblasts. In this comparison, statistically significant differences are noted in 396 genes (Rinn et al., 2006). The differences concern particularly the fibroblasts' expression of a number of signaling molecules, such as interleukins IL-6, IL-8, the transforming growth factor TGF-β, the hepatocyte growth factor (HGF), and especially the keratinocyte growth factor (KGF), which is essential for dermal fibroblasts in terms of their participation in wound healing (Nolte et al., 2007).

The heterogeneity of a tissue fibroblast's phenotype is manifested by their uneven response to mechanical stress. Upon exposing the culturing fibroblasts derived from the cornea, skin and tendon to mechanical stress, the differences between them have been detected in the expression of about 350 genes. The differences were predominantly related to the genes associated with the synthesis of the extracellular matrix and focal adhesions' components, enzymes that are responsible for matrix remodeling, and cytokines and other signaling molecules (Mackley et al., 2006). It should be recalled that, among all fibroblast specialized types, tenoblasts/tenocytes are closest to universal fibroblasts and are often referred to as fibroblasts.

The significant molecular biochemical phenotype differences are noted in fibroblasts of the connective tissue stroma of various visceral organs. These differences are reflected in the definition of tissue fibroblasts as "organ-specific".

For example, morphologically identical fibroblasts of the heart stroma and those of the lungs manifest a different fibro-proliferating response to the effect of cerium. This response, having a mitogenic character, is evident in the cardiac fibroblasts but it is almost absent in the lung fibroblasts; this specificity of cardiac fibroblasts' response is due to the intensive intracellular production of active oxygen radicals. In cerium-induced pneumoconiosis, lung fibrosis also occurs but the lung fibroblasts neutralize oxygen radicals by means of N-acetyl-L-cysteine production; therefore the developing fibrosis has a different pathogenesis (Nair et al., 2003).

With their morphologic similarity, periodont fibroblasts differ from those of the dermis by more active expression of the signaling molecules–hepatocyte growth factors (HGF) and keratinocytes (KGF) in a combined culturing with keratinocytes. This explains the peculiarities of chronic periodont disorders (Gren et al., 2002).

The phenotypic differences between typical tissue fibroblasts of the dermis and similar cells of dense connective tissue types, such as tendons and joint capsules are great. These cells (tenoblasts/tenocytes) are often referred to as fibroblasts but they differ from fibroblasts resident in other localities by a number of signs and chiefly by their capacity for intensive expression of so-called FACIT type XII (Zhang et al., 2003) and XIV (Young et al., 2000) collagens (see section 3.1.1.1), especially in embryogenesis, which are involved in the formation of the mechanical properties of the fibers of type I collagen and the extracellular matrix on the whole. The fibroblasts of the periodontal ligament significantly differ from gingival fibroblasts, which are morphologically close to them in the expression of 163 genes: the former have a higher expression of genes related to cell cycle regulation, i.e. the ability to proliferate, whereas genes encoding the cytoskeleton and

transmembrane proteins are more active in the latter (Han & Amar, 2002). These phenotypic differences in the fibroblasts of tendons and ligaments are determined by the peculiarities of gene transcription regulation. The transcription factor Scleraxis, a member of the bHLH (basic helix-loop-helix) domain-containing protein superfamily, is one of the leading transcription regulators in tendon cells (Lejard et al., 2007).

Synoviocytes B in the synovial membrane, which meet all the criteria of fibroblasts, are another example of a special cell population (Edwards, 2000). The synovial fibroblasts of the membrane internal layer, which directly contact with the synovia (synovial fluid), express VCAM-1 (vascular cell adhesion molecule), the enzyme UDPGD (uridine diphosphoglucose dehydrogenase) and DAF (decay-accelerating factor) with increased activity.

The concept of fibroblasts' heterogeneity is significantly broadened upon its consideration at the second level–upon comparing all populations of tissue (resident) fibroblasts on the one hand, and the aforementioned **active (reparative)** fibroblasts' functioning in those connective tissue regions where they are in an activated state on the other hand.

Several types of reparative fibroblasts are known. The first type consists of cells originating from the resident (tissue) fibroblasts and performing their main function–the expression and secretion of extracellular matrix macromolecular components in a maximally intensified mode. The reparative fibroblasts are close to differentiated embryonic fibroblasts in their functional activity, but their difference from the resident fibroblasts is not only quantitative (in the sense of intensity of biosynthetic processes). The qualitative difference, as has already been stated, is that it is the reparative (activated) fibroblasts that exhibit the prominently marked expression of specific markers–vimentin, HSP47, FSP1/S100A4, FAPα.

The reparative fibroblasts in their majority refer to a special cell population–myofibroblasts. The **myofibroblasts**, which have been discussed in detail in section 2.2.1, are a group of various cells that are between the fibroblasts and smooth muscle cells in terms of their phenotypic characteristics. In other words, these cells exert activity intrinsic for typical fibroblasts, which is targeted at the biosynthesis of the extracellular matrix components and, at the same time, contain structural intracellular proteins that are characteristic for smooth muscle cells; these proteins provide myofibroblasts with their contracting ability.

This contracting ability, which is especially evident in the contraction of wound scars and fibrosis-sclerotic intermediate layers, does not cover myofibroblasts' functions. They are present, albeit in a small amount, in normal tissues and are involved in the physiologic remodeling of the extracellular matrix and in the regulation of the interstitial fluid volume and pressure (McAnulty, 2007). The myofibroblasts exert prominent paracrine signaling activity, which is somehow different from that of the fibroblasts, by expressing a great deal of molecules of local (short-distance) action (see section 4.2), such as growth factors, cytokines, chemokines and inflammation mediators, including mediators of a lipid nature regulating the progress of both normal and pathologic tissue reactions (Powell et al., 1999).

The myofibroblasts differ from smooth muscle cells in the peculiarities of transcription intracellular regulation of one of the contracting system's main proteins–α-actin (α-SMA). Specifically, they employ a transcription factor–the protein RTEF-1 (TEAD-4), binding to the promoter element MCAT, whereas the factor TEF-1 (TEAD-3) acts in interaction with the same element in smooth muscle cells (Gan et al., 2007).

The main factor initiating and then stimulating the differentiation of fibroblasts into myofibroblasts is the leading member of the transforming growth factor β superfamily (TGF-β), the factor TGF-β1, which exerts pronounced proinflammatory activity (Demoulliére et al., 2005).

Along with this, other factors present in the extracellular matrix affect myofibroblasts' differentiation in the same direction. The matrix glycoproteins–fibronectins and vitronectin (see section 3.2.1.1)–affecting the cells as ligands of relative specific receptors, integrins α5 and αv, are necessary to initiate the enhanced expression of α-SMA and to perform the contracting function (Lygoe et al., 2007). The multifunctional cytokine **osteopontin**, which is intensely expressed in the tissues of healing wounds and in fibrosis foci, is also essential; switching off the osteopontin-encoding gene OPN discontinues myofibroblast differentiation (Lenga et al., 2007).

Myofibroblasts' induction (the beginning of differentiation) is stimulated by the vasoconstrictor peptide endothelin-1 and thrombin (coagulation factor IIa) (Demoulliére et al., 2005). The action of mechanical factors is also of importance (Tomasek et al., 2002).

The proliferation of tissue fibroblasts and their differentiation into myofibroblasts actively occur at the edges of a skin wound. The influence of paracrine molecular factors, which are expressed by the epidermis cells–keratinocytes–is of great importance to induce and stimulate this process. In particular, the keratinocytes are a source for the epidermis growth factor (EGF), the platelet-derived growth factor (PDGF) and the transforming growth factor α (TGF-α), which actively affect myofibroblast differentiation (Werner et al., 2007). The uPA/uPAR system serves as one of the established molecular mechanisms mediating the differentiation. This system consists of the extracellular protease–urokinase (plasminogen activator) (uPA), which is essential for matrix remodeling and cell migration, and a receptor of this enzyme (uPAR). The fibroblasts actively express uPA and uPAR; the receptor, which is of a glycoprotein nature and also known as the CD87-antigen, is present on the surface of their cytoplasmic membrane. The uPAR receptor extracellular domain is shortened in myofibroblasts and it has been established that protease inhibition, which breaks

down this domain, prevents myofibroblasts' differentiation. Therefore, the uPAR breakdown is a critical step in differentiation (Bernstein et al., 2007).

The chemokines CCL2 and CCL3 and specific pro-fibrotic interleukins Il-12 and IL-21 promote the involvement of myofibroblasts into the foci of fibrous tissue formation (Wynn, 2008).

During differentiation, a myofibroblast undergoes a proto-myofibroblast stage, where the cells contain only β- and γ-cytoplasmic actins. The differentiation can discontinue at this stage and smooth muscle actin α (α-SMA) originates only in a mature myofibroblast (Tomasek et al., 2002).

A myofibroblasts' population is heterogeneous. Myofibroblasts differentiated in different organs originate from different cells, referring to a fibroblastic differon (Hinz et al., 2007), and therefore retain some specific markers. For example, myofibroblasts that are formed from so-called stellate cells (they normally play a role of a vitamin A reservoir) in fibrosis-sclerotic processes in the liver carry a marker that distinguishes them from other myofibroblasts: it is the membrane glycoprotein Thy-1 (CD90-antigen) bond to a cell membrane lipid component–glycophosphatidylinositol (Dudas et al., 2007). The myofibroblasts of atheromatous plaques are formed not only of resident fibroblasts of the vascular wall medial and adventitial layers, but are also formed of smooth muscle cells. Upon differentiating into myofibroblasts, these cells start expressing collagens and α-SMA. However, at the same time, they retain the ill-marked expression of smooth muscle myosin (Hinz et al., 2007).

Circulating (mobile) **fibrocytes** are common progenitors of reparative fibroblasts, including fibroblasts' differentiation into myofibroblasts. The cellular hematopoietic elements of bone marrow–cells that comprise a small subpopulation of the white blood cells (WBC)–can be one of the fibrocyte progenitors. These progenitors have WBC typical markers–CD34, CD45, CD13. At the same time, they exhibit plasticity, which enables their further differentiation, and express the chemokine receptors CXCR4 and CCR7, facilitating extravascularization (Gomperts & Strieter, 2007). As a result of differentiation, they take on a number of phenotypic features of reparative (active) fibroblasts, such as vimentin expression, the intensive biosynthesis of type I and III collagens and fibronectins, while retaining some features of their progenitors (Bucala et al., 2004). They adjoin activated tissue fibroblasts in the foci of proliferative reparative connective tissue reactions, contribute their share towards the formation of an extracellular matrix and, moreover, intensively express signaling molecules–TGF-β1 and the connective tissue growth factor (CTGF, see 4.2)–which exert a stimulating effect on biosynthetic activity of tissue fibroblasts (Wang J.F. et al., 2007).

These activated circulating fibrocytes are capable of continuing differentiation. Many of them take on myofibroblast functions and markers, including the main marker α-SMA (Bellini & Mattoli, 2007). The growth factor TGF-β1 plays the main regulating role at this stage of fibrocyte differentiation. With the participation of the enzymes serine/threonine protein kinase (SAPK) and mitogen-activating JUN protein kinase (JNK MAPK), it activates the intracellular proteins SMAD2 and SMAD3, which enter the nucleus and affect the transcription of the genes essential for the differentiation (Hong et al., 2007).

Various cells of ectodermal origin undergoing the program of **epithelial-mesenchymal transition** (EMT) or, in other words, **transdifferentiation** can serve as another progenitor of reparative fibroblasts (or fibroblast-like cells) (Iwano et al., 2002; Kalluri & Nielson, 2002). The most prominent manifestation of this transition is that the epithelial cells lose the polarity and mutual adhesion specific for them, and the intercellular contacts (desmosomes) break. Organized cell layers disintegrate. The cells become isolated in the midst of the extracellular matrix and relatively motile, which is intrinsic for most mesenchymal cells.

The EMT, which also occurs in normal morphogenesis, is based on interactions of a complicated complex of molecular mechanisms, starting with the earliest stages of embryonic development and in different pathological processes. The superfamily TGF-β signaling molecules serve as the main trigger factor of the molecular mechanisms of transdifferentiation (as in fibrocyte differentiation) (Zavadil & Böttinger, 2005).

TGF-β binding with its receptor on the surface of an endothelial cell's cytoplasmic membrane initiates intracellular signaling cascades, leading to the transcription repression of the main desmosome component – E-cadherin (see section 3.6.3). Snail/Slug family factors, along with the proteins Twist, SIP1, LIV1, MTA3, and δEF, play the leading role in this repression. E-cadherin (epithelial) destruction is carried out by the enzyme γ-secretase and the contacts between the cells are destroyed.

Under the influence of TGF-β, the protein guanine nucleotide exchange factors (GEF) activate guanosine triphosphatase of the Rho family (Fan et al., 2007), which leads to switching in other signaling cascades, which involve the proteins Smads, Notch, Wnt and β-cathepsin, NFκB and in which the Ras, ERK, MAP families' kinases act. These signaling cascades enable the remodeling of the cytoskeleton. An epithelial cell desmosomes-bond keratine network is substituted for a network of vimentin-rich fibers, which are connected with the forming focal contacts, providing cells' interaction with the extracellular matrix (Kokkinos et al., 2007). The expression of integrins and other numerous proteins comprising the focal contacts is activated herein.

At the same time, TGF-β, along with one of the fibroblast growth factors, FGF2, enhance the expression of the metalloproteases (see section 3.7.1) MMP2 (gelatinase A) and MMP9 (gelatinase B), which perform the proteolysis of type IV collagens. The destruction of basement membranes occurs, representing one of the obstacles to cell mobility.

Influenced by TGF-β, the epithelial cells lose not only E-cadherin but also other proteins, which are specific for them – MUC1, ZO-1, desmoplakins, and cytokeratin 18. The expression of the proteins intrinsic for mesenchymal cells – vimentin, the fibroblast specific protein 1 (S100A4/FSP1) and α-SMA – in the differentiation into myofibroblasts starts.

As a result of TGF-β-produced intracellular interactions, in which a lot of other proteins – signal transmitters and transcription factors – are involved, the expression of so many genes is changed, radically altering the epithelial cells' phenotype. Such an alteration is referred to as a change of "**transcriptome**" (this notion, a derivative of the notion "genome" combines all genes' transcripts formed in a cell) (Venkov et al., 2007). The phenotype becomes fibroblast-like ("fibroblastoid") or takes on features of the myofibroblast phenotype. The most essential consequence thereof is that the transdifferentiated cells start expressing great fibrous type I and III collagens and other macromolecular components of the connective tissue extracellular matrix.

The possibility of the epithelial-mesenchymal transition of ectodermal cells cultured *in vitro* might be considered as strongly supported. Convincing evidence suggests such a possibility in a number of settings *in vivo*; for example, in liver fibrosis, developing where active fibroblasts originate not only from so-called stellate cells, which are connective tissue cells in nature, but also from mature hepatocytes (Zeisberg et al., 2007). In kidney fibrosis, up to one-third of the total number of fibroblasts involved in the process originate from a tubule's epithelium (Kalluri & Nielson, 2002). As already mentioned, fibroblasts that have undergone the epithelial-mesenchymal transition retain the particular phenotypic features of their progenitors. These data confirm the importance of the EMT as a significant factor of fibroblastic differon phenotypic heterogeneity.

However, despite the marked heterogeneity, all fibroblasts manifest very significant general peculiarities of the phenotype.

The expression and secretion of numerous **enzymes**, along with the structural macromolecular components, into the extracellular matrix are among the properties uniting all types of fibroblasts. The enzymes carry out the final stages of post-translation processing of proteins synthesized by fibroblasts and the assembly of supramolecular structures within the matrix. Enzymes secreted into the matrix also provide a catabolic stage of constant matrix remodeling, which is essential for the maintenance of its mechanical stability. The matrix catabolism, moreover, eliminates obstacles to the normal course of such steps in morphogenesis processes such as cell proliferation and migration, which is especially important in embryogenesis. In this aspect, the role of some metazinsin family collagenolytic enzymes – MT-metalloproteases MT1/MMP-14 and MT3/MMP-16, which catabolize great fiber-forming type I, II and III collagens, is especially important. Switching off the genes encoding the synthesis of these cell membrane-bound enzymes induces a delay in growth, a decline in mesenchyme cells' viability, and the disturbed development of all connective tissue types in mice embryos (Shi et al., 2008).

The effect the fibroblast-secreted enzymes exert on extracellular matrix components has one more aspect. The peptide fragments of structural macromolecules (collagens, elastin, fibronectins) formed with their participation become free protein molecules, which are sometimes comparatively large, and take on the role of short-distance (local) regulators in a number of cases. In this role they attach to numerous signaling molecules, which are expressed by the fibroblasts (Smith, 2005) and influence the functions of the fibroblasts themselves, as well as other cells.

For example, a collagen type I carboxyterminal propeptide cleaved from the corresponding procollagen' macromolecule by C-proteinase is a molecule with a molecular mass of 120 kDa, which inhibits this subsequent procollagen synthesis and exerts a chemotaxic effect in relation to the endothelium cells that facilitate angiogenesis. Type XV and XVIII collagen C-terminal domains, cleaved by elastase and cathepsin L, have the opposite, anti-angiogenic effect. An arginine-rich propeptide of the lysyl oxidase enzyme exerts prominent anti-tumor activity (Trackman, 2005). The fragments of elastin and fibronectin macromolecules exert a chemotaxic and mitogenic (proliferation stimulating) influence on the cells involved in inflammatory reactions.

As a general property, uniting all fibroblasts and fibroblast-like cells, the extremely close interaction (crosstalk) of cells cytoskeleton with the extracellular matrix should be emphasized (Geiger et al., 2001). The interaction whose external manifestation, especially when observed *in vitro*, is an adhesion of cells to the matrix (Berrier&Yamada, 2007), is provided by numerous transmembrane receptors, among which specialized molecular machines (complexes)–**focal adhesions (FA)** (focal contacts in the other words) are especially important. **Integrins** (see section 3.6.3), heterodimeric transmembrane proteins, are the central link in these sophisticated complexes. Each integrin macromolecule consists of two subunits (α and β), encoded by individual genes. Every cell has integrins; fibroblasts' main integrins are $\alpha1\beta1$, $\alpha2\beta1$, $\alpha5\beta1$, $\alpha v\beta5$.

The integrin $\alpha v\beta5$ is a receptor for TGF-β, which, as already mentioned, induces fibroblasts' differentiation into myofibroblasts and it is this increased integrin expression that intensifies this differentiation of dermal fibroblasts (Asano et al., 2006).

All numerous proteins of these molecular machines, transmitting the signals perceivable by the integrins to the cytoskeleton, are somehow important in the focal contacts' functioning. In turn, some proteins of the cytoplasm influence FA proteins.

For example, the cytoplasm phosphoprotein N-WASP, involved in the regulation of actin polymerization, enhances the adhesion of fibroblasts to the matrix and in particular, to fibronectins, enabling the formation of integrin clusters that contain the subunit $\beta2$ and the accumulation of vinculin, one of the FA components, in FA (Misra et al., 2007). The protein WIP, which interacts with N-WASP, controls its functions; the over-expression of WIP inhibits adhesion (Lanzardo et al., 2007).

The large (with a molecular mass of more than 150 kDa) cytoplasmic protein **palladin** provides adhesive interactions of the fibroblasts and the extracellular matrix: it maintains the normal architectonics of the actin cytoskeleton and stabilizes integrins' β-subunits. In the absence of paladin, these subunits are exposed to destruction (Liu et al., 2007).

The most important fibroblast functions are related to focal contacts and primarily to integrins. Adhesion of the matrix structural macromolecules and supramolecular formations, for example collagen fibers or fibronectin microfibrils, to a fibroblast cell membrane has a strictly arranged character. Adhesion is an attachment ("sticking") of a certain macromolecule domain, rather than the entire macromolecule, to a particular integrin. Owing to this, the macromolecule occupies a spatial-oriented locality in the matrix, which further regulates the localization of other macromolecules that are not in direct contact with the membrane. Thus, a fibroblast does not simply provide the materials for the construction of the extracellular matrix, but as an architect, coordinates the formation of its structural organization (structuralization).

This fibroblast function, which depends on the integrins, is directly related to the formation of matrix mechanic properties. The blocking of the rat skin fibroblasts' integrin subunits $\alpha2$ and $\beta1$ through the intradermal administration of specific antibodies resulted in the skin becoming thicker and its elasticity reduced (Fujimura et al., 2007).

It should be emphasized that the functional connection of fibroblasts and the extracellular matrix, mediated by the focal contacts and all other receptors, is bilateral. The FA integrins, as transmembrane receptors, provide the transmitting of diverse signals within a cell. These signals can be small signaling molecules (local regulators) penetrating through the matrix to the cell membrane. Growth factors of the transforming growth factors superfamily β TGF-β (without brackets), which stimulate fibroblasts' functional activity and induce their differentiation into myofibroblasts, exert the most powerful effect on fibroblasts, as has been shown.

A connective tissue growth factor (CTGF), also known as CCN2, is also essential for the fibroblasts' function, especially in the embryonic period. Switching off the gene encoding this factor causes changes in the fibroblast proteome–the expression of the proteins with anti-adhesive, anti-inflammatory and anti-angiogenic effects such as interleukin- (IL-5), ceruloplasmin, thrombospondin-1, lipokalin-2 and syndecan-4 is inhibited (Kennedy et al., 2006).

The extracellular matrix, in total, affects the fibroblasts via transmembrane receptors. In experiments with fibroblasts cultured *in vitro*, it has been established that the cells' normal differentiation is feasible only in a 3D medium most similar to a natural one; the differentiation is impaired in flat (2D) media, which are usually used while working with cell cultures. The expression of genes of the cell (cytoplasmic) membrane proteoglycan syndecan-4 (syndecans are involved in the interactions "cell–matrix" as integrins' co-receptors) is enhanced in a 3D medium. The expression of glycoproteins and proteoglycans of the differentiation center (cellular antigen) CD44, which serves as receptor of hyaluronan and many other ligands of the extracellular matrix, is also enhanced (Sawaguchi et al., 2006). When cultured in a 3D medium, only fibroblasts and myofibroblasts derived from the tumor stroma, retain *in vitro* their desmoplastic activity (the capability to continue the formation of a fibrous stroma). It is only in 3D medium that the fibroblasts retain the ability to produce a sufficient amount of type I collagen, to provide cross-linking and an organized nature for the fibronectin microfibril network, and maintain the expression of α-SMA, which is characteristic for myofibroblasts (Amatangelo et al., 2005).

Individual structural macromolecular components of the extracellular matrix also influence the fibroblasts by means of receptors. For example, macromolecules of a fibronectin isoform, in which the ED-A domain is present, bind to the end regions of the intracellular actin fibers under the influence of TGF-β. The size of focal contacts increases herein, the expression of one of the main adhesion protein kinases–FAK–is enhanced, and additional molecules of protein-contacts, vinculin and paxillin transfer from the cytoplasm and imbed into focal contacts. Thus, new transmembrane structures are formed with the participation of fibronectin; these structures facilitate the differentiation of fibroblasts into myofibroblasts, particularly α-SMA expression (Dugina et al., 2001).

A with matrix polysaccharide–**hyaluronan**–affects fibroblasts' functions (see 3.2.1.1). Hyaluronan possesses adhesive properties, and the fine hyaluronan-rich cytoplasm layer coating a cell provides the primary adhesion of a fibroblast and the matrix, which later changes by a stronger adhesion, mediated by integrins and forming focal contacts (Zaidel-Bar et al., 2004). Under the influence of TGF-β1, the enhancement of the expression of hyaluronan synthases HAS1 and HAS2, the enzymes providing the synthesis of the extracellular hyaluronan, is intrinsic for the fibroblasts of skin wounds, which heal with the formation of fibrous scarring tissue. The increase of hyaluronan synthesis, influenced by TGF-β1, does not occur in fibroblasts of the oral mucous membrane, the wounds of which heal without scarring, i.e. without excessive collagen accumulation. Therefore, the hyaluronan layer that fibroblasts create around themselves regulates the cell's biosynthetic activity and actually controls its phenotype (Meran et al., 2007).

The small proteoglycans **decorin** affects a phenotype of the cultured myofibroblasts. Enhanced decorin expression causes a decrease in α-SMA expression and an inhibition of myofibroblast activity in fibrous reactions, whereas the inhibition of decorin expression causes the opposite effect (Nakatani et al., 2008).

By means of the whole set of transmembrane receptors, fibroblasts receive signals from the extracellular matrix, which inform the cells upon mechanical exposure to tissues and organs. These mechanical signals transform mechanic events ongoing within the matrix into molecular signals transmitting inside the fibroblasts, modeling many cell functions and eventually influencing gene expression. Arising changes in the genes' expression are directed towards an increase in matrix resistance to mechanical stress, but these changes can take on a pathologic nature at a certain level (Wang J.H. et al., 2007). Therefore, the mechanical influence is of importance as one more control factor over fibroblasts on the part of the extracellular matrix.

Although fibroblasts are matrix "architects and builders", the matrix's manifold influence on fibroblasts is so significant that the fibroblasts' relationships with the matrix should be considered as interdependence rather than interaction.

Another general feature is intrinsic for the fibroblastic differon. It can be defined as a phenotype **plasticity** or **lability**. The described differentiation of a tissue (resident) fibroblast into an active myofibroblast is an example of the phenotype lability.

The fibroblasts can take on the phenotypic features of other connective tissue cells, for example, by taking the way of chondrogenic differentiation. Such a phenotype alteration occurs when culturing mature dermal fibroblasts *in vitro* in a medium containing a great concentration of the cartilaginous tissue large proteoglycan, aggrecan, under the influence of the insulin-like growth factor 1 (IGF1). Under these conditions, the cells start expressing the main chondrocyte marker–type II collagen (French et al., 2004). The transdifferentiation of fibroblasts into bone tissue cells–osteoblasts–is also known.

The cells of a fibroblastic differon undergo the most radical phenotype changes in the case of **mesenchymal-epithelial transition**, (MET), a phenomenon which is the opposite of the aforementioned epithelial-mesenchymal transition (EMT) (Chaffer et al., 2007). This phenomenon is common in the early stages of embryogenesis and a little later when, for example, the cells of the metanephric (circumrenal) mesenchyme–potential fibroblasts' progenitors–differentiate into epithelial cells of renal tubules. MET also originates in somite formation. The MET regulation in nephrogenesis involves the fibroblast growth factors FGF1, FGF3, FGF7, the bone morphogenetic protein BMP7, the Wnt family' morphogens (Wnt4 is especially active), the transcription factors Pax2, Pax3, Pax8, Foxc1, Foxc2, Foxd1, and the Rho family's guanosine triphosphatase (GTPase). In somitogenesis, the signals of Notch family molecules and the transcription factors Osterix, Msp1 and Msp2 join the Wnt signals. As a result of these factors' action, the expression of many genes that are active in mesenchyme cells, including genes coding vimentin, N-cadherin, is inhibited. Simultaneously, the expression of a number of genes, whose high activity is specific for epithelial cells, commences (Plisov et al., 2000); the expression of the cadherins E-cadherin, R-cadherin and cadherin-6, which provides mutual adhesion and the fixation of cells, is activated.

The versican isoform, the large chondroitin sulfate proteoglycan expressed by fibroblasts, is one of the MET inductors of mature differentiated fibroblasts. Switching the expression from "mesenchymal" N-cadherin to "epithelial" E-cadherin is a marker of this fibroblast transdifferentiation, reproducible in vitro (Sheng et al., 2006).

The transdifferentiation of human mature dermal fibroblasts into hepatocyte-like cells occurs upon applying a particular combination of activating factors in an experiment in vitro. In the intravenous administration of these cells in mice, they are concentrated in the liver, express hepatocyte markers (α-fetoprotein, albumin, cytokeratin 18), and exert activity that is intrinsic for hepatocytes (e.g. glycogen deposition, urea synthesis) (Lysy et al., 2007).

There is a strong presumption that the mesenchymal-epithelial transition of differentiated fibroblasts occurs in vivo in the process of carcinogenesis and tumor dissemination. However, this fact cannot be considered as being conclusively proven (Hugo et al., 2007).

The main functions common to all cells of the fibroblastic differon—the expression and secretion of extracellular matrix components—are the subject of the discussion regarding the biosynthesis of these macromolecules in the corresponding sections of Chapter 3.

2.3. ADVENTITIOUS CELLS

These are poorly differentiated cells that accompany blood vessels. They are flattened or spindle-shaped and have a poorly developed basophilic cytoplasm and an oval nucleus. During the differentiation process, the cells appear to develop into fibroblasts, myofibroblasts, lipocytes, i.e. they can act as stem cells of a fibroblastic differon.

2.4. ADIPOSE CELLS (LIPOCYTES, ADIPOCYTES)

Adipose cells (lipocytes, adipocytes) are the cells that can accumulate large amounts of reserve fat. As a rule, lipocytes can be found in loose fibrous irregular connective tissue near blood vessels; they are more frequently located in groups than separately. Large agglomerates of these cells are called adipose tissue (**AT**). Being a type of connective tissue, the AT performs the same functions but on the basis of the peculiarities of its structure. The *trophic function* consists of: 1) the accumulation of lipids, which serve as reserve sources of energy for metabolic

reactions and thermogenesis in an organism, and 2) the storage and release of water as a result of lipids' accumulation and disintegration, accordingly. The *biomechanical function* entails that the AT surrounds various organs and fills the space between them, acting as a dampening structure, thereby protecting them from mechanical exposure and maintaining their particular spatial relationship (position). The AT's *heat-maintaining function* consists of saving heat (AT acts as a heat insulator), which is released in tremulous and non-tremulous thermogenesis. The latter is provided by brown adipose tissue, a type of the AT. The *regulatory function* is performed as a local or systemic (distant) influence on the various processes ongoing in an organism. Locally, bone marrow adipose cells create an optimal environment for hematopoiesis by creating a microenvironment for the proliferation and differentiation of formed blood elements. The production of estrogens and cytokines (leptin, resistin, adiponectin or visfatin) by adipocytes indicates their possible influence on important endocrine and immune functions. The AT's *protective function* can be considered a manifestation of a complex of AT's properties targeted at protecting an organism from the destructive influence of various factors (infectious, toxicochemical, mechanical, etc.).

There are two types of adipose tissue in mammal and human organisms–**white adipose tissue and brown adipose tissue**, which differ both structurally and functionally.

2.4.1. Histophysiologic characteristic of adipose cells

A mature white adipose cell (adipocyte) is spherical in shape and ranges in size from 25–250 μm in equivalent diameter (*Fig. 2.13a,b,c*). The cells normally contain one large droplet of neutral lipid, occupying the whole central part of the cell and surrounded by a thin cytoplasmic limbus whose thickened part contains a nucleus. Part of the cytoplasm includes small lipid droplets, which can fuse with the large droplet. Besides, there is a small amount of other lipids–cholesterol, phospholipids, and free fatty acids. Lipids are well-stained in orange with sudan-III, or in black or brown with osmium tetroxide. There are rod-shaped and threadlike mitochondria with densely packed cristae, a smooth endoplasmatic reticulum, a small vesicular lamellar complex, and threadlike structures in the cytoplasm adjacent to the nucleus, and sometimes in the thinner opposite part. Numerous pinocytic vesicles can be found in the cell's periphery.

Lipocytes possess a high level of metabolism. The amount of fat in them and the number of cells considerably fluctuate in smooth fibrous connective tissue. In the connective tissue of an adult organism, new adipose cells can develop in intensive nutrition when anabolic processes prevail over catabolic ones or when dysmetabolism is present. The adipose cells can lose fat if the organism does not receive sufficient amounts of nutrients or when the metabolism' level is increased. Thus, the adipose cells heavily decrease in size and become scarcely visible under a microscope. Four functional states are typical for mature white adipocytes.

1) With maximum fat accumulation in a cell cytoplasm, there is one large lipid droplet filling almost its entire volume and pushing the nucleus and few organelles towards one of the cellular poles. The rest of the lipid droplet directly adjoins the cytoplasmic membrane. There are no small droplets.

2) With fat accumulation, its large droplet does not occupy the entire cytoplasm. It is surrounded by a rather wide cytoplasm layer with various organelles and numerous smaller lipid droplets, located independently or at different stages of fusion with the large central droplet.

3) The large lipid droplet is surrounded by a wide limbus of the cytoplasm with a nucleus and organelles. There are no smaller lipid droplets. Such a state can be regarded both as the stabilization of fat accumulation, and as a stage of its partial utilization.

4) Adipose cells which lost fat wholly or partially.

The population of the adipose cells in animal and human organisms is apparently maintained in the same way as for the whole CT-differon. It is assumed that the adventitious cells located around vascular capillaries and the fibroblast-like cells located between adipose cells can be organ-specific stem cells and an "operative reserve" of committed precursors that replenish the population of adipose cells. In the case of the physiological depletion of this reserve or a considerable loss of adipose tissue in destructive processes, its replenishment is possible due to stem mobile (circulating) CT-cells. Hong et al. (2005) have demonstrated the possibility of such circulating precursors (fibrocytes) differentiating into cells that express adipocyte-specific markers and genes, and the possibility of them storing intracellular lipids and synthesizing leptin.

Fat deposition in a young adipocyte begins with the accumulation of its soluble components (fatty acids, short chains of fatty acid esters). As a lipid droplet increases in size, the RER and the lamellar complex are reduced and the nucleus is compressed and flattened. The nature of the cells in which the lipocytes are transformed in the case of fat loss is insufficiently studied. There is also another point of view stating that lipocytes' progenitors are an independent line.

Adipose cells can be derived from an adipose tissue (for example from subcutaneous fat) with the help of collagenase and cultured under cultural conditions. However, when isolated, the lipocytes with one large lipid droplet in the cytoplasm are not retained. Lipocytes (medium size of 30×100 µm) whose cytoplasm contains numerous lipid droplets of varying size, ranging from 0.5–20 µm, are present in the culture. The droplets of a small diameter–1–3 µm–prevail (*Fig. 2.14 a*). That the droplets are stained with a selective "oil red" dye confirms their lipid specification (Fig. 2.14 b). In these cells' division, lipid droplets are distributed throughout daughter cells and therefore, their number is gradually reduced (*Fig. 2.14 c*). The fusion of small droplets into larger ones is possible, but lipid neo-formation is unlikely to occur, as in 2–3 passages, only small droplets are retained in those cells and their qualitative composition cannot be determined without the special staining of fixed cells. Besides lipocytes, the culture includes a great number of fibroblast-like cells containing numerous small lipid droplets (*Fig. 2.14 d*). Committed (adapted) CT-progenitors for the subcutaneous fat and dermis are likely to be present among them.

A lot of animals and humans have **brown adipose tissue (BAT)**. BAT is widely represented in all regions of the body during the first 10 years of development. Its large conglomerates are located in the interscapular region, at the aorta and around the cardiac vessels, between muscles in the neck axillary regions and in the axilla, around the costal and mediastinal vessels, between the esophagus and the trachea, at the adrenal glands, little less around the kidneys, in the mesenterium of the small intestine and in other regions (Heaton, 1972). With aging, the subcutaneous BAT (between the scapulae, in the anterior abdominal wall, etc.) gradually diminishes or disappears. At the same time, it remains in the more deeply located regions of an organism for up to 70–80 years.

In macroscopic examinations, the BAT looks like lobular, irregular brown distinctly localized formations. Large amounts of iron-containing enzymes–cytochromes in BAT cells–make it brown. The color intensity, ranging from beige to brown, depends on age, environmental conditions, nutrition, season, the BAT's functional state, blood hemoglobin and hemoporphyrin levels. This tissue closely interacts with many large vessels (Afanasiev & Kolodeznikova, 1995).

Brown adipocytes are considerably smaller in size (25–40 µm) than white adipocytes (*Fig. 2.15*). There are numerous invaginations and pinocytic vesicles on the membrane surface. Deep invaginations form the channels connecting a cell surface with the smooth endoplasmic reticulum, which possibly delivers substances, particularly fatty acids, to the cell (Blanchette-Macrie, 1983). In the brown adipocytes of adult rats, most of the cytoplasm is occupied by one large lipid droplet and several small lipid droplets that are undergoing the stage of lipid synthesis and subsequently, will probably fuse with the large droplet. The brown adipocytes have oval or circular nuclei, and 1 or 2 nucleoli. Chromatin is represented by euchromatin and heterochromatin. A unique feature of brown lipocytes is that their cytoplasm contains a considerable quantity of mitochondria of various forms and size, as well as numerous small lipid inclusions (*Fig. 2.16*). There is a poorly developed rough endoplasmic reticulum and smooth endoplasmic reticulum (RER and SER) between the mitochondria. Most ribosomes and

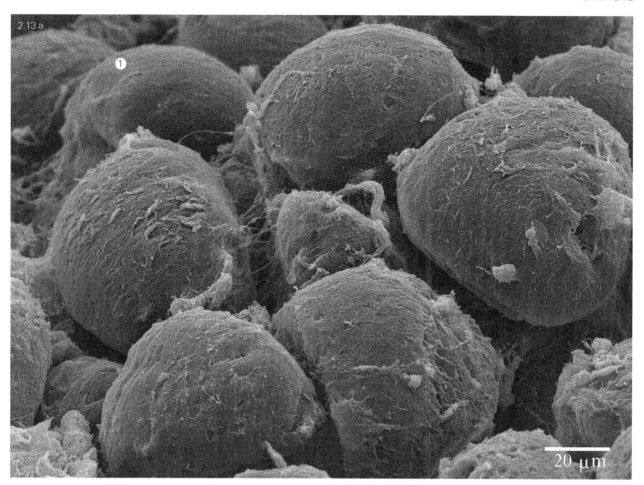

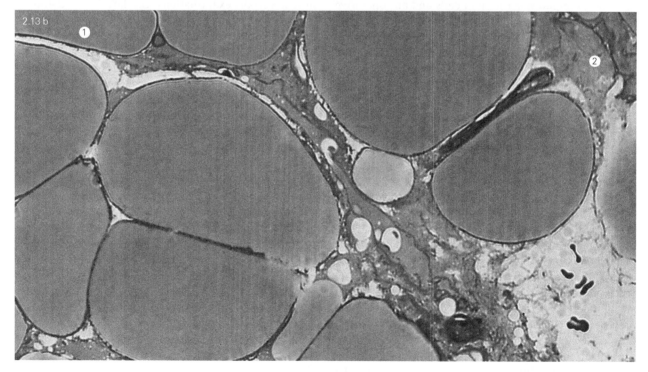

Fig. 2.13.
White adipocytes (1)
of the subcutaneous
adipose tissue.
The loose fibrous irregular
connective tissue between
adipocytes (2).

Lipid droplets (3)
and nucleus (4)
in white multicameral
adipocyte
a,c – SEM-micrograph.
a x 700; c x 1,400
b – LM-micrograph.

A light optic microscope Ni
Nikon (Japan).
Contrasting with an OsO4
solution in fragments and
staining of the section with
methylene blue + azure II,
counterstaining with basic

fuchsine, x 700
(see color insert)
d – TEM-micrograph.
Contrastin of ultrathin
sections g with lead citrate
and uranyl acetate.
x 20,000

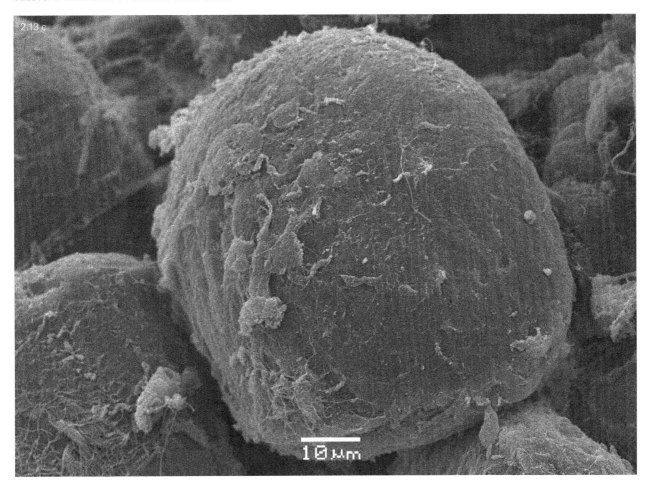

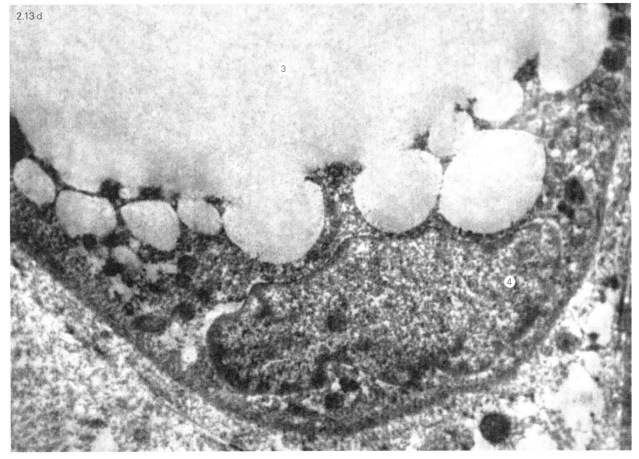

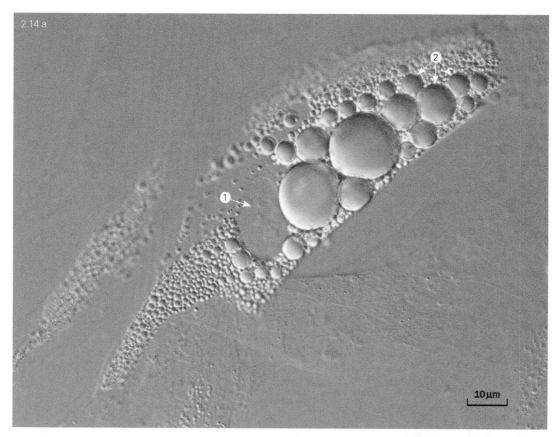

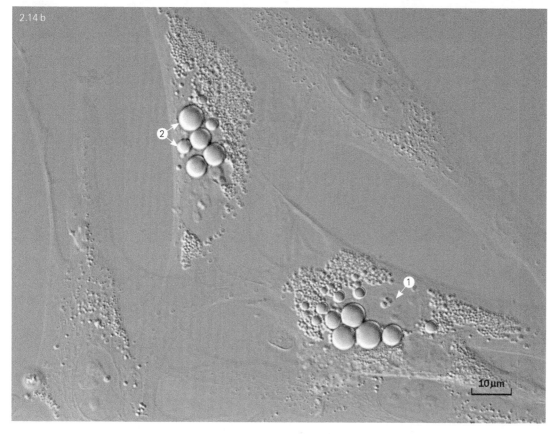

Fig. 2.14.
Multicameral adipocytes (lipocytes) of the subcutaneous fat in culturing.

a, b, c – a multicameral adipocytes with large, medium and small lipid droplets.

b – two daughter cells after adipocyte division.
d – fibroblast-like cells containing small lipid droplets.

A nucleus with nucleoli (1).
Lipid droplets (2).
Cytoskeleton microfilaments (4).

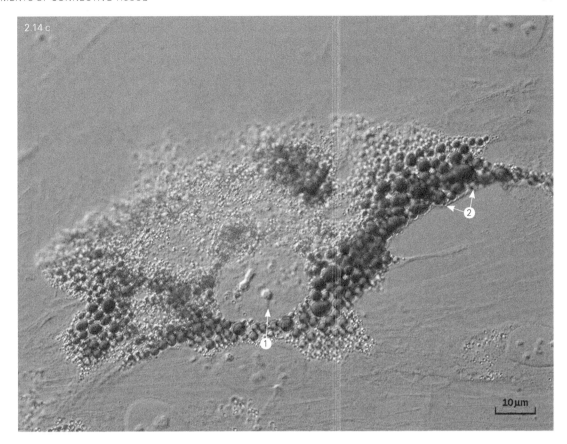

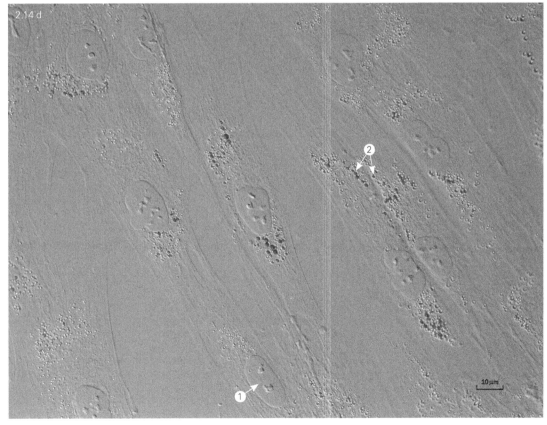

a, b – LM-micrograph.   Nomarsky (differential)   Cultured cells after fixation   a – x 900
A light optic inverted   interference contrast (DIC).   and staining with Oil Red.   b, c, d – x 600
microscope Ti Nikon (Japan)   c, d – LM-micrograph.   *(see color insert)*
integrated with an incubator.

polysomes are located freely, without connecting to membranes. The SER in the form of vacuoles of various sizes is more often located around the lipid inclusions; it is possibly associated with the synthesis of fatty acids in these organelles. The lamellar complex, lysosomes and peroxisomes are poorly developed.

Chromatin is distributed equally throughout the entire nucleoplasm in the brown adipocytes of adult rats (*Fig. 2.17*). Fat is represented by simple small lipid inclusions. At the same time, most of the cytoplasm is occupied by medium sized mitochondria. These seem to be still immature adipocytes, which have not accumulated the reserve fat observed in adult animals.

Lipids are accumulated in the brown adipocytes for subsequent use in heat generation during non-tremulous thermogenesis under adverse conditions (hypothermia) or settings (hibernation). The great number of mitochondria in such cells' cytoplasm should be noted. It is many times greater than the number of mitochondria in white adipocytes. In this connection, the fat accumulated in the brown adipocytes is utilized directly within them during heat generation, warming the blood in capillaries surrounding the brown adipocytes. During the BAT activation period, for example upon being exposed to cold, the lysosomes and peroxisomes increase in size and number. Glycogen can constantly be found in the brown lipocytes, but its quantity varies (Kolodeznikova, 1971; Sculls & Johnston, 1971).

The BAT is sufficiently vasculated. Each cell is covered by plenty of haemocapillaries from several sides. A well-developed microcirculatory bed and the high speed of the blood stream provide the brown adipocytes with oxygen and essential substrates for energy generation, and also create necessary conditions for the output of the heat produced. With cooling of an organism the lipids "burn" quickly, and the released heat energy is not accumulated but used for blood heating. Such thermogenesis, which is called non-tremulous

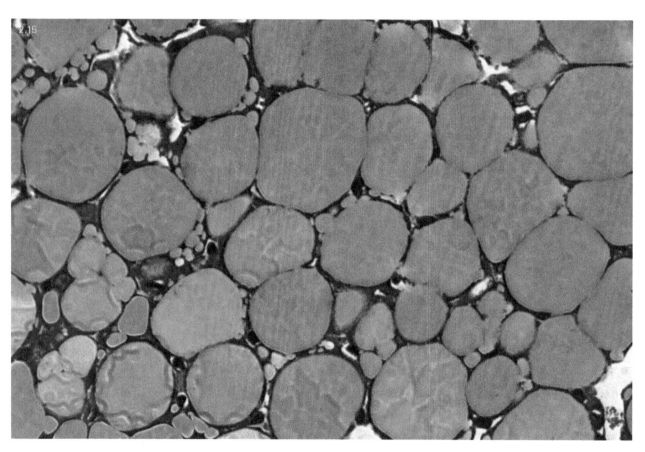

Fig. 2.15.

Fig. 2.15.
Brown adipocytes (1) of brown adipose tissue from the interscapular region of an adult rat. The loose fibrous irregular connective tissue (2) between adipocytes. LM-micrograph. A light optic microscope Ni Nikon (Japan). A semifine section. Contrasting with an OsO4 solution in fragments and staining of the sections with methylene blue + azure II, counterstaining with basic fuchsine. x 400.

Fig. 2.16.
Brown adipocytes of the brown adipose tissue of newborn rats. A nucleus (1). Mitochondria (2). Lipid inclusions (3). TEM-micrograph. contrasting of ultrathin sections with lead citrate and uranyl acetate. x 10,000.

Fig. 2.17.
A fragment of a brown adipocyte of an adult rat's brown adipose tissue. A nucleus (1). Mitochondria (2). Lipid droplets (3). TEM-micrograph. contrasting of ultrathin sections with lead citrate and uranyl acetate. x 30,000.

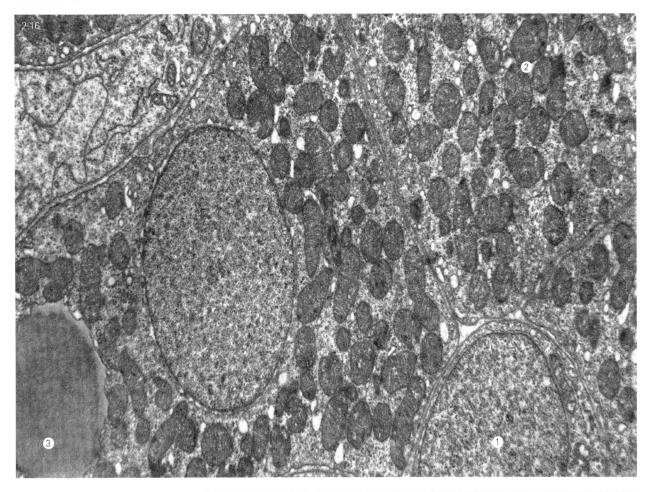

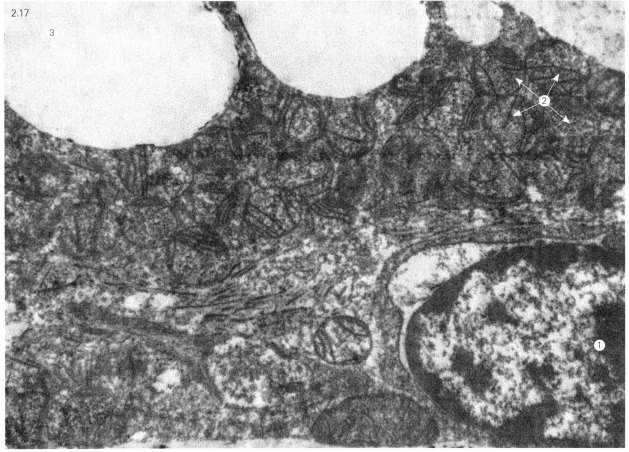

thermogenesis, is typical in early childhood as well as in hibernating animals.

The BAT is characterized by a rather rich sympathetic innervation. Brown adipocytes' cytolemma contains a large amount of α- and β-adrenoreceptors. These receptors are concentrated around the sympathetic nerve terminals. This tissue contains more noradrenalin than all other tissues and organs (Sidman et al., 1962).

A number of morphological characteristics indicate the organ composition of BAT. Its separately located clusters (for example, in the interscapular region) are covered with a connective-tissue capsule, the branches of which divide it into lobules deep in the BAT. In turn, a lobule consists of several types of adipocytes reflecting the stages of maturation and cells' functional activity. There are some manifestations of a holocrine secretion type. The BAT is not only highly vasculated but it is also innervated and contains intramural ganglia.

At the same time, the intensity of blood supply, the speed of response to environmental temperature changes (exposure to cold), and the relative independence of metabolism of the whole organism make it possible to describe the BAT as a peculiar heat-producing organ, whose peculiarity is non-tremulous thermogenesis (Afanasiev & Kolodeznikova, 1995).

2.4.2. Biochemical and biomolecular characteristics of adipose cells

Adipose cells (**adipocytes**) differ from their prototype, a fibroblast, by the presence of large lipid droplets consisting of neutral **triglycerides** (triacylglycerols, TG or TAG). A white adipocyte contains one large droplet, occupying almost the whole volume of the cell; a brown adipocyte can contain several smaller lipid droplets distributed throughout the cytoplasm, depending on the maturity and functional state.

Eukaryotic organisms keep necessary energy stores mostly in fatty acids, which are attached to three alcohol hydroxyl groups of glycerol by means of ether bonds (esterified). These compounds (TG or TAG) differ by the nature of the fatty acids composing them. In terms of energy conservation, the triglycerides represent the most effective molecules with hydrophobic properties that lead to their encapsulation in droplets, which are insoluble in the hydrophilic cytosol (the liquid phase of the cytoplasm). By the energy concentrated per unit of volume, the lipid droplets are 10 times larger than those of carbohydrates or proteins (Wolins et al., 2006). Given an energy deficiency in an organism, triglycerides release fatty acids by means of lipolysis, and, in combination with blood serum albumin, they are delivered to the energy-deficient cells, primarily to muscle cells, where they are used as energy suppliers.

The smallest lipid droplets (LD), also called lipid bodies or adiposomes, are present as inclusions in the cytoplasm of almost all cells. Particularly large amounts of these inclusions are present in cardiac and skeletal muscles. In some cells, LD contains cholesterol along with triglycerides. Large droplets, which are characteristic for adipocytes, are a special LD type, and their formation, stabilization and utilization follow the same regularities, which relate to all these dynamic **organelles** (Martin & Parton, 2005).

Any neutral lipid inclusions (of a hydrophobic nature) can exist in the cytosol, which is an aqueous solution of proteins and other hydrophilic molecules and which is physically incompatible with them, with the exception of an interaction with specific proteins. This interaction begins from the moment of LD generation in the endoplasmic reticulum, in the same place where lipid biosynthesis takes place.

The initial impulse to lipid biosynthesis comes from the protein factors–**fat-inducing transcripts** FIT1 and FIT2–localized in the membrane of an endoplasmic reticulum. The genes encoding these factors are extremely conservative–they remain practically unchanged during eukaryotes' evolution from yeast to mammals and humans (Kadereit et al., 2008).

To be more precise, caveolae, the crypts of the endoplasmic reticulum's membrane, are considered as a site of LD biogenesis. In the caveolae area, there are clusters of transmembrane proteins involved in LD generation and formation–**adipophilin** (this protein will be described later) (Robenek et al., 2006) and **caveolin-1**; caveolin is associated with LD movement to its localization in the cytoplasm (Pol et al., 2004). **Stomatin**, an endosome protein, is also involved in the regulation of LD migration (Umlauf et al., 2004).

The lipid droplets continue to be present in the cytoplasm given that they have membranes composed by special proteins, which are turned to the cytoplasm with hydrophilic domains, and with lipophilic (hydrophobic) domains to lipids within the droplets. These proteins are also present in the droplets' depth, maintaining their stability and providing their additional structural properties (Robenek et al., 2005).

Proteins of the **perilipin** family (otherwise known as **PAT**) are the main structural material for membranes of any lipid droplets (both large adipocyte droplets and small lipid inclusions of other cells) located in the cytosol (Robenek et al., 2005). The family consists of 5 members. They are adipophilin (or **ADRP**, adipose differentiation-related protein), TIP47, OXPAT/MLDP [myocardial **LD** protein], SS-12 and perilipin. Perilipin A, a phosphoprotein with a molecular mass of about 56 kDa encoded by the gene *PLINA*, quantitatively prevails in a membrane of adipocytes' lipid droplets (Brasaemle, 2007). Apart from perilipins, a droplet's membrane contains the recently identified protein **FSP27/Cidec** (Puri et al., 2007). The functions of these proteins are oppositely directed in a dynamic structure like a lipid droplet's membrane. Along with the function of separating lipid and water phases and lipid protection against the untimely action of cytosol lipases, perilipins act as a substrate for protein kinase A (PKA), an enzyme that is activated in lipolysis.

PKA phosphorylates the perilipins, thereby providing lipids access to lipases. Triglycerides deposited in adipocytes are mobilized in such a way. On the contrary, FSP27 stimulates adipogenesis (fat accumulation, increase of lipid droplets) and inhibits lipolysis.

The expression of the transmembrane (one-pass, i.e. crossing a cell membrane once) protein, **adipogenin**, which is specific for adipocytes, is significantly intensified in the adipogenesis process (Hong et al., 2005). (In mice this small molecule, with a mass of about 9.5 kDa, is also called a **small adipocytes factor 1**, SMAF-1).

Thus, adipocytes differ from other cells, firstly, by their particularly high content of lipids and, secondly, by the presence of significant amounts of specific proteins, which are essential for the creation and maintenance of lipid droplets' stability.

In this regard, the phenotype of adipocytes differs from that of fibroblasts by the active expression of genes related to transportation (of both lipids and the metabolites used in their biosynthesis) and to lipid synthesis (lipogenesis) and their utilization (catabolism, lipolysis) (Granemann & Moore, 2008).

Adipocytes, for example, are characterized by the intensive expression and high enzymatic activity of fatty acids synthase (**FAS**), a multifunctional cytoplasmic enzyme, and a phosphoprotein with a molecular mass of 273 kDa, consisting of 2511 amino acid residues. The expression of a cytoplasmic protein, called an adipocyte protein or a fatty acids binding protein (**aP2** or **FABP4**), is also intensive (Rosen & Spiegelman, 2000).

Genes of several lipolytic enzymes, lipases, are actively expressed. Among them, the hormone-sensitive lipase (**HSL**), a phosphoprotein localized in the cytoplasmic membrane that moves into a cytosol under the influence of insulin and performs the initial stage of the hydrolysis of lipid droplets' triglycerides, is worthy of mention. Lipase **ABHD5** (CGI-58) exerts esterase–lipase activity and is located in the cytosol, mainly on a surface of lipid droplets. Monoglyceridlipase (MGL, HU-K5), which acts like serine esterase, releases free fatty acids from monoglycerides.

The adiponutrin family, which includes **adiponutrin, desnutrin** (ATGL), GS2, GS2-like and PNPLA1, comprises an important group of adipocyte lipases (Lake et al., 2005). All proteins of this family are united by the presence of a domain similar to that of the one of potato proteins, patatin. They are multifunctional enzymes that combine the activity of triglyceride lipases, phospholipases and acylglyceroltransacylases. They are localized on the cell membrane and inside the cell on the surface of lipid droplets. Desnutrin is actively expressed, especially in the case of starvation, when it is necessary to mobilize reserve lipids.

The second peculiarity of the adipocyte phenotype is the active expression of the genes encoding proteins associated with lipid droplets' formation and functioning.

Both phenotypic peculiarities of adipocytes develop gradually. The transcription profile (activity of gene expression) is changed in the course of differentiation from a mesenchymal, fibroblast-like, progenitor through the stage of a pre-adipocyte into that of a mature adipocyte (Gregoire et al., 1998). A specific adipocyte proteome is formed as a result of these changes (Brasaemle et al., 2004).

A decline in the expression of the cytoskeleton proteins actin and tubulin is one of the early manifestations of the pre-adipocyte stage. The expression of type I and III collagens sharply decreases (by 80–90%), and the synthesis of fibronectins is inhibited. At the same time, the expression of type IV collagen and other components of basement membranes (entaktin/nidogen, laminins) begins. Type VI collagen emerges and the expression of the large chondroitin sulfate proteoglycan–versican–increases (Gregoire et al., 1998).

Upon passing to the stage of a differentiated adipocyte, the transcription of the genes directly or indirectly related to lipid exchange takes priority. The expression of the genes *GLUT4* (a transmembrane glucose transporter), *aFABP* (a fatty acid binding protein), *SCD1* (an enzyme essential for acetyl coenzyme A synthesis), *ATGL* (an enzyme of adipocyte triglyceride lipase), *GPDH-C* (glycerolphosphate dehydrogenase) and several others is increased. In comparison with preadipocytes, the expression of some genes is depressed, including genes coding catenin-β1, an inhibitor of serine/cysteine peptidase f1, and thrombospondin-2 (Kim et al., 2007).

The rearrangement of a mesenchymal progenitor cell phenotype, which ends at the stage of an adipocyte differentiation (adipogenesis), is controlled by a complex system of local specific regulating factors. The transcription factors encoded by the genes of two families –the C/EBP factor's family and the family of the peroxisome proliferator-activated receptor (PPAR)–are essential in this complex (Mandrup and Lane, 1997).

The factors of the first family, the **C/EBP** proteins (CAAT/ enhancer binding protein), are transcription factors binding to the sequence of 4 (CAAT) nucleotides in the conservative genes' enhancer domain (activator)–the sequence of nucleotides GGX**CAAT**CT. Three representatives of this family, CAATα, CAATβ and CAATδ, conjointly participate in the induction of the PPAR factors' expression. It is their main function.

PPAR (peroxisome proliferator activated receptors) are simultaneously nuclear receptors of hormones and transcription factors, which directly influence adipogenesis factors and, thus, play a central role in a complex system of transcriptional events in adipogenesis (Mandrup and Lane, 1997). The mechanism of their action involves binding to a DNA response element (PPRE)–a consensus sequence of nucleotides AGGTCAXAGGTCA.

One of these receptors, **PPAR**γ (especially its isoform PPARγ2), which regulates the expression of key genes determining the adipocyte's phenotype including the genes regulating lipid exchange, exerts the most expressed adipogenic activity (Kershaw et al., 2007). PPARγ controls the choice of a differentiation way for a multipotent mesenchymal progenitor cell: upon switching off the gene encoding PPARγ, there is no adipocytogenesis, but osteoblastogenesis is intensified (Akune et al., 2004). The stated system of adipogenesis regulation factors is considerably complicated by a greater number of other factors supplementing the action of C/EBP and PPAR.

If this system is considered as a downstream cascade of signals distribution (see section 1.2), the protein encoded by the imprinted (transferred with the paternal allele) gene *peg10* occupies the top position in this cascade. This protein is essential to induce the expression of the first main adipogenesis regulator–C/EBP. This is evidenced by the inhibition of C/EBP expression in switching off *peg10*, which makes it possible to consider it as a key factor in adipocyte differentiation (Hishida et al., 2007).

Adipogenesis is not only the differentiation of a cell leading to fat accumulation therein and the hypertrophy associated with this accumulation, but also an increase in the number of cells exposed to such differentiation. This phenomenon is called clonal or mitotic expansion. Under the influence of adipogenesis-inducing factors (for example, hormonal, see below) during the first 24-hour period, the expression of nuclear proteins of the pRB-family, p107 and p130, increases; these proteins regulate a cell cycle, i.e. cells' replication (Ross et al., 2008).

Some more factors act on the top steps of the regulatory cascade, "above" a progenitor cell's transition into a pre-adipocyte.

The expression of the actin-bound protein (phosphoprotein) **ENC-1** is considerably enhanced for a short period of time at the initial stage of differentiation. This expression, preceding the expression of C/EBP, is obviously necessary for the cytoskeleton rearrangement that takes place in adipogenesis (Zhao et al., 2000).

A phosphoglycoprotein called **Klotho** facilitates the beginning of the differentiation of adipocyte precursors. This transmembrane protein exerts the enzymatic activity of glycoside hydrolase. The expression of its mRNA in progenitor cells is intensified upon achieving its maximum on the 3rd day, after which it decreases. The overexpression of Klotho stimulates adipocytogenesis (Chihara et al., 2006).

At the same time, the autocrine (produced by adipocytes themselves) **preadipocyte factor-1 (pref-1)** is active; this factor is a protein, which exists in transmembrane and soluble isoforms. Its molecule contains amino acid repeats, which are typical for the epithelium growth factor (EGF). Pref-1 affects a cell by means of its own receptor, transmitting the signals coming from the extracellular matrix; its action, as a counter to the aforementioned factors, is directed at inhibiting the effect of the factors stimulating adipocyte differentiation and delaying adipogenesis (Wang Y. et al., 2006). The transcription factor **GATA2**, a protein with "zinc fingers", which binds to the nucleotide sequence AGATAG in a DNA macromolecule, exerts a similar adipogenesis-inhibiting effect; GATA2 overexpression terminates the differentiation of an adipocyte (Okitsu et al., 2007).

Thus, pref-1 and GATA2 control the number of adipocytes.

Epigenetic (indirectly influencing gene expression) mechanisms are involved in the adipocyte differentiation process at the stage of a cell's transformation from a pre-adipocyte into a differentiated adipocyte. One such mechanism is the modification of nuclear chromatin proteins included in a complex with DNA contained in the chromosomes. For example, adipogenic factors cause the demethylation of the histone H3K4a, a chromatin component, and this insignificant alteration of chromatin composition affects the expression of the factors involved in adipogenesis (Musri et al., 2007).

Chemerin, a small (18 kDa) signaling molecule secreted by pre-adipocytes, is involved in the process of pre-adipocyte's transition into an adipocyte as a stimulator (adipokine). By employing its own receptor to act on cells, chemerin induces the activation of some kinases and lipases (Roh et al., 2007).

In the downstream stage of the cascade of adipogenesis-regulating signals, PPARγ activity is manifested in interaction with a retinoic receptor **RXR**, localized in the nucleus. PPARγ reacts with DNA, building a heterodimer complex with RXR, whose activity as a transcription factor is controlled by an enzyme called poly (ADF-ribose) polymerase-2 (PARP-2) (Bai et al., 2007). Depending on particular peculiarities of a heterodimer structure, it can have not only a stimulating, but also a suppressing effect. With heterodimer formation, there is competition for the receptor RXR between PPARγ and the retinoids; this explains adipogenesis' inhibition by retinoic acid.

Along with all the aforementioned specific factors of adipogenesis' local regulation, numerous nonspecific regulators of both local and systemic action influence this process. The effects of these factors cannot always be unequivocally estimated. In experiments *in vitro*, the effect's target depends on the cell line used, the stage of their differentiation, and nutrient solution. In studies *in vivo*, several factors are of importance: nutritive conditions, gender and the animal's housing conditions, as well as the anatomic position in an organism of cells exposed to adipogenesis. This latter circumstance resembles the topographical heterogeneity of fibroblasts.

Despite such a discrepancy in experimental results, it is possible to consider that glucocorticoid hormones (dexamethasone is therefore widely used in experimental settings for adipocytogenesis' induction), insulin and the insulin-like growth factor 1 (IGF-1) are positive effectors of adipogenesis. Steroid sex hormones modulate the expression of this factor's receptor (IGF1R) and indirectly influence pre-adipocytes' differentiation–estrogens have a positive influence, while androgens have a negative one (Diedonne et al., 2000). The thyroid hormone triiodothyronine, which affects specific DNA sites (thyroid-reactive elements, TRE), stimulates the proliferation of pre-adipocytes and lipogenesis (Obregon, 2008). Prostaglandin PGI2 (prostacyclin) and various factors, which promote an increase in the intracellular level of cyclic adenosine monophosphate (cAMP), exert a positive influence on adipogenesis (Gregoire et al., 1998).

Many cytokines, growth factors of the TGF-β family, the transforming growth factor α (TGF-α), and an epithelium growth factor (EGF) have a negative (inhibiting) effect on adipogenesis. The morphogens of the Wnt/β-catenin signaling system have the same effect (Prestwich and MacDougald, 2007).

The extracellular matrix surrounding differentiating cells undoubtedly influences adipogenesis, but data concerning the direction of the influence of the separate matrix components is contradictory. Only the influence of fibronectins is estimated as unequivocally negative (Gregoire et al., 1998).

A mature differentiated adipocyte, the basic cell form of **white adipose tissue** (WAT), is a cell fully adapted to perform its main function–the accumulation, storage and utilization, as required, of a lipid deposit as the energy reserve of an organism. In the final stage of differentiation, transcription mechanisms provide the maximum contents and activity of proteins–enzymes, which carry out the metabolism of triglycerides (triacylglycerols, TAG), and of lipoproteins. The conditions essential for this metabolism, such as the expression of a sufficient quantity of glucose transporters and insulin receptors, are also created.

Along with the function of lipid storage, the mature adipocytes, mainly white ones, also have an important secretory function, which transforms adipose tissue distributed throughout the organism into an integrated **endocrine** organ.

Adipocytes produce and secrete a number of protein and peptide signaling molecules: leptin; adipsin; resistin; an acyl group transfer-stimulating protein; angiotensin II, the transforming growth factor α (TGF-α); prostaglandins; a macrophage migration inhibitory factor; the fasting-induced adiposity factor (FIAF); adiponectin (Acrp30, AdipoQ, AgM-1); Agouti; and acidic cysteine-rich protein (osteonectin, SPARC) (Gregoire, 2001). **Leptin** is a hormone that regulates the needs for food; it is highly important in the regulation of morphogenesis and functions of the bone tissue. The influence of the whole complex of adipocyte-secreted factors (adipocyte "secretome") falls outside the limits of the connective tissue and extends to many organs and systems. It includes the regulation of energetic homeostasis, insulin sensibility, the course of immune reactions, the development of vascular diseases and other functions of an organism.

The third typical feature of adipocytes' phenotype–the active expression of genes, which encode the proteins involved in the biosynthesis of the biologically active factors secreted by adipocytes, is associated with white adipocytes' endocrine function.

Adipocytes of **brown adipose tissue (BAT)**, as well as WAT adipocytes, are energy reservoirs, but the energy stored as a protons' concentration gradient in the internal membrane of their abundant mitochondria (the abundance of mitochondria makes BAT adipocytes brown) is used differently than the energy accumulated in white adipocytes.

In white adipocytes, the process of lipid oxidation is associated with the formation of adenosine triphosphoric acid (ATP); this process is called oxidative phosphorylation. The concentration gradient-associated movement of protons from the intermembranous space (a mitochondrion coat is comprised of two membranes) into the mitochondrial matrix occurs in the interaction with the transmembrane protein of the internal membrane, which is a channel for protons and, at the same time, is the enzyme ATP-synthase. The protons' movement activates the enzyme that carries out ATP synthesis; adenosine triphosphate acts as the main energy carrier in an organism. This energy can then be used in different metabolic reactions.

In brown adipocytes, this association of lipids' oxidation with phosphorylation can be dissociated, and the energy released by oxidation is dissipated in the form of heat. Thermogenesis (heat generation) is brown adipocytes' main function (Cannon & Nedelgaard, 2004).

The main factor making oxidation and phosphorylation dissociation possible is presence of other transmembrane protein–**uncoupling protein** (UCP1 or SLC25A7) in the same internal mitochondrial membrane (Skulachev, 1998). The expression of this protein, which is also called **thermogenin**, is a unique feature of brown adipocytes.

The signal as to the organism's need to produce heat comes from the sympathetic nervous system, which strongly influences brown adipocytes. The mediator noradrenalin, secreted by sympathetic nerve terminations, stimulates their proliferation and differentiation and inhibits their apoptosis, acting upon β3-adrenoreceptors of a brown adipocyte's cytoplasmic membrane. The activation of receptors is the initial step in the intracellular signaling cascade. The next step is the activation of the enzyme adenyl cyclase, which transforms ATP into cyclic adenosine monophosphate (cAMP). The cAMP activates the protein kinase A, which, in turn, activates triacylglycerol lipase (triglyceride lipase). This enzyme releases fatty acids, and the oxidation of fatty acids is accompanied by energy production; thermogenin is simultaneously activated.

The activation of thermogenin (a protein consisting of 307 amino acid residues) by free fatty acids consists in the formation of homodimeric macromolecules. Each of these macromolecules is a transmembrane channel enabling the easy movement of protons from the intermembranous space to the mitochondrial matrix without involving the ATP-synthase macromolecule. This setting (figuratively compared to a short circuit in an electrical network) leads to the termination of oxidative phosphorylation, oxidation and the formation of ATP dissociate, and all the energy released in fatty acids' oxidation is released by brown adipocytes in the form of heat.

The brown adipocytes differentiate with the participation of the same regulating factors, which are effective in

WAT differentiation. In both cases, transcription factors of the C/EBP and PPAR families, primarily PPARγ, play the leading role. However, despite a high similarity, the brown and white adipocytes represent two various types of cells; their phenotype is formed independently, and the possibility of transdifferentiation has not been proven (Moulin et al., 2001).

The activity of a complex of factors determines the occurrence of phenotypic differences between the two types of adipocytes (Rosen and Spiegelman, 2000). They include members of the PPAR family – PPARα PPARβ and PPARδ – the deficiency of which leads to a decrease in UCP1 uncoupler expression. Owing to the ability to stimulate the biogenesis of mitochondria, the nuclear protein PPRC1 (or PGC-1), a cold-induced protein similar to a coactivator of peroxisome proliferator activated receptor γ, directs the differentiation towards a brown adipocyte. The balance between BAT and WAT is regulated in the same direction by nuclear proteins – a steroid receptor coactivator 1 (**SRC-1**) and a transcription intermediate factor 2 (**TIF-2**) (Picard et al., 2002). One of the cellular cycle proteins, a protein of retinoblastoma (**pRB**) (Hansen et al., 2004) and the transcription factor **GATA 2**, which was already mentioned as an adipogenesis inhibitor (Tsai et al., 2005), are very likely to take part in the regulation of adipocytes' phenotype (white or brown) formation. Both latter factors act as negative regulators of brown adipocyte differentiation. The thyroid gland hormone triiodothyronine (T3) has a stimulating effect on brown adipocyte differentiation (Obregon, 2008).

2.5. CELLS ASSOCIATED WITH CONNECTIVE TISSUE

2.5.1. Macrophages

Macrophages or macrophagocytes are a specialized heterogeneous cell population that carries out the function of clearing an organism from naturally degraded tissues and those destroyed under the influence of a destructive factor, or that of protective, metabolic (trophic), reparative and other functions.

The macrophages develop from a bone marrow stem hematopoietic cell. Macrophage (mononuclear phagocyte) formation involves three stages:

1) the differentiation of bone marrow monocytes from a polypotent hematopoietic stem cell;
2) the specialization of monocytes, which enter a respective tissue microenvironment, their adaptation to the medium and transformation into organ-specific and tissue-specific macrophages; and
3) the activation of the latter.

The aforementioned stages are key ones in generating the heterogeneity of macrophages' population. It should be noted that the intensity degree of cell differentiation is not the same at all given stages. The division of stem bone marrow hematopoietic cells occurs rather rarely. At the same time, bone marrow monocytes possess a high proliferative potential, which they constantly realize. Part of these cells enters the blood, where they become circulating monocytes and play the role of multipotent progenitors (Seta & Kuwana, 2007). They comprise 5–10% of the total white blood cell number in human blood. It used to be supposed that these circulating CD14-positive monocytes, the derivatives of hematopoietic bone marrow stem cells, were the progenitors only for phagocytes such as macrophages and dendritic cells. However, investigations in recent years have significantly widened the range of the possible differentiation of the circulating CD14-positive monocytes. Seta & Kuwana (2007) described multipotent cells as monocyte-derivatives that demonstrate a fibroblast-like morphology and a phenotype that is positive for CD14, CD15, CD34 and type I collagen, i.e. it is characteristic for both phagocytes and non-phagocytes (endothelial cells and the cells of mesenchymal origin). It is obvious that the differentiation of circulating CD14-positive monocytes into macrophages and other cells mainly depends on the respective tissue microenvironment in which they come.

Phagocytosis is the initial function or the most reliable criterion of macrophages' identification and classification (Dijkstra & Damoiseaux, 1993). The mechanism that the macrophages employ to take in particles (usually less than 0.5 µm) is detailed well (Dijkstra & Damoiseaux, 1997). There are markers that identify particular macrophage populations, but not all macrophages. However, the macrophages are extremely heterogeneous in gene expression and cell activity. There is no marker that recognizes all allocated types of macrophages (Arlein et al., 1998).

There are two groups of macrophages: free macrophages and fixed (resident) macrophages. Each group is represented by several varieties. The following macrophages are deemed as free (migrating) ones: the macrophages of loose connective tissue (histocytes), the macrophages of serous cavities, those of inflammatory exudates and alveolar macrophages. These cells are capable of being motile in an organism. The group of resident macrophages comprises the macrophages of the liver (the Kupffer cells), the spleen, bone marrow, lymphatic nodes, intraepidermal macrophages (the Langerhans cells), those of the central nervous system (microglia), endocrine glands, the thymus, placenta (the Hoffbauer cells) and others. The resident macrophages are long-lived cells. However, their different populations differ by lifespan, morphology and phenotype. These cells usually do not proliferate but they retain the ability to express mRNA and proteins (Male et al., 2012).

The macrophages' size and form vary depending on their maturity and functional state. The cells can be flattened, circular, elongated or irregular. The most characteristic macrophage morphologic peculiarity is the presence of various cytoplasm projections through which these cells grasp foreign particles (*Fig. 2.18*). The number of processes significantly increases in activated cells.

A glycosaminoglycan-containing supramembranous complex, with a width of 0.8–0.16 nm, is noted on a macrophage plasmolemma surface. There are numerous receptors of different hormones (insulin, glucagon and others), biologically active amines, tumor cells and red blood cells, T- and B-lymphocytes, antigens, and immunoglobulins on the plasmolemma and in the cytoplasm. The presence of the receptors to all immunoglobulin classes (CD16, CD23, CD32, CD64 and so on) among membrane proteins stipulates the involvement of macrophages in immune response. The presence of the CD80 and CD86 co-receptors in macrophages confirms their antigen-presenting properties. The macrophage employs the CD14 receptor in engulfing microbes. The macrophages contact with extracellular matrix components and other cells that are present therein by means of integrin group receptors (GDI la/CD18, GDI lb/CD18, CD49 and so on) (Taylor et al., 2005).

The macrophages also express various receptors for chemotaxic agents (fMLP, C5α-receptor, LTB4, PAF-receptor, CCR1, CCR2, CCR5, CXR1, CXCR2, CXCR3 and others). In expressing the CX3CR1 and CCR2 receptors of the transmembrane ligand fractalkine (cX3cL1), the monocytes differentiate into inflammatory or resident macrophages. At the same time, the macrophages are liable to the influence of their microenvironment. The macrophage colony-stimulating factor (M-CSF) is the main selective growth factor of macrophage differentiation and vitality. The cytokines IFNγ, TNFα, IL-4, IL-13 cause macrophages' activation; the chemokine CCL4 induces their migration, while fibronectin causes their adhesion, phagocytosis and involvement in the process of antigen presentation. The vasoactive interstitial peptide (VIP), leucotriene B4 (LTB4) and prostaglandin E2 (PGE2) cause the modulation of various functions (Male et al., 2012).

A "cell periphery" is distinguished in the macrophage cytoplasm; it provides the ability to recognize a material, which is amenable to phagocytosis, to move and take in the cytoplasm microprocesses, and to perform endocytosis and exocytosis. A network of actin microfilaments with a diameter of 5 nm and microtubules with a diameter of 20 nm, which attach to the cytoplasm, is located immediately beneath the plasmolemma. The microtubules extend radically from the cell center towards a cell periphery and play an important role in the intracellular dislocation of lysosomes, micropinocytotic vesicles and other structures.

Another specific morphologic feature of macrophages is the presence (in their cytoplasm) of a significant number of different vesicular structures associated with endocytosis and degradation of the material entering the cell, and all kinds of lysosomes, which synthesize enzymes for the intracellular and extracellular breakdown of foreign material, antibacterial and other biologically active substances (proteases, acidic hydrolases, interferons, lysozyme and others) (*Fig. 2.18*). Mitochondria, GER, and the Golgi complex are moderately developed in mac-

rophages' cytoplasm. The macrophage nuclei are small in size and have an oval or bean-like form.

Multinucleated giant cells, for example "giant cells of foreign bodies" are one macrophage variety. They are symplasts containing 10–20 and more nuclei, originating either by the fusion of mononuclear macrophages or by endomytosis without cytotomia. The multinucleated giant cells contain a developed synthetic and secretory apparatus and plenty of secretory granules. The cytolemma forms numerous folds.

The above-described macrophage structure ensures the performance of the aforementioned functions.

The resorption of collagen structures in any wound, including one to the skin, is the main function of macrophages (Serov & Shekhter, 1981). According to these authors' data, collagen fibrils are exposed to destruction and lysis in the immediate vicinity of the macrophages under the influence of collagenolytic enzymes secreted by a cell; the breakdown products are then phagocyted by a cell. Polypetides and peptides, which are capable of stimulating collagen synthesis in fibroblasts, are the result of further degradation. Shekhter et al. (1977) found direct cell contacts between macrophages and fibroblasts in skin wounds, which are more often found at the beginning of the inflammation proliferative phase.

The macrophages' protective function is manifested as follows:

1) the engulfment and subsequent breakdown or isolation of foreign material;

2) its neutralization in an immediate contact;

3) transfer of information on foreign material to the immunocompetent cells, which are capable of neutralizing it, and exerting a stimulating effect on another cell population of the organism protective system. The macrophages exert this effect by means of the cytokines they secrete (IL-1, IL-6, TNF, IL-8, IL-12, IL10, TGF), which activate DNA synthesis in lymphocytes and immunoglobulin production by B-lymphocytes; they also stimulate the differentiation of T- and B-lymphocytes, cause the chemotaxis of T-lymphocytes and the activity of T-helpers, and of cytolytic factors, which selectively destroy tumor cells and other cells. The macrophage's contact with antigens abruptly enhances the processes of oxidation, glucose consumption, lipid exchange and phagocytic activity therein (Harnett, 1994).

Macrophages synthesize and secrete growth factors of autocrine regulation and for regulating other cells, chemokines for various cells, which enable the adhesion of white blood cells to the vessel endothelium and subsequently, transendothelial migration (TNF, IL-8, and other chemokines) (Harnett, 1994).

Apart from the protective function, macrophages are involved in homeostasis maintenance. By affecting the connective tissue extracellular matrix hydrophilic proteoglycan complex by lysosomal enzymes, they thereby decrease its hydrophilia and cause the inflow of the released structural water in the circulation. There is an

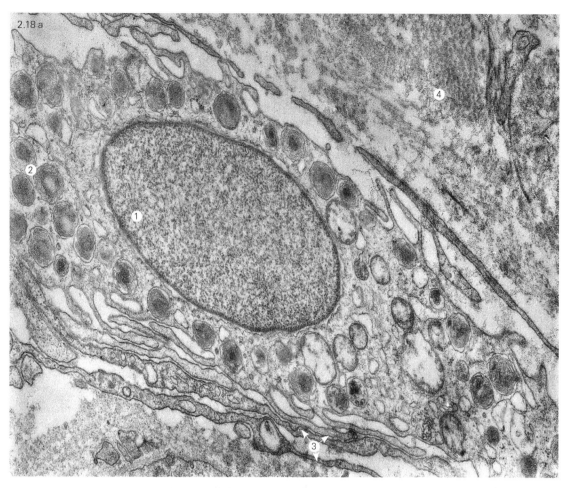

2.18 a

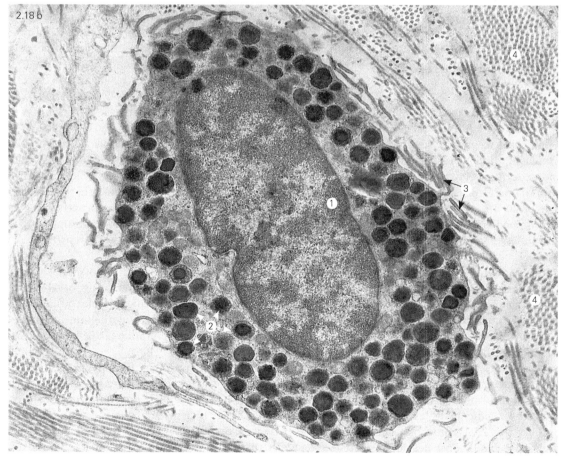

2.18 b

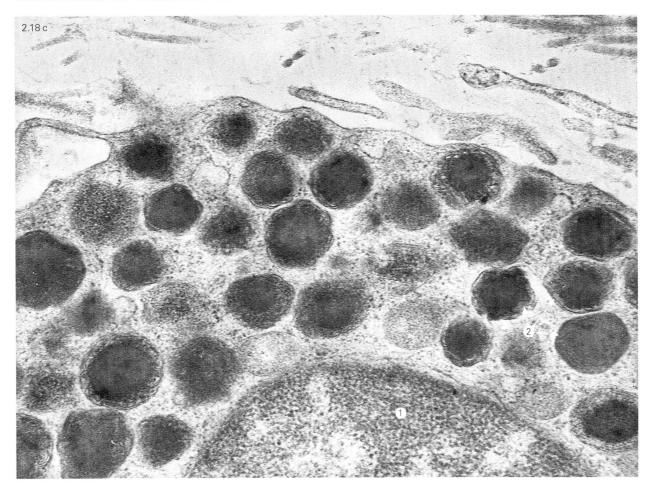

2.18 c

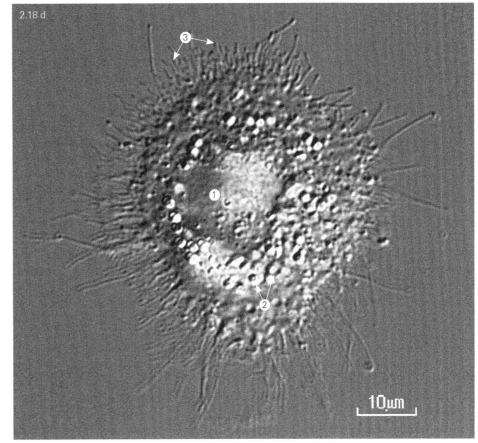

2.18 d

Fig. 2.18.
I. A macrophages of fibrous
loose connective tissue.
a – young macrophage;
b,c – mature macrophage;
A nucleus (1).
Phagolysosomes (2).
Cell processes (3).
Collagen fibers of the
extracellular matrix (4).
TEM-micrograph.
contrasting of ultrathin
sections with lead citrate
and uranyl acetate
a, b – x 10,000.
c – x 30,000.
II. Human bone marrow cells
in a cultural medium.
a – Macrophage attached to the
bottom of the cultural flask.
Nucleus (1).
Phagolysosomes (2).
Cell processes (3).
b – Macrophage (M)
in a cultural medium
(in a suspension) immediately
after isolation.
Erythroblasts (E).
LM-micrograph.
A light optic inverted
microscope Ti Nikon (Japan)
integrated with an incubator.
Nomarsky differential
interference contrast (DIC),
a, b – 800.

10μm

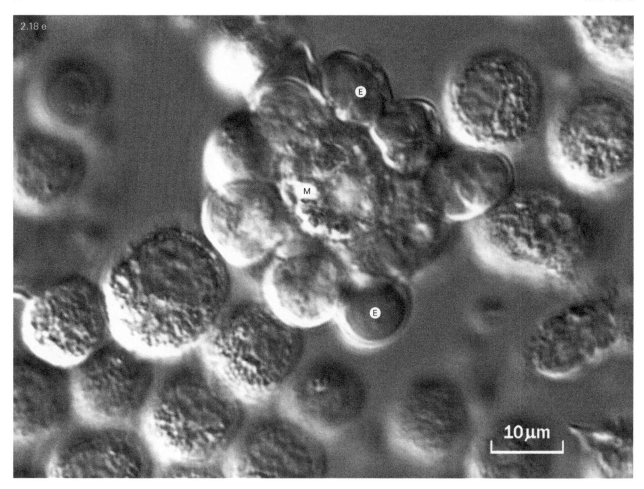

2.18 e

10 μm

intensive "burning" of the lipids mobilized from fat depositions in the macrophages, as a result of which metabolic water originates. This leads to some normalization of the internal medium and facilitates the organism's survival in the case of dehydration (Vinogradov et al., 1981).

Being part of the stromal microenvironment in the bone marrow, the macrophages interact with hematopoietic cells that perform the trophic function and eliminate the degenerating cells and red blood cells nuclei therein (Male et al., 2012).

It has also been determined that macrophages are able to express many growth factors, including the fibroblast growth factor (Leibovich & Ross, 1975; Simpson & Ross, 1972; Rappolee et al., 1988; Harnett, 1994), and thereby stimulate their proliferation.

Investigations of recent years have found wider capabilities of macrophages in wound healing and fibrosis, making it possible to suppose the presence of a phenotypic succession between macrophages and fibroblasts i.e. the overlapping of functions and phenotypes of a classic macrophage and fibroblast (Arlein et al., 1998; Betrand et al., 1992; Chesney et al., 1997; Labat, 1994; Vaage & Harlos, 1992; Vaage & Lindblad, 1990).

Not only can the fibroblasts be "non-professional" phagocytes, but also the capabilities of the cells manifesting hematopoietic markers differentiate into a collagen-generating phenotype spoken about.

2.5.2. Mast cells (tissue basophiles) (MC)

Mast cells (tissue basophiles) (MC) are a specialized cell population which is involved in providing the local homeostasis of connective tissue, maintaining certain parameters of organisms' functional systems (blood clotting and others), and in protective reactions (inflammation, immunogenesis).

The mast cells are present in the connective tissue surrounding small blood and lymph vessels; they can also be found near glands and under the epithelial layers, especially under those more often exposed to antigens – under the epithelium of the respiratory pathways, the digestive tract and the epidermis (Metz et al., 2008). The number of mast cells in healthy individuals' tissues is relatively stable, but this homeostasis is impaired in a number of pathologic conditions (Kitamura et al., 1981). Their number increases abruptly due to inflammations, allergies and so on (Gibson et al., 1993; Viegas et al., 1987). The mast cells differ in the organism's various tissues morphologically and by gene expression. They are not found in the blood flow (Pinheiro et al., 2007).

Mast cells originate from a bone marrow progenitor. However, the mast cells normally do not mature until they leave the bone marrow, and upon leaving it, they can circulate in the blood as immature progenitors. These polypotent progenitors of basophiles, mast cells and eosinophils are present in the blood, multiply under the influence of interleukin-3, and give origin to two types of cells: a progenitor of basophiles and eosinophils, and that of mast cells. The progenitor of basophiles and oesinophils is acted upon by colony-stimulating factors (CSF), as a result of which respective lines are formed (Okayama, 2006).

In humans, the progenitors of mast cells circulate as mononuclear white blood cells, which lack characteristic secretory granules (Castells et al., 1996). They express CD13, CD33, CD38, CD34 and Kit, and less often HLA-DK (Kirshenbaum et al., 1999; Kempuraj et al., 1999; Rottem et al., 1994).

Under interleukins' influence, the mast cells' progenitors give origin to typical and atypical tissue basophiles. A cell phenotype is determined by microenvironment conditions, and particularly by the factors that fibroblasts and other cells secrete. Interleukin-3 (IL-3) stimulates the proliferation of the bone marrow progenitors of mast cells and their vital activity in connective tissue (Nakahata et al., 1986; Tsuji et al., 1990).

The main factor, which facilitates and directly stimulates the proliferation and development of mast cells, is the stem cell factor (SCF) (Sawai et al., 1999; Copeland et al., 1990; Chabot et al., 1988), also known as the Kit ligand, which binds the Kit receptor on the surface of mast cells' committed progenitors. Along with the SCF, there is a group of cytokines (Il-3, 4, 5, 6; Il-9,10; INF-y; NGF; TGF-β; GM-CSF; TPO) that influence the development of the mast cells' progenitors via the respective receptors on their plasma membrane (Okayama et al., 2006).

The signals required to attract the mast cells' reproduction into different tissues are also provided by SCF binding to Kit. In various experimental states, the membrane-bond SCF and/or its soluble form is a chemotaxic factor for mast cells and their progenitors; SCF not only induces the adhesion of mast cells to other cells and components of the extracellular matrix, but also facilitates their proliferation and maintains their differentiation, maturation and vital activities (Okayama et al., 2006).

Chemokine-receptors, which are expressed by MC progenitors and the mast cells of mature tissues, most likely induce the transfer of MC progenitors from the circulating blood into the tissues, where they maturate. Mature mast cells express a set of chemokine-receptors, which differ by the certain degree from that which is expressed by their progenitors, and their expression is also different in mast cell subtypes (Ochi et al., 1999).

There exist two subpopulations of mast cells: mucous membrane mast cells (MMC) and connective tissue mast cells (CMC). The MMC contain tryptase, but no chymase, while the CMC have chymase and tryptase. By the ratio of these proteases, the mast cells are subdivided into subpopulations, which are differently represented in human tissues. These enzymes can break down mediators or exert activity in relation to fibroblast growth factors (Galli, 1993; Miller & Schwartz, 1989). The differences of these cells in the morphology and response to pharma-

ceutical agents indicate their non-identical functions *in vivo*. The mast cells of mucous membranes play a significant role in helminthiases and possibly in allergic response. They have smaller sizes and a shorter lifespan than the mast cells of connective tissue; their function depends on T-cells, they carry more Fc RI-receptors, and IgE is present in their cytoplasm. The granules of both cell types contain histamine and serotonin. The main metabolites of arachidonic acid – prostaglandins and leukotrienes – are formed in the cells of both types in a different amount. The ratio of the leukotriene LTC4 and prostaglandin PGD2 is equal to 25:1 in MMC and 1:40 in CMC. The therapeutic substances have a different affect on the degranulation of both type cells. Sodium kromoglycate and theophylline inhibit a release of histamine from the CMC but not from the CMC. This is of importance in terms of curing asthma. It should be noted that some of the data provided has been obtained in rodent experiments and are not applicable to humans. The basophiles contain an extremely small amount of both proteases (Galli, 1993; Miller & Schwartz, 1989).

Mast cells have various forms. They can be oval, irregular, spindle-shaped, sometimes with wide short processes. In humans, the size of these cells ranges from 4–14 µm in width and up to 22 µm in length. Their nuclei are relatively small and are usually round or oval in form with densely located chromatin, which is more concentrated on the periphery. The mitochondria, lamellar Golgi complex, GER have a structure, which is common for these organelles. The presence of microfilaments under the plasmolemma, as well as microtubules in the perinuclear regions near the centrioles and plasmolemma is described in the mast cells' cytoplasm. The presence of specific large (0.3–1 µm) granules, which are metachromatically stained and occupy its most part in the mast cells' cytoplasm is their characteristic feature. Some granules are stained orthochromatically with azure and are lysosomes. The tinctorial properties of the mast cells' granules and their structure depend on the degree of maturation, functional state, localization of a mast cell and its type specificity, and the presence or absence of substance exocytosis. The mature granules are dense and more homogenous, and the immature ones exhibit more polymorphism. The mature granules may consist of smaller "telescopic" structures. They have a stratified organization and circular form in cross sections. A stratified constitution is retained in their lengthwise sections. It is obvious that such an organization of granules indicates the specificity of their chemical composition (*Fig. 2.19*). The process of granule formation may depend on an animal species or the mast cells' localization. The formation begins in the region of the lamella complex, where progranules (approximately 70 nm in diameter) are formed, which is surrounded by a membrane. Then several progranules fuse, forming a specific granule with a coarse-grained structure within a transparent matrix; the organization of an amorphous fine-granular mate-

2.19 a

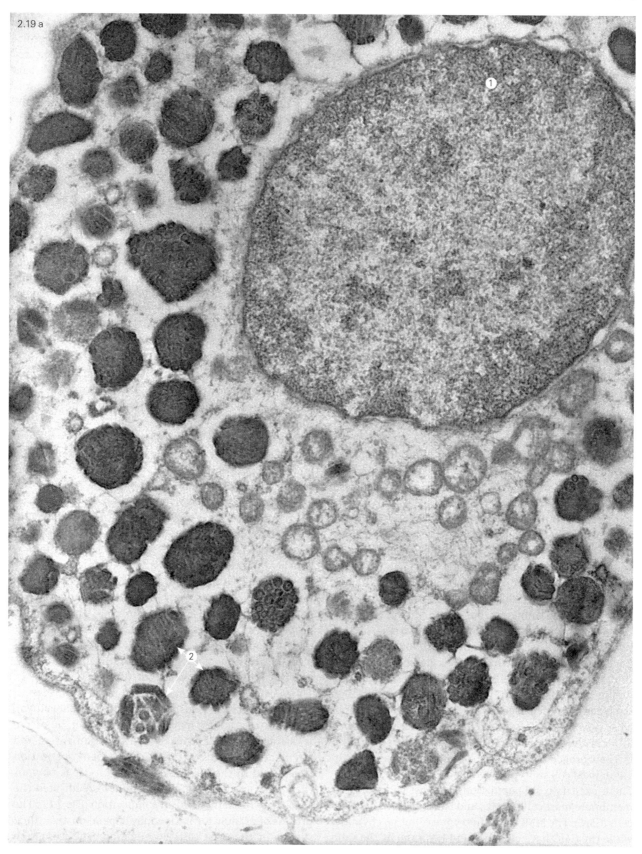

Fig. 2.19.
A mast cell of fibrous loose
irregular connective tissue.
A nucleus (1).
Specific granules (2)
at various formation stages.
Spiral-shaped, stratified,
concentric structures in the
granules' composition (3).
TEM-micrograph.
Contrasting with lead
citrate and uranylacetate.
a – x 10,000; b – x 50,000
c – x 100,000.

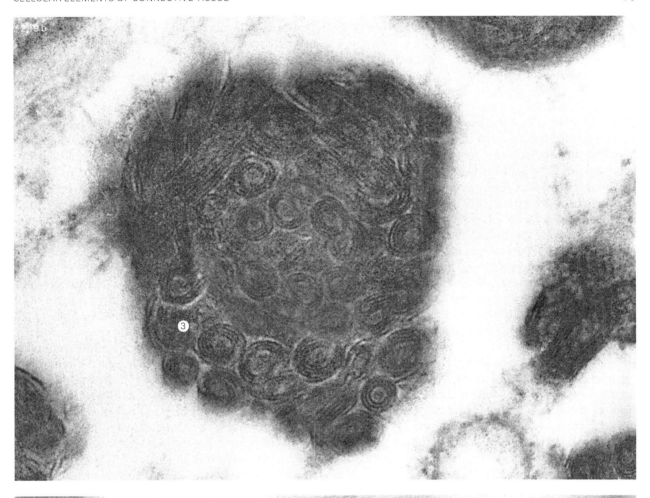

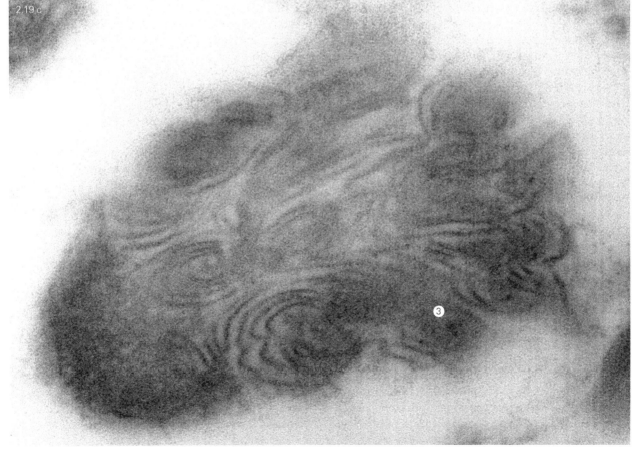

rial into more arranged stratified concentric structures occurs later in this granule.

Granules' composition determines the functional capabilities of mast cells. They are mainly biologically active substances that are mediators, through which the mast cells exert influence on their microenvironment–the permeability of microvasculature vessels and the functions of connective tissue and blood cells.

Mast cells' preformed mediators and secondary or newly-generated mediators are distinguished. The preformed mediators are synthesized by resting mast cells and accumulated in their granules. The secondary or newly-generated mediators are only synthesized by stimulated mast cells (during the process of their degranulation); there are no secondary mediators in resting mast cells. Biogenic amins (histamine, serotonine), glycosaminoglycans (herapin and chondroitin sulfates) and enzymes (triptase, chymase, hydrolase and others) are the preformed mediators, while prostaglandin D2, a platelet-activating factor, and others are newly-generated mediators (Sim, 2006).

Histamine causes a spasm of smooth musculature, dilatation of capillaries and an increase in their permeability, which results in the swelling of tissue and a drop in blood pressure. Histamine enhances the secretion of the salivary, bronchial, lacrimal glands, the stomach mucous coating and the endocrine part of the pancreas. The histamine concentration in mast cells depends on an animal species or the mast cells' localization.

Histamine, which is synthesized and accumulated in mast cells, and other biologically active substances are released under various exposures, such as those that are physical (mechanical irritation, trauma, cold, heat and so on) and chemical (alkalis, polymers, lymphokines, neuromediators and others). The ability of mast cells to secret histamine and a number of other biologically active substances in response to the antigen-antibody reaction on their surface and therefore, their ability to play an important pathogenic role in all diseases with an allergic component, is determined by the expression of high-affinity receptors to IgG and IgE on their surface (Bischoff, 2007).

Serotonin causes the contraction of smooth muscle cells of the internal organs and vessels, reduces the bleeding time. Heparin, an acidic sulfated glycosaminoglycan, is the most important carbohydrate compound. Upon releasing from the mast cells, heparin exerts both general and local effects. It is a direct-acting anticoagulant, i.e. it affects blood-clotting factors, which are immediately in the blood. The heparin pharmacologic properties vary depending upon the animal species. Neutral proteases are attached to histamine and heparin proteoglycan of the mast cell granules as the third main granule component. The oxidative enzymes superoxide dismutase and peroxidase also bond to granules' heparin. The proteases, which are capable of activating kallikrein, prekallikrein and exhibit the properties of elastase and cathepsin C, are found in the mast cells' granules.

Dopamine–dihydroxyphenylethylamine, one of the nervous system mediators, a progenitor of noradrenalin, is synthesized in the mast cells of some animal species. The degranulation process of mast cells and basophiles has type peculiarities. For example, in rats, degranulation occurs non-synchronously and each granule functions individually. In humans, there is a tendency towards granule fusion and simultaneous degranulation. The latter starts with the phase of a granule membrane's fusion with an outward cell membrane. As a result, the granule membrane becomes part of the cell membrane. The granule contents rapidly dissolve and are excreted, with the cell remaining viable after complete or partial degranulation. In most cases, this process is initiated by the cross-binding of two specific surface IgE-molecules of the receptor by means of an allergen. Herein the transduction signal–via the receptor γ-chains–causes calcium inflow, which initiates both the degranulation and synthesis of new mediators (Galli, 1993; Galli et al., 2005).

The mediators are released from basophiles and mast cells with the help of this mechanism. The preformed mediators are released rapidly, and the metabolites of arachidonic acid–leukotriene D4 (LTD4) and prostaglandin D2 (PGD2)–are released slower. Opiates, radiopaque substances, the antibiotic vancomycin and the complement components can also induce degranulation. Acute response reactions, which are not associated with Ig-E-antibodies, are called anaphylactoid (Miller & Schwartz, 1989; Dahl et al., 2004).

The functional peculiarity of mast cells is their ability to uptake biologically active amines, which they have previously synthesized from the integrating buffer metabolic medium of connective tissue surrounding cells. The local homeostasis is regulated in such a manner (Bachelet et al., 2006).

2.5.3. Plasma cells (plasmocytes)

Plasma cells (plasmocytes) are representatives of the immunocyte group, which synthesize and secret immunoglobulins (antibodies) in response to an antigen appearing in an organism. Mature plasmocytes are circular or oval in form and are 7–20 μm in size. The nuclei are relatively small with a circular or oval form and, in general, are located eccentrically. The cytoplasm of plasma cells is basophilic apart from a small region near the nucleus. This pale zone, called an areola, only contains centrioles and a hypertrophic Golgi apparatus. Mitochondria are diffusely located along the periphery of the pale zone. The cytoplasm basophilia is due to a well-developed GER with numerous ribosomes on its membranes' surface and a great number of small vacuoles. A high rate of antibodies synthesis and secretion is characteristic for plasma cells. This distinguishes them from their progenitors. A well-developed secreting apparatus provides synthesis and secretion of several thousand molecules of immunoglobulins per second.

The plasmocytes are usually found in the connective tissue of the proper plate of the intestine mucous coat and respiratory organs, in interstitial connective tissue of various glands (mammary, salivary and so on), and in bone marrow, the spleen, lymphatic nodes, and the omentum. The number of plasmocytes increases in the case of various infectious allergic and inflammatory rheumatic diseases, cancer, hepatic cirrhosis and others. Plasma cells have a multistage development, which is characterized by the progenitors' ability to act as independent immunocompetent cells.

A bone marrow hematopoietic stem cell, which differentiates into B-lymphocytes, gives rise to a clone of plasma cells. This occurs in lymphoid organs under the conditions of a peculiar inducing microenvironment. The intermediate stages of B-cells' differentiation are associated with the changing expression of various cell surface proteins, which are essential for B-lymphocytes' interaction with other cells. These interactions largely determine the ways of B-cells' dissemination in an organism, their replication and differentiation. Early (maturating) and mature B-cells express the specific antigens CD19 and CD20 and later synthesize surface immunoglobulins (sIg) and cytoplasmic immunoglobulins (Ig). The activation of B-cells' transition into antibody-producing cells occurs under the influence of antigens, with the help of T-cells and with the participation of macrophages and stromal cells, which create the necessary microenvironment. The hyperplasia of GER occurs in the B-lymphocytes after the antigen's interaction and the cooperation process for immunocompetent cells, wherefore the cells become more basophilic and pyroninophilic, taking on the features of an early plasma cell. At the same time, the surface expression of specific B-cell markers is retained in this cell. Losing the latter and gaining CD38 and CD56 expression indicate the completion of plasma cells' differentiation into mature cells (Hillman & Ault, 1995).

[1] Tryptase is a tetramer with a molecular mass of 134 kDa, which comprises up to 25% of a mast cell protein.

[2] Chymase is a monomer with a molecular weight of 30 kDa.

Chapter 3

EXTRACELLULAR
MATRIX
OF CONNECTIVE
TISSUE.
HISTOPHYSIOLOGY,
BIOCHEMISTRY
AND MOLECULAR
BIOLOGY

3.1. FIBROUS STRUCTURES

The main structural elements of connective tissues (including bone tissue) by means of which their biomechanical function is performed are fibrous elements and integrating buffer metabolic medium (ground substance). Each of these extracellular matrix components, whose combination largely specifies the biomechanical potential of any organ, has its own specific properties.

3.1.1. Collagenous fibrous structures

Being part of human and animal connective tissues, the collagenuus structures are their most common components, forming a complex organization hierarchy (Omelyanenko, 1984.) The main component of all collagenous structures are fibrillar proteins–collagens, which are responsible for their exact identification. A collagenous protein is identified biochemically by presence of typical unique amino acid composition and the sequence of amino acid residues therein localization. An X-ray diffraction pattern and collagen molecule parameters are specific for "classical" (see section 3.1.1.1) collagens in physical chemistry. A reliable morphologic feature of these collagens fibrous structures is an electron microscopic image of a collagen fibril in the axial view with an exact frequency of similar 60–70 nm repeats (periods) along its length. Inside these periods, there are fine cross lines or disks in 3D reconstruction, detected when contrasting with heavy metal salts. The physical chemical and morphologic characteristics are determined by primary and secondary structures of collagen macromolecules and the pathway of their aggregation into supramolecular formations.

3.1.1.1. Biochemistry of collagenous proteins. collagen classification. collagen biosynthesis

Collagen, a protein from which collagen fibrils of the extracellular matrix are built up and which gelatinizes when boiled in water, has been known since the first half of the 19th century. It was spoken of as a single protein in mammalian collagen biochemistry until the end of the 1960s. In 1969, it was constateted that collagen structures (fibrils) of the cartilaginous tissue are made of collagen, which somehow differs from that of other tissue fibrils by its amino acid composition. This collagen was referred to as type II collagen and the previously known one was called type I collagen. In such a way, a concept of collagen types appeared; they were numbered with Roman numerals. Soon, type III collagen was identified in collagen fibrils of embryo tissues, which is similar to type I collagen in composition and the structure of macromolecules. The main feature, common for all the first three (nowadays called "classical") collagens, is the presence in a macromolecule of a peculiar large uninterrupted domain, which consists of three linear polypeptide chains with an α-type helix coiled in a rigid triple helix.

The next discovered collagen type, type IV, appeared to be absolutely different from classical collagens. Type IV collagen is not comprised in collagen fibrils and fibers but is involved in forming a reticular structure of various basement membranes. Its triple helical domain consists of small fragments linked by the domains of another, non-fibrillar structure, which makes the entire macromolecule significantly flexible. Then a large number of other collagens was identified, among them only two– types V and XI collagens–although they do not form independent collagen fibrils, but are part of fibril composition as minor (small) components. All other collagens are not included in the composition of fibrils. They radically differ from large **fiber-forming** collagens by their macromolecule structure and functions. The main characteristic that combines all the **collagenous proteins** is the presence of more or less extended triple-helical ("collagenous") domains in their macromolecule. A concept of a superfamily of collagenous proteins appeared. At present, the term "collagen" (singular, without specifying type) can be used only collectively.

Collagenous proteins comprise not less than 30% of the total protein mass in mammal and human organisms; a human adult body contains, on average, about 4 kg of collagens.

Plants do not contain collagens, but all animal multicellular organisms have collagens. Their appearance during phylogenesis coincided with the origination of first multicellular organisms and occurred 500 million to 1 billion years ago.

Collagens of invertebrates, especially of inferior ones, usually known by other names (for example, spongin in Spongia, actinin in Actinia and so on) differ from those of vertebrates, especially in the case of mammalian collagens. Various fish and reptile collagens are significantly different from mammalian ones as well. Nonetheless, the general principles of collagen-encoding genes, macromolecular structure peculiarities, cell secretion, assembling (aggregation) into chemically and mechanically stable supramolecular structures remain unchanged for all collagenous proteins at all the stages of phylogenesis, starting with spongia and coelenterata right through to a human being (Kadler, 1995; Kadler et a!., 1996).

The most significant peculiarities of the triple helical ("collagenous") domains of collagenous proteins are as follows:

1) Amino acid residues in polypeptide α-chains are arranged into one-type, **regular tripeptides (triplets)**. The structure of these triplets is presented by the formula:

Gly-Xxx-Yyy,

wherein, the first position must be occupied by glycine residue (glycyl), meaning that about 1/3 of the total amount of amino acids residues in these domains is glycine. It is much more more than in any other protein. Xxx is very often a proline (prolyl) residue, Yyy can be a residue of any amino acid, but comparatively often, the residue of hydroxyproline (hydroxyprolyl) occupies this position. All collagen polypeptides also contain significant amounts of hydroxylysine residues compared to other proteins.

2) The second peculiarity of the amino acid composition of collagenous domains is the complete lack of tryptophan residues, an extremely low content of aromatic amino acid (phenylalanine and tyrosine) residues, and a comparatively low amount of histidine residues. On average, 1/4 of the residues in these domains are prolyls and 1/7 are hydroxyprolyls. The number of proline and hydroxyproline residues in different collagen types is more variable than is the case for glycyls.

Special attention should be paid to **hydroxyproline**. In animal and human proteins, this **imino acid** is present only in collagens and (in a very little amount) in elastin. In the triple helical domains of collagen macromolecules, hydroxyprolyls play an important role in stabilizing the secondary structure.

A relatively high and almost equal content of hydroxyprolyl in most common collagen types has allowed using an assay of hydroxyprolyl concentrations in tissues as is much more of collagenous proteins total concentrations therein. It should also be kept in mind when addressing hydroxyproline that this imino acid, specific for collagenous proteins, is not among the 20 amino acids encoded in DNA and does not immediately reflect genetic information: it appears only as a product of the post-translational processing of already assembled polypeptide chains.

3) Collagen polypeptide α-chains gain a secondary structure (conformation) of a polyproline-type left-side helix due to a peculiar primary structure (amino acid composition). On average, there are three amino acid residues on every wing of such a helix.

These three polypeptide α-chains are coiled into a triple (right-side) helix, i.e. a helix of the second order. A developed system of intramolecular cross-links between α-chains provides the strength and rigidity of triple helical domains. Triple helical domains are so specific for collagenous protein macromolecules that they are called "collagenous" (COL), as opposed to domains without a triple helix structure. The latter are referred to as "non-collagenous" (NC); their proper definition would be "non-triple helical".

However, collagens are considered to be only those proteins meeting the aforementioned conditions that: a) are within the connective tissue extracellular matrix, and b) play a special structural role in the matrix. This criterion is required insofar as a number (not less than 20) of proteins (ficolin, conglutinin, ectodysplasin, acetylcholinesterase, one of macrophage receptors, mannan-binding protein collectin others) becomes known, whose macromolecules contain small, collagen-typical triple-helical domains, but they are not related to the connective tissue extracellular matrix and have non-structural functions in an organism.

In mammals' organisms, including human beings, there are 29 known proteins, which are considered to be collagenous according to all the above criteria. Macromolecules of a number of collagens are heterotypic – they contain non-identical α-chains. Roman numerals denoting collagen types are included (in brackets) in polypeptide-chains names, composing relevant collagen type macromolecules; α-chains, in turn, are numbered with Arabic numerals. All collagenous proteins known so far, comprising the collagen superfamily, are shown and presented as families in *Table 3.1*.

The structure of a type XXVI collagen macromolecule, identified only in ovaries and testicles, has been insufficiently studied, which does not allow attributing this collagen to any subfamily (Sato et al., 2002).

Macromolecules of 29 collagen types specified in *Table 3.1* contain, in total, at least 47 various polypeptide α-chains, every one being a product of an individual gene expression.

Pursuant to *Table 3.1*, the superfamily of collagenous proteins is divided into two families based on their macromolecule structure and the structure of the supramolecular formations they generate, their properties and functions.

The first family is **fiber-forming (fibrillar)** collagens; there are five of them. The second diverse family, consisting of several subfamilies and containing 24 proteins, embraces the remaining proteins classed as collagenous. These collagens **not forming fibrils** are referred to as **non-fibrillar** ones.

The family of fiber-forming or fibrillar collagens is subdivided into two subfamilies. The first subfamily includes collagenous proteins comprising the basic mass of an organism's collagens (not less than 90% of the total mass). Among these collagens, types I, II and III ones prevail quantitatively, with type I collagen in first place.

These collagens are called large, implying their total mass and the size of the supramolecular structures (collagen fibers) they form. They are also called "classical" (Kühn, 1987), as best known and well studied (the most typical structural peculiarities of the entire collagen superfamily are present in their macromolecules) or interstitial (Latin *interstitio* – intermediate). These collagens play a leading role in the formative and biomechanical functions of the connective tissue.

As follows from their common name, large collagens form fibers in an organism, in the connective tissue extracellular matrix that can be seen using a light-optical microscope. Type I collagen is the main component of these fibers. Type I collagen is relatively easily extracted from tissues, which makes it available for comprehensive study. It is in studies of type I collagen, where the essentials of large collagens macromolecular structure, biosynthesis and properties, a mechanism of collagen fiber formation, in particular, have been gained. It was type I collagen that was considered as a single collagen before the discovery of other collagenous proteins and is considered as a prototype of the structure and functions of typical elements of all other collagens macromolecules. The most significant peculiarities of the macromolecule structure of large collagens, revealed when studying

Table 3.1.

Collagen types: polypeptide chains, molecular formulae, localization in organism

Types	Polypeptide chains	Molecular formula	Localization
Fiber-forming collagens			
Large Fiber-Forming Collagens			
I	$\alpha1(I)$, $\alpha2(I)$	$[\alpha1(I)]_2\alpha2(I)$	Spread in solid and soft tissues, the basic protein in bones, derma, tendons
		$[\alpha1(I)]_3$	Some tumors
II	$\alpha1(II)$	$[\alpha1(II)]_3$, see also type XI	Hyaline cartilaginous tissue, vitreous humour, nucleus pulposus of intervertebral disc
III	$\alpha1(III)$	$[\alpha1(III)]_3$	Soft tissues, hollow organ walls; widespread in an embryonal period
Small fiber-forming collagens			
V	$\alpha1(V)$, $\alpha2(V)$, $\alpha3(V)$	$\alpha1(V)\alpha2(V)\alpha3(V)$, $\alpha1(V)]_2\,\alpha(V)$	Soft tissue, blood vessel walls, placenta, chorion; $\alpha2(V)$ can substitute $\alpha2(XI)$ in vitreous humour
XI	$\alpha1(XI)$, $\alpha2(XI)$, $\alpha1(II)$	$\alpha1(XI)\alpha2(XI)\alpha1(II)$ $\alpha1(XI)\alpha2(V)\alpha1(II)$	Hyaline cartilaginous tissue, vitreous humour
Collagens similar to fiber-forming collagens in gene and macromolecule structure			
XXIV	$\alpha1(XXIV)$	$[\alpha1(XXIV)]_3$	Bone tissue and embryo cornea
XXVII	$\alpha1(XXVII)$	$[\alpha1(XXVII)]_3$	Hyaline cartilaginous tissue
Fiber non-forming (non-fibrillar) ollagens			
FACIT-collagens			
X	$\alpha1(IX)$, $\alpha2(IX)$, $\alpha3(IX)$	$\alpha1(IX)\alpha2(IX)\alpha3(IX)$	Hyaline cartilaginous tissue, vitreous humour, nucleus pulposus of intervertebral disc
XII	$\alpha1(XII)$	$[\alpha1(XII)]_3$	Fibrous tissues, bone tissue
XIV	$\alpha1(XIV)$	$[\alpha1(XIV)]_3$	Fibrous tissues
XVI	$\alpha1(XVI)$	$[\alpha1(XVI)]_3$	Various
XIX	$\alpha1(XIX)$	$[\alpha1(XIX)]_3$	

XX	$\alpha1(XX)$	$[\alpha1(XX)]_3$	
XXI	$\alpha1(XXI)$	$[\alpha1(XXI)]_3$	Cardiac and skeletal muscles, stomach, kidneys, placenta
XXII	$\alpha1(XXII)$	$[\alpha1(XXII)]_3$	Cardiac and skeletal muscles, derma

Collagens forming mesh-like structures

Basement membrane collagens

| IV | $\alpha1(IV)$, $\alpha2(IV)$, $\alpha3(IV)$, $\alpha4(IV)$, $\alpha5(IV)$, $\alpha6(IV)$ | $[\alpha1(IV)]2\alpha2(IV)$ $[\alpha3(IV)]_2\alpha4(IV)$ $[\alpha1(IV)]_3[\alpha3(IV)]_3$? | Various basement membranes |

Short-chain collagens

| VIII | $\alpha1(VIII)$, $\alpha2(VIII)$ | $[\alpha1(VIII)]_2\alpha2(VIII)$ | Cornea, endothelium |
| X | $\alpha1(X)$ | $[\alpha1(X)]_3$ | Hypertrophic zone of epiphyseal cartilages |

Collagen of attaching fibrils

| VII | $\alpha1(VII)$ | $[\alpha1(VII)]_3$ | Fibrils on the border of derma and epidermis |

Collagens of microfibrils (forming beads-like structures)

VI	$\alpha1(VI)$ $\alpha2(VI)$, $\alpha3(VI)$, $\alpha4(VI)$, $\alpha5(VI)$, $\alpha6(VI)$	various heterotrimer	Microfibrils in different tissues
XXVIII	$\alpha1(XXVIII)$	$[\alpha1(XXVIII)]_3$	Mainly peripheral nerves; skull bones
XV	$\alpha1(XV)$	$[\alpha1(XV)]_3$	Cells of endothelium

Multiplexins

| XVIII | $\alpha1(XVIII)$ | $[\alpha1(XVIII)]_3$ | Cells of endothelium |

Transmembrane collagens

XIII	$\alpha1(XIII)$	$[\alpha1(XIII)]_3$	Cell membranes
XVII	$\alpha1(XVII)$	$[\alpha1(XVII)]_3$	Cell membranes of epidermis
XXIII	$\alpha1(XXIII)$	$[\alpha1(XXIII)]_3$	Heart, retina, some tumors
XXV	$\alpha1(XXV)$	$[\alpha1(XXV)]_3$	Along with amyloid fibrils in Alzheimer's disease

type I collagen, are a) **continuity of a triple helical domain,** formed by three spiralized polypeptide α-chains, in particular, the domain typically considered as "collagenous" occupies the prevailing part of the macromolecule length, and b) **cross-striation** of collagen-forming fibrils, which is revealed in electron microscopy after special fibril staining (treatment).

As has already been mentioned, the primary structure of collagenous protein polypeptide α-chains is characterized by triplet repeats of the amino acid residues Gly-Xxx-Yyy. As the triple helical structure is uninterrupted in the central ("collagenous") domain, its general formula is (Gly-Xxx-Yyy)$_n$ in fibrillar collagens.

As the first position in triplets must be occupied by glycyl, all differences in the central domain's primary structure of various large fibrillar collagen types are due to variations in amino acid residues occupying the second and third positions.

The role of glycyl, the smallest amino acid residue, is especially important. The regular repetition of glycyls provides the possibility for three α-chains to be folded into a triple helical structure. Point mutations (single base change), where at least one glycyl was replaced by any other amino acid residue, result in impairments of the triple helical conformation in the macromolecule main domain of fibrillar collagens, not uncommon with severe consequences for all the supramolecular architectonics of the connective tissue extracellular matrix.

The presence in triplets of **imino acid** residues (prolyl and hydroxyprolyl) forming intrachain and intramolecular bonds is of significant importance for stabilizing both the secondary (helical) structure of α-chains and especially the triple helical (tertiary) structure. The special significance of hydroxyprolyl in this aspect has been established in studying engineered type I collagen, where macromolecules of all the proline residues remained non-hydroxylated. Such collagen, produced by genetically modified plants (tobacco) (Perret et al., 2001), was distinguished by the increased flexibility (reduced rigidity) of macromolecules and decreased temperature of heat denaturation.

The extent of various tripeptides' influence on the stability and rigidity of collagen macromolecules depends on their composition in the following manner:
Gly-Pro-Hyp>Gly-Pro-Yyy>Gly-Xxx-Hyp.

The alternation of these triplet types makes various α-chains dissimilar rigid. The most rigid is the carboxyl terminus of the α1(I)-chain central domain, which is "sealed", in the words of Kühn (1987), with the most rigid sequence of Gly-Pro-Hyp repeating five times. On the contrary, the only locus of the same chain, which is attacked in collagenases breaking down large fibrillar collagens (see section 3.7.1), is characterized by the presence of triplets, which have neither residues of proline nor those of hydroxyproline. The less rigid triplets make the polypeptide chains of fiber-forming collagens flexible to some extent (Silver et al., 2002).

In a type I collagen macromolecule, two of three polypeptide chains denoted as α1(I) are identical. The third one, α2(I), is a product of another gene expression; it has some peculiarities of the primary structure. Therefore, the type I collagen macromolecule is a **heterodimer.**

Besides an extended central triple helical domain consisting (in an α1(I)-chain) of 1014 amino acid residues, the type I collagen macromolecule contains short non-helical domains referred to as **telopeptides** (terminal peptides) on both ends of each polypeptide chain. A N-terminal (**amino-terminal**) telopeptide consists of 16 amino acid residues, while a C-terminal (**carboxyl-terminal**) telopeptide contains 25 residues (Miller, 1984).

The macromolecule, assembled of three chains (triple helical) and referred to as **tropocollagen,** coiled into a rigid helix for most of its length, is about 300 nm long and 1.5 nm wide (Darnel et al., 1990).

The second principle peculiarity of large fibrillar collagens studied in detail in type I collagen, is cross striation, which can be seen in the electron microscopy of collagen fibrils. Its appearance, which is accepted for comparison with a bar code, is detected by a contrasting technique using salts of heavy metals. Salts of phosphotungstic acid react with positively charged side groups of amino acid residues, while uranyl acetate reacts with negative-charged side groups (Kühn, 1987).

As the binding of contrasting reagents with collagens, which provide a picture of cross striation, is due to the interaction of these substances with amino acid side groups, there is a correlation of striation with the amino acid sequence of polypeptide chains. This allows elaborating the chemical nature of every stria (*Fig. 3.1*).

Under certain conditions *in vitro* (temperature, osmotic pressure, ionic strength and others), when adding adenosine triphosphate (ATP) to a solution at pH 2.8, containing connective tissue derived macromolecules of one of large fibrillar collagens, the lateral aggregation of macromolecules takes place. They are arranged parallel to each other in such a way that their homonymous ends are located on the same line (it is assumed to say that macromolecules "are in register"). The process is addressed as crystallization; the formed cylindric "crystallite", whose length (280–300 nm) corresponds to that of a

Fig 3.1.
Separate collagen fibrils
of human skin dermis.
a – collagen fibril.
Microfibrils (1).
A fibril period (2) –
primary striation.
Dark (3) and light (4)
regions of the period.
TEM-micrograph.
Contrasting of suspension
of native (unstable) collagen
fibrils with phosphotungstic acid
(PTA) solution
at pH 7.2 (negative
contrasting according
to Brenner and Horne, 1959).

b – collagen fibril on the
longitudinal section.
A fibril period (2).
Lines of thin cross- striation
in the period.
(5) – secondary striation.
TEM-micrograph.
Ultrathin section.
Contrasting with uranyl
acetate solution and PTA
(pH 1.8)
a, b – x 120,000.
(according to
Omelyanenko, 1984).

macromolecule, are referred to as segments long spacing (SLS) as the total segment length contains one period of specific non-repetitious cross striation (Wiedemann, 1975).

It is obvious that the formation of SLS-segments occurs due to the ATP blocking positive charges of collagen macromolecules, while negative ones are inhibited as a result the low pH value in the system. Thus, the repulsive interaction of molecules which prevents their aggregation is eliminated, with forming contacts within zones containing similar charges. At the same time, the precise mechanism of such aggregation is not clear. An electron microscopic examination of ultrathin sections of SLS-segments, contrasted with phosphotungstic acid (PTA) and uranyl acetate, detected 58 fine cross lines, differing in contrast thickness and intensity. Every line seems to reflect the combination of negative and positive charges concentrated in this area, as PTA in an acidic environment interacts with the basic groups in lysine, hydroxylysine, arginine and histidine residues, while uranyl acetate is fixed by carboxyl groups. The appearance of the cross striation of SLS-crystallites, prepared from types I and III collagens, are generally very similar and have only insignificant differences (Wiedemann, 1975).

SLS are not stable. For example, when heated up to 30°C or upon increasing salts concentrations in the system, they degrade into initial collagen molecules. Nevertheless, a less detailed examination of SLS cross-striation appeared to be most useful in decoding the primary structure of large fibrillar collagens.

Cross striation of native collagen fibrils differs from that of SLS. It has a different, so-called D-periodicity, where the D-period length is 67 nm.

It is supposed that assembling collagen molecules into a fibril *in vivo* occurs with an axial stagger of macromolecules relative to each other on their length quarter (to be precise, a little less, on 1/4,4) rather than in the "register" as in SLS, due to electrostatic hydrophobic-hydrophilic interactions between side groups of amino acid residues. Such a stagger is possibly to occur due to distribution of preferably charged areas of collagen molecules into four approximately equal regions: positive–negative–positive–negative. Thereby a period of cross striation with the length of 1/4,4 length of macromolecules, packed into fibrils, is formed (it should be remembered that this length is 300 nm). One D-period contains 234 amino acid residues. This axial stagger of tropocollagen macromolecules is so regular that fibrillar collagens are referred to as D-staggered.

One of consequences of the axial contact of α-chains in the triple helix is the generation of **intramolecular** cross-links between chains. These links play the most impor-

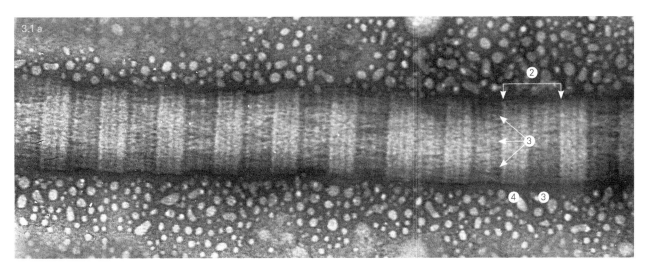

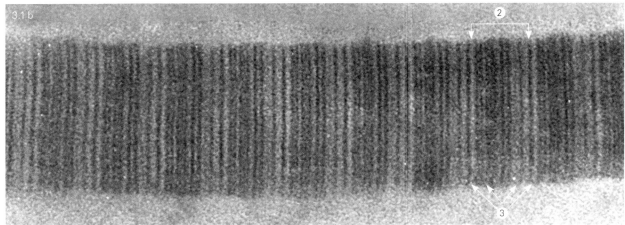

tant role in the structural stabilization of a tropocollagen macromolecule. Intramolecular cross-links are only a part of the cross-link network of supramolecular collagen structures; its second part is **intermolecular** cross-links, similar to intramolecular ones in terms of chemical composition and formation mechanisms.

The presence of gaps (non-filled space), between the ends of successively located tropocollagen macromolecules is a most interesting structural peculiarity of collagen fibrils, especially those assembled as described. These gaps are of significance for the structural interactions of collagen fibrils with other components of the extracellular matrix.

The presence of gaps between tropocollagen macromolecule ends means that collagen fibrils have no intermolecular axial links. This fact seems paradoxical as the main biomechanical function of classical (cross-striated) collagen fibrils is to provide tissues with tensile and breaking **strength**. This paradox is solved by the fact that the developed system of intermolecular cross-links is enough to provide collagen fibers with such axial strength, comparable to that of a steel wire of the same diameter.

The above data on the collagen macromolecule structure, obtained through studying type I collagen, can, in their majority, be overspread to both other large fibrillar collagens–type II and III. In particular, the similarity of structural properties (homology) of all three large collagen macromolecules manifests itself as a marked similarity of the fibril cross-striation picture.

At the same time, fiber-forming type II and III collagens exhibit certain differences from type I collagen. Unlike type I collagen, whose macromolecule is **heterotrimeric**, the macromolecules of type II and III collagens are **homotrimeric**: they are formed from three similar $\alpha1(II)$ or $\alpha1(III)$ polypeptide chains, respectively. There are also differences in the amino acid composition (for example, the central helical domain of the $\alpha1(III)$-chain consists of 1,023 amino acid residues, i.e. it is 9 domains residues longer than the relevant $\alpha1(I)$-chain domain), as well as in all levels of the supramolecular structural organization, up to fibers and fiber bundles. Another peculiarity of type III collagen is the presence of disulfide cross-links.

Type III collagen is present in small amounts, along with type I collagen in many types of the connective tissue, particularly as a part of **reticular** (reticuline) fibers. These fibers, stained in black in silver (argentum) impregnation (this property is referred to as **argyrophily**), are collagen fibers whose superficial layers consist of type III collagen. Argyrophily is most often observed in loose non-shaped connective tissue. The fact that sometimes reticular fibers are an immediate prolongation of collagen fibers is, inter alia, indirect evidence of the collagen nature of reticular fibers (Ortega, 2002; Ushiki, 2002).

In adult human and animal organisms, type III collagen is found, along with type I collagen, mainly in the walls of arteries and hollow organs. In the embryonal period, it is the main interstitial collagen, a product of the mesenchymal cells, which appears in forming connective tissue structures earlier than type I collagen does.

Type II collagen is the major and largely specific collagen of hyaline cartilaginous tissue; it will be addressed in detail in the relevant section of chapter 7.

The second subfamily of fiber-forming (fibrillar) collagens is comprised by collagens whose molecules, like those of large collagens, have an extended uninterrupted triple helical domain and cross striation of aggregates obtained *in vitro*. But these collagens do not independently form fibrils or moreover, fibers. In an organism, they are exhibited in smaller amounts than large collagens. According to these features, they are called small fibrillar collagens.

Two small (also called "minor") fibrillar collagens are known: type V and type XI (Kadler at al., 1996). Everything said about the macromolecule structure of large collagens essentially refers to these two collagens. However, this similarity, which is particularly manifested as cross striation of SLS-aggregates, is only revealed to the full extent when studying aggregates generated *in vitro*. *In vivo*, they are present in complex collagen fibers, where large collagens prevail in amount. Thus, with good reason, type V and XI collagens can be characterized as fiber-forming.

Type V collagen is present mainly inside fibrils, essentially consisting of type I collagen (Birk, 2001).

Type XI collagen, very similar to type V collagen in its primary structure, occupies a similar position in collagen fibrils, between molecules of type II collagen in the hyaline cartilaginous tissue. Moreover, type XI collagen can, *in vivo*, form short homogenous fragments (a sort of "alloy" with type I collagen) in some normal and pathologically altered tissues. These fragments serve as cores, around which fibrils of type I collagen are formed (Hansen & Bruckner, 2003).

In recent years, two more types of collagen have been identified–types XXIV and XXVII, which have a large uninterrupted central domain, like fibrillar collagens.

The expression of **type XXIV collagen** (Koch et al., 2003) in mice takes place in embryogenesis during the development of bone tissue and eye tissues, along with type I collagen. This collagen contains a uninterrupted triple helical domain consisting of 931 amino acid residues. However, the Gly-Xxx-Yyy triplet is replaced with a STVL tetrapeptide in this domain, between residues 649 and 652. An amino acid sequence of such a sort is intrinsic for invertebrate collagens (for example, spongia). Based on this and taking into account some peculiarities of the primary structure of C-propeptide, the phylogenetic old age of type XXIV collagen has been suggested.

At first, **type XXVII collagen** was characterized at the level of its gene (Pace et al., 2003). The gene structure is similar to that of a type XXIV collagen gene. A triple helical domain contains 994–997 amino acid residues (at a total length of the polypeptide chains in 1845 residues, estimated by the mRNA length) and, in mammals, has no interruptions, being no different from other fibrillar collagens in this respect (Boot-Handford et al., 2003). The expression of a COL27A1 gene is found in cartilaginous tissue as well as in tissues of eye, ear, teeth, lungs, stomach, large intestine and gonads.

It is supposed that type XXIV and XXVII collagens are ancient products of collagen evolution; similar to them, collagen, whose macromolecule triple helical domain has a small interruption, has been found in the ancient fish *Fugu rubripes* (Boot-Handford et al., 2003). Genes of these collagens are considered as possible phylogenetic precursors of the genes of the modern large fiber-forming collagens of vertebrates (Aouacheria et al., 2004). Therefore, it is proposed that these collagens be included in the subfamily of minor fiber-forming collagens (Wada et al., 2006). Yet nothing is known on the interaction of type XXIV and XXVII collagen macromolecules with those of large fiber-forming collagens; they are subdivided into a special subfamily in *Table 3.1*.

Collagenous proteins' non-forming fibers, whose discovery and studying became possible only due to using molecular biological methods, are subdivided into several families, as presented in *Table 3.1*.

a) The first family includes collagens, whose macromolecules are located on the surface of fibrils formed by large fibrillar collagens, but are not involved in their formation and that, in their majority, are non-covalently bound with fiber-forming collagens. The name of this family–**fibril-associated collagens with interrupted triple helices,** abbreviated as FACIT–implies their localization in the extracellular matrix and the interruption of triple helical regions. Type IX, XII, XIV, XVI, XIX, XX, XXI and XXII collagens comprise this family (Fitzgerald & Bateman, 2001; Koch et al., 2001; Chou & Li, 2002; Tuckwell, 2002).

b) Collagens with a mesh-like appearance of supramolecular structures. This family includes two subfamilies: a subfamily of type IV collagens, the basic collagens of basement membranes (Hudson et al., 1993) (see 3.3.2), and a subfamily of short-chain collagens, including type VIII and X collagens (type X collagen is expressed only by chondrocytes during the final stage of their differentiation).

c) One collagenous protein–type VII collagen, which forms special microfibrils that attach the cells to basement membranes, is singled out for inclusion into a separate family. In particular, these microfibrils play a significant role in the structural interaction of the derma and epidermis (Burgeson, 1987).

d) The next family includes collagens, which form the microfibrils of another structure–fine, necklace- or beads-like (types VI and XXVIII collagen). Microfibrils of type VI collagen, formed by uniting four macromolecules (tetramerization) and the sequential ("tandem") junction of tetramers (Knupp et al., 2006), are present in many tissues. Microfibrils of the most re-

cently identified type of collagen–type XXVIII collagen (Veit et al., 2006)–are found in skull bones and in peripheral nerve membranes.

e) It should be particularly emphasized that collagen microfibrils formed by type VI, VII, XXVIII collagens have nothing in common with fibrillar microfibrills, whose main components are fibrillins.

f) Type XV and XVIII collagens are combined into a family referred to as **multiple triple-helix**, **multiplexins**. This name reflects a structure of macromolecules that contain small, albeit numerous (more than 10), interrupted triple helical domains. Multiplexins are bound with cellular and basement membranes. By proteolytic cleavage of the C-terminal domain of multiplexin macromolecules peptides, endostatins, are released, which are able to delay the proliferation of endothelium cells and, thus, inhibit angiogenesis.

g) The last family includes collagens, which possess a transmembrane domain and thus are part of the cellular membrane structure. Part of a macromolecule of these collagens is located inside the cell cytosol (XIII, XVII, XXIII, XXV types) (Franzke et al., 2005). Essentially, these proteins must be classified as transmembrane receptors (see section 3.6.3); unlike the majority of transmembrane receptors, they enter the extracellular matrix with their C-terminal rather that N-terminal domain.

The peculiarities of the distribution of triple helical ("collagenous") and non-triple helical ("non-collagenous") domains in the macromolecules of several fiber non-forming (non-fibrillar) collagens are outlined in Fukai et al., 1994 .

Manifold supramolecular formations, are formed by collagens, as well as other proteins containing "collagenous" (triple helical) domains (Myllyharju & Kivirikko, 2004).

All **collagens are synthesized by fibroblasts** and cells that are specialized types of connective tissue cells–osteoblasts, chondroblasts and others. Each of the polypeptide α-chains listed in *Table 3.1* is, as already mentioned, is a product of an individual gene expression.

The sizes of the polypeptide chain genes of fiber-forming (fibrillar) collagens, localized on different chromosomes, range from 39,000 nucleotide pairs in a chicken α2(I)-chain to 18,000 pairs in a human α1(I)-chain. Encoding sequences (exons), comprising 10–30% of the total gene length, are interrupted with numerous introns. It should be underlined that the number and size of exons are similar in all the genes of fiber-forming collagens.

The main peculiarities of the genetic regulation of collagen polypeptide chain biosynthesis have been more thoroughly studied in type I collagen. It has been determined that the gene region encoding the central helical domain of the α1(I)-chain is divided into 42 exons (Kühn, 1987). Two more exons encode the domains directly flanking this largest domain.

The most interesting peculiarity of helical domain exons is that the number of base pairs therein must be a multiple of 9 – in full conformity with the triplet nature of the amino acid sequence in α-chains (we recall that a codon of every amino acid residue consists of base pairs in DNA). The majority of exons (21) contain 54 base pairs each, nine more exons containing 108 pairs each, and one exon that has 162 pairs.

The opinion exists that the evolution of a collagen gene started with a primary gene exactly 54 pairs long (Burgeson & Nimni, 1992). The amplification (enlarging, or extending by forming additional copies) of this exon, in combination with a number of other alterations in genome DNA, firstly resulted in the elongation of the triple helical domains of polypeptide chains, and, secondly, in the generation of collagen type diversity.

Every exon with a 54 base pair length encodes a polypeptide containing 18 amino acid residues; in turn, the length of such a polypeptide corresponds to 1/13 of D-period of collagen fibril cross striation (Kühn, 1987).

Transcription of collagen genes is controlled by complex programs, including the involvement of cis-regulating elements (regulating DNA segments, non-incorporated into genes) and the action of trans-regulating elements (protein transcription factors). The number of protein factors directly or indirectly interacting with DNA, thereby involved in regulating the transcription of a type I collagen gene, includes:

Herein, it is in the case of type I collagen that coordination of all these factors' activity is extremely important as this collagen macromolecule is a heterodimer – it consists of two α1-chains and one α2-chain, whereas the genes encoding these chains are located on different chromosomes, and the transcription and further translation of genetic information for both polypeptide chains have to be coordinated in intensity and in time. In achieving such coordination, a significant role is played by the zinc-containing c-Krox factor, capable of binding with gene promoters of both α-chains (Galera et al., 1996).

Polypeptides called **prepro-α-chains** are primary translation products of the collagen messenger RNA (mRNA), which takes place at ribosomes.

In the very beginning (in the amino- or N-terminus), where the assembly of an assembling α-chain begins, a short hydrophobic **signal** peptide is formed; this is essential for the further penetration of the entire chain into the cisterns of the granular endoplasmic reticulum. Here the signal peptide is cleaved by a peptidase, bound to the reticulum membrane, as a result of which a prepro-α-chain is transformed into a **pro-α-chain**. The latter differs from a future ready α-chain by the presence of two end (terminal) peptides – amino terminal and carboxyterminal (Kühn, 1987). The removal of the signal peptide is the first **co-translational** modification of synthesized collagen (i.e. ongoing before the translation is completed).

Almost simultaneously to the removal of the signal peptide (it is also referred to as **pre**peptide, unlike terminal **pro**peptides) within the carboxyterminal propeptide, disulfate bonds are formed, connecting the other pro-α-

chains closest to each other; in such a way, this provides an optimal mutual arrangement of three α-chains, facilitating their further assembly into a single triple helical collagen macromolecule. As an elongating pro-α-chain advances into a cistern of the granular reticulum, hydroxylating enzymes become involved in this organelle: one of them transforms some strictly specified proline residues (prolyls) into 4-hydroxyprolyls, and the other one (far less often) transforms them into 3-hydroxyprolyls.

Prolyl-4-hydroxulase (P4H) is a tetrameric protein known in at least two isoforms, the structure of which is denoted by the formula $\alpha_2\beta_2$. Both α-subunits of the enzyme have a catalytic (hydroxylating) activity (Myllyharju, 2003).

Prolyl-4-hydroxulase acts only on prolyls, positioned as Yyy in the Cly-Xxx-Yyy triplets specific for the primary structure of collagen polypeptides. Therefore, 4-hydroxyprolyl always occupies the third position (Yyy) in triplets in collagens.

Another enzyme, prolyl-3-hydroxylase (P3H) (Vranka et al., 2004), hydroxylates only prolyl in the second position (Xxx), provided that prolyl in the nearby, the third (Yyy), position has already been transformed into 4-hydroxyprolyl. Such strict conditions result in 3-hydroxyproline being detected only in the singular in an α1(I)-chain in the unique triplet Gly-3Hyp-4Hyp; this only residue of 3-hydroxyproline, as opposed to 4-hydroxyprolyl, destabilizes a collagen macromolecule's rigidity to some extent (Jenkins et al., 2003) (Darnell et al., 1990).

For the formation of an uninterrupted triplet helix of a type I collagen macromolecule stable at 37°C, at least 90 residues of 4-hydroxyproline have to appear in every α-chain. These residues are essential for the further inclusion of water molecules into the triple helix between α-chains and for forming hydrogen bridges supporting helical conformation. Afterwards, the spiralization (spiral folding) of pro-α-chains and their further splicing into a triplet helix occur. The non-hydroxylased prolyls and lysyls remaining become unavailable for hydroxylase action from this time and hydroxylation terminates. Herein, it should be kept in mind that **all** hydroxyprolyls contained in collagens are formed only at the stage of the post-translation processing of pro-collagen α-chains already assembled at ribosomes, by means of the hydroxylation of a part of prolyls. Hydroxyproline is not among the animal amino acids encoded in the genome; the hydroxyproline messenger RNA is also unknown. Due to this, the free hydroxyprolyl, found in tissues, cannot be utilized in collagen biosynthesis. It, as well as small hydroxyprolyl-containing peptides contained in tissues and biologic fluids, are considered as breakdown products of incompletely mature collagen macromolecules; a certain part of newly synthesized macromolecules of procollagens, in which the system of cross links is not completely developed undergoes such decomposition breakdown. Not coincidentally, therefore, free hydroxyprolyl is found mostly in tissues, intensely expressing collagens.

The transformation of proline, included in a polypeptide chain, into hydroxyproline is a phenomenon specific for the biosynthesis of collagenous proteins, as well as the presence of hydroxyprolyl in these proteins. Therefore, the appearance of protein-bound hydroxyproline in tissues synthesizing *in vivo* and *in vitro* can serve as (and it is widely used in analytic practices) an indication of collagen biosynthesis, and the intensity of radioactive (C^{14}) hydroxyproline accumulation after radioactive proline has been administered into an organism (or into a tissue culture) serves as evidence of the quantitative aspect of this biosynthesis.

Simultaneously with the hydroxylation of proline residues, some lysyl residues are hydroxylated by the enzyme lysylhydroxylase (PLOD), known in three isoforms (Mercer et al., 2003). Lysyls predominantly located in hydrophilic peptides, where acidic amino acid residues prevail, undergo hydroxylation (Risteli et al., 2004).

Both prolylhydroxylases and lysylhydroxylases act solely on substrates that satisfy special general requirements. An amino acid residue subject to hydroxylation has to already be included into a polypeptide and to occupy a definite position in its amino acid sequence. The pro-α-polypeptide chain should not have a helical conformation by the moment of hydroxylation, and the formation of the triple helix should no to have started by this time (obviously, otherwise the enzyme has no access to a substrate).

The hydroxylation of peptidyl lysyl with the formation of hydroxylysine residues makes one more modification possible–the anchoring of monosaccharides to some of these residues. Two specific enzymes–galactosyl transferase and glucosyl transferase–catalyze these reactions of pro-α-chains glycosylation, also ongoing in endoplasmic reticulum cisterns. At first, the first enzyme anchors galactose to hydroxylysyl, then the second one attaches glucose to the formed galactosyl hydroxylysyl. Both transferases carry saccharides in an active state–in a form of compounds with uridine diphosphate.

As like hydroxylases, these transferases can only act on non-spiralized pro-α-chains. Triple helical conformation creates irreducible obstacles for transferases. Therefore, glycosylation is supposed to start shortly after the N-terminal of the assembling pro-α-chain has entered the granular reticulum cistern and the first residues of hygroxylysyl have appeared. Glycosylation can possibly continue after the assembled pro-α-chain has been released from a ribosome, but discontinues after the chain's spiralization and triple helix formation.

The glycosylation of pro-α-chain C-terminal polypeptides occur in a different way. In this case, the already assembled mannose-rich oligosaccharide, activated by attaching to dolichol phosphate, is carried to an asparagines residue located in the Asn-Xxx-Thr-sequence. In this particular case, the glycosylation mechanism does not differ from that of many other glycoproteins.

As already mentioned, the synthesis of disulfide bonds binding, C-propeptide domains, is one more step of intra-cellular modifications of pro-α-chain peptides performed by an enzyme disulfide isomerase (Wilson et al., 1998).

It is from these domains that the formation of the triple helical macromolecules of **procollagen**, folding three α-chains together, begins. Triple spiralization spreads from the carboxyl terminus of the chain to the amino one (Hulmes, 2002). This process, in which the initiation the C-terminal globular (G2) domain of the α2(I)- chain plays the leading role (Malone et al., 2005), is compared with fastening a "zipper". The folding process takes place extremely fast, which can be explained by the effect of an enzyme peptidyl prolyl isomerase (PPI), a member of the prolyl isomerase family, catalyzing the macromolecule folding of many proteins (Schmid, 1995).

The role of the amino terminal peptide, being rather conservative in the phylogenetic aspect, in particular the role of a small triple helical domain formed herein, remains unclear in this process (Bornstein, 2002).

The macromolecules being produced are accompanied by special escorting proteins–**chaperons**–from the moment of assembling polypeptide α-chains on the ribosomes (translation) until the assembly of a procollagen triple helical molecule, also ongoing in granular endoplasmic reticulum cisterns, is completed. The chaperon function is to prevent the improper processing of newly synthesized polypeptide chains. Chaperons serve to hinder the premature proteolytic cleavage of α-chain terminal regions; they prevent spiral conformation before hydroxylation is over, prevent formation of redundant links with other components, and enable the proper folding of a triple helix. It is obvious that several chaperons are involved in collagen processing; in particular, the above protein, disulfide isomerase, acts as a chaperon and is, at the same time, a component of prolyl-4-hydroxylase. Hsp47, also called **colligin** (the name Hsp designates another function of these proteins–heat shock proteins) (Nagata, 2003), is considered to be a chaperon most specific for collagens. The fact that the experimental switching off of this protein gene in mice is accompanied with absolute embryo mortality shows how significant the role of Hsp47 is in post-translational collagen processing.

The assembled triple helical collagen macromolecules move from the cisterns of the endoplasmic reticulum via the cytosol into cavities of a lamellar complex. The mechanisms of this movement of long and rigid macromolecules, as well as the further movement within the lamellar complex and then from this to the cellular (cytoplasmic) membrane, have not been fully clarified (Canty & Kadler, 2005). It is known that the transfer process involves proteins of two coating complexes, COPI and COPII, as well as some other proteins, including the so-called "molecular motors" **dynactine** and **dynein**, generating energy for molecule motility along the system of microtubules (Watson et et al., 2005).

Having undergone all stages of the intracellular processing, procollagen macromolecules are secreted into the extracellular matrix, where the cleavage of retained propeptides occurs. Various proteolytic enzymes, whose action is not dependent on each other, carry out the cleavage of aminoterminal and carboxyterminal propeptides. Zinc-containing metalloproteases, members of the **tolloid** family (the so-called bone morphogenetic protein BMP-1 is also part of this family), exhibit C-protease activity. Members of ADAMTS, the adamalysin subfamily, namely ADAMTS-2, -3 and -14, play a role as N-proteases (Canty & Kadler, 2005). A certain specificity of proteinases to every type of large collagen is most likely to occur. The cleavage of N-peptide is known to be ahead of that of C-propeptide.

As a result of the entire complex of intra- and extracellular modifications, a completed collagen macromolecule, called **tropocollagen** (this name was proposed even when only type I collagen was known, and it is applicable only to this collagen), appears to be significantly shortened compared to polypeptide α-chains, the immediate products of procollagen mRNA translation.

The prepro α-1(I)-chain, escaping from the ribosome, consists of 1,464 amino acid residues, of which 22 form a signal peptide, removed even inside the cell; 139 residues comprise the aminoterminal propeptide, while 246 comprise the carboxyterminal propeptide. 1,218 amino acid residues are retained in a polypeptide chain, ready for assembly into a triple helix: 1,014 residues comprise the main triple helical domain built up by typical triplets, 17 residues then are retained as an aminoterminal telopeptide, and 26 as a carboxyterminal telopeptide.

Thus, the synthesis of fiber-forming collagen macromolecules is not completed with the translation–assembly of polypeptide α-chains. Polypeptide chains undergo a number of modifications–co-translational, i.e. ongoing when assembly is not completed, and post-translational, to which already assembled polypeptide chains are exposed. This means that the biosynthesis of functionally comprehensive macromolecules involves coordinated expression and the activation of not only the structural genes, directly encoding collagen propeptide α-chains, but also the genes encoding the enzymes essential for the above modifications. Not less than 20 of these enzymes (including isoenzymes) are known (Myllyharju & Kivirikko, 2004).

After conversion into tropocollagen, the macromolecules are ready for fibrillogenesis. The formation of a **cross**-link system is an important part of this process, ongoing in the extracellular matrix.

After C-propeptide cleavage, along with which the triple helical molecule loses intramolecular disulfide bonds (it does not refer to type III collagen), three tropocollagen macromolecule-forming polypeptide chains are retained together for a short time only by relatively weak, but numerous non-covalent hydrogen bonds. These bonds, binding the hydrogen atom of the glycine NH group with the pentatomic pyrrolidone cycles of prolyl and hydroprolyl residues located on the triple helix external side of the same or neighboring α-chain, retain their significance in maintaining the stability of a collagen macromolecule's triple helical structure after other stronger links have been formed.

At the same time, the assembly of the primary aggregates of tropocollagen macromolecules begins, which is an initial stage of collagen fibril formation and is a spontaneously ongoing process, whose biochemical mechanisms will be discussed a little later. Such aggregates, however, are not perfect biomechanically, nor are tropocollagen macromolecules perfect; they are stabilized only with weak hydrogen bonds.

For the formation of full-fledged fibrils that are chemically stabile and mechanically strong, the dual covalent cross-linking of polypeptide α-chains must occur. Firstly, this is the cross-linking of α-chains between them inside one triple helical macromolecule (**intramolecular binding**). Secondly, this is the cross-linking of the adjoining macromolecules comprising aggregates (**intermolecular binding**).

At present, the covalent cross-links of three types are known to occur in fiber-forming collagens (Eyre & Wu, 2005).

Cross-links of the first type are **disulfide** bonds. There are few of them. They are formed in C-terminal propeptides in type I and II collagens. In type III collagen, in all three polypeptide chains, one cysteine residue is retained in the last triplet before the C-terminal telopeptide. Two of these cysteyls can form a disulfide bridge between two α-chains within a single macromolecule, which occurs involving the same protein disulfide isomerase that catalyzes the formation of similar disulfide bonds in the type I collagen C-propeptide. Unlike type I collagen, a disulfide bond is retained after the proteolytic cleavage of the type II collagen C-propeptide. The cysteyl of the third polypeptide chain might be used to form a disulfide bond with the α-chain of an adjoining molecule. Thus, in type III collagen, disulfide bonds can be intra- and intermolecular.

Covalent cross-links of the second type, present in every fiber-forming fibrillar collagen, are **reducible bonds**, formed from lysyl and hydroxylysyl aldehydes. Their formation takes place in two stages.

In the first stage, a copper-dependent enzyme–**lysyl oxidase** (the full name is protein-lysine 6-oxidase)–acts on collagen macromolecules secreted into the extracellular matrix and is assembled into microfibrils (Smith-Mungo & Kagan, 1998). The lysyl oxidase (LOX) family is known (Csiszar, 2001). Lysyl oxidase performs the oxidative deamination of lysine residues localized in the non-helical (telopeptide) domains of α-chains, transforming these lysyls into lysyl aldehydes (**allysine**, the full chemical name is 2-amino-6-oxo-hexanoic acid or 2-aminoadipate semialdehyde).

To perform its function, lysyl oxidase is bond with the amino acid sequence Hyl-Gly-His-Arg-, which is common for all fibrillar collagens and is contained in the helical domain of one of the collagen polypeptide α-chains. Positioned in such way, the enzyme acts on the only lysyl lo cated in the non-helical (N-terminal) domain of the adjoining polypeptide α-1-chain. Such an interaction does not occur in the C-terminal domain, possibly due to steric hindrance. There is no lysyl in the N-terminal telopeptide of the α1(I)-chain; therefore, we are only talking about two lysyls and only these two lysyls, contained in two α1(I)-chains, can react with each other as they are in immediate contact. We recall that the collagen macromolecules located nearby are staggered in length, relative to each other, inside a fibril (to be exact, a collagen microfibril). In other words, only an intramolecular cross-link can be formed in the given setting.

This link – **allysine aldol** – arises as a result of the spontaneous reaction of two allysines which does not require enzyme participation.

The appearance of aldol covalent cross-links leads to two α-chains being converted into a two-chain β-component, stable in extraction with an acetic acid weak solution and in the thermal denaturation of collagen (gelatination), when hydrogen bonds are disrupted and helical α-chains are transformed into chaotic tangles. But for the mechanical strength of collagen fibers, there is no evidence as to the significance of aldol links due to their intramolecular nature – they do not band macromolecules in fibrils.

Intermolecular cross-links provide the basic mechanical effect. Their formation also begins with the oxidative deamination of lysyl in a telopeptide, i.e. from converting lysyl into allysyl under the effect of lysyl oxidase.

In the formation of intermolecular links, allysine (spontaneously, without enzyme participation) reacts with a nearby hydroxylysine ε-amino group in the locus where, as already mentioned, the lysyl oxidase is affixed at the amino acid sequence Hyl-Gly-His-Arg- of the triple helical domain, in an α-chain of the adjoining molecule. The so-called Schiff base, serving as a cross-link, is formed in this reaction. The full name of this **aldimine** is dehydrohydroxylysinonorleucine (lysine lacking the ε–amino group is called norleucine). As follows from the formula, it contains a double link between an atom of amino nitrogen in one molecule and an atom of carbohydrate aldehyde in the other.

In some fibrillar collagens (this refers to type I collagen of mineralized tissues and to type II collagen), all telopepdite lysyls are hydroxylated (converted into **hydroxylysyls**). Lysyl oxidase acts upon these amino acid residues in the same way as upon lysyls, exposing them to oxidative deamination. In this case, the same spontaneous interaction of formed aldehyde with the ε–amino group of oppositely localized hydroxylysyl of the adjoining macromolecule takes place. A dihydroxylated Schiff base – dehydrohydroxylysinonorleucine – is formed.

This base undergoes a spontaneous rearrangement (Amadori rearrangement). A cross-link transformed in such a way – oxoimine – is called hydroxylysino-5-oxonorleucine.

We once again recall that macromolecules in fibrils are arranged parallel, but with a staggered length (along a fibril) of 1/4,4 of their length. Such an arrangement is of great biomechanical significance: it prevents the appearance of potentially weak sites, where cross treaks could have occurred in overstretching.

It also leads to intermolecular cross-links being localized between amino acid residues, unequally distant from the ends of polypeptide α-chains. For example, one of the reducible bonds arises between hydroxylysyl-930, not far from the triple helical domain C-terminus of one of the chains and lysyl-5^N in the N-telopeptide of another α-chain. In turn, lysyl-16C in the C-telopeptide is bound by a reducible cross-link to hydroxylysyl-87, localized near to the triple helical domain N-terminus of the other α-chain.

Reducible cross-links are formed during the intense biosynthesis of collagen and its deposition in the extracellular matrix, i.e. mainly in the period of an organism's growth. Their amount is strictly limited by the number of lysyl and hydrolysine residues exposed to oxidative deamination. Therefore, later, under physiologic conditions, the amount of reducible cross-links is unable to increase. Moreover, the number of reducible cross-links determined by chemical methods decreases with the age.

Meanwhile, it is known as the organism "matures" that the indices of the chemical and structural stability of fibrous collagens alter, depending on the maturity degree of cross-links: mechanical strength increases, while extractability decreases. This contradiction is explained by the fact that links of the third type, **non-reducible** cross-links, also called mature ones, join reducible cross-links. A significant number of mature links arises through the additional complication of reducible links so the number of the latter seems to be actually declining; they cannot be determined by the methods used to detect reducible links but they are retained in a new capacity, included into tri- and tetrafunctional bonds, integrating three and sometimes four polypeptide α-chains.

One such non-reducible cross-link arises between an imidazole group of histidyl and norleucyl (generated as a result of lysyl oxidative deamination), which, in turn, is bound to a hydroxylysyl amino group. Such a complicated cross-link is called histidinohydroxynorleucine (Tamura & Ishikawa, 2001).

Another complicated cross-link intrinsic for type II collagen, a product of interaction of the oxoimine bond and hydroxyallysyl, is a fluorescent compound pyridinolin (Ureña & De Vermejoul, 1999). It can integrate three α-chains, comprising two or three adjoining molecules.

There is evidence about other covalent cross-links. This data requires further verification but the set of cross-links in fiber-forming collagens is most likely not limited to those discussed here (Robins, 2007).

This is followed by a final stage of the formation of collagen fibrous structures. Regardless of the morphological aspects of tropocollagen macromolecule aggregations into microfibrils, fibrils and finally fibers, as seen under a light optical microscope, only key data on biochemical factors influencing this process are to be given.

The aggregation of tropocollagen macromolecules into microfibrils and then into fibrils in physiologic conditions occurs spontaneously, as already mentioned. The process is ongoing in the interaction of polypeptide chains of adjoining macromolecules, with this interaction being mainly of an electrostatic nature. In addition, as a consequence of the non-uniform arrangement of the positively and negatively charged side groups of amino acid residues along a macromolecule length, the macromolecules are staggered relative to each other in length. The information required for this interaction is localized in the central triple helical domains of macromolecules; telopeptides only catalyze the process (Kuznetsova & Leikin, 1999).

Covalent cross-links between tropocollagen macromolecules are generally thought to exist only inside microfibrils. Covalent cross-links between the macromolecules of microfibrils integrated into larger fibrils and fibers are not likely to occur and this gives evidence to the assumption that, under certain circumstances, microfibrils can be released from fibers and be reutilized for the formation of new fibers.

In many cases, collagen fibrils are **heterotypic**, i.e. they are built up by macromolecules of various types of collagens – two and, less often, three types. A combination of type I and III collagens is very common, with molecules of these two types bound to each other by covalent cross-links. Type III collagen usually localizes on fibril surfaces, whose main mass consists of type I collagen. Type V collagen, not uncommonly (in particular, in the cornea) comprising heterotypic fibrils along with type I collagen is, on the contrary, localized in fibrils core. Mutations interrupting the expression of type V collagen lead to restraining the formation of fibrils based on type I collagen, particularly in the skin derma (Wenstrup et al., 2006).

It is possible that structural peculiarities of type V collagen macromolecules (retaining of the N-terminal propeptide) are such that their presence inside fibrils restrains its lateral growth. Similarly, in the cartilaginous tissue, type XI collagen comprises fibrils, whose main components are type II collagen.

Molecules of non-fibrillar FACIT collagens are located on collagen fibril surfaces (see *Table 3.1*). Covalent links do not remain affixed on the fibril surface, the one exception being type IX collagen. FACIT collagens are assigned a significant role in fibril interaction with non-collagen components of the extracellular matrix, but they cannot be regarded as fibril components.

The process of collagen fibril formation is significantly affected by proteoglycans comprising the family of small (leucine-rich) proteoglycans (SLRP), such as decorin, biglycan, fibromodullin and some others. Macromolecules of these proteoglycans are located, like those of FACIT-collagens, on fibril and fiber surfaces. They are involved in their interaction with components of the extracellular matrix ground substance, and they also promote the stabilization of a collagen fibril supramolecular structure (Matheson et al., 2005). Switching off SLRP genes ("null" mutations) in an experiment is accompanied by a serious distortion of large collagen fibrillogenesis (Ameye & Young, 2002).

The presented regularities of type I collagen biosynthesis are extended in slightly different terms to the biosynthesis of type II and III collagens. In general, these regularities can be extended to the biosynthesis of minor fiber-forming type V and XI collagens.

The mechanisms of the biosynthesis of non-fibrillar (fiber non-forming) collagens are less studied; the biosynthesis of type IV collagens (basement membrane collagens) has been better investigated than others.

The genes of non-fibrillar collagens, along with typical exons encoding the triple helical ("collagenous") domains of macromolecules, contain a large number of exons encoding "non-collagenous" domains, the consequence of which is that the number of exons increases (Fukai et al., 1994). For example, the gene of type VII collagen contains a total of 118 exons (Byers, 2000), whereas their number in genes of fiber-forming collagens ranges from 51 to 66. Potential mutations of such numerous exons and possible splicing variations of the mRNA they encode make the generation of numerous isoforms intrinsic for non-fibrillar collagens unavoidable.

Some details on the post-translational processing and assembly of macromolecules and supramolecular structures, where non-fibrillar collagens differ from fiber-forming collagens, are known.

For example, in macromolecules of some non-fibrillar collagens, which have completed processing, amino terminal and/or carboxyterminal "non-collagenous" domains, which are sometimes rather large, are retained. This indicates the total or partial absence of their proteolytic cleavage.

Heptad (consisting of 7 amino acid residues) subdomains, exhibiting a secondary structure of a coiled coil and containing two hydrophobic residues, have been found in "non-collagenous" domains, which separate "collagenous" ones in non-fibrillar collagens. These subdomains signal the onset of the folding of the triple helix in a "collagenous" domain immediately adjoining the subdomain N-terminus. As in fiber-forming collagens, folding occurs in every domain in the direction from the C-terminus to the N-terminus (McAlinden et al., 2003). Other subdomains with the similar secondary structure and function are also found (Latvanlehto et al., 2003).

The molecular mechanisms of the supramolecular structure formation of fiber non-forming collagens remain virtually unstudied.

3.1.1.2. Collagen fibrillogenesis and fiber formation

The formation of a fibrous basis of connective tissues, including skeletal tissues, can be conditionally divided into two stages:
1) the intracellular biosynthesis of a collagenous protein and proteoglycans (glycosaminoglycans) and
2) the aggregation of molecules into supramolecular structures, ongoing outside the cell, in the extracellular space. The biosynthesis of collagenous protein by cells of a connective tissue differon is stimulated by: embryonic and postnatal cellular induction; growth factors and morphogenetic proteins released from destroyed tissues during physiological regeneration (renewal of the "worn" tissues) and reparative regeneration; and long-term fixed change of the fibrous structures' form.

As a result of biosynthesis, a connective tissue cell (fibroblast, osteoblast, etc.) delivers rod-shaped collagen macromolecules about 300 nm long and 1.4 nm thick, consisting of 3 polypeptide α-helices, and molecules of various glycosaminoglycans (GAG) into the extracellular space. The second stage begins with the cleavage of end peptides from collagen molecules and consists of consecutive stages of collagen molecules' aggregation into supramolecular structures: protofibrils and microfibrils, the latter aggregating into fibrils, and fibrils into fibers. This process is completed through the formation of a fibrous framework of the extracellular matrix, typical for each type of connecting tissue.

The assumption of spontaneity of self-assembly of the above-mentioned collagen supramolecular fibrous aggregates (Chapman et al., 1966) is probably a result of the lack of convincing data on the mechanisms of collagen molecules' extracellular aggregation. The analysis of works (Mikhailov, 1971, 1980), which indicates the possibility of collagen molecules' aggregation and control over this process in a cell-free medium, allowed making up a hypothetical scheme of the stages of intercellular fibrous framework formation and determining the mechanisms affecting this process.

The formation of fibrous structures begins in the extracellular medium after the cell secretion of tropocollagen molecules and the cleavage of end procollagen fragments interfering with molecules' intracellular aggregation. Tropocollagen molecules are not allocated across the entire volume of an intercellular ground substance, and form molecular clumps or mesophases near the cell, where collagen molecules are arranged parallel to each other and liquid layers remain between them. Such systems are referred to as tactoids or liquid crystals. They contain rod-shaped tropocollagen molecules with an asymmetric surface, for which such a spatial orientation or mutual relation to each other is, energetically, the most efficient one. The molecules' form plays a significant role in stabilizing the liquid-crystal state, along with the energy of molecular-kinetic movement, electro-

static forces, and the effect of colloids' interaction with a surrounding liquid phase. Disperse particles are in equilibrium in a liquid medium only provided that the forces promoting their mutual approach and repulsion are balanced. Although the parallel focused asymmetric disperse molecules of tropocollagen within tactoids are tens of nanometers from each other in distance, they continue interacting amongst one another. The formation of supramolecular aggregates from collagen molecules present in tactoids is only possible when they approach each other to a distance where intermolecular forces act. This can happen when increasing the concentration of collagen molecules near the cellular surface due to their additional synthesis, as well as GAG synthesis and their release into the extracellular space in close proximity to collagen tactoids. GAGs, possessing a higher affinity to water, absorb the water from collagen tactoids osmotically, thereby enabling collagen molecules to approach the point where intermolecular cohesion forces act. The occurrence of these forces between tropocollagen molecules leads, at first, to the formation of supramolecular structures–protofibrils–monomolecular strands of 4–5 collagen molecules that link to each other endwise for 30 nm.

The next stage is the formation of microfibrils, thread-like structures with a typical periodic striation pattern serving as their specific morphological marker. Microfibrils are formed from 4–5 protofibrils by their lateral aggregation, with the axial stagger to each other by a 1/4,4 molecule length. Such a stagger probably occurs for the following reasons. The amino acids are located throughout the length of each collagen molecule so that they form four regions of almost identical length, where positive or negative charges prevail. These regions alternate. Approaching each other with the side surfaces, the molecules will be linked to each other with oppositely charged sites; this will result in their axial stagger relative to each other by a quarter. In the same way, the subsequent thickening of a microfibril will increase to 4–5 molecules. It is obvious that such a thickness of the supramolecular aggregate essentially changes the character and axial distribution of the cumulative charge along its long axis and is also the reason for the selective adsorption of glycosaminoglycans on the surface of mainly positively charged regions. The glycosaminoglycans enable microfibrils to integrate into fibrils–the next structural fibrous element of connecting tissue. At the given stage, the interaction of microfibrils occurs along identical regions of GAG accumulation.

The process of fibril formation is highly labile and depends on a great number of factors and conditions. Nevertheless, it can be reproduced in model experiments *in vitro* with the generation of collagen fibrils and even fibers. We have outlined the main conditions of artificial fiber formation in a scheme (*Fig.3.2*). By changing the conditions of a medium, it is possible to generate either "abnormal" forms of collagen molecular aggregates, i.e.

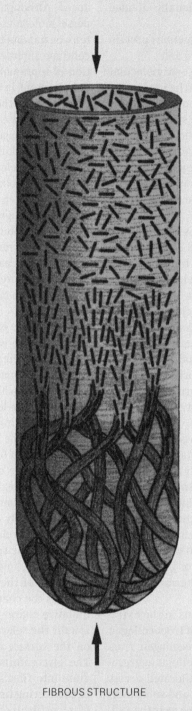

TROPOCOLLAGEN MOLECULES

CONDITION COLLAGEN
FIBRILLOGENESIS
AND FIBER FORMATION

REAGENTS EXERTING
INFLUENCE
ON FIBER FORMATION

1. MEDIUM WATER

1. PROTEOGLYCANS

2. TROPOCOLLAGEN
MOLECULES
CONCENTRATION

2. COMPLEX
FORMING
IONS

3. OSMOTIC PRESSURE

3. ATP – (ADENOSINE
TRIPHOSPHATE)

4. TEMPERATURE

4. ASCORBIC ACID

5. pH

5. ALDEHYDES

6. IONIC FORCE

6. GLYCOLYTIC ENZYMES

7. MEDIUM MOBILITY

FIBROUS STRUCTURE

Fig. 3.2.
Image of fibrous structure
reconstruction from a collagen
macromolecule solution
(according to Omelyanenko,
2005).

separate long spacing segments (SLS), where collagen molecules are aggregated without the stagger by 1/4,4, or fibrils consisting of such segments (FLS) (Mikhailov, 1971; Hilkin et al., 1976).

Fibrils are integrated into fibers by means of the same mechanisms as the microfibrils' integration into fibrils. Proteoglycans of large molecular weight are possibly involved in the osmotic elimination of water, which separates the generated fibrils. Other proteoglycans of smaller molecular weight adsorbed on collagen fibrils' surfaces, as well as the membranes forming them, bind fibrils by means of autohesion in a uniform functional complex – a fiber. The integrative role of proteoglycans is confirmed by the results of processing fibrous connecting tissue with glycolytic enzymes. Being exposed to hyaluronidase, papain, and others' collagen, fibers disintegrate into separate fibrils, which herein retain their membranes as a complex of collagenous protein and proteoglycans. A similar process of collagen fibers' disintegration can occur in the connective tissue by autolysis. In this case, glycolytic enzymes released by cellular destruction cause disintegration of proteoglycans.

The characteristics of forming collagen fibers (thickness, fibril number, form) are determined by the type of collagenous proteins, an organ biomechanical function (mechanical mobility, strength etc.), a chemical composition of the environment, and properties of components comprised into a fiber structure. An organ framework is made of fibrils and fibers.

Collagen fibrils and fibers make up an organ framework. During its formation remodeling or "adaptation" of the framework, construction takes place according to the functional features of the organ. At this particular time, the biomechanical factor or **dynamic structuring** is critical. It means external mechanical effects (in the body – muscle contraction, pulsatile blood flow, fluid osmotic shift, etc.), which influence final formation of the fibrous framework (orientation of fibrous elements, fixation of their form and others) (Mikhailov, 1980).

The role of dynamic structuring is significantly confirmed by a comparative morphological analysis of the architectonics of animal and human fibrous frameworks with known mechanical stress. Moreover, the fact that mechanical factors affect the fibrous framework formation has been proven by experimental data on the effects of vibration on a tropocollagen solution during the period of fibril and fiber formation *in vitro* (Mikhailov, 1980). In this case, the largest part of fibrous structures being formed was oriented along the direction of vibration exposure. Collagen structures formed in a motionless solution had no prevailing orientation. The presence of proteoglycans in the solution enhances the effect of dynamic structuring.

Thus, based on the aforementioned, it follows that the process of organ fibrous framework formation is multistage and is influenced by various factors; and there is a critical possibility to control this process and even to create fragments of fibrous frameworks *in vitro*. During the period of fibril and fiber formation, a complex structural hierarchy of fibrous (collagen) elements from a molecule to a fibrous framework (*Fig.3.3*) is generated, which is classified according to appropriate organization levels. The term "fibrous" means all supramolecular collagen aggregates: microfibrils, fibrils, and fibers.

3.1.1.3. Composition of collagen fibrous structures

The distinctive feature of collagenous proteins is that molecules of various collagen types, secreted by cells into the extracellular space, exist there in several forms (see section 3.1.1.1). Supramolecular aggregates account for their majority.

Molecules of the collagenous protein represent the molecular level. They can be located directly around a cell, as well as in other places of an integrative-buffer EM metabolic medium, alone or as a part of supramolecular aggregates (*supramolecular level*). The first of them is a *microfibril*. A microfibril is an ultra-microaggregate of collagen molecules, interacting on generatricies of the oppositely charged sites of the surface.

This is a thread-like element 3.5–5.0 nm thick, with a 64 nm axial periodicity (repetition) structural organization. The most accurate way to identify microfibrils in the collagen fibrils present in suspension (*Fig.3.1a*) is through the negative contrasting method (Brenner & Horne, 1959).

The next fibrous elements of collagen, *representing the fibrillar level*, are collagen fibrils – microaggregates interacting on geneatrices of microfibrils in accordance with similar zones and lines of periods (*Fig. 3.1a,b*). Fibril diameters in different connective tissues range widely, from 20–400 nm. However, only a few organs show a uniform distribution of fibrils with different diameters. In the majority of connective tissues, fibrils of one or several sizes prevail. So, the main part of fibrils in the derma reticular layer has an equivalent diameter of 90–100 nm. The tendon and fibrous cartilage contain fibrils with the following diameters: 150–200 nm (thick fibrils) and 30–50 nm (thin fibrils). It can be assumed that the distribution of fibrils by a size depends on the functions of an organ or its part containing the connective tissue. The presence of a numerous group of thick fibrils in a tendon is probably related to the significant mechanical stress it undergoes in the limited mobility of collagen fibrils. In this case, thin fibrils appear to serve for the denser arrangement of all collagen fibrils in a tendon and fibrous cartilage. Fibrils branch out and are helix-shaped. At the cross-section, the fibril is basically round- or oval-shaped.

Another important characteristic of collagen fibrils, which has already been mentioned above, is their periodicity, i.e. the repetition of identically arranged structural fragments throughout the fibril entire length (*Fig.3.1 a,b*). The period length is about 64 nm (60–70 nm),

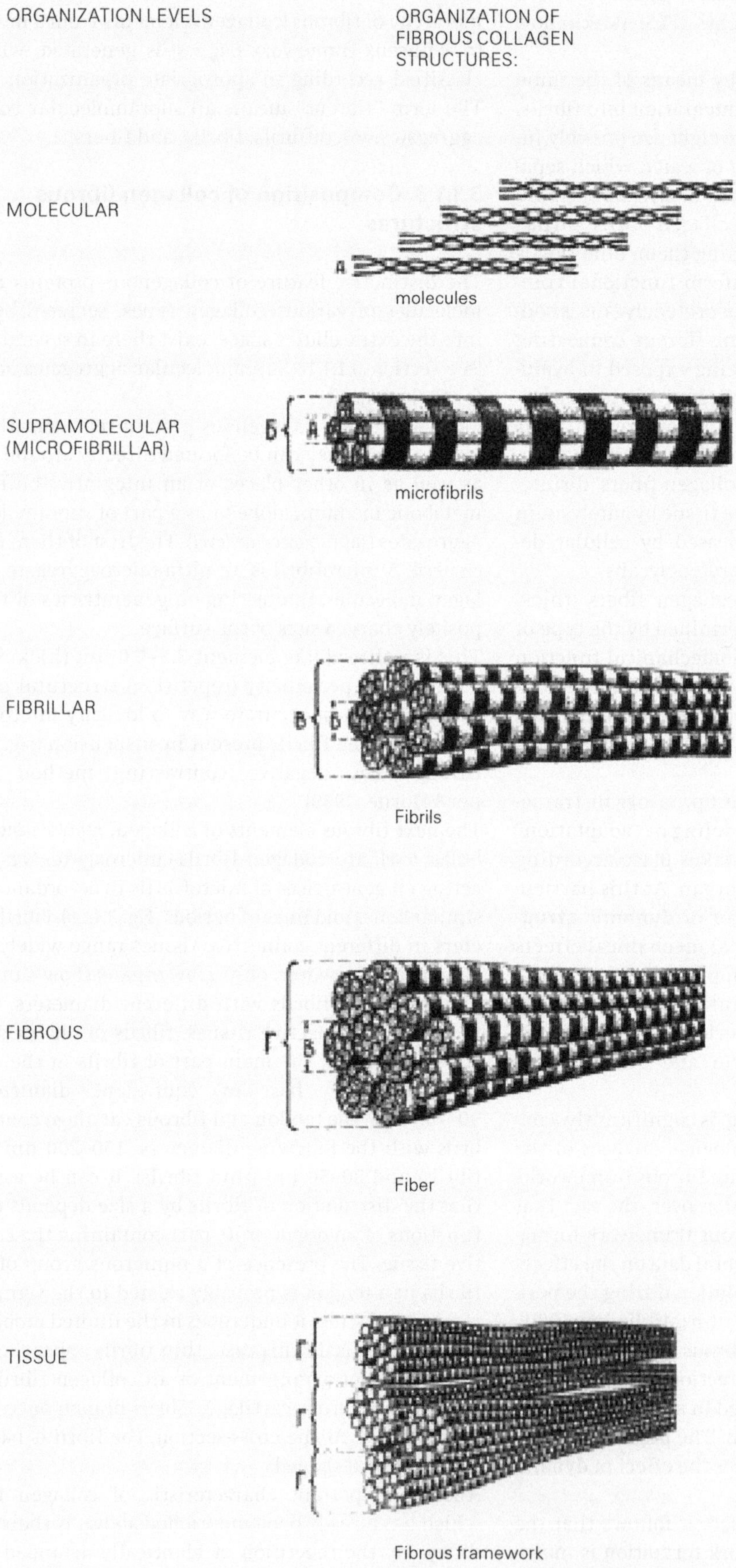
ORGANIZATION LEVELS
ORGANIZATION OF FIBROUS COLLAGEN STRUCTURES:
MOLECULAR
A
molecules
SUPRAMOLECULAR (MICROFIBRILLAR)
Б
A
microfibrils
FIBRILLAR
В
Б
Fibrils
FIBROUS
Г
В
Fiber
TISSUE
Г
Г
Г
Fibrous framework

Fig. 3.3.
Organizational hierarchy of collagen fibrous structures (according to Omelyanenko, 1984).

and the number of cross-sectional lines within one period varies from 2–12.

Based on numerous data obtained when studying the chemical composition of collagenous proteins and, particularly, when studying the primary structure of the polar and non-polar regions of collagen molecules, it can be considered that the cross-striation of collagen fibrils is determined by a specific sequence of amino-acid residue location in the polypeptide chains of collagen molecules and by an arrangement pattern of molecules during the formation of microfibrils and then fibrils (Mark et al., 1970; Ramachandran and Reddi, 1976). Dark bands show the location of polar sites – the most reactive areas of collagen molecules comprising a fibril, whereas light bands are associated with non-polar areas (Borasky, 1967). Differences in a number of the cross-striation lines revealed obviously depend on the character of contrasting substances used or staining conditions. Letter symbols, from "a" to "f", were introduced for cross-lines within the same period, considering the differences in cross-striation lines' thickness, their electron density or contrast degree (i.e. intensity of the contrasting agent adsorption on fibril corresponding sites), and the non-uniformity of distribution within the period (Schmitt & Gross, 1948; Hodge & Scmitt, 1960).

An examination of the serial ultrathin sections of collagen fibrils leads to the assumption that their cross-section lines (light and dark) constitute a kind of disk in the whole fibril.. In the dark disks, the polar amino acid residues prevail, which is why the anions of heavy metals react with them. In the light disks, the non-polar less reactive amino acid residues prevail. It should be noted that these regions contain electron-dense granules, evidencing the presence of some quantity of polar amino acid residues therein.

Fluctuations in the period length obviously depend mainly on the state of the tissue studied. For example, the fibrils of a native non-changed tissue are 64 nm long, whereas the disintegration of collagen fibers into separate collagen fibrils, either mechanically or by enzymes, leads to some, but naturally following increase in the period up to 70 nm (i.e. by 10–15%). Mechanical stress is shown to lead to a period increase by 10–15% without damaging their structure (the structure of cross-striation lines remains unchanged) (Flint & Merrilless, 1977). This facilitates an assumption that the collagen fibrils present in fibers are in a somewhat compressed (apparently spiralized) state, which gives them certain mechanical mobility. Being released of contact with adjacent fibrils probably causes partial despiralization (an unfolding of the helix) of fibril structural elements, which results in a period increase. However, it is still impossible to precisely define which level's (or all together) elements are partially despiralized: polypeptide chains in collagen molecules, molecules themselves as a part of microfibrils, or microfibrils in a fibril.

One more argument in favor of the spiralization of fibril structural elements is the change in their structure by fibril bending. If the angle of bending is more than 90°, the structure and balance of fibril cross-striation lines do not change. However, the fibril period length is slightly more on the convex side. Obviously, it is due to the unfolding of spiralized structural elements of the fibril on the convex side and some compression on the concave side. If this angle is less than 90° at the site of the collagen fibril's bending, the periodicity and cross-section lines are not detected. The fibril has a homogeneous structure at this site. Microfibrils are also not detected. Therefore, the elongation potential of fibril structural elements through despiralization is limited. It is obviously related to the interruption of intermolecular cross-links between collagen molecules, the consequence of which is that the spatial relationship between microfibrils in a fibril is disrupted.

In the periphery, the collagen fibrils are surrounded by proteoglycans adsorbed on their surface. Herein when glycosaminoglycans contact with collagen molecules of a fibril surface layer, a special boundary (separating) membrane or coat of collagen fibrils is formed, separating a protein-collagen from a polysaccharide – glycosaminoglycan. The literature pays reference to the formation of similar membranes on the border of contact beween two chemically different compounds – protein and polysaccharide (Thiale, 1967). The other part of adsorbed proteoglycan does not interact directly with collagen.

Fibrils can exist independently, incorporated into fibers (Fig.3.4, 3.5). In the latter, proteoglycans present on a fibril surface and not comprised in the boundary membrane ("coat") structure, are involved in integrating fibrils into fibers, forming "contact zones".

In the destruction of these proteoglycans by glycolytic enzymes, the fibers will disintegrate into separate fibrils, thus identifying the involvement of PG in maintaining the structural integrity of collagen fibers. Proteoglycan-collagen coats are resistant to hyaluronidase action; this is apparently a result of the strong interaction between protein and the polysaccharide substrates comprising this coat.

Usage of various study methods (TEM, SEM, AFM) and techniques of tissue samples' preparation allow characterizing the different "sides" and details of collagen fibril structure. Investigations of native (non-processed) connective tissue by means of AFM (atomic force microscopy) confirm the segmental (periodic) structure of the superficial part of collagen fibrils (Zeveke et al., 2004; Guschina et al., 2007).

The latter certainly depends on a periodic (but not segmental) organization of collagen macromolecules within collagen fibrils.

Certain contrasting methods indicate special "bridges" or "linkers", or "binding filaments" between collagen fibrils, apart from adsorbed proteoglycans. It can also be one of the mechanisms of integrating fibrils into a fiber. "Opposite directionality" or "anti-parallelism" is another peculiarity of the relationship of collagen fibrils in collagen fibers (Gieseking, 1962; Braun-Falco & Rupec, 1964). Neither of the two terms used by different authors exactly reflects the implication of the phenomenon discovered, which is characterized as follows. In the adjacent fibrils comprising a fiber, the cross- striation lines are located in the reverse order, i.e. if one (randomly chosen) fibril has cross-striation lines located according to the classification from "a" to "f", the next adjoining fibril will have them classified from "f" to "a". Such fibrils, with a different order in its arrangement, are conditionally designated as R and L (right and left). It is easy to imagine that each R-fibril is surrounded by four L-fibrils. The significance of this phenomenon has not been specified exactly. The possible participation of the fibril R-L structure in maintaining collagen fiber integrity is only assumed.

Therefore, collagen fibers are aggregates of collagen fibrils interacting on geneatrices as a result of proteoglycan adhesive action. Fibers have an equivalent diameter of 500–20,000 nm. Their length is not determined. They represent a more sophisticated level of collagen organization – the *fiber level* (Fig. 3.5, 3.6).

An elongated helical form is an attribute of fibers. At the same time, they can be cylindrical (Fig.3.7), flattened (Fig.3.8) or flat (Fig. 3.9). The last classification of fibers is made on the basis of circumference ratios (P-perimeter) and the maximum cross-sectional size (L) on the sections perpendicular to the fiber axis, i.e. cross-sections. If the P/L ratio is close to 2.0, the fibers are flat; if it is close to ϖ-value, they are cylindrical; if the P/L ratio ranges from 2.3 to 3.14, the fibers are flattened (Omelyanenko, 1984).

An analysis of the structural organization of fibrous elements of various connective tissues reveals a number of general patterns in their structure. One of them is a spiral form of fibrous elements. Spirality is noted at the molecular level in polypeptide chains and collagen molecules (Ramachandran and Reddi, 1976). The helical form of microfibrils and fibrils is also confirmed in a number of investigations. Especially accurately the spirality of collagen fibers is demonstrated when studying fibrous connective tissue by means of SEM (Fig.3.7; 3.8.) (Omelyanenko et al., 1977).

Other general regularity of collagen fiber structure is branching of fibrous elements or their integration. The general concept for these two peculiarities is redistribution of fibrous structures inside the framework. Fibrils can divide in two or more branches in one location or along a fibril length. Further, thin fibrils or branches can merge, forming larger branches, and, thus, it is possible to say about unity of the whole fibrous framework of an organ and even an organism. Neither beginnings nor ends of collagen fibrils have been discovered, and interruption in their integrity is related to some damage. The extent of fibril branching can be various. It can be estimated according to the length of fibril non-branched regions. Such regions are the shortest in the cartilage and the longest in the skin dermis. Especially demonstrative branching is seen on the fiber level. Collagen fib-

ers divide into thinner branches, which form new fibers by assembling with other collagen fibers.

It is necessary to note that, among the main part of collagen fibrils comprising fibers and arranged parallel to each other, there exist fibrils or their small aggregates (small thin fibers consisting of several fibrils), which have tangential or cross orientation towards the longitudinal axis of collagen fibers (Fig.3.10). By orientation, such fibril distribution is probably one of the mechanisms supporting fiber's structural integrity.

Along with collagen and elastic fibers, a mixed form of fibers (collagen-elastic and elastic-collagen) is present in the connective tissue. This depends on the prevalence of one or another substrate in the given site of contact. The mixed fibers are probably sites of interaction sites of limited length between collagen fibers and elastic fibrils with the help of proteoglycans by forming "contact zones". These sites are located along fibers, alternating with independently (not linked) located sites of collagen and elastic fibers. Such an interaction sums up two properties: strength of collagen fibers and elasticity of elastic fibers.

During the increase of collagen fiber length, the unfolding of their spiral form (probably the spirality of other structural elements as well) occurs. Fully straightened collagen fibers and fibrils cannot be stretched without resulting in structure damage. Having a certain strength, collagen fibers provide this strength to those organs of which they comprise a part. When an organ is stretching, the collagen fibers straighten, and the elastic fibers or fibrils attached to them in several sites (i.e. in a discrete way) are also stretched.

Having eliminated the stress (exertion-stretching) of the elastic structures, which exhibit the properties of elastomer, they contract, thereby returning collagen fibers to their initial (spiral) state. The system of binding fibers and the ground substance also participate in restoring the normal form of fibrous structures and their relationship, i.e. the three-dimensional structure of the entire fibrous framework.

Fig. 3.4.
Fragment of collagen fiber of human skin dermis. Collagen fibrils tightly adjoin to each other.
The surface of fibrils has fine-granular relief.
It shows regularly (periodically) repeating thin "hoops" of round-shaped granules (1) as well as irregularly located granules (2).
TEM-micrograph.
Method – freeze cleaving.
A carbon-platinum replica of native (unfixed) tissue (dermis).
x – 120,000 (according to Semkin).

Fig. 3.5.
Fragment of collagen fiber of human skin dermis.
Collagen fibrils tightly adjoin to each other (1).
Their surface has segmental structure.
One segment (2) constitutes the thickened (light) part and the interval (dark) part.
Segments periodically repeat, evidently reflecting the internal periodic (but non-segmental) organization of collagen macromolecules.
SEM-micrograph.
Gold flashed of the native dehydrated (lyophilized) sample.
x – 50,000.

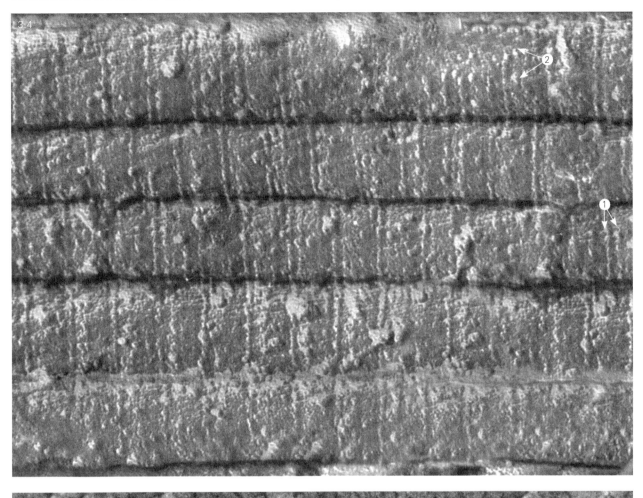

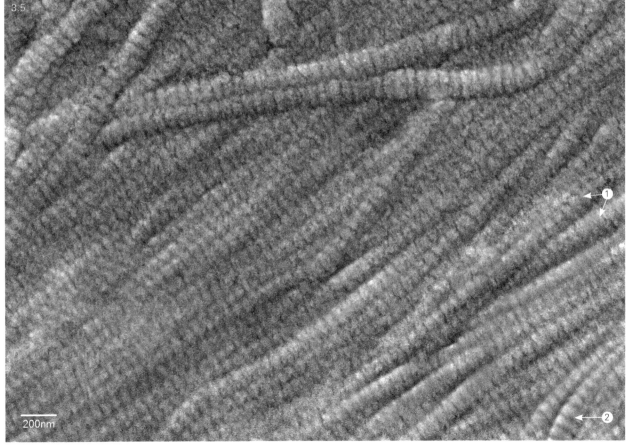

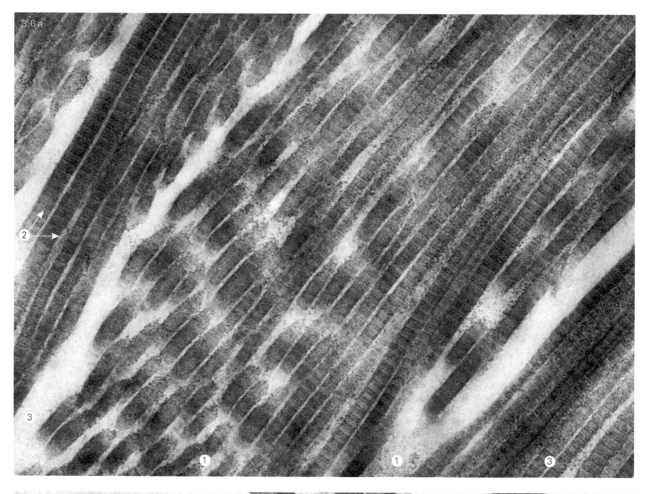

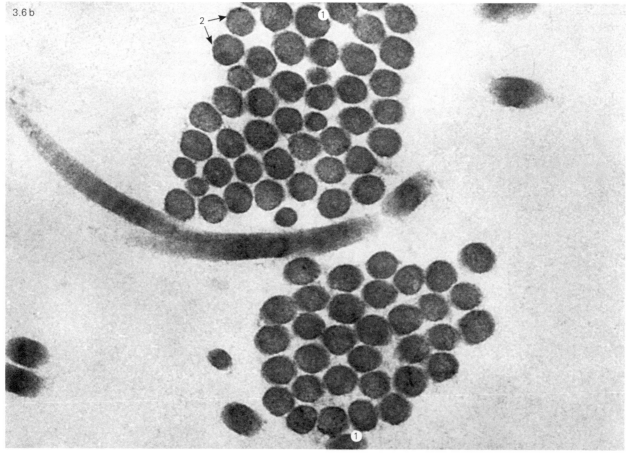

However, if fibrous structures remain in a straightened (non-spiral) state for a long time, i.e. under the influence of exertion-stretching forces, this results in the remodeling of collagen and elastic fibers. There is an increase in the quantity and activity of fibroblasts in the remodeling area. The spiral form of collagen fibers is restored, and elastic fibers are stretched. Therefore, the exertion–stretching is eliminated from the fibers, and they turn out to be in a more favorable (or "steady") energy state.

The last and most complex level of organization of connective tissue fibrous elements is the *tissue level*. It is represented by a fibrous framework, which is a spatial composite of mobile cooperating fibers and fibrils, surrounded by the integrating buffer metabolic medium of the connective tissue (the ground substance).

There are three types of frameworks identified according to the ratio of fibrous elements they contain. In the *fiber framework*, there is a substantial prevalence of collagen fibers over individual collagen fibrils comprising its structure. The *fibrillar framework* basically consists of individual collagen fibrils. In the *fiber-fibrillar framework*, fibers prevail quantitatively, but, besides that, a substantial part of fibrous elements constitutes individual collagen fibrils (Omelyanenko, 1990).

On the basis of a computer quantitative orientation analysis of SEM-images using a specially developed program (Tovey, 1980; Sokolov, 1988) for fibrous frameworks of various connective tissues, four types of fibrous frameworks may be detected, depending on the degree of fibrous elements' orientation: *oriented, slightly oriented, non-oriented and mixed types.*

In the oriented type of framework, the majority of fibrous structures is located parallel to each other. The anisotropy factor is 20–50% and higher. The slightly oriented type has an anisotropy factor of 7 to 20%. The non-oriented type of framework is formed by fibrous structures, located without any prevailing orientation. The anisotropy factor does not exceed 7%. The mixed-type frameworks have a stratified structure: one layer exhibits an oriented-type structure with a certain predominant (prevailing) direction of fibrous elements' location; the other adjacent (adjoining) layer is organized with another direction of the predominant orientation vector. An alternation of several layers by the framework thickness is possible (Omelyanenko, 1990).

The fibrous elements of fiber and fiber-fibrillar frameworks can be subdivided into two groups. One group (the largest) is comprised by fibers with equivalent diameters of 500–20,000 nm, oriented along one of the potential lines of force. These fibers play the main role in performing the connective tissue's biomechanical function. Another, the smallest, part of fibers and separate fibrils, with a diameter of approximately 200–2,000 nm, is located perpendicular or at another angle to the fiber long axis, these being binding or bound elements. Separate regions of thin fibers or individual fibrils can be located along a surface of main collagen fibers or interspersed into main fibers as a continuation of binding fibrous elements or change their orientation to be parallel to the main fiber long axis (*Fig. 3.10*).

Fig. 3.6.
Fragment of collagen fibers
of human skin dermis (1).
The collagen fibrils that
are part of their structure (2).
Interfibrillar intervals (3).
a – longitudinal section;
b – cross-section.
TEM-micrograph.
Contrasting of ultrathin
sections with uranyl acetate
and lead citrate.
x 60,000.

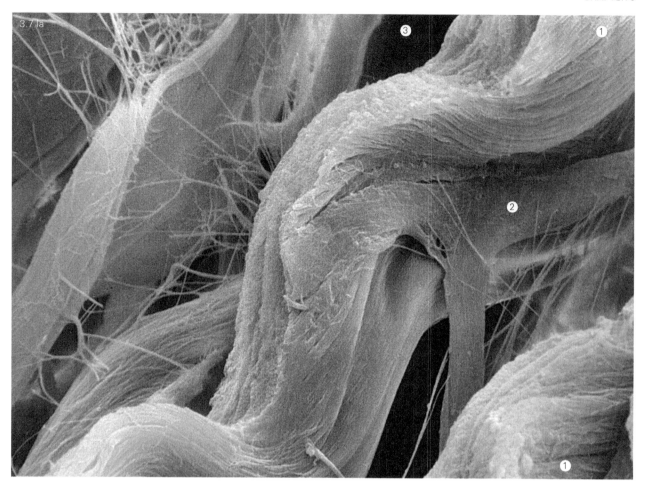

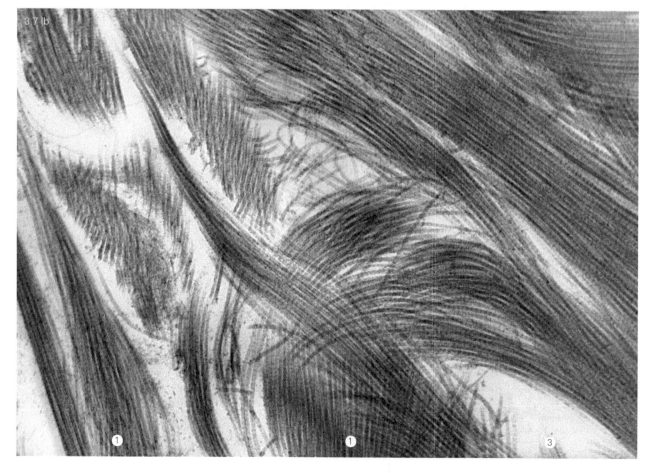

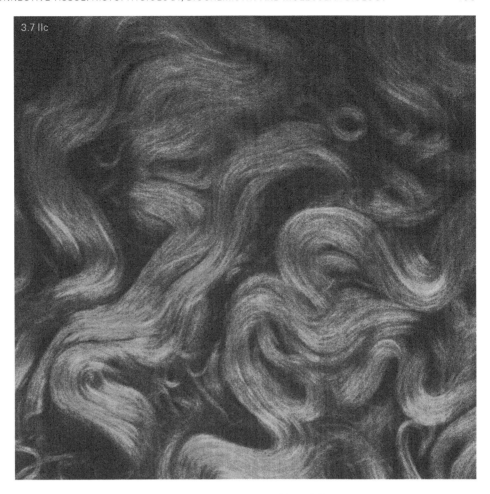

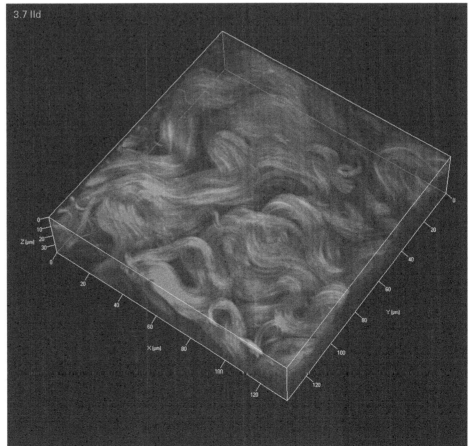

Fig. 3.7.
I.a, b – Fragment of human skin dermis.
Collagen fibers (1).
Elastic fiber (2).
Interfibrillar intervals (3).
a – SEM-micrograph.
b – TEM-micrograph.
Contrasting of ultrathin sections with uranyl acetateand lead citrate.
a – x 2,000;
b – x 10,000.
II.c, d – Unfixed and unstained living specimens of human skin dermis.
Collagen fibers (1) are a source of tissue second-harmonic generation and twophoton excited autofluorescence characterized by emission maxima at 500 and 560 nm.
d – a three-dimensional view of collagen fibers (1).
Multiphoton laser confocal microscopy.
a, b – x 900.

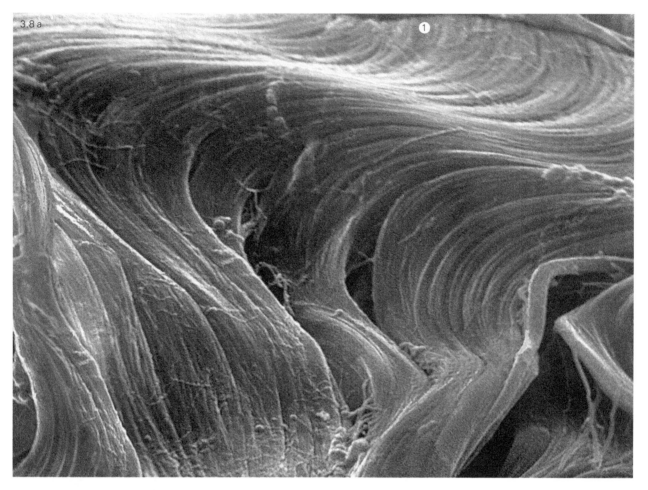

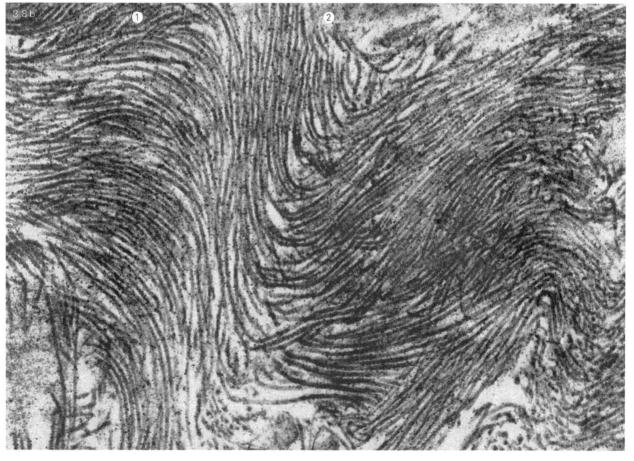

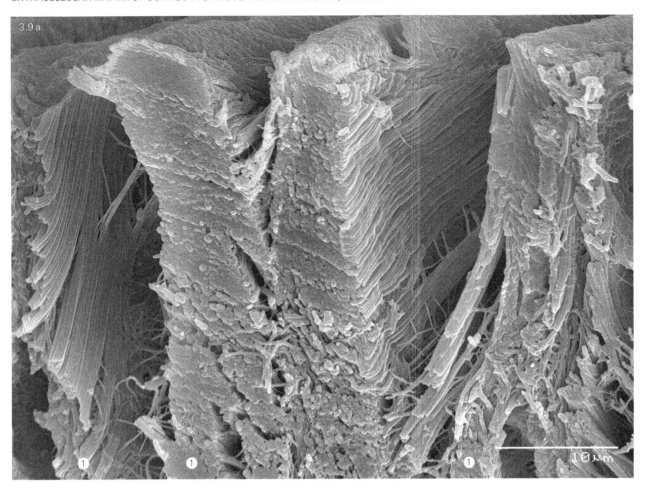

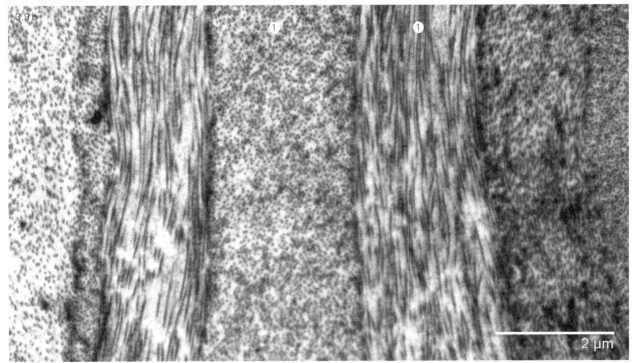

Fig. 3.8.
Flattened collagen fiber
of a spiral form in the
adventitia of human aorta (1).
Fragment of elastic fiber (2).
a – SEM-micrograph.
TEM-micrograph.

Contrasting of ultrathin
sections with uranyl
acetate and lead citrate.
a – x 3,000;
b – x 10,000.

Fig. 3.9.
Fragments of flat collagen
fibers of sclera (1).
a – SEM-micrograph.
b – TEM-micrograph.
a – x 3,000,
b – x 10,000.

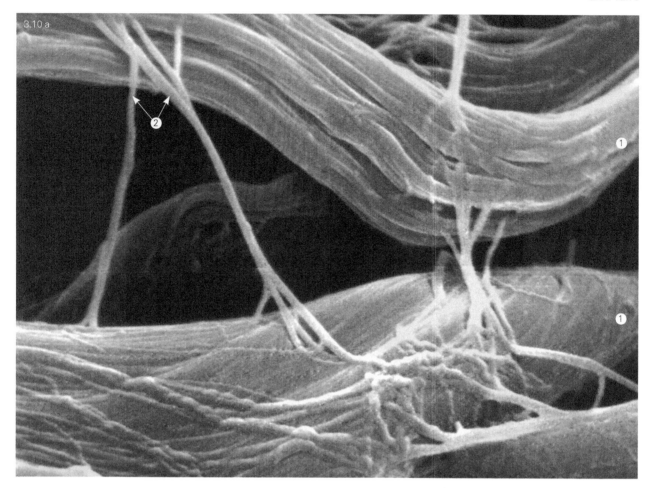

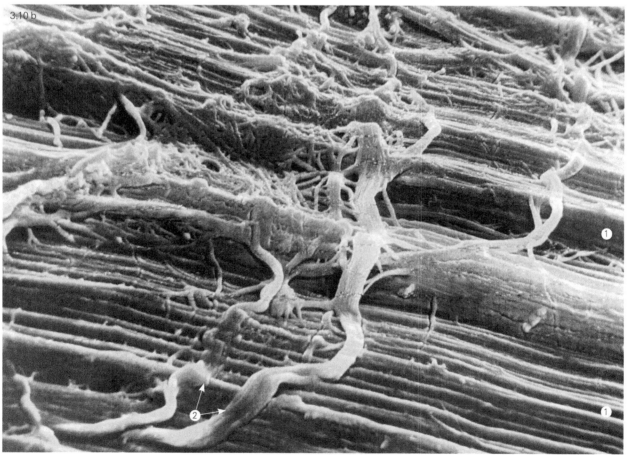

3.1.2. Elastic fibrous structures

Elastic fibrous structures are essential components of the extracellular matrix of connective tissue types whose main properties are elasticity and reversible deformability, resembling rubber properties (Gosline, 1976). They can be deformed even with little force, but completely restore their initial size and shape after significant deformities. It is this property that determines their position in the structure of organs liable to straining deformations during the performance of their vital activities (the dermis, vessel membranes, tendons, ligaments and others).

The connective tissue contains two elastic structures.

The first is a phylogenetically old and comparatively functionally less effective system of microfibrils with a diameter of 10–12 nm, seen only under an electron microscope (Rosenbloom et al., 1993; Kielty et al., 2002a; 2002b). It is mainly composed by fibrillins (fibrillin microfibrils). The literature previously referred to them as elastic glycoproteid microfibrils.

The second fibrous elastic system, also known as "elastic fibers" exhibits a more complicated structure. It is formed by elastic fibers, comparable in size to collagen fibers, as seen under a light-optical microscope. Electron microscopy shows that the same fibrillin microfibrils constitute one of two intrinsic parts (the "reinforcing" framework) of elastic fibers. However, about 90% of the elastic fibers' mass, comprising their core, accrues a comparatively new (phylogenetically) protein – **elastin** (see section 3.1.2.2.). It forms an amorphous substance or component (amorphous in the sense that it has no external signs of structural properties like the cross-striation of collagen fibrils, for example).

There are elastic fibers in those tissues and organs whose function depends on a high degree of elasticity. Along with elastic fibers, the same tissues contain fibrillin microfibrils that do not comprise elastic fibers, which form mesh-like structures. What is especially important is that some tissues, which do not contain elastic fibres, contain well-developed fibrillin microfibrillar structures. This indicates that the fibrillin microfibril system maintains an independent role in the connective tissue extracellular matrix.

Elastic fibers principally differ from collagen ones. It should be noted that collagen fibrils are based on molecules of the same chemical nature – macromolecules of fiber-forming collagens and those of other collagen types. Elastic fibers that contain both elastin and about 10% of fibrillins (comprising microfibrils) constitute at least a two-component system. Microfibrils are also heterogenic in their composition, containing not only fibrillins, but also other glycoproteins. Moreover, elastic fibers comprise other glycoconjugates that are not microfibrils-related (Pasquali-Ronchetti & Baccarini-Contri, 1997; Kielty et al., 2002a; 2002b), making these fibers even more complex structures.

3.1.2.1. Biochemistry of fibrillin microfibrils

The main material that comprise the microfibrils forming a framework of elastic fibers is a non-collagenous protein called **fibrillin** (Kielty et al., 2005),

Two fibrillin isoforms have been characterized in detail – fibrillin-1 (FBN-1) and fibrillin-2 (FBN-2). Fibrillin-3 (FBN-3) is less studied, its gene is found in humans and birds, but is absent in rodents (Corson et al., 2004).

A polypeptide chain of fibrillin-1, a translation immediate product, consists of 2,871 amino acid residues. This very long linear macromolecule is flexible; therefore, in a natural state, its length is equal to 148 nm, which is less than otherwise would be expected.

The molecular structure of fibrillin-1 is a complex multidomain one (Ramirez & Pereira, 1999).

Domains that consist of two types of repetitive sequences, like to the primary structure of the epidermal growth factor (EGF), occupy the central position in the macromolecule. There are 47 such repeats, 43 of which are a special variant of a calcium-binding (cb) EGF-motif (cbEGF-motif). The ability to attach Ca^{2+} is of significant importance in the formation of the secondary structure of fibrillin macromolecules and microfibrils' mechanic properties (strength) (Handford, 2000; Eriksen et al., 2001).

Fibrillins are rich in cysteine. The EGF-motif contains 6–8 cysteine residues in every repeat. In total, a fibrillin-1 macromolecule has about 13% of cysteine residues including cysteils contained in some other repeats.

The fibrillin-1 macromolecule has at least 15 sites containing asparagine residues and each of them can be used to attach carbohydrate groups by N-glycosylation. Three of the sites of potential N-glycosylation are localized in the C-terminal domain.

A proline-rich residue domain is localized in the central part of a fibrillin-1 macromolecule, a little closer to the N-terminal domain. In the same place, fibrillin-2 (FBN-2) has a domain rich in glycine residues. In fact, this is the main difference between the two fibrillins, as they are similar to each other in all other respects. In general, a fibrillin-2 macromolecule has the same architectonics and consists of 2,918 amino acid residues. Each macromolecule contains one adhesive RGD-sequence.

Microfibrils are not only comprised of fibrillins. They also comprise several glycoproteins, among which **microfibril-associated glycoprotein-1** (MAGP-1) primarily pretends to be essential for microfibrils' structural integrity. It is found in microfibrils of almost every tissue selectively localizing in their "beads" (Henderson et al., 1996).

Fig. 3.10.
The basic collagen fibers (1) of human skin dermis (a) and human Achilles tendon (b). Ligamental collagen fibers (2). SEM-micrograph.
a – x 5,000; b – x 2,000.

The MAGP-1 molecular mass is 31 kDa; it contains 183 amino acid residues allocated into two domains: the molecule N-terminal region is rich in proline residues, and it also has an aggregation (cluster) of glutamine residues. The C-terminal region has 13 cysteine residues, which seem to be used to form disulfide bonds with fibrillin macromolecules.

The second **microfibril-associated glycoprotein, MAGP-2**, has a molecular mass of 25 kDa, consisting of 170–173 amino acid residues. It differs very little from MAGP-1 in its primary structure, especially in the central region; it has more serine and threonine residues (Segade et al., 2002).

Fibrillins and the glycoproteins that, together with them, comprise microfibrils are expressed by fibroblasts as all the structural biopolymers of the connective tissue extracellular matrix.

Although the degree of homology between fibrillins 1 and 2 is very high, chromosome localization of their genes in human differs: these are chromosomes 15 and 5 respectively. The gene of the insufficiently studied fibrillin-3 is localized in chromosome 19.

Secreted into the extracellular matrix, these genes' translation products are assembled into microfibrils. The molecular mechanisms of this process have been insufficiently studied. It is known (Lin et al., 2002) that both homotypic and heterotypic interaction between fibrillin-1 and fibrillin-2 is possible to occur. Binding takes place according to a "head to tail" type, i.e. the N-terminus of one molecule is attached to the C-terminus of the other with the formation of both homotypic microfibrils, containing only fibrillin-1 and the heterotypic ones comprising both fibrillins (Kielty et al., 2002a; 2002b).

The homotypic binding of fibrillin-2 N- and C-terminal peptides appeared to be impossible, and it remains unknown how microfibrils that are only made by fibrillin-2 grow in length.

The peculiarities of microfibrils made only of fibrillin-2 manifest themselves in that, during the postnatal period, they are found in the only localization – in peripheral nerves membranes, although both fibrillins interact effectively with each other during the embryonic period (Charbonneau et al., 2003).

As for microfibrils' growth in thickness, such growth occurs due to the formation of inter- and intramolecular cross-links. Two types of cross-links are known in microfibrils. The first type is disulfide bonds. It is supposed that one of the intermolecular disulfide bonds can be formed involving cysteyl-204 in a fibrillin-1 molecule and cysteyl-233 in a fibrillin-2 molecule (Reinhardt et al., 2000). The fact that there are plenty of cysteine residues in fibrillin molecules provides the potential for the further formation of intermolecular, as well as intramolecular, disulfide bonds, thereby enhancing conformation stability.

The second type is homotypic intermolecular cross-links between fibrillin-1 molecules, which are formed with the participation of a transglutaminase enzyme. Trans-glutaminase can also create links between fibrillin-1 and MAGP-1 (Quian & Glanville, 1997).

Microfibril-associated glycoprotein MAGP-2 can interact with both fibrillins, but those cbEGF-like repeats of amino acid residues which MAGP-1 reacts to are not involved in this interaction. In the case of interaction with MAGP-2, these are the repeats located closer to the C-terminal region of fibrillin molecules (Penner et al., 2002).

Fibrillins form the core of microfibrils. In addition to that, microfibril-associated glycoproteins and other proteins similar to these glycoproteins are involved in microfibril formation. Moreover, a number of macromolecules are found in microfibrils; these macromolecules are obviously not their integral components and are not involved in the formation of a microfibril supramolecular structure, but are located in close contact with them, interacting with other components of the extracellular matrix.

For example, the binding of the fibrillin-1 N-terminal sequence is determined to occur with the C-terminal domain of one of large proteoglycans – versican (Isogai et al., 2002), which enables the strengthening of the microfibril's position in the extracellular matrix. The binding of MAGP-1 with the small proteoglycan, biglycan, is also known.

Using 3D electron tomography in combination with the detailed immune electron-microscopic localization of fibrillin molecule epitopes, revealed by means of a complex of antibodies, has allowed for proposing a model of the microfibril supramolecular organization (Baldock et al., 2001; Kielty et al., 2002a; 2002b). According to this model, microfibrils consist of fibrillin filaments, each of which consists of eight fibrillin molecules, as can be seen in a cross-section. Herein a fold originates in every molecule (Lu et al., 2005). Molecules stacking into linear aggregates form complex folds, seen as thickenings in an electron micrograph. These thickenings form microfibrils' shape like threads studded with beads. The folding formation in fibrillin macromolecules results in their axial stagger in relation to each other by 1/3 of their length and the generation of a 56 nm interval periodicity. This interval corresponds to 1/3 of the stretched out molecule length (about 145–160 nm).

The proposed model does not address a number of issues, for example, on the role of MAGP-1 in a fold (bead) structure, where the molecules of this glycoprotein are located. This model is mainly effective for fibrillin-1; the peculiarities of the supramolecular organization of microfibrils made by fibrillin-2 have not been ascertained.

However, due to the above small differences in the primary structure of both fibrillins, the peculiarities of microfibrils, whose core consists of fibrillin-2, are apparently of great functional significance. They manifest in the differences in the interaction of molecules between themselves and with other microfibril components, with tropoelastin molecules, and the surrounding matrix, as well as in the differences of fibrillin-1 and fibrillin-2 tissue localization (Charbonneau et al., 2003).

The area of distribution of fibrillin microfibrils in connective tissue is not limited to their participation in the elastic fiber structure. Immune electron microscopic examinations have revealed their presence in all tissues and organs studied (e.g. the skin, skeletal muscles, cardial muscles, bone and cartilage, tendons and ligaments, kidneys, tissues of the liver, lungs, walls of blood vessels, eyes) as **independent** microfibrils, which are located outside elastic fibers.

Fibrillin microfibrils have the capacity for reversible (elastic) stretching, which is elasticity although it is less effective than that of elastin containing fibers. The molecular mechanism of microfibril elasticity includes the unbending of the molecule within a fold (bead) upon applying stretching strain and upon restoring the folding after its removal (Kielty et al., 2002a; 2002b). Elasticity is the main biomechanical property of fibrillin microfibrils; therefore, their prevailing distribution, along with elastic (containing elastin) fibers, seems to be natural in tissues sustaining repeated shape alterations such as blood vessels, lungs, the skin, and tendons.

The fibrillin microfibrils making tissues elastic are a very old structure, which originated in phylogenesis significantly earlier than elastic fibers. Microfibrils are found in arthropods, in holothurians ("sea cucumbers") and even in medusas. Being so conservative, microfibrils appear early in embryogenesis – during the fifth week in a human embryo – and obviously play a certain morphogenetic role in tissue and organ development (Quondamatteo et al., 2002).

The elasticity of fibrillin microfibrils is more limited than that of elastin-containing fibers. When demands as to elasticity (in combination with strength) of some tissues (primarily, aorta walls due to an increase in systolic pressure) increased during evolution and a significantly more perfect elastin elastomer appeared, elastic fibers' formation began on the basis of a previously formed fibrillin microfibrillar framework.

But fibrillin microfibrils did not lose their independent significance and have been retained in tissues and organs that do not possess marked elasticity and do not contain elastic fibers such as, for example, in the bone tissue and eye tissues. We can suppose that every biological tissue needs some minimal elasticity to ensure which microfibril elasticity will be sufficient.

The functional significance of the fibrillin microfibril system is supported by pathological alterations, which develop with molecular genetic impairments in microfibrils, known as **microfibrilopathy** or **fibrillinopathy** (Hubmacher et al., 2006). Marfan's syndrome is the most common microfibrilopathy. This syndrome, caused by mutations of the *FBN1* gene, has a pleiotropic clinical picture observed as defects in skeleton formation, resulting in the development of marked deformities of the bone system, impairments of the cardiovascular system and visual functions. While the role of fibrillin in elastogenesis can account for defects in blood vessels in the case of Marfan's syndrome, pathological alterations in bone and eye tissues that do not contain elastic fibers are a direct indication of the independent function of microfibrils. Mutations of the *FBN2* gene encoding fibrillin-2 cause another microfibrilopathy – Beal's syndrome, which is manifested in particular as congenital joint contracture. Such alterations indicate the involvement of microfibrils in normal joint development (Jordan et al., 2006).

The role played by fibrillin microfibrils in connective tissue structural organization is not solely mechanical. Numerous potential interactions of fibrillins with other components of the extracellular matrix are also of great functional significance (Ramirez et al., 2004).

Based on the similarity in domain structures and common localization in tissues, some representatives of so-called latent ligands, binding signaling molecules of the transforming growth factor beta superfamily (TGF-β-LTBP), are referred to as members of the fibrillin superfamily and therefore, as microfibril components (Oklu & Hesketh, 2000). One of these ligands, LTB2, is possibly an integral component of microfibrils (Hubmacher et al, 2006). Owing to this, microfibrils gain the ability to control the dynamics and activity of the TGF-β superfamily signaling molecules, including bone morphogenetic proteins and thereby, the capability to influence the cell function, morphogenetic processes and homeostasis of connective tissue structures (Ramirez & Dietz, 2007).

Thus, the system of fibrillin microfibrils, characterized by a high degree of conservatism (more precisely, they should be referred to as fibrillin-rich microfibrils due to the complexity of their composition) (Ramirez et al., 2008), is reasonably considered as the third **independent fibrous system** within the structure of the connective tissue extracellular matrix, along with collagen and elastic fiber systems.

3.1.2.2. Elastin biochemistry

Elastin is one of the comparatively few elastomeric (rubber-like) proteins, i.e. proteins that are characterized by elasticity, the ability to sustain significant deformity like stretching with a subsequent return to the object's initial, relaxed state without residual deformation. Additional energy consumption is not required for this return (Urry et al., 2002). In elastin, elasticity indicating significant strength is combined with a small degree of rigidity, as well as with some features of viscosity as is the case, for example, with the formation of blunt ends in the rupture of elastic fibers (Lillie & Gosline, 2002).

Due to the practically absolute insolubility of elastic fibers, the initial information on the elastin molecular structure was limited to its total amino acid composition. This composition appeared to be peculiar. Elastin is rich in glycine (33%) and proline (10–13%) no less than collagens, but what is more specific is that hydrophobic (non-polar) amino acids comprise approximately 44% of the total number of amino acid residues.

The following investigations, which became possible due to molecular genetics methods (isolation and cloning of complementary DNA) on the one hand, and research on a soluble elastin precursor–**tropoelastin**–on the other hand, showed that this protein has a rather arranged structural organization at the molecular level in spite of an elastin amorphous appearance.

The orderliness of the elastin structure, first of all, consists of the domain nature of the primary structure of polypeptide chains. The latter are made by two types of domains. Hydrophobic domains, i.e. those saturated with hydrophobic amino acid residues, sharply prevail in number. Moreover, there are hydrophilic domains repeated at definite, relatively short intervals (Tatham & Shewry, 2000).

Secondly, peculiarities of the hydrophobic domain primary structure also indicate an orderliness. Aliphatic amino acid and glycine residues are not located irregularly within them but preferably as repetitive sequences. VPGVG and VGGVG pentapeptides are repeated remarkably often (Li & Daggett, 2002).

Thirdly, tropoelastin shorter hydrophilic peptides (relative to hydrophobic peptides) also follow a certain regularity of structure: all of them contain lysine residues, often paired and mostly located following di-, tri- and polyalanyl sequences (Debelle & Tamburro, 1999). These peptide domains have an α-helical conformation.

Fourthly, like collagens, elastin possesses a well-developed system of intermolecular cross-links. All these links are formed by involving lysine residues, comprised in hydrophilic domains, and are located with distinct regularity–at intervals of 60–70 residues in a polypeptide chain. All of them are products of lysyls enzymatic oxidation and subsequent aldol and aldimine condensations. Difunctional cross-links similar to those of collagens are known, such as dehydrolysinonorleucine and allysine aldol, connecting two polypeptide chains between them (P and P'). There is also a three-functional link–**dehydromerodesmosine**–that can connect three chains (P, P' and P''). The final products of lysyl residues' condensation–the tetra-functional bonds, **desmosine** and **isodesmosine**–are theoretically able to connect four chains, but they most likely bind two pairs of twin lysyls of two polypeptide chains.

The majority of lysyls are involved in cross-links' formation; of the 34–38 lysyls (the number varies with species differences) contained within a tropoelastin macromolecule; only 4 to 6 remain unbound in mature, cross-linked elastin. Cross-links make hydrophilic domains rigid and transform aggregates of elastin macromolecules within elastic fibers into an organized three-dimensional network.

Elastin is the protein that specifies the biomechanical properties of elastic fibers. Therefore, its molecular and supramolecular organization has served as a subject for multiple attempts to develop a hypothesis capable of explaining the nature of elastin elasticity at the molecular level (Tamburro et al., 2005).

Without amplifying the essence of theoretical assumptions proposed in this respect, it can be noted that all of them are based on the same general idea, which can be expounded in the following way. The repetitive hydrophobic domains of elastin polypeptide chains, where aliphatic amino acid residues such as valine, proline, leucine, isoleucine and alanine as well as the residue of glycine's smallest amino acid molecule (with the marked prevalence of valyl and glycyl) prevail, are characterized such that in the sequences comprising them, small amino acid residues possess a high degree of motility around peptide bonds in the absence of external strain. This movement is largely chaotic. From the thermodynamic point of view, such a state is maximally entropic (Keeley et al., 2002).

During the application of an external stretching effort, the entire structure becomes more organized (Pollard & Earnshaw, 2002).

Spatial restrictions of molecular motility arise, and movements of molecules become more ordered. At the same time, the energy accumulates and the system's entropy decreases. It is therefore natural that the system immediately returns to the condition of maximal entropy following the removal of external strain; thus, the energy balance remains invariable.

It is interesting that amino acid sequences of hydrophobic domains, which actually provide elastin with its elasticity, are characterized by appreciable interspecific distinctions in relation to their size and amino acid composition. It follows from this that the exact adherence of amino acid sequences, providing that the same set of amino acids is maintained, is not critical for a macromolecule's adequate biomechanical functioning. Evidently, any or almost any sequence of amino acid residues P, V, L, I, G, A provides them with the freedom of movement sufficient for maintaining the above-mentioned transitions from one energy condition to another. At the same time, the total length of a polypeptide chain, which was strongly preserved within 750–800 amino acid residues during its evolution, is probably functionally important The rigid hydrophilic sites of elastin polypeptide chains, where intermolecular cross-links are localized, act as mobility restrainers. They prevent elastic fibers both from a rupture-threatening excessive stretching and from an excessive relaxation, which could have transformed the organized three-dimensional network of elastin macromolecules into a tangled chaotic ball.

The fibroblast-synthesized tropoelastin macromolecule is an immediate product of an elastin gene expression. (Rosenbloom et al., 1993).

Some distinctions in cDNA in different mammals species have been established. For example, in humans, as can be seen in the scheme, there are no 34th and 35th exons, which are present in the carboxyl terminus in bovine elastin cDNA. The circumstance that gene encoding regions (exons) corresponding to complementary DNA, in their total extent (about 2,200 base pairs) are many times less than the total gene extent (about

44,000 base pairs) common for all species. In other words, the elastin gene is characterized by a very low – 1:20 – exon/intron ratio. A consequence of this is the rather intensive splicing of premRNA (premessenger premature RNA), providing the possibility for tropoelastin isoform macromolecules to originate (Jacob et al., 2001).

A specific peculiarity of an elastin gene is that the amino acid sequences of hydrophobic domains (i.e., those domains providing elastin with its elastic properties) and the amino acid sequences of hydrophilic domains, specified to form cross-links, are encoded by different exons. Thus, the domain structure of a protein macromolecule directly reflects the organization of gene exons.

The tropoelastin primary structure as this macromolecule is assembled on mRNA in a human granular endoplasmic reticulum, consists of 792 amino acid residues with a molecular mass of 69,094 Da is presented. Elastin macromolecules similar in size (about 70 kDa) are expressed in other vertebrates.

The assembled tropoelastin macromolecules pass further than the common way for all secreted proteins via a lamellar complex system (Goldgi apparatus) into the extracellular matrix. The process for the assembly and intracellular transport of macromolecules takes approximately 20 minutes.

Unlike collagens, tropoelastin is not exposed to somehow significant proteolytic effects, coupled with shortening of polypeptide chains. The length of an elastin mature macromolecule practically does not differ from that of tropoelastin. The similarity to collagens' posttranslational processing is seen in the intracellular hydroxylation of some proline (mostly those which directly follow glycyls) and lysine residues. The same enzymes as in collagen carry out this hydroxylation; the role of lysyl oxidases is particularly essential in the subsequent formation of cross-links (Kagan & Li, 2003). Two representatives of the lysyl oxidase family – LOX1 and LOXL – have been found to be in direct contact with elastic fibers in a tissue.

The number of hydroxylised prolyls in tropoelastin is significantly less than is the case in collagens; the content of hydroproline ultimately does not exceed 1.5g/100g in elastin. The functional significance of a hydroxyproline residue in elastin is not known; in any case, prolyl hydroxylation inhibition is not accompanied by interference in secretion and elastin condensation in the extracellular matrix between fibrillin microfibrils.

The transformation of tropoelastin into mature elastin occurs extracellularly. It includes both changes in tropoelastin macromolecules (maturation) and the assembly of elastic fibers. In the assembly mechanism, a hydrophobic sequence of a tropoelastin polypeptide chain, encoded by the exon 30, located in the gene C-terminal region, play a special role. Elastin assembly does not occur in mice lacking this exon (Kozel et al., 2003).

Changes in tropoelastin itself consist in the formation of the intermolecular cross-link system. The formation of

this system, as has already been mentioned, transforms individual tropoelastin polypeptide chains into a highly extensible organized three-dimensional structure. As in collagens, cross-linking begins with the participation of copper-dependent peptidyl lysyl oxidase (it is this copper-dependence of the enzyme that accounts for the extractability of soluble tropoelastin from tissues in cases where the organism is copper deficient), which catalyzes the deamination of lysine to allysine (α-aminoadipate β-semialdehyde). The further stages of cross-link formation involve a series of spontaneous condensation reactions that do not demand enzymes' participation.

Like collagen secretion, that of tropoelastin – starting with the propagation of a tropoelastin molecule within the cell's synthesizing right through to the completion with inclusion of the already-formed cross-linked insoluble elastin into elastic fibers in the extracellular matrix – occurs accompanied by a transport protein – chaperon (in this case a chaperon with a molecular mass of 67 kDa). The chaperon prevents the improper structural conformation of tropoelastin and nonspecific and premature binding with the "wrong" glycosylated proteins. These functions of elastin chaperons do not differ from those of collagen, but tropoelastin's 67 kDa-chaperon performs one additional function: its macromolecule is fixed on the external surface of a tropoelastin-producing cell membrane. Along with it, the tropoelastin macromolecule is fixed, so the localization of an assembly process of elastic fibers in the pericellular zone is specified (Jacob et al., 2001).

Cross-linked elastin, as indicated by electron-microscopic examinations, is deposited by coacervation (Mithieux & Weiss, 2005) as an amorphous mass into an already-completed framework, formed by fibrillin microfibril aggregates. Gradually, elastin becomes an elastic fiber component prevailing in mass. During the assembly of elastic fibers, there is an insertion of a number of other macromolecular components into their structure other than amorphous elastin and fibrillin microfibrils. An immune electron-microscopic examination has revealed the third component of elastic fibers, presented by several isoforms of one more representative of glycoproteins – **fibulin** (see section 3.2.1.1). Fibulin-1 is localized in the amorphous (elastin) substance of elastic fibers and is no way associated with fibrillin microfibrils. Fibulin-2, found in blood vessel walls, on the contrary, possesses a high affinity not only to elastin, but also to fibrillin, and it is detected in elastic fibers in the contact area of microfibrils and amorphous elastin (Sasaki et al., 1999). Another fibulin isoform – fibulin-5, is located on the external surface of elastic fibers. It is considered to be one of the components of the external framework structure of elastic fibers (Yanagisawa et al., 2002). Moreover, fibulin-5 (also called DANCE) is involved, along with fibulin-2, in linking elastic fibers with other proteins of the extracellular matrix and with cells. Fibulin-5 performs this latter function as a ligand of αVβ3, αVβV and α9β1 integrins located on the cell surface (Nakamura et al., 2002). It is possible that fibulins contribute to maintaining the elastic properties of elastin fibers and/or are involved in their fibrillogenesis.

Like fibulin-2 **emilin** molecules (emilin-1 and emilin-2), members of the new glycoprotein family (Emu) are located at the interface between fibrillin microfibrils and elastin as the amorphous substance of elastic fibers' framework (Leitmeister et al., 2002) The functional significance of emilins in elastic fibers remains unknown at the present time.

Thus, the concept of elastic fibers as a two-component system made by two main constructive components – amorphous substance and fibrillin microfibrils – is true only in the first approach. In fact, the system of elastic fibers is much more complicated, and this complexity increases even more owing to macromolecules that are located on the fibers' external surface and that mediate their interaction with other components of the extracellular matrix and with cells.

Two small (leucine-rich) proteoglycans – biglycan and decorin – are found to be in immediate contact with elastic fibers (Pasquali-Ronchetti & Baccarani-Contri, 1997). Both of them are bound (by their core proteins but not by glycosaminglycan chains) with tropoelastin macromolecules, and biglycan forms a triple complex also comprising the MAGP-1 glycoprotein mentioned earlier (Reinboth et al., 2002). Apparently, these macromolecules contacting the elastic fibers take part in the inclusion of fibers into the supramolecular archetictonics of the extracellular matrix.

3.1.2.3. Formation of elastic fibers

The assembly of elastic fibers from synthesized components takes place in the extracellular space. Elastic (fibrillin) microfibrils originate first during embryogenesis and the physiological renewal of the connective tissue. Further deposition of cross-linked elastin begins by means of coacervation as an amorphous substance in an already completed framework formed by microfibrils, i.e. between them, in several sites (Mithieux and Weiss, 2005). The amount of elastin gradually increases, the amorphous substance coacervates into a homologous mass. At the same time, microfibrils appear to be embedded into the amorphous substance and are not revealed as independent structures. However, the majority of mature elastic fibers have free microfibrils on the periphery. Besides amorphous substance, a number of other macromolecular components are inserted into elastic fibers during their assembly (see section 3.1.2.2).

The sequence of the origination of microfibrillar and amorphous components indicates that one is a predecessor of the other. Originating first, elastic (fibrillin) microfibrils can possibly play a role in specifying both the form and direction (orientation) of elastic fibers (Ross, et al., 1985). This assumption is based on the fact that, in the nuchal ligament and the tendon, originating microfibrils immediately simulate a form of cylinder, which mature elastic fibers here, containing both components (microfibrils and amorphous substance), then have. The same occurs in the formation of elastic fibers and membranes in the aorta wall, where microfibrils form a framework of a window-form bed, i.e. elastic fenestrated membranes.

Similar dynamics of elastic fibers architectonics takes place in the skin dermis. The aggregation of a part of elastic microfibrils into larger supramolecular formations – "skeletal fibrils" with a thickness of 15–180 nm – is an additional stage. In the deposition of amorphous substance in intermicrofibrillar spaces, "skeletal fibrils" are not pushed aside on the fibers periphery, but are distributed throughout the entire volume of the amorphous substance (Hashimoto and Di Bella, 1967).

3.1.2.4. Structure of elastic fibers

Elastic fibers and fibrils are the generally accepted names for elastic structures. When they have an oval or round shape in a cross section they retain this name. When the fibers and fibrils are flat, they are denoted as lamellar-fibrous formations or elastic membranes.

The aforementioned elastic structures are seen in the connective tissue by means of selective staining methods: by orcein, fuchsilin, and others.

Elastic fibers, as well as elastic membranes, consist of two components. Most of the fiber (about 90%) consists of an amorphous substance with low electron density when studying fibers under a transmission electron microscope (TEM) (Fig. 3.11, 3.12). The fiber peripheral part exhibits a higher electron density; therefore, it is referred to as the cortex part. Thin thread-like formations – fibrillin (elastic, glycoproteid) microfibrils – branch from the fiber surface. These microfibrils also have a more dense peripheral part in a cross-section, a 4–14 nm diameter, and rosary-like 15–20 nm periodicity in the axial section (Kadar, 1979). It should be noted that the number and length of microfibrils on an elastic fiber's surface is largely variable. A portion of fibers can lack them completely. In the end regions of some microfibrils, there can be even thinner threads with a thickness of 1–1.5 nm (microfibrillar filaments). The amorphous substance structure contains fibrillar inclusions denoted as "skeletal fibrils" (Hashimoto and

Fig. 3.11.
Elastic fibers (fibrils) of the human skin dermis. Amorphous substance (1). Fibrillin microfibrils (2). "Skeletal fibrils" (3). a – a lengthwise section; b – a cross-section. TEM-micrograph. Contrasting of ultrathin sections with uranyl acetate and lead citrate. a – x 20,000; b – x 50,000.

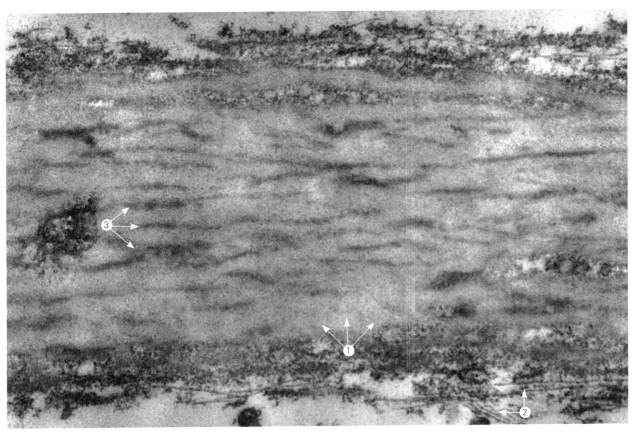

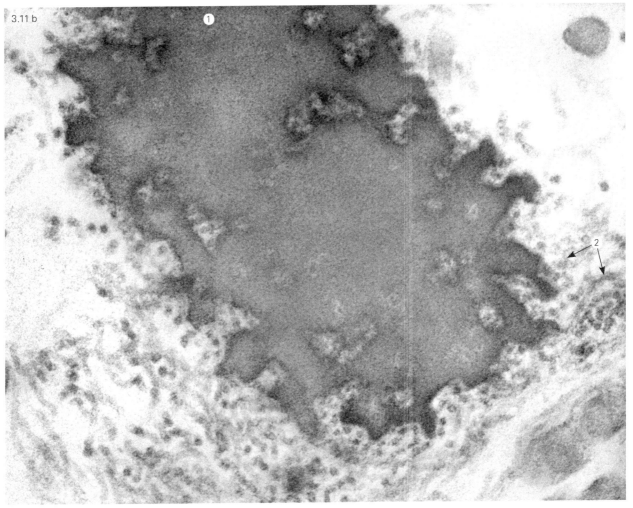

3.12 a

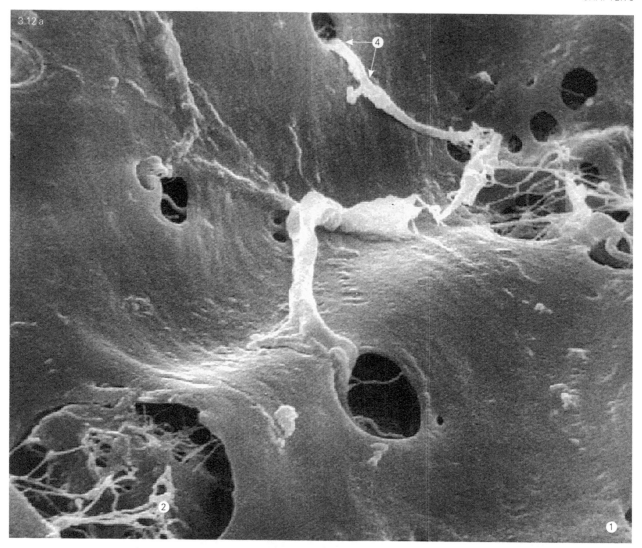

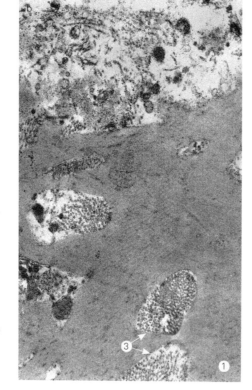

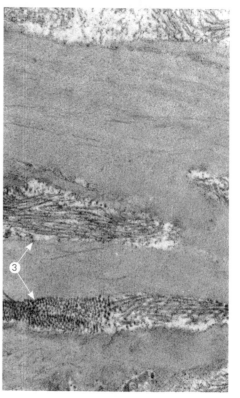

Fig. 3.12
Elastic fenestral membranes
(EM) of the human aorta wall (1).
Fenestras ("windows") (2).
Collagen (3) and elastic (4)
fibers and fibrils in fenestras
and interfibrillar (intermembranous) spaces.
a – SEM-micrograph;
b, c – TEM-micrograph.
b – a section perpendicular
to the EM plane.
Contrasting of ultrathin sections
with uranyl acetate and lead
citrate.
a – x 5,000;
b – x 10,000.

Di Bella, 1967). Depending on the tissue type specificity of elastic fibers, "skeletal fibrils" range in thickness from 15 to 80 nm and exhibit a rosary-like cross-striation with 45–65 nm periodicity in some parts. Apparently, skeletal fibrils are aggregates of elastic microfibrils, which are formed in deposition of the amorphous substance between microfibrils during elastic fibers' formation. In individual cases, their thickness has reached 110–130 nm (Kewley et al., 1977).

The amorphous substance structure is not entirely homogeneous. There exist cavities in various shapes, as well as canals communicating with the fiber surface. Therefore, the latter is not smooth or a plane but has a marked relief, formed by crypts or protrusions of the fiber cortex layer as well as peripheral microfibrils. The elastic fiber amorphous substance has a granular structure. TEM has determined granules are 3–3.5 nm in size (Gotte & Volpin, 1974). Upon exposing tissue homogenates containing elastic fibers with ultrasound and negative contrasting, TEM demonstrated that long thin filaments arranged mostly parallel to the fiber's long axis comprised most of the elastic fiber's amorphous substance. The mean diameter was 3–3.5 nm. Regarding the structure's 3–3.5 nm periodicity, it was also noted that its filaments consist of globules or the above-mentioned granules (Gotte & Volpin, 1974). Therefore, the filamentous organization of elastic is quite real and does not contradict the available data (Cox & Dell, 1966), according to which elastin exhibits a globular nature. Globules, as an elastin morphologic structure and having a diameter of 2.8 nm and density of 1.23, may possibly form linear rows, i.e. filaments, elastin's supramolecular structure. During "maturation" and functioning involving exposure to mechanical stress, it is possible that additional inter- and intramolecular links are formed in elastic fiber components. They determine the greater stability of these structures in the direction of a prevailing stress vector (structural anisotropy). Upon being exposed to ultrasound, disintegration of the amorphous substance occurs along the less resistant intermolecular links. It may be due to this that elastic filaments form as supramolecular aggregates, which do not exist independently within the elastic fiber's structure.

Depending upon the ratio of the elastic microfibrils and the amorphous substance, four types of elastic fibers are determined:

1) proper (mature) elastic fibers;
2) oxytalan elastic fibers;
3) elaunin fibers; and
4) pre-elastic fibers.

The structure of proper or mature elastic fibers is presented above. Oxytalan fibers are formed by bundles of elastic glycoproteid (fibrillin) microfibrils, with a thickness of 15–16 nm in thickness, located parallel, which are similar to the elastic glycoproteid microfibrils that make up elastic fibers, though their diameter is slightly greater (*Fig. 3.13 a, b*) (Carmichael & Fullmer, 1966). The

quoted authors have used the name "elastic glycoproteid microfibrils". The modern name is fibrillin microfibrils. A comparative analysis of elastic, pre-elastic and oxytalan fibers led to the conclusion that oxytalan fibers are immature or specifically altered elastic fibers (Fullmer, 1960). The term "pre-elastic fibers" is proposed to define elastic-like fibers in the connective tissue of those organs where these fibers have never been transformed into definitive elastic fibers (Fullmer, 1960). The term "pre-elastic fibers" has been used to determine developing (maturing) elastic fibers. However, it is impossible to distinguish pre-elastic and oxytalan fibers morphologically (*Fig. 3.13 a, b, c*).

As a rule, oxytalan fibers are present in those regions where significant mechanical loading appears, for example, in the periodont, walls of blood vessels and tendons, (Fullmer & Lillie, 1958). These fibers might be functionally related to mechanical resistance.

Elaunin fibers are an intermediate form between oxytalan and proper elastic fibers. Their significant part is comprised of fibrillin microfibrils, between which islets of the amorphous substance are located in separate sites (*Fig. 3.13 c, d*).

An interaction analysis of all the determined types of elastic fibers shows that they are parts of an integral system of elastic structures in the organs where they are present.

With age, elastic fibers undergo definite changes. A significant part of fibers is fragmented, resulting in the impairment of the structural integrity of the organ's entire elastic framework. Obviously, this affects the biomechanical properties of both the organ's elastic and connective tissue framework. Another manifestation of ageing degradation is the formation of aggregations at the site of the elastic fibers or aggregations of material that have been stained with selective dyes for elastic fibers. These aggregations can occupy a significant space, and, naturally, impair the construction and mechanical properties of the elastic framework. This phenomenon is referred to as hyperelastosis (Zherebtsov, 1960) or elastosis (Uitto, 2008).

Degradation of elastic fibers in autolysis occurs through the destruction of the amorphous substance and microfibrils gradually from the periphery towards the fiber center taking into account fibers' superficial relief, which becomes more pronounced. Fibers' lysis involves a definite reverse stage-by-stage process in relation to their formation. Degradation of the amorphous substance occurs with some advance of microfibrils disintegration (that is quite logical); therefore, there are some regions where there is an increased number of "bare" microfibrils.

3.13 a

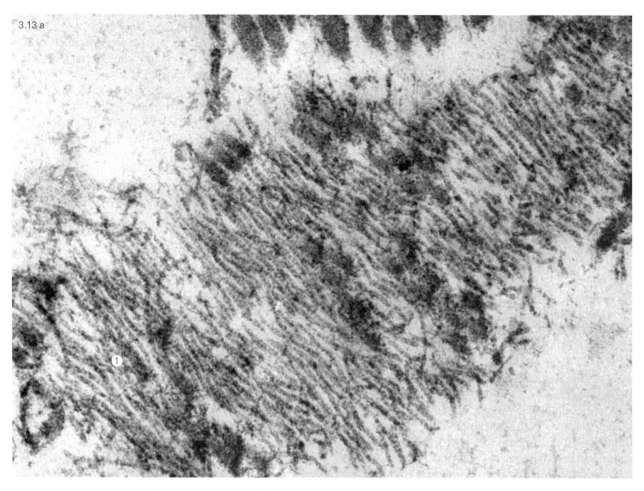

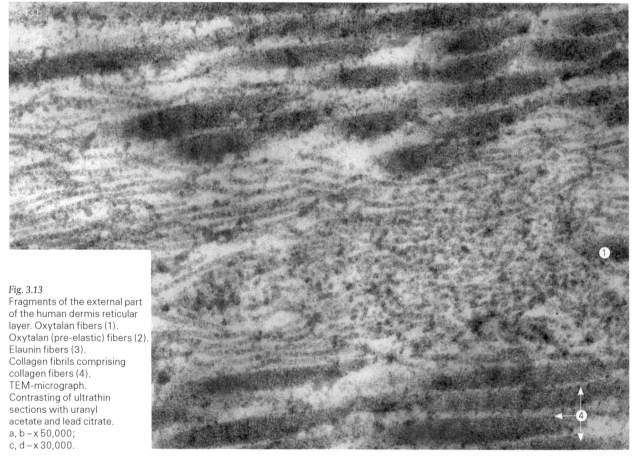

Fig. 3.13
Fragments of the external part
of the human dermis reticular
layer. Oxytalan fibers (1).
Oxytalan (pre-elastic) fibers (2).
Elaunin fibers (3).
Collagen fibrils comprising
collagen fibers (4).
TEM-micrograph.
Contrasting of ultrathin
sections with uranyl
acetate and lead citrate.
a, b – x 50,000;
c, d – x 30,000.

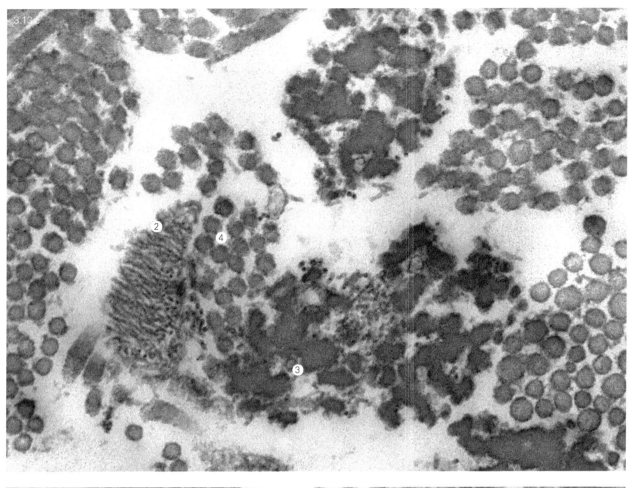

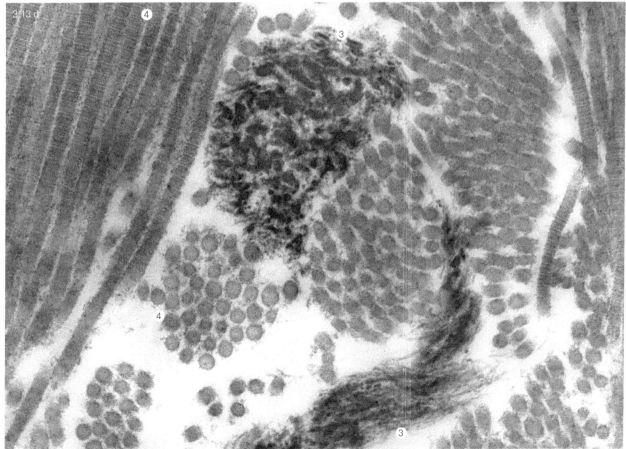

3.1.2.5. Organ peculiarities of elastic fibers structure

Comparing the organization of elastic fibers of the nuchal ligament, dermis, vessel wall, cartilage, perichondrium and others it can be said that the structure of microfibrillar and amorphous-filamentous components and their relationship are not apparently different in mature elastic fibers of various organs. Organ peculiarities of these fibrous structures begin to manifest only at the level of a whole fiber and construction of an elastic system of an organ connective tissue. A 3-dimensional construction formed by elastic fibers within an organ is a common principle of an organ's organization of the elastic fiber system. Its character differs in various organs and depends upon the peculiarities of the biomechanical function they perform in an organ, together with collagen structures, in resisting a stretching stress (peculiar buffering), and restoring a deformed organ or a part thereof to its initial state without permanent deformities after the stretching force action discontinues. The greater part of elastic fibers or membranes in an organ can be oriented along a dominant force vector. Another, smaller part of fibers is located tangentially, acting as bonding elements. These fibers can be branches (organic part) of main fibers or can interact with the latter by means of proteioglycans. Thus, the integrity of the whole elastic structure originates.

Cylindrical elastic fibers prevail in the dermis (Fig.3.14). The fibers branch. Within the reticular layer, the majority of fibers is located parallel to the skin surface (Fig.3.14a,c). Another part is perpendicular to the surface. These fibers connect the parallel ones. Proper elastic fibers are mainly present within the reticular layer. Within the papillary layer, elastic fibers are significantly thinner (Fig. 3.14 b). There is a great number of oxytalan (possibly pre-elastic) and elaunin fibers (Fig. 3.13). On the one hand, their microfibrils are in contact with the basement membrane; on the other, upon gaining an amorphous substance, they merge into deeper layers and become proper elastic fibers. Elastic fibers proceed to move from the reticular layer to the adipose (subcutaneous fat) layer.

Within elastic type a vessel walls, a significant part of the elastic framework is comprised of elastic membranes. Part of them are flattened elastic fibers, i.e. an integral structure made by amorphous and microfibrillar components (Fig. 3.12). Most fibers have a spiral or undulated configuration, where the wavelength and amplitude can vary significantly. Obviously, such a structure is necessary in the aorta's widening during the passing of a pulse wave (Fig. 3.15, 3.16). Elastic membranes can either laminate (a special branching) or combine. Another part of membranes is an aggregate of several cylindrical or flattened elastic fibers. Besides membranes, there are elastic fibers of a cylindrical form within blood vessel walls. The elastic framework is a layered construction,

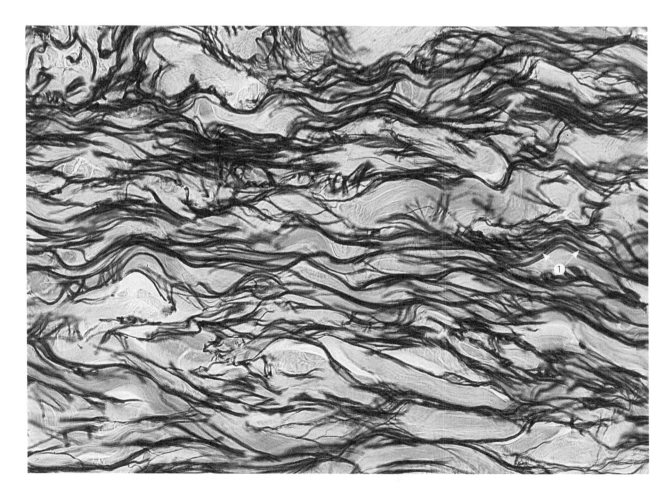

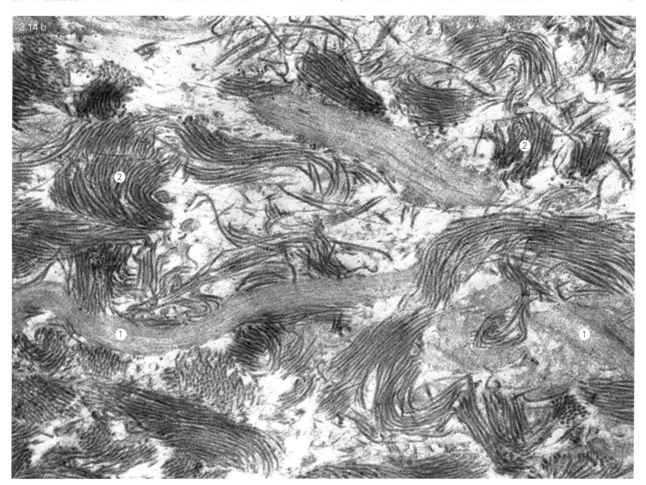

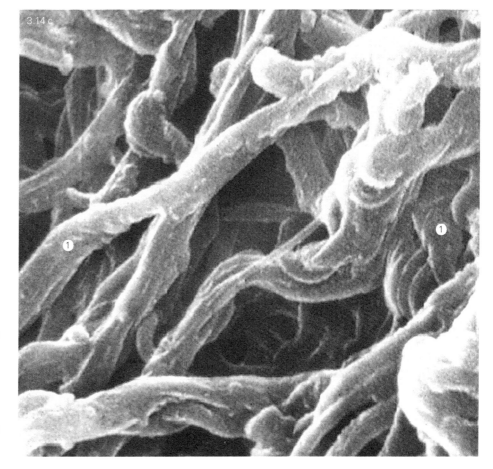

Fig. 3.14
Elastic fibers of the human
dermis reticular layer (1).
a – a significant portion
of elastic fibers is oriented
parallel to the skin surface.
LM-micrograph.
Selective staining with
orcein for elastic fibers.
x 250
b – dermis papillary layer.
Elastic(1) and collagen fibers(2);
c – dermis elastic fibers (1)
remained after the enzymatic
destruction of collagen
fibers by collagenase.
c – SEM-micrograph,
x 2,000;
b – TEM-micrograph.
Contrasting of ultrathin sections
with uranyl acetate and lead
citrat, x 20,000;

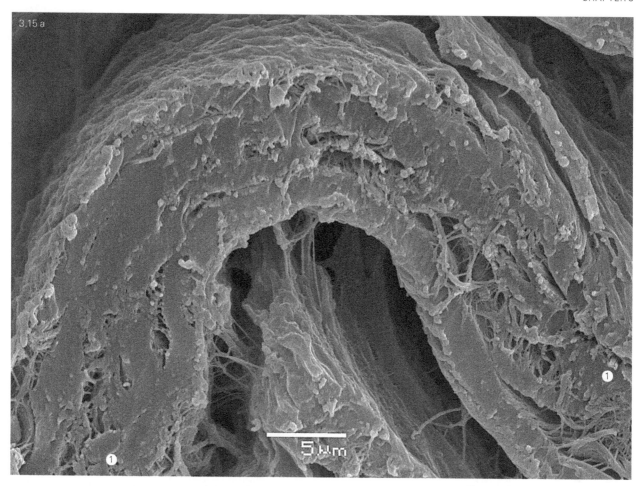

3.15 a

5 μm

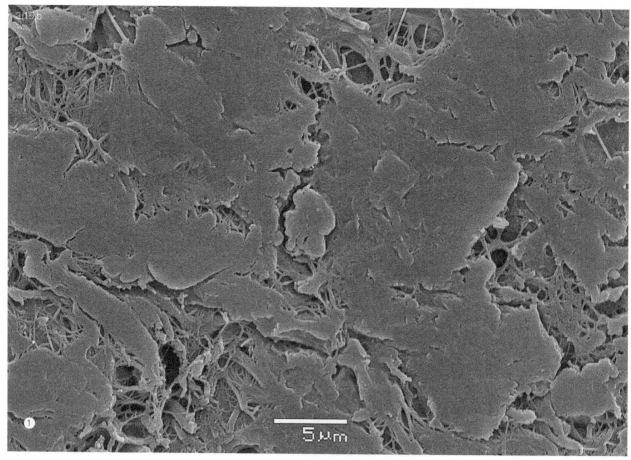

3.15 b

5 μm

whose elastic membranes (layers) are combined by perpendicularly arranged the elastic fibers and collagen fibrous structures (fibrils and fibers) located between them (*Fig. 3.16*). The given data is integrated into the scheme depicted in *Fig. 3.17*.

The elastic framework of the human nuchal ligament is mainly formed by cylindrical and flattened elastic fibers. Their prevailing orientation is along the longest ligament axis (*Fig. 3.18*).

Based on analogous collagen structures, elastic ones can also be classified according to the levels of their structural organization, thereby permitting a comparison of both types of connective tissue fibrous structures.

The *molecular level* of the elastic structures' organization is represented as molecules of an elastic protein, fibrillin (elastic glycoprotein) and other minor molecules.

The *supramolecular level* is represented as an amorphous-filamentous substance and fibrillin microfibrils. The first, most representative in mass, component consists of an elastin protein, whose molecules exhibit a globular form (the most common, but not the only point of view). Globules form a 3-dimensional construction with the presence of individual linear aggregates called filaments. Fibrillin microfibrils are composed by filaments, possibly by two of them (Baldock et al., 2001), which are not independent structures but are an intermediate stage of fibrillin molecule aggregation in microfibrils' formation.

A complex of fibrillin microfibrils and amorphous-filamentous substance represents the *fibrillar level* of elastic structures' organization. It is quite logical that this fibrous complex should be called an elastic fibril (based on the analogous organization level of a collagen fibril). However, in the literature, the term "elastic fiber" is used. It is apparent that such a name is associated with the sizes of these elastic structures–0.5–20 μm, which are comparable with collagen fiber sizes. Elastic fibrils as collagen fibrils can be varied in size, including cylindrical, flattened and flat (membranes).

The *fibrous level* elastic fibrils as collagen fibrils can be aggregated, forming elastic fibers. However, unlike collagen fibers, such aggregates contain fewer elastic fibrils: 2–5. One of the two types of elastic membranes can be formed by several dozen elastic fibrils.

The *tissue level* is a spatial construction of elastic structures forming an integrated framework with a component composition specific for every organ or anatomical formation.

The aforementioned multi-level structural hierarchy is presented in a scheme (*Fig. 3.19*).

Fig. 3.15
Fragments of elastic
membranes (EM)
of a sheep aorta (1),
a – a section perpendicular
to the EM plane;
b – a section parallel
to the EM plane.
SEM-micrograph, x 3,000.

3.2. INTEGRATING THE BUFFER METABOLIC MEDIUM (GROUND SUBSTANCE) OF THE CONNECTIVE TISSUE EXTRACELLULAR MATRIX

All the cellular and fibrous elements of the connective tissue are surrounded by a gel-like substance which, on the one hand, participates in their integration, and, on the other hand, interferes with their contact and aggregation. This substance is an intermediate in metabolic processes between blood and cells that are out of vasculature. This substance is thereby defined as an integrating buffer metabolic medium of the connective tissue (Omelyanenko, 1984), known in the literature as a ground substance. Gel concentration or density depends on its localization. For example, in the interfibrillar space of a loose non-formed connective tissue, the substance is liquideous, and in the hyaline cartilaginous tissue it determines the marked viscoelasticity of the cartilage enabling its amortization.

The ground substance is a multicomponent system for which the main components are glycoconjugates (glycoproteins, proteoglycans) and water. Proteoglycans form a gel structural basis, and water serves as a dissolvent for substances it contains and participates in the amortization mechanism by moving along "channels" or "capillaries" of an interstitial space–the second link of microvasculature (Kupriyanov et al., 1975). This water permanently contains inorganic ions, blood proteins and urea, metabolic products of parenchymatous, myeloid and connective tissue cells, synthesis products of connective tissue cells: soluble forms of fibrous proteins, proteoglycans, glycoproteins and the complexes they form (Montagna & Parakkal, 1974).

3.2.1. Biochemical characteristics of glycoconjugates and their classification

The integrating-buffer metabolic medium of the connective tissue (ground substance) includes an extremely wide range of macromolecules varying in structure and functions that are collectively referred to as **glycoconjugates**. This term (the name **glycoproteids** earlier used to be common) covers all the proteins whose macromolecules contain larger or smaller carbohydrate fragments **covalently** attached to polypeptide chains.

As a rule, glycoconjugates are **secreted** proteins, i.e. proteins expressed by cells to be released into the extracellular space. The majority of intracellular proteins–proteins of cellular organelles, cytosol proteins and proteins contained in the nucleus–are not glycoconjugates. On the contrary, in eukaryotes, almost all extracellular matrix proteins (i.e. proteins of extracellular matrix) carry attached oligosaccharide groups and, thus, are glycoconjugates.

The attachment of carbohydrate fragments to protein macromolecules–one of the stages of posttranslational processing–takes place in Golgi apparatus cisterns,

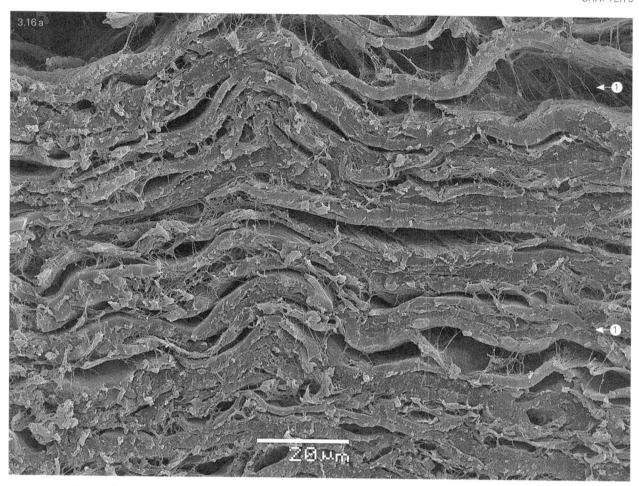

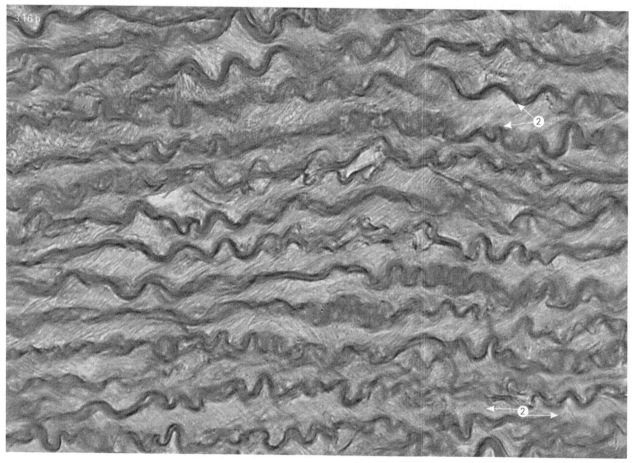

3.17

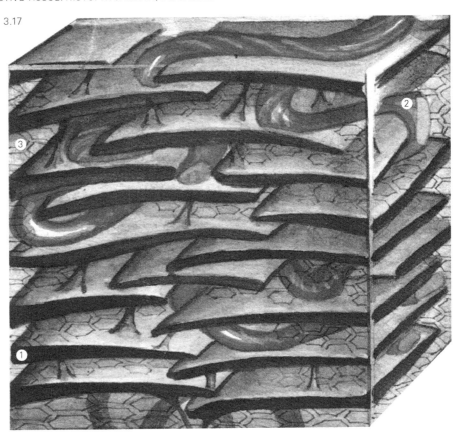

Fig. 3.16
A fragment of the aorta wall
of a male sheep.
A sample made perpendicular
to the wall plane.
Elastic membranes (1).
Collagen fibers and fibrils (2).
a – SEM-micrograph, x 800;
b – LM-micrograph.
Orcein staining. x 250.

Fig. 3.17
Image of an elastic-collagen
framework of the aorta wall.
Elastic membranes (1).
Collagen fibers (2).
Structured proteoglycans of the
integrative-buffer metabolic
medium (3) (according
to Omelyanenko, 1984).

Fig. 3.18
A fragment of the human
nuchal ligament elastic
framework. Elastic fibers (1).
Collagen fibers (2).
SEM-micrograph. x 800.

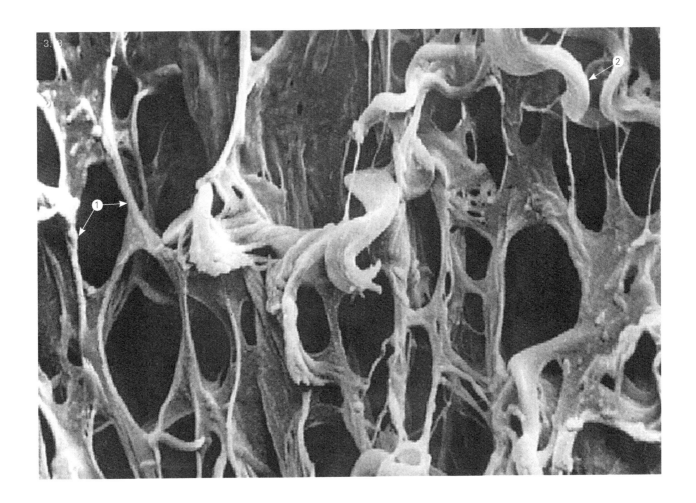

Organization levels	Organization of fibrous elastic structures
Molecular	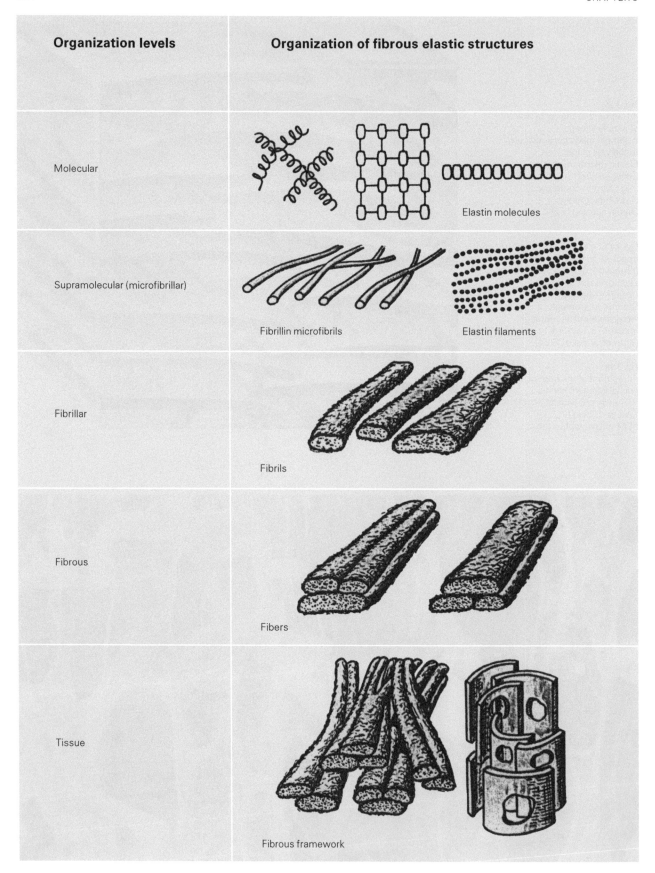
Supramolecular (microfibrillar)	
Fibrillar	
Fibrous	
Tissue	

Fig. 3.19
A scheme of the elastic
fibrous structure organization
hierarchy (according to
Omelyanenko, 1991).

through which the secreted proteins pass from the site of polypeptide chain assembly on polyribosomes of the rough endoplasmic reticulum to a cell membrane. The attached carbohydrate fragment is believed to serve as a signal or "identifier" for protein to be released from a cell.

It should be noted that many proteins of fibrous and microfibrillar structures of the extracellular matrix, including some collagens and fibrillins, are glycoconjugates. At the final stages of posttranslational processing, some secreted proteins lose most attached carbohydrates, retaining only very small oligosaccharide fragments; and some secreted proteins are fully released from carbohydrates. But the secreted proteins incorporated into the supramolecular structures of the extracellular matrix are still glycoconjugates after the processing is over. Their carbohydrate fragments play an essential role in their interactions with other macromolecules of the matrix and cells, as well as in other functions.

Moreover, not only structural components of the ground substance, but also many enzymes acting in the ground substance and also signaling molecules, are glycoconjugates.

Glycoconjugates are usually divided into glycoproteins and proteoglycans.

Glycoproteins contain small carbohydrate fragments–oligosaccharides–of a various, often branched structure. Their total mass is insignificant in comparison with that of a polypeptide component.

As a matter of fact, **proteoglycans** are a special class of glycoproteins which, **along** with typical oligosaccharides, contain **glycosaminoglycans** (formerly known as "mucopolysaccharides") –linear (not branched) polysaccharides usually containing sulfate groups (sulfated); these polysaccharides are comprised of amino sugars. In some proteoglycans, the cumulative mass of a macromolecule glycosaminoglycan component can exceed that of a glycosaminoglycans-carrying polypeptide. It is glycosaminoglycans in these not numerous proteoglycans that determine their functions.

3.2.1.1. Glycoproteins: Structures and functions

The main difference of glycoproteins from other proteins is the presence of carbohydrate (oligosaccharide) fragments in macromolecules. These fragments, which vary in their structure, are divided in two large groups depending on the way and site of attachment to a polypeptide chain.

O- and N-linked oligosaccharides are substantively different in structure and composition **O-linked** oligosaccharides are small in size and contain only one to four monosaccharide residues in most cases. They are attached by means of an O-glycosidic bond to the hydroxyl group oxygen of one of three amino acid residues–serine, threonine and hydroxylysine (the last case only in collagens). The attachment to seryl and threonyl is real-

ized by a galactose or N-acetylgalactosamine residue. **N-linked** oligosaccharides are larger, consist of at least five monosaccharide residues, and have a branched structure. They are attached to asparagine nitrogen by a N-glycosidic bond with N-acetylglucosamine..

Oligosaccharides of glycoproteins perform several functions. Firstly, as has already been mentioned, they act as a signal distinguishing proteins intended to be exported from a cell into the extracellular matrix or to be used as integrated components of a cytoplasmic membrane, but not to be used inside a cell. With glycosylation failure, glycoprotein polypeptide cores are not able to leave a rough endoplasmic reticulum where their synthesis takes place, or lamellar complex cisterns where their assembly is completed. Mainly N-linked oligosaccharides act as a signal ("admission"), providing glycoprotein normal transport.

Secondly, given N-linked oligosaccharides' deficiency in a molecule of glycoprotein secreted into the matrix, its molecule becomes unnecessarily sensitive to the destructive influence of proteolytic enzymes. It is established particularly in relation to fibronectin, which is one of the matrix's widespread structural glycoproteins. This essentially means that oligosaccharides enhance glycoprotein stability.

Thirdly, N- and O-linked oligosaccharides are essential for glycoprotein macromolecules to achieve the proper conformation and electric charge.

The basic structural glycoproteins of the connective tissue extracellular matrix are presented in *Table 3.2*.

The table covers glycoproteins which are part of the interfibrillar and interfiber ground substance of the extracellular matrix; it does not include glycoproteins of fibrous structures or glycoproteins present selectively only in separate types of connective tissue.

All glycoproteins listed in *Table 3.2* are adhesive ("sticky"), i.e. they easily bind with cells and other components of the matrix. But having adhesive properties does not mean that these properties appear in all circumstances and that the functions of these glycoproteins are limited to structural ones. The same glycoprotein can perform absolutely different functions in various tissues. Under certain conditions, adhesive molecules can gain antiadhesive activity; sometimes antiadhesive molecules also acquire opposite properties. Such functional versatility on the part of matrix glycoproteins causes the allocation of a glycoprotein special group called **matricellular proteins** (Bornstein & Sage, 2002). The properties determining the inclusion of glycoproteins in this group are provided in *Table 3.3* (including trombospondines-1 and 2, SPARC, tenascins-C and–X, osteopontin).

Table 3.2

Basic structural glycoproteins of connective tissue

Glycoproteins	Description	Interacting ligands
Fibronectins	Products of one gene expression; alternative splicing makes 235–270 kDa isoforms ; dimeric molecules linked via disulfide bond; consist of 12 FN-I domains, 2 FN-II domains, 15–17 FN-III domains; contain 4–5% of N- and O-linked oligosaccharides	Fibrinogen, heparin, collagen, integrins
Tenascins	Products of one gene expression; alternative splicing makes isoforms weighing 190, 200 and 230 kDa; a molecule contains 14 EGF-domains, 8–11 FN-III- domains and fibrinogen-like domains; 6 polypeptide chains are linked via disulfide bonds	Integrins, proteoglycans
Thrombospondins	Macromolecules that weigh 400–420 kDa; contain EGF-domains, procollagen and complement-like domains	Integrin $\alpha v\beta 3$, syndecan, heparin, Ca^{2+}
Fibulins	Products of one gene expression; alternative splicing makes at least 5 monomeric isoforms; molecules contain various number of EGF-domains and complement-like domains; contain N- and O-linked carbohydrates; are present in blood plasma	Fibronectins, elastin, proteoglycans, fibrinogen, Ca^{2+}, integrins
Vitronectin	Product of one gene expression, 75 kDa; contains N-linked carbohydrates; phosphorylated; sulfated	Integrin $\alpha V\beta 3$, collagens, heparin, glass, plastics
Matrilins	Homotypic and, less frequently, heterotypic oligomeric macromolecules; monomers with length of about 580 amino acid residues consist of EGF-domains, domains similar to the domain A of von Willebrand factor, and α-helical domain	Collagens I, fibrillin-2, fibronectins, laminin-1 and nidogen-1
SPARC (osteonectin)	Product of one gene expression; a 32 kDa monomer; especially typical for bone tissue	Collagens I, III, IV and V, hydroxyapatite, cells
Osteopontin	Monomer consisting of about 300 amino-acid residues; phosphorylated; contains N –and O-linked carbohydrates, including sialic acid; typical for bone tissue	Hydroxyapatite
Glycoproteins of basement membranes		
Laminins	Macromolecules are made of one 200 –400 kDa α-chain, one 200 kDa β-chain, one 200 kDa γ-chain; several isoforms of each chain are known; contain poly-N-acetylgalactosamin	The network formed by laminin macromolecules is linked through nidogen in basement membranes to a network formed by collagen IV
Nidogens (entactins)	Products of one gene expression; a 140 kDa monomer; contains 8 EGF-domains and 2 EF-domains; contains N- and O-linked carbohydrates	Binds collagen II and laminin in basement membranes

Table 3.3.
The main features of matricellular proteins

They are expressed in significant amounts mainly during the development and in reparative processes.

They do not play an essential role in the structural organization of the extracellular matrix, but function as modulators of cells and matrix interactions.

They bind many receptors of the cytoplasmatic membrane, extracellular matrix components, growth factors, cytokines and proteases.

Unlike the majority of matrix structural glycoproteins, they cause the de-adhesion, rather than adhesion, of cells.

In most cases, switching off the genes of matricellular proteins is accompanied by insignificant phenotypic defects.

According to Bornstein & Sage (2002).

The properties listed in the table show that matricellular proteins act, at least in certain cases, as regulators (modulators) of cell functions, with their adhesiveness paling into insignificance. Moreover, they exhibit an opposite, de-adhesive or antiadhesive, activity. Cells influenced by matricellular proteins pass into a state defined as partial or intermediate adhesion (Murphy-Ulrich, 2001). During this transition the cell loses a part of cytoskeleton actin fibrils; a radical rearrangement of focal contacts mediated by intracellular mediators takes place: vinculin and α–actinin proteins involved in cell adhesion are lost, with other proteins–talin and transmembrane receptors-integrins–retained in contacts. It is assumed that these alterations of cells' adhesive properties are of adaptive significance. The cells gain additional abilities to express genes involved in the processes of morphogenesis and in response to tissue damage.

The majority of extracellular matrix structural glycoproteins simultaneously have both adhesive properties and those typical for matricellular proteins. Certain properties are exhibited depending on circumstances.

This duality of properties is distinct in **fibronectins**, i.e. glycoproteins, which are present in significant amounts in the matrix at certain stages of its formation. The main function of these glycoproteins is to bind cells with various, mainly fibrillar components of the extracellular matrix. This adhesive function is reflected in their name (Lat. *fibra–a fiber, necto*–to bind), but it is manifested only after fibronectin macromolecules have formed fibronectin microfibrils.

Fibronectins macromolecules are dimers of two identical polypeptide chains, connected at an acute angle (Karp, 1999) by two di-sulfide bonds located in the C-terminal region.

Each chain has a molecular mass of about 250 kDa, is about 60–70 nm long and about 2–3 nm thick, and consists of 6 functional domains differing by the specificity of interaction with extracellular matrix structural components, which are ligands in relation to fibronectin (collagens, proteoglycans, heparin, fibrin), as well as with cells.

Domains have a modular structure: they consist of three different types of modules (repeats of amino acid sequences)–12 modules of the FN-I type, 2 modules of the FN-II type, and 15–17 modules of the FN-III type (Mosher et al., 1991). The FN-I module contains about 40 amino acid residues and two disulfide bonds, the FN-II module–about 60 amino acid residues and two disulfide bonds; the FN-III module comprises about 90 residues, but no disulfide bonds (Pankov & Yamada, 2002).

More than 20 isoforms of fibronectin polypeptide chains (monomers) have been identified. They differ from each other by the number of FN-III modules and some peculiarities of the amino acid composition of all modules. All of them are products of alternative splicing of the same gene RNA-transcript.

Fibronectins of the connective tissue extracellular matrix are mainly expressed by fibroblasts. They accumulate at the fibroblasts' surface as individual dimeric macromolecules. Fibronectin determined in the circulating blood (see below) is synthesized by hepatocytes.

Fibronectins act as ligands in relation to the cells. A "sticky" (adhesive) tripeptide arginine-glycine-asparaginic acid (RGD), comprised in the FN-III10 module, binds with one of the transmembrane receptors–**integrins**; herein, integrin α5β1 exhibits a specific activity. Some amino acid residues from adjacent modules are also involved in the consolidation of the bond formed. Many other amino acid sequences of fibronectins interacting with various integrins, in particular with the integrins α4β1 and α4β7, are adhesive as well.

At the same time, integrin-bond fibronectin macromolecules become an object of the active influence of intracellular processes (Wiezrbicka-Patinowski & Schwarzbauer, 2003).

The case is that, with the participation of the complex of proteins forming so-called focal adhesion (or adhesion locus, focal contact), integrins exert a decisive exposure on the conformation of macromolecules of the cytoskeleton main protein–**actin**. The direction and tension degree of actin fibers, also known as "stress-fibers", are altered; the cell form and cell membrane configuration change accordingly (Baneyx et al, 2002). At the same time, integrin receptors migrate in the plane of the cell membrane and their assembly in clusters occurs, enhancing the possibilities of additional binding of fibronectin dimers (Wierzbicka-Patinovski & Schwarzbauer, 2003).

Fibronectin's influence on intracellular processes, where the matricellular properties of these globulins manifest, is, at the same time, a mitogenic factor promoting cell reproduction (Danen & Yamada, 2001).

Moreover, the integrin-mediated fixation of fibronectin dimers on the cell membrane surface represents the beginning of fibronectin fibrillogenesis.

Changes in the cytoskeleton structure caused by the binding of fibronectins with integrins, and due to dynamic changes of the cell membrane are accompanied by stretching or unfolding, and the straightening of fibronectin V-shaped dimeric macromolecules fixed on the membrane surface; N-terminal domains, the binding of which is unlikely, are located on both ends of such straightened dimers.

But dimers' stretching results in the revealing of epitopes previously concealed in globular macromolecule modules; epitopes interact with the adjacent macromolecules. This creates the conditions for the formation of fibronectin microfibrils and their thickening, as well as for the generation of cross-bonds between macromolecules inside microfibrils. Presumably this can be disulfide bonds and/or bonds, the formation of which is catalyzed by transglutaminase as it takes place in fibrillin microfibrils (see section 3.1.2.4). The elongation of microfibrils occurs, probably due to a longitudinal shear of macromolecules relative to each other in the same way that it occurs during the fibrillogenesis of collagens. A fibronectin microfibril's diameter does not exceed 12 nm (Chen et al., 1997); therefore, they can be also called nanofibrills (Pompe et al., 2006).

Thus, fibronectin microfibrils are formed around cells; these fibronectin microfibrils possess a certain elasticity mainly due to the reversible unfolding of type III globular modules (Abu-Lail et al., 2006). These microfibrils are subsequently combined into a three-dimensional network; it can be assumed that the changeable spatial structure of this network is organized due to the migration of cells along with the microfibrils attached to them.

It should be emphasized that the aforementioned patterns of fibronectin fibrillogenesis, as a process directly related to intracellular processes, were discovered mainly during *in vitro* studies using fibroblast cultures. These cultures produce an extracellular matrix; and this process is considered to be a paradigm of connective tissue matrix assembly *in vivo*, as an experimental model reproducing the processes that occur in the formation of a new matrix during ontogenesis or in matrix restoration (remodeling) if necessary. In these processes, fibronectin microfibrils regulate cell migration and matrix composition, maintain the stability of the matrix structure and its bonds with cells (Sottile and Hocking, 2002; Mao and Schwarzbauer, 2005).

The studies *in vivo*, the objects of which were the forming and differentiating embryo tissues (Jingui, 2003; Davidson et al., 2004) or a granulation-fibrous tissue, developing in the course of wound healing and in other prolif-erative -reparative reactions of the connective tissue, indicate the presence of a developed fibronectin microfibril network in these objects. But this network, indicating intensive fibrillogenesis at these stages of morphogenesis, is obviously not stable. Unlike collagens, elastin and fibrillins, fibronectins are not resistant to proteases' action and are exposed to proteolytic splitting, which occurs both in the extracellular matrix (Ray et al., 2006) and inside cells, in lysosomes (Sottile & Chandler, 2005). Fibronectin peptides, resulting from proteolysis, stimulate cell migration, which promotes morphogenesis (Yamada, 2000). The half-life of fibronectin is estimated in months, and the network of fibronectin microfibrils is maintained by cells' biosynthetic activity only until it is necessary.

When differentiation processes of newly formed or remodeling tissues are completed, fibronectins can be continuously identified, mainly, only near the basement membranes. In this localization fibronectins stabilize the contact surface of two tissues of different origin (mesenchymal and epithelial), regulating invasion into the extracellular matrix of cells foreign for it (Armstrong and Armstrong, 2000).

It should be added that fibronectin, in the form of a soluble isoform, was originally isolated from blood plasma as early as 1948 and was called "insoluble in cold globulin". The first fibronectin possibly enters a blood clot in a wound site together with plasma.

In this connection, the assessment of a fibronectin concentration in the circulating blood has been applied in clinical and laboratory practices and has a diagnostic value. Hypofibronectinemia develops after severe traumas and extensive surgical interventions, in the case of burn injuries and sepsis, as well as in disseminated intravascular coagulation. It is observed in tumor dissemination. Blood fibronectin falling below the critical level (100 μg/ml) is a prognostically adverse factor.

Along with fibronectins **tenascins**–a family of oligomeric glycoprotein macromolecules (consisting of 3 or 6 polypeptide chains)–are widespread glycoproteins of the connective tissue extracellular matrix. Tenascins are inherent only to chordates, indicating the phylogenetic youth of this family (Tucker et al., 2006). In vertebrates, the family of tenascins comprises six paralogical glycoproteins: tenascin-C, tenascin-R, tenascin-W, tenascin-N, tenascin-X and tenascin-Y, encoded by individual genes–products of intraspecific mutations of the same gene (Chiquet-Erisman, 2004; Hsia & Schwarzbauer, 2005). Tenascin-Y and tenascin-N appear to be genetically very close to tenascin-X and tenascin-W, accordingly. The polypeptide chains of each tenascin consist of several modules, assembled in the same sequence. The N-terminal spiralized domain contains a conservative, sequence of 7 amino acid residues (heptades), common to all tenascins and essential for trimer formation. It is followed by some modules inherent for epidermal growth factor (EGF), and further by large fibronectin modules FN-III. The C-terminal domain, also common for all tenascins, is similar to the fibrinogen C-terminal globular domain (Hsia & Schwarzbaue, 2004).

Three identical polypeptide chains (subunits) agglomerate in trimers by uniting into a triple helix of N-terminal helical domains. A six-membered tenascin-C macromolecule (hence its second name– **hexabrachion**, which sometimes is applied to all tenascins), is formed as a result of disulfide binding of two trimers between cysteine residues occupying the 64th position in the N-terminal domains. (Sakakura & Kusano, 1991).

27 isoforms of a tenascin-C polypeptide chain are known due to mRNA alternative splicing. Isoforms differ by the number of modules and degree of glycosylation; the molecular weight of chains ranges from 200–300 kDa.

Like fibronectins, tenascins, tenascin-C in particular, is actively expressed in the embryo developing connective tissue, as well as in all cases of tissues' *de novo* formation and remodeling. The intensive expression of tenascin-C in the stroma of tumors has attracted the special attention (Orend, 2005).

Like fibronectins, tenascin-C actively binds with cells owing to FN-III modules by interacting with integrins; this interaction exerts a significant influence on intracellular processes. Therefore, tenascin-C is considered to be a matricellular protein.

On the contrary, tenascin-R has adhesive-structural functions. It binds with large proteoglycans, with versican particularly, employing their lectin-like domains. This binding occurs through "protein-protein", interaction involving fibronectin modules of tenascin and without the participation of carbohydrate components. This results in proteoglycan aggregates' additional fixation in the matrix.

Polypeptide chains of tenascin-R are shorter than those of tenascin-C; their molecular mass does not exceed 160–180 kDa. Tenascin-C is expressed, along with tenascin-R, in the nervous system, and phenotypic changes in null mutations of both these tenascins' genes manifest mainly in the impairment of nervous system functions.

Tenascin-X has the longest polypeptide chains, containing more than 18 EGF modules and more than 29 FN-III modules; their molecular mass exceeds 400 kDa. Tenascin-X macromolecules form trimers, rather than hexamers. This tenascin is intensively expressed in many tissues during the embryonal period; later it is mainly expressed in muscular tissue, tissues of the skeleton and in the dermis. In the dermis, tenascin promotes the formation of type I collagen fibers (Minatami et al., 2004); the absence of this influence results in skin's overstretching. According to effects targeting, tenascin-X is assigned to matricellular proteins (Bornstein & Sage, 2002).

Tenascin-W, which is inherent to fish, has short polypeptide chains. It is actively expressed in the developing tissues of the skeleton and partially coincides with the expression of tenascin-C.

Although many varied adhesive, as well as matricellular individual effects, of tenascins have been discovered, their general biological value remains rather unclear.

Fibulins are a family consisting of six glycoproteins of the connective tissue extracellular matrix, where they are bound with such supramolecular structures as elastic fibers, basement membranes, fibronectin microfibrils, proteoglycan aggregates; fibulins also bind with the integrin receptors of cell membranes (Argraves at al., 2003; Chu & Tsuda, 2004).

Fibulins are also present in blood plasma, where their concentration is about 30 µg/ml.

Most fibulins are synthesized by fibroblasts. Each fibulin (phylogenetically very ancient proteins) is encoded by an individual gene, with the genes localized on different chromosomes. The macromolecule primary structure is characterized by noticeable differences, but has essential common features as well.

The main common features are a continuous number of EGF-modules (which amino acid motifs create conditions for calcium binding) and an original large globular C-terminal domain called a fibulin module, which is obligatory for all fibulins. Another common feature is the high content of cysteine residues, enabling fibulins to form oligomers linked by disulfide bonds. All fibulins contain both O- and N-linked oligosaccharides, which are rich in galactose residues in the N-terminal region.

During the embryonic period, fibulins are especially clearly revealed by immunohistochemical methods in zones of epithelium and mesenchyma contact and interaction.

The main structural role of fibulins in the extracellular matrix is their participation in the fibrillogenesis of elastic fibers. Fibulins 1, 2 and especially actively, fibulin-5, also known as EVEC/DANCE, bind with tropoelastin. Fibulin-2 is found in elastic fibers between amorphous elastin and fibrillin microfibrils. In the absence of fibulin-5 (EVEC/DANCE), a disorganization of an elastic fiber's structure is observed (Nakamura et al., 2002); fibulin-5 interaction with integrins of cell membranes enables the spatial stabilization of elastic fibers within the matrix.

Fibulins are involved in the formation and stabilization of a variety of other extracellular matrix supramolecular structures; this involvement is essential for the structure of a cardiac valves (Timpl et al., 2003). Most interactions of fibulins with other macromolecules require calcium participation. Therefore, it is no coincidence that their name is derived from Latin *fibula* – a fastener, buckle.

At the same time some fibulins exhibit matricellular activity. For example, fibulin-1 has a pronounced anti-adhesive effect, manifesting as an inhibition of cell adhesion to fibronectins (Twai et al., 2001).

Vitronectin (the name is derived from Latin *vitrum* – glass; other names are protein S or spreading factor) is a multifunctional glycoprotein (Schvartz et al., 1999).

After the cleavage of a signal peptide, a vitronectin macromolecule contains 459 amino acid residues, including eight sulfated residues of tyrosine and one of phosphoserine, as well as five intramolecular disulfide bonds and at least three potential loci of oligosaccharide attachment. Within the polypeptide chain's middle part, there are two modules similar to hemopexin in the primary structure. Vitronectin discovered in blood serum is present in the extracellular matrix and has marked adhesive properties, in particular due to a RGD-sequence (residues 64–66). It binds with cells by means of a specific integrin receptor αVβ3, and with collagens, proteoglycans, heparin and other matrix structural components.

Upon coming into contact with a glass or plastic surface of a cultural flask, vitronectin dissolves in a culture medium, spontaneously precipitates in a densely fixed residual matter, and attaches cells to this surface; attachment is accompanied by cell spreading. This activity explains vitronectin's name and underlies the assumption about its important role as an adhesive protein in biologic tissues' interaction with implanted synthetic polymeric biomaterials.

However, vitronectin exhibits also properties intrinsic for matricellular proteins. It regulates not only cell's attachment and shape changes, but also their migration. It also regulates the activity of the matrix proteolytic enzymes and growth factors present in the matrix (Schoppet et al., 2002), and is involved in immune response.

The vitronectin content in the matrix, assessed under normal conditions using immunohistochemical methods, is not very large. Its expression increases sharply in tissue damage, inflammatory (granulation-fibrous) processes and tumor growth, indicating its importance in connective tissue proliferation.

Multifunctionality, as a specific peculiarity of matricellular proteins, is intrinsic for **thrombospondins**. The first of the thrombospondins was discovered in thrombocyte α-granules, from which it is released in thrombocyte activation at the beginning of blood clotting. Hence, they derived the first part of their name; the Latin word *spondeo* means forecast or ensure; it implies that thrombocytes' activation is a trigger mechanism of the processes developed following blood clotting.

The family of thrombospondins (TSP) consists of five glycoproteins and is divided into two subfamilies: the subfamily A comprises thrombospondin-1 and thrombospondin-2, the B-subfamily including TSP-3, TSP-4 and TSP-5; the latter (TPS-5) is also known as **COMP** (cartilage oligomeric matrix protein). Macromolecules of the A subfamily thrombospondins are homotrimers, while those of the subfamily B are homopentamers.

Thrombospondins are synthesized by megakaryocytes, by monocytes and by the smooth muscle cells of blood vessel walls, fibroblasts, choondrocytes and osteoblasts (Adams & Lawler, 2004).

TSP-1 and TSP-2 polypeptide chains with a molecular mass of about 130 kDa each (about 10 kDa of which are of oligosaccharides) have the same modular structure (Bornstein & Sage, 1994).

Globular domains are located on both chain ends. The N-terminal globular domain is immediately followed by a module whereby the intrachain disulfide bonds binding chains are formed into trimers; this is followed by a PC module that is homologous to the corresponding one of the type I procollagen α1-chain. The next are three repeats of a peculiar TSP module (in the other words module I); then there are three repeats of an EGF-like module (module II); and seven repeats of a calcium-binding module (module III), the last of which contains tripeptide RGD and the C-terminal globular domain.

The incorporation of three identical polypeptide chains of both subfamily A thrombospondins into a trimeric macromolecule significantly increases their matricellular activity, which manifests as enhancing their influence on cytoskeleton organization, cell spreading and migration (Anilkumar et al., 2002). The matricellular activity of thrombospondins 1 and 2, mediated by their interaction with many receptors of the cytoplasmic membrane, also manifests as an effect on cell proliferation and apoptosis. Influence upon the endothelial cells' apoptosis is considered to have a leading role in the mechanism of the antiangiogenic effect of these thrombospondins.

Repeats of the TSR-I module, specific for thrombospondins 1 and 2 (there are three tandem repeats of this module in each polypeptide chain), are detected in the macromolecules of many proteins of the extracellular matrix. All these proteins are involved in the regulation of the matrix organization, interaction of cells and the matrix, interaction of cells between themselves, and cell migration. Some proteins exhibit an enzymatic activity. Thrombospondins 1 and 2 are therefore considered as members of a numerous protein superfamily TSR (thrombospondin type I repeat), which is very important in cell biology (Tucker, 2004).

Thrombospondins of the subfamily B lack the TSP(I) module; they also have no the PC module. "Shortened" polypeptide chains of these thrombospondins do not form trimers, but form five-membered macromolecules–homopentamers with a total molecular weight of about 550 kDa. Globular terminal domains of polypeptide chains play a leading role in the formation of the olygomeric macromolecules of all thrombospondins (Engel, 2004).

The functions of thrombospondins 3 and 4 have not been studied well; they exhibit predominantly matricellular activity, regulating the action of various factors on cells. TSP-4 binds heparin. TSP-5 (COMP) is present mainly in cartilaginous tissue.

In all thrombospondins, matricellular activity is combined with adhesive and structural functions. All thrombospondins are present in the connective tissue extracellular matrix as structural components; their accumulation is especially marked in the matrix during embryogenesis (Iruela-Araspe et al., 2005). The expression of TSP-2 is specific for organized types of connective tissue–the dermis, ligaments, perichordium, pericardium, and meninges–during their formation. The adhesive function of thrombospondins is due to the presence of the RGD amino acid sequence in their molecules. The molecular mechanisms of thrombospondins' involvement in the matrix supramolecular structure have not been determined.

Matrilins are a family consisting of 4 extracellular matrix glycoproteins, whose molecules are formed by modules of the same type: one (matrilin-3) or two (matrilins -1, -2, -4) large domains similar to the von Willebrand factor (vWF) A-domain and from one (matrilin-1) to 10 (matrilin); 2) domains similar to a domain of the epithelial growth factor (EGF-domain); a CC (coiled coil) –domain is located in the C-terminal region of all the matrilins. The molecular mass of matrilin-2 is about 107 kDa, while that of other matrilins ranges from 52 to 64 kDa.

Matrilin-1 and matrilin-3 are present only in skeletal tissues, mainly in cartilaginous tissue, while matrilin-2 and matrilin-4 are also present in many types of connective tissue (Piecha et al., 2002).

Matrilin macromolecules are able to interact with each other. This interaction, mediated by the CC-domain (Frank et al., 2002), results in di-, tri- and tetramer macromolecules. The latter can be united into microfilaments (Klatt et al., 2000), which participate in the formation of a matrix supramolecular structure. They can bind with collagen fibers and fibrils, proteoglycans and cells. Herein, hydrophobic interactions, which involve vWF-domains, are of importance. It is obvious that matrilins are (true) structural adhesive glycoproteins in the proper sense of the word; they are called adapter proteins, uniting matrix components and "adjusting" them to each other (Wagener et al., 2005).

SPARC (secreted protein, acidic and rich in cysteine) was discovered in bone tissue; in adults, its content is higher in bone tissue. Due to this fact, it obtained its initial name – **osteonectin**. As the name implies, at the time of its discovery, it was considered as a specific structural adhesive glycoprotein of the bone tissue. Traditionally knowledge on osteonectin's molecular structure is provided along with the biochemistry of the bone tissue.

Later it was revealed that this glycoprotein is present in the matrix of not only bone tissue, but also in other connective tissue types, the predominant distribution was called SPARC, which does not designate a location. Less often another name is also used – BM-40 – implying its presence in basement membranes. SPARC appeared to be a multifunctional protein with adhesive activity. For example, SPARC *in vitro* inhibits the adhesion of cultured endothelial cells, caused by the activity of such an adhesive glycoprotein as vitronectin.

Studies performed on SPARC null mutant mice (this mutation did not cause impaired embryonal development) detected that glycoprotein exerts a variety of effects on cell functions. Such effects on the interaction of extracellular matrix and cells are specific for matricellular proteins.

The total collagen concentration in the dermis of these mice decreased 2-fold when compared to the control animals. Collagen fibers were thinned and their location within tissue was disorganized. Tissue breaking strength was also approximately twice less. At the same time, mRNA expression of the quantitatively prevailing type I collagen in the dermis was not altered; therefore, this points to the intensification of this collagen catabolism rather than its synthesis depression (Bradshaw et al., 2003).

In mice with SPARC deficiency, the closure of small (diameter of up to 6 mm) dissected skin wounds is enhanced. This phenomenon is due to the fact that the delayed formation of collagen fibers facilitates wound contraction. The healing of large (25-mm diameter) wounds is delayed mainly due to the impairment of cell migration. The course of another proliferative reparative response of the connective tissue, i.e the encapsulation of foreign bodies implanted into subcutaneous fat, is also altered. Capsules developing around implants are thinner; their collagen fibers are thinner than in control animals and non-uniform in thickness (Puolakkainen et al., 2003).

SPARC inhibits cell proliferation, arresting cell cycle in a growth phase (G-phase), and regulates expression of a number of growth factors (PDGF, FGF-2, VEGF) by cells (Brekken & Sage, 2000), in addition to modulating cell response to growth factors and cytokines.

It can be supposed that disorganization of the connective tissue extracellular matrix is a cause of enhanced tumor growth, as observed in SPARC null mutant mice (Brekken et al., 2003).

It was found while studying yeast cells that there is also SPARC inside cells, particularly in a Golgi apparatus. Moreover, it was detected in a cell nucleus matrix by means of immunochemistry methods (Yan & Sage, 1999). Therefore, SPARC not only affects the cells from the side of the extracellular matrix, but also exhibits direct intracellular effects. It acts as a transcription factor and, at the same time, its N-terminal domain interacts with a number of proteins (Sodek et al., 2002). These intracellular effects provide an additional explanation to the numerous changes of the phenotype observed in mice that lacked SPARC.

All these data allow full consideration of SPARC in extraosseous localizations, predominantly as a matricellular protein rather than an adhesive one. SPARC of bone tissue also possesses matricellular properties.

Like other matricellular glycoproteins, SPARC is expressed especially intensively during the growth and development of an organism and in tissues where the rearrangement of the connective tissue extracellular matrix occurs for one reason or another (e.g. wound healing, tumor dissemination). SPARC is one of five members of the related glycoprotein family similar to it in domain structure. Especially similar to SPARC is the **SC1** protein isolated from a rat brain, and its analogue **hevin**, detected in humans (Yan & Sage, 1999). Hevin slows down inflammatory reactions and inhibits angiogenesis in combination with SPARC (Barker et al., 2005).

SMOC-1 and **SMOC-2** (secreted modular calcium-binding proteins) proteins somehow differ from these two glycoproteins; nonetheless, they are included in this family (Vannahme et al., 2002; 2003). The presence of a homologous calcium-binding domain aligns them with glycoproteins of the SPARC family. SMOC are found in basement membranes and in the extracellular matrix.

Osteopontin, which is mainly found in bone tissue, is also referred to matricellular glycoproteins.

Specific glycoproteins of basement membrane – laminins and nidogens – are discussed in section 3.3.2.

The **biosynthesis of glycoproteins** differs from that of other proteins in the attachment of oligosaccharides, which takes place after a polypeptide chain has been assembled. Herein high-energy intermediates – mono- or diphosphate nucleosides of monosaccharides – are used. There are various mechanisms of binding of O-linked or N-linked oligosaccharides to a polypeptide chain. In the formation of glycoproteins carrying O-linked oligosaccharides, sugars are sequentially attached to a polypeptide one by one; the transfer of every monosaccharide is catalyzed by a **glycosyltransferase**. For example, in assembling of disaccharide bound with collagen (galactose-glucose), initially the first glycosyltransferase transfers galactose from a UDP-galactose molecule to a hydroxylysine residue. Thereafter, another glycosyltransferase catalyzes glucose attachment to galactose. Glycosyltransferases carrying out the assembly of O-oligosaccharides are integral proteins of endoplasmic reticulum membranes or those of a lamellar complex, with their active zones inverted inside these cavities. Nucleoside derivatives of sugars are synthesized inside the cytosol from ATP and phosphosugars and are transported via membranes involving special enzymes – **permeases**. The process of O-oligosaccharide assembly is known to be completed some minutes before a ready glycoprotein approaches a cell membrane.

The assembly of glycoproteins carrying N-linked oligosaccharides occurs differently. Oligosaccharides are assembled in cavities of the lamellar complex, and each of them can serve as a precursor for a number of glycoprotein N-linked oligosaccharides. These precursors, called oligosaccharide cores, are assembled within the rough endoplasmic reticulum from a glucose molecule, N-acetylglucosamine and mannose, with some excess of mannose compared with future assembled oligosaccharides. Branched oligosaccharides-precursors are attached via a pyrophosphate-mediated bond to large hydrophobic molecules of a lipid nature. The most prevalent among these lipids is **dolichol** – an unsaturated alcohol with a long (75–95 C atoms) carbon chain.

The complex dolichol-pyrophosphate-oligosaccharide is located in such a way that its lipid component is strongly fixed in a reticulum membrane, while oligosaccharide is in the lumen. An assembled oligosaccharide-precursor (core) is transferred **entirely** on a polypeptide chain of a growing polypeptide by means of the enzyme **oligosaccharidetransferase**. Tripeptides Asn-Xxx-Ser or Asn-Xxx-Thr, where Xxx is any amino acid residue except proline, are loci recognizing N-oligosaccharides.

Immediately after the oligosaccharide-precursor attaches to a polypeptide, its rearrangement starts, wherein it loses some glucose and mannose residues. Rearrangement continues while glycoprotein passes via a lamellar complex, where residues of N-acetylneuraminic (sialic) acid and, in some cases, those of fucose are attached to the oligosaccharide. A special enzyme catalyzes every reaction that removes an excessive monosaccharide, as well as every reaction that attaches additional monosaccharides. As a result of the sum of these reactions, which an oligosaccharide previously attached to a protein is exposed to, manifold ready oligosaccharides are formed, namely those specific for a given glycoprotein. (Karp, 1999).

3.2.1.2. Proteoglycans: structures, properties and biosynthesis

Proteoglycans are a superfamily of various glycoproteins, which differ from other glycoproteins by a presence of **glycosaminoglycans** in macromolecules in addition to O-linked and N-linked oligosaccharide fragments. Glycosaminoglycans are a kind of linear polysaccharides, covalently bound to a polypeptide chain.

Glycosaminoglycans of the vertebrate connective tissue are linear non-branched polysaccharides formed by repeated disaccharide units. Each unit consists of monosaccharides (monoses) – N-acetylated hexosamine (glucosamine or galactosamine) and a hexuronic acid (D-glucuronic or L-iduronic). Keratan sulfate is the only one in which another monose – galactose – is located instead of hexuronic acid.

All glycosaminoglycans, except hyaluronan, contain linked sulfate groups (sulfate ester). For the most part, the number of sulfate groups is equimolar to that of monoses, but the degree of sulfation is one of the most variable features of a glycosaminoglycan structure.

A detailed analysis of tissue-derived glycosaminoglycans reveals monosaccharides' marked heterogeneity, sometimes even within the same polysaccharide chain. This heterogeneity can be entirely explained by peculiarities of the glycosaminoglycan biosynthesis mechanism. The assembly of every glycosaminoglycan is a strict repetition of identical disaccharide units, but subsequent modifications (sulfation and desulfation, epimerization and others) are largely liable to contingencies. These contingencies are determined by the peculiarities of modifying enzymes' expression and specificity (Habuchi et al., 2004).

As a result, the occurrence of glycosaminoglycans' various disaccharide units becomes possible. For example, 16 variants of keratan sulfate disaccharide units might theoretically exist, 10 of which have been really found in tissues. The number of possible variants of keratan sulfate polymer molecules, per an average length of this glycosaminoglycan in 30 disaccharide units, approaches astronomical quantities as high as 10^{45} (Scott, 1995). The primary structure of another glycosaminoglycan–heparan sulfate–is also very variable, enabling the interaction of heparan sulfate-containing proteoglycans with many proteins of the extracellular matrix (Iozzo, 2001) and participation in the regulation of different signaling pathways in morphogenesis processes (Lin, 2004). Scott (1995) considered a certain sequence of not quite identical disaccharide units in each glycosaminoglycan as a significant functionally important property of its structure.

Having determined the actual and most potential multiplicity of the glycosaminoglycans' primary structure by the diversity of their disaccharide units, all glycosaminoglycans comprising proteoglycans have two common peculiarities.

The first peculiarity is the essential presence of ester sulfate groups, giving these polysaccharides a distinct anion nature.

The second is that all glycosaminoglycans comprising proteoglycans have a common "skeleton"; all of them are made by alternative galactose and glycose residues in a cyclic form. This "skeleton" becomes apparent if coupled functional groups–acetamide (CH_3CONH-) and sulfate ($-OSO_3$-) ones–are ignored; from this point of view, glycosaminoglycans are modified polylactoses (Scott, 1995). A polylactose skeleton, common for all sulfated glycosaminoglycans, provides the same secondary–spiral–conformation of their macromolecules, both in aqueous solutions and in tissues. It also provides the general potential for supramolecular structures' formation–double-layer helices which are stabilized by intramolecular hydrogen bonds, as well as acetamide and sulfate groups (Scott, 1995).

Hyaluronan significantly differs from all the glycosaminoglycans discussed. The name "hyaluronan" replaced the previously generally used name "hyaluronic acid", as this macromolecule is present *in vivo* as a polyanion rather than as an acid. Hyaluronan is not exposed to sulfation. It does not form covalent bonds with proteins and therefore, is not involved in building proteoglycan macromolecules. Both monosaccharide residues composing hyaluronan are glucose ones, provided with additional functional groups. Therefore, polyglucose rather than polylactose forms a hyaluronan "skeleton" (Scott, 1995).

A disaccharide, which hyaluronan is made from, called a **hyalobiuronic acid**, consists of D-glucuronic acid and D-N-acetylglucosamine residues linked by regularly alternating β-1,4- and β 1,3-glycoside bonds, the same as in sulfated glycosaminoglycans.

The disaccharides' number in a hyaluronan macromolecule is, in general, very high, reaching 10,000 and higher. Therefore, a hyaluronan molecular mass (the mass of one disaccharide is about 400 Da) can exceed 4,000 kDa. The length of one disaccharide is approximately 1 nm; so the hyaluronan macromolecule length in a strained state is about 10 μm at such a mass, which is comparable to the diameter of a human red blood cell.

In an aqueous solution, which an extracellular matrix essentially is, a hyaluronan macromolecule gains a dynamic tertiary structure of a chaotically coiled, twisted tape (Furlan et al., 2005). With such a structure, one gigantic giant hyaluronan macromolecule occupies a very large hydrodynamic volume in a solution, with the mass of hyaluronan itself being only 0.1% in this volume.

This practically means that, with hyaluronan concentrations of 1 mg/ml and more, solution volumes occupied by hyaluronan individual molecules overlap each other. A relatively stable and arranged tertiary structure formed as plates and tubes appears (despite the fact that hyaluronan macromolecules are constantly moving in a solution). The structure is seen when studying hyaluronan solutions with MRI methods (Scott & Heatley, 1999). The tertiary structure is supported by intramolecular hydrogen bonds, providing the macromolecule with distinct rigidity and promoting the formation of hydrophobic plaques on its surface. These plaques make the cross-linking of adjacent macromolecules possible, as well as interaction with a cell membrane and other lipid structures.

The structural organization of hyaluronan solutions gives them **viscoelastic** properties and provides such hyaluronan functions in the matrix as a space-occupying function, that of filtering, and a lubricating functions (Tammi et al., 2002).

However, functions of hyaluronan, the only matrix macromolecule of a carbohydrate nature, are significantly wider than these biomechanical tasks. Having appeared in multicellular organisms shortly before the first vertebrates' origin during evolution, hyaluronan is present in the connective tissue of all vertebrates; it is essential for the differentiation, migration, adhesion and normal functioning of cells specific for vertebrates (Spicer & Tien, 2004). Hyaluronan maintains these roles during all stages of ontogenesis (McDonald & Camenish, 2002).

Hyaluronan is a dominating matrix component of most proliferating tissues, as well as those undergoing the differentiation stage, including all differentiating connective tissue structures. Hyaluronan (HA) is stated to be present inside proliferating cells, where it is bound to intracellular **HA**-binding proteins (**IHABP**) (Lee & Spicer, 2000). Intracellular HA is supposed to participate in RNA processing and chromosome rearrangements.

Hyaluronan promotes the maintenance of tissues' water homeostasis (hydration), which is essential for their normal vital activities.

HA also plays the role of a signaling molecule, affecting many cell functions via cytoplasmic membrane specialized receptors and some intracellular signaling pathways (Lee & Spicer, 2000). This informational function is especially marked in hyaluronan oligomeric fragments, which are formed during the initial phase of its catabolism (Stern et al., 2006). In particular, hyaluronan exerts a regulating effect on the functions of cell involved in body immune responses (Mummert, 2005).

Hyaluronan is predominantly produced by cells of a mesenchymal origin. In adults, the highest amount of hyaluronan is in the skin's dermal layer (about 50% of the total 15 g, i.e. approximately 7–8 g). The hyaluronan concentration is very high in the synovia, vitreous body and umbilical cord. In a rat's body, 56% of the HA total amount is in the skin, 27% in supportive tissues, 8% in muscles and 9% in visceral organs (Fraser et al., 1997).

As has been already emphasized, hyaluronan, the only glycosaminoglycan, does not form covalent bonds with proteins, and therefore is not included in proteoglycan macromolecules. However, *in vivo* it can bind via stable electrostatic (ionic) bonds with various proteins combined in a large family of **hyaladherins** (hyaluronan-binding proteins) (Knudson & Knudson, 1993; Day & Prestwich, 2002). They are subdivided into extracellular matrix hyaladherins and those of the cytoplasmic membrane; moreover, the above intracellular HA-binding proteins (IHABP) are also hyaladherins.

Thus, within the extracellular matrix, there are three metabolic pools of HA, which differ very little from each other in the half-life period, which is 1–3 days. These pools are:

1) matrix hyaladherins-linked hyaluronan,
2) cell membrane hyaladherins-linked hyaluronan, and
3) free hyaluronan. Each of the two first pools accounts for not more than 1% of the hyaluronan total amount, and the remaining hyaluronan is free in the matrix.

The hyladherin modules active in hyaluronan binding differ in size and conformation. The most common peculiarity for these modules is the presence of clusters of basic amino acids–arginine, tyrosine, and lysine. They form ionic bonds with the carboxyl groups of hexuronic acid residues in a hyaluronan macromolecule. The minimal sizes of HA domains interacting with various hyaladherins are 6–10 disaccharides.

Within the extracellular matrix, the role of hyaladherins is primarily played by the core proteins of large proteoglycans, in which a binding module is located in the N-terminal domain. Small molecules of special link proteins, which also exhibit hyaladherin properties, harden the bond being formed. This interaction is intrinsic for all large proteoglycans; this is studied in detail in aggrecan, a cartilaginous tissue large proteoglycan. In binding a great number of aggrecan macromolecules, hyaluronan organizes and maintains the stability of the cartilage matrix supramolecular organization. A number of other matrix hayladherins is also known, which are not proteoglycans.

The hyaladherins of a cell membrane are transmembrane receptor proteins. They include RHAMM, BRAL1, SPACRAN, and LYVE-1 (Day & PrestwIch, 2002). The receptor LYVE-1 is a lymphatic vessel endothelial receptor. It is involved in penetrating a part of hyaluronan macromolecules into the lymph and then into the blood stream.

The CD44 receptor is the most widespread and important as a hyaladherin; it is a heparane sulfate proteoglycan similar to members of the transmembrane proteoglycan family–syndecans. CD44 possesses a certain degree of homology (up to 40%) with matrix hyaladherins. This receptor transfers a signal from hyaluronan to intracellular signal systems, via which the information reaches a cell nucleus. In such a way, a hyaluronan signaling function is provided (Turley et al., 2002). At the same time, in binding hyaluronan macromolecules located nearby cell surfaces, CD44 renders a pericellular matrix organized..

The CD44 receptor plays a decisive role in hyaluronan catabolism. The case is that **hyaluronidases**, enzymes that break down hyaluronan, are active only in an acid medium and that is why they cannot act in the extracellular matrix neutral medium. Therefore, hyaluronan catabolism may take place only intracellularly, unlike that of matrix protein components. This means that ~~the~~ an intensive hyaluronan **endocytosis** (or **internalization**, absorption) by cells takes place. Endocytosis occurs with the involvement of transmembrane receptors, predominantly in the participation of CD44 (Knudson et al., 2002).

The CD44 numerous molecules linking a very long hyaluronan macromolecule are concentrated in clusters on the walls of a cell membrane crypt, the so-called **caveola**, trapping hyaluronan into the caveola. The caveola edges close–the molecular mechanism of this phenomenon remains unclear; but the fact itself is certain. An **endosome** is formed; it is a transitory organelle, inside of which hyaluronan is exposed to the membrane phospholipids-bound hyaluronidase Hyal2, which breaks the hyaluronan macromolecule down to large fragments weighing about 20 kDa. Then the endosome is fused with a **lysosome**, an organelle in whose acid inner medium the more active hyaluronidase Hyal1 and two exoglycosidases–β-N-acetylglucosaminidase and β-glycuronidase–complete hyaluronan breakdown to very small fragments; these fragments, consisting predominantly of 4 disaccharides, enter the blood and are excreted with urine from the body. This is the unique way of hyaluronan catabolism (Stern, 2004).

Not all internalized hyaluronan enters lysosomes and undergoes immediate degradation. There are 4 intracellular **HA**-binding proteins (**IHABP**) inside cells. Hyaluronan, in the interaction with IHABP, is involved in RNA processing (Lee & Spicer, 2000).

Except hyaluronan, all other glycosaminoglycans are components of **proteoglycans'** protein–carbohydrate macromolecules; even their synthesis is directly associated with these macromolecules protein components.

The first studied proteoglycans were those whose greatest part of the macromolecule mast is provided by the glycosaminoglycan component. Such was the case with cartilaginous tissue essential proteoglycan, later called aggrecan. Therefore, it was accepted to consider a molecule carbohydrate part as functionally main, assigning a glycosaminoglycan-carrying polypeptide a passive, secondary role (it was called a core one). Such an understanding is reflected in the very name of proteoglycans:

Table 3.4

Main representatives of large proteoglycans

Proteoglycan	Core protein (kDa)	Glycosaminoglycans (type and chain number)
Versican	265–370	Chondroitin sulfate (10–30)
Aggrecan	220	Chondroitin sulfate and keratan sulfate (about 1,000)
Neurocan	136	Chondroitin sulfate (3–7)
Brevican	100	Chondroitin sulfate (1–3)

the ending "glycan" emphasizes the molecule carbohydrate nature.

Later it became apparent that the functionally main components of the vast majority of proteoglycan macromolecules are polypeptide chains of core proteins rather than glycosaminoglycans with all their doubtless importance. This was not only because genetically determined amino acid sequences and therefore, core proteins' secondary structures, play a decisive role in determining a composition, size (length) and the number of glycosaminoglycans connected to them. It is also relevant that core proteins that have a complex domain structure actively participate in the formation of the extracellular matrix supramolecular organization, interacting with interfibrillar substance other components and with fibrous structures and cells. Both core proteins and the glycosaminoglycans connected to them are equally important for molecular interactions, facilitating proteoglycan functions (Cattaruzza & Perris, 2006).

The superfamily of proteoglycans, comprised of not less than 60 members, is divided by their localization in tissues into the following classes:

a) proteoglycans of the extracellular matrix; this class is subdivided into two groups–big large and small proteoglycans, depending on the molecular mass;

b) proteoglycans of basement membranes; to the same degree as basement membranes differ from the extracellular matrix by special functions, their proteoglycans appear special;

c) proteoglycans of cell (cytoplasmic) membranes; these proteoglycans are actively involved in cell interactions with the extracellular matrix;

d) intracellular proteoglycans, generally contained in secretory granules; such granules are particularly found in blood cells.

Large proteoglycans are named such for several reasons. First of all, their core proteins have a large molecular mass (ranged from 100–370 kDa); secondly, these proteins, as a rule, carry a large number (up to 100) of long glycosaminoglycan chains. Thirdly, due to such an abundance of glycosaminoglycans, they occupy large spaces within the extracellular matrix. The last property gives grounds for another name for large proteoglycans' class–**space-occupying proteoglycans**. Another peculiarity of large proteoglycans is that their main weight mass is composed by chondroitin sulfates. The main members of the large proteoglycan class are listed in *Table 3.4*. Macromolecules are structured according to the same scheme and have a one-type triple-domain structure.

End domains are responsible for the stabilization of a proteoglycan macromolecule location within the matrix. The N-terminal domain is responsible for binding with hyaluronan. The C-terminal domain is close in primary structure to lectins, proteins which selectively react with some glycoproteins of cell membranes. The presence of such C-terminal domains, linking proteoglycans with cells, explains another name for large proteoglycans–**hyalectans** or **lecticans**.

An extensive central domain carrying glycosaminoglycan chains, connected by O-glycoside bonds to serine residues, is located between the N- and C-terminal domains. Some specific regions, including those carrying oligosaccharide groups, interrupt this domain.

Two large proteoglycans–neurocan and brevican–are only found in connective tissue structures of the central nervous system and synthesized by neuroglia cells. Aggrecan dominates in the extracellular matrix structure of cartilaginous tissue. Here we will describe the main general characteristics of large proteoglycans, with the example of **versican** (also called **PG-M**) common for many connective tissue types.

Several versican isoforms are known–V0, V1, and V2. They are expression products of the same gene, their origin being the result of alternative splicing. V0 and V1 are expressed by fibroblasts and chondrocytes; keratino-cytes express only V1, while the cells of some tumors express V2.

A versican core protein is the largest among the core proteins of all large proteoglycans. The total length of its core protein polypeptide chain in humans, evaluated by its gene structure (*VCAN*), comprises 3,396 amino acid residues, 20 of which fall on a signal peptide removed in post-translation processing. The most common isoform–V1 core protein–consists of 2,389 amino acid residues. The molecular mass of this versican isoform is 263 kDa.

As in other hyalolectans, the N-terminal domain of a versican core protein facilitates its binding with hyaluronan. Interactions involving globular domains of the core protein C-terminal region are more manifold. One of these domains–a C-lectin-like one–is most likely to perform a link with glycoprotein oligosaccharide groups of cells cytoplasmic membrane, as well as with the extracellular matrix glycoproteins. Due to this interaction, mesh-like structures are formed, facilitating a space fixation of versican macromolecules (Olin et al., 2001). Other domains specific for versican (absent in other hyalectins) are characterized by repeats of amino acid residues similar in structure to that of an epidermal growth factor (EGF). They can exert effects on cell differentiation, organization, migration and adhesion in histogenesis processes, as well as cell functions, including transcription factors' activity (Rahmani et al., 2006). These effects are considered very important in mesenchymal epithelial interactions (Sheng et al., 2006).

The central extended domain of a versican core protein contains 14 Ser-Gly and Gly-Ser dipeptides, serving as loci for chondroitin sulfates conncetion. A versican macromolecule contains 14 chondroitin sulfates, which are rather tightly diffused along the central domain length. There are no other glycosaminoglycans in versican.

The versatility of versican functions accounts for its name (Wight, 2002).

Besides hyalectans, proteoglycans of basement membranes also have large (up to 500 kDa) macromolecules. These proteoglycans will be discussed in section 3.3.2.

Large proteoglycans are united in a single family, not only because of similar macromolecule sizes and uniform principles of their structure. A molecular genetic analysis (Schwartz et al., 1999) shows that the genes encoding the core proteins of this macromolecules' group represent a family originating from the same progenitor. Their inner congeniality is reflected in common motives, both at the level of an expressed proteins' primary structure and at the level of mRNA nucleotide sequences. Their genome organizations are almost identical, especially in those regions that encode polypeptide chain terminal (globular) domains. There are some more differences in the exon structure in those gene regions encoding central–linear–domains, serving as glycosaminoglycan carriers; it is certain that these differences have developed gradually during evolution.

Small leucin-rich proteoglycans (**SLRP**) comprise the majority of connective tissue extracellular matrix proteoglycans. The molecular mass of their core proteins ranges from 35–59 kDa, with the number of glycosaminoglycan chains ranging only from 1–5 (Iozzo, 1998). Like large proteoglycans, they also carry attached oligosaccharide groups apart from glycosaminoglycans and therefore, are not only proteoglycans, but also glycoproteins.

The matrix contains glycoproteins, whose polypeptide chains correspond to the model of a SLRP core protein structure, but lack glycosaminoglycans. Their functions (to the extent they have been clarified) are similar to those of small proteoglycans, and they are included in the SLRP family.

In accordance with the encoding genes' assumed evolution and structure, as well as with the type of glycosaminoglycans connected, the SLRP family is subdivided into three classes, as presented in *Table 3.5.*

The first class comprises **decorin** (synonyms: proteoglycan I or PG-S1), usually carrying one glycosaminoglycan chain, and **biglycan**, which is also known as proteoglycan II, PG-S2 or PG-40 and have two glycosaminoglycans. Both of them are dermatan/chondroitin sulfate proteoglycans. Together, they comprise up to 95% of the total mass of fibrous connective tissues, i.e. rich in fiber-forming collagens.

The main peculiarity of decorin and biglycan core proteins' primary structure is the presence of a linear region consisting of 10–12 amino acid repeats in the polypeptide chain central domain. Each repeat contains 24 amino acid residues, at least 6 of which are leucine residues (or isoleucine and valin ones similar to leucine by amphipathic properties). Hence the name of these repeats–**LRR** (leucine-rich repeats). The total number of leucin and similar amino acids repeats in a protein exceeds 20%.

Proteoglycans of the second class contain keratan sulfate as a glycosaminoglycan component. This class comprises proteoglycans of the cornea–**lumican**, **keratocan** and **fibromodulin**, which are related to providing its clarity (moreover, fibromodulin is found in cartilaginous tissue), and **osteoadherin**, contained in bone and cartilaginous tissues. **PRELP** (proline arginin-rich end leucine-rich repeat protein), which bind basement membranes with the underlying connective tissue, also belongs to this class (Bengtsson et al., 2002).

The third class subdivided on the basis of evolution and genetic considerations (Iozzo, 1998) includes **osteoglycin**, a dermatan/ chondroitin sulfate proteoglycan also found in bone tissue, and **epiphycan**, a keratan sulfate proteoglycan expressed only by epiphyseal cartilage cells.

There are globular domains from which small linear polypeptide endings protrude on central linear domains; both ends of their core proteins each carry several N-oligosaccharides attached to an asparagines residue. In decorin and biglycan, glycosaminoglycans are

Table 3.5
Main representatives of small (leucin-rich) proteoglycans

Proteoglycans	Core protein (kDa)	Glycosaminoglycans (chain type and number)
Class I		
Decorin	40	Dermatan/chondroitin sulfate (1)
Biglycan	40	Dermatan/chondroitin sulfate (2)
Class II		
Fibromodulin	42	Keratan sulfate (2–3)
Lumican	38	Keratan sulfate (3–4)
Keratocan	38	Keratan sulfate (3–5)
PRELP	44	Keratan sulfate (2–3)
Osteoadherin	42	Keratan sulfate (2–3)
Class III		
Epiphycan	35	Dermatan/chondroitin sulfate (2–3)
Osteoglycin	35	Keratan sulfate (2–3)

connected to such a N-terminal ending. In fibromodulin and lumican, an N-terminal fragment is slightly longer and differs by the presence of several tyrosine sulfated residues, while the only glycosaminoglycan chain is connected to the central linear domain (Svensson et al, 2001).

The N-terminal domain of decorin and biglycan (but not of other small proteoglycans) has one other distinuishign factor: the terminal region with a length of 41 amino acid residues most actively connects zinc ions (Zn^{2+}). This activity is associated with the presence of 4 cysteine residues in the N-domain. Thus, decorin and biglycan are metalloproteins. The connection of zinc ions alters their molecules' configuration (a secondary structure), which is obviously reflected in their function (Yang et al., 1999).

Both the degree of core protein primary structure homology and that of their mRNA structure leave no doubt that the genes of all small proteoglycans originate from the same progenitor. The genes of small proteoglycans contain an identical module in their promoter zones, providing the possibility for their coordinated expression (Tasheva et al., 2004).

Small proteoglycans interact with large (fiber-forming) collagens. Biglycan and decorin, to a lesser degree, influence the process of collagen fibril formation regulating their diameter and fibrillogenesis rate; SLRP bind especially actively with type II collagen (Douglas et al., 2006). SLRP also increase collagen fibrils' resistance to the collagenases activity (Geng et al., 2006). Interaction with collagens is reflected in the names of small proteoglycans, such as fibromodulin and decorin (this proteoglycan "decorates" a surface of collagen fibrils). Small proteoglycans are also referred to as collagen-binding proteins (Svensson et al., 2001).

At the same time, they interact with other matrix structural proteins and enzymes, as well as with signaling molecules, particularly with growth factors (Moreno et al., 2005). They, especially dermatan sulfate-containing SLRP (Trowbridge & Gallo, 2002), affect cell proliferation and functions actively. Therefore, they are considered to play a controlling and organizing role in tissue growth, including the growth of malignant neoplasms (Kresse & Schönherr, 2001; Naito, 2005). In all these interactions, not only small proteoglycans glycosaminoglycan components is of great importance for the formation of extracellular matrix supramolecular architectonics, but also, to a large degree, core proteins are involved.

Most **proteoglycans connected with a cell (cytoplasmic) membrane** (also called pericellular) are transmembrane proteins. Their core proteins consist of three domains. Small endodomains, located in the cell cytoplasm, have a similar primary structure to the entire group of these proteoglycans. Domains passing via the lipid cell membrane (transmembrane) are also uniform; in these domains, hydrophobic amino acid residues prevail. On the contrary, the outstretching from cells into the extracellular matrix ectodomains, to which few chains of glycosaminoglycans are attached, is highly varied (Elenius & Jalkanen).

The ectodomains of some plasma membrane proteoglycans contain a few chondroitin sulfates. But heparan sulfate is a glycosaminoglycan prevailing in these proteoglycans, with its chain structure being of a wide variety, as has been mentioned.

Syndecans are transmembrane heparan sulfate proteoglycans. Their name originates from Greek *syndein*–to bind together. This family consists of 4 proteins in vertebrates (Zimmermann & David, 1999). These proteins significantly differ from each other by their molecular mass (ranged from 19.5–30.6 kDa) and by peculiarities of a structure of heparan sulfate chains connected to them. Syndecans have a peculiar function in transducing signals from the extracellular matrix to a cell. They can be considered as cytoplasmic membrane signal receptors owing to their transmembrane structure, the endodomains bonds with a cytoskeleton and the ability to alter the conformation of these domains when contacting with ligands (Simons & Horowitz, 2001) and to activate intracellular phosphorylation. The diversity of structural motives in syndecan heparan sulfates increases the number of potential ligands (signaling molecules) in the matrix, with which the syndecans can interact (Park et al., 2000). This number increases more due to the proper structure features of each syndecan core proteins (Oh & Couchman, 2004; Lopes et al., 2006).

At the same time, due to the diversity of heparan sulfates, syndecans are able not only to translate signals themselves, but to regulate signaling molecules (growth factors, cytokines) ability to contact with other receptors. In other words, syndecans modulate signal activity and function as co-receptors of other factors (Rapraeger, 2000).

Such a complex function determines syndecans' role in regulating cell's vital activities, particularly cell proliferation and the ability for adhesion with the matrix and other cells. The fact that, in animals with switched off genes, which encode enzymes essential for heparan sulfates' synthesis, non-survivable phenotypic changes develop (e.g. dwarfism of the heart, lungs, kidneys) indicates the importance of this role (Forsberg & Kjellén, 2001). This is supported by the pronounced phylogenic conservatism of syndecans–drosophila and earthworm genes are homologous to those of vertebrate syndecans, have the same origin (orthologs), and are similar to them in structure.

A receptor protein, called CD44, partly discussed above and known in at least 10 isoforms, has a special place among heparan sulfate proteoglycans. Alternative splicing of shared gene transcripts accounts for their origin (Goodison et al., 1999). A molecule of this transmembrane proteoglycan consists of four rather than three domains–its ectodomain is subdivided into two subdomains (Goodison et al., 1999).

The first of them, the distal (N-terminal) domain, contains a cluster of 4 essential amino acid residues (Arg41, Arg42 и Tyr78, Tyr79), with which hyaluronan of the extracellular matrix binds.

The second proximal subdomain, where alternative splicing is most commonly noticed, serves as a locus for heparan sulfate connection. Not every isoform contains a glycosaminoglycan; therefore, CD44 is called a "partial" proteoglycan. The transmembrane domain is similar to analogous ones of other transmembrane proteins; a small (70 amino acid residues) endodomain contacting with cytosol proteins transfers signals coming from a cell to the entire proteoglycan molecule for their further transmission into the extracellular matrix. Thus, signal transduction via the CD44 receptor occurs in both directions.

The special position of CD44 among transmembrane proteins is due to this receptor playing a central role in hyaluronan catabolism. This function is carried out by the most common isoform–CD44H. The functions of receptor other isoforms, called CD44v1-v10, are various; generally these functions are associated with intercellular interactions (Fuchs et al., 2003).

Not every proteoglycan connected with a cytoplasmic membrane is a transmembrane membrane. **Glypicans** core proteins, comprising a family of 6 heparan sulfate proteoglycans, lack transmembrane and cytoplasmic domains. Glypicans are connected to a cell surface on the outward side via the C-terminal domain-bond glycosylphosphatidylinositol (GPI); GPI is inserted into a cell phospholipid membrane (Filmus & Selleck, 2001). An interesting peculiarity of glypican core proteins is the presence of 14 cysteine residues, forming several intra-molecular disulfide bonds in all their isoforms. Heparan sulfates are attached to the C-terminal domain nearby a cell membrane. Such a location of heparan sulfates allows them to regulate the interaction of different signaling molecules with transmembrane receptors. Moreover, glypican-1 acts as a transporter protein, circulating between the extracellular matrix and the cytoplasm (Fransson et al., 2004).

Cells express both transmembrane heparan sulfate proteoglycans and glypicans especially actively during morphogenesis processes (Song & Filmus, 2002).

Before discussing **proteoglycan biosynthesis**, it should be noted that a proteoglycan complex macromolecule is a product of the coordinated synthetic reactions system comprising:

a) the expression of a core protein;

b) the subsequent connection of oligosaccharide groups specific for glycoproteins to the core protein, and finally;

c) the assembly of glycosaminoglycan polymeric chains connected to the core protein appropriate loci. Based on data on the aggrecan molecular mass, it has been estimated that, to perform the entire complex of these reactions and to produce one finished aggrecan macromolecule, approximately 25,000 covalent bonds should be formed, not including the bonds generated in forming biosynthesis by-products, as well as the information macromolecules and enzymes involved in the process.

Enzymes, responsible for **glycosylation**, i.e. transformation of a core protein into a glycoprotein (see section 3.2.1.1) are fixed on granular (rough) endoplasmic reticulum membranes. Glycosylation precedes **glycosamino-glycanation**.

The first step of glycosaminoglycan chain assembly is addition of a monosaccharide **xylose** to a serine residue hydroxyl group in the core protein (**O-glycosylation**). For this purpose, definite rather than any serine residues are used. As a rule, a connection locus for a glycosaminoglycan chain is a tetrapeptide S-G-X-G, where seryl is followed by two glycyls, separated by any amino acid residue X; this sequence is usually preceded by some residues of acidic amino acids. Some other variants of serine residue of immediate surroundings are also known (Kjellén & Lindahl, 1991).

Glycosylation starts with a xylose transfer from its nucleotide derivative – uridine diphosphate xylose. The transfer is performed by a specific enzyme – **xylosyltransferase**, the first enzyme from the glycosyltransferase series involved in glycosaminoglycan synthesis as xylose always is the monosaccharide connecting a glycosaminoglycan to a core protein.

The activity of all glycosyltransferases comprising this series of enzymes follows the general principles. Firstly, in every reaction, these enzymes catalyze the nucleotide derivatives of monosaccharides – **uridine diphosphate nucleotides** serve as their donors. Glucose is a precursor of these derivatives, their formation occurs in the cyto-sol. As a result of connecting to a nucleotide, the monosaccharide residue is activated, facilitating its inclusion in the glycosaminoglycan chain and its further enzymatic transformation into glycosaminoglycans' structural units – uronic acids and hexosamines.

Secondly, the effects of all glycosyltransferases comply with the principle "one bond – one enzyme". This principle implies the specificity of every enzyme in relation to a monosaccharide being transferred, the core protein acceptor locus and the arising bond anomeric configuration. The specificity in relation to the anomeric configuration is of an absolute nature: if there were no configuration, the assembly reproducibility of hydrogen macromolecules would be impossible.

The first transferase – xylosyltransferase – mentioned above is characterized in detail. An enzyme macromolecule, isolated from a chicken embryo cartilaginous tissue, consists of two pairs of different subunits with a molecular mass of 23 and 27 kDa. This enzyme plays an important role in regulating proteoglycan synthesis. The case is that UDP-xysole appeared to be an inhibitor of some enzymes related to UDP-glucose transformations. Therefore, an inhibition or knockdown of a xylosyltransferase gene, resulting in an unused UDP-xylose accumulation in the cell, is accompanied by a deficiency of other UDP-monosaccharides, the result of which is the discontinuance of the entire assembly of glycosaminoglycans.

Connected to a core protein, a xylose residue is the first link of the so-called **connection region** of a glycosaminoglycan chain. This region's next is a galactose residue connected to that of xylose. This second reaction is catalyzed by the enzyme **galactosyltransferase I**. In this case, a nucleotide derivative UDP-galactose is a donor, while O-β-D-xylosyl-L-serine, formed as a result of xylose addution to a core protein, is a receptor.

Further elongation of a glycosaminoglycan binding region occurs by connecting a second galactose residue to the first one (catalyzed by **galactosyltransferase II**) and the subsequent addition of the uronic acid first residue to the second residue of galactose, for example, in the case of assembling chondroitin sulfate, it is a glucuronic acid. The transfer of the first glucuronic acid residue is catalyzed by **glucuronic acid transferase I**, which differs from transferase, which carries glucuronic acid residues during the subsequent growth (elongation) of a chondroitin sulfate chain. On this basis, the first residue of glucuronic acid is considered as the final link of the connection region which thus consists of four monosaccharide residues: xylose – galactose – galactose – glucuronic acid. Both galactosyltransferases and glucuronic acid transferase I are bound with the granular endoplasmic reticulum membrane.

Following the completion of the connection region assembly, glycosaminoglycan elongation begins. In chonrdoitin sulfate biosynthesis, this occurs by means of transferring N-acetyl-galactosamine and glucuronic acid residues from associated UDP-nucleotides. In this process, two specific glycosyltransferases–**N-acetylgalac-tosamine transferase and glucuronic acid transferase II**–act. The assembly of other glycosaminoglycans occurs in the same way.

As this assembly takes place in the absence of matrices, as opposed to polypeptide chains translation assembly, the glycosyl transferases' specificity is the only factor determining the sequence reproducibility (regular alteration) of monosaccharide units in a glycosaminoglycan chain. The lack of other controlling factors might explain arising failures in this regularity, leading to the occurrence of glycosaminoglycan polymorphism.

Essential for chondroitin sulfates and dermatan sulfates biosynthesis, galactosamine originates by means of the epimerization of glucosamine formed from glucose. Even before the completion of glycosaminoglycan assembly, the N-acetylgalactosamine residues inserted therein are exposed to **sulfation**–sulfate groups are added to them. These groups are preactivated by the formation of 3-phospho-adenosine-5-phosphosulfate (**PAPS**) (in adenosinephosphate and sulfate interaction). PAPS serves as a donor of sulfate groups transferred by several specific **sulfotransferases** (Habuchi et al., 2004). For example, in assembling two chondroitin sulfate isoforms, chondroitin-4-sulfate and chondroitin-6-sulfate, two different sulfotransferases–chondroitin-4-sulfotrans-ferase and chondroitin-6-sulfotransferase–act. The specificity of these enzymes is that they use either the 4th or 6th hydrogen atom of N-acetylgalactosamine as a sulfate acceptor. It is not entirely clear which mechanisms determine the usage of one or another enzyme in each specific case. It is not completely clear whether separate glycosyltransferases are, in fact, individual proteins or if they are a uniform protein complex exhibiting manifold enzymatic functions (Sugahara & Kitagawa, 2000).

These patterns of large proteoglycans' biosythesis are amplified to that of small proteoglycans and cytoplasmic membranes, as well as the biosynthesis of basement membrane proteoglycans as described below (see section 3.3.2). The genes of each of these proteoglycans families have the same origin.

Hyaluronan biosynthesis requires a separate discussion. Hyaluronan biosynthesis principally differs from that of other glycosaminoglycans in that it is not in a covalent bond with a protein; therefore, there can be no mention of a specific locus within a polypeptide chain that could serve as an information carrier to initiate glycosaminoglycan assembly. Furthermore, a huge hyaluronan macromolecule (in vertabrates, it is comprised of 10,000 disaccharides on average) consumes tremendous energy from a cell for its assembly (up to 50,000 eqivalents of adenosine triphosphate, 20,000 NAD-cofactor molecules and 10,000 acetyl coenzyme A molecules) (Lee & Spicer, 2000).

Hyaluronan is synthesised on the cell membrane's internal surface, unlike other glycos-aminoglycans, whose assembly is ongoing on a granular endoplasmic reticulum membrane (DeAngelo, 1999) and which remain bound

with core proteins after assembly has been completed. Glycosyltransferases that assemble hyaluronan as a linear polysaccharide and are referred to as **hyaluronic acid synthases (HAS)** are integral components of the cell membrane (Toole, 1998).

There are three HAS isoforms known. Amino acid residues Asp242, Asp344 and Trp384 (Lee & Spicer, 2000) are critical for the enzymatic activity of all isoforms. HAS also have the ability to translocate assembled hyaluronan into the extracellular matrix. Mice with the knockdown genes Has1 and Has3 are totally viable, while switching Has2 off results in severe embryogenesis defects, especially in cardiac malformations (Tammi et al., 2002).

It is possible that some undetermined sequence of amino acid residues of one transmembrane protein of the cytoplasmic membrane, which is also undetermined, plays the role of a specific locus, promoting an initiation of hyaluronan assembly. But later the assembled hyaluronan polypeptide chain separates from the protein and continues elongating, being in a free state within the extracellular matrix.

3.2.1.3. Structural organization of connective tissue integrating buffer metabolic medium (ground substance)

In describing the morphology of the integrating buffer metabolic medium's structured components, it should be kept in mind that only those proteoglycans (PG) that might be detected by means of morphological investigations are discussed. In the PG composition, the glycosaminoglycans (GAG) linear, non-branched polymers composed by repeated disaccharide units and being of a polyanion nature due to the presence of anion groups in them, are concentrated and regularly located along the length of each molecule and are responsible for their histochemical properties. It is these anion groups that interact with various cationic dyes such as toluidine blue, alcian blue, colloid ferrous hydroxide, safranin O and others. Using different controls (enzymatic, chemical, various pH levels and so on), various glycosaminoglycans can be differentiated. However, PG investigations at the light optical level are rather informatively limited and can reveal only their presence by specific staining. In staining the histologic samples of various connective tissue types with cationic dyes, the latter are adsorbed in the extracellular matrix mainly on collagen and elastic fibers; as a rule, stained structures are not detected in interfibrous, interfibrillar and intercellular spaces. It is obvious that, in the fixation aldehyde proteoglycans that are not a part of a fiber structure (i.e. are the ground substance components), they are destroyed (protein coagulation and GAG cleavage) and largely washed out. Hyaline and elastic cartilaginous tissues are the connective tissue types where most of the ground substance PG is retained. This is due to a rather dense location of their fibrous structures and their organization level (these connective tissue types will be described in detail in Volume II). Despite the wide variety of dyes available, the light optics resolving power cannot provide the exact localization of polysaccharide substances in a structure of fibrous elements, let alone detect their ultra-structural organization. This can be done by means of electron histochemistry when PG determination is based on their polyanion electrolytes' properties. Unlike routine histochemistry, "electron dyes" or contrasting substances are to be cationic dyes and have a high charge electron density. Such contrasting agents include lanthanum salts (Revel & Karnovsky, 1967), bismuth salts (Smith & Serafini-Fracassini, 1968), phospho-wolframic acid (Pease & Bouteille, 1971) and others. The Luft method for applying ruthenium red (ruthenium is a hexavalent cation) (Luft, 1965, 1971, 1971) seems theoretically most reasonable. The application of this method provided the most exact, complete and reproducible information on a proteoglycan structure at each morphologically registered level of connective tissue fibrous elements' organization, including the interstitial space.

However, despite the Luft method's general theoretic propriety (Luft, 1965, 1971a, 1971b), there were significant disadvantages in its practical feasibility. For example, the primary fixation of tissues with a mixture of glutarol aldehyde and ruthenium red in a cacodylate buffer disallowed reliance on an adequate fixation and the ensuing integrity of the structured proteoglycans' 3-D organization, especially in the integrating buffer metabolic medium of the extracellular matrix. These doubts are due to the fact that a glutarol aldehyde molecule is only based on two hydrogen atoms. Its molecular weight is manifold less than that of ruthenium red. Hence, it is obvious that glutarol aldehyde penetrates tissues significantly more rapidly than does ruthenium red and fixes a proteoglycan protein part, thereby inducing their structural organization damage. Therefore, subsequent ruthenium red attachment to such glycoconjugates does not reflect their true morphologic picture. It largely refers to intercellular and interfibrous space proteoglycans. Nevertheless, a modification of the Luft method, taking into account the above considerations, facilitated better proteoglycan structural organization integrity. In the advanced procedure, the initial stage consisted of tissue samples' exposure in a ruthenium red solution alone in a cacodylate buffer for 0.5–2.0 h (depending on the sample size and density). It promoted a dye penetration into the tissue and its attachment to glycosaminoglycans. The further stages of the staining were in complete compliance with the Luft method. This modified procedure enabled the widening of the morphologic scale of ruthenium-positive structures of a proteoglycan nature and brought our understanding of a structured proteoglycans' tissue composition close to the one truly existing in native tissues. Moreover, the data obtained thereby made it possible to combine all evidence available on a connective tissue's PG structure into a general system (Omelyanenko, 1978; 1984; 1991).

This means that collagen microfibrils within a fibril are surrounded by an intrafibrillar amorphous (fine-granular) substance of a proteoglycan nature (Pease & Bouteille, 1971). There is a more dense and concentrated proteoglycan location on the collagen fibril's periphery imitating a peculiar proteoglycan membrane, with a thickness of 20 nm. Large proteoglycan granules (20.0–30.0 nm), located in intervals of 60–70 nm along the fibrils' surface at the level of period d-bands, can be detected over membranes. In cases when collagen fibrils form fibers, the majority of interfibrillar spaces are filled with fine-granular amorphous substance of a proteoglycan nature (Fig. 3.20 a, b). A similar substance is found between fibrous elements and the muscle cells in their clos.e vicinity. Narrow interfibrous gaps, the width of which does not exceed that of one collagen fibril (i.e. up to 200 nm), are filled in with the same substance. In wider interfibrous or interfibrillar spaces, a mesh-like structure of a proteoglycan nature can be detected (Fig. 3.20 a, d). Its structural components–threads and "nodal" thickenings to which they are attached–vary significantly in size depending upon a connective tissue type or kind of "dye". However, the principle of forming interfibrous structural proteoglycans as a mesh-like structure is retained. When collagen fibrils are the main fibrous structure (for example, in a hyaline cartilage) where the distances between them are more than interfibrous gaps in fibers, but are significantly less than interfibrous spaces, then structured proteoglycans will be of a mixed form in such interfibrillar spaces, i.e. the regions of the mesh-like structure will be altered with the amorphous fine-granular substance (Omelyanenko, 1978; 1984; 1991). The complex biochemical and electron-microscopic investigations of separate cartilage, dermis and other fractions confirm the reality of a mesh-like organization of the gel-like ground substance framework in interfibrous spaces (Gregory, 1974; Thyberg, 1977). The dried residue of sodium hyaluronate in redistilled water had a structure of branching and anastomosing threads 5–20 nm wide (Gross, 1948).

Based on the literature's definition of the ground substance as an extravascular, extrafibrous, extracellular phase of the connective tissue (Montagna & Parakkal, 1974), the proteoglycans found within the aforementioned limits should be referred to as ground substance PGs. This assignment is certain to be conditional as all the connective tissue structured proteoglycans form an integral system, united with the fibrous framework.

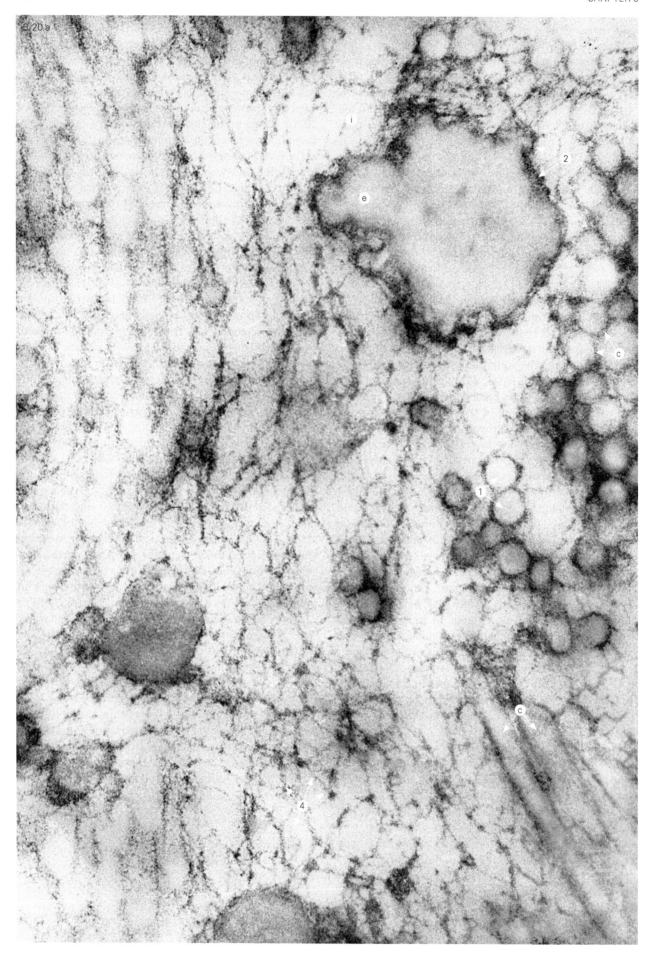

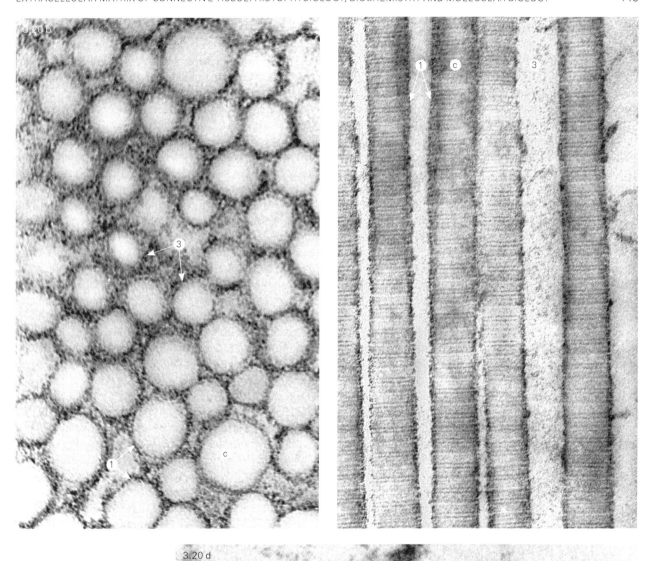

Fig. 3.20.
A fragment of a reticular
layer intercellular matrix
of the human skin dermis.
Collagen fibrils (c) comprising
individual fibers.
Elastic fibers (fibrils) (e).
Interstitial space (i).
Ruthenium-positive structures
of a proteoglycan nature:
collagen fibril coats (1);
an elastic fiber (fibril) coat (2);
fine granular amorphous
substance (3);
mesh-like/reticular
structure (4).
TEM-micrograph,
Staining: ruthenium red.
a − x 50,000;
b, c − x 80,000;
d − x 200,000

3.3. BASEMENT MEMBRANES

3.3.1. Structure of basement membranes

A basement membrane (**BM**) is a specifically organized part of the extracellular matrix of the connective tissue, separating it from epithelial, muscular and partly nervous tissues. BM serves as a support for the cells that attach to it, and plays the role of an additional coating for the cells it surrounds, and serves as an integrating structure for connective and other tissues. BM regulates the nutrients passing from blood vessels to epithelial and muscular cells and, in part, nerve cells, as well as cellular metabolic products to the vessels. The similarity of the BM functions corresponds to the general character of their architecture of various topography and organ specificity: in the skin–between the epidermis and dermis; in the cornea–between the epithelium and Bowman's membrane; under the endothelium–Descemet's membrane, under the respiratory, gastrointestinal, urinary epithelium, and that of the renal tubules, Malpighian glomerulus–a membrane covering peripheral nerves and muscular fibers, and so on.

A basement membrane looks like an electron-dense streak (in TEM-imaging) outlining the cells and connecting to it. A basement membrane ranges from 30–120 nm in thickness (*Fig. 3.21*). It consists of a fine-granular material where fine microfibrils without any preferable orientation are seen. A routine TEM-investigation reveals an electron-transparent structureless gap with a width of 10–40 nm between the BM and the cells adjacent to it. When contrasting the test skin with ruthenium red (a relatively selective dye for proteoglycans and glycoproteins), the BM was thicker and immediately adjacent to basal keratinocytes. There was no electron-transparent structureless gap. Obviously there are two layers in the BM. An external layer adjacent to basal keratinocytes mainly consists of proteoglycans and glycoproteins and it is not detected in routine contrasting (lead citrate or uranyl acetate). An internal, denser layer along with proteoglycans contains a network of collagen microfibrils; therefore, it is stained with protein dyes. The external layer is likely to provide cell adhesion to the basement membrane. It is entirely possible that this connection is added by hemidesmosomes between cell and basement membranes. Worthy of attention is the presence in the hemidesmosome of an electron-dense structure as a fine band in a plasmolemma-thickened plate with the same length. There is a light gap of 10–20 nm between these structures. In this gap there are cross-located microfibrils connecting both electron-dense plates. The peculiarity of BM structural organization in capillaries is its periodic cleavage into two equivalent constituents as a duplication, between which pericytes are enclosed. In the cornea, BMs have a thickness significantly higher than that in other organs. Collagen fibrils of the connective tissue underlying the basement membrane can interact with it either by means of proteoglycans as an amorphous ruthenium-positive fine-granular substance or by anchor fibrils, or else it can entwine into the BM microfibrillar structure. All of the above mechanisms make the interaction of BM with the underlying connective tissue rather coherent. Therefore, when separating the epidermis from the dermis, BMs always remain with the latter.

A part of the cells surrounding the basement membrane provide its organization and its constant renewal, the maintenance of its physiologic structural and functional state, which depends on an organ specificity. In the skin, fibroblasts and keratinocytes mutually regulate the synthesis of the components comprising a basement membrane and their organization into a distinct structure (Fleischmajer et al., 1993; Marinkovich et al., 1993; Smola et al., 1998; Moulin et al., 2000). Type IV and VII collagens and laminin-1 are produced by fibroblasts found in the line of the derma-epidermal connection (DEC). Keratinocytes also produce and organize type IV and VII collagens, laminin-5, other laminins and perlecan (Marinkovich et al., 1993). Fibroblasts are shown to be main sources of entactin/nidogen (Contard et al., 1993; Fleischmajer et al., 1995).

The combined culture of fibroblasts and keratinocytes modifies the activity of both types of cells. The keratinocytes induce the expression of the transforming growth factor TGF-β2 in dermal fibroblasts (Smola et al., 1994). The fibroblasts regulate the production of laminins and type VII collagen by keratinocytes, possibly via TGF-β2 (Konig & Bruckner-Tuderman, 1991; Konig & Bruckner-Tuderman, 1994; Monical & Kefalides, 1994).

However, not all dermal fibroblasts interact similarly with keratinocytes in basement membrane formation (Moulin et al., 2000). Differentiated fibroblast populations are supposed to be in the skin DEC; these fibroblasts produce basement membrane components and assist keratinocytes in their organization (Marinkovich et al., 1993).

3.3.2. Biochemistry of basement membranes

Basement membranes are, phylogenetically, the oldest structures of the connective tissue. The macromolecules of basement membranes and those providing mutual cell adhesion originated between the period of first eukaryotic cells generation (this occurred about 2 billion years ago) and that of the multicellular organisms origin (metazoa) about 0.8 gigayears ago. This was concluded on the basis of a complete mapping of an earthworm genome–nematoda Caenorhabditis elegans. In C.elegans genes of the BM, most components were found; moreover, these genes appeared to be quite conservative; they differ little from the present genes. But C.elegans had neither genes of fibrillar collagens, nor elastin, nor fibronectines, i.e. the typical biopolymers of the connective tissue extracellular matrix; these connective tissue genes, in a form similar to the present one, only appeared in vertebrates (Hutter et al., 2000).

The macromolecular components of a basement membrane have a different origin. Specific components of the lamina basalis are expressed by the ectodermal cells located therein. The cells of the connective tissue express components of a reticular structure, non-separated from the connective tissue matrix.

The main macromolecular components of basement membranes are type IV collagens, specific glycoproteins, as well as specific proteoglycans.

The collagens of basement membranes are presented by six isoforms of **type IV collagen** polypeptide α-chains: α1(IV), α2(IV), α3(IV), α4(IV), α5(IV), and α6(IV). These chains, with a little difference in the amino acid composition from each other, are encoded by the 6 respective genes: *Col4α1, Col4α2, Col4α3, Col4α4, Col4α5,* and *Col4α6.* The genes are localized in pairs in three different chromosomes; they are also expressed in pairs, as each pair of genes shares the same promoter (Sado et al., 1998).

The polypeptide chains α1(IV) and α2(IV) are seen throughout basement membranes. They compose a collagen macromolecule having the formula $[\alpha1(IV)]_2\alpha2(IV)$. The remaining four isoforms of polypeptide chains are less common; they are seen only in the basement membranes of some organs and form macromolecules in various combinations, both homomeric and heteromeric.

Demands to the mechanical properties of type IV collagens are less strict in comparison with those to fibrillar collagens. This accounts for the possibility of numerous interruptions in the triple-helic domains, providing macromolecules with certain flexibility in polypeptide chains. Mutations causing these alterations are most likely to have originated long ago, even in invertebrates; then the genes' altered exon composition was firmly fixed.

At the same time, the extraordinary importance of basement membranes in the earliest stages of ontogenesis, which is evidenced by the above-mentioned gene's phylogenetic conservatism, resulted in the extreme stability of genes of the most common collagen of basement membranes–collagen $[\alpha1(IV)]_2\alpha2(IV)$. Mice with null mutation of this type IV collagen isoform failed to be generated. Such mutations are fatal and animals die at the very beginning of embryogenesis.

The remaining four isoforms of the polypeptide chains of more specialized type IV collagens are very liable to mutagenic exposure. More than 200 mutations of these collagens are already known.

In all polypeptide chains of type IV collagens, there are numerous (at least 20) structural defects of the triplets Gly-Xxx-Yyy essential for collagens: any other amino acid residue substitutes glycine residue. When building a triple helical macromolecule, such a substitution is followed by an interruption of the triple helix, since any amino acid residues in this position, other than glycyl, are not packed in the triple helix. Therefore, type IV collagen is considered a non-fibrillar collagen. At points of interruption, the molecule loses its rigidity and gains a certain flexibility. This, in turn, creates obstacles for macromolecules' regular arrangement in fibrils, which is specific for fiber-forming collagens and manifests as their cross-striation; type IV collagens have no cross striation.

Type IV collagens contain about 10% (in weight) carbohydrates–glucosamine, glucose, galactose, mannose, fucose and sialic acid–in attached di- and oligosaccharides. Such a content of carbohydrates is higher than that found in most other collagens.

Type IV collagen macromolecules look like a flexible thread about 40 nm long. In a long central domain of collagen $[\alpha1(IV)]_2\alpha2(IV)$, the triple helix has 26 interruptions; these small interruptions are located irregularly but in various species, the interruption's location is rather conservative, indicating the definiteness of such a location. The C-terminal domains of three polypeptide chains, consisting of 227–229 amino acid residues including 6 cysteine residues, form a globular structure stabilized by intramolecular disulfide bonds.

The N-terminal domain of type IV collagen macromolecules (the data provided herein refer to the α1(IV)-chain) starts with a non-spiralized sequence of amino acid residues, including 4 cysteine and 2 lysine residues. Then follows a triple helix domain consisting of 39 typical collagen tripeptides, which is separated from the central triple-helix domain by a larger interruption compared with the subsequent one (Martin, 2000).

The molecular mass of polypeptide chains (165–180 kDa), synthesized by cells, changes insignificantly during post-translation processing. Both the N-terminal and C-terminal domains are almost completely retained and are used in the formation of supramolecular structures. Synthesized macromolecules leave the cell in approximately 100 minutes since the beginning of a polypeptide chain assembly (translation takes 10 minutes and the hydroxylation of proline and lysine residues and glycosylation take 40 minutes). This is significantly longer than the time interstitial collagen macromolecules stay in a cell, which does not exceed 20 minutes. Such a difference owes to the delayed formation of triple helical conformation, which is due to multiple errors in the amino acid sequence regularity.

Having reached the necessary localization nearly the cells expressing them, the secreted macromolecules of type IV collagens serve as material for the self-assembly of peculiar aggregates in a net-like formation (Khasigov et al., 2004), forming a base for the entire complex supramolecular architectonics of basement membranes and supporting its stability (Poschl E. et al., 2004).

Besides type IV collagens, type XVIII collagen is found in some basement membranes; it comprises a special family of non-fibrillar collagens called **multiplexins** (proteins with **multiple** triple-helix domains and interruptions), along with type XV collagen (see *Table 3.1*) (Erickson&Couchman, 2000).

Three isoforms of type XVIII collagen are known. This collagen is of interest in two aspects. First, it is a proteoglycan, notably a heparan sulfate proteoglycan. Second,

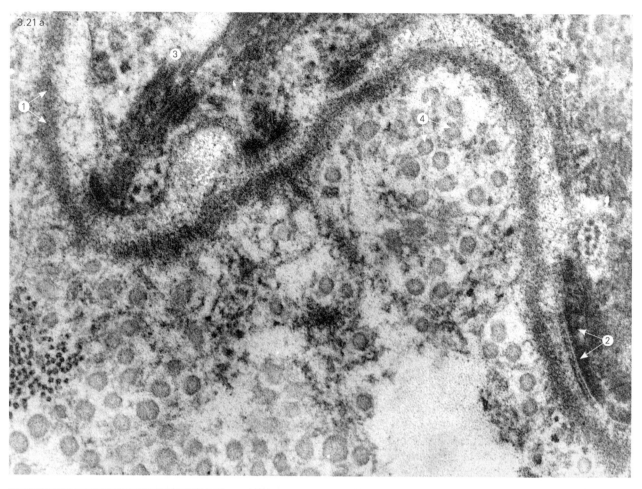

3.21 a

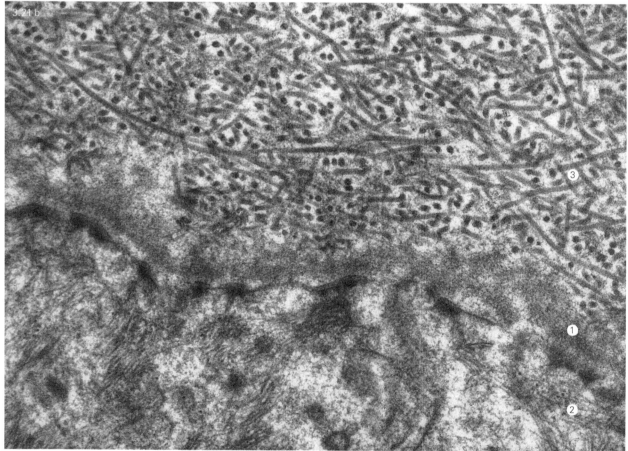

3.21 b

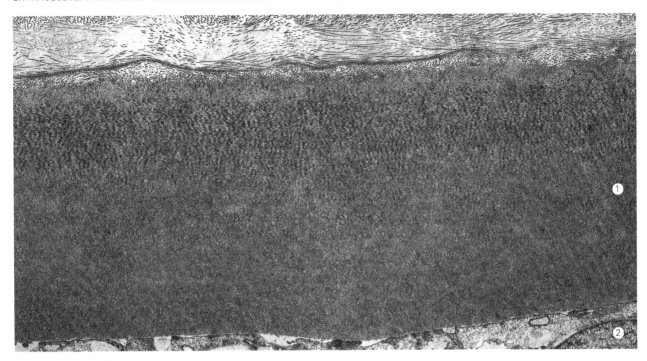

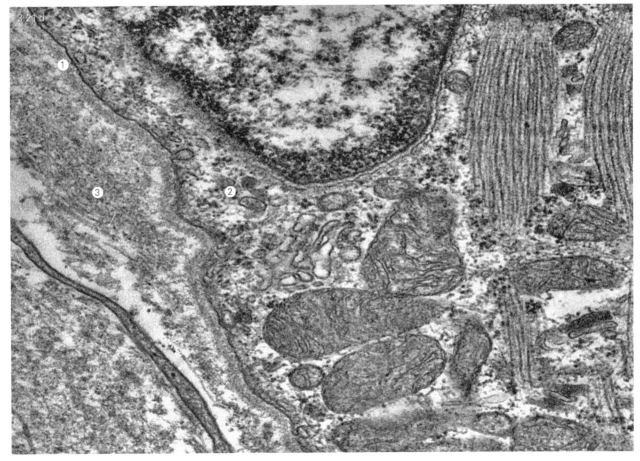

Fig. 3.21.
Fragments of basement membranes.
a – a human skin basement membrane (1).
Hemidesmosome (2) A part of a keratinocyte (3)
Keratinocyte tonofilaments (4).
Collagen fibrils (4) of the dermis subepidermal plexus (according to V.I.Semkin).

b – anterior basement membrane(1) of the cornea – between the epithelium(1) and Bowman's membrane. Collagen fibrils of Bowman's layer (3).
c – posterior basement membrane(1) of the cornea (Descemet's membrane) (under the endothelium(2)).

d – basement membrane(1) in skeletal (striated) muscular tissue between skeletal myocyte(2) and connective tissue(3).
e – a glomerulus basement membrane (1).
Podocyte processes (2).
Bowman's space (Urinary space) (3).

Endotheliocyte processes (4)
A capillary's lumen (5).
A part of a red blood cell (6)
TEM-micrograph.
Contrasting of ultrathin sections with uranyl acetate and lead citrate.
a, b – x 50,000, c – x 1,500,
d – x 20,000, e – x 5,000.

being the only collagen carrying heparan sulfate chains adds to the list of heparan sulfate proteoglycans of basement membranes. What is of special interest is that its carboxyterminal domain contains an antiangiogenic peptide with a molecular mass of 22 kDa, called **endostatin** (which delays blood vessel growth by inhibiting the proliferation of endothelium cells). Moreover, endostatin also exhibits an anti-tumor activity possibly associated with its antiangiogenic effect.

Type XVIII collagen is found in the basement membranes of striated muscle, the cardiac muscle, kidneys and in other localizations. Its function there is unknown.

Among the glycoproteins of basement membranes, **laminins** occupy the central place. fifteen laminins' isoforms are known.

The large macromolecules of laminins are cross-like in form. Two small globules are located on each arm of the crossbar of this structure. Two similar globules are located on the upper region of the longitudinal bar; sometimes the third, smaller globule is also detected here. The largest globule is located at the base of the long bar. Laminins' macromolecules have a heterotrimeric structure: each one consists of three polypeptide chains encoded by individual genes. According to one of the established nomenclatures, the polypeptide chains are named α, β and γ with the addition of a digital symbol of the laminin isoform; for example, in laminin-1, it would be α1-, β1-, γ1-chains, and the relative genes would be called *Lama1*, *Lamb1* and *Lamc1*.

Five isoforms of the α-, 4 β- and 3 γ-polypeptide chains of

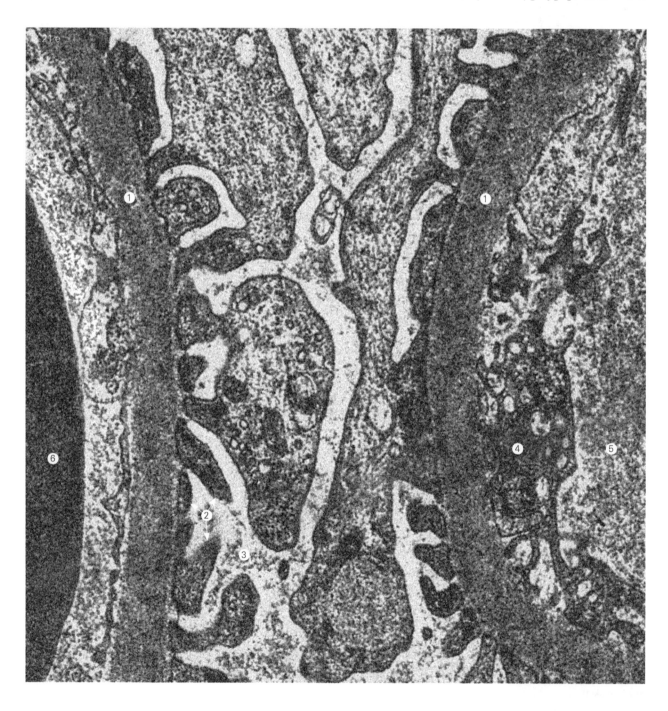

laminins and at least 15 isoforms of heterotrimeric macromolecules, composed by various combinations of these chains, are known (Hallmann et al., 2005). Such a diversity of laminin isoforms is one of the factors providing the structural and functional peculiarities of basement membranes in different tissues and organs.

The length of the longitudinal ("vertical") bar, passing the basement membrane entire thickness, is about 120 nm. The length of this bar upper region and of both, not fully identical arms of the crossbar, is about 40 nm. The total molecular mass of the laminin-1 macromolecule is approximately 800–850 kDa, more than 400 kDa of which comes to the α-chain and approximately 200 kDa for each of shorter β- and γ-chains. (Lodish et al.,2003).

In the longitudinal bar, all three polypeptide chains are untied into a triple helix, stabilized by disulfide bonds in the region of an intersection, and, in the large globule, localized at the bar base.

Laminins' macromolecules have a multidomain structure. A large number of cysteine-rich EGF-like modules is a peculiarity of the linear interglobular domains of polypeptide chains. A part of domains is specialized for self-assembly functions and for stabilizing the macromolecules themselves and their binding to each other; the other domains' function is in selective binding to other components of basement membranes and cells (Suzuki et al., 2005). Thus, laminins are adhesive glycoproteins.

Laminins' macromolecules contain a significant amount (12–15% in weight) of carbohydrates as N-linked, structurally various oligosaccharides.

A number of glycoproteins, related to laminins in their functions in basement membranes and structured homologically to laminins, is known although their differences from laminins are somehow more prominent than those between laminin isoforms. They are **merosin, kalinin, nicein,** and **epiligrin. Netrins** are also included in this superfamily. These are laminin-like glycoprotein molecules that, along with laminins, are found in basement membranes (Koch et al., 2000).

The expression of laminins' isoforms and the glycoproteins related to them is strictly genetically determined (Aberdam et al., 2000).

The domain structure of laminins provides for their multifunctionality, with the functions of individual isoforms being specific. The main common functions of laminins are determined by their ability to interact with cells and modulate their behavior, on the one hand, and, on the other hand, by their interaction with other macromolecule components of basement membranes, particularly with type IV collagen.

Laminins' binding to cells is mediated by specialized membrane receptors–integrins (see 3.6.3). A number of integrins (α1β1, α2β1, α3β1, α6β1, α7β1, and α6β4) serve as laminins' receptors in many cell types (Belkin & Stepp, 2000). The transmembrane receptor protein **dystroglycan** and other receptors of a cell membrane are also involved in interactions with laminins (Colognato & Yurchenko, 2000).

Binding to laminins mediates cell attachment to a reticular framework of the basement membrane formed by type IV collagens, as the direct connection of cells to these collagens is impossible.

Laminin-5 (the molecular formula is α3β3γ2) performs a special function in a skin basement membrane. It is bound to epithelial cells (keratinocytes) given the participation of integrin α6β4. Together with the phosphorylated protein **plectin** and a variety of other proteins (BP230, BP180 and others), this laminin forms hemidesmosomes, multicomponent adhesive complexes binding epithelial cells to the extracellular matrix and basement membranes (Borradori & Sonnenberg, 1999). At the same time, laminin-5 binds to the N-terminal "non-collagen" domain of type VII collagen (Borradori & Sonnerberg, 1999), which forms fine, so-called anchoring fibers holding the epidermis and dermis together. This binding is done by the laminin-5 β3-chain (Nakashima et al., 2005). Without type VII collagen, a separation of the skin's epidermal layer from the dermal layer occurs (Sitaru et al., 2005). Thus, along with type VII collagen, laminin-5 provides the structural integrity of the skin's epidermal and dermal layers.

One of globular modules (LG4) of the laminin-1 α1-chain is essential for the normal morphogenesis of epithelial structures (Ekblom et al., 2003).

The multiple interactions, which laminin macromolecules can enter into, determine the laminins' leading role in assembling basement membranes.

Besides laminins and the glycoproteins related to them, other glycoproteins are essential components of basement membranes.

One such glycoprotein is **osteonectin** (SPARC) (see section 3.2.1.1), also known as BM-40 (basal membrane-40). It is located on the endodermal surface of the basement membrane. Among the manifold interactions of SPARC with proteins, it interacts with type IV collagen. The absence of osteonectin, caused by null mutation in mice, negatively affects the structural integrity of basement membranes and, for instance, manifests as a lens capsule disruption.

Nidogen-1 (entactin) is a dumbbell-like macromolecule with a molecular mass of 150 kDa, which consists of 1,217 amino acid residues and is about 30 nm long. The macromolecule contains about 5% carbohydrates, part of which is sulfated. There are three thickenings–globular domains (G1, G2, G3) in the macromolecule; G2 and G3 domains are connected by a rigid rod-like structure built by 5 EGF-like domains. Nidogen-1 actively binds to laminins via its C-terminal G3 domain; the laminin γ1-chain is involved in forming this bond. Nidogen also binds to type IV collagens; the center for collagen binding is located in the G2 domain.

The second nidogen isoform has been discovered and characterized–nidogen-2 (Kohfeldt et al., 1998). In all, 46% of amino acid sequences of this isoform are identical to nidogen-1. A nidogen-2 molecule, also comprising 3 globular domains, is a little bigger than that of nido-

Table 3.6
Proteoglycans of basement membranes

Proteoglycan	Core protein (kDa)	Glycosaminoglycans (type and number)
Perlecan	400–467	Heparan/chondroitin sulfate (3)
Agrin	250	Heparan sulfate (3)
Bamacan	138	Chondroitin sulfate (3)

gen-1; it consists of 1,375 amino acid residues with a molecular mass of 200 kDa. Nidogen-2 contains a great number of N- and O-linked carbohydrate groups. It interacts with type I and IV collagens and is very active as a cell adhesion factor. Its adhesiveness is associated with the presence of RGD-sequences in both nidogen macromolecules (Erickson & Couchman, 2000).

Besides the glycoproteins here listed, basement membranes contain some other ones.

The main proteoglycans contained in basement membranes are listed in *Table 3.6*.

The **agrin** and **bamacan** listed in the table are present only in some basement membranes. Agrin is characterized as an organizer of the post-synaptic membrane of the neuromuscular junction. It is also found in the cartilaginous extracellular matrix and possibly plays a certain role in endochondral ossification. The less-studied bamacan is found in the embryo basement membrane, separating the trophoblast from the parietal entoderm.

Perlecan is practically universally spread in basement membranes. Its macromolecule resembles a chain of pearl beads in electro-microscopic imaging; hence its name.

A perlecan polypeptide chain carries three glycosaminoglycan chains. All three chains are attached to the N-terminal end. The polypeptide chain is very long and, has a complex multidomain structure. (Olsen, 1999).

The first N-terminal domain, rich in acidic amino acid residues, contains three SGD tripeptides used to attach heparan sulfate chains (in some tissues perlecan heparan sulfate is entirely or partially displaced by chondroitin sulfate). The same domain has six residues of serine (or threonine) to which galactosamine-containing O-oligosaccharides are connected, and one asparagine residue, carrying N-oligosaccharide.

Domains II, III and IV possess a significant degree of homology to laminin polypeptide chains and, in total, the structures of perlecan and laminins' macromolecules are very similar.

The longest domain IV encoded by 40 exons contains 21 repeats of amino acid residues, which are homologous to immunoglobulins.

A perlecan gene, along with genes of other components of basement membranes, belongs to the phylogenetically oldest genes. It is found in the earliest stages of embryogenesis. A little later, perlecan deposition occurs in each and all basement membranes of vascularized organs. However, the distribution of this proteoglycan is not limited by basement membranes. It is detected in the connective tissue extracellular matrix, mostly in the matrix's pericellular zones. A lot of perlecan is in the tumor stroma. Unlike the other macromolecules of basement membranes, perlecan is mainly synthesized by fibroblasts.

Modified variants of perlecan macromolecules are found in a number of localizations; these variants are likely to be alternative splicing- mediated isoforms or result from extracellular proteolysis. The variants where heparan sulfate is substituted by chondroitin sulfate are also known.

The main function of perlecan is to bind to other components of basement membranes, in particular, to laminins and nidogens and, thus, to organize a process of membrane self-assembly.

However, perlecan functions are not limited to its participation in the basement membrane structure. A multidomain structure of the perlecan macromolecule manifests in prominent multifunctionality (Knox & Whitelock, 2006). Perlecan binds to many other components of the extracellular matrix and to cells. The ability to bind to cells, which is mediated by integrin β1 and β3 components, depends on the C-terminal domain of the perlecan polypeptide chain. This process is also influenced by perlecan glycosaminoglycans connected to the N-terminal domain. As a result of all these interactions, perlecan takes on the role of an extracellular framework involved in cell adhesion and in binding growth factors as, for example, fibroblast growth factors FGF-2 and FGF-7, as well as the platelet-derived growth factor

PDGF-β, and a variety of morphogens. This perlecan function regulates the activity of signaling molecules and modulates various signaling pathways in the extracellular matrix. The role of the perlecan framework also expands to apoptosis regulation (Farach-Carson & Carson, 2007).

Besides perlecan, basement membranes contain other proteoglycans, including those containing heparin or chondroitin sulfates, other than heparansulfate. A part of glycosaminoglycans are present in basement membranes in proteoglycan molecules that are smaller than in perlecan. Their role can be attributed to the filtering function of basement membranes.

Type XVIII collagen, which contains heparan sulfate as it has already been noted above, is one of basement membranes' proteoglycans.

The building of basement membranes as morphologic structures occurs by means of **self-assembly** of laminin and type IV collagen macromolecules' aggregates. Initiators of this process are laminins (Sasaki et al., 2004) and, in some cases, netrins related to laminins (Yurchenco & Wadsworth, 2004). Here the central role is played by laminin-1, the only laminin that is present in all germ layers in the earliest stages of embryogenesis (in mice starting from the 7th day) (Gersdorff et al., 2005). The expression of glycoprotein SMOC-1 (secreted modular calcium binding protein-1), from the SPARC family (osteonectin), is evident equally as early as in forming basement membranes (Gersdorff et al., 2006).

Laminin, at first oligomeric and then polymeric aggregates, are assembled owing to the interaction of the end regions of both macromolecules' short and long arms. Electron-microscopic imaging shows that each arm can simultaneously interact with more than one adjacent arm.

The significance of laminins in initiating the formation of basement membranes was seen in experiments on animals with switched-off genes. In null mutation of a laminin-5 γ1-chain gene mice die by the 6th day of embryonic development due to a complete lack of basement membranes in the organism (Schneider et al., 2006). The null mutation of the widespread α5-chain is fatal; other membrane components–type IV collagens and perlecan–are herein found in the extracellular matrix as spontaneous clusters (Erickson & Couchman, 2000).

Aggregates of laminin macromolecules are assembled into a network interacting with another net-like structure, formed by type IV collagens. The N-terminal regions of four collagen molecules overlap each other in parallel, are bidirectional, and are fixed by disulfide bonds and the intermolecular links typical for collagens, whose buildup is catalyzed by lysyl oxidase. This tetramer region is sometimes called a 7S-domain. Intermolecular links originate between the globular C-terminal domains of two macromolecules. The lateral association of triple helix regions of these domains leads to the formation of a more complex supercoiled structure. As a result of all these intermolecular interactions, the regular aggregates of a reticular (or net-like) supramolecular structure originate.

Both networks–laminin and macromolecules' aggregates assembled from type IV collagen–are interwoven. This united supramolecular structure, to which type XVIII collagen macromolecules connect, forms the base of basement membranes. The spatial localization of both networks to each other is determined firstly by immediate bonds between collagen macromolecules and laminin arms and, secondly, by the inclusion of nidogen molecules into the double network. The C-terminal domains of nidogen molecules can bind the triple helix domains of collagen macromolecules and γ-chains of the laminin macromolecules between them. Nidogen molecules, which actively connect with the amino acid sequence Asp-Asn-Val (Mayer et al., 1998), thereby become binding bridges between the two networks.

Obviously the formed construction possesses mechanical properties (strength and flexibility) sufficient to ensure the mechanical functioning of basement membranes–the support for epithelial or parenchymatous cells. But as theoretical calculations have shown, the sizes of double network cells are too large to provide the second function of basement membranes–the function of a molecular "sieve" or filter, regulating access for various molecules from the extracellular matrix to the cells. These sizes are not an obstacle for molecules whose size approaches that of an albumin molecule.

Such obstacles are formed owing to the connection of perlecan and other heparan sulfate proteoglycans to the network. Laminins serve as the main site for proteoglycan connection, but proteoglycans are also able to bind to collagens. Large hydration spheres, creating additional obstacles for molecule motion, surround the glycosaminoglycan chains of proteoglycans. Electrical charges of heparan sulfate are also obstacles. Eventually the basement membrane gains the properties of an anion filter, enabling its effective control of cell metabolism (Iozzo, 2005).

The results of experiments on mice with nil mutation of the perlecan gene indicate how perlecan is essential for the normal assembly and normal functioning of basement membranes (Costell et al., 1999). Homozygous mice with this mutation are nonviable, 70–80% of them die before the 12the day of embryogenesis due to the underdevelopment of basement membranes in the cardiac muscle, which leads to hemorrhaging into the pericardium. In mice that sustained this period, fatal malformations of the central nervous system develop a little later due to defects in the meninges' basement membranes. Later, disturbances of chondro- and osteogenesis due to alterations in the dynamics of chondrocyte differentiation are detected in those animals that survived (Olsen, 1999).

A hypothetical image of the supramolecular architectonics of a typical basement membrane is provided by Yurchenco & Schittny, 1990.

3.4. INTERSTITIAL (INTERFIBROUS AND EXTRACELLULAR) SPACE OF CONNECTIVE TISSUE

An interstitial space is the second link of microcirculation and represents a system of interconnected interfibrous spaces, which are filled with an integrating buffer metabolic medium. The shift of fluid and the substances dissolved therein considerably depend on the form and sizes of these spaces. The interstitial space is most studied in the bone tissue, where it is presented by the system of canals and lacunae, which have distinct borders.

From a physical-chemical point of view, the interstitial space of bone and other connective tissues is a porous space, and the canals are pores. Porosity is defined as free volume per unit of the total volume of the sample studied (Martin, 1986). A specific surface is the area of an internal surface per unit of the volume of the sample studied. Various physical and chemical methods, such as mercury and centrifugal oil porosimetry, gas adsorption, pycnometry and others are used to study porosity and the internal surface (Gregg & Sing, 1982). At the same time, an investigation of porosity and a specific surface of the compact bone tissue can be carried out by taking the graphic measurements of bone canals by means of a specially developed mathematical model (Martin, 1986). Morphological methods of investigation provide some information on the forms, spatial relationships, and orientation of the interstitial spaces. A complex methodical (morphological and physical-chemical) approach makes it possible to establish the comparative correlation between the visual and quantitative data.

According to the organization levels of fibrous structures, an interstitial space is classified into intermolecular, intermicrofibrillar (intrafibrillar), interfibrillar (intrafibrous), and interfibrous (tissue).

In comparing differential porograms, i.e. the size distributions of the interstitial spaces of various connective tissues, it is possible to track the similarity and differences in their characteristics. First of all, this implies the percentage of spaces ("canals") with various equivalent diameters. The porograms of cartilaginous and dense (regular and irregular) connective tissues differ mostly. "Canals" with equivalent diameters of 50–150 nm make up the greatest part in the former and, in the latter, they are about 6,000 nm. It is obvious that such a difference is due to the structural differences of the fibrous base. The distinct conformity between the sizes (equivalent diameters) of fibrous elements and interstitial canals has been established after studying various types of the connective tissue (Omelyanenko, 1991; 2005). The "structure" of the interstitial space of the connective tissue will be discussed in detail for each particular type.

3.5. STRUCTURAL PECULIARITIES OF CONNECTIVE TISSUE VARIOUS TYPES AND THEIR ORGAN SPECIFICITY

3.5.1. Morphological characteristics of connective tissue of various types

The structure and biochemistry of fibrous elements, their orientation and volume ratio to the interfibrous and intercellular spaces, as presented above, form the basis for allocating the fibrous tissue as follows: loose irregular, dense regular (oriented), and dense irregular (non-oriented) connective tissues (CT). Each of the above-listed types of CT has the peculiarities of a cell composition.

A fibrous loose irregular connective tissue has a collagen-elastic fibrillar fibrous framework (base) *(Fig. 3.22)*. The collagen fibers are spiralized, have a circular form in cross-sections, and a thickness ranging from 1 to 10 µm. The collagen fibrils comprising the fibers are circular in form, and most of them have an equivalent diameter or thickness of 70–90 nm. The fibril branching is rarely seen. The fibers' surface has a distinct longitudinal relief, formed due to a superficial layer of collagen fibrils, comprising fibers and segregating fibrillar aggregates in their composition, i.e. smaller fibers. A system of binding cross fibrils is prominent. The collagen fibers are located without any distinct preferable orientation within a framework, confirming a low anisotropy factor (less that 7%) (Omelyanenko, 1981; 1983; 1991). It is intrinsic quantitative orientation characteristics (in the given case, it is the absence of preferable orientation) that underlie the "irregularity" (to be precise – non-orientation) of this type of connective tissue, which was previously distinguished solely by a visual evaluation of histologic specimens when comparing them to other types of connective tissue.

Elastic fibers (fibrils) are circular in form, without prominent spirality; the thickness ranges from 0.5–3 µm (it is mainly 1.5 µm); the surface relief is not distinct and is not arranged. The fibers are located without orientation. There are areas (zones) of immediate contact with collagen fibers or fibrils via proteoglycans. These contact zones are obviously of significant functional importance in maintaining the structural integrity of the entire fibrous framework and its 3D construction, which corresponds to the middle of the physiologic mobility structural range of a particular organ topographic type of connective tissue. *The range of structural physiologic mobili-*

Fig. 3.22.
A fragment of fibrous loose irregular connective tissue externally surrounding the connective tissue coat of eye coating (sclera) of sheep.
Collagen fibers and fibrils (1).
Elastic fibers (fibrils) (2)
SEM-micrograph. x 1,200.

ty is an interval between the extreme (opposite) limits of a structure deformity (distention, compression, twisting) (considering the duration of its deformation process) when the natural (physiologic) organization of a cell, tissue, organ is not damaged or altered, and when exposure to the deforming factor is discontinued, the structure returns to its initial condition in a self-induced (spontaneous) manner.

As a rule, in deformations within a range of physiological mobility, the conditions are created for returning a deformable object into the initial state without residual deformation.

"Distention" (deformation) of the connective tissue framework under the adequate load is associated with straightening of collagen fibers and fibrils, i.e. with the peculiar despiralization of fibrous elements probably of all structural levels of organization. However, the molecular organization of collagen fibrils is essentially not changed. For elastic fibers (fibrils), the alteration of a spatial form under the load is obviously the cause of the conformation molecular alterations (but not damage), leading to a change (augmentation) in the structure energy state (entropy reduction). When the load is removed, the elastic fibers, like an elastomer, revert to the initial state without residual deformation (if the load was not out-of-limit and has not caused structural damage). Considering the local, but regular link between elastic and collagen fibers, the latter also restore their natural form con-

siderably due to elastic fibers. When glucoamilase or hyalunidase destroy the proteoglycans binding collagen and elastic fibers or when elastase selectively dissolves elastic fibers, a form of collagen fibers is restored only partially after relieving load–stretching and this process occurs very slowly.

The maximal distances between the adjacent collagen fibers can exceed their maximal thickness. A network of individual collagen fibrils, collagen, fibrillin, fibronectin or other microfibrils is located in spaces between collagen and elastic fibers. Interfibrous and intercellular spaces of the loose connective tissue (as well as its other types) are filled with the integrating buffer metabolic medium, whose structural base is formed by proteoglycans and glycoproteins organized in different structural forms. Relatively large spaces, exceeding 100–200 nm, are filled with a reticular structure *(Fig. 3.23)* (described in detail above, along with others structured proteoglycans, see section 3.2.1.3).

The "looseness" of the connective tissue type discussed, also defined earlier by the comparative visual estimation of a connective tissue in histologic specimens, has been fairly quantified. This estimation is the quantitative characteristic of the interfibrous, intercellular (interstitial) space by means of physical-chemical methods, in combination (comparison) with TEM and SEM findings (Omelyanenko, 1978; 1991). For example, a specific vol-

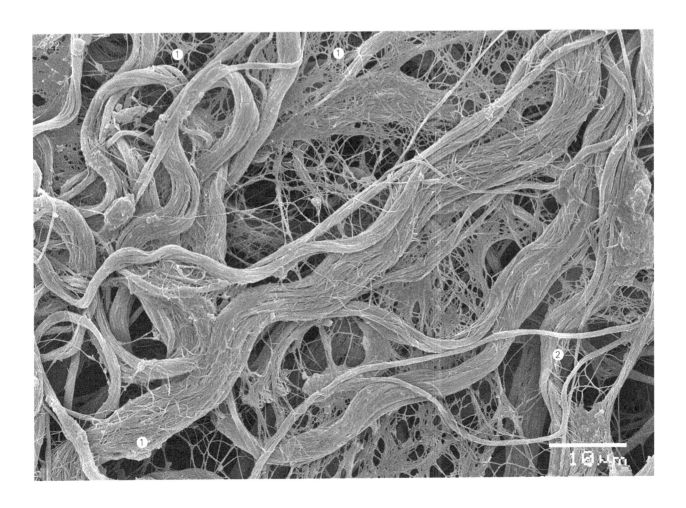

ume (SV) of the interstitial space, reflecting the density of connective tissue, is 2.1 cm³/g. The size of interfibrous gaps in equivalent diameters ranges from 0.15–120 µm. There are 80% of equivalent diameters ranging from 10–50 µm among them.

All of the aforementioned is integrated in the image seen in *Fig. 3.24*. The structural organization of fibrous loose irregular connective tissue determines the intensity of its trophic function in relation to the organs it comprises or surrounds. At the same time, it acts as a peculiar "reductor" or a mediator between organs with a different composition of a fibrous framework and therefore, with different mechanical properties.

In fact, the CT cells of a fibroblastic differon are rather regularly distributed throughout the interstitial space. Associated cells of the connective tissue are also present there.

A fibrous dense irregular connective tissue has a collagen-elastic, fiber-fibrillar non-oriented fibrous framework *(Fig. 3.25)*. The collagen fibers are spiralized, have a circular form at the cross-sections, i.e. they are cylindrical or flattened, and their thickness ranges from 1–20 µm. The collagen fibrils comprising the fibers are circular in form at the cross-sections, and most of them have an equivalent diameter or thickness of 90–110 nm *(Fig. 3.1; 3.4; 3.5; 3.6)*. The fibril branching occurs rarely. The structure of collagen and elastic fibers and their re-

lationship *(Fig. 3.7)* are, for the most part, similar to those in the loose irregular connective tissue. Structured proteoglycans of the integrating buffer metabolic medium are also present as several morphologic formations *(Fig. 3.20)* (Omelyanenko, 1978; 1991). The ratio of the fibrous part of the extracellular matrix to the interstitial space is the main difference between loose and dense irregular connective tissue. The special volume (SV) of the interstitial space indicates the density of connective tissue is 1.17 cm³/g inertly dehydrated tissue in the dense irregular connective tissue when compared to SV 2.1 cm³/g for the loose CT, i.e. it is nearly twice as dense. It is obvious that this represents narrower interfibrillar spaces, for which the size of equivalent diameters ranges from 0.15–100 µm and, what is more important, 85% of the spaces with equivalent diameters range from 3–37 µm. Therefore, in addressing the image in *Fig. 3.24*, for it to be considered a model of fibrous dense irregular connective tissue, the number of fibrous structures therein can increase (be added).

The structural difference of the two types of connective tissue discussed shifts the functional emphasis from the dense irregular connective tissue to the supportive (including mechanical protective) functions, herein retaining the trophic and other functions.

The fibrous dense regular connective tissue has a collagen-elastic, fiber-fibrillar or fibrous, oriented frame-

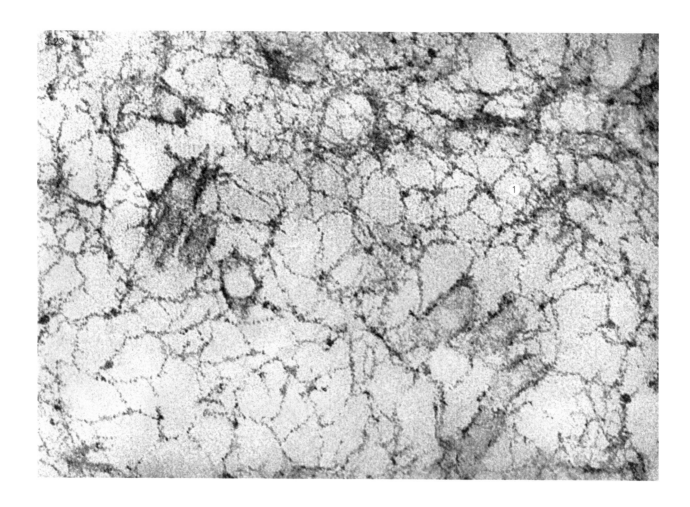

work *(Fig. 3.26).* The collagen fibers have a circular or multiangular form at the cross-sections, and range in thickness from 1–50 μm; their spirality is less prominent than in collagen fibers of the loose and dense irregular connective tissue. The collagen fibrils, comprising part of the fibers, are circular in form. The fibrils' equivalent diameters can vary considerably, from 30–150 nm, and can be homogeneous or be distributed as several size groups; the degree of branching varies depending on organ specificity. The fibers' surface has a distinct longitudinal relief formed due to a superficial layer of collagen fibrils, comprising fibers. The system of binding cross fibers or fibrils is evident. The collagen fibers are closely adjacent to each other. They have a primary orientation corresponding to a vector or vectors of the forces affecting the connective tissue. This confirms a high anisotropy factor (more than 50%) (Omelyanenko, 1983; 1991). The primary character of orientation determines the "regularity" (to be more correct–directivity) of the given connective tissue. There are elongated fibroblasts between the collagen fibers.

The elastic fibers (fibrils) are circular, their spirality is not prominent, and they range from 0.5–3 μm (mainly 1.5–2 μm) in thickness; the superficial relief is distinct and is not arranged. Most of the fibers are spatially oriented along collagen fibers. The relationship of elastic and collagen fibers is similar to that of the above-mentioned types of connective tissue. The interfibrous spaces are filled with the integrating-buffer metabolic medium, the structural base of which is formed by proteoglycans and glycoproteins, organized mainly in a fine granular amorphous substance.

The "density" of this type of CT, also defined earlier by a comparative visual evaluation of the ratio of interfibrous interstitial space to fibrous structures of the connective tissue in histologic specimens, now has a characteristic specific volume (SV) of 0.46 cm^3 (Omelyanenko, 1991). The comparison of this data to the specific volume of the dense irregular connective tissue (SV – 1.17 cm^3/g) shows that the oriented structures "are packed" more densely than non-oriented ones and therefore, have more strength in stretching forces towards the long axes of collagen fibers.

The allocation of the three CT types described above is conditional to a certain degree and represents only the general, most typical structural features of both of the comprising individual components of the connective tissue and their composition as a whole. There can be many transitive variants of the CT structure in an organism, which cannot exactly be assigned to any of the classified tissues. In such cases, it is desirable to describe their structure according to those signs that have been presented, and to specify the approximate degree of conformity to one or another type of connective tissue.

3.24

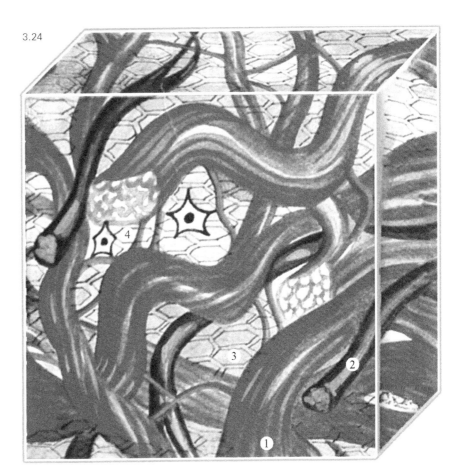

Fig. 3.23.
A ruthenium-positive reticular structure of a proteoglycan nature (1) filling up the interfibrous and intercellular space in fibrous loose irregular connective tissue. TEM-micrograph. Staining with red ruthenium. x 50,000.

Fig. 3.24.
Image of the structural organization of fibrous loose irregular connective tissue. Collagen fibers (1). Elastic fibers (2). Integrating buffer metabolic medium (3). Cell elements (4) (according to Omelyanenko, 1984).

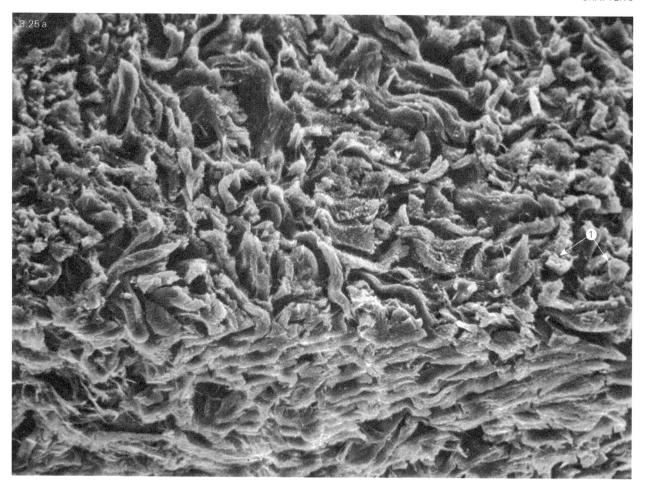

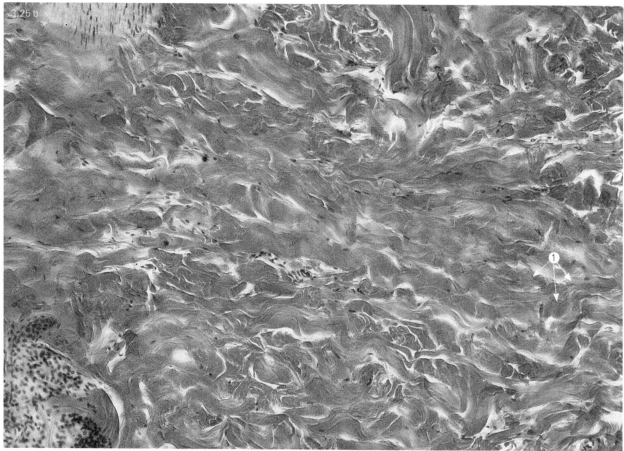

The organ specificities of the connective tissue's structural organization are certainly determined by the function of a particular organ and, consequently, the connective tissue can be classified by functional significance into three types:
1) the connective tissue performing the basic function in an organ or its part,
2) additional functions, and
3) combined functions.

3.5.2 Peculiarities of organ structure of fibrous connective tissue

The skin dermis mainly consists of the connective tissue. The reticular layer is made by the fibrous dense irregular CT, which, as described above, is exemplified by the dermis (Fig. 3.25); thus, its description is not provided here. The papillary layer is formed by the fibrous loose irregular CT. The dermis' deep layer, without interruption, passes into the loose irregular connective tissue of the subcutaneous fat. Therefore, the dermis' fibrous framework is an integrated structure, though it is made up of two types of fibrous connective tissue (Omelyanenko et al., 1977; Omelyanenko & Zerebtsov, 1987).

The structural organization of the connective tissue logically differs in the dermis of the skin integument's different topographical areas. These peculiarities primarily relate to the construction of a fibrous framework and proteoglycan composition, which primarily indicate the mechanical (supporting) function of the connective tissue in these areas.

A unique property of connective tissue is its ability to grow under stress conditions such as distortion. If a human or animal skin is stretched, i.e. to get its fibrous framework into one of the extreme conditions of the physiologic mobility scale and hold it in such a state for a long time, there will be a remodeling of collagen and elastic fibers and fibrils towards their elongation and inversion of the initial spirality that was lost when stretched. Re-stretching will have the same effect. This property has distinct clinical relevance as it facilitates the creation of a skin "reserve" for autotransplantation. On the other hand, this property prevents the long-term effect of plastic surgery on the face skin ("lifting") in order to eradicate wrinkles and to produce the visibility of rejuvenation.

Fig. 3.25.
A fragment of fibrous dense irregular connective tissue.
A reticular layer of the human skin dermis.
Collagen fibers (1).
a – SEM-micrograph.
An angled section of the dermis sample. x 300.
b – LM-micrograph.
Histologic section.
Staining with hematoxylin and eosin. x 300.

Achilles tendon. The base of the Achilles tendon base is comprised of fibrous dense regular connective tissue, which, as described above, is exemplified by the Achilles tendon; thus, its description is not provided here. The fibrous framework is fibrillar, collagen-elastic, and oriented (Fig. 3.26). The peculiarity of the Achilles tendon CT is the intensity of the collagen fibrils' branching and their allocation into two main groups by the following diameter sizes: 30–70 nm and 150–200 nm (Fig. 3.27). Most of the collagen fibers are located parallel to each other along the tendon's long axis. Their borders are defined by elongated fibroblasts and the fibrocytes located in narrow interfibrillar spaces (Fig. 3.26) (Omelyanenko et al., 1981; Omelyanenko, 1983).

Densely and parallel located collagen fibers are united into bundles of the first order. Each bundle has a connective tissue membrane and is separated from the adjacent one by narrow spaces, where there are fibrous loose connective tissue and cells of a fibroblast differon. Several bundles of the first order, surrounded by a shared connective tissue membrane, comprise bundles of the second order. The latter are also separated from each other by wider spaces, filled in with fibrous loose connective tissue. In sites characterized by the convergence of several bundles, there are spaces filled with the fibrous loose connective tissue where the blood vessels and nerves pass. Smaller interlayers spring into the interfascicular spaces, as well as thinner blood vessels, and nerves branch from this loose connective tissue perpendicularly to the direction of the longitudinal vessels.

Thus, two types of connective tissue combine in the Achilles tendon, one of which performs the main biomechanical function, while the other has an accessory function that is both integrating and trophic.

The fibrous dense regular connective tissue also prevails in **the nuchal ligament**. The fibrous framework is collagen-elastic, fibrillar, and oriented. However, the equivalent diameter of collagen fibrils is more homologous and is 60–70 nm. Fibril branching occurs rarely.

The connective tissue in **skeletal (striated) muscles** is organized the same way as in the tendon connective tissue, which performs an integrating function, combining main collagen and elastic fibers into structural and functional units. The connective tissue surrounds every muscle fiber (endomysium) (Fig. 3.28), bundles of muscle fibers (perimysium), and muscle as a whole (epimysium). Meanwhile, it also (loosely) fills in the spaces between the above-listed muscular elements. This connective tissue supports the structural organization of the muscle tissue and muscles, and provides their interaction and necessary synchronicity in contraction. The fibrous elements of the endomysium, perimysium and epimysium connective tissue are arranged in different directions, creating a particular framework for muscular elements that prevent the possible destructive consequences of intense contractions. The blood vessels and nerves providing trophism and the regulation of the muscle tissue pass in the connective tissue, filling the gaps between

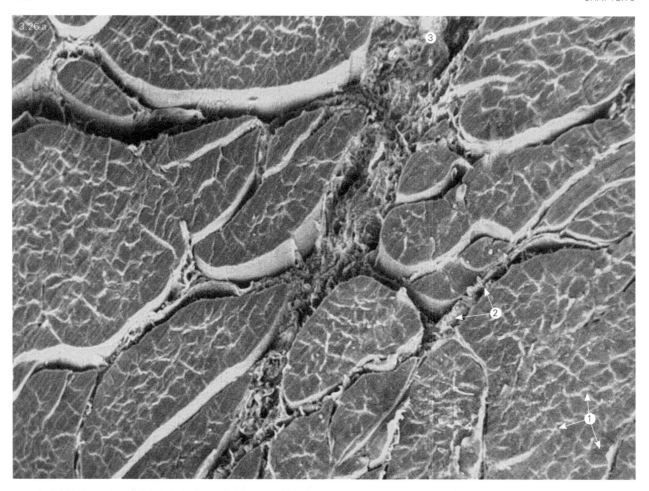

3.26 a

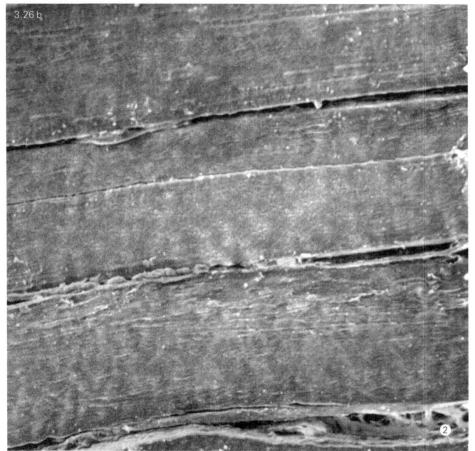

3.26 b

Fig. 3.26.
A fragment of the human
Achilles tendon.
Collagen fibers and their
bundles comprising dense
regular connective tissue (1).
Connective tissue interlayers
between the bundles
of collagen fibers of the first
and second orders (2).
Fibrous loose irregular
connective tissue surrounds
blood vessels and nerves
in the interbundle spaces (3).
Tenoblasts and tenocytes (4).
a, c – a tendon cross-section;
b, d – a longitudinal section;
a, b – SEM-micrograph.
x 100.
c, d – LM-micrograph.
Histologic sections.
Staining with hematoxylin
and eosin. x 100.

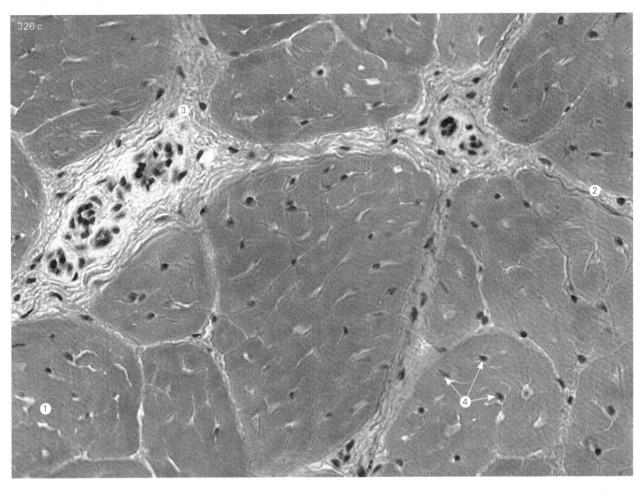

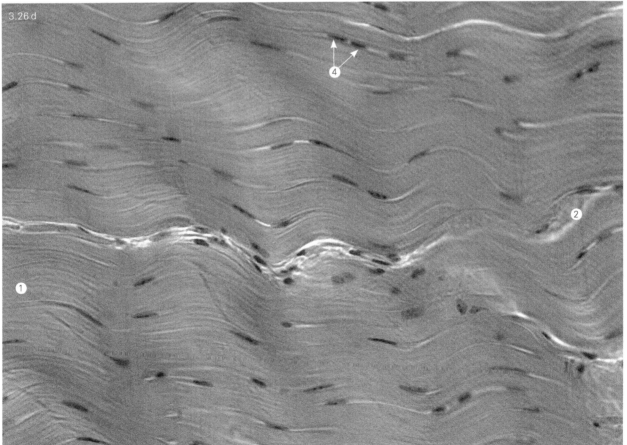

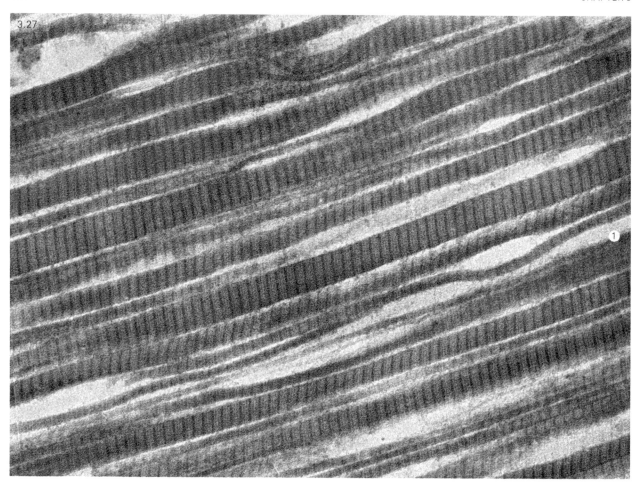

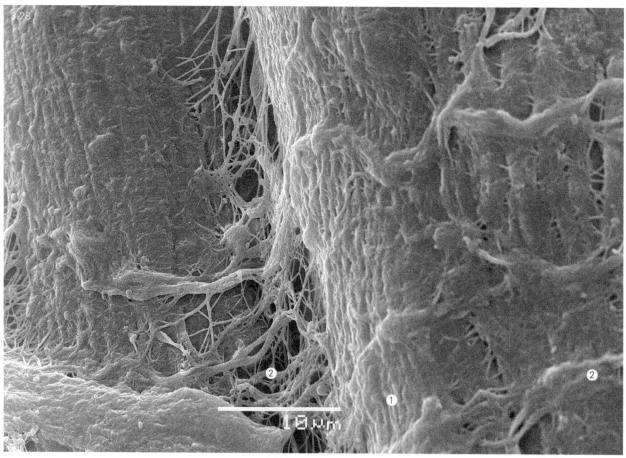

muscle fibers, their bundles and muscles. Muscles' long-term contracting or inflammation can lead to the rearrangement of the muscles' fibrous framework, wherein the range of its physiologic mobility does not correlate to that of the muscles. Therefore, the restriction of natural movement and pains arise therein both in human and in animals.

Cornea and Sclera. A fibrous dense regular connective tissue is the base of the eye bulb connective tissue membrane. Its fibrous framework is mainly composed of flat or flattened collagen fibers, which are arranged in several layers and oriented parallel to the eye bulb surface. In this plane, the collagen fibers' orientation is determined by the uniaxial arrangement of collagen fibrils therein, making the fibers apparently anisotropic (the anisotropy factor is more than 50%). This feature distinguishes adjacent collagen fibers from each other.

Despite the general principles of the architecture, the structure of the cornea fibrous framework differs from that of the sclera. The thickness of the human adult cornea is 550–600 µm at the "pole" (the most protruding part) and 600–700 µm at the periphery. Outside the cornea fibrous framework is separated from multilayer flat non-squamous epithelium the basement membrane (with a thickness of 90–110 nm), the main structural element of which is type IV collagenous protein *(Fig. 3.29 a)*. The basement membrane borders with a Bowman's (anterior border) layer *(Fig. 3.29 a, 3.21 b)* that is 8–10 µm thick. That this membrane is comprised of separately located (i.e. non-forming fibers) collagen fibrils is its specific peculiarity. Type I and III collagenous proteins make up the fibrils' base. The fibrils have no preferred orientation, i.e. they are non-orderly located. The fibril thickness and diameter is 20–40 nm. The fibrils of the Bowman's layer do not branch and are comprised of flat or flattened collagen fibers of the cornea's main fibrous layer *(Fig. 3.29 f, 3.29 e)*. They retain the same diameter as in the l Bowman's ayer but they have a prominent general preferred orientation; that is, they are located parallel to each other, thereby determining the anisotropy of the cornea fibrous layer. The cornea collagen fibers may consist of one layer of parallel located and similarly oriented collagen fibrils. The thickness of such fibers is 0.8–4 µm. Part of the fibers can have several fibrillar layers. In this case, their thickness is 4–10 µm *(Fig. 3.39 f,e)*. At the same time, the direction of fibrils of the same layer is, as a rule, perpendicular or tangential to the di-

rection of fibrils of the adjacent layer. The same angular orientation of the configuration takes place between adjacent collagen fibers *(Fig. 3.29 g, 3.29 h)*.

For the cornea, the flattened collagen fibers have 3D undulation *(Fig. 3.29 c,d,e,g,h)*. The "undulation" does not coincide in adjacent fibers; therefore, cavities are formed between the fibers; these cavities provide high porosity in the cornea.

The cavities' size is not the same from the bowman layer towards the descemet membrane *(Fig. 3.29 c, 3.29 d)*. In the external quadrant, the cavities' size at sections ranges from 7×10 µm to 15×45 µm (the largest part is 15×25 µm). In the second quadrant, the cavity size ranges from 7×10 µm to 30×65 µm (the largest part is 15×45 µm). The cavity size in the third quadrant ranges from 15×40 µm to 50×120 µm (the largest part is 30×50 µm). In the inner quadrant, the cavity size is from 15×35 µm to 30×120 µm (the largest part is 30×60 µm). In this cornea area, the cavities exhibit a more elongated form with the long axis located parallel to the cornea's surface.

The structured proteoglycans filling these interstitial spaces retain the water in them, which is obviously one of the factors determining the cornea's transparency. The branching and integration of the collagen fibers are intense in the cornea; they look more like the lamination and fusion of the flat fibers.

Collagen fibrils of the cornea's inner quadrant fibers contact directly with the Descemet's membrane *(Fig. 3.21 d, 3.29 b)*. Part of them is surrounded by the granular substance comprising the membrane. There are no collagen fibrils in its structure. Threads or filaments, the base of which is comprised of type IV collagen, generally make up the membrane. Cells of the endothelium *(Fig. 3.21 d, 3.29 b)* are adjacent to (in direct contact with) the Descemet's membrane from the other side. The aforementioned peculiarities indicate that the Descemet's membrane is a peculiar basement membrane that has a thickness of 8–10 µm, as well as specific structural features.

The transition of the cornea into the sclera (a limbus area) or visa versa gradually occurs. The cornea "overlaps" the sclera from the eye globe outside. Within the limbus center, the thickness ratio of the cornea and sclera is approximately equal. The sclera terminates (or starts) at the border between the limbus and the cornea. From the limbus' other side (i.e. along its border with the sclera), the cornea starts (or terminates). This transition (the limbus) is somehow thicker than the cornea and sclera. Changes in the structural organization do not result in the disintegration of the whole construction of the fibrous framework of the eye connective tissue's coat as collagen fibrils or the fibers of conditionally divided eye parts are continuous formations and pass from one part into another. Therefore, the aforementioned general principles of their structure are retained.

Thicker flat collagen fibers, the absence of evident undulation, the close contact of fibers to one another and the resulting very small interfibrillar spaces, low porosity

Fig 3.27.
A fragment of a human tendon collagen fiber.
Collagen fibrils (1) are of differing thickness; they branch, and are oriented parallel and along the tendon long axis.
TEM-micrograph.
Contrasting of the ultrathin sections with uranyl acetate and lead citrate.
x 60,000.

Fig. 3.28.
A fragment of the striated (skeletal) muscular tissue of sheep.
Muscle fibers (1).
Fibrous loose irregular connective tissue on a surface of muscle fibers (endomysium) and in the spaces between them (2).
SEM-micrograph.
x 2,500.

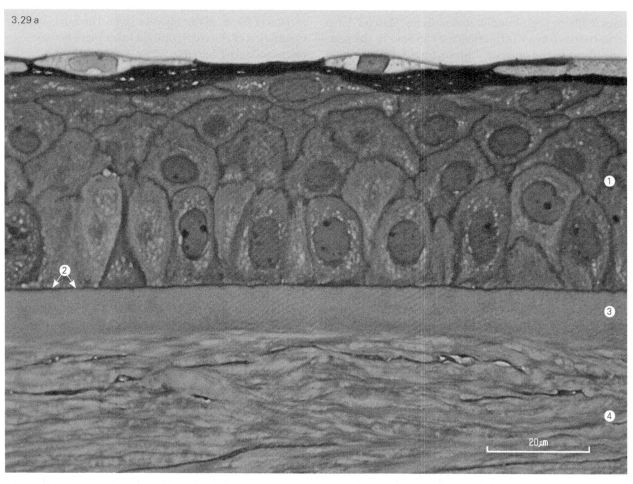

3.29 a

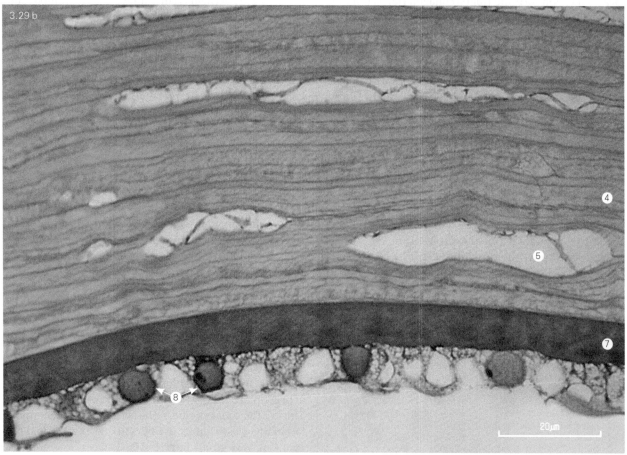

3.29 b

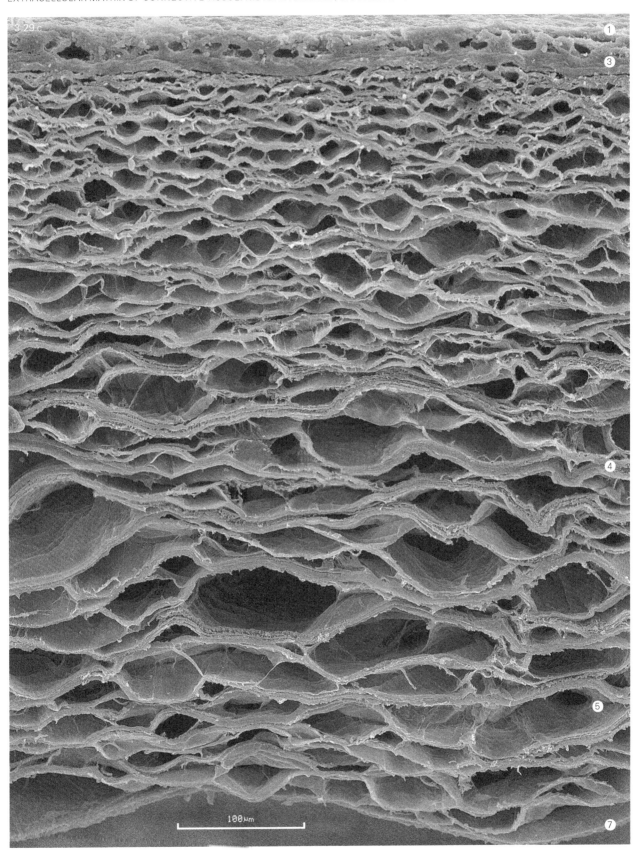

Fig. 3.29.
A connective tissue coat of
a human eye – the cornea.
a,b,c,e,f – a perpendicular
section of the cornea surface.
d – an angled section of the
cornea sample.

g, h – a parallel section
of the cornea surface.
Cornea epithelium (1).
Basement membrane (2).
Bowman's layer (3).
Flat collagen fibers (4).
Interfibrillar cavities (5).

Collagen fibrils (6).
Descemet's membrane (7).
Endothelium (8).
a, b – LM-micrograph.
Histological slices.
Staining with azur eosin.
x 1,000.

c, d, e, g, h – SEM micrograph.
c, d, g, x 250. e – x 1,200.
h – x 2,000.
f – TEM-micrograph.
Contrasting with lead
citrate and uranyl acetate.
x 50,000.

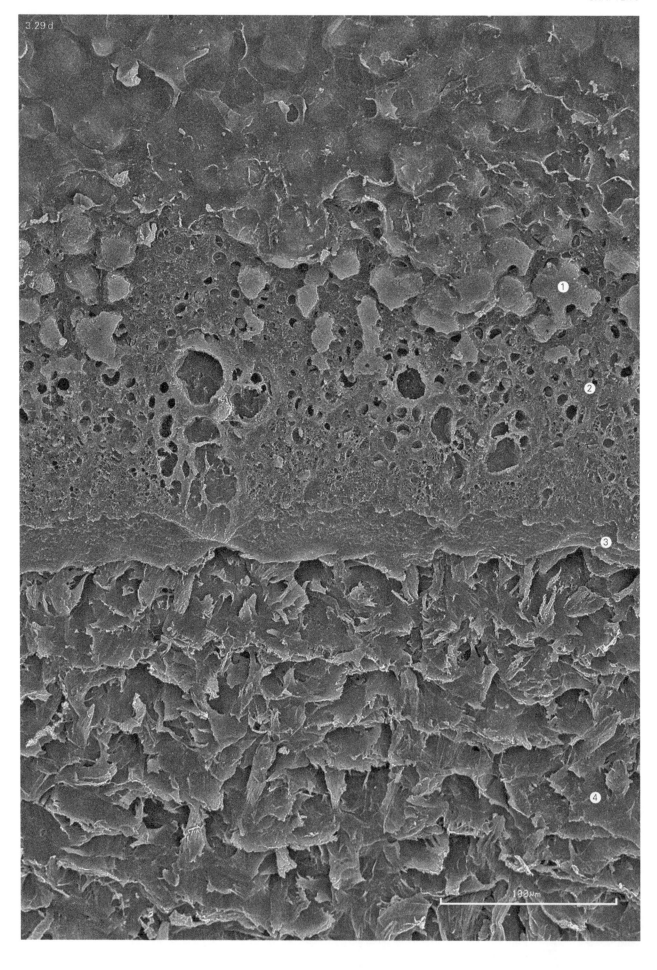

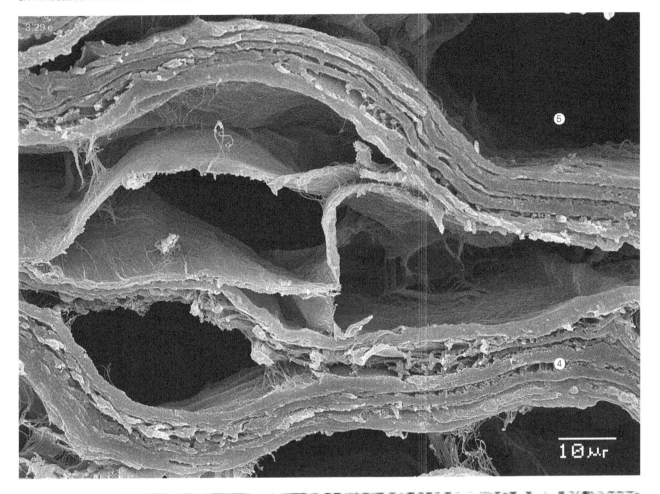

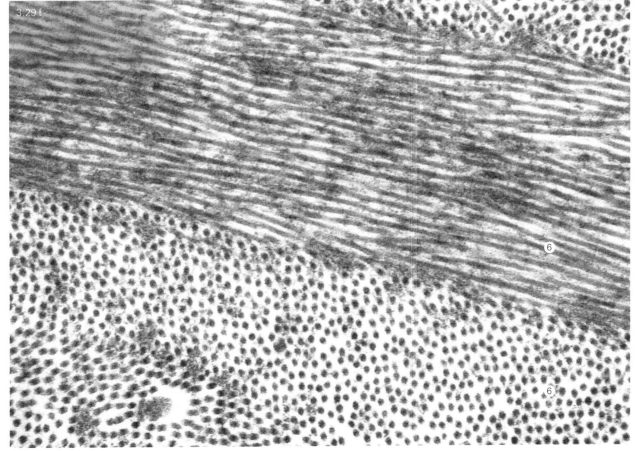

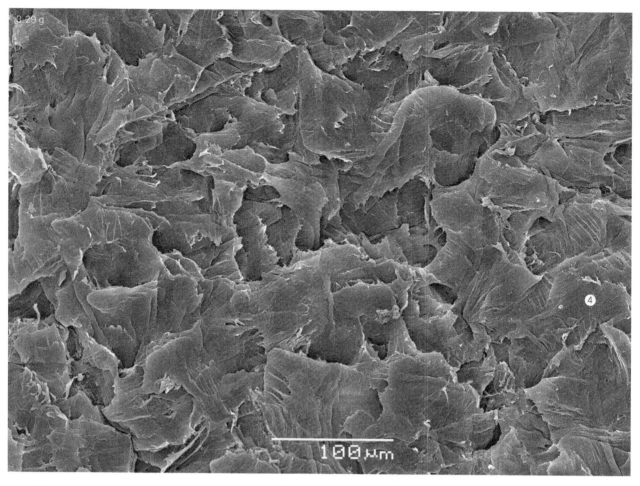

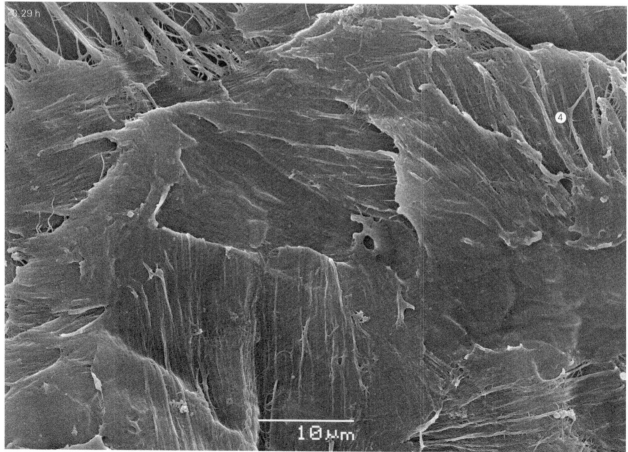

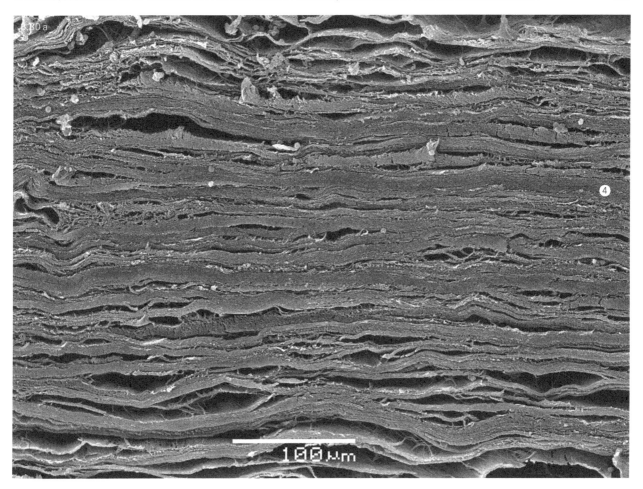

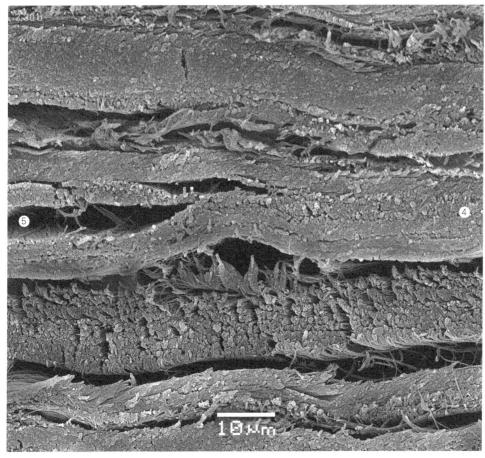

Fig.3.30.
A connective tissue coat
of a human eye – the sclera.
a, b – a perpendicular section
of the sclera surface.
c, d – a parallel section
of the sclera surface.
Flat collagen fibers (1).
Interfibrillar cavities (2).
SEM-micrograph.
a, c – x 250.
b – x 1,200.
d – x 2,500.

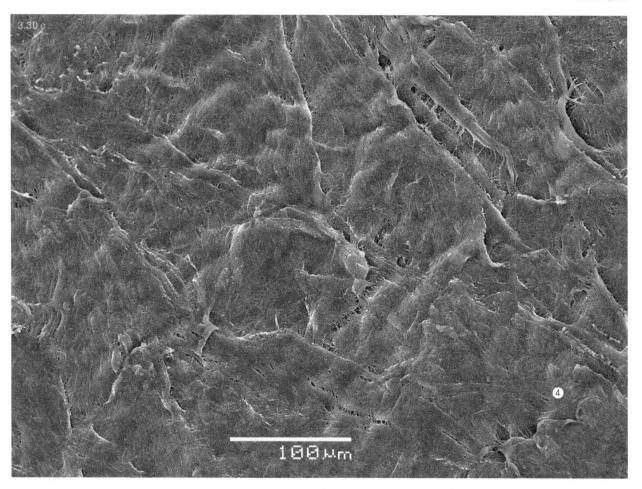

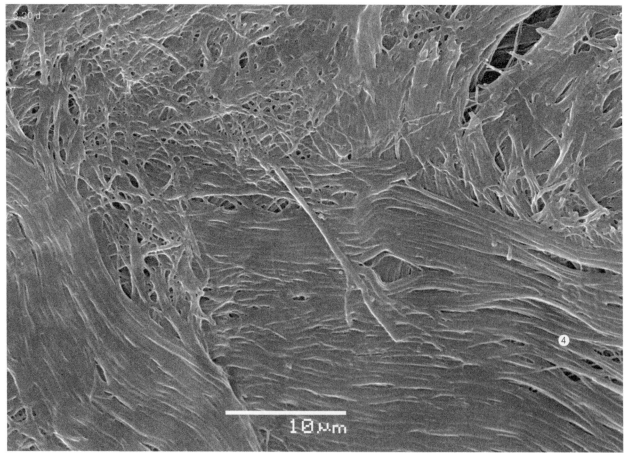

and high density significantly distinguish the sclera from the cornea *(Fig. 3.29 b)*. It is obvious that such a construction provides the sclera with light-tightness.

The determined differences between the sclera and the cornea are as follows: the sclera's thickness is 300–400 µm, which is significantly less than that of the cornea (Fig. 3.30 a); in turn, sclera flat collagen fibers are 5–15 µm thick, which is thicker than in the cornea *(Fig. 3.30 a,b)*. The fibers' undulation is not pronounced and is not very evident; the collagen fibrils are more loosely located within the fibers. At the same time, the gaps between the fibers are narrow; therefore, the fibers are densely adjacent to each other, indicating the low porosity and high density of the sclera structure.

The eye connective tissue coat is an integrated fibrous system, which maintains an eye globe oval form, limiting the pressure of the eye inner fluid medium. This is provided by the circular location of fibers at different angles to each other.

Outside the sclera, collagen fibers pass into thinner flat collagen fibers. These fibers, in turn, pass into the fibers (of a circular form at cross sections) of loose irregular connective tissue, which entirely surrounds the eye globe from the side of the orbit. Some sclera thickening and the formation of a peculiar outgrowth from loose irregular connective tissue by fibrous connective tissue are observed at these sites of muscle attachment to the eye globe. The inner part of the sclera fibrous framework borders with the vascular coat. The circular-linear (meridional-parallel) orientation of the collagen fibers of the sclera and loose irregular connective tissue takes place around the optic nerve leaving the eye globe.

There are also species-related differences in the structure of the eye bulb connective tissue membrane. This is especially specific for the cornea. In sheep, the general principle of the fibrous framework structure described for the human cornea applies. However, there are distinctly outlined cavities with a prominent internal surface resembling that of the endothelium that lines the cornea's internal surface in sheep cornea. The lamination of the internal lining of these cavities from the walls limiting them is evident in several regions. The cavity size can reach 500×300 µm. These cavities are capable of communicating with one another, forming a system of interstitial canals. Another type of cavity (of a significantly smaller size, 150×30 µm), which is only possibly gaps, contains internal partitions dividing the cavities or interfibrillar gaps into individual compartments. These partitions are also flat collagen fibers, but they are thinner than the main ones. The sheep sclera differs less from the human one, although numerous but small canals are also found therein.

Fibrous Membranes. They include fascia, aponeurosis, the tendon center of diaphragm, dura matter, sclera, perichondrium, periosteum, as well as the perididymis, joint capsules and others. A fibrous dense regular connective tissue forms their base.

Fibrous membranes are little stretched. The collagen fibers have indistinct spirality and are located densely, in a particular order, in several layers, one above another. In each layer, the collagen fibers and their bundles pass parallel to each other and are oriented in the same direction, but they do not follow the direction of the adjacent layers. Individual bundles of fibers pass from one layer to another, binding them to each other. Apart from the collagen fibers, elastic ones are also present in fibrous membranes.

Solid (parenchymal) organs generally contain loose irregular connective tissue, which performs form-supporting, integrating and trophic functions.

Based on an analysis of the structural organization of fibrous elements and the integrating buffer metabolic medium of different types of connective tissue described above, a number of regularities of their structure have been distinguished.

The fibrous elements of all types of human and animal connective tissue have five levels of structural organization *(Fig. 3.3)*. Every level is represented by one element or groups of them with an identical structure as follows:

1) the molecular level – molecules of different types of collage, such as elastin, fibrillins, glycoconjugates and others; the qualitative and quantitative composition is genetically determined and is regulated by the microenvironment of CT-synthesizing cells, as well as local and systemic regulation factors;

2) the supramolecular (microfibrillar) level is presented by collagen protofibrils, microfibrils, fibrillin microfibrils and an amorphous-filamentous substance; the structural organization of elements of this level is determined by the spatial relationship and specific interaction of the macromolecules involved in their construction; the formation and maintenance of the structural integrity is provided and regulated by the microenvironment conditions and components;

3) the fibrillar level consists of collagen and elastic fibrils; the fibril structural organization is determined by the spatial relationship and the interaction of both elements of the previous levels (macromolecules and microfibrils) involved in their composition and the fibrils amongst themselves; the formation and maintenance of the structural integrity is provided and regulated by microenvironment conditions and components, as well as dynamic structuring factors;

4) the fibrous level – collagen, elastic and combined (collagen-elastic and elastic-collagen) fibers; the fibers' structural organization is determined by the spatial relationship and the fibrils' (collagen and elastic) interaction with the participation of glycoconjugates in fibers' composition, by the interference of the adjacent fibers incorporated in the upper organization level and the integrating buffer metabolic medium surrounding the fibers; the formation and maintenance of the structural integrity is provided and regulated by microenvironment conditions and components, as well as dynamic structuring factors and functional remodeling;

5) the tissue level is presented by fibrous frameworks with a varied composition of fibrous elements (colla-

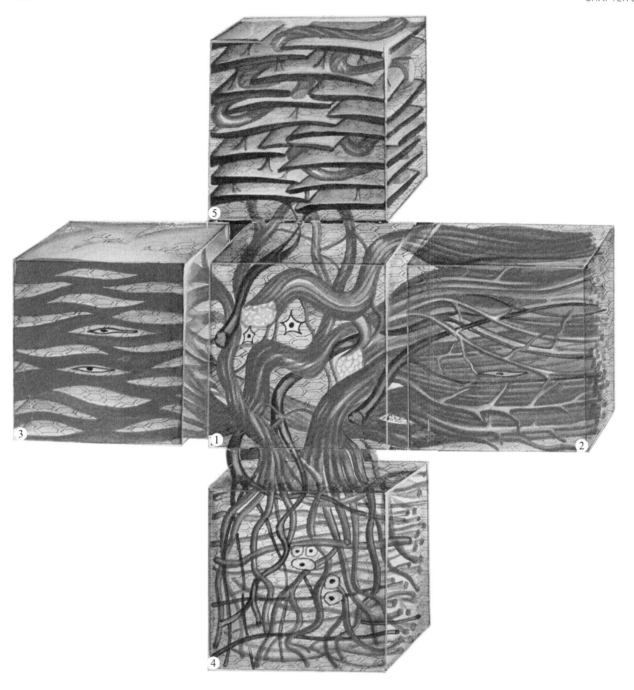

Fig. 3.31.
A summary image of the structural organization of different connective tissue types, their relationship, and the constructive transformation of the fibrous elements and frameworks in transitioning from one type to another. (according to Omelyanenko, 1984). *(see color insert)*

1 –fibrous loose irregular CT, collagen-elastic, fiber-fibrillar, non-oriented type of a fibrous framework.

2 –fibrous dense regular CT, the collagen-elastic, fibrillar, oriented type of a fibrous framework (tendon).

3 –fibrous dense regular CT, the collagen, fibrillar, combined in orientation type of a fibrous framework (cornea).

4 –hyaline cartilaginous tissue. The collagen, fibrillar non-oriented type of a fibrous framework (hyaline cartilage).

5 –the elastic-collagen, fibrillar combined type of a fibrous framework (the aorta middle layer).

gen, elastic, combined; fibrous, fibrous-fibrillar, fibrillar) and by construction (oriented, poorly oriented, non-oriented, combined); the frameworks' structural organization is determined by the qualitative and quantitative composition of their fibrous elements, the character of the spatial interaction and relationship, organ functional peculiarities, interorgan junctions, the integrating buffer metabolic medium of the extracellular matrix;

the specificity (diversity) of the extracellular matrix fibrous frameworks' structural organization depends on the functions of the organ, which the connective tissue is a part of, or its topographic specificity; the formation and maintenance of the structural integrity is provided and regulated by microenvironment conditions and components, as well as dynamic structuring factors and functional remodeling.

Physiological renewal (regeneration) and reparative regeneration are enabled by the synthesis activity of the CT cells, the microenvironment conditions and components, and factors of dynamic structuring and functional remodeling.

The fibrous structures of connective tissues are composed according to general principles such as:

1) collagen structures in all organization level have a spiral conformation and superspirality;

2) they branch and merge, i.e. they rearrange, thereby creating the integrity of the organ's fibrous framework or part thereof;

3) two types of fibrous structures, such as essential and accessory ones, are distinguished by their functional (biomechanical) relevance. Essential collagen fibers are thicker and oriented along the potential stress vector(s) when performing their biomechanical function. Accessory fibers play a binding role, providing for interaction of the essential fibers and maintaining their spatial interrelations and the structural integrity of the fibrous framework.

Adjacent fibrous frameworks of contiguous organs or their parts, differing in their construction, are united by means of passing a part of collagen and elastic fibers from one organ into another directly or via fibrous loose irregular connective tissue (*Fig. 3.31*). The latter mechanism provides a peculiar functional "yawn" for organs with different mechanical mobility.

Several forms, such as a reticular structure, amorphous substance, membranes of collagen and elastic fibrils and others represent structured proteoglycans (SPGs) of the CT integrating buffer metabolic medium (ground substance). All SPGs are interrelated and transform into each other, forming a continuous system, which has structural integrity with elements of the fibrous framework.

The interstitial (intercellular and interfibrous) space is represented by an integrated system of tissue microcanals, which have a particular form, orientation, shape and size distribution. The microcanal parameters are in certain conformity with the organization of fibrous structures of particular types of connective tissue. Therefore, considering the levels of their organization, the interstitial spaces can be classified as follows:

1) intermolecular;

2) intermicrofibrillar (intrafibrillar);

3) interfibrillar (interfibrous); and

4) interfibrous or interfascicular (intratissular). The volume ratio of interstitial spaces and fibrous structures provides a quantified characterization of connective tissues' density.

Components of the extracellular matrix represent an integrated system of all connective tissues of humans and animals. The specificity of their organ-tissue structural organization is determined by a complex of the qualitative and quantitative composition of fibrous elements and the integrating buffer metabolic medium, such as quantitative differences in the fibrous structure orientation, the volume and size distribution of an interstitial space, the equivalent diameters of collagen fibrils, fibers, their bundles, as well as the intensity of qualitative indicators such as the composition and construction of the fibrous framework, the branching and spirality degree of fibrous elements, and the form of structured proteoglycans, among others. Such a complex makes it possible to establish the identification of non-cellular components with a particular type of connective tissue.

3.5.3. Biochemical and molecular biological characteristics of fibrous dense regular connective tissue

Fibrous dense regular connective tissue includes tendons, ligaments, and joint capsules involved in the construction of the locomotor apparatus, along with bone, cartilaginous and muscular tissues.

A tendon cell – a **tenoblast**, whose mature form is called **tenocyte** – is one type of fibroblast and has all the functional (biochemical and molecular biological) properties specific for resident fibroblasts (see section 2.2.1). A tenocyte is not infrequently called a tendon fibroblast. These cells synthesize all components of the extracellular matrix.

At the same time, the tenoblasts differ from other fibroblasts by some functional peculiarities, in particular, by their response to various types of mechanical stress. These peculiarities are largely associated with tenoblast interaction with a specific extracellular matrix produced by this cell (Benjamin et al., 2008).

Tenomodulin, which has several synonymous names, including tendin, myodulin and ChM1L, is a specific marker of tenoblasts' differentiation. This is a transmembrane (one-pass) glycoprotein that contains 317 amino acid residues, 30 of which comprise the cytoplasmic domain, while 266 make up the extracellular one; two N-linked oligosaccharides are connected to the extracellular domain. Tenomodulin is very close to chondromodulin-1, an angiogenesis inhibitor in the cartilaginous tissue. The expression of tenomodulin by tenoblasts is significantly more intensive than its expression by the cells of other tissues. It is essential for the proliferation of tenoblasts/tenocytes, whose number decreases upon switching off the gene encoding tenomodulin; it is also important for the normal fibrillogenesis of tendon collagens (Docheva et al., 2005).

The expression of tenomodulin is stimulated by the protein **scleraxis**, a transcription factor localized in the nucleus (Shikumani et al., 2006). This protein is one of the transcription factors' TF 1.2 family, which has a specific motif bHLH (basic helix-loop-helix). The bHLH motif, comprising the polypeptide chain region from the 88–128th amino acid residues (in total the molecule consists of 201 residues), is preceded by a cluster of basic amino acid residues (from the 73rd–87th residues), which carries out DNA binding. Scleraxis is essential for the morphogenesis of all structures of mesodermal origin; switching off the gene *Scx* encoding this factor in mice results in the absence of the mesoderm and the very premature (on the 8th and 5th day) death of embryos. In the later stages of embryogenesis, scleraxis is only involved in tendon and ligament morphogenesis. Its selective expression is prominent in somites and limb buds, from which tendons are formed (Brent et al., 2003). Therefore, like tenomodulin, scleraxis is considered as a specific marker of tenoblast (tenocyte) differentiation (Schweizer et al., 2001). In tenoblasts, the main function of these cells – the synthesis of fibrillar collagens – is regulated by Scleraxis interacting with DNA, together with another transcription factor, NFATc4, (Léjard et al., 2007).

During tendon formation (tendogenesis), the expression of scleraxis essential for tenoblast differentiation, is stimulated by fibroblast growth factor-4 (FGF-4), which originates in developing muscles. This fact indicates the coordination of tendo- and myogenesis (Edom-Vovard et al., 2002). The expression of scleraxis is also coordinated in an experiment with the expression of the transcription factor Sox9, which plays the central role in regulating chondroblast differentiation (Asou et al., 2002).

The differentiation of the tendons transmitting the force emanating from muscles to skeleton bone elements suffers from a deficiency of scleraxis in embryogenesis. The tendons, whose function is limited to attaching muscles to bones (for instance, tendons attaching intercostal muscles to ribs), as well as ligaments, develop normally. Herein, the molecular differences of tendons, associated with the peculiarities of their functions, manifest themselves (Murchison et al., 2007).

Smad8, one of the intracellular signaling pathway proteins, a member of the growth factor superfamily TGF-β, plays a certain role in choosing the differentiation way of mesenchymal stem cells (MSC) towards a tenoblastic phenotype. The artificially induced excessive expression of Smad8 increases the efficacy of the tenoblastic differentiation of cultured MSCs (Hoffmann et al., 2006).

Besides tenomodulin and scleraxis, the proteins encoded by the genes *EphA4, Six1 and Six2, Eya1* and *Six2, Fst*, as well as the growth factor FGF8, stimulating scleraxis expression, and the transforming growth factor TGF-β2 are considered as specific markers of tenoblasts, particularly those forming extremity tendons. Although used as a tenoblast marker, tenascin C is less specific as its expression in embryogenesis is seen in some other cells (Schweizer et al., 2001).

A zinc fingers-containing protein 537, encoded by a *TSHZ3* gene in a human, is involved in tenoblast differentiation and tendon formation. This is one of three transcription factors TSH ("teashirt") that control a general body pattern, together with Hox-factors (Manfroid et al., 2006).

All dense types of connective tissue contain few cells. These cells from the fibroblast family possess a significant biosynthetic potential. The not numerous tenoblasts manifest their biosynthetic potential, producing and renewing the tendon extracellular matrix, which provides for the performance of the biomechanical function of these structures.

The matrix main component responsible for performing tendons' and ligaments' biomechanical function is, as already mentioned, the great fibrillar **type I collagen**. It comprises the matrix basic mass and, in fact, it comprises the basic mass of the entire tissue due to the fact that there are few cells in it.

However, as in any other type of connective tissue, the extracellular matrix of tendons and ligaments is a complex multicomponent system. The components comprising this system create the conditions essential for the formation of collagen fibrils and fibers, and for their functioning. The extracellular matrix composition is, in general, provided in *Table 3.7*.

Significant variations of the data in the table are noticeable. Several factors can explain this phenomenon.

Firstly, different tendons are not similar in their chemical composition. Secondly, the tendons' biochemical quantitative parameters change with ageing. Thirdly, there are significant differences between the regions of the same tendon – the regions located along the tendon differ from those attached to a bone or muscle. Fourthly, the tendons' biochemical parameters largely depend on the physical exercise they are exposed to; therefore, they reflect the results of tendon tissue adaptation to functional training. We will describe these factors later.

The supramolecular collagen structures of tendons (collagen microfibrils, fibrils, fibers and their bundles) are, in general, comprised of type I collagen. They mainly perform the tendons' biomechanical function – the transmission of muscular effort to skeletal bone elements. The macromolecular organization of type I collagen is obviously adequate to perform this function, which involves such components as resistance to stretching, dispersion and absorption of the tension originating

Table 3.7
Main quantitative characteristics of biochemical composition of tendon tissue

Components	Content (g/100 g of tissue)
Water	55–70
	G/100 g of a dried tissue residue
Collagens:	60–85
Type I collagen	55–70
Type II collagen	0–10
Type IV collagen	~2
Type V and VI collagens, FACIT-collagens	<1
Elastin	~2–3
Fibrillins	~1
Total Glycoproteins and Proteoglycans	1–5
Decorin	<1
COMP	<1
Fibromodulin, Biglycan	0,5–1,0
Other Glycoproteins and Proteoglycans	<1
Inorganic Components	<0,2

in stretching (Franchi et al., 2007). The presence of small amounts of the more flexible type III collagen in the tendons' collagen structures enables them some flexibility (Silver et al., 2002).

The properties of fibrils mainly comprised of large collagens, in particular, of the collagen fibrils and fibers of tendons formed during fibrillogenesis, largely depend on the heterotypical state of their structure (i.e., they depend on the presence of macromolecules of another collagen–type V collagen, one of small fibrillar collagens influencing lateral growth. Hence, the fibril diameter in a fibril structure, along with macromolecules of the prevailing collagen type, in this case it is type I collagen (see section 3.1.1.1).

Moreover, collagen fibrils' properties are influenced by the accompanying macromolecules of non-fibrillar collagens located on their surface, which are, however not in all cases, bound to them by covalent bonds. These are

so-called FACIT-collagens (fibril-associated collagens with interrupted triple helices). Two FACIT-collagens of XII and XIV types are associated with type I collagen, comprising the basic mass of collagen fibrils of fibrous dense connective tissues.

Type XII collagen is a homotrimer with the molecular formula $[\alpha 1 \, (XII)]_3$. Its macromolecule consists of two interrupted triple helix ("collagen") domains (COL1 and COL2) and three non-spiralized ("non-collagen") domains (NC1, NC2, NC3).

The triple helix domains, comprising about 10% of the macromolecule's weight (313 amino acid residues), are located in the macromolecule carboxyterminal region. NC3, together with the NC1 and NC2 domains, forms a region responsible for binding (association) to collagen fibrils. The NC1 domain is known in two variants – long (74 amino acid residues) and short (19 residues) ones – originating as a result of alternative splicing (Kania et al.,

1999). The type XII collagen isoform with a long NC1 domain is predominantly present in tendons and ligaments, while the isoform with a short NC1 prevails in other types of dense connective tissue. The tissue specificity of isoforms' distribution indicates some functional role of the certain domain.

At the N-end of the COL2 domain, there is a globular thickening, from which the NC3 domains of three α-chains, branching as three twigs, begin comprising a significant part of the macromolecule length. Like the NC1 domain, the NC3 domain is also not similar in two known isoforms if type XII collagen (collagen XIIA and collagen XIIB), and these differences also originated as a result of the alternative splicing of the gene first transcript. (Fukai et al., 1994).

A very long NC3 domain of each α-chain of the XIIA isoform consists of four modules (domains) of A type intrinsic for a von Willebrand factor (vWFA), and 18 fibronectin modules FNIII. This isoform of type XII collagen is predominantly expressed by fibroblasts cultured in vitro. The significantly shorter (by 1,165 amino acid residues) NC3 domains of the isoform XIIB, which is present in tissues in vivo, each have two modules of the von Willebrand factor A and 10 FNIII modules.

Unlike the fibril-associated area, NC3 non-collagen domains do not adjoin to the surfaces of large collagen fibrils but project over their surface into the extracellular matrix. Such a location enables NC3 active interactions with other fibrils, cells and non-fibrillar components. Proteoglycans, particularly decorin, are involved in NC3 interactions with cells and matrix non-fibrillar components. The structural glycoprotein tenascin X, one of the tenascin family members (see section 3.2.1.1), occupies a central place in interactions with other fibrils. Tenascin X is bound to NC3 in vitro and co-localized with it in tissues in immuno-histo-chemical investigations. Owing to such a bond with type XII collagen, tenascin X affects the distance between collagen fibrils and thus is involved in regulating the formation of supramolecular architectonics of type I collagen-rich tissues. This role of type XII collagen is especially significant in tendons and ligaments, as well as in the periosteum, endosteum and perichondrium (Veit et al., 2006).

Another FACIT–**type XIV collagen**, associated with fibrils, whose base is comprised of type I collagen, also binds to tenascin X (Lethias et al., 2006). This collagen is known in three isoforms, which resulted from alternative splicing. Is similar to type XII collagen in macromolecule structure. Each α1 (XIV)-polypeptide chain also contains two small (277 amino acid residues in total) triple helix domains (COL1 and COL2) in the C-terminal region; the homology degree of the amino acid composition of both collagens' triple helix domains exceeds 60%. (Tzortzaki et al., 2006).

Non-collagen domains comprise the main part of α (XIV)-chains (the total length is 1,768 amino acid residues after the signal peptide cleavage). Like similar domains of type XII collagen, these non-collagen domains contain modules, which are present in macromolecules of structural connective tissue glycoproteins–fibronectin, laminin, tenascin and others. These modules (vWFA, FNIII and others) carry the attached oligosaccharide groups; therefore FACIT-collagens are glycoproteins (Gerecke et al., 1993).

A "non-collagen" (glycoprotein) part of the type XIV collagen macromolecule had been isolated before the whole macromolecule had and it was called undulin. **Undulin** is known as a large glycoprotein, forming collagen fibril-associated undulated structures seen in electron microscopy (the name undulin is derived from Latin undula–a wavelet). After small collagen domains were discovered in this macromolecule, the name "undulin" and "type XIV collagen" are accepted as synonymous (Ehnis et al., 1997).

The expression of type XII and XIV collagens is tissue-specific. Type XIV is a prevailing FACIT-collagen in the dermis, where it is associated with the fibrils whose base is comprised by type I collagen. On the contrary, the expression of type XIV collagen is not too large in tendons and ligaments where type XII is mainly concentrated. There are also peculiarities in the expression dynamics of both FACIT-collagens in different localizations during embryogenesis (Wälchli et al., 1994). An exchange of type XIV collagen isoforms, involving the NC1 domain, is noticed at the entry of large collagen fibrils into the maturation stage (Young et al., 2000).

Despite the differences, the similarity in macromolecules' structure and their similar localization on the surface of large collagen fibrils determine the common functions of FACIT-collagen of the XII and XIV types. These general functions are referred to regulating the organization process of the collagen structures of fibrous dense connective tissue types, including the formation of bonds ("bridges") between fibrils, as well as the regulation of the fibril's diameter.

The functions of maintaining the fibrils' stability, including biomechanical (deformative) properties, in their interactions with cells and non-fibrillar components of the extracellular matrix, are also common for both FACIT-collagens (Tzortzaki et al., 2006).

The NC3 domains of type XII and XIV collagens are involved in maintaining the fibril's biomechanical stability. In an experiment in vitro, the conformation alterations of these domains induced the activation of fibroblasts' motility in collagen gel while, at the same time relieving the stabilizing effect on collagen fibrils, thereby decreasing their rigidity (Akutsu et al., 1999). These data correlate with the findings of another experiment: exerting the stretching force to tendons resulted in enhancing the expression of type XII collagen by cells (Chiquet, 1999).

Besides the collagens described, the tendons contain a microfibrillar heterotrimeric **type VI collagen**. This collagen is found in bovine tendon tissue along the entire length of the tendon; its concentration is especially high (reaching 3.3 mg/g of fresh tissue) in those regions that are exposed to compression and have the structure of fibrous cartilage. The microfibrils of type VI collagen are involved in the structural organization of the pericellular matrix in these regions (Carvalho et al., 2006). Like FACIT, type VI collagen's function in the extracellular matrix is also associated with tenascin X. In the absence of tenascin X (in switching off of the encoding gene), the expression level of type VI collagen mRNA decreases (Minamitani et al., 2004).

The participation of tenascin X in the functions of FACIT and type VI collagen is one manifestation of this glycoprotein's advanced interactions network with collagen structures. Tenascin X, which is present in tissues *in vivo*, mainly as a homotrimer, is also bound to type I, III and V fibrillar collagens, and finally takes on a critical role in the general structural organization of the fibrillar collagen-containing extracellular matrix (Lethias et al., 2006). This role is shown in an experiment on mice, with the knock-out of the tenascin X encoding gene *Tnx*, to become evident between the E15 and E19 days of the embryonic development, i.e. when the initial stages of fibrillogenesis are over, at the stages of maturation and the stabilization of collagen fibrils and elastic fibers (Egging et al., 2006).

Clinical observations confirm the FACIT-collagen-mediated role of tenascin X in the formation of fibrillar structures. Mutations of the gene *TNX* induce the inhibition of fibrillar collagens' expression, disturbances in fibrillogenesis, and the maturation of collagen structures, manifested as one form of the so-called Ehlers-Danlos syndrome. The symptoms of this syndrome form include overstretching of the skin and pathologic excessive joint mobility (Egging et al., 2006).

Tendons and ligaments contain small amounts of **elastin** in elastic fibers, varying in different tendons and in different regions of the same tendon. The elastin concentration evaluated by cross-links–desmosines specific for this protein – is 1–3 g/100 g of dried dehydrated tissue. The elastin concentration is higher in ligaments than in tendons, and the highest concentration is seen in the nuchal ligament and the lumbar yellow ligament. The elastin content decreases with age (against the background of the increasing content of inorganic components, calcium and phosphorus), with this reduction being more prominent in men than in women (Osakabe et al., 2001).

Fibrillins (fibrillin-1 and fibrillin-2) forming a fiber microfibrillar framework, and the microfibril-associated glycoproteins MAGP-1 and MAGP-2 are present in the elastic fibers of tendons, along with elastin. According to immuno-histochemical findings obtained in the investigation of the deep flexor tendon of fingers, all components of elastic fibers are present in all regions of tendons. The content of fibrillin-2 is more inside the tendon, while fibrillin-1 prevails in the superficial layer. The content of both MAGP is higher in the region of the tendon's attachment to a bone, where the tendon tissue takes on

some similarity with cartilaginous tissue (Ritty et al., 2002).

Fibrillin microfibrils are not only present in tendon elastic fibers. As in many other types of connective tissue, they exist as independent microfibrillar structures, mainly pericellularly, around tenoblasts of the tendon's inner layers.

These tenoblasts, forming small rows between the bundles of collagen fibers, are surrounded by a peculiar matrix, containing fibrillin-2 microfibrils, as well as type VI collagen microfibrils and versican. The microfibrils are oriented along the tendon axis, suggesting fibrillins' participation in the formation of weak elasticity, which is attributable to tendons, along with elastic fibers, taking fibrillin's elastic properties into account (Ritty et al., 2003).

The collagen fibers comprising the basic mass of the tendon's extracellular matrix and carrying the major functional load leave little space for interfibrous ground substance. The total content of **proteoglycans**, a qualitatively prevailing component of this substance, in the tendon tissue, as in other structures formed by fibrous dense types of connective tissue, is not very large (see *Table 3.7*). The main representatives of proteoglycans, which are present in tendons, are listed in *Table 3.8*.

As it follows from the table, most of tendon proteoglycans are members of the family of small leucin-rich proteoglycans (SLRP). The concentration of other proteoglycans is extremely small in the region (zone of stretching) exposed to the stretching force.

Decorin, carrying one (more often) or two glycosaminoglycan chains in the amino terminal domain, which can be dermatan sulfate or chondroitin sulfate, is of the greatest quantity amongst SLRP in this zone. Decorin binds to fibrillar collagens of different types. The glycosaminoglycan and the central domain of the core protein are involved in binding. Its main functions are regulating fibrillogenesis (limiting a fibril diameter) and maintaining the stability of fibrillar collagen structures, which become fragile in the case of decorin deficiency. Moreover, decorin serves as a filter regulating the movement of signaling molecules, in particular of growth factors TGF-β and EGF in the matrix.

Biglycan, falling into the same SLRP class as decorin, performs similar functions. In switching off of the biglycan gene, the tendon's collagen fibrils become thin and weaker; sometimes the ectopic ossification of tendons occurs.

Fibromodulin and **lumican**, close to it in molecule structure, are SLRP of another class. They carry only keratan sulfate chains localized in the central domain and bind to type I collagen by this domain. Unlike decorin and biglycan, fibromodulin and lumican facilitate fibrils' thickness and maturation. Fibromodulin can substitute lumican in the case of a deficiency of the latter, but the inverse substitution in the fibromodulin deficiency, which results in reducing tendon rigidity, appeared to be impossible.

Table 3.8
Main proteoglycans of tendons

Proteoglycans	Properties and functions
Decorin	Binds to fibrillar collagens, inhibits collagen fibrillogenesis, and binds the growth factors TGF-β and EGF
Biglycan	Binds to fibrillar collagens
Fibromodulin	Binds to type I collagen, facilitates the maturation of large collagen fibrils, modulating their tensile strength
Lumican	Binds to type I collagen, restrains the growth of collagen fibrils, and modulates their mechanical properties
Aggrecan	Forms aggregates united by hyaluronan, makes tissue compression-resistant, is primarily present in areas exposed to compression
Versican	Binds to hyaluronan, present in small amounts in the tendon regions exposed to stretching and in more amounts in regions exposed to compression, improves tissue viscoelasticity, and facilitates the retention of the cell form

The large proteoglycan **aggrecan**, the main proteoglycan of the cartilage extracellular matrix's ground substance, is present in those tendon zones that are exposed to compression in bending due to anatomic localization. These zones are localized near the connection of a tendon with a bone and take on the properties of fibrous cartilage, including the presence of type II collagen. Aggrecan aggregates, united by hyaluronan, provide water retention in the tissue (hydration), making the tissue compression-resistant and viscoelastic (Vogel&Peters, 2005).

Another large proteoglycan, **versican**, also predominantly present in the same tendon zones as aggrecan, provides tissue viscoelasticity. Moreover, it maintains the cells' form, optimal for their functions.

The peculiarities of the zonal distribution of small and large proteoglycans indicate biochemical heterogeneity of the extracellular matrix within the same tendon. They also evidence the adaptation of the matrix molecular and supramolecular structure to a biomechanical load–the tendons' main function. The functional adaptation also plays a not less significant role in the formation and maturation of the tendons' entire collagen structure (Zhang et al., 2005) and the expression of the **COMP** (cartilage oligomeric matrix protein) glycoprotein involved in regulating tendon collagens' fibrillogenesis (Södersen et al., 2005).

The functional adaptation of the tendon extracellular matrix to mechanical loads represents unity with the functional adaptation of muscles. The load effects are mediated by the involvement of the system of regulating factors. This system includes the growth factors TGF-β, CTGF, FGF, IGF and binding IGF-proteins, interleukins IL-1 and IL-6 (see section 4.2) (Kjaer, 2003). There is increased expression of these signaling molecules by tenoblasts/tenocytes and the cells of the tissues surrounding tendons. Tenocytes' total metabolic activity increases, which is evidenced by the enhancement of glucose utilization. Collagen synthesis de novo and the remodeling of collagen structures are intensified (Kjaer et al., 2006). From a practical point of view, it should be stated that some regulating factors, such as glucocorticoid hormones for instance, exert opposite, inhibiting effects to the tendon functional adaptation; proteoglycan expression in particular is inhibited (Toricelli et al., 2006).

The remodeling of collagen structures, which is a manifestation of the tendons' functional adaptation, is provided by the metalloproteases MMP-2 and MMP-9 expressed by tenocytes, whose activity is regulated by the tissue inhibitors TIMP-1 and TIMP-2. The metalloprotease activity abruptly increases in tendon damage (ruptures) when the remodeling necessity is especially high (Karousou et al., 2008).

The data provided on the biochemical characteristics of tendons make it possible to formulate the general biochemical peculiarities of dense types of connective tissue. They are as follows:

The marked presence of the extracellular matrix, whose basic mass consists of collagen fibers, mainly comprised of "classic" fibrillar type I collagen;

The involvement of the non-fibrillar FACIT collagens in the formation of the entire system of collagen structures;

The dominant prevalence of small proteoglycans (SLRP), regulating collagen fibrillogenesis in the extracellular matrix ground substance;

The marked adaptation ability of the extracellular matrix to biomechanical functions, provided by effective remodeling mechanisms.

These peculiarities manifest in ligaments to the full extent but, at the same time, even in comparing the biochemical values of such similar structures as tendons and ligaments, the features of their organ specificity should be noted. In ligaments, there are more cells, which are closer to resident fibroblasts than tenoblasts, but exhibit higher metabolic activity than tenocytes (Comerford et al., 2005). The content of the extracellular matrix ground substance is more, the collagen total concentration is lower and the content of type III collagen is higher in the ligaments. As well, the expression of type II collagen occurs in some ligaments, for example, in the knee anterior cruciate ligament. As already mentioned above, some ligaments have an increased content of elastin and elastin-bound proteins. In using tendons for the plasty of damaged intra-articular ligaments, the tendons eventually undergo pronounced molecular alterations, the designation for which the term "ligamentization" has been proposed (Roseti et al., 2008).

The biochemical and molecular organ specificity of fibrous dense types of connective tissue is distinctly seen in specialized structures involved in joint formation – a fibrous joint capsule, menisci, and disks.

3.6. GENERAL REGULARITIES OF MOLECULAR AND SUPRAMOLECULAR ORGANIZATION OF CONNECTIVE TISSUE EXTRACELLULAR MATRIX. MOLECULAR MECHANISMS OF CELLS AND MATRIX INTERACTIONS

3.6.1. Main general peculiarities of macromolecular components of extracellular matrix

A complex **domain** structure of the extracellular matrix protein macromolecules is their common peculiarity. Herein many domains are **modules**, standard sequences of amino acid residues (peptide fragments), a kind of building blocks, a set of which is used by the cells in assembling polypeptide chains; the same modules are found in proteins, which differ in their functions and the pattern of macromolecules' structure.

A modular principle of the extracellular matrix polymers' construction is employed not only in structural components. The same principle is realized in the macromolecular structure of many enzymes functioning in the matrix. It makes many proteins multifunctional, si-

multaneously rendering them the members of protein families, whose functions are absolutely different. The multifunctionality determines the proteins "social" properties, and their capability to be involved in various interactions with other proteins (Luo & Wan, 2006).

For example, the enzyme protein disulfide isomerase (PDI) appears to be multifunctional. Several catalytic functions have been revealed in this enzyme, which catalyzes the formation of disulfide bonds in protein molecules: it is one of the components of prolyl-4-hydroxylase and a protein–triglyceride carrier in microsomes. Moreover, it acts as one of the chaperones (one of the foldases) in the fibrillogenesis of type I collagen (Wilson et al., 1998).

Some enzymes have functions, which are intrinsic for structural proteins, along with their enzymatic function. For example, being members of the adamalysin family (see section 3.7.1), N-procollagen proteases, cleaving the aminoterminal peptide during the fibrillogenesis of large collagens, contain domains in the macromolecule that are homologous to the thrombospondin motifs; thus, the enzyme is able to bind to other proteins of the extracellular matrix and to the cells owing to these domains.

An enzyme can exert various enzymatic activities due to the presence of modules with various functions in matrix enzyme macromolecules. For example, C-procollagen proteinase, an enzyme that selectively cleaves a C-peptide from procollagens during posttranslational processing, is identical to the bone morphogenetic protein BMP-1 (Li et al., 1996) and exerts a wider proteolytic activity. Such as activity is attributable to tolloids, zinc-containing metalloproteases from the astacin family (see section 3.7.1); BMP-1 is also part of the tolloid family. Some modules take on an independent functional role after proteolytic cleavage from structural macromolecules. **Chondrocalcin**, a small protein involved in the mineralization of the extracellular matrix of cartilaginous tissue during endochondral osteogenesis, appears to be a C-peptide of type II procollagen (Kirsch & Pfafle, 1992).

The multiplicity of isoforms is another common peculiarity of molecular components of the extracellular matrix. This multiplicity, which is due to two factors such as the existence of related genes, united by the common origin, and alternative splicing, is of biological significance. It creates the possibility for the mutual compensation of the functions of different proteins in defects or the absence of their expression. Due to this mutual compensation, the phenotypical consequences of experimentally-induced mutations (so-called "null mutation", "gene knockout"), which lead to a total absence of the proteins encoded by the relevant genes in an organism, appears to be less severe in many cases that could be expected on the basis of the concept of these proteins' functional purpose (*Table 3.9*). If the fatal mutations, totally inconsistent with embryogenesis' completion, are excluded, the postnatal development of mutant animals

Table 3.9

Phenotypic alterations of mice in experimental mutations of the extracellular matrix proteins

Mutated polypeptide chain	Consequences of mutation	Characteristics of a phenotype
Collagen α1(I)	L	Vascular defects
Collagen α1(II)	L	Chondrodysplasia, defects of the intervertebral disks
Collagen α1(III)	L	Vascular defects, skin defects
Collagen α1(IV)	L	Renal insufficiency, progressive glomerulonephritis
Collagen α2(V)	L+V/F	Skin fragility, deformities of the skeleton
Collagen α1(VI)	V, F	Mild muscle dystrophy
Collagen α1(VII)	L	Skin blistering
Collagen α1(IX)	V, F	Degenerative changes in articular cartilages
Collagen α1(X)	V, F	Insignificant deformities of the skeleton
Collagen α1(XI)	V, F	Hearing loss
Elastin	L	Vascular defects
Fibrillin-1	L	Vascular defects
Proteoglycan binding protein		L. Chondrodysplasia
Decorin	V, F	Skin fragility, alteration of collagen fibrils and fibers
Biglycan	V, F	Osteoporosis
Fibromodulin	V, F	Altered tendons
Fibronectin	L	Mesodermal and cardiovascular defects, disorders of embryogenesis (somite deficiency)
Tenascin C	V, F	Insignificant neurological abnormalities and behavior disorders, inhibition of hematopoiesis, abnormal response to skin injury
Tenascin R	V, F	Defects of the central nervous system
Tenascin X	V, F	Decreased amount of collagens in the skin, enhanced invasion and dissemination of tumors, increased activity of tissue metalloproteases MMP2 and MMP9
Thrombospondin-1	V, F	Hyperplasia of epithelial and smooth muscle cells, increase in activity of the TGF-β1 factor. Increased vascularization, inflammations in the lungs, defects of the pancreas and hematopoiesis
Thrombospondin-2	V, F	Increased bone vascularization and density, disorders of fibroblast adhesion, abnormal collagen fibers, impairment of platelet function (hemorrhages), enhanced skin wound healing
Fibulin-1	L + V/F	Vascular, renal and pulmonary defects

Matrilin-1	V, F	Phenotypic abnormalities have not been revealed
Vitronectin	V, F	Phenotypic abnormalities have not been revealed
Laminin α2	L	Muscle dystrophy
Laminin α3	L	Skin blistering
Laminin α5	L	Encephalic abnormalities, placentopathy, impaired genesis of the renal glomerulus, syndactylia
Laminin β2	L	Defects of the central nervous system, the nerve-muscular system and kidneys
Laminin γ1	L	The absence of entoderm differentiation, basement membranes are not formed
Osteonectin (SPARC)	V, F	Cataract formation, osteopenia, decreased bone formation, immature collagen fibers, enhanced fibrovascular response to injury and accelerated wound healing, enhanced fat deposition
Osteocalcin	V, F	Increased bone formation
Matrix Gla-protein	L	Abnormal calcification of the cardiovascular system and cartilages
Osteopontin	V, F	Delayed bone resorption, appearing of the foci of dystrophic calcification, impairment of wound healing, inhibition of T-cell mediated immunity

Note.
V – Animals are viable,
F – Animals are fertile,
L – Animals are not viable (lethal phenotype),
L+V/F – Few animals are viable and fertile.
According to Gustafsson & Fässler (2000) and Bornstein & Sage (2002).

which have no one or another protein, often go on with the insignificant impairment of the phenotype only. Such tolerance of an organism to genetic abnormalities confirms the capability of the extracellular matrix to compensatory rearrangements.

At the same time, switching off the expression of some genes or posttranslational alterations (alternative splicing) leads to the generation of unexpected features. This can be explained by the forced rearrangement of the entire system of intermolecular interactions in the extracellular matrix. Sometimes, as follows from the table, the functions of some proteins, which were not supposed before, are revealed in experimental mutations.

One more peculiarity of many extracellular proteins is the presence of specialized modules (domains) containing amino acid sequences, which provide the proteins with adhesive properties ("stickiness"). The most common sequence among them is the repeatedly mentioned tripeptide RGD (arginine-glycine-asparagine). The adhesive sequences are of significant importance for matrix assembly and for matrix interactions with cells.

3.6.2. Interaction of extracellular matrix macromolecular components and morphogenetic role of these interactions

The integrating buffer metabolic medium of the extracellular matrix is a gel, in which the macromolecules of structural components and enzymes are in such a high total concentration that they should come into constant interaction with each other. The possibility of occurrence of such chemical interactions increases even more because many macromolecules are in movement, which is especially intensive during morphogenesis when the matrix components, expressed by cells in considerable amounts, proceed to their target sites.

This creates potential hazards of the occurrence of unnecessary chemical reactions, for instance, of proteolytic cleavage or immature or improper aggregation. Protective mechanisms have been developed to prevent these hazards. These mechanisms are the presence of carbohydrate fragments in macromolecules, the presence of the macromolecules blocking or restraining the activity of proteases, and the above-mentioned transportation of macromolecules (this refers to collagens, elastin and proteoglycans) in the participation of accompanying proteins–**chaperons.**

However, close contact of various macromolecules is the most important condition for the processes of **self-assembly** of tissue supramolecular structures of the connective tissue extracellular matrix, and its general structural organization.

This self-assembly follows the principles, which Scott (1995; 2002) named the laws of the chemical morphology of connective tissue:

a) The matrix composition is determined by specific interactions of the macromolecules involved in its formation.

b) The form of a tissue object (organ) is determined by the form and spatial position of the macromolecules forming this object. This means that the tissue's total volume is filled by interacting macromolecules in such a manner that the tissue eventually takes on its intrinsic form.

c) The structure and functions (including the biomechanical properties) of the tissue depend on interactions between the matrix macromolecules (Scott, 2001).

The process of self-assembly represents an arranged and systematized combination of homophilic and heterophilic reactions (reactions between similar and different macromolecules correspondingly). The formation of homopolymeric and heteropolymeric complexes of a strictly determined biochemical composition occurs so that their architectonics appear to precisely match the functional needs, as well as requirements of the form. The initially emerging unstable (electrostatic and hydrogen) bonds between molecules are changed into stable covalent ones if necessary.

Numerous examples of both homophilic and heterophilic interactions of this kind have been provided in the previous sections. It is possible to recall the fibrillogenesis of collagen fibrils from tropocollagen macromolecules, including heteromeric fibers composed by several types of collagens, the assembly of multicomponent elastic fibers consisting of elastin, fibrillins and other glycoproteins, the assembly of proteoglycan aggregates, and the assembly of basement membranes from such different components as type IV collagen, laminin and perlecan.

Adhesive glycoproteins, in particular fibronectins, are involved in heterophilic interactions more often than other matrix components. The fibronectins have several different adhesive domains (modules), which react with different ligands. They serve as the basis to which these various ligands bind. Fibrillar fibronectin aggregates are sometimes so large that they can be seen under a light-optical microscope. This central role of fibronectins in the assembly of the extracellular matrix is especially significant in the processes of morphogenesis, in both the stage of embryonic development and reparative connective tissue reactions.

The processes of heterophilic self-assembly, involving collagen fibrils and fibers, are of particular interest. The proteoglycan macromolecules interacting with large collagens in the final stages of fibrillogenesis play a morphogenetic role, influencing the formation and stabilization of the spatial organization of collagen fibrils and fibers, as well as their strength.

Collagen fibrils whose base is composed by type I, II and III collagens possess special sites for binding with the glycosaminoglycan components of proteoglycans. These sites, which contain homologous amino acid sequences (with a length of 11 residues), are localized in particular areas marked by "bars" of cross-striation of collagen fibrils, namely on bars **e**, **d**, **c** and **a**. The last two loci are occupied only in the cornea collagen, where keratan sulfate (contained in the SLRP proteoglycans fibromodulin and lumican) attaches to them. The loci **e** and **d** are used in various tissues; proteoglycans containing dermatan sulfate and chondroitin sulfate bind to them. (Scott, 1995).

The rigid molecules of decorin, in the form of a horseshoe, are positioned as bridges, strictly orthogonally (perpendicularly) to the axis of collagen fibrils; the interval between decorin bridges is 64–68 nm in the type I collagen prevailing in tendons (Redselli et al., 2003). A mechanically created exposure is transmitted from fibril to fibril, and the fibrils are held in a position fixed to each other due to these bridges. The maintenance of a required tissue configuration is provided in such a manner. Decorin molecules act as formative modules in this situation while dermatan sulfate chains, which possess sliding properties, provide fiber sliding (Scott, 2003). The bond between collagen macromolecules and decorin dermatan sulfate is very strong and is not destroyed *in vitro* even in a significantly aggressive chemical medium. Decorin production is regulated by hevin, a matricellular glycoprotein from the SPARC-family; hevin is thus indirectly involved in the regulation of collagen fibril formation (Sullivan et al., 2006).

Decorin also has other organizing-binding functions: decorin dermatan sulfate binds to one of the tenascin-X domains (FN-III) and mediates the bond of this tenascin isoform with collagen fibrils. This interaction with collagens enables the mechanical-chemical role of tenascin-X in the extracellular matrix (Elefteriou et al., 2001). Moreover, this role manifests in the necessity of tenascin-X for the normal fibrillogenesis of elastic fibers/fibrils and fibrillin microfibrils (Zweers et al., 2004).

Besides decorin, other SLRP (biglycan, fibromodulin, lumican) are significant for providing the structural integrity of the connective tissue extracellular matrix. The phenotypes of mice with "null" mutations of these proteoglycan genes (i.e. with a deficiency of these genes in an organism) appeared interesting *in vivo* experimental models of some pathologies of the connective tissue (osteoporosis, osteoarthrosis, Ehlers-Danlos syndrome) in humans (Ameye & Young, 2002). These disorders obviously may be the consequences of not only mutations of the genes of large collagen proteins, but also disturbances of collagen fibrillogenesis due to SLRP deficiency (Douglas et al., 2006).

Matrilin-2 is actively involved in the matrix self-assembly. It binds to type II, III, IV, V collagens, but especially actively with type I collagen. Sometimes one molecule of matrilin-2 connects two collagen macromolecules (Piecha et al., 2002). Matrilin-2 even more actively binds to fibronectins and a laminin-nidogen complex. The supramolecular aggregates, providing additional bonds between collagen fibrils, basement membranes and the components of an interfibrillar substance, are formed in such a way.

A large proteoglycan, versican, whose role is especially significant in the morphogenesis of connective tissue, interacts with fibrillin-1 (Isogai et al., 2002) and fibulin-2 (Olin et al., 2001) via the C-terminal (lectin) domain of its core protein. Both interactions are calcium-dependent and are important in the self-assembly of elastic fibers and fibrillin microfibrils.

As a result of the whole combination of supramolecular aggregates' self-assembly processes, the extracellular matrix becomes an integrated organized system, whose properties provide:
1) the effective performance of the metabolic and biomechanical functions of the matrix itself; and
2) the optimal conditions for interactions with the cells.

3.6.3. Proteins of cell (cytoplasmic) membrane. cells' interactions with extracellular matrix

The extracellular matrix is produced by the cells, which secrete all matrix-comprising structural macromolecules and all enzymes functioning in the matrix, as well as their inhibitors, and all signaling molecules transported via the matrix to other cells (Zhu & Scott, 2004). In turn, the extracellular matrix is a medium where the cells function. The materials essential for biosynthesis processes enter the cells from the extracellular matrix. The matrix also provides the cells with information, which determines cells' topographic differentiation (specificity of the genes' expression depending upon the cell localization in an organism) (Chang et al., 2002) and their response to the normal and pathologic processes ongoing in the organism and in the surrounding tissues in particular.

Therefore, intensive continuous interaction must occur between the cells and the extracellular matrix. However, this interaction is restrained by a two-layer phospholipid cell (cytoplasmic) membrane, which is permeable for the natural, gradient-concentration-determined diffusion of O_2, N_2, CO_2 and few lipid-soluble molecules only, such as ethanol and steroid hormones, for instance. Even the transport of water and urea through the cytoplasmic membrane is rather limited; the membrane is impermeable for ions and bid molecules (both for those that are non-carrying, such as glucose for example, and those carrying the electric charge, such as amino acids, proteins, ATP).

The feasibility of bilateral interaction between the cells and the matrix is ensured by the presence of numerous

transmembrane proteins in the cytoplasmic membrane, which are the membrane' integral components, the macromolecules of which overpass (penetrate) through both membrane phospholipid layers. Many transmembrane proteins are not diffused throughout the membrane, but rather are concentrated in special areas of the membrane–rafts that project over its surface, and **caveolae** (*Latin* caveola–a little cave) representing clefts in the membrane (Simons & Toomre, 2000). The peculiarities of the phospholipid composition distinguish the rafts and caveolae from the remainder of the membrane.

The functions of the transmembrane proteins are manifold. Among them, there are proteins forming canals, which are open (open if necessary) for the diffusion of particular molecules. **Aquaporins** are among these proteins. Each aquaporin macromolecule is a canal that facilitates water supply to the cell due to its conformation in the membrane mass (Verkman & Mitra, 2000).

The macromolecules of two transmembrane protein families–**RyR** and **TRCP**–form canals appropriate for movements of the calcium ions providing the dynamic balance between the contents of these ions in the matrix and within the cells (Lee et al., 2006).

The **transport** proteins (transporters) attach particular molecules and carry them across the membrane. For example, glucose transporters comprising the **GLUT** family, have a connection center that is open towards the extracellular matrix. Upon the glucose molecule's connecting, the GLUT macromolecule conformation is altered, the center opens inside the cell and the glucose molecule enters the cytoplasm, after which the macromolecule primary conformation is restored. Transporters of the **SGLT** family, carrying sodium ions along with glucose, act in the same manner (Wood & Trayburn, 2003). Some transmembrane transporters carry molecules and ions in both directions.

Numerous **CAM** (cell adhesion molecules), connecting cells with each other and with the extracellular matrix, occupy a significant place among the integral proteins of the cytoplasmic membrane. The main groups of proteins connecting the cells with each other are cadherins, selectins and proteins from the immunoglobulin superfamily.

The superfamily of **cadherins**, consisting of more than 30 single-chain transmembrane glycoproteins that are similar in structure, includes "classical" cadherins and proteins similar to them (protocadherins, desmocollins, desmogleins and others). The cadherins are components of the desmosomes of complex adhesive structures, which provide contacts between the cells, unlike hemidesmosomes (hemidesmosomes are involved in binding the cells with the extracellular matrix) (Green & Jones, 1996). The cadherin macromolecules consist of 720–750 amino acid residues. Their extracellular domains (ectodomains) are formed by 3–5 repeated subsequent (tandem) subdomains, each 110 amino acid residues in length. The N-terminal domain plays a leading role in cadherins' adhesive function and in determining the adhesion specificity (Leckband & Prakasam, 2006). The ectodomains' conformation is stabilized by the calcium ions attached to them. The cadherins' adhesive activity is therefore calcium-dependent, which is reflected in their name (cadherins). A cadherin short cytoplasmic domain, connected to the ectodomain via a transmembrane domain that is 24 amino acid residues long, interacts with proteins of the catenin family; the catenins (Latin catena–a chain) connect the cadherins with the cytoskeleton proteins.

In most cases, a certain type of cells possess the cadherins that are specific for them; these cadherins bind to the same cadherins of the same type of cells (such a bond is called homophilic).

Cadherins, whose expression is controlled by hormone and growth factors, play an important role in regulating cell migration, proliferation and differentiation, as well as in tissue morphogenesis and the maintenance of the multicellular structures' integrity.

The **selectins** (E-, P- and N-selectins) comprise the second family of calcium-dependent transmembrane adhesive glycoproteins. The selectines are the members of the lectine superfamily (this is reflected in their name), proteins which recognize and selectively bind to glycoproteins' monosaccharide and oligosaccharide groups. The selectins' large domains perform this lectin role, due to which the selectins of the same type of cells bind to glycoproteins located on the surface of another type of cells (such a bond is called heterophilic). For instance, platelet selectin (selectin P) binds to a glycoprotein on the surface of endothelial cells, which is therefore a ligand specific for this selectin (P-selectin glycoprotein ligand-1, **PSGL-1**) (Vestweber & Blanks, 1999). These interactions are of significant importance in the pathogenesis of thromboses and inflammatory reactions.

Some members of the immunoglobulin family are calcium-independent adhesive transmembrane glycoproteins (**IgCAM**), whose macromolecules contain an immunoglobulin domain (Ig) (Pollard & Earnshaw, 2002). The multiplicity of these proteins is mainly due to the alternative splicing of some mRNA. They form both homophilic and heterophilic bonds between cells. The Ig-CAM are subdivided into several groups. The following have been studied in detail: NCAM, which act primarily between nerve cells; ICAM, which binds white blood cells with endothelium cells but are also present in the epithelial cells; and VCAM, functioning in the endothelium cells.

The families of **nectins** and **nectin-like** transmembrane macromolecules, functioning in many interacellular connections, are close to immunoglobulins in structure and their adhesive function (Ogita & Takai, 2006).

The role of adhesive proteins connecting cells to one another in cell bonds with the extracellular matrix is mediated. This role is generally determined by adhesive proteins' influence on cell differentiation, proliferation and metabolic functions. The immediate interaction of the cells and the matrix is determined by other, numerous and various **transmembrane receptors**, which bind the cells with macromolecule components of their immediate surrounding.

The large family of **integrins** is most significant among these receptors; the integrins are integral proteins of the cytoplasmic membrane, which are vitally essential for all multicellular organisms (Metazoa) from the spongi to the human being (Hynes & Zhao, 2001). Although some integrins interact with CAM on the surface of adjacent cells, the extracellular matrix protein components are the main ligands for most integrins. Mostly these ligands contain "sticky" amino acid sequences (the aforementioned sequence arginin–glycine–aspartic acid (**RGD**) and some others). The integrins' main function is to provide the cell's stable adhesion to the matrix.

The integrins are heterodimers consisting of two molecular subunits–one α type polypeptide chain (with a molecular mass of 130–200 kDa) and one β type polypeptide chain (90–130 kDa) interconnected by non-covalent bonds only. At least 18 different α-subunits and 8 different β-subunits have been identified; some subunits exist in several isoforms. The formation of 128 pair combinations of α- and β-subunits is theoretically feasible, however, only 24 variants of integrins have actually been detected; they are specifically distributed along individual cell types. Many cells possess various integrins, and many integrins are present on the surface of several cell types; some ligands can bind to several different integrins (Berman et al., 2003).

Each integrin subunit consists of a long (700–1,100 amino acid residues) ectodomain, a short transmembrane domain, and a short (40–70 amino acid residues) endodomain (cytoplasmic domain) (the exception is a very long endodomain in subunit β4). The sites of binding to the extracellular components–ligands–are located in the ectodomains' N-terminal region (Karp, 1999).

Both subunits are involved in binding each ligand. The sites determining integrin specific activity belong to the β-subunits, which is why the integrin family is subdivided into subfamilies in dependency of the β-subunits.

Integrins having a β1-subunit generally bind to matrix proteins–collagens, laminins, fibronectins. β2-integrins are present in white blood cells and bind to the ICAM receptors of endothelial cells. Integrins β3 co-act with αIIb- or αV-subunits; the integrin αIIbβ3 is preset in platelets, which employ it during blood clotting, while the integrin αVβ3 serves as a vitronectin receptor and is involved in angiogenesis. The integrin α6β4 binds hemidesmosomes to laminin and plays a central role in hemidesmosome formation. αVβ5, αVβ6, αVβ8, as well as α4β7 and αEβ7 are essential for cell participation in immune response.

The function of α-subunits is to recognize proper amino acid sequences in a ligand macromolecule and to provide the fidelity of its contact to the site of a β-subunit binding (Takagi, 2004).

For example, the β1-subunit binding site of the integrin α5β1 is connected with the RGD-sequence of a surface of the fibronectin macromolecule III domain FN-module (see 3.2.1), while the α5-subunit binding site connects with the adjacent, 9th module of the same domain.

The N-terminal regions of the integrins' extracellular domains have a crystal structure; an alteration of this structure in contact with the ligand is a primary signal inducing adhesive interactions (Humphries, 2004). The interaction of ligands with integrins occurs with the participation of divalent cations–calcium and magnesium. These cations are supposed to play a role in providing the necessary conformation for the integrins' extracellular domains. The integrins are glycoproteins and their activity depends on the degree of their glycosylation, among other factors (Gu & Taniguchi, 2004).

The mutual chemical affinity of the integrins and their macromolecular ligands is low; the stability of their binding is achieved due to their multiplicity rather than due to the strength of the arising bonds. In a cell interaction with the extracellular ligand, the proper integrins, which are capable of migrating within a membrane plane as other transmembrane proteins do, collect in aggregates (clusters). Such a gathering of integrins enables the formation of many cells' bonds with a fibronectin microfibril for example.

The endodomains of the clustered integrins are comprised of transitory organelles specialized in cell adhesion–hemidesmosomes and desmosomes (Litjens et al., 2006), as well as **focal contacts** (FC). The focal contacts have been studied in detail in cells cultured *in vitro* where they are formed if necessary. The initial stage of this complex process is mediated by a fine layer of hyaluronan covering the cell surface, which is bond by a glycoprotein CD44, a hyaluronan specific receptor (see section 3.2.1.2). Point **focal complexes** are formed, which transform into integrin-containing stronger FC and then into **focal adhesions** (FA, or **adhesion loci** in the other words) as bonds with a cytoskeleton are established. Hyaluronan facilitates cell recognition (Cohen et al., 2006).

The dynamics of focal contacts' formation and their subsequent transformation into focal adhesions is largely determined by bilateral mechanical interactions between the cells and a substrate on which the cells are cultured. The integrins receive and transmit mechanical impulses (stretching, fluid mobility) in both directions (Katsumi et al., 2004). This integrins' activity is called **mechanotransduction**. There is significant evidence to suppose that focal contacts and focal adhesions are formed in the cells *in vivo* in the same manner (Brakebusch & Fässler, 2003).

The integrins' main functions are firstly to bind a ligand to the cytoskeleton, whose basic protein is actin–changes in the cytoskeleton architectonics influence the cells' form and migration–and secondly, to activate the intracellular signaling pathways of the signals forthcoming from the extracellular matrix; this second function of the integrins is directed at modulating the cell metabolic activity. The starting signal to perform these functions is ligand interaction-mediated alteration in the conformation of both integrin macromolecules (subunits), which is transmitted from the ectodomain to the cytoplasmic domain (endodomain). The subsequent signal transmission to the final targets is mediated by the integrin endodomain' interaction with a complex of proteins concentrated in the focal contacts, as well as in the hemidesmosomes and desmosomes (Green & Jones, 1996).

These complexes, which can be considered as **molecular machines**, are extremely complicated; the total number of proteins involved in integrins' adhesive and signaling functions reaches 65 (Zamir & Geiger, 2001; Lo, 2006). The focal contacts contain:

a) **structural proteins** related to the cytoskeleton (**actin, α-actinin, talin, ezrin, filamin, fimbrin, moesin, nexilin, palladin, parvins (α and β), profilin, ponsin, radixin, tensins, tenuin, vinculin, vinexin** and others);

b) **adapter** proteins, binding other proteins to each other and transmitting signals between them (**paxillin, PINCH, migfilin, syntenin, caveolin-1** and others); it should be noted that it is difficult to strictly distinguish structural and adapter proteins;

c) **enzymes**–different **kinases**, activating proteins by means of phosphorylation (**protein tyrosine kinases**, including **FAK** (focal adhesion kinases), **protein serin/threonine kinases**, including **ILK, PAK** and others), **protein phosphatases**, modulators of **guanosine triphosphatase**, and **proteases**, including cysteine proteases–**calpains**.

All these proteins enter into various interactions between themselves; hereby, different active complexes affecting adhesion and signal transmission are generated. For example, a triple complex called PIP, which consists of proteins (PINCH and parvin-α) and the kinase ILK (integrin-linked kinase), is the central effector in one of several possible ways to establish the bonds between integrins and actin, the main structural protein of the cytoskeleton (Sepulveda & Wu, 2006).

At the same time, some proteins of the focal contacts affect integrins; this influence determines their functional state. The interaction of integrin endodomains with talin, which occurs involving one of calpains, causes such changes in the integrins' conformation (increasing the distance between subunits, ectodomain straightening), which modulate integrins' binding to the ligands. This influence of talin is characterized as the activation of **integrins**; it should be noted that null mutations of the talin's gene are fatal (Calderwood, 2004).

Activating ligands' binding by the integrins influenced by signals from the focal contacts results in changes in the extracellular matrix; the integrins' signaling function is therefore bilateral (Qin et al., 2004).

A number of members of the β1-subunit-containing integrin subfamily is specialized to bind to collagen. They are α1β1, α2β1, α10β1 and α11β1 integrins. The N-terminal region of these integrins' α-subunit domains contains a special module (subdomain 1 or I, inserted) that is involved in collagen binding (Eble, 2005). The sequence GER (glycine–glutamic acid–arginine) is a "sticky" ("recognizing") amino acid sequence in fiber-forming collagen macromolecules; the "stickiness" is enhanced in the composition of a GFOGER hexapeptide (glycine–phenylalanine hydroxyproline-GER) (Siljander et al., 2004). The binding activity of the A-subdomain of different integrins is not identical in relation to different collagens: the A-subdomain of the α2-subunit is more tightly bound to type I-III collagens, whereas the A-subdomain of the α10-subunit selectively binds type IV and VI collagens (Tulla et al., 2001).

In general, interations of integrins with ligands is characterized by a high specificity. This specificity manifests in the diversity of the phenotypic alterations originating in null mutations of each integrin (Hynes, 2002).

Thus, the functions of integrins are manifold. Firstly, integrins form stable adhesions between cells and the extracellular matrix or the substrate on which cells are cultured. Secondly, integrins act as signaling receptors, which carry information from the matrix inside the cells; this information can affect the expression of particular genes. Thirdly, they play a significant role in cell migration and in regulating the cells' form. Fourthly, the integrins transfer the information back from the cells to the matrix, which is reflected in the process of matrix assembly. Moreover, they are essential to provide the cells' polarity and their viability.

Integrins' adhesive and signaling functions are coordinated with those of other receptors. There is evidence that integrins interact with the receptors of cell adhesion, cadherins, with the participation of paxillin and kinase FAK (Schaller, 2004), as well as by means of the protein Rap1 (Retta et al., 2006). These interactions affect cell migration.

Also, the integrins' adhesive function is coordinated with the function of **syndecans**, transmembrane proteoglycans in whose macromolecules heparan sulfates prevail, between the glycosaminoglycans. The syndecans are not only signal but also adhesive receptors (Couchman et al., 2001). The ability of syndecan-1 to bind type I, III and V collagens, fibronectins, thrombospondins and tenascins has been established. This ability enables cell fixation.

It is supposed that, as adhesive receptors, syndecans do not compete with integrins; on the contrary, they are **co-receptors**, which enable the formation of ligand complexes with integrin receptors.

Both the adhesive and signaling transmembrane receptors binding the cells to collagens are especially important for the optimal interaction of cells and the connective tissue extracellular matrix. Along with integrins containing β1-subunits, the **discoidin domain receptors**, DDR1 and DDR2 and their isoforms, carry out this binding (Vogel et al., 2006). These receptors are among the superfamily of the receptor tyrosine kinases (RTK); they contain an ectodomain, which is homologous to *Dictyostelium discoideum* mold-derived lectin, hence their

name. Not only collagen native triple helical macromolecules, but also formed collagen fibrils, are ligands for the discoidin domain-containing receptors; this provides the cells with information on the integrity of the matrix supramolecular structure.

In a dimeric state, DDR1 is activated by all type I-VII collagens tested in an experiment. DDR2 is especially effectively bond to type I collagen. In this binding, the metalloprotease MMP-1 is activated; it breaks down this collagen and its fibrillogenesis is impaired (Mihai et al., 2006). Two members of the subfamily of **transmembrane collagens**–type XIII and XVII collagens, can also be attributed to cell adhesion molecules. Theh short cytoplasmic N-terminal domains of these collagens are parts of cell adhesive organelles (the C-terminal domain is cytoplasmic in all other transmembrane proteins). Type XVII collagen is a hemidesmosome component, connecting the epithelial cells with the basement membrane. Type XIII collagen is involved in the formation of **focal adhesions** in fibroblasts cultured *in vitro*. The large C-terminal ectodomains of both collagens stabilize cells' spatial localization (Franzke et al., 2005).

Along with the listed adhesive and signaling receptors, as well as those mentioned above (dystroglycans, glypicans), the cytoplasmic membrane contains many **receptors of signaling molecules**. Unlike signaling receptors, whose ligands are mainly structural macromolecules of the extracellular matrix and which can also perceive the mechanical impulses, it is with the signaling molecules that the receptors of signaling molecules are specialized to interact. It should be emphasized that the specialization of these numerous receptors is very narrow. Each of them transmits a signal into the cell, selectively interacting with any one biologically active signaling molecule or with families of signaling molecules, which are very similar to each other in both structure and function.

In all the diversity of the "links" interconnecting the cells and the extracellular matrix, in general the connection between them is dynamic. The matricellular glycoproteins (see section 3.2.1.1), exhibiting anti-adhesive activity, enable this dynamism; some other fragments, which are the products of proteolytic degradation of the matrix structural proteins, exhibit anti-adhesive activity (Sage, 2001).

The integrin-supported bonds are particularly dynamic. These bonds, especially those between the integrins and fibronectins, are easily disintegrated and at once interchanged by new bonds with nearby integrins and adjacent "sticky" modules on the fibronectin microfibrils. Employing transitory adhesions as supporting points, the cells herewith move along the fibrils; owing to this, the cells are able to secrete the structural macromolecular components of the matrix in proper localizations. At the same time, fibronectin microfibrils migrate; their growth and movement influence the matrix's general supramolecular organization (Dallas et al., 2006). All these dynamic events are especially evident in morphogenetic processes.

It can be stated that the relationship between the cells and the extracellular matrix is vitally essential for cells. In a number of settings, the impairment of this relationship results in cell death. This phenomenon is regarded as one of the forms of natural programmed cell death–**apoptosis**–and is denoted by the special term **anoikis** (from the Greek *anoikis*–the state of being without a home) (Grossmann, 2002). Anoikis, which does not principally differ from apoptosis in either its biochemical mechanisms and morphologic manifestations, is of importance for the processes involved in the tissue's normal development, the maintenance of tissue homeostasis, and the pathogenesis of some diseases.

3.7. CATABOLISM OF MACROMOLECULAR COMPONENTS OF THE EXTRACELLULAR MATRIX

3.7.1. Metalloproteases (metalloproteinases)

The physiologic state of metabolic balance, being the prerequisite of normal vital activities of an adult organism, implies the mutual balance of anabolic (biosynthesis) and catabolic (degradation) processes. Although the stability of most biopolymers of the extracellular matrix, defined by their half-life period, is generally significantly higher than it is intrinsic for many components of the parenchymatous organs, the degradation of connective tissue biopolymers still constantly occurs even to a significantly less degree.

This normal constant degradation is significantly more intensive in the period of an organism's growth until the completion of the organs' and tissues' morphogenesis (examples of this degradation include a tadpole tail absorbing in its metamorphosis into a frog and the annual re-growing of deer antlers) and in embryogenesis, especially when the formation of some tissue and organ structures is associated with the replacement of some tissues by the transubstantiation of others.

Other examples of intensified normal (physiologic) degradation include the postpartum involution of the uterus, the peeling of the endometrium during menstruation, and the embryonic trophoblast's insertion into the uterus wall. Here, the processes of degradation of the biopolymers in their replacement by others occurring in wound-healing dynamics should also be mentioned. The prevalence of the physiologic catabolic process over anabolic reactions is observed in an organism's ageing involution.

Unlike the anabolic reactions mostly specific for the expression of each of the biopolymer classes, catabolism regularities are of a more general character despite the existence of numerous partial differences. Therefore, we will combine our consideration of the enzymatic mechanisms of the catabolic reactions related to various structural components of the extracellular matrix.

Numerous proteins, which are present in the matrix and exhibit proteolytic properties, are involved in the catabolism of the extracellular matrix. The activity of these enzymes (**proteinases** or **proteases**) is **endopeptidasic**, breaking down the inner peptide bonds in the polypeptide chains of proteins-substrates. The enzyme macromolecules, just as those of the structural proteins, have a multidomain structure; among the domains, there is an **active center** (catalytic domain) that directly exerts a proteolytic effect on the substrate. By the character of their active centers, the proteases are subdivided into metalloproteases, serin proteases, threonine proteases, cystein proteases, and asparagine proteases (Hooper, 2002).

Enzymes of the metalloprotease (MP) family play a central role in all physiologic and pathologic catabolic processes in the connective tissue extracellular matrix. The presence of the metal **zinc** in their active center is common for all members of this family, accounting for their other combining name–**metazincins**.

The metazincin superfamily is further subdivided into families: matrixins or matrix metalloprpoteases (MMP) adamalysins (reprolysins)–metalloproteases with disintegrin domain (ADAM), astacins. The adamalysin family comprises the ADAMTS subfamily.

Besides the aforementioned mandatory presence of zinc in the catalytic center, all metalloproteases (metzincins) are combined by the following common properties: they have a similar amino acid composition; the catalytic domain, which is about 170–180 amino acid residues in length, contains the motif HExxHxxGxxH (where x can be any amino acid residue, while three histidine residues bind zinc ions) in common for all these enzymes (Lee & Murphy, 2004). They are secreted by cells into the extracellular matrix in a latent form (as zymogens) and take on their proteolytic activity only after activation.

The metalloproteases are glycoproteins. The presence of oligosaccharides in their macromolecules prevents the enzymes from the proteolytic activity of other proteases, and provides enzyme macromolecules with a most appropriate conformation for exhibiting catalytic action, thereby regulating their activity (Visse & Nagase, 2003).

The family of homologous endopeptidases–**matrixins** or matrix metalloproteases (**MMP**)–is one of the most numerous families of this superfamily. There are at least 28 MMP in the vertebrates (Flannery, 2006). The main members of this family are listed in *Table 3.10*.

The matrix metalloproteases exhibit a multidomain structure of macromolecules as other metzincins. The mechanism of domain assembly into enzymes' multidomain macromolecules was formed in the early stage of evolution. (Mort & Billington, 2001).

The N-terminal signal sequence of amino acid residues, which is intrinsic for all proteins secreted by the cells, is common for all MMP. There is an autoinhibitory propeptide between this signal peptide, cleaved after secretion, and the cataleptic domain. This propeptide contains a very conservative cysteine residue bond to the zinc atom in the catalytic domain. Proteolytic removal of the autoinhibitory propeptide activates MMP transforming a pro-

Table 3.10
The family of matrix metalloproteases (matrixins) (MMP)

Enzyme	Basic substrates	Activators	Inducers
MMP-1/interstitial collagenase	Type I, II, III, X collagens, gelatin	Plasmin, MMP-3, -7, -10	TNF-α, IL-1β, PDGF EGF
MMP-2/gelatinase A	Gelatin, laminin, fibronectin, elastin, I, II, IV, V, VII type collagens	MT-MMP, MMP-1, -13	TGF-β
MMP-3/stromelysin	Proteoglycans, fibronectin, gelatin, proMMP-1, III, IV, V, IX	Plasmin	TNF-α, IL-1β, EGF
MMP-7/matrilysin	Gelatin, fibronectin, type IV collagen, proteoglycans, proMMP-1	Plasmin	LPS
MMP-8/collagenase-2	Type I, II, III collagens, gelatin	MMP-3, -7, -10	TNFα, IL-1β,
MMP-9/gelatinase B	Gelatin, proteoglycans, elastin, fibronectin, type IV, V, VII collagens	Plasmin, MMP-3, -13, -26	TGF-β, TNF-α, IL-1β, LPS, EGF
MMP-10/ stromelysin-2	Gelatin, fibronectin, proMMP-1, type III, IV, IX collagens	Plasmin	TGF-α, EGF, TNF-α
MMP-11/ stromelysin-3	Gelatin	Furin	TGF-β, EGF, IL-6, PDGF
MMP-12/metalloelastase	Elastin, type IV collagen, laminin		TNF-α, IL-1β, PDGF
MMP-13/collagenase-3	Type I, II, III collagens, aggrecan	Plasmin, MT-MMP, MMP-2, -3, -10	LIF, TNF-α, IL-1β
MMP-14/MT1-MMP	Type I, II, III collagens, ProMMP-2, ProMMP-13		TNF-α, IL-1β, EGF
MMP-15/MT2-MMP	ProMMP-2, fibronectin, gelatin		Stretching
MMP-16/ MT3-MMP	ProMMP-2, type III collagen, gelatin		
MMP-17/ MT4-MMP	Gelatin, fibrin, fibronectin		
MMP-18/collagenase-4	Type I, II, III collagens		
MMP-19	Gelatin, type IV collagen, laminin		Phorbol ester
MMP-20/enamelysin	Amelogenin, gelatin		Stretching
MMP-21			
MMP-22	Gelatin		
MMP-23/MMP			
MMP-24/MT5-MMP	ProMMP-2, gelatin, fibronectin		
MMP-25/MT6-MMP	ProMMP-2, type IV collagen, gelatin		IL-8
MMP-26/matrilysin-2	Gelatin, type IV collagen, fibronectin		
MMP-28		Furin	

enzyme into an active enzyme. A regulatory domain determining the MMP specificity in relation to the substrates in located closer to the macromolecule C-terminal region of most MMP.

MMP-14 and MMP-15, MMP-16 and MMP-17, which are close to it in structure and their functions possess a transmembrane C-terminal domain, whereby they attach to a cell membrane. These MMP (also called MT-MMP) are activated and exhibit their enzymatic activity without being cleaved from the cells.

The synonymic names provided in *Table 3.10* give a general idea on the substrates of every matrixin functioning in the extracellular matrix in neutral pH. MMP-1, -8, -13, -14 are interstitial collagenases that break down not only great type I, II and III collagens, but also type VII and X collagens. The action of interstitial collagenases is highly specific and precisely targeted. They break down great collagens in the only locus disrupting the $\alpha1$(I), $\alpha2$(I) and $\alpha1$(II) polypeptide chains between the Gly775 and Ile776 residues and the $\alpha1$(III) polypeptide chain between the Gly784 and Ile785 residues. The matrixin's impact is as precisely targeted to other substrates (Flannery, 2006).

The mechanisms of this specificity and the exactness have not been entirely clarified. The catalytic domain's ability to break down a collagen triple helix (triple helical peptidase activity) is especially important for the specificity of collagenase action. The enzyme C-terminal domain destabilizes the triple helical molecule and optimally orients it in relation to the enzyme (Lauer-Fields et al., 2002).

Gelatinases (MMP-2 and MMP-9) break down type IV (in triple helix domains), V and VII collagens, elastin, fibronectins and gelatin. Stromelysins, matrilysin and metalloelastase act upon a wide number of substrates, including the non-spiralized regions of type IV collagens, fibronectins, laminins and proteoglycans. Moreover, MMP break down osteonectin (SPARC), cytokines, growth factors and other proteins (Malemud, 2006).

Mice lacking the genes of any matrixin are quite viable, indicating the functional substitution of these enzymes. At the same time, the response targeting of such animals towards different external exposure is abruptly altered. For example, mice with an impaired expression of MMP-12 (macrophage elastase) exhibit tolerance to tobacco smoke, which causes emphysema in normal mice. In the absence of MMP-12, the destruction of lungs' elastic fibers, which is usual for normal mice, does not originate under the influence of smoke, accompanied by inflammatory events.

The second numerous metalloprotease family is comprised by adamalysins (reprolysins), which are **ADAM** (a disintegrin and matrix metalloproteases), sometimes also called **MDC** (metalloprotease/disintegrin/cysteinerich). More than 30 gene-encoding ADAM are known (Primakoff & Myles, 2000).

The ADAM macromolecules posses a domain structure that is similar to the structure of matrixins, but with some significant differences. The catalytic, zinc-containing domain is followed by a domain, resembling disintegrins in the primary structure, which is reflected in the name of this enzyme group (disintegrins are small monomeric protein molecules contained in snake venom; owing to the presence of the RGD-sequence, disintegrins bind to cell receptors – integrins, destroying their interaction with ligands). Then the cysteine-residue rich domain is located; this domain is similar in primary structure to an epithelium growth factor (EGF). ADAM are firmly attached to the cell membrane by a special transmembrane amino acid sequence followed by a short C-terminal cytoplasmic domain. In the other words, ADAM, as well as MMP-14, -15, -16 and –17, are transmembrane enzymes.

ADAM cleave the extracellular domains of a number of proteins bound to the cell membrane (the enzymes exhibiting such activity are called **sheddases**). Some of these released extracellular domains are important signaling molecules, such as the tumor necrosis factor (TNF-α) and the transforming growth factor (TGF-α). The importance of the signaling system regulation, conditioned by ADAM, is indicated by the fact that mutations involving the ADAM-17 gene lead to animals' death even in the stage of embryonic development.

ADAM also are involved in cell adhesion and fusion, including such a significant phenomenon as a sperm fusing with an ovum in fertilization.

ADAMTS (a disintegrin and metalloproteases with thrombospondin motifs) comprise a special adamalysin subfamily (Jones & Riley, 2005). The enzymes of this family, which are also called **aggrecanases** (due to the ability of some of them to break down a large proteoglycan of the cartilaginous tissue – aggrecan), contain all the main domains intrinsic for ADAM enzymes, as well as a domain resembling thrombospondin-1 by its repeats of amino acid sequences. It is located between disintegrin-like and cysteine-rich domains. Moreover, thrombospondin-like repeats are present in the molecule C-terminal region. This C-terminal thrombospondin-like motif is essential for aggrecanases, for aggrecanase-1 (ADAMTS4) in particular, for recognition of the substrate – aggrecan – by its glycosaminoglycan component and for binding to it, since binding to keratan sulfate determines the enzyme specificity in relation to aggrecan.

Another difference between ADAMTS and ADAM is the absence of a transmembrane domain; the ADAMTS enzymes are not bond to cells and are free in their motility in the extracellular matrix as most matrixins.

The ADAMTS4 (aggrecanase–1) enzymatic activity, as possibly in other aggrecanases, manifests only after the post-translation processing of a synthesized macromolecule. The processing consists of removing a propeptide and part of the C-terminal domain (Gao et al., 2002).

20 ADAMTS enzymes are known in humans (Porter et al., 2005). The most studied members of the ADAMTS subfamily with their functions are listed in *Table 3.11*.

ADAMTS enzymes carry out the catabolism of all proteoglycans acting as proteases (proteinases) on their core

Table 3.11
Some ADAMTS enzymes

Name	Synonyms	Functions
ADAMTS-1	METH-1, KIAA1346	Involved in inflammatory reactions, angiogenesis and morphogenesis
ADAMTS-2	Collagen N-proteinase	Procollagen processing
ADAMTS-3	KIAA0366	
ADAMTS-4	Aggrecanase-1, KIAA0688	Aggrecan and brevican breaking down
ADAMTS-5	Aggrecanase-2, ADAMTS11	Aggrecan breaking down
ADAMTS-8	METH-2	

Table 3.12
Some TIMP properties

	TIMP-1	TIMP-2	TIMP-3	TIMP-4
Molecular weight (kDa)	28	21	24/27	21
Number of N-glycosylated sites	2	0	1	0
Localization in tissues	Soluble	Soluble/Bond to cell membrane	Soluble	Soluble/Bond to cell membrane
Inhibition of MMP	MT1-MMP MT2-MMP MT3-MMP MT5-MMP MMP-19	–	–	–
Inhibition of ADAM and ADAMTS	ADAM10 ADAM-17 ADAM-19 ADAMTS-4 ADAMTS-5	– –	ADAM-12	–
Effect on tumor development	Inhibition	Inhibition	Inhibition	Inhibition

proteins. ADAMTS-1, -4, -5, -8, -9 and –15 enzymes exhibit pronounced aggrecanase activity. This process occurs in the extracellular matrix. The glycosaminoglycan chains hereby released are exposed to further degradation up to monosaccharides by the hydrolytic enzymes, which are present in the matrix. ADAMTS-2, -3, -14 are procollagen N-proteases, cleaving the N-terminal propeptide from type I, II and III procollagens.

The expression of individual ADAMTS-proteases exhibits a particular tissue specificity. Switching off their genes impairs the cleavage of an amino terminal propeptide, leading to phenotypic consequences that are not identical (Le Goff et al., 2006).

The third family of metalloproteases functioning in the connective tissue extracellular matrix are **astacins**. More than 20 members of this family have been identified. As previously mentioned, the bone morphogenetic protein-1 (BMP-1/tolloid) is also an astacin. Other astacin members – **meprins** – are involved in the catabolism of basement membrane components – type IV collagens, nidogens and fibronectins (Kruze et al., 2004). Astacins also exert their influence on cell differentiation and tissue formation by activating the latent transforming growth factors of the TGF-β superfamily (see 4.2).

According to some data, the proteolysis of extracellular matrix proteins, of collagens in particular, is feasible in some cases without the participation of metalloproteases (Song et al., 2006). For example, in the osteoclastic resorption of bone tissue, collagen is broken down by cathepsins acting in an acidic medium.

The intensity of catabolic as well as proteolytic processes is not uniformly distributed throughout the entire extracellular matrix space. This space is compartmentalized in a particular manner i.e. it is subdivided into zones that differ from each other by protease activity. The highest enzymatic activity is concentrated in the nearby vicinity of the cells secreting these enzymes; within these zones, the proteases can act effectively even in the presence of inhibitors (Basbaum & Werb, 1996).

Many peptide fragments of the matrix's structural components, which are formed in proteolysis, exhibit biologic activity that is not intrinsic for intact protein macromolecules. The fragments of elastin, interstitial collagens and basement membranes' collagens actively affect the cell production of proteases, cell proliferation, migration and apoptosis. It has been proposed that these peptides, taking on the role of signaling molecules, be called matrikines (Maquart et al., 2005).

The only matrix structural macromolecular component that is not exposed to protease action is hyaluronan. The catabolism of this glycosaminoglycan, which is not comprised in the proteoglycan macromolecules, occurs inside cells rather than in the matrix. This principally distinguishes hyaluronan catabolism from that of other matrix polymers.

3.7.2. Inhibitors of metalloproteases

Under physiologic conditions, the catalytic activity of matrix metalloproteases correlates with the tissue's state. This correspondence is maintained by the intensity of enzyme expression, which is regulated at the transcription and post-transcription levels by the activity of different signaling molecules.

Their binding to cell surface proteins, particularly to some integrins and syndecans and to matrix protein structural components, to thrombospondin in particular, also regulates metalloprotease activity. This binding results in enzyme inhibition (Baker et al., 2002; Lee & Murphy, 2004).

TIMP (tissue inhibitors of metalloproteases) play the most important role in metalloprotease inhibition.

4 TIMP are known in mammals (see *Table 3.12*) (Baker et al., 2002). They are small protein molecules with a molecular mass of 21–28 kDa; TIMP-1 and TIMP-3 are glycoproteins. They are secreted by the cells into the extracellular matrix but can act, being bond to the cytoplasmic membrane. All TIMP are homologous in primary structure; they contain 6 disulfide bonds each and inactivate all metalloproteases by binding firmly with their catalytic domains. A common to all TIMP region of the N-terminal domain, starting at Cys3 and ending at Cys13, is of critical significance for their inhibitory activity. A selectivity of TIMP actions towards individual metalloproteases depends on the differences in structure of the C-terminal domain. The selectivity is only obvious in TIMP-3, which is able to inhibit ADAM and ADAMTS proteases (Woessner, 2001). The selectivity of TIMP activity can be enhanced through point mutations of the N-terminal region (Nagase & Brew, 2003), which offer the challenge of employing these modified metalloproteases inhibitors in clinical practice.

The expression of TIMP by cells, like that of metalloproteases, is under the control of regulating factors. In most tissues, the expression intensity of TIMP enables the maintenance of metalloprotease activity at low rates, which even creates methodical difficulties in their determination. The exception is present tissues with enhanced rearrangement.

In a number of pathological conditions, the imbalance between the MMP and TIMP activities arise, and the MMP's unrestricted activity leads to tissue destruction. For example, upon switching off the TIMP-3 gene in mice, pulmonary emphysema develops. Therefore, significant efforts have been made to develop pharmaceutical products designed to inhibit the MMP activity and catabolic reactions in the matrix they catalyze. Synthetic low-molecular analogues of TIMP delay the growth and dissemination of some experimental tumors by preventing the basement membranes from degradation by metalloproteases.

Chapter 4

REGULATION
OF CONNECTIVE
TISSUE METABOLIC
FUNCTIONS

4.1. SYSTEMIC FACTORS OF REGULATION

The main types of compounds regarded as systemic factors influencing molecular and biochemical processes in the connective tissue are:

a) **Hormones**–the regulatory (signaling) molecules of varying chemical nature, which are produced by specialized cells found in the endocrine glands and by certain types of cells scattered in various tissues, and released into the bloodstream and transported throughout the body to the target cells on they exert their influence. The effects caused by hormones are diverse and differ in various types of connective tissue.

b) **Vitamins**–molecules that are essential (indispensable) participants of certain metabolic reactions. In these reactions, vitamins play the role of catalytic cofactors or substrates for enzymes. The organism does not produce vitamins or produces them only under specific conditions, and therefore should obtain them with food or from the bacterial flora of the intestine (only true for few of them). Vitamins may be viewed as systemic regulatory factors since their presence ensures the optimal performance of biochemical processes in many tissues and organs.

Vitamin C, or **L-ascorbate** (the ascorbate ion is the active principle of ascorbic acid) is of utmost universal significance to the entire connective tissue system; obtaining sufficient amounts of ascorbate from food is absolutely essential for the human body.

Unlike most mammals (except for primates and guinea pigs), humans lack the *GULO* gene encoding the enzyme gulonolactone oxidase, which is required to convert glucose into ascorbate (Parsons et al., 2006). Animals that have the ability to synthesize ascorbate may develop an intracellular vitamin C deficiency due to a deficiency in the transmembrane glycoproteins SVCT1 and SVCT2, the co-transporters enabling the transport of hexoses and ascorbate across the plasma membrane (Savini et al., 2007).

Ascorbate serves as a cofactor for eight enzymes, three of which are enzymes of the post-translational processing of collagens and therefore, are especially important in the connective tissue biochemistry. These include procollagen prolyl-4-hydroxylase (P4H) and prolyl 3-hydroxylase (P3H), the enzymes responsible for the hydroxylation of the proline residues, which are already incorporated into the polypeptide chains of procollagens, by converting them into 4-hydroxyprolyl and 3-hydroxyprolyl respectively. Hydroxyprolyls are essential for the formation and stabilization of collagen macromolecules and for the supramolecular organization of collagen structures (see section 3.1.11).

The third enzyme, working with the help of ascorbate, is the procollagen lysyl hydroxylase (PLOD), which transfers the hydroxyl groups to the lysine residues; the subsequent glycosylation of hydroxylysyl constitutes one of the stages in cross-linking that increases collagen structures' stability.

The role of the ascorbate ion in the biosynthesis of collagens is not limited to its participation in the enzymatic hydroxylation of prolyls and lysyls. Ascorbate stimulates the production of type I and III collagens in cultured human fibroblasts by enhancing the transcription and messenger RNA stability for these proteins. The same effect is achieved in human skin through the local application of vitamin C, with an additional effect of increasing the activity of carboxy- and amino-terminal proteinases of procollagens (Nusgens et al., 2001).

In addition, in *in vivo* studies of guinea pigs and *in vitro* studies of human fibroblasts ascorbate deficiency was shown to not only to disturb the helix formation in collagen polypeptide α-chains but also the formation of the triple-helix conformation of type IV collagen macromolecules; the latter abnormality is due to suppressed formation of temporary disulphide bonds between the α-chains (Yoshikawa et al., 2001).

The inferior quality of collagens formed in the presence of vitamin C deficiency particularly strongly affects those connective tissue structures that are characterized by intensive metabolism in adults. Thus, the common symptoms of scurvy (a disease caused by the absence of ascorbate in food), such as loss of teeth and the dehiscence of previously healed wounds, are due to the short half-life period of collagens in the periodontal ligament and scar tissue respectively.

In addition to the ascorbate's effects on collagen metabolism, its anti-oxidant action is also important for metabolic processes within the entire connective tissue system, as it protects cells and components of the extracellular matrix against oxidative stress (the destructive influence of active oxygen radicals).

In guinea pigs, vitamin C deficiency leads to the increased expression of IGFPB1 and IGFPB2 proteins binding the insulin-like growth factors (IGFs). Such binding inhibits the actions of IGFs, which are implicated in the regulation of the normal growth of connective tissue.

Another vitamin known for its universal role as a systemic regulator of connective tissue is **vitamin A (retinol)**. An alcohol by its chemical nature (which enters the body as part of animal fats), it is converted, through the action of two dehydrogenases (ROLDH and RALDH) and some other enzymes, into active metabolites such as **retinaldehyde**, **retinoids** and the especially active **retinoic acid**, known in the form of several isomers. Retinoic acid is mostly formed within those cells that need it (Maden, 2000). Such an endogenous origin of the most active forms of vitamin A makes this regulating factor (similar, in these terms, to vitamin D) close to hormones (Reichrath et al., 2007).

Retinoic acid binds with specific binding proteins in the cytoplasm, constituting one of the mechanisms used to regulate its activity in the cell. Free retinoic acid (hydrophobic in its nature) penetrates into the nucleus, where it binds to RAR nuclear receptors comprised by three isotypes; there are also three isotypes of RXR nuclear receptors whose ligands are retinoids. This results in the formation of "ligand-receptor" complexes acting as transcription factors on specific elements (RARE) of genes responding to retinoic acid and retinoids (Marill et al., 2003). The inactivation of genes encoding enzymes, involved in the formation of retinoic acid, is accompanied (when such inactivation occurs at the earliest stages of embryogenesis) by major impairments in the morphogenesis of a number of organs and systems in experimental animals. The development of nervous system, the eye, the ear, and the cardiovascular and urogenital systems are especially vulnerable. Apart from cardiovascular system defects, the essentiality of retinoic acid for the normal morphogenesis of connective tissue structures is demonstrated by abnormalities in trunk and limb growth, and deformations in the cranio-facial skeleton, vertebrae and ribs (Maden, 2000). On the other hand, if the inactivation of enzymatic mechanisms for the formation of vitamin A active metabolites occurs in adulthood, the regeneration and reparative processes involving the connective tissue is supressed, along with abnormal changes in the eye (Maden and Hind, 2003).

The peculiarity of the action of vitamin A (or, more precisely, of its most active metabolite, retinoic acid) is the fact that its excess in the body produces toxic effects very similar to developmental abnormalities caused by its deficiency. This suggests that cells (especially those of the embryo) must have a mechanism for the tight regulation of the endogenous synthesis of retinoic acid, maintaining optimum levels (Maden, 2000).

We shall return to the effects of systemic regulators such as hormones and vitamins when we discuss the metabolic functions of specific types of connective tissue.

4.2. LOCAL FACTORS OF REGULATION

The regulation of cell functions (including those of all forms of connective tissue) by such systemic regulators as hormones and exogenous vitamins (as well as other components of food such as micronutrients) represents a higher level of regulation compared to the regulatory effects of local biochemical mechanisms. The basic level of cell function regulation in multicellular organisms is a highly organized system of signals transferred directly from cell to neighbouring cells, as well as from cells to the extracellular matrix and from matrix to cells.

The material substrate for these local (sometimes referred to as "short-distance") regulatory mechanisms is a special group of **signaling molecules**. They provide the cell to cell and cell to matrix information exchange, enabling cells' functional interactions.

The transfer of the biological information involves various types of molecules. Signaling molecules, in a wider sense of this term, should also include systemic hormones of various chemical nature, released by specialized cells in the endocrine glands and carried with the bloodstream throughout the body. The cells also receive information from the structural protein macromolecules of the matrix (such as collagens and fibronectins),

which can also be considered as signaling molecules. The signaling role is carried out by neurotransmitters (the low-molecular-mass transmitters of nervous impulses, such as catecholamines and acetylcholine), and even by such a simple molecule as nitric oxide.

Information signals are transmitted by numerous intracellular carrier proteins ("signal transducers"), which transfer a signal arriving into a cell to the cell nucleus, initiating the use of part of the genetic information required for adequate cell response. These protein molecules, varying in size and structure, such as STAT (signal transducers and activators of transcription) or SMAD, can transform (amplify, attenuate or qualitatively modify) the transferred signal by involving other proteins in the process, so that transduction occurs in a cascade-like manner.

However, by commonly accepted convention, only small (with a molecular mass of five to several hundred kDa), hydrophilic (water-soluble) **secreted** peptide or protein (polypeptide) molecules are viewed as signaling molecules responsible for the local regulation of cell functions; they are often glycoproteins. They are expressed by a wide variety of cells (in addition to other functions of these cells), and not just by endocrine gland cells dedicated to the biosynthesis of certain hormones. These molecules are released not into blood but into extracellular matrix, and the scope of their action is mostly limited to the tissue areas nearest to the expressing cells.

The secreted signaling molecules affect the nearest surrounding cells; this action is called **paracrine**. They may exert their regulating influence on the cell in which they have been produced; such an influence is called **autocrine**. However, in many cases, they may move far enough within the intercellular space, using various mechanisms and sometimes even passing through cells (Zhu and Scott, 2004). In such cases, their influence does not differ from the **endocrine** action of systemic hormones.

In this (narrower) sense, only four groups of peptides and larger polypeptides should be considered as signaling molecules:

1) growth factors,
2) cytokines,
3) neuropeptides and
4) morphogens. However, it should be noted that the above grouping is largely arbitrary since the distinctions between these groups are not always clearly definable. The contradistinction of growth factors and cytokines is especially controversial.

Growth factors are protein signaling molecules produced by many cells and acting mainly to stimulate the proliferation and differentiation of cells, including those of the connective tissue. At the same time, the effect of most growth factors is pleiotropic (multifunctional) in nature: it is aimed at various types of cells and various aspects of cell functions, including those unrelated to proliferation, such as growth and reproduction. In addition, in many known instances, the same activity is displayed by several growth factors.

Also pleiotropic is the action of **cytokines** (Ozaki & Leonard, 2002). Their molecules are often (although not always) smaller than those of growth factors. The presence of four closely spaced cysteine residues in the amino-terminal region is seen as the formal structural characteristic of cytokine molecules (Fernandez & Lolis, 2002). Many cytokines are expressed by haemopoietic cells, and their activity often primarily affects blood cells. Hence the names of several cytokine families, such as **interleukins** (a cytokine family comprised of 33 members), whose main function was believed to be the regulation of interactions between leukocytes shortly after the discovery of cytokines. However, it was subsequently established that interleukins also affect other cells and are expressed (as well as other types of cytokines) by many other cells. The role of cytokines is especially important in inflammatory reactions and in normal and pathologic immune responses. Cytokines belonging to the large family of **chemokines** induce chemotaxis; the specific aspects of activity of individual chemokines are determined by the number and collocation of cysteine residues in the amino-terminal regions of their molecules. Cytokines play an important role in a number of cellular interactions during embryogenesis.

The considerable functional and structural similarity between growth factors and cytokines has justified the merging of these two groups of signaling molecules. It has been proposed that the term "cytokines" be used as the general name for both groups, covering all protein signaling molecules expressed by any one cell to affect the functions of another cell. However, the collective name of **"growth factors/cytokines"** should be currently recognized as the most appropriate, preserving (largely as a matter of tradition) the separate terms "growth factor" and "cytokine" for those molecules whose characteristics are uncontroversial.

Morphogens are signaling molecules whose concentration gradient, formed as a result of their spreading from the expressing cell across a developing tissue, determines the structural arrangement of tissues and organs during embryogenesis (in particular, the positions of certain cell types within the tissue). Some morphogens, such as Wnt-proteins, also affect cells after the completion of the morphogenetic processes in a way similar to the action of growth factors (Baron et al., 2006). On the other hand, many growth factors/cytokines are able (like morphogens) to spread over considerable distances from the secreting cells. These facts blur out much of the distinction between morphogens and growth factors/cytokines.

Growth factors/cytokines can also enter the bloodstream and thereby exert their activity in regard to cells within tissues and organs remote from the source of local signals. This blurs the boundaries between the functions of signaling molecules and hormones, and therefore, many molecules are seen as both growth factors/cytokines and systemic hormones. The term histohormones has been proposed to designate signaling molecules with a basi-

cally local action (N.N. Mushkambarov and S.L. Kuznetsov, 2003).

Neuropeptides are peptides expressed mainly by neurons. There are about 100 known neuropeptides; hypothalamic neurons play a considerable role in their expression. Different groups of neurons produce different neuropeptides, transmitting information from neuron to neuron. Some neuropeptides (such as oxytocin and vasopressin) stimulate the expression of pituitary hormones and subsequently act as hormones themselves after entering the bloodstream. The neuropeptides somatomedin C and somatomedin A are expressed not only by neurons but also by liver cells; they are known as insulin-like growth factors IGF1 and IGF2 respectively. These growth factors stimulate the growth of cartilaginous and bone tissues. The neuropeptide Y in the hypothalamus is the major mediator of the effects of leptin, a hormone produced by fat cells and involved in regulating the metabolic functions of bone tissue cells (osteoblasts). Therefore, as with other short-distance signaling molecules, it is not possible to define a clear boundary between neuropeptides, growth factors/cytokines and systemic hormones.

Like systemic protein hormones, peptide (hydrophilic) short-distance signaling molecules can exert their actions on cells, with very few exceptions (Planque, 2006), only via transmembrane receptors in the cellular (cytoplasmatic) membranes. The inactivation of receptor-encoding genes or pharmacological blockade of receptors blocks the effects of signaling molecules.

Receptors that transmit into the cell information originating from their interactions with short-distance signaling molecules acting as ligands belong (like the receptors of systemic peptide hormones) to the class of metabotropic (influencing the cell metabolism) receptors. They vary in structure and functions. The most common of them are: a) G protein coupled receptors (also known as serpentine, heptahelical or 7TM receptors), the long twisting central domain of which crosses (traverses) the cell membrane seven times; and b) receptors whose intracellular domain exhibits the enzymatic activity of the tyrosine kinase.

The receptors for short-distance signaling molecules are characterised (as well as their ligands) by a marked pleiotropy. In most cases, each ligand has its own receptor expressed by the cell; yet, not infrequently, the same receptor is used by several ligands related in structure and functions (growth factors/cytokines) and belonging to the same family. This suggests a certain redundancy in receptors for signaling molecules (Ozaki & Leonard, 2002).

The mechanisms regulating the magnitude of responses initiated by signals become activated even before contact between signaling molecules and their receptors occurs. One of these mechanisms is the binding of signaling molecules by structural macromolecules of the extracellular matrix, such as proteoglycans. This deposition of signaling molecules is especially pronounced in bone tissue. Another regulatory mechanism is the existence of specific binding proteins that transport signaling peptides in an inactive (latent) state from cell to cell. Finally, one more mechanism is the activity of competing ("decoy") receptors. Decoy receptors, which may be secreted (soluble) or membrane-bound, are similar to true receptors in molecular structure but lack their functional associations. They "intercept" some number of ligand molecules, preventing their interaction with true (functional) receptors (Levine, 2004). All three mechanisms (binding of signaling molecules by structural components of the matrix; binding with specific soluble binding proteins; and blocking by decoy receptors) attenuate signals' effects on cells, apparently in accordance with immediate physiological conditions.

The regulation of the magnitude of a cell's response to information transferred by a receptor then continues along intracellular signal transduction pathways. As already mentioned, these multiple pathways (some of which will be addressed below when discussing the functions of individual short-distance regulators) include signal transducer (carrier) proteins and enzymes, mainly kinases. The complex interactions of signaling pathway components offer possibilities for both amplifying and attenuating signals. The attenuation of cytokine signals is mediated by specialized SOCS (suppressor of cytokine **signaling**) proteins. This family includes seven proteins whose expression increases in response to the action of various cytokines, and their influence applies to most components of signaling pathways (Krebs & Hilton, 2001).

Short-distance peptide signaling molecules are extremely numerous, and their number still increases as new members of this class are discovered. Based on the similarity of their molecular structures, they may be grouped into a number of families. The names of these families mostly reflect the function established for the first known member of the family or the source from which it was obtained. But the functions of most signaling peptides are generally characterised by pleiotropy (orientation of its effects at different aspects of cell activity), and subsequent studies have demonstrated the diversity of effects displayed by members of many families. It has also been shown that their sources of origin may differ. Therefore, it should be kept in mind that the names of most families are largely conventional.

For instance, the name of one growth factors family, the **fibroblast growth factors** (FGF), reflects their role in the regulation of connective tissue, although, as will be shown below, the functions of FGFs are not limited to stimulating the fibroblast growth.

The name of another growth factor, the **connective tissue growth factor** (CTGF), also contains an express reference to its effect on the connective tissue, which is not the case with the name of the family (CCN) of six proteins including CTGF (Rachfal & Brigstock, 2005). This factor, also known by other names (Hcs24, ecogenin), is a polypeptide consisting of 349 amino-acid residues, 38 of which are cysteine residues. CTGF is expressed by many cells and has a stimulating effect on many types of connective tissue, especially on the proliferation and differentiation of bone tissue cells (osteoblasts) and, in wider terms, on skeletal growth (Takigawa et al., 2003). CTGF also stimulates the synthesis of structural components of the extracellular matrix by connective tissue cells, thus promoting the development of fibrotic disorders that cause the excessive deposition of collagens in tissues (Leask & Abraham, 2003). These and other effects of CTGF mediate the action of signals from growth factors of the TGF-β superfamily, such as bone morphogenetic proteins (BMPs).

On the other hand, for a number of families of growth factors/cytokines, the participation of their members in the regulation of connective tissue is regarded as their main function (Henry & Garner, 2003), yet this is not reflected in their names. These are **platelet-derived growth factor** (PDGF), **epidermal growth factor** (EGF), **vascular endothelial growth factor** (VEGF), and the **transforming growth factor-β superfamily** (TGF-β).

Table 4.1 outlines the brief characteristics of the main families of local signaling molecules involved in the regulation of connective tissue.

Short-distance signaling molecules collectively form a highly organized regulatory system. In exerting their influence on cells, they interact with each other, showing antagonisms and synergies in their effects. They interact with systemic regulatory factors and with structural components of the extracellular matrix; the latter interactions result in the modification of their effects on cells.

Table 4.1.

The main families of growth factors/cytokines involved in connective tissue regulation

Members	Characteristic and functions
I. Transforming growth factor-β superfamily (TGF-β) [1]	This superfamily consists of about 100 members with a similar (at least 35–40% similarity) primary structure; they affect the cells via receptors (serine/threonine kinases) and use a SMAD protein system for intracellular transducing of signals.
1. Transforming growth factors-β	Stimulate the proliferation of undifferentiated mesenchymal cells; produce an anti-inflammatory effect (exerted by suppressing cytokine production and macrophage and lymphocyte proliferation); promote wound healing and stimulate fibrotic reactions.
2. Bone morphogenetic proteins (BMPs); cartilage-derived morphogenetic proteins, growth and differentiation factors (CDMP/GDF)	Regulate the differentiation and functions of mesenchymal cells since the early stages of ontogenesis; activate the differentiation of mesenchymal cells in chondrocytes and osteoblasts; influence skeletal morphogenesis.
3. Activins	Regulate the growth and differentiation of many cells; promote wound healing.
II. Fibroblast growth factor family (FGF) [2-4]	Many FGFs and some FGFRs are known in several isoforms.
1. FGF1–FGF10 subfamily	Play an important role in the differentiation of skeletal tissues during embryogenesis; use tyrosine kinases as receptors (FGFR).
2. FGF11–FGF14 subfamily	These FGFs do not act as ligands for FGFRs but penetrate into the cell (and, subsequently, into the nucleus) by way of endocytosis; they are of great importance in the early stages of embryogenesis (3); they are basically active in the morphogenesis of the nervous system, and are also known as FGF homologous factors (FHF).
3. FGF15–FGF23 subfamily	Participate in the regulation of angiogenesis, chondrogenesis and osteogenesis; the mechanisms of their action are not sufficiently understood.
III. Cell colony stimulating factors (G-CSF, GM-CSF, M-CSF)	Involved in hematopoietic processes. The macrophage colony-stimulating factor (M-CSF) is required for osteoclastogenesis.
IV. Epidermal growth factor (EGF) family	In addition to EGFs as such, the family encompasses 10 homologous proteins including the transforming growth factor-α (TGF-α), greatly differing in structure from the TGF-β superfamily.
1. EGF	Acts via an EGFR receptor that exhibits tyrosine kinase activity. EGF family factors stimulate cell growth, proliferation and differentiation, as well as protein biosynthesis.

V. Platelet-derived growth factor (PDGF) family	The PDGF-family consists of 5 peptides that act via two tyrosine-kinase receptors and stimulate angiogenesis, as well as cell growth and division.
VI. Tumour necrosis factor (TNF) superfamily [5]	Most TNFs are expressed by macrophages. The family also includes the osteoblast-produced RANKL.
1. RANKL	The 11th member of the superfamily of TNF-ligands, and one of the factors required for osteoclast differentiation.
2. TNF-α (also described under the names of cachexin or cachectin)	Causes apoptosis (not only in tumour cells) and plays a role in the morphogenesis of connective tissue structures; it is also involved in the regulation of immune processes.
VII. Vascular endothelial growth factor (VEGF) family [6]	This factor exists in seven known isoforms produced by alternative splicing. In addition, several related proteins are known, which exhibit similar activity. The VEGFs are potent mitogens required for the growth of blood vessels, including those found in connective tissue structures. They play a significant role in bone tissue morphogenesis and in the wound-healing process.
VIII. Insulin-like growth factors (IGF1 and IGF2)	IGF-1 and IGF-2 are highly similar to the hormone insulin in their structure but more actively stimulate cell growth and proliferation and hinder cells' apoptosis. These factors act as part of the so-called IGF "axis", including the growth hormone (GH), the IGF and six IGF binding proteins (IGFBP). They circulate in the blood plasma like hormones and are especially important in the morphogenesis of cartilaginous and bone tissues. These factors are highly similar to the hormone insulin in their structure but more actively stimulate cell growth and proliferation and detain cells apoptosis.
IX. Interleukins (IL) [7]	This collective name describes 33 cytokines (IL-1 – IL-33). Some IL types (such as IL-1, IL-6 and IL-10) are in fact families of genetically related molecules. One of the many functions of interleukins reflected in their name is the exchange of information between leukocytes. Interleukins are not only expressed by leukocytes, but also by other cells of the haemopoietic system and immunocompetent cells, as well as by cells of other tissues. Interleukins play an important role in regulating immune, inflammatory and proliferative processes. The effects of specific interleukins on the connective tissue are diverse, ranging from proinflammatory or catabolic (destructive) to anti-inflammatory (protective). Often, the nature of an interleukin's effect depends on the initial state of the cell, on the expression of receptors and the interactions of several interleukins among themselves and with other signaling molecules. Interleukins can mediate the effects of other signaling molecules or promote their expression. Some interleukins possess the properties of chemokines.
X. Interferons (IFN) [7]	Cytokines produced by macrophages and fibroblasts. Stimulate antiviral immunity and other immune processes. Interferon-α is involved in the pathogenesis of some systemic disorders of the connective tissue.

[1] Herpin et al., 2004;
[2] Ornitz & Itoh, 2001;
[3] Böttcher & Niehrs, 2005;
[4] Olsen et al., 2003;
[5] Locksley et al., 2001;
[6] Ferrara, 2004;
[7] Thibault & Utz, 2003.

Chapter 5

BIOCHEMICAL
AND MOLECULAR
MECHANISMS
AND MANIFESTATIONS
OF CONNECTIVE
TISSUE AGING

The natural (normal or physiological) changes in the connective tissue, designated by the general term **"aging"**, are currently characterized by the following features (Freemont & Hoylan, 2007):

- a reduction in tissue mass due to a disbalance between the synthesis and degradation of the extracellular matrix;
- a decrease in cells' biosynthetic activity;
- a reduction in the number of active progenitor cells;
- a change in the molecular structure of the matrix, caused by changes in the expression of genes and post-translational modifications, especially pronounced in fibrillar proteins such as collagens and elastin, but also affecting other numerous macromolecular components;
- accumulation of degraded macromolecules in the matrix;
- a decrease in the functional efficiency of all tissue elements;
- changes in the levels of the regulatory factors (hormones and local-action signaling molecules), as well as in cells' ability to respond to these factors and
- changes in how the tissue responds to the applied loads.

These are the signs through which aging is manifested in all types of connective tissue. Of course, in each of its types, aging has its peculiarities depending on the cellular and molecular structure of the tissue and its properties.

The aging process actually develops throughout ontogenesis and is primarily governed by the action of internal (intrinsic, endogenous) factors. These factors, regulating the process at the molecular level, are subdivided into two groups: genetic and epigenetic.

Genetic factors entail the influences of genes that define the program for overall cell activity and control its execution.

Epigenetic (from Greek *epi*–over, after) factors include the influence of gene-encoded products and modulating of the functioning through various mechanisms, and also act in the extracellular matrix after getting out of direct control of genes.

During its lifetime, the endogenous factors of connective tissue aging are accompanied by exogenous factors, i.e. the environmental influences, the physiological and pathogenic effects of which are difficult to demarcate. Of all exogenous influences, the effect of light (or, more precisely, of the ultraviolet spectral region), which plays an important role in the aging of the dermal layer of exposed skin areas, should be mentioned in the first place. This role is reflected in special terms such as the "light aging", "actinic aging" or "photoaging" of skin.

The molecular mechanism of light aging, superimposed upon the effects of natural (chronological) aging and accelerating its development, includes, as its main component, the formation, under the influence of ultra-violet radiation, of **reactive oxygen species (ROS)**, which destroys the tissue's antioxidative protective systems. The ROS subsequently causes the activation of a number of transmembrane receptors for growth factors and cytokines, which, in turn, activate the intracellular signaling cascades. Arriving at the cell nucleus, the signals cause changes in genes' expression; in particular, there is an increase in the expression of NADPH-oxidase by macrophages, which leads to the increased production of one of the most active ROS, hydrogen peroxide. In the resident fibroblasts (the cells responsible for the formation, maintenance, remodeling and degradation of the extracellular matrix), the expression of genes encoding the polypeptide chains of large fibrillar type I and III collagens, as well as that of elastin and other components of elastic fibrils, become suppressed. The expression of proteolytic enzymes, including some metalloproteinases, is concurrently increased. Long-term exposure to UV radiation makes these changes in the fibroblast genome irreversible (Fisher, 2005).

The direct action of ROS on the extracellular matrix, along with their effects on the cells, leads to an aging-specific decrease in collagen protein levels in the dermis. This decrease affects the large fibrillar type I and III collagens and microfibrillar type VII collagen, with levels of microfibrillar type VI collagen remaining practically unchanged (Watson et al., 2001). Also of great importance are mechanical stimuli (such as gravity) altering the configurations of cellular (cytoplasmatic) membranes. These configuration changes affect membrane receptors' functions and the condition of the so-called "phosphate relay" (the receptor-associated kinases, i.e. enzymes transporting phosphatic groups from protein to protein) activating the intracellular signaling pathways. This results in impairments in mechanochemical transduction, i.e. the transfer of mechanical and chemical signals originating in the extracellular matrix to the cells. Changes in the cell function produced by this mechanism are involved in the aging process (Silver et al., 2003).

Genetic factors play a leading role in the development of age-dependent changes in the cells. These changes, as shown in the example of tendon fibroblasts (tenoblasts), are so significant that they may be viewed as a fundamental rearrangement of their entire phenotype (Arnesen & Lawson, 2006). Fibroblasts from old mice have low mobility and proliferation; the organization of their cytoskeleton and its interaction with focal contact proteins are impaired; the expression of GADD153 (growth arrest and DNA-damage inducible protein) is activated.

These dramatic changes in phenotype, reflected by the term "cell aging", result from the execution of their genetic program, defining the genome stability and the dynamics of expression of various genes at various stages of ontogenesis. Cells' biosynthetic activity changes in accordance with these dynamics. A sharp decrease in the biosynthetic activity of human fibroblasts starts to occur in the second decade of life; this decline continues at a slower rate into old age. In some cell populations, the execution of their genetic program includes **apoptosis**, the natural death of cells. The apoptosis-induced loss of cells is only partially compensated for due to age-dependent changes in the progenitor mesenchymal stem cells (MSCs) remaining in the tissue. Due to these processes, the number of anabolically active cells decreases with age (Freemont & Hoylan, 2007).

The genetic program dictates a decrease in the production of structural components of the extracellular matrix and the activity of the enzymes involved in biosynthetic processes (both acting inside the cells and secreted for the post-translational processing of the matrix proteins). This drop in activity affects, in particular, such collagen processing enzymes as prolyl and lysyl hydroxylases and glycosyl and galactosyl transferases (see section 3.1.1.1) (Schofield & Weightman, 1978).

The suppression of anabolic processes in old age is accompanied by the activated catabolism of extracellular matrix structural components, caused by the hyperexpression of some proteolytic enzymes, including metalloproteinases such as MMP-1, with a simultaneous decrease in the production of their inhibitors. Changes in the catabolic activity of cells are also considered as genetically-defined aging mechanisms. The proteolytic degradation of collagen fibrils, consisting mainly of type I collagen, intensifies. In the dermis, where the action of genetic factors is accompanied by the influence of ultra-violet radiation, the proteolysis also affects type VII collagen microfibrils (Uitto, 2008).

While quantitative changes in collagen levels, caused by insufficient expression and excess proteolytic degradation, are genetically determined, the qualitative changes in collagen structures observed in old age are mainly due to epigenetic factors. Epigenetic changes develop mainly at the level of collagens' post-translational modifications and are seen, in particular, in the intermolecular cross-linking system (Bailey & Knott, 1999).

The age-specific dynamics of this system differ in long-lived and short-lived organisms, as well as in different parts of the connective tissue (Reiser et al., 1987). However, a general pattern that has been revealed is that the main changes occur at an early stage of the life cycle. Even before the end of the body's growth, the number of reduced difunctional cross-links (connecting two adjacent macromolecules), including dihydroxylysinonorleucine, declines. The trifunctional hydroxy pyridinium and similar cross-links are more stable. At a later age, the changes in cross-linking become less regular, but the tendency to reduction in number of lysyl oxidase mediated cross-links remains.

The endogenous changes in collagen structures developing in young and middle adulthood are controlled by regulatory factors (hormones and local molecular regulators) (Freemont & Hoylan, 2007). Among these factors, of primary importance is the so-called GH-IGF1 (pituitary growth hormone/insulin-like growth factor-1) axis (see 4.1), whose influence becomes insufficient in old age due to an increase in the serum levels of proteins that bind and inactivate IGFs. The second most important factor (not only in females but also in males) consists of estrogenic hormones, whose levels decline in old age. The aging of collagens is promoted by multifunctional cytokines (interleukins) IL-1 and IL-6, the serum concentrations of which increase in old age. In an aged body, cells develop a resistance to the effects of regulatory factors (hormones and local regulation factors), which effectively control cells' metabolic activity at a younger age. This resistance is attributed to the decreased expression of the corresponding receptors by cells.

During the aging process, the number of natural intermolecular cross-links typical for normal collagen fibrils does not increase compared to middle age but does decrease compared to the body's growth period. The partial proteolytic degradation of collagen fibrils is also observed, accompanied by certain changes in the properties of collagen structures, with a tendency to an increase in their stiffness and resistance to enzymes' action. These changes are caused by the formation of new cross-links of a different origin and a different chemical structure (Robins, 2007).

New intermolecular cross-links form in long-lived proteins, including fibrillar collagens, as a result of their long-term (over the entire lifetime) contacts with reducing sugars, primarily with glucose but also with ribose and others. The complex of reactions occurring in such contacts is collectively termed a Maillard reaction.

The aldehyde group of a reducing sugar bonds covalently, without the involvement of enzymes, to one of the free amino groups of the protein's macromolecule (usually to those of lysine or arginine residues). This reaction differs fundamentally from the enzymatic glycosylation of collagens that occurs during their post-translational processing. After a series of chemical conversions (also occurring without the assistance of enzymes), the sugar attached to the protein binds to another protein macromolecule, forming an intermolecular cross-link. This process is known by the term "glycation" which may be interpreted as "non-enzymatic glycosylation", and the newly formed compounds taking on the role of cross-links are referred to as **AGEs** (advanced glycation end-products).

There are about 20 known AGEs. Among them, the ones that are quantitatively dominant are **glucosepane** (Sell et al., 2005), α-diketone and lysine-dihydropyridinium-lysine (Susic, 2007). Some AGEs impart a yellowish-brown colouring to proteins; others, such as **pentosidine**, exhibit a characteristic fluorescence. Although pentosidine occurs in small amounts, it circulates in blood together with other AGEs and can be used, due to its fluorescence, as a marker for the Maillard reaction. The formed AGEs are highly stable and enzyme-resistant.

The accumulation of AGEs reaching considerable concentrations in old age causes two types of changes in collagen structures.

First, there occurs the formation of new intermolecular cross-links that are uncharacteristic to young and middle adulthood. Unlike the organized, strictly regulated enzymatic cross-linking in a growing body, the AGE-induced cross-linking has a chaotic nature. The newly formed bonds may connect two lysine residues or a lysine residue and an arginine residue from the adjacent macromolecules. An especially important distinction is the fact that these bonds are located not in the telopeptides (non-helical end regions), but in the central triple-helical domains of macromolecules. Such localization has a much stronger impact on the physical properties of collagen fibrils. Their solubility declines, with a concurrent increase in the stiffness, thermal denaturation temperature and resistance to proteolytic effects of metalloproteinases, such as stromelysin and gelatinase; AGE have a direct inhibiting effect on MMP-2.

Secondly, there are modifications in the side-groups of amino-acid residues to which AGE attach. These modifications alter their electrical charge, which leads to impaired interactions between the macromolecules within collagen fibrils. Thus, the modification of arginyls within the "sticky" RGD and GFOGER sequences affects the collagen-cell interactions involving the $\alpha1\beta2$ and $\alpha2\beta1$ integrins.

Both types of changes deteriorate the properties of collagen fibrils that are essential for their biomechanical functions and for control over the cell-matrix interactions exercised by them (Avery & Bailey, 2006). The changes affect fibrils' binding with heparin and keratan sulfate-containing proteoglycans, disrupting the adhesion and migration of cells (Reigle et al., 2008).

The AGEs also affect the cells themselves, irrespective of the changes in the matrix. The suppression of cell proliferation is observed upon adding AGEs to a culture of fibroblasts, and apoptosis occurs given the long-term contact of AGEs with cells (Peterszegi et al., 2006). Changes also occur in genes' expression profiles: the expression of proteolytic enzymes (metalloproteinase-9 and serpin-1) is elevated, while the expression of the collagen-, cadherin- and fibronectin encoding genes is suppressed (Molinari et al., 2008). Another manifestation of AGEs' influence on cells is the impaired differentiation of mesenchymal stem cells, observed in fatty, cartilaginous and bone varieties of connective tissue (Kume et al., 2005). These effects are mediated by specialized receptors, whose expression by cells is induced by AGEs and by TNF-α (Lohwasser et al., 2006). There are five known receptors of this type; this fact may be interpreted as indirect evidence of organisms' phylogenetic adaptation to AGE formation. It should be noted that the collagen macromolecules tightly packed in the native fibrils are largely protected from non-enzymatic glycosylation. Hence, it should be preceded by other age-related changes in collagen structures, caused by both genetic and epigenetic factors (Slatter et al., 2008). Along with large interstitial fibrillar collagens, the structures especially affected by AGE accumulation are basement membrane collagens (type IV collagens. Modeling studies involving the prolonged incubation of the isolated domains of placental type IV collagen with sugars have revealed the formation of intermolecular cross-links unknown under normal conditions and character-

ised by pentosidine-like fluorescence. In addition, impairment was observed in the ability to bind the triple-helical and non-helical domains of macromolecules during the formation of supramolecular structures, as well as in the conformation and thermal stability of macromolecules (Raabe et al., 1996). The effect of AGEs appeared to be more complicated in a study involving cultured type IV collagen-producing mesangial cells. The AGEs not only create excess cross-links between the existing type IV collagen macromolecules, but also promote the hyper-expression of these collagens. The AGE-induced stimulation of type IV collagen expression is associated with the increased expression of Smad1 protein, which is part of the intracellular SMAD signal transduction pathway (see section 4.2) and interacts with the *Col4A* gene promoter. At the same time, the expression of ALK1 kinase, associated with one of the receptors for TGF-β superfamily growth factors, is activated. These signaling molecules stimulate the biosynthesis of collagen proteins (Abe et al. 2004). This intricate mechanism of AGE action constitutes one example of how the function of the genetic apparatus is influenced by epigenetic factors.

The over-expression of type IV collagens, which promotes their increased accumulation in basement membranes, together with redundant cross-linking and changes in the conformations of macromolecules, leads to the thickening of basement membranes (in particular, those of capillaries) and to the reduced permeability of membranes.

The processes caused by the Maillard reaction are considerably accelerated and intensified in diabetes mellitus, where the fibrillar components of connective tissue are continuously exposed to high glucose levels. These processes, especially the developing changes in basement membranes, become the reason for diabetic complications such as nephropathy and retinopathy.

The aging of the second fibrillar system of connective tissue – the elastic fibers – results from the action of an even more complex set of molecular mechanisms than in the case of collagen structures. It involves changes in both elastin and all components of elastic fibers: fibrillin microfibrils and other fiber-associated proteins.

The basic age-related changes in elastic fibers, especially pronounced in the walls of the large arterial vessels and

Fig. 5.1.
Fragments of human skin.
a – normal skin;
b – hyperelastosis (elastosis).
Epidermis (1).
Papillary dermis (2).
Reticular dermis (3).
Elastic fibers (4).
Aggregates of elastic material (5).
Histologic sections.
Orcein stain.
SM-micrograph,
a, b – x 250.

in the skin, including the enhanced binding (fixation) of calcium and lipids and in proteolytic degradation (Robert et al., 2008).

Calcium levels in humans reach their maximum at 75–80 years of age, approaching 7% of the mass of purified elastin. An excess of calcium induces changes in conformations of elastin polypeptide chains, which leads to the opening of the lipid binding loci for various lipid classes, primarily for cholesterol esters. The binding of calcium and lipids compromises the elastic properties of fibers/fibrils.

The proteolytic degradation of elastin is performed by several elastases that possess an endopeptidase activity, primarily the metalloproteinases MMP-2 and MMP-9, and by a bound to the cell membranes by serine elastase. The total expression of the elastolytic endopeptidases increases during aging; this increase is promoted by the accumulating lipids.

The pathogenetic significance of the proteolysis-induced age-dependent degradation and fragmentation of elastic fibrils is not limited to the deterioration of the elastic properties of the fibrils and or those of the connective tissue as a whole. The matter is that, in the elastolytic peptide fragments of elastin macromolecules, such sites

(loci) of the large polypeptide chains become exposed which are hidden in the native conformations of the whole macromolecules. These opening loci endow fragments called **matricriptins** (also known as **elastokines** due to their cytokine-like activity), a biological activity uncharacteristic to the whole native elastin molecules. Due to the metabolic stability of elastin (an extremely long-lived protein), its fragments appear "alien" to the body, which has no effective mechanisms to control their activity (Labat-Robert, 2003).

The elastin fragments interact with cells using a transmembrane receptor known as S-Gal (a variant of the enzyme galactosidase) or a 67-kDa elastin-binding and laminin-binding protein (Mecham et al., 1991). The most effective ligands for this receptor are fragments that contain repetitions of the VGVAPG hexapeptide.

Elastokines' effects on cells are diverse. They cause the further upregulation of elastases, creating a vicious circle in which the aging process is promoted through increased proteolysis. The elastokines also stimulate the formation of free oxygen radicals, damaging the structural macromolecules of the matrix. In addition, they induce the chemotaxis of leukocytes, stimulate the proliferation of fibroblast and smooth

5.1 a

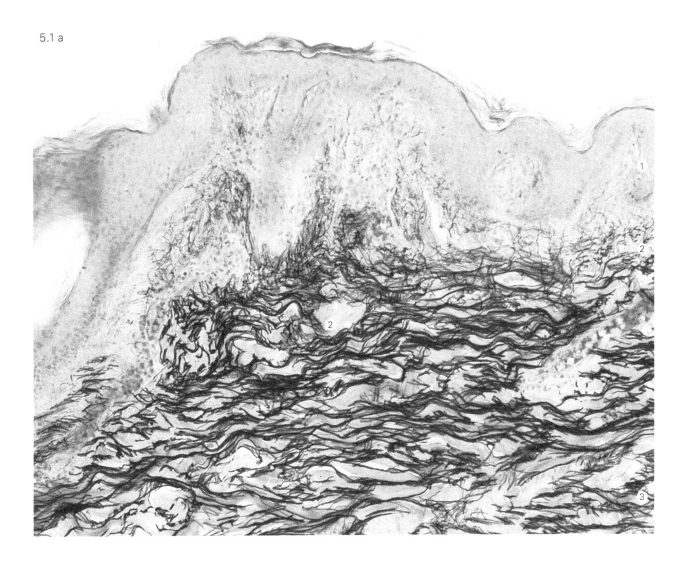

muscle cells, and exhibit pronounced angiogenic activity. Due to these phenomena, especially occurring in the aorta and dermis, the aging process exhibits the characteristics of a progressive chronic inflammation (Antonicelli et al., 2007).

The metabolic stability of elastin makes its no less susceptible than long-lived fibrillar collagens to interactions with reducing sugars (the Maillard reaction). The advanced glycation end-products (AGEs), similar to the AGEs found in collagens, upon accumulating in elastin, promote aging-specific changes such as an increase in stiffness and a reduction in elasticity of elastin structures, as well as the formation of free oxygen radicals (Robert et al., 2008).

As for exogenous factors, their role in elastin aging is the most significant in developing age-related changes in open (sun-exposed) areas of skin. UV radiation promotes the proteolytic degradation of elastic fibrils and, at the same time, causes a paradoxical phenomenon called elastosis, i.e. the massive accumulation and deposition of elastin (referred to as elastotic material) in the upper and middle dermis, characterized by impaired supramolecular organization and hence, by compromised elastic function (*Fig. 5.1*). This phenomenon is explained by the

stimulating influence of UV radiation on the elastin gene promoter, which is manifested by an increase in its expression (Uitto, 2008).

The abnormalities in elastin fibrillogenesis seen in elastosis (which is sometimes characterized as the accumulation of degenerated elastic fibers) are associated with the age-dependent decline in the expression of **fibulin-5**.

This glycoprotein (also known as Evec/DANCE) is associated with elastic fibers/fibrils and is required for elastogenesis *in vivo* (Nakamura et al., 2002). The expression of fibulin-5 in the dermis progressively decreases with aging and under the influence of UV radiation. In elastosis, it is partially restored but, apparently not to a degree sufficient for the normal formation of elastic fibers/fibrils (Kadoya et al., 2005).

There are two more proteins that are involved in the development of elastosis. **Elafin** is a small protein with a molecular mass of about 12 kDa, which is an elastase-specific inhibitor (hence its other name, ESI). In elastosis, it binds with elastin, protecting it from proteolytic degradation. In this way, elafin promotes elastin accumulation in the dermis (Muto et al., 2007).

Another protein (glycoprotein), **clusterin**, performs a chaperon-like function in regard to elastin in elastosis

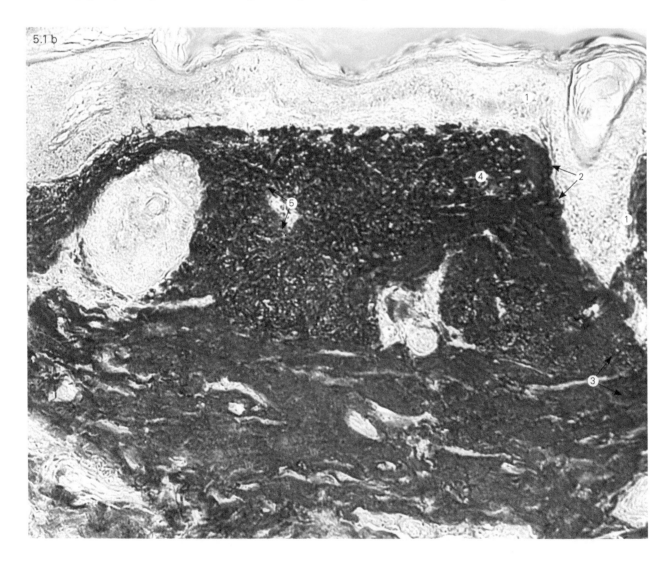

5.1 b

(see section 3.1.1.1). Clusterin, a multifunctional protein circulating in blood serum, preferentially associates with conformationally disturbed proteins. Associating with defective elastic fibers/fibrils in elastosis, it inhibits their aggregation, restricting the formation of elastosis-specific elastin depositions within the dermis (Janig et al., 2007).

The aging of elastic fibers/fibrils affects not only elastin but also all the components of fibers. Along with the reduction in elastin levels in tissues, proteolytic degradation leads to the destruction of the fibrillin microfibrillar structural scaffold of elastic fibers/fibrils.

This destruction is attributed to the proteolysis of fibrillins, mediated not by elastases but by metalloproteinases (MMP), actively expressed during aging (Ashworth et al., 1999). The increase in proteolysis during aging affects not only microfibrils of elastic fibers/fibrils but also the microfibrils that form the third (independent) fibrillar system of connective tissue.

A reduction in the overall levels of fibrillin-1 and glycoprotein MAGP-1 coexisting with it in fibrillin microfibrils' structure has been confirmed in the elastotic material accumulating during the light-aging of skin (Ohnishi et al., 2000). This reduction undoubtedly plays a role in the degeneration of elastic fibers/fibrils in elastosis.

The proteolysis activated during aging promotes the release of peptide fragments from the macromolecules of large glycoproteins of the extracellular matrix and basement membranes (fibronectins and laminins). Like elastin fragments (elastokines), fibronectin and laminin fragments become biologically active through the exposure of cryptic sites within the native macromolecules, thus becoming **matrikines**. Matrikines affect fibroblasts using the same S-Gal receptor as elastokines do. This results in a similar effect, i.e. the activation of such fibroblast functions (proteolytic enzyme expression and ROS formation) that promote the progression of matrix aging-specific changes (Labat-Robert, 2003).

An important role in the functions of proteoglycans, as the main component of the integrative buffer metabolic medium of the connective tissue extracellular matrix, is played by carbohydrate polymer chains (glycosaminoglycans) that are part of their macromolecules. The role of glycosaminoglycans is especially important in large proteoglycans, the core proteins of which have dozens of glycosaminoglycan chains, representing up to 50% of the macromolecule's total mass. Glycosaminoglycans are required to maintain the physicochemical and biomechanical properties of the matrix, as well as for the transduction of signals required for cell functions to the cells. In the aging process, this defines the significance of changes in glycosaminoglycans, along with changes in the core proteins of proteoglycans.

Like other carbohydrate polymers and unlike proteins, glycosaminoglycans are by-products of genes; their biosynthesis is not directly controlled by genetic information, but by the coordinated activity of enzymes, mainly the glycosyltransferases and sulfotransferases responsible for the assembly of their molecules (see section 3.2.1.2). Such a complex control system (Kobata, 2003) enables the occurrence of vast number of variations in the structure of glycosaminoglycan chains unspecified by the genetic program. These variations affect such structural characteristics as the glycosaminoglycan chain length, the degree of sulfation, the location of sulfate groups and the epimerization of uronic acid residues. Since the intense exchange of proteoglycans enables repeated renewals of macromolecules throughout life, the accumulation of variations altering the "glycomic" pattern of the tissue occurs with aging (the term **glycome**, meaning the carbohydrate structure of tissue, has been proposed by analogy with the terms genome and proteome). Proteoglycans' interactions with other structural components of the matrix, as well as with signaling molecules and cells, are changed accordingly (Hitchcock et al., 2008). The resulting impairments of cell functions become an additional reason for the development of even more dramatic and extensive changes in all extracellular matrix components.

The age-related changes in the glycosaminoglycans of cartilaginous tissue (where the main proteoglycan is the large hyalectan aggrecan, especially rich in glycosaminoglycans) may, to some degree, be considered as characteristic of the entire connective tissue system. These changes include:

a) quantitative changes in the balance between the various glycosaminoglycans contained in aggrecan macromolecules (an increase in keratan sulfates with a concomitant decrease in chondroitin sulfates);

b) changes in glycosaminoglycan chain lengths (longer keratan sulfate chains and shorter chondroitin sulfate chains);

c) changes in the disaccharide pattern of glycosaminoglycans (increased chondroitin-6-sulfate levels); and

d) the double sulfation of the terminal disaccharide of chondroitin sulfate (Dudhia, 2005).

The same type of changes occurs to glycosaminoglycans in skin. Thus, in the process of aging, the single glycosaminoglycan chain of decorin shortens, which reduces the distance between the adjacent collagen fibrils (Nomura, 2006).

The core proteins of proteoglycans are affected by age-related changes to no less an extent than are glycosaminoglycans.

The changes to core proteins in cartilaginous tissues are represented by:

a) a reduced aggrecan core protein length due to the shortening of its C-terminal domain;

b) the reduced sizes of supramolecular aggrecan aggregates with hyaluronan;

c) the decreased expression of the link protein of aggregates (which diminishes aggregate stability); and

d) the decreased extractability of proteoglycans from the tissue, indicating the strengthening of intermolecular bonds between the macromolecules of proteoglycans and between proteoglycans and other structural components of the matrix, such as collagens (protein-protein bonds) (Dudhia, 2005).

The age-dependent changes in the protein components of proteoglycans are brought about by the same factors and mechanisms as those causing changes in collagens and elastins. The genetic factor undoubtedly plays the leading role in the gradual decline in the expression of small leucine-rich proteoglycans (SLRPs), such as lumican (Vuillermoz et al., 2005) and fibromodulin (Bevilacqua et al., 2005) by fibroblasts of the dermis during aging. The epigenetic factor, i.e. the hyperactivity of metalloproteinases such as MMP-12, underlies the qualitative changes in the core protein of a major proteoglycan of the dermis, versican, impairing its hyaluronan-binding ability. However, this is also accompanied by the action of an exogenous factor, the UV radiation stimulating the expression of proteolytic enzymes (Hasegawa et al., 2007).

Although the core proteins of proteoglycans are not so long-lived as fibrillar collagens and elastin, some of their domains undergo a Maillard reaction during aging. Nonenzymatic glycosylation end products (AGEs), including the characteristic marker of this process, pentosidine, accumulate in the link protein and G1-domain of aggrecan (Dudhia, 2005). This affects the conformations of macromolecules and increases their stiffness.

All of the aforementioned aging-specific changes in the connective tissue are associated with the fibroblast function. Another type of age-related change, which plays a major role in the regulation of life expectancy, affects fat cells (adipocytes), their function and regulation.

The volumes of fat depots and their distribution within the body change throughout life. The overall mass of fat reaches its maximum in middle age but declines in old age. This is accompanied by the slowed differentiation of adipocytes from the mesenchymal stem cell-derived preadipocytes present in adipose tissue and, representing 15–20% of the total amount of all cells in the tissue (Cartwright et al., 2007). This suppression of adipogenesis, occurring during the transition from middle age to old age, is attributed to the action of several molecular factors.

These factors include the C/EBP homologous protein (CHOP). This protein, whose expression by preadipocytes increases in old age, blocks the activity of adipogenic factors of the C/EBP family and raises the preadipocytes' resistance to adipogenesis (Tchkonia et al., 2007). The expression of CHOP is stimulated by TNF-α growth factor, which, along with a number of other inflammation mediators such as IL-1β and IL-6 interleukins and COX-2 cyclooxygenase, is more actively produced by preadipocytes in old age (Wu et al., 2007).

Another factor that suppresses adipogenesis in old age that uses a similar mechanism in its action is the CUGBPl protein. Like CHOP, this protein, whose levels in the adipose tissue increase over the years, acts to restrict the activity of C/EBP adipogenic factors (in particular, of

C/EBPα) and, furthermore, of the PPARγ factor that is especially important to adipogenesis (refer to 2.4.2) (Karagiannides et al., 2006).

The activity of PPARγ is repressed by the action of still another factor–protein sirtuin 1 (SIRT1). Under the influence of sirtuin 1 (as a result of this repression), the accumulation of fat in adipocytes is inhibited. The gene encoding this protein is the mammalian ortholog of the *Sir2* gene, known for its ability to increase the lifespan in invertebrates. Consequently, SIRT1, along with other members of the sirtulin family, apparently acts as a molecular link between fat metabolism and lifespan (Picard and Guarante, 2005).

In the process of aging, the influence of all of the above factors impairs certain links in the metabolism of fat acids, which acquire a paradoxical toxicity in respect to preadipocytes, stimulating the mechanisms of their apoptosis (the activity of caspases and the *Bax* and *p53* genes). This results in a decrease in the number of mature adipocytes within the body (Gao et al., 2007).

Chapter 6

BONE – AN ORGAN
OF THE SUPPORT
AND LOCOMOTOR
APPARATUS
CONTAINING
ALL TYPES
OF CONNECTIVE
TISSUE

6.1. OVERVIEW OF BONE STRUCTURE AND FUNCTIONS

The structural foundation of **bone**, as an **organ** (BO), consists of bone proper, the periosteum and endosteum, together with the bone marrow, blood vessels and nerves (*Fig. 6.1*).

The constituents of bone are composed of all types of connective tissue: bone, cartilage, fibrous and adipose.

The functions and properties of bone are determined by its components: biomechanical (integrating, supporting, protective and locomotor), plastic, morphogenetic, metabolic, hematopoietic and immune.

Each bone component performs its specific function or functions, and is also involved in supporting the functions of other components. These interactions or cooperation make bone an independent organ.

Owing to its multifunctional capabilities, bone participates in the activities of an organism's vital functional systems (Anokhin, 1975): the maintenance of a certain level of minerals in the blood, the pH of blood, its cellular composition, etc.

Individual bones are integrated in a support system – the bone skeleton – with the help of various types of connections: continuous (fibrous (synarthrosis)), discontinuous (diarthrosis (synovial)) and transitional (hemiarthrosis), providing them with physiological mobility during locomotion.

All forms of bone connections are realized through various types of connective tissue: fibrous dense regular, cartilaginous and osseous. The extent of involvement of a particular type of connective tissue is determined by the shape of the connections, and the degree and nature of their movements.

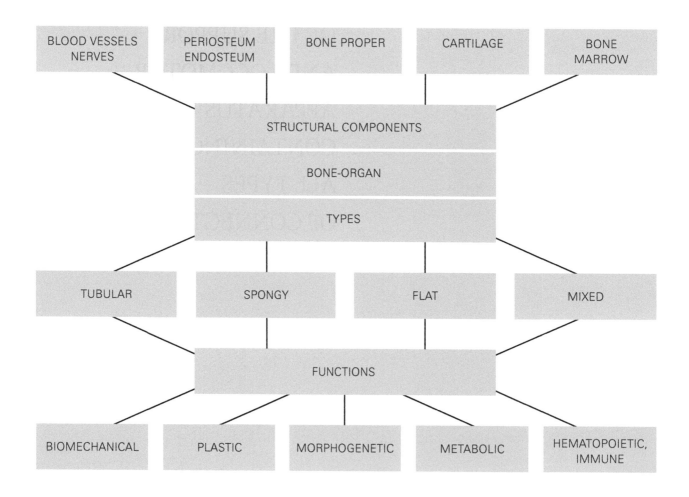

Fig. 6.1.
Schematic representation of the structural and functional organization of the bone organ (according to Omelyanenko).

6.2. GENERAL STRUCTURAL AND FUNCTIONAL CHARACTERISTICS OF BONE COMPONENTS

Bone proper, the main part of **bone organ**, is made up only of bone tissue (see Chapter 8). It determines the bone shape, its mass, biomechanical, and physicochemical properties. The remaining components of the bone organ are involved in supporting the normal vital activity of bone proper.

Bones themselves are built of compact and spongy osseous tissue, whose ratio in bones determines the characteristics of their general structure, shapes, properties and functions. Bones are classified as tubular, spongy, flat and mixed.

The **periosteum** is a thin layer of fibrous connective tissue that covers most of the outer surface of bone proper. The periosteum connects the bone to the surrounding tissues and participates in its blood supply, innervation, growth, renewal and reparative regeneration after bone injuries. These features are reflected in its structural organization. Two layers (without clear boundaries) are distinguished in the periosteum (*Fig. 6.2*). The outer fibrous layer represents dense fibrous regular connective tissue, which contains numerous blood vessels and nerves, forming multilevel plexuses. The vessels and nerves branching out of these plexuses enter the bone proper. The second, deeper, inner layer of the periosteum is called fibroelastic or cambial. It is a continuation of the outer layer, but the fibers are less oriented and more loosely arranged. It contains more elastic fibers than the outer layer. A large amount of osteoprogenitor cells are present in the border zone of this layer, adjacent to the bone. Fasciae, ligaments, tendons, fibers and fascicles attach to the periosteum, extending into its fibrous framework. Some of these fibers pass through the periosteum and proceed into the fibrous foundation of bone.

The inner part of bone proper, on the side of the marrow cavity (channel), is represented by a thin layer of non-mineralized bone matrix (osteoid). Its surface relief is formed by collagen fibrils and numerous channels (*Fig. 6.3*). Apparently, the latter are responsible for feeding this layer and its mineralized extension into bone proper from the bone marrow. Osteogenic cells and their progenitors are found in the osteoid.

In turn, a thin layer of loose fibrous connective tissue adheres to this layer; it exhibits an uneven thickness and the characteristic fibrous structures (fine collagen fibers and fibrils), cellular elements (fibroblasts, reticular cells, osteoprogenitor cells and osteoblasts) and integrating buffer metabolic medium (*Fig. 6.4*). This layer is called **endosteum**. It is not continuous and is absent in some places, whereby the bone marrow can be in direct contact with the surface of bone proper. The structure of the endosteum varies depending on bone remodeling, bone region, and age dynamics. The endosteum represents the boundary structure between the bone marrow stroma and bone. Its morphology is discussed in detail in recent literature (Denisov-Nikolsky, 2005).

Cartilage is an anatomical structure built of cartilage tissue (see Chapter 7) or cartilaginous and fibrous dense regular connective tissue (perichondrium), which exists either autonomously (extraosseous) or as a part of bone (organ). The types of cartilage and its functions are shown schematically in *Fig. 6.5*.

In accordance with this classification, there are three types of cartilage or cartilage tissue, which are distinguished by appearance (hyaline), by the presence of elastic protein and its supramolecular structures in the composition of the cartilage (elastic), and by the characteristics of the structural organization (fibrous).

Cartilages can have perichondrium or lack it. The former contain both cartilage proper and a perichondrium. The perichondrium is similar in structure and function to the periosteum. It is composed of nerves and blood vessels, which are responsible for feeding the cartilage tissue of cartilage proper. The blood vessels and nerves do not penetrate the cartilage tissue, and therefore, the nutrients enter it by diffusion. Metabolites are removed from the cartilage tissue in the same way. The feeding of articular cartilages (that lack perichondrium) occurs through the synovial fluid bathing their surface. Besides the mechanism of nutrients' passive diffusion into the cartilage tissue and of metabolites out of it, their shifts in opposite directions also occur due to the movement of portions of the synovial fluid into and out of cartilage during its deformations, resulting from alternating loading and relaxation. Therefore, the normal vital activity of the cartilage depends on the intensity of the latter movements. The subchondral bone is another source of nutrition for the cartilage. The mechanisms of nutrient intake from the subchondral bone and metabolite removal in the opposite direction will be discussed in Chapter 7.

Cartilage exhibits elastic and isotropic properties, generated by the special structural organization (fibrillar non-oriented framework) (see Chapter 7). As an anatomical structure within the bone organ, articular hyaline cartilage performs biomechanical functions. Among these, amortization provides the "damping" or "dispersion" of shock loads occurring during movements. A second one – tribological – ensures the optimal sliding of one articular surface relative to another with minimal friction. Third – the function of plastic congruence complements the anatomical congruity of articulating bone ends, thereby enabling their closer interaction at the micro level, i.e. it provides the best match between adjacent contacting surfaces.

Cartilages within bone connections provide the links between individual bones, integrating them into one system – the skeleton. In many cases, hyaline cartilages participate, along with fibrous cartilages, in these connections (continuous), damping the mutual pressure of bones.

Cartilages, as autonomous (extraosseous) anatomical structures, play a role in maintaining shape. This largely

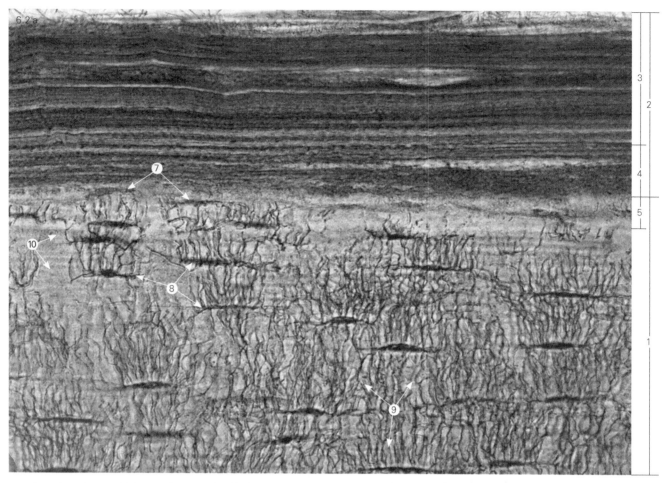

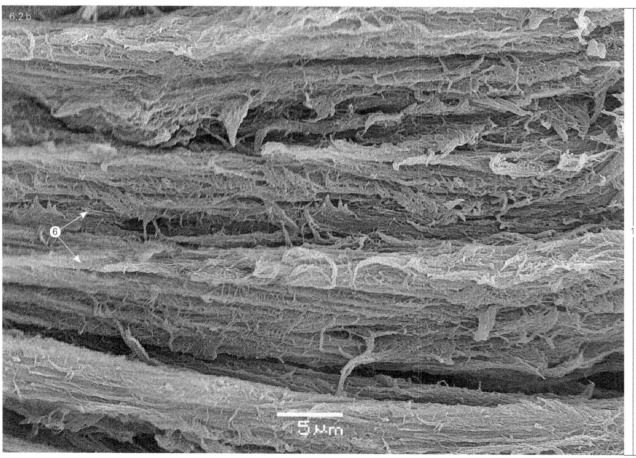

determines people's facial features (ear and nose cartilages – hyaline and elastic), and the tubular non-collapsing shape of the airways (larynx, epiglottis, trachea, bronchi – elastic and hyaline cartilages).

Temporary (transitory) cartilages (hyaline) mediate bone formation during embryogenesis and the early postnatal period – hyaline cartilage models, and the growth and development of bones (epiphyseal cartilages, cartilage end-plates of the intervertebral discs).

Bone marrow is a tissue complex composed of fibrous loose irregular connective tissue (stroma), hematopoietic cells, mature blood corpuscles (parenchyma), blood vessels and nerves, which fills in bone marrow cavities (*Fig. 6.6, 6.7, 6.8*). Bone marrow performs a number of functions in the body such as hematopoietic, immune and endocrine functions, supplying energy, supplying a bone with osteogenic cells, maintaining the connective tissue cell population in any type of connective tissue within an organism by releasing circulating (mobile) connective tissue multipotent progenitor-cells into the blood.

As all other types of connective tissue, the bone marrow stroma consists of cellular elements of mesenchymal origin and an extracellular (intercellular) matrix. The cellular elements comprise stem connective tissue multipotent cells (SCTMC), circulating (mobile) connective tissue multipotent progenitor-cells, reticulocytes (bone marrow fibroblasts), adventitial cells (poorly differentiated cells of a fibroblastic type), adipocytes, osteogenic cells, and macrophages.

Stem connective tissue multipotent (polypotent) cells (SCTMC), present in bone marrow, are poorly differentiated CT-cells capable of self-reproduction and maintaining the CT-cells of several differons therein: fibroblastic (reticular cells, reticulocytes), osteochondrocytic and adipocytic (*Fig. 6.9*). In SCTMC division, one of their daughter cells retains stem properties, while the other takes on the way of differentiation and the formation of one of the aforementioned differons.

The SCTMC are involved in maintaining similar connective tissue differons in connective tissues outside bone

Fig. 6.2.
A fragment of the cortical
part of bone proper (1)
with the periosteum (2).
Outer layer (3)
and inner layer (4)
of the periosteum. Osteoid (5).
Collagen fibers (6).
Preosteoblasts/osteoblasts (7).
Osteocytes (8).
Canaliculi (9).
Bone matrix (10).
a – LM-micrograph.
A light optic microscope
Ni Nikon (Japan).
Histological section.
Schmorl staining,
x 400.
b – SEM-micrograph.
x 2,700.

marrow and in the formation of fibroblastic differons in reparation foci via their derivatives – multipotent mobile CT-cells entering the blood and constantly circulating therein (*Fig. 6.10*).

Reticulocytes (bone marrow fibroblasts) exhibit a structural organization similar to that of fibrous connective tissue fibroblasts. The form, sizes, the development of organelles and their number in the reticular cell cytoplasm depend on the degree of their differentiation and functional state (*Fig. 6.11*). The reticular cells (reticulocytes) interact with each other and with other CT-cells by means of their long and short processes forming a cellular network, which is similar to the syncytium.

Adventitial cells are poorly differentiated CT-cells of a fibroblastic differon. It is supposed that they can be SCTMC. They are located near blood vessels and cover a significant part of the external surface of sinusoid capillaries. The adventitial cells contain microfilaments, which, upon contracting, change their location, resulting in the alteration of the sinusoid area covered by an adventitial layer. The processes of adventitial cells spring deep inside the bone marrow, where they bind with the reticulocyte processes involved in an integrated stromal cellular network (Weiss, 1976).

Osteogenic cells in a bone marrow cavity (preosteoblasts and osteoblasts) are mainly located on the inner surface of a bone proper, comprising a non-mineralized superficial layer (osteoid) and endost. These cells are described in detail in Chapter 8.

Adipocytes (lipocytes) are adipose cells that can be part of bone marrow as separate cells or in small groups involved in the formation of a microenvironment for hematopoietic parenchyma cells, which prevail in number, thereby creating an optimal medium for hematopoiesis. These adipocytes have the same progenitors as reticular, osteogenic and adventitial cells. They retain all the functions and structure peculiarities of adipose cells, as described in Chapter 2 (2.4).

There are mature (unicameral) adipose cells and immature (multicameral) fibroblast-like adipose cells (preadipocytes) in the bone marrow adipose tissue. The former contain large lipid droplets occupying almost the entire cytoplasm volume and comprise the base for adipose tissue. The latter are fibroblast-like adipose cells containing numerous lipid droplets of varying size in their cytoplasm (Shigematsu et al., 1999).

Differentiated (unicameral, mature) bone marrow adipose cells are stationary cells, which lose their proliferative ability in an adult organism. However, the derivation of differentiated adipose cells from bone marrow and their subsequent culturing in a 3D collagen gel matrix induces their de-differentiation and transformation into multicameral fibroblast-like adipose cells, which actively proliferate. A delay or halting of this process occurs due to contact inhibition, i.e.it depends on cell density. Herein the re-differentiation of multicameral adipose cells into unicameral ones occurs (Shigematsu et al., 1999).

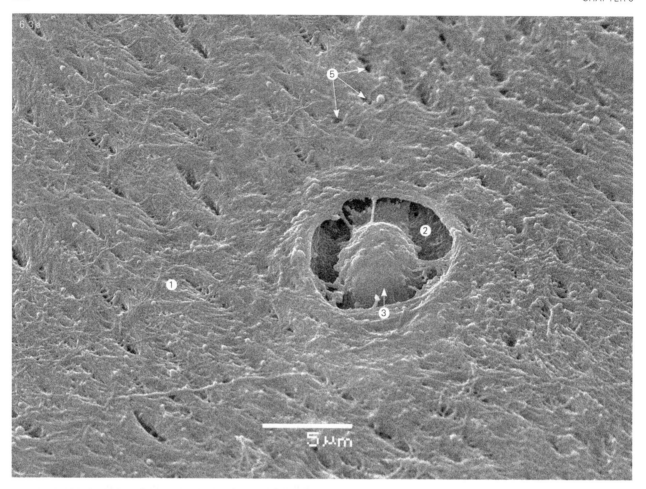

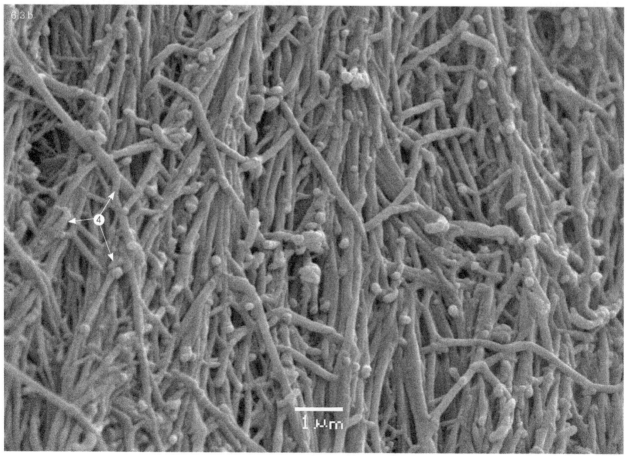

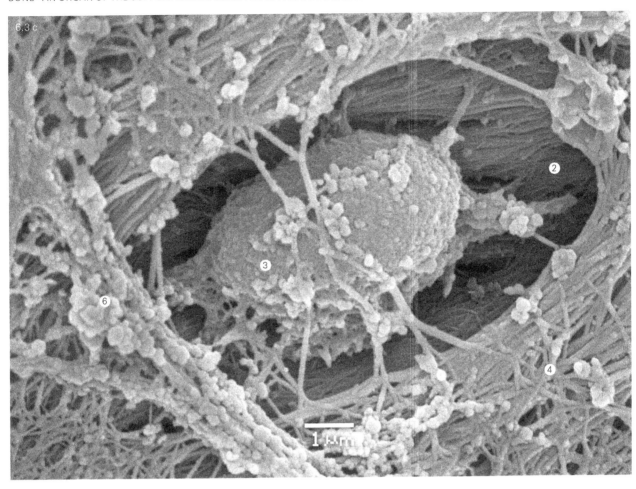

Fig. 6.3.
The inner part of bone proper on the side of the marrow cavity (channel). Surface of the osteoid layer (1).
Cell lacuna (2).
Preosteoblast/osteoblast (3) in the lacuna.
Fibrillar structure of the lacuna walls and the osteoid layer (4).
Channels (5).
Endosteum segment (6).
SEM-micrograph.
a – x 3,700,
b – x 7,000,
c – x 10,000

Bone marrow adipose cells are considered to perform five main functions (Gimble et al., 1996) as follows:
1) a passive (supportive) role–they fill free space in a bone marrow cavity;
2) an active role in lipid systemic metabolism (unicameral adipose cells possess a lipogenic and lipolytic potential);
3) a local source of energy in bone marrow;
4) a direct participation in hematopoiesis stimulation (Bookkoff, 1982; Hirata et al., 1988);
5) direct participation in osteogenesis (including a reparative one) stimulation (Mizuno et al., 1997).

The adipocytes express receptors to a growth hormone, mediating a direct effect on lipolysis (Vikman et al., 1991; Yang et al., 1996). The growth hormone can also exert a direct influence on the adipocytes' number as it influences the differentiation of preadipocytes/adipocytes demonstrated in vitro (Green et al., 1985; Hansen et al., 1998).

The bone marrow adipocytes are a source of paracrine factors, which possibly regulate osteoblastogenesis, osteoclastogenesis and hematopoiesis. At present, the peripheral adipocytes are considered as a source of several regulatory factors, some of which also play important local roles with their high concentration in bone marrow (Trayhurn & Beattie, 2001; Manolagas & Jilka, 1995). Leptin is a most striking instance; it is known to be produced by bone marrow adipocytes (Laharrague et al., 1998) and can enable differentiation of human mesenchymal stem cells into osteoblasts rather than adipocytes (Thomas et al., 1999).

The bone marrow adipocytes do not undergo any changes in starvation, associated with lipid loss, unlike adipose tissue of the other localization.

With the hematopoietic part prevailing over the lipid one in bone marrow, it is called red bone marrow. In the case of lipid tissue prevalence, it is called yellow bone marrow. The ratio of yellow and red bone marrow in a human body and mammals can change depending on

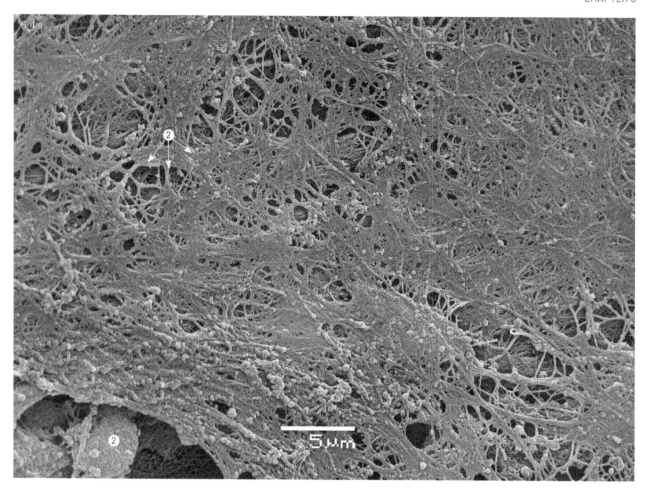

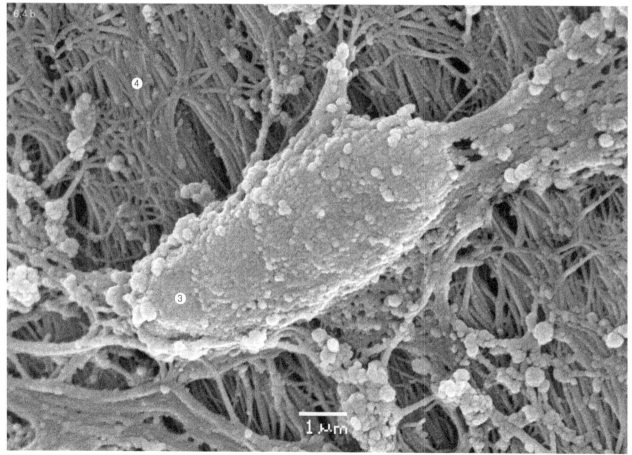

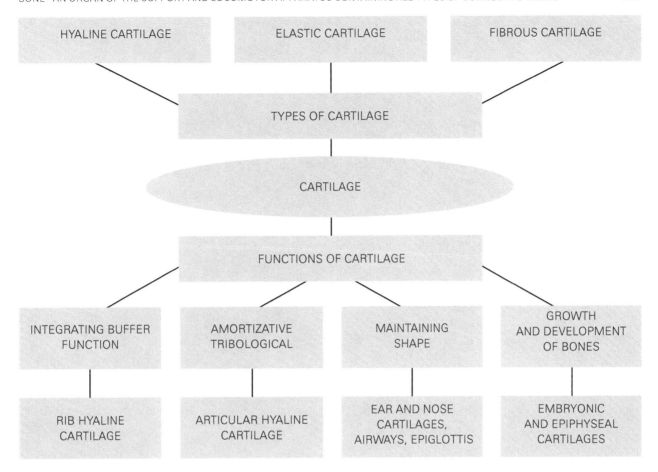

Fig. 6.5.
Schematic representation of the structural and functional organization of cartilage (according to Omelyanenko).

age, nutrition conditions, as well as nervous, endocrine and other factors.

Under normal conditions, yellow bone marrow performs functions intrinsic for adipose tissue and does not carry out hematopoiesis. In extreme settings (large blood loss, some pathologies), myelopoesis foci appear in adipose bone marrow, possibly due to the differentiation of local SCTMC and hematopoietic cells or else due to their migration from red bone marrow.

Bone marrow connective tissue(stromal) and hematopoietic cells in cultura.

The aforementioned types of CT-cells of all CT-differons can be derived from bone marrow by culturing bone marrow cells isolated from punctuates or bone bioptates. A primary (null) inoculation (passage) is performed with all bone marrow nuclear cells. Therefore, a cell suspension isolated and transferred into a cultural medium is polymorphic (Fig. 6.12; 6.8). Most of the cells are ball-shaped and 10–12 µm and 2–5 µm in diameter with a clearly visible surface relief. A nucleus, which occupies a significant part of the cytoplasm, and numerous circular granules that are 0.1–0.2 µm in size (apparently mitochondria, lysosomes, lipid droplets and others) are present inside the cell.

The second group is comprised of cells that are irregular and constantly change their form. This is accompanied by nucleus form changing and cytoplasm relocation along with organelles from one part of the cell to another. A cell membrane has numerous folds. The cells actively relocate and constantly contact with a flask bottom by the extended part of a cell, temporarily attaching locally by "sliding" along the flask bottom, then detach, "drift" and re-attach and so on. The attachment mechanism is similar to that of fibroblasts, which are placed in a cultural medium (see section 2.2.1), and takes place due to the secretion of a transparent gel-like substance (obviously of a glycoconjugate nature), "leaking" over the bottom by a cell apical part, which contacts with the flask bottom. Later, the cells attached with the help of a gel intermediate layer relocate in the same manner as in the case of fibroblasts. Changes in the gel-like secretion dur-

Fig. 6.4.
A fragment of the endosteum.
Fibrillar structure (1).
Preosteoblast/osteoblast (2) in a lacuna and on the surface of the osteoid (3).
Osteoid collagen fibrils (4).
SEM-micrograph.
a–x 3,000,
b–x 10,000.

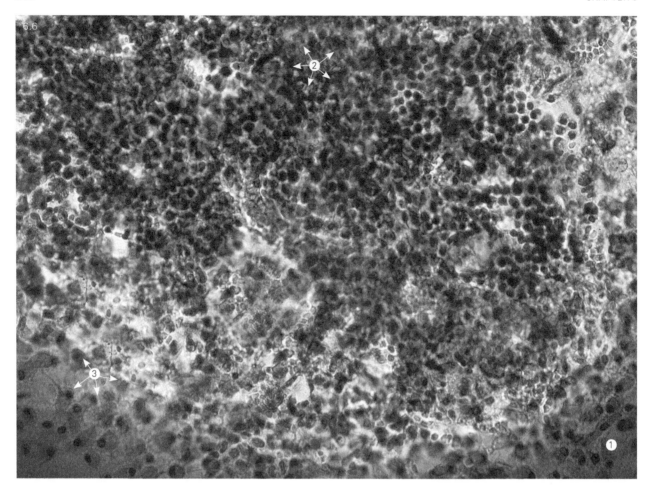

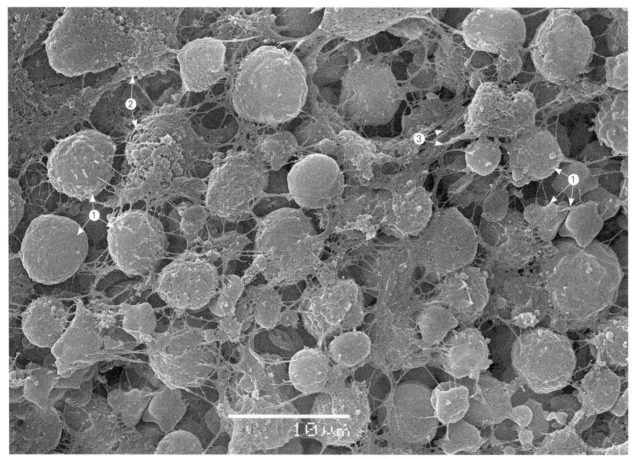

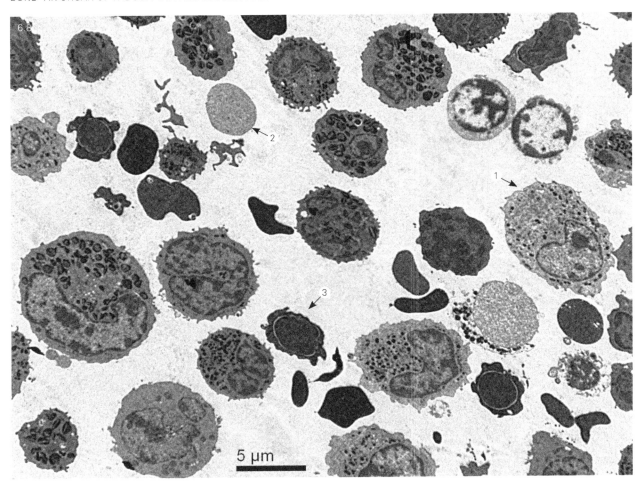

ing the attached cells' vital activities result in its partial shrinking and the formation of folds like cell processes around them. Cell attachment to a flask bottom starts as soon as 15–20 min after the primary passage and can continue for several days. This seems to reflect their various functional state, the degree of differentiation and structural differences.

The third group of cells consists of small (micro-) cells that are 2–5 μm in diameter. A fine band of the cytoplasm with single organelles surrounds the nucleus of such a cell. These cells are rarely found in some individuals; in others, there can be aggregations of these cells. Four types of microcells, which can be stem cells, have been described in the literature (Kucia et al., 2008; Domaratskaya, 2011).

The fourth group is represented by erythroid cells, which are nuclear (erythroblasts, normocytes, etc.) and enucleated (reticulocytes and red blood cells shaped as biconcave disks).

Platelets with a specific discoid form and one or several processes are cell structures, i.e. cell parts in the whole isolated cell fraction. They move between the cells or attach to irregular cells. The platelet number in a bone marrow cell suspension depends on the individuals from whom the bone marrow was obtained. The highest platelet count is observed around megakaryocytes or on their surface (*Fig. 6.12 a, b*).

Irrespective of the cells' belonging to any distinguished group they have the cytoplasm vacuolated to a varying degree and a "rarefied" nucleus in some cells that obvi-

Fig. 6.6.
A fragment of red bone marrow in an intertrabecular space.
Parts of bone trabeoules (1)
Hematopoietic cellular elements (2).
Preosteoblasts/osteoblasts (3).
LM-micrograph.
A light optic microscope
Ni Nikon (Japan). A histological slice. Staining with hematoxylin and eosin. x 200.

Fig. 6.7.
A fragment of red bone marrow in an intertrabecular space.
Hematopoietic (1) and stromal (2) cellular elements.
Fibrous structures (3).
SEM-micrograph.
x 2,500.

Fig. 6.8.
A suspension of bone marrow-derived cells.
Metamyelocyte (1).
Erythrocytes (2).
Proerythrocyte (3).
TEM-micrograph.
Ultrathine sectione.
Contrasting with lead citrate and uranyl acetate.
x 3,000.

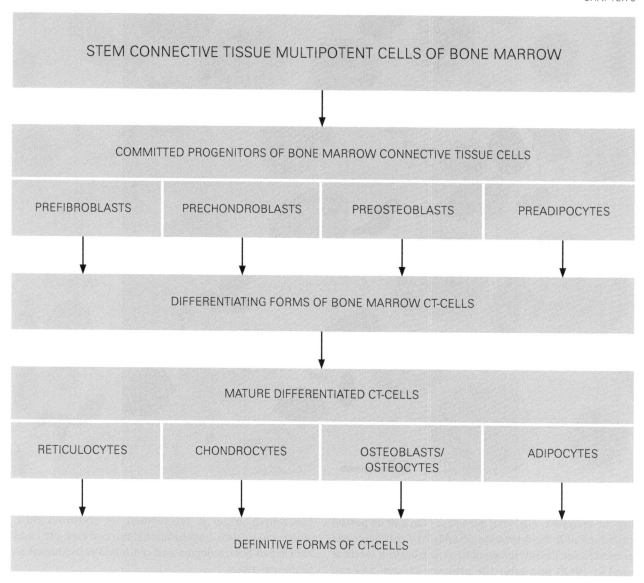

STEM CONNECTIVE TISSUE MULTIPOTENT CELLS OF BONE MARROW

COMMITTED PROGENITORS OF BONE MARROW CONNECTIVE TISSUE CELLS

| PREFIBROBLASTS | PRECHONDROBLASTS | PREOSTEOBLASTS | PREADIPOCYTES |

DIFFERENTIATING FORMS OF BONE MARROW CT-CELLS

MATURE DIFFERENTIATED CT-CELLS

| RETICULOCYTES | CHONDROCYTES | OSTEOBLASTS/ OSTEOCYTES | ADIPOCYTES |

DEFINITIVE FORMS OF CT-CELLS

Fig. 6.9.
A hypothetical image
of the hierarchy of bone
marrow CT
(according to Omelyanenko).

ously results from watering of the cells entered a cultural medium(*Fig. 6.12 c, d*)

A further examination was carried out after replacement of the cultural medium which was done in 5, 10, 15, 30, 60 minutes, 2,4,8,12,24 hours after the primary inoculation. An average inoculum density was used in this time window. At the same time non-adherent cells were removed (discarded). Nonetheless, approximately 1–0.5% of the total amount of the passaged core cells remained on the bottom of the flask. It is obvious that the remaining cells attached (to a varying degree) possess adhesive properties (*Fig. 6.13*). Among them there may be

bone marrow stromal cells (BMSC) which are a cluster of connective tissue cells of a mesenchymal origin including bone-cartilage progenitor-cells in varying stages of differentiation as well as multipotent stem cells. Among the attached cells there might also be those of a monocytic differon including macrophages and osteoclasts, which might have been eliminated from the culture in 2–3 passages or were not detected due to a relative decline in their number. According to the preliminary data most of the attached cells (approximately 85–90%) have a mesenchyme hematopoietic origin i.e. they refer to hematopoietic differons.

The distribution of the cells attached to the flask bottom is irregular and their number depends on the total amount of bone marrow nuclear cells inoculated and the time duration when the first medium exchange is carried out after the primary passage. A longer period from the primary passage to the first "discharge" enables the attachment of more cells or else a stronger attachment. The range of structurally different cells widens.

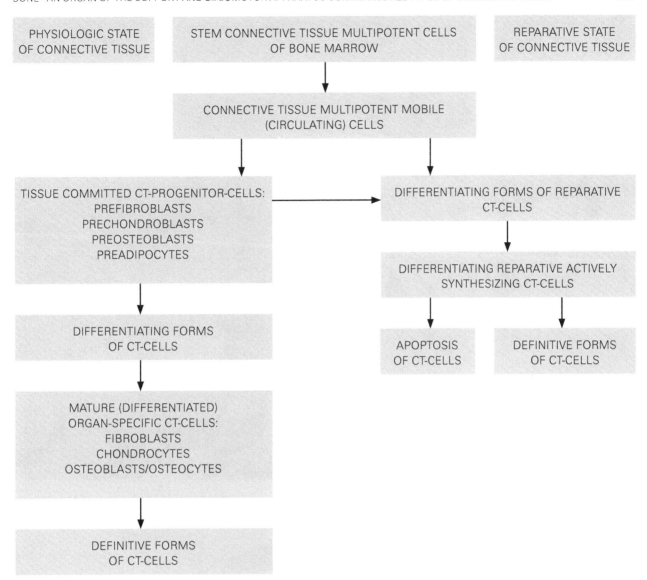

Thus, a range of structurally different cells increases. However, most of the cells attach within the first 4 hours and subsequently their number does not significantly increase. Part of the cells attached becomes flattened at once. A cell volume is then not distinctly changed. A gel secret is seen round the attached and flattened cells. The cells can be circular (10–20 μm in diameter), oval-elongated or narrow elongated (10–15 μm in thickness and 20–30 μm and more in length) (*Fig. 6.2*). Microcells retain: circular (2–5 μm in diameter) and elongated (2–5 μm in

thickness and 10–15 μm in length) ones. Part of the microcells is located independently, another part of the cells attaches to larger cells and constantly accompanies them by being attached to their surface and performing a role of specific satellite cells.

Cell attachment should not be identified with cell fixation as the cells continue to move, i.e. they move on the bottom of the flask with varying speed by employing the mechanism of gel secretion, and they can elongate or contract. Fragments of time-lapse photography of this process in one cell are presented in *Fig. 6.14*.

2–3 hours after the exchange of the cultural medium, the detachment of the part of the cells that were attached solely by their apical parts is observed. Later, in approximately 24 hours, part of these cells can attach by employing the above-described mechanism.

The cells that were not detached also respond to the medium exchange. They contract slightly. This is indicated by processes that resemble thin threads, which are radially located around a cell. They are likely residues of a gel-like substance, by means of which cells attach to the

Fig. 6.10.
A hypothetical image of the participation of multipotent mobile (circulating) connective tissue cells, which are derivatives of SCTMC, in maintaining tissue connective tissue differons outside the bone marrow (according to Omelyanenko).

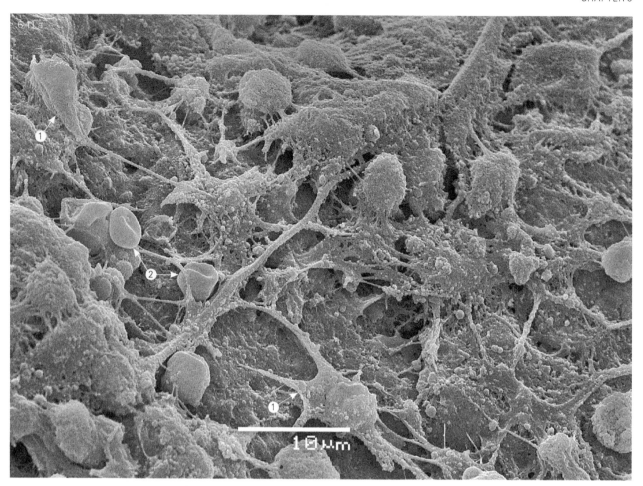

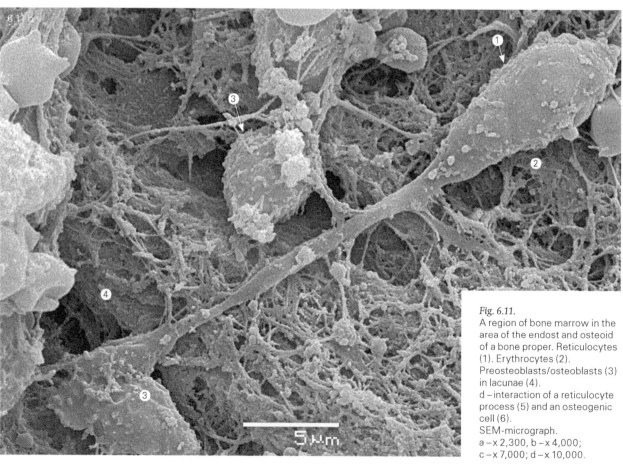

Fig. 6.11.
A region of bone marrow in the area of the endost and osteoid of a bone proper. Reticulocytes (1). Erythrocytes (2). Preosteoblasts/osteoblasts (3) in lacunae (4).
d – interaction of a reticulocyte process (5) and an osteogenic cell (6).
SEM-micrograph.
a – x 2,300, b – x 4,000;
c – x 7,000; d – x 10,000.

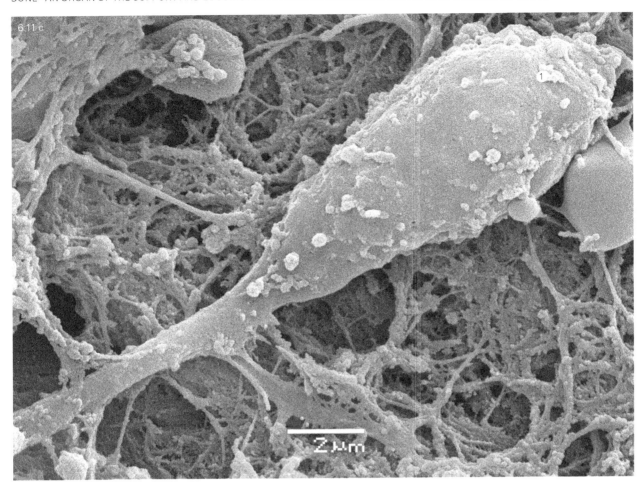

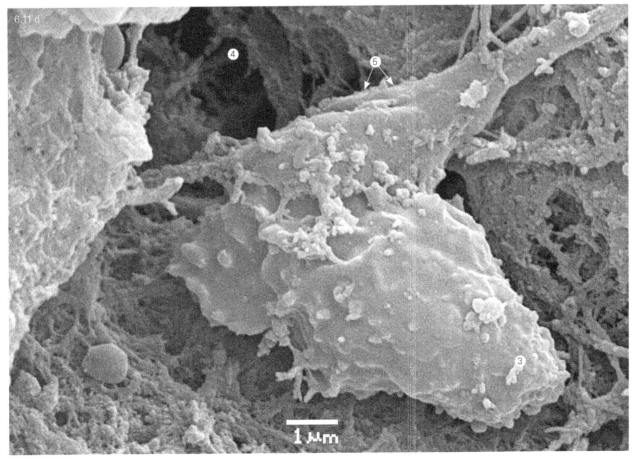

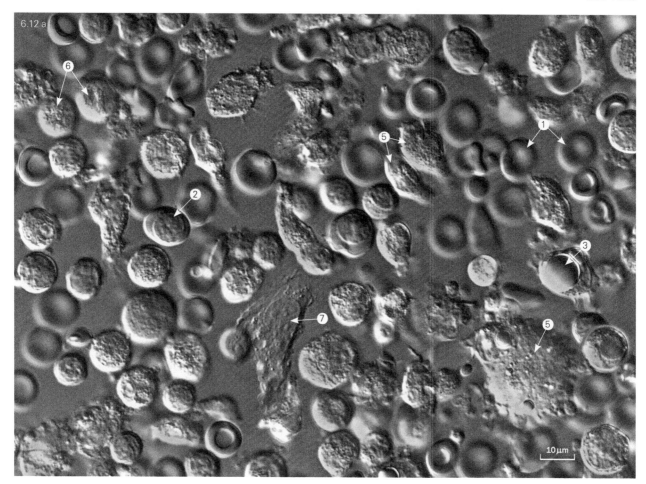

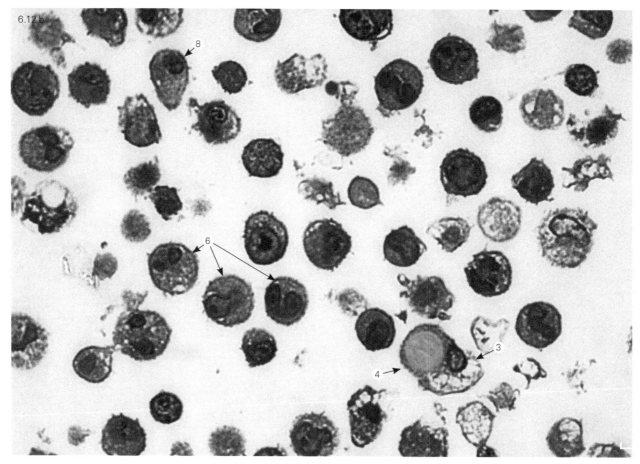

6.12 c

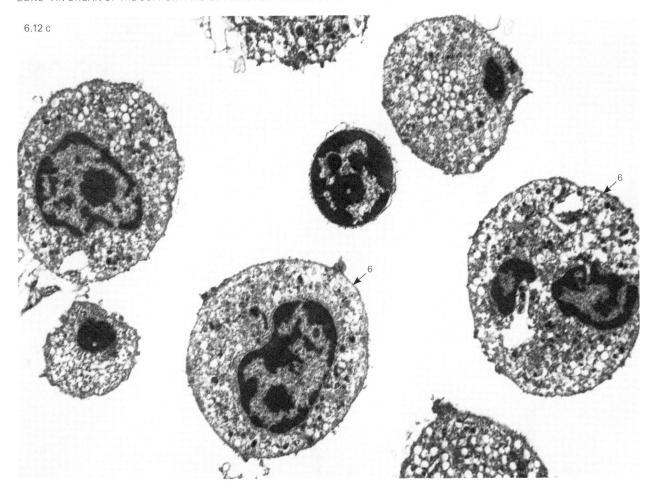

Fig. 6.12.
Human bone marrow cells
immediately upon isolation:
a –in a cultural medium;
b –semi-thine sectione;
c, d –.ultrathine sectione.
Red blood cells (1).
A normocyte (2).
A lipocyte (3).
A drop fat(4).
A megakaryocyte (5).
White blood cells (6)
Attached and flattened
adhesive cells(7).
Cells changing their form (8).
A nucleus (9).
The cytoplasm (10).
A vacuol (11).
a –LM-micrograph.
A light optic inverted
microscope Ti Nikon (Japan)
integrated with an incubator.
Nomarsky differential
interference contrast (DIC),
a –x 800.
b –LM-micrograph.
A light optic microscope
Ni Nikon (Japan).
Semi thine sectione.
Azur-eozin.
x 800.
(see color insert)
c, d –TEM-micrograph.
Ultrathine sectione.
Contrasting with lead citrate
and uranyl acetate.
c –x 4,000, d –10,000.

6.12 d

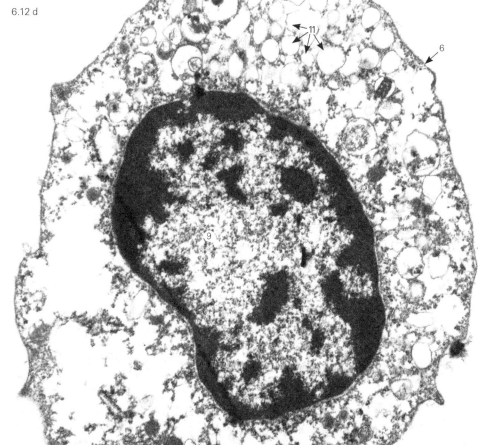

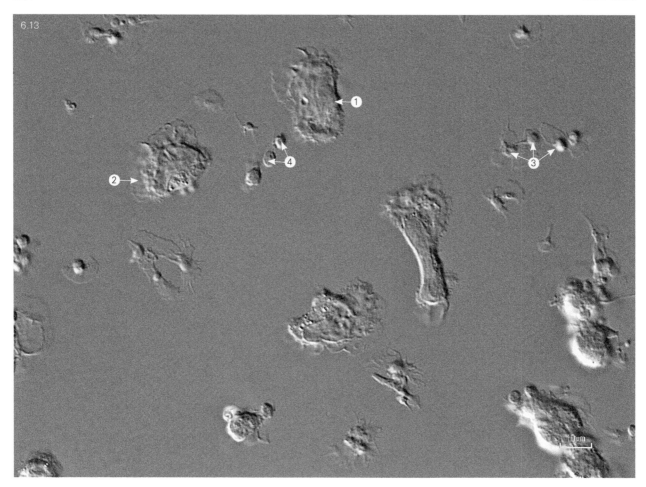

bottom of the flask. However, a gel intermediate layer is not completely destroyed in a larger contact area.

In approximately 18–24 hours, the cells restore their initial state and begin the next stage of vital activities of cultured cells, which is generally known as spreading. It should be noted that the form and sizes the cells take on, as well the rate of this process, are not the same. This has made it possible to distinguish several groups of the cells. Spreading begins with flattening, through which the height of cells' protrusion over the surface of the flask bottom declines, and an oval, circular and slightly elongated form is maintained. The following characteristics are common for all cells at this stage of life: a decline in

Fig. 6.13.
Human bone marrow cells adhesive attached to the bottom of the cultural flask when placed in a cultural medium.
Attached and flattened adhesive cells (1) and the gel-likel substance in the periphery (2).
Microcells (3).
Platelets (4).
LM-micrograph.
A light optic inverted microscope Ti Nikon (Japan) integrated with an incubator.
Nomarsky differential interference contrast (DIC), x 800.

the number of cytoplasmic membrane folds (i.e. the membrane is straightened and its surface becomes smoother); the nuclei, endoplasm with granules-organelles, small ectoplasm and a gel-like substrate on the cell periphery, which varies in width is visualized. The cells continue to secrete the gel at intervals, which is obviously associated with cells' relocation and their adaptation response to the conditions of a cultural medium. The continuous motility of the granules-organelles in the cells' cytoplasm should be noted. Some granules do fluctuating motions only around a single point, while the others move to other regions of the cell. There are platelets on the surface of many attached and spread cells.

Cells of an oval or irregular form with several nuclei (from 3 to 8) and the sizes such as cross–30–40 μm and longitudinal–80–120 μm which are rarely seen spread reaching their final size before the others (in 12–24 hours). These cells are likely to be osteoclasts (*Fig. 6.15*). They constantly changed their form and moved.

By this time the sizes of other circular cells somewhat increased (25×40 μm, 20×60 μm, 30×30 μm and others), that respectively increased their coverage area of the bottom surface of the flask.

A subsequent cell flattening (in 48 hours or more) manifested in the development of the aforementioned tendency in changing their form. Part of the cells became circular with an equivalent diameter of 30–50 µm. A circular nucleus surrounded by the endoplasm occupied their central part, with the ectoplasm having a peculiar "fringe" occupying the peripheral part (*Fig. 6.16 a*). Such cells resembled "rosettes" in form.

Another part of the cells gained an elongated form (resembling a "racket" form) in which an average cross size (10–20 µm) was several times less than the longitudinal one (30–100 µm and more). One end of these cells could be oval with a cross size of 30–50 µm, the other one being 5–15 µm (*Fig. 6.16 b*). A cell enlarged part is surrounded by a "fringe" in its periphery. It indicated the direction of cell motion. A large peripheral part of the cell enlarged region is the ectoplasm. An oval nucleus with nucleoli surrounded by the endoplasm is located in the cell central part. A cell's opposite part is narrow. It is followed by fine threads, which are obviously the residues of a gel-like substance. A cell was moving by means of contraction-extension. There are cells which are transient in form. A time-lapse examination determined the possibility of cell form changing in the range of the aforementioned forms.

Rod-like cells with a length of 100–120 µm and a relatively uniform width of 5–10 µm along the entire length of a flat-angulated cell can be another variation of spreading (*Fig. 16 c*). An oval slightly elongated nucleus with nucleoli was located in the center of a cell. Its cross-size corresponded to a cell width almost completely. There was ectoplasm on each side of the nucleus. The peripheral parts of the cell are the ectoplasm. A gel-like substance locally secreted by a cell is seen in some regions. Needle-shaped cells which central part's thickness can reach 15–20 µm may be distinguished in this group of cells.

In a long-term observation by means of time-lapse photography it was determined that sizes of "rosettes", "rockets" and their intermediate forms were gradually increasing with the cultivation time (2–3 weeks) likely due to flattening and a growth. However, the division of these cells has not been detected.

Part of the cells has a narrow small body and thick processes which constantly changed their length and orientation (*Fig. 6.16 d*). These cells look like dendritic antigen-presenting cells of a bone marrow origin (xxx). The cells of this group exerted the highest activity in motion and form changing. The above-described groups of cells comprised most of the attached cells.

Among the attached cells there is another small group of cells (approximately 5–10%), which completely spread in 12–24 hours after the primary inoculation (*Fig. 6.17*). The spread cells have a length of 110–140 µm. A cell central part is the widest – 20–30 µm. An oval elongated nucleus (8–10 µm) with nucleoli and endoplasm is located in it. The ectoplasm with granules-organelles is in the narrower (10–15 µm) peripheral part. The granules-organelles move from the endoplasm into the ectoplasm. Fluctuating motion of these structures also occurs. A cell cytoskeleton in the form of fine threads is well-visualized. The number of the spread cells of the last group does not increase in 24 hours owing to the remaining attached cells (before proliferation starts). It is in the cells of this small group that the division started.

All processes, such as attachment, flattening, spreading and division, do not occur simultaneously in different cells. Therefore, in the culture, such cells are at varying stages of their life cycle.

The absence of contact inhibition, which stabilizes the influence of the environment and the natural tissue microenvironment, the presence of an adequate nutritional medium and the potential capability to multiply are favorable conditions for starting division. However, only the cells of the last, less numerous group exhibit the ability to divide.

The division process for cells of the last group begins in 36–72 hours after inoculation and had a number of peculiarities.

1. The division of cells started not simultaneously in various cells.

2. The division of daughter cells had an asynchronous character. In some cases one of the daughter (divided for the first time) cells could return to a non-spread oval form and discontinue noticeable motions (and division) for a long time (or completely). At the same time another daughter cell being completely spread could move relatively far away from another daughter cell and continue dividing further also asynchronously. The time difference between subsequent divisions of two daughter cells could be of several hours. The daughter cells could also remain in a close proximity contacting with each other. A mechanism of such a behavior of dividing cells is still unknown.

The detailed structural dynamics of this process, presented in successive fragments of time-lapse photography, is, in general, similar to fibroblasts' division (*Fig. 6.18*).

The first stage, the preparation for division (*Fig. 6.18 a*), initially starts with a cell contraction in the width along its long axis. Its peripheral parts on the site of the spread ectoplasm contract and take the form of several thick long processes ranging from 2–5 (more often two with opposite poles) with a width of 5–10 µm and a length of 20–50 µm. When the cell retains two processes with opposite poles, it becomes spindle-shaped. Fine threads in the form of rays perpendicularly branch from the processes. They might be residues of a gel substance, by means of which the cell attaches and fixes on the flask bottom. Later the processes contract in length approaching to the cell's central part. Their contraction can be uneven. One process (or processes) contracts quicker, while others do so more slowly. The aforementioned ray-like fine threads remain after the cell's contracted parts. The cell's central part also changes form. It becomes less spread and more prominent and circular. The radiating threads are left on the cells' sides. The cell rises more prominently over the flask bottom surface. The processes (more often two processes with opposite poles are left) become narrowed (2–3 µm) in width and shorter (10–30 µm). It should be noted that the processes are not drawn

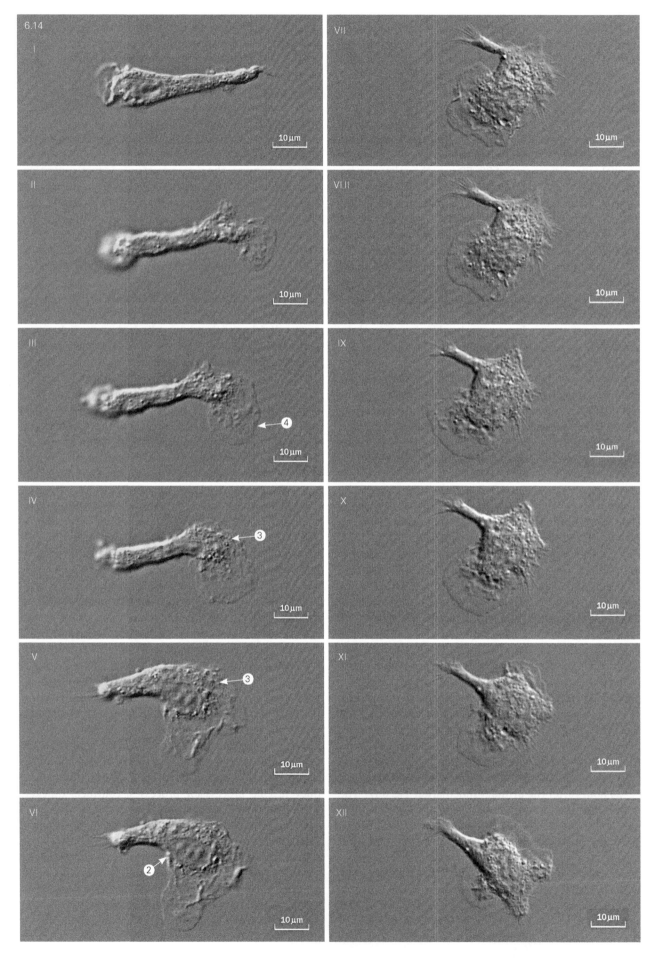

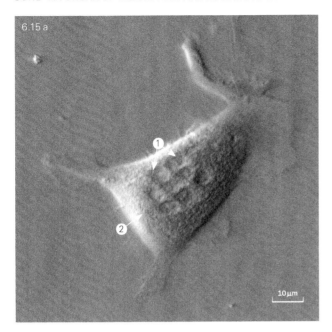

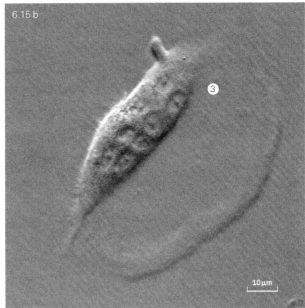

into the cell completely and are not detached from the flask's bottom, holding the cell in a certain position.

The aforementioned changes comprise the stage of mitosis – the prophase. Then the cell enters the next stage – the metaphase. It becomes circular-oval or ball-shaped and 20 × 30 μm in size, significantly rising over the flask bottom. The cell nucleus is not detected in such a state. Only granules-organelles in the cytoplasm and chromosomes along a cell's equatorial plane forming a metaphase plate or a mother star can be seen. Then the stage of division proper follows. A cell becomes oval-elongated and the chromosomes are pulled toward opposing poles (the stage – anaphase) (*Fig. 6.18 b*). Immediately after that, a division constriction appears on the cell's equator. The cell looks like a dumbbell. The constriction widens. The cell enters the telophase in such a manner, the significant event of which is cytotomia (*Fig. 6.18 c*). Numerous protrusions of the cytoplasmic membrane, which can pull in and appear on other sites, arise on the two forming daughter cells. Their size ranges from 1–5 μm. The protrusion reaches its maximal size as the constriction deepens. Part of the cytoplasm with granules-organelles

moves in the protrusions formed. In the period of generating protrusions, the future daughter cells take on an irregular bizarre form. This is a relatively short period of time, in which the cell's surface becomes relatively smooth and the cell starts to spread. In the division process, a fine cleavage furrow or a cell cytotomia bridge resembling an umbilical cord is retained between future independent cells. Such a state is defined as incomplete cytokinesis as the communication between the daughter cells' cytoplasm is retained via the bridge (Danilov & Klishov, 1995). Later the protrusions are reduced in size and number. The daughter cells become more circular. Nuclear lines appear. The cells approach and come into close contact to one another. Then occurs the cells' slow elongation, and the process or processes by means of which cells are fixed to the flask bottom is maintained. Part of the cytoplasm migrates into them. If the process completely pulls in any daughter cell during contraction, a cytoplasmic membrane starts to protrude on the site of the former process in this cell, i.e. in an apical pole region, and part of the cytoplasm migrates into this protrusion. Before that, a cell produces a gel-like secretion, along which the protruding part of a cell spreads. The same mechanism that is observed in cell motility, flattening and spreading is reproduced. At first a gel is secreted, then a cell membrane protrusion is layered and the cytoplasm migrates into it and so on. The elongation of daughter cells continues and they start moving in opposite directions. Herein a disruption of the retained fine cell bridge occurs, i.e. cytotomia is complete. The cells move apart. They can spread or become elongated and spindle-shaped. In the latter case, local protrusions appear and disappear quickly on the surface of spindle-shaped cells along their entire length. Irrespective of which cell starts spearing earlier, both cells spread eventually and continue dividing, albeit not simultaneously. As a rule, the first to start the following division is the

Fig. 6.14.
A adhesive attached flattened cell (1).
A nucleus (2).
The cytoplasm (3).
Dynamics of form changing, movement and secretion of a gel-like substance (4).
Fragments of time-lapse photography (I–XII).
LM-micrograph.
A light optic inverted microscope Ti Nikon (Japan) integrated with an incubator.
Nomarsky differential interference contrast (DIC), x 800.

Fig. 6.15.
Large spread multinucleated cells, possibly osteoclasts.
A nucleus (1).
Endoplasm (2).
Ectoplasm (3).
LM-micrograph.
A light-optic inverted microscope Ti Nikon, (Japan) integrated with an incubator.
Hoffman modulation contrast.
x 400.

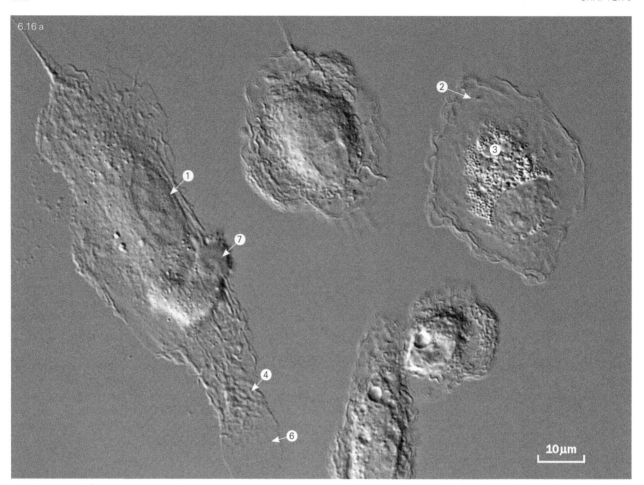

6.16 a

10 μm

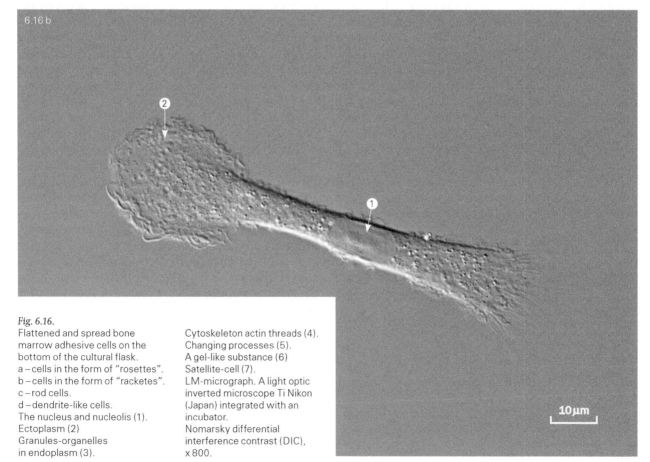

6.16 b

Fig. 6.16.
Flattened and spread bone
marrow adhesive cells on the
bottom of the cultural flask.
a – cells in the form of "rosettes".
b – cells in the form of "racketes".
c – rod cells.
d – dendrite-like cells.
The nucleus and nucleolis (1).
Ectoplasm (2)
Granules-organelles
in endoplasm (3).

Cytoskeleton actin threads (4).
Changing processes (5).
A gel-like substance (6)
Satellite-cell (7).
LM-micrograph. A light optic
inverted microscope Ti Nikon
(Japan) integrated with an
incubator.
Nomarsky differential
interference contrast (DIC),
x 800.

10 μm

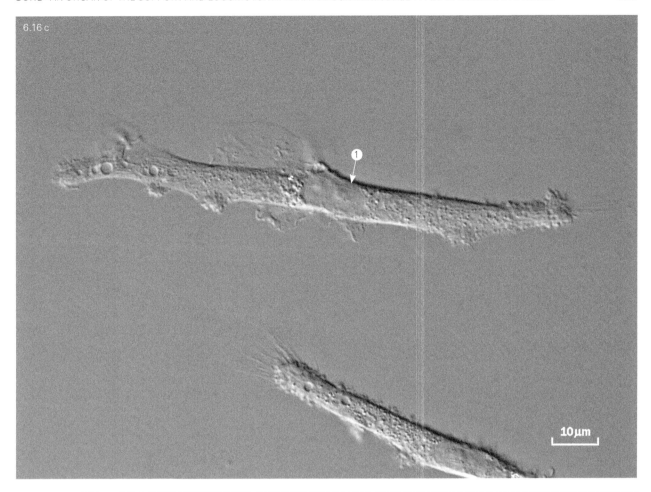

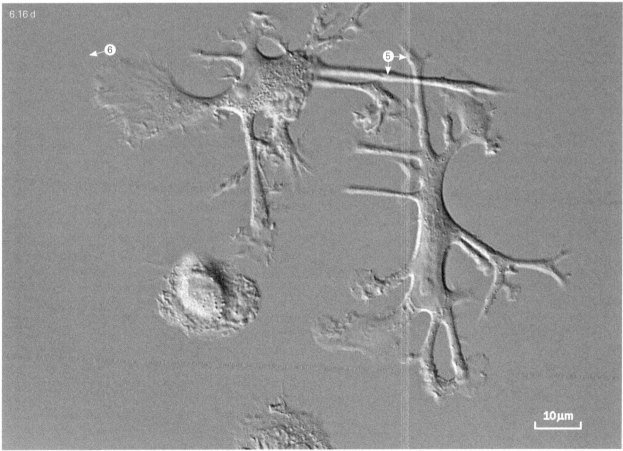

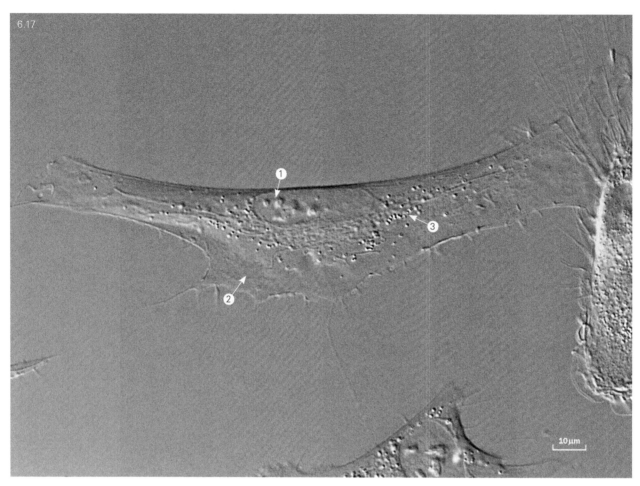

Fig. 6.17.
A spread fibroblast-like cell in a cultural medium on a bottom of the cultural flask. The nucleus and nucleolis (1). Ectoplasm (2). Granules-organelles in endoplasm (3).

Cytoskeleton actin threads (4). LM-micrograph. A light optic inverted microscope Ti Nikon (Japan) integrated with an incubator. Nomarsky (differential) interference contrast (DIC), x 800.

daughter cell that has spread earlier. The division of the second cell can be delayed. The spread cells can take on various forms–elongated, multiangular, triangular. At the same time, the cells' form can constantly change. The adjacent cells contact (interact) with each other by their numerous processes ('examine" or "inspect") or else temporarily overlap each other and form a cell association similar to a syncytium (Fig. 6.19 a).

The division rates of fixed and spread cells is not the same. Therefore, the rate of increasing cell clones also differs. This indicates the varying proliferative potencies of the cells, which depend on the degree of their development (differentiation) at the moment of their transfer into a culture, attachment and spreading. It is evident that a synthetic apparatus is to be formed in cells with a high proliferative potential to provide vital activities, to form a cell itself and its attachment to the bottom of a cultural flask by means of a gel-like secretion. At the same time, a highly differentiated or definite cell pos-

sesses less proliferative potencies. On the other hand, a relatively long stay in a cultural medium is required for a non-differentiated or poorly differentiated cell to form a synthetic apparatus, which is essential for the synthesis of a gel-like substance, by means of which the cell can attach to a cultural flask bottom and to cell proteins, which are essential for subsequent proliferation The continuous irregular proliferation of the cells results in uneven clone growth (i.e. monoclonal colonies) and the fusion of large clones with small ones with the formation of polyclonal colonies, which represent a combination of several clones.

In colony formation, due to proliferation, the cells gradually fill in the free space by limiting the range of their motion or movement therein and by affecting (changing) their form in spreading, i.e. the shape of newly formed cells and previously formed ones.A gradual increase in the number of cells results in a reduction of these spaces and in changing the cell form associated with their mutual pressure. The latter seems to cause contact inhibition and to delay cell proliferation. Thus, a continuous or confluent monolayer is being formed in which cells with a higher division rate will prevail. In this monolayer, the interaction of cells with each other will lead to most of the cells become elongated and are arranged in complexes, in which they are parallel or fan (radial) oriented (Fig. 6.19 b, c). The thread-like or granular structures forming a cytoskeleton are clearly visible in the cells. It seems that contact inhibition, delaying cell proliferation, manifests in the interaction involving the mutual pressure of the cells forming a continuous monolayer. The prevailing direction of cell orientation is different in adjacent complexes. There are sites where the cells are multiangular (not elongated). Complexes of elongated cells surround the accumulations of such cells. The aforementioned cells include spindle-shaped small cells or microcells that are 15–20 μm along the long axis and 3–5 μm along the cross axis. No division of these cells has been observed.

It should be noted that cell division does not discontinue completely. The cells will overlap the walls or each other on the flask's edges

The spreading of all attached cells does not occur simultaneously, nor does their attachment. Therefore, on the flask bottom, there are cells at varying stages of adaptation to cultural conditions or in varying morphologic states, in which the cells exist in native bone marrow.

The form the cells take on after being suspended appears to be similar, to a certain extent, to the form the cells exhibited in the bone marrow extracellular matrix by contacting directly with fibrous elements, the integrating buffer metabolic medium and other cells or by exchanging with signals. The dendritic cells exert the most activity in moving and changing form.

The formation of a continuous(entire) monolayer can occur in several ways. With a seeding low density, the spread and potentially dividing cells are located far from each other and when dividing, each of them can form clone colonies, which reach significantly large sizes and fuse with each other to form a continuous monolayer. The colonies grow uneven, which is due to the uneven onset of cell division and the rate of their further proliferation. The colonies also differ from each other in terms of the arrangement density of the cells forming them (dense or loose) and by size. Some colonies can be multilayered. The continuous monolayer formation will be long enough.

With a moderate density of seeding and the presence of a great number of cells, which are potentially capable of division and located not far from each other, colonies are formed of several small clones of primary (inoculated) cells with their division and the origin of only several daughter cells. In this case, the colonies will be formed from several clones, i.e. they will be multiangular.

With a dense inoculation, the dividing cells will be distributed rather regularly and be located close to each other; therefore, there will be no formation of clearly separated colonies. A continuous monolayer will form rapidly. With a very dense seeding, the attached cells can form aggregates. The division of the cells with proliferative potential will be abruptly delayed. This seems to be associated with a living space limitation. The passage of this densely inoculated culture provides the possibility for the appropriate cells to exert their proliferative capabilities and form a continuous monolayer.

Non-dividing cells will prevail among the attached cells in any inoculum density. Their number will be about 90% of the total number of the cells attached.

After the continuous monolayer is fully formed, vacuoles that are larger than granules-organelles start accumulating in the cells. This appears to be associated with an increase in the concentration of collagen and glycoconjugates in a cultural fluid. The death of some cells is possible in further culturing.

The ratio of dividing and non-dividing cells will change for the former. Their number will suddenly prevail. The same trend is observed in terms of the size ratio. Despite some increase in the sizes of the cells that have been attached but are not dividing, their sizes are significantly less that those of dividing cells. In passaging the grown cell culture, the proliferative process will continue. Meanwhile, the number of non-dividing cells will decline.

Upon detaching, the cells contract, becoming ball-shaped or circular like those cells that are preparing to divide. Unlike the latter, these cells are completely detached from the flask bottom. They are more homologous in structure and in size that in the null passage (*Fig. 6.20 a, a1, a2*). Their diameter is 20–25 μm, which is twice more than that of most cells of the primary culture (null passage). The cells that are transferred into flasks with a fresh nutritive medium are suspended for some time. Their entire surface consists of small or large circular protrusions of the cytoplasmic membrane. These protrusions constantly "pulsate", i.e. they increase or decrease. It is obvious that these protrusions are a peculiar optimal form of the cytoplasmic membrane's arrangement of a spread cell in its contraction upon detachment from the flask bottom. During the time that they are in a cultural medium from the time of their primary passage, the BMSC have undergone significant changes as, being suspended, they significantly differ from primary BMSC. Cytoplasm hydration is observed in such cells. They contain a great number of vacuoles of varying size. In general, the structural state of such cells is identical to that of fibroblasts placed in a cultural medium after their monolayer has been detached from the primary passage (see Chapter 2). The attachment of cells passaged to a flask bottom starts in 10–15 minutes and, in 2–3 hours, almost every cell has already been attached, flattened or partially spread (*Fig. 6.20 b*). Subsequent spreading follows rapidly, in which a few processes at first originate in the cells. Then, the cells take on a large size (*Fig. 6.20 c*). Nuclei are clearly visible in them, which also become flat. They are clearly separated from the cytoplasm by the nuclear membrane. Some nucleoli are well determined therein. In turn, the cytoplasm is divided into two parts: the inner–endoplasm and outer–ectoplasm. Most of the granules-organelles are present in the endoplasm. The ectoplasm contains only single granules. Thin filaments of the cytoskeleton are present in the cytoplasm of the whole cell. In spreading, part of the cells takes on various forms (including multiangular

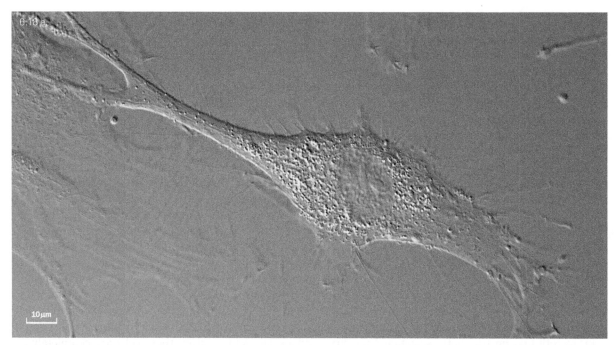

6.18 a.

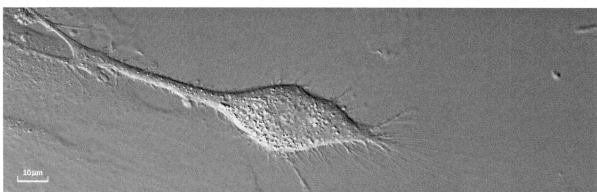

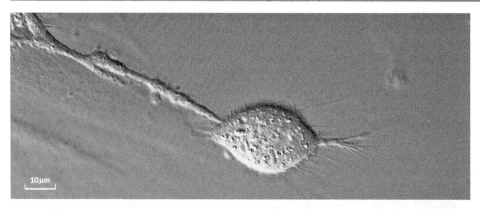

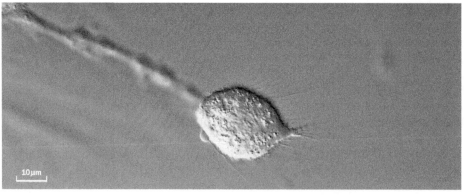

Fig. 6.18.
The division dynamics
of a adhesive spread bone
marrow stromal cell under
cultural medium conditions
on the bottom of a cultural
flask.
a – a cell's preparation for
division – contraction of the
spread cell to circular-oval
(the stage of mitosis –
the prophase);
b – division proper – distribution
of chromosomes and cell
organelles into two daughter
cells (the stages of mitosis –
the metaphase, anaphase,
telophase), incomplete
cytokinesis;
c – division completion –
complete cytokinesis, daughter
cells' disjunction and spreading.
Fragments of time-lapse
photography.
LM-micrograph.
A light optic inverted
microscope Ti Nikon (Japan)
integrated with an incubator.
Nomarsky differential)
interference contrast (DIC),
x 800.

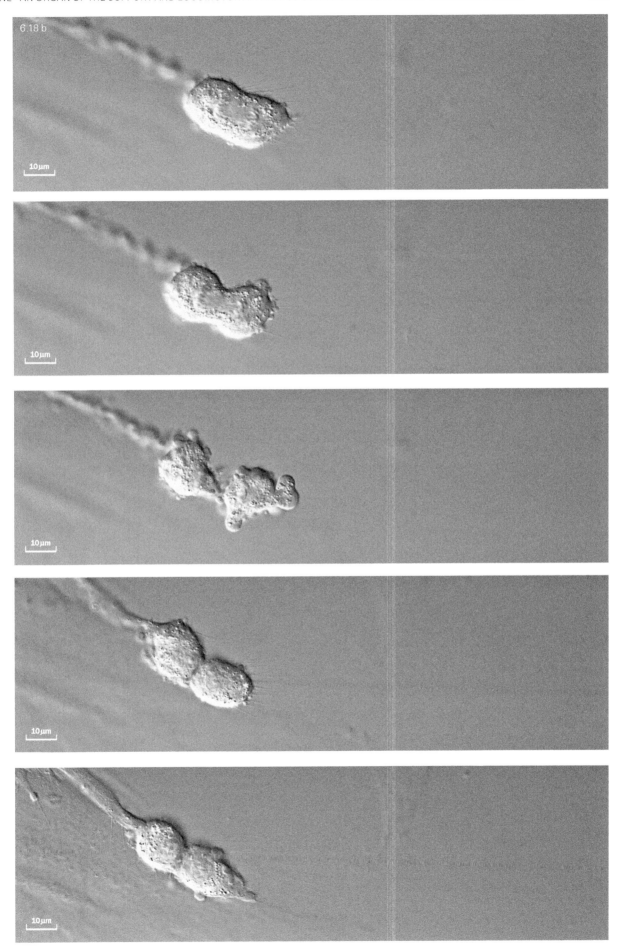

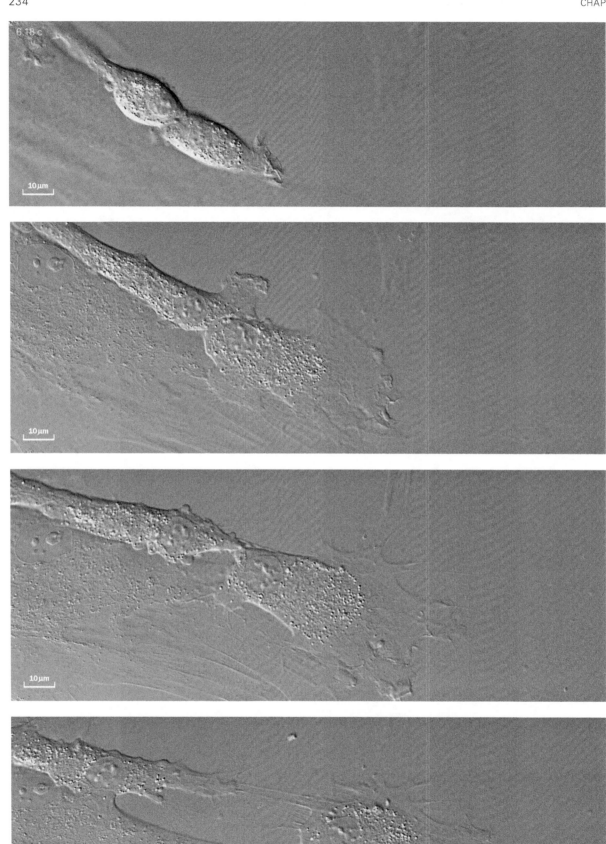

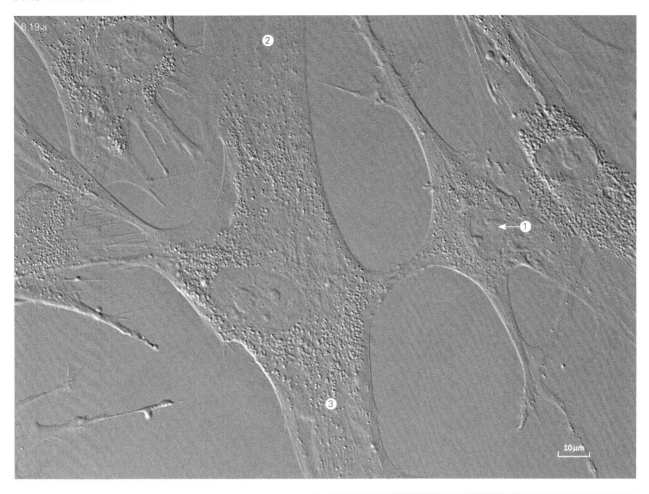

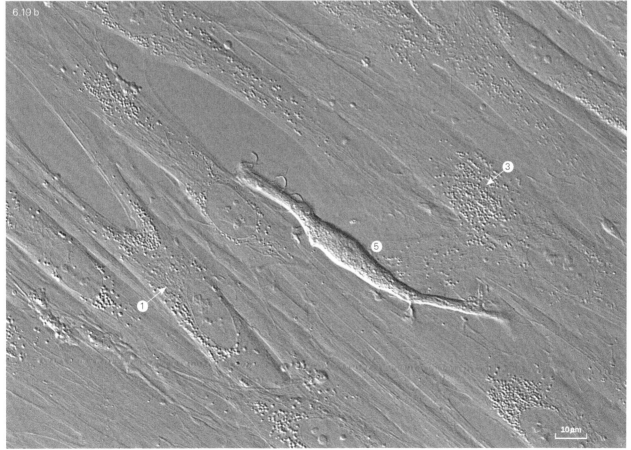

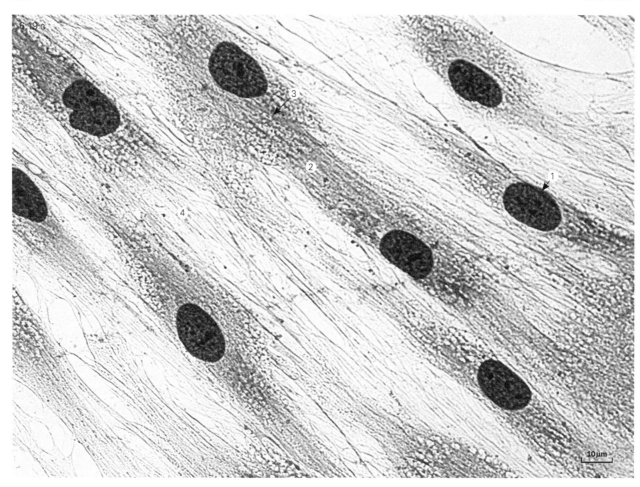

6.19 c

3

2

1

4

10 µm

Fig. 6.19.
A monolayer of a bone
marrow stromal cell culture.
a – a non-continuous
monolayer;
b – a continuous (confluent)
monolayer.
A nucleus and nucleoli (1).
Ectoplasm (2).
Granules-organelles
in endoplasm (3).

Actin filaments (4).
An elongated microcell (5).
LM-micrograph.
A light optic inverted
microscope Ti Nikon (Japan)
integrated with an incubator.
a, b – Nomarsky (differential)
interference contrast (DIC),
c – Staining with azur eosin.
a, b, c – x 800.

or triangular one) and sizes in planes, which are not found in the bone marrow in its natural state. This particularly refers to the ectoplasm. This process occurs in the vast majority of cells with a small time difference. The first division starts in most cells in 24–30 hours, and in 72 hours, a continuous monolayer, which is ready to be subcultured, may form (*Fig. 6.20 d*). This process is completely identical to that of the null passage. Undoubtedly, the time staging depends on many factors such as: the number of cells seeded, the quality of bottles (plastic or glass), the age of patients who have donated the bone marrow cells, etc. Non-dividing cells are found among the cells of the first inoculation, but in a much smaller amount than in the null passage. Subsequently, their number is even further reduced. Most of the cells of a confluent monolayer (more than 90%) are the cells of a mesenchymal connective tissue origin.

As in fibroblasts, there are certain differences in the structure of the cultured BMSC in different passages.
The cultured BMSC can grow on different scaffolding material. A demineralized bone matrix (DBM) is the most favorable material for their growth (*Fig. 6.21*).
Culturing of the BMSC under various conditions is of general theoretical importance, as is the ensuing practical application of the BMSC as cell-based therapy. This use is the most common in terms of experimental and clinical orthopedics and traumatology.
The main mechanism of reparative bone regeneration is the proliferation and differentiation of osteogenic progenitor cells, which are located in the periosteum and endosteum, near the zone of bone damage, and the subsequent synthesis of the extracellular matrix by the bone cells. In this regard, the mechanism of action on reparative osteogenesis is the prolonged stimulation of resident osteogenic progenitor cells in the area of bone damage. Implantation (on a matrix, or by injection) into the damage area of autologous and allogeneic BMSC (progenitor cells of connective tissue differons, including osteogenic ones) derived from bone marrow and multiplied in a culture can be applied.
However, cells that have been cultured under ideal conditions prior to their transplantation are unlikely to survive, differentiate into osteogenic cells, and function adequately at the site of inflammation with its intrinsic

acidosis, hypoxia, and the presence of numerous lytic enzymes released in leucolysis (the destruction of leucocytes). The optimal conditions for the manifestation of BMSC osteogenesis-stimulating properties include the absence of components of the inflammatory response in the damaged area in the form of acidosis, hypoxia and leukocyte infiltration (lytic enzyme activity) on the one hand, and the beginning of their own (resident) bone formation (osteogenesis) on the other hand. Stimulating the latter results in the restoration of damaged bones, even in critical defects, i.e. when the bones do not recover spontaneously. This approach laid the basis for using autologous BMSC to stimulate distraction regenerates when carrying out a surgical correction of congenital limb-length discrepancy in children.

At the same time, after the inflammation stage is over and its own osteogenesis commences, injections of an autologous BMSC suspension into experimental bone defects stimulated the latter, leading to the restoration of the damaged bones, even in the case of critical defects, i.e. when the bones do not recover spontaneously (Omelyanenko et al. 2005b). This approach laid the basis for using autologous BMSC to stimulate distraction regenerates when carrying out a surgical correction of congenital limb-length discrepancy in children.

The distraction regenerate has virtually none of the aforementioned adverse inflammatory factors and its own (possibly not significantly distinct) osteogenesis occurs. Autologous BMSC implanted in injections appeared in a favorable microenvironment, including an unmineralized fibrous framework where they could exert their potential capabilities directed at optimizing reparative osteogenesis. The feasibility of these capabilities could occur in several ways. First, the BMSC, as a whole complex of connective tissue cells' differons (including the osteoblastic one) at various stages of differentiation, could differentiate into osteogenic cells, adding to a pool of local primary osteoblasts involved in the formation of primary (reticulofibrous) bone tissue. Second, part of the implanted stromal cells could die and then act as a feeder ("a food") for the remaining cultured and resident osteogenic cells, promoting cell proliferation, differentiation, and more active vital activities. Third, part of the implanted cells could survive (function) in the area of regeneration for some time, secreting numerous growth factors, thereby exerting a stimulating effect on all the resident cells of an osteoblastic differon. As the regenerate forms and maturates, these cells die.

Autologous BMSC were implanted in the distraction regenerate both in the distraction period and upon its termination (Mironov et al., 2011a, c).

The results obtained strongly suggest that cell-based therapy has had a marked stimulating effect on the formation and "maturation" of distraction regenerates in children when surgically correcting leg-length discrepancies.

This effect is manifested primarily in terms of a significant reduction in the ossification time of the forming distraction regenerates of elongated limbs, in comparison to patients who had not received cell-based therapy; this allowed the dismantling of distraction devices much earlier (40%), thereby avoiding possible complications associated with the long-term fixation in an apparatus. In turn, earlier disengagement of the limbs operated from external fixation constructions provided an opportunity to carry out rehabilitation with a full axial load. As a result, the limbs' functional recovery in those patients who had undergone cell-based therapy surpassed recovery levels in patients who had not yet received it; this has had a positive effect on the quality of life and the subsequent social adaptation of children who have undergone operations. It should be noted that, after cell therapy had been carried out, the correction results were sustained longer in the extended segment: as a child grew, the length discrepancy was less evident than that in the control subjects. This observation makes it possible to suggest that the application of BMSC had a stimulating effect on the growth of a "dysplasia" segment, bringing the rate of its length increase to the physiological one. BMSC-based therapy was applied in 16 patients. The patients' follow-up lasted for six years. No complications or irregularities in the structure of the distraction regenerates were observed during adaptive remodeling.

The similar evident stimulating effect of cell-based therapy has been observed in the surgical treatment of congenital pseudarthrosis (Mironov et al., 2011b).

The duration of fixation in an Ilizarov apparatus ranged from 5–7.5 months. The consolidation of bone fragments occurred without an evident callus in all four patients who had received cell-based therapy. In addition, these patients underwent the simultaneous or delayed extension of the operated limb to compensate for its length, which developed during a pseudarthrosis resection. The patients' follow-up lasted for 3–5 years. A recurrence of pseudarthrosis and defects of a medullary canal reconstruction has not been observed in any case.

Bone marrow **macrophages** are heterogeneous in their structural and functional properties. Nevertheless, their main characteristics fit into the spectrum described in section 2.5.1. A characteristic feature of bone marrow macrophages is their involvement in erythropoiesis within the erythroblastic islands, which represent clusters of erythroid cells surrounding central macrophages. With the help of their processes, which penetrate through the walls of sinusoidal capillaries, the latter absorb iron compounds (transferrin) and pass them on to the maturing erythroid cells. Furthermore, macrophages facilitate the entry of erythropoietin and erythropoietic vitamins (vitamin D3) into erythroblasts.

Endothelial cells (endotheliocytes) form the inside walls of blood vessels, including the sinusoidal capillaries. They can come into contact with hematopoietic and stromal cells, since the capillary basement membrane is not continuous. The endotheliocytes making up the thin continuous lining of blood vessels are flat, their periphery being especially thin. Organelles are scarce.

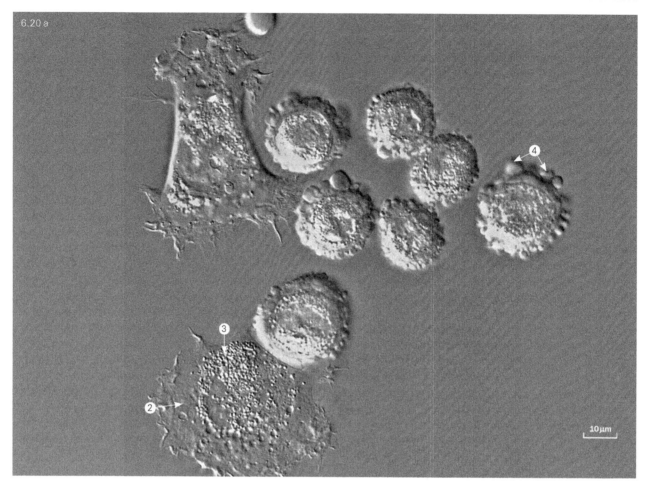

6.20 a

Fig. 6.20.
Bone marrow stromal cells
(BMSC) in a cultural medium
after the primary passage:
a, a1, a2 – after 2 hours –
non-attached and attached
flattened BMSC ;
b – after 4 hour – attached
flattened BMSC;
c – after 24 hours – spread cells
of a non-continuous monolayer;
d – after 72 hours – BMSC of
a continuous monolayer.
A nucleus (1). Ectoplasm (2).
Granules-organelles
in endoplasm (3).
Protrusions of the BMSC
cytoplasmic membrane with
cytoplasm (4).
Protrusions of the BMSC
cytoplasmic membrane with
cleavage from the cytoplasm
structural part (5).
A gel-like substance (secretion) (6).
Folds of a gel-like substance (7).
A vacuol(8).
LM-micrograph. A light optic
inverted microscope Ti Nikon
(Japan) integrated with an incubator. Nomarsky (differential)
interference contrast (DIC),
x 800. a1 – LM-micrograph.
A light optic microscope
Ni Nikon (Japan). Semi-thine
sectione. Azur-eozin. x 800.
a2 – TEM-micrograph.
Ultrathine sectione.
Contrasting with lead citrate
and uranelacetate. x 4,000.

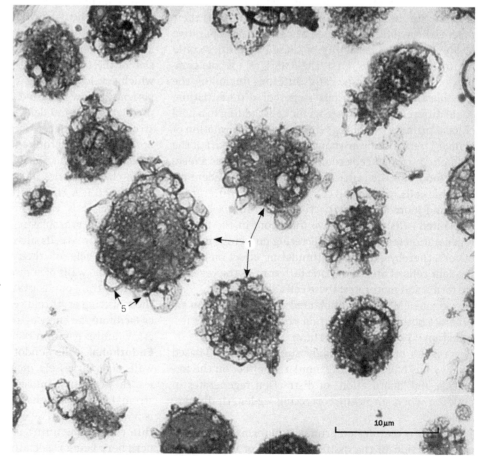

6.20 a2

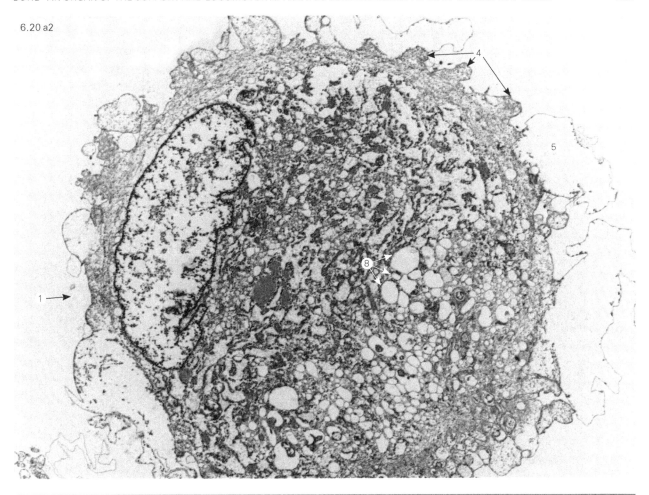

6.20 b

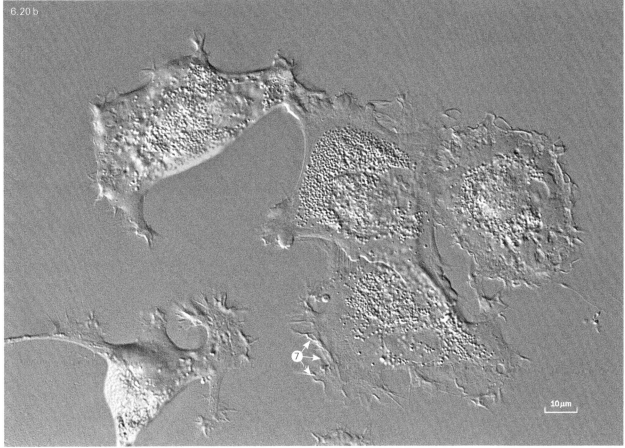

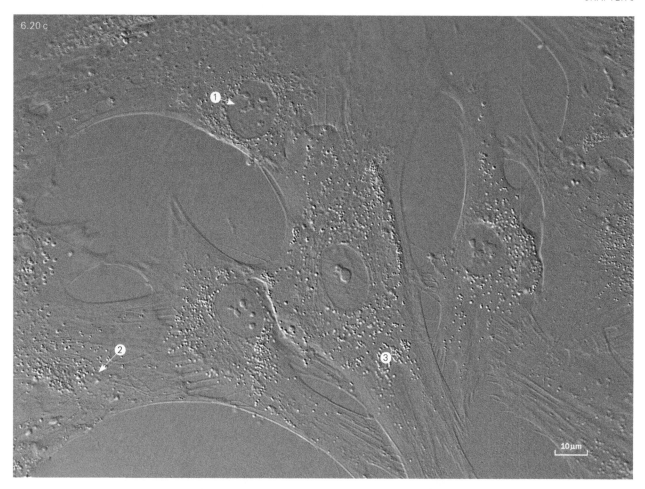

6.20 c

10μm

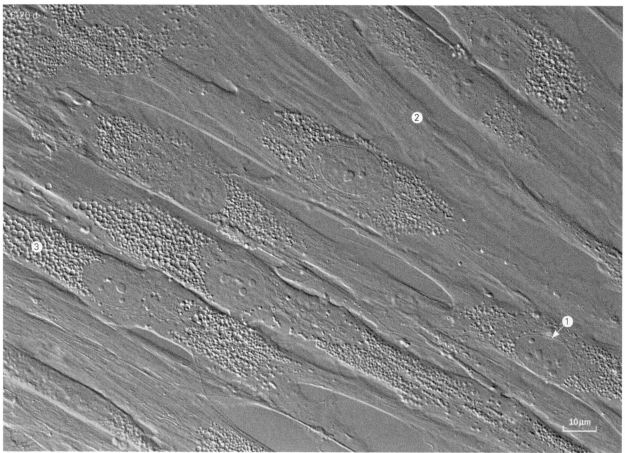

6.20 d

10μm

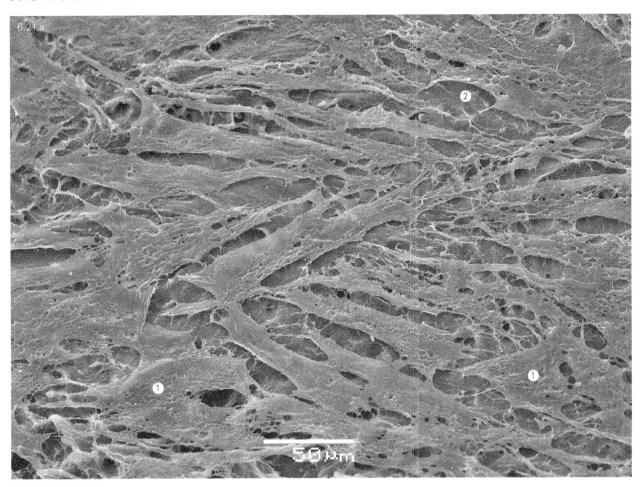

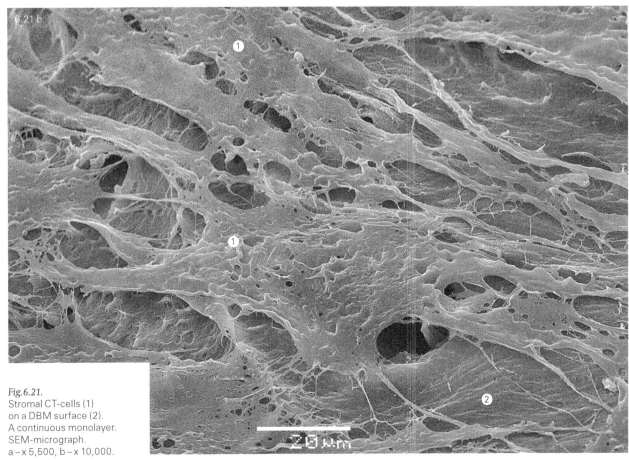

Fig.6.21.
Stromal CT-cells (1)
on a DBM surface (2).
A continuous monolayer.
SEM-micrograph.
a – x 5,500, b – x 10,000.

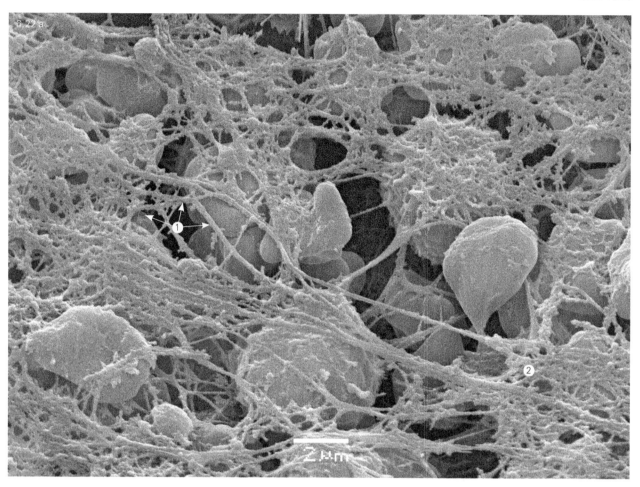

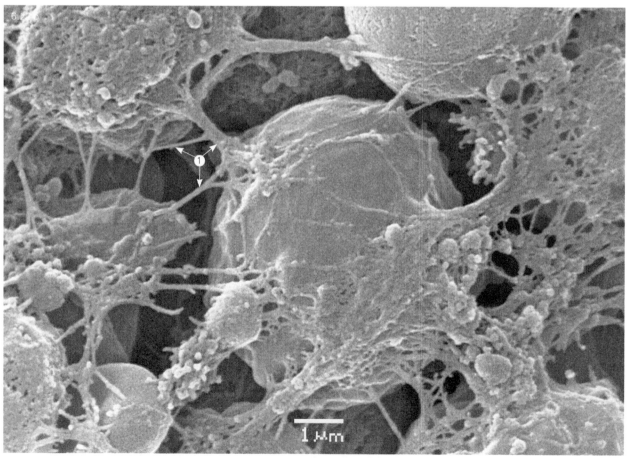

The cells synthesize type IV collagen, hemopoietin and colony-stimulating factor (CSF) – a factor that stimulates the formation of colonies.

Sinusoidal endothelial cells form a continuous layer. Mature blood cells exit through an endotheliocyte. During the time of the hematopoietic cell's passage, a temporary aperture forms in a region of the endothelial cell where it is not connected to the basement membrane and to adventitial cells.

The **extracellular matrix** (EM) of the stroma connective tissue is made up of loosely arranged thin collagen and elastic fibrils and fibers forming a meshwork, which interacts with the network of reticular and adventitial cells. This network is of general significance, integrating a large amount of hematopoietic cells and forming local plexuses on their surfaces (*Fig. 6.22 a*). Furthermore, these cells, which lie adjacent or nearby, are connected to each other by thin short fibers and fibrils, which unravel into separate fibrils at the cell surface and attach to the cell membrane (*Fig. 6.22 b*). Therefore, there is a general and local (dual) system of intercellular integration. These fibrous and cellular structures of the stroma, as well as the hematopoietic elements, blood vessels and nerves, are surrounded by the integrating buffer metabolic medium (ground substance) (see 3.2), which mediates all the metabolic and regulatory processes in the bone marrow.

Thus, the bone marrow stroma, forming the hematopoietic microenvironment, performs maintenance and trophic functions with regard to the hematopoietic elements. However, its regulatory function is no less important. The regulation of hematopoiesis occurs at two levels (Chertkov & Gurevich, 1984). Hematopoietic progenitor cells that have lost their pluripotency are controlled by systemic regulatory factors of an organismal nature, i.e. by special hormones. However, the hematopoietic stem cells are regulated locally by stromal cells. The combination of these two levels of regulation allows the maintenance of hematopoietic stem cell populations, while simultaneously meeting the need for such cells in blood formation. Therefore, differentiation is accompanied by a change in the type of regulation.

The tissues in bone marrow are characterized by specific spatial architectonics of the arrangement of hematopoietic elements. Granulocyte progenitors are positioned in the center, far away from the sinusoid. They move toward the sinusoid wall in the course of differentiation and approach it in the metamyelocyte stage. In contrast, megakaryocytes surround the wall, and thrombocytes are formed from strips of cytoplasm

pinching off when already in the lumen of the sinuses. It is important to note the contacts between cells of the hematopoietic tissue and the stromal elements. Reticulocytes are associated with the granulocyte progenitors. Erythroid cells surround a macrophage, which embraces them with its protrusions, thus forming an erythroblastic island (Vessis, 1958). The macrophage probably regulates their differentiation, or represents a feeder cell for the erythroblasts.

The **hematopoietic tissue** represents the bone marrow parenchyma. It hosts the continuous production and differentiation of peripheral blood and immune system cellular elements. In 1910, Maksimov (1925) proposed a hypothesis for the monophyletic origin of blood cells, according to which all the varied forms of peripheral blood cells represent the progeny of a single parent cell, arising through division and differentiation. Subsequent studies using radiation hematology, tissue culture, cytogenetic and molecular biology methods have fully confirmed these ideas (Chertkov & Friedenstein, 1977). According to the modern scheme of hematopoiesis, a pluripotent, morphologically unidentifiable cell, resembling a lymphocyte, lies in its foundation (Abramov & Vorobiov, 2002). This is either an embryonic stem cell, or an adult hematopoietic stem cell (HSC) repopulating the bone marrow for a long period of time. Multipotent stem cells arise as a result of its differentiation, repopulating the bone marrow for a short period of time. In the course of further differentiation, committed progenitors of the lymphoid and myeloid lineages are formed. These cells are capable of producing colonies of different cellular composition; however, their progeny already specialize into a particular cell type, generating a specific blast. The blast cell is the first morphologically identifiable element undergoing mitotic divisions and producing daughter cells, which differentiate strictly into a specific type of peripheral blood cells. The morphological characteristics of a blast cell are a fairly large size and a large nucleus with a "fine" structure. The nucleo-cytoplasmic ratio is considerably biased toward the nucleus, which is surrounded by only a thin cytoplasmic rim. One or more nucleoli are usually visible in the nucleus. Myeloblasts, erythroblasts, megakaryoblasts, monoblasts and lymphoblasts can be distinguished among the blast cells, giving rise to the corresponding hematopoietic lineages.

Myeloblasts can be neutrophilic, basophilic and eosinophilic. The latter two types normally are extremely rare in bone marrow.

The next differentiation stages of the myeloid lineage are promyelocyte, myelocyte and metamyelocyte. The latter differentiates without dividing into a band granulocyte (neutrophil, eosinophil, basophil), whose nucleus is in the form of an elongated rod or is bent in a horseshoe shape. Then follows the final stage of the granulocytic series – segmented neutrophil, eosinophil or basophil. The nucleus is divided into several segments connected to each other by thin filaments.

Fig. 6.22.
A bone marrow fragment. Hematopoietic and stromal cells are surrounded by a meshwork of fibrous structures (1) forming plexuses on the cell surfaces,

(2) and individual fibers and fibrils,
(3) connecting adjacent or nearby cells.
SEM-micrograph.
a – x 5,500,
b – x 10,000.

The erythroblast is the first morphologically definable cell type of the erythroid lineage. It differentiates into a pronormocyte.

The next stage in the erythroid series is the normocyte. There is a gradual accumulation of hemoglobin in the cytoplasm, determining its color. The basophilic normocyte with a blue cytoplasm appears first, followed by the polychromatic normocyte, which takes in both acid and basic dyes and has a purple cytoplasmic tint; finally comes the oxyphilic normocyte with a pinkish cytoplasm. The nucleus undergoes involution in the course of normocyte differentiation.

The oxyphilic normocyte loses its nucleus through pyknosis and turns into a mature cell–an erythrocyte, which then enters the peripheral blood. Reticulocytes containing basophilic meshwork substance often enter the blood in anemia. They lose the reticular substance within two days of circulation in the blood, thus becoming mature erythrocytes.

The monoblast is the first cell of the monocytic series. The promonocyte represents the next stage in differentiation. The monocyte is the final stage in differentiation of the monocytic lineage. Macrophages are considered derivatives of monocytes. The osteoclast is probably a type of macrophage. The megakaryoblast is a committed megakaryocyte progenitor. Its nucleus is round in shape. The cytoplasm is basophilic and does not contain grains. The megakaryoblast turns into a megakaryocyte by passing through the promegakaryocyte stage.

The megakaryocyte, a giant cell, reaching 60–120 μm in size, is a source of thrombocytes (platelets), which emerge as cytoplasmic fragments, 2–4 μm in diameter, pinching off megakaryocytes. Platelets are not cells in the full sense of the word. They have a centrally located granulomere, which stains in a purple-red color, and a peripheral part, hyalomere, which has a basophilic color. The differentiation of cells of the lymphoid series also takes place in the bone marrow. Its progenitor cell is the lymphoblast, the diameter of which is 15 μm or more. The nucleus is round and the cytoplasm is basophilic with a clear perinuclear zone. The lymphoblast differentiates into a prolymphocyte, which is smaller in size and has a lower nucleo-cytoplasmic ratio. In turn, the prolymphocyte becomes a lymphocyte: a B lymphocyte or a T-lymphocyte progenitor. The latter moves to the thymus, where it undergoes terminal specialization. The B lymphocyte can exist as a terminally differentiated cell, or can continue to differentiate into a plasmablast, proplasmacyte, and a plasmacyte (plasma cell).

The **blood supply of bones** is largely dependent on the specifics of their shape, internal structure and levels of various functions. The following represent common features. A significant portion of the blood supply to all bones is provided by the vessels located in the periosteum. These vessels penetrate the cortical part of bones through the bone canals, branch, and the finest branches are found in the Haversian and Volkmann's canals of the osteons. In the diaphyses of long bones, the periosteal vessels spread only in the surface layer of the cortex, which is relatively thick. In the spongy and flat bones, the periosteal vessels can pass through the thin cortical layer and enter the interstitial spaces filled with bone marrow, thereby participating in its blood supply too. Another source of blood supply is the regional feeding arteries, representing the branches of nearby arteries (main, muscular, and fascial). In diaphyses, a.nutritia penetrates the medullary canal through a similarly named opening in the diaphyseal cortex and forms a well-developed intramedullary vasculature. The latter participates in supplying blood to both the contents of the medullary canal (the bone marrow) and the cortical diaphyseal plate, thereby anastomosing with the vessels branching out of the periosteal network. Thus, the diaphysis is supplied with blood by both the intramedullary and periosteal networks. The microcirculation of the cortical plate is presented by arterioles, precapillaries, capillaries, postcapillaries and venules. The microvessels of the medullary cavity form an integrated vascular system.

The metaphyseal vessels are represented by numerous small arterioles running through the depth of the synovial and fibrous membranes, as well as the intra-articular ligaments. There is a wide looped network of arterioles and precapillaries in the metaphyseal spongy bone, composed of metaphyseal vessels and the anastomosing branches of feeding arteries. A dense capillary network surrounds the bone trabeculae (Onoprienko, 1993).

The venous outflow from bones is carried out by vessels, which generally follow throughout the arterial system. The numerous venules of the medullary cavity form larger veins, matching the organization of the branches of the feeding arteries, thereby resulting in one or two stems of feeding veins. The latter flow into a nearby main venous stem after leaving the bone.

The capillary network densely covers the bone trabeculae in spongiose bone, giving rise to postcapillaries and venules. These, in turn, generate numerous veins, some of which form branches of the medullary venous system. However, most reach the venous system on the bone surface, which is connected to the vessels of the surrounding tissues.

Bone innervation is closely linked to its blood supply. Bone nerves are a continuation of the periosteal nerves and the branches of the nerve stems running along the bone. They accompany blood vessels both in the periosteum and in the bone (bone canals, interstitial spaces, and on the surface of bone trabeculae), as well as in the bone marrow, forming plexuses, similar to the vascular ones. Bone nerves contain sensory (afferent) and vagal (efferent) nerve fibres. The sensory fibers terminate with structurally different nerve endings that are either free or encapsulated.

Chapter 7

CARTILAGE –
CARTILAGINOUS
TISSUE:
STRUCTURAL,
BIOCHEMICAL
AND MOLECULAR
BIOLOGICAL
CHARACTERISTICS

7.1. OVERVIEW OF STRUCTURE AND COMPOSITION OF CARTILAGE TISSUE

Cartilage tissue is a peculiar type of connective tissue; it plays an important role in the organization and formation of the vertebrate skeleton, as well as of some extraskeletal structures. Three different types of cartilage tissue – hyaline, elastic and fibrous – are present in the organism, forming the hyaline, elastic and fibrous types of cartilage, respectively. Despite their significant morphological and biochemical differences, these have in common the predominant presence of two main macromolecular components in the extracellular matrix – the large type II fibrillar collagen and the large proteoglycan, aggrecan. These two components, expressed by cells of the specific chondroblastic differon, impart unique biomechanical properties to cartilage tissue that define its biological significance.

The morphological, biochemical and molecular-biological characteristics of cartilage tissue are most clearly represented in hyaline cartilages, also called "true". The biochemical and molecular-biological characterization of cartilage tissue in this chapter is therefore based primarily on studies of hyaline cartilages, more specifically, articular cartilage, which have been studied in great detail. It should be emphasized that, despite some differences among the different types of cartilage, the outlined concepts, to a significant degree, apply to the elastic and, to some degree, to the fibrous cartilages as well. The presence of elastic fibers in the extracellular matrix distinguishes elastic from hyaline cartilages, and imparts elasticity upon the structures comprised of such cartilages.

Fibrous cartilages are complex fibrous structures built mostly of dense fibrous connective tissue, which contain regions or zones of hyaline cartilage tissue. These regions contribute to the biomechanical properties of fibrous cartilages.

The formation of virtually all bones of the axial skeleton (except for parts of the clavicle), and of all limb bones, proceeds through the stage of cartilage models. The models are formed from mesenchymal condensation cells undergoing chondroblastic differentiation (see section 10.2.2). The models' cartilage tissue – called provisory (from the Lat. *provideo* – to foresee) or transitory, i.e. preliminary, temporary – is substituted by bone tissue at

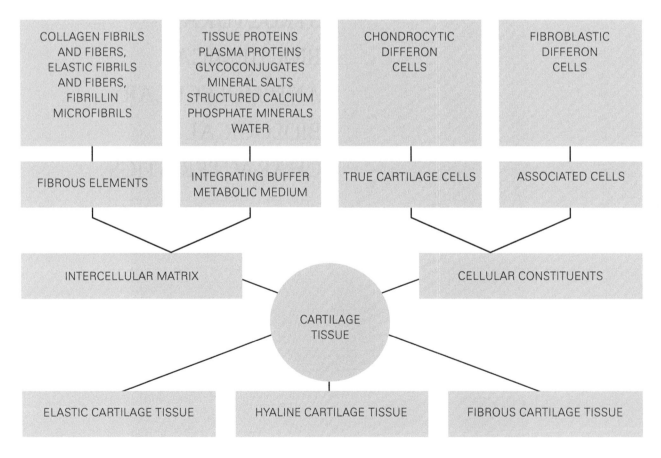

Fig. 7.1.
Hyalin cartilagefibrous cartilage.
Diagram of cartilage tissue
organization and classification.
(According to Omelyanenko)

Table 7.1

Quantitative biochemical parameters of human femoral head articular cartilage

Components	Concentration (g/100 g dried fat-free tissue)
Hydroxyproline	6,30 ± 0,8
Hexuronic acid	3,29 ± 0,66
Hexosamines	5,65 ± 1,17
Non-collagenous proteins*	16,2 ± 0,9
DNA	0,57 ± 0,07
RNA	0,16 ± 0,03

*The term "non-collagenous" proteins refersto all proteins of non-collagenous nature. Their content is calculated based on the ratio between the hydroxyproline and tyrosine concentrations.

birth, and persists only in the so-called growth plates (metaepiphyseal cartilage of long bones) (see 10.3) during the postnatal period until the onset of puberty and until the organism completes growth. The transitory cartilage tissue resembles hyaline cartilage in terms of its structural and biochemical characteristics.

All types of permanent cartilage tissue – hyaline, fibrous and elastic (*Fig. 7.1*) – possess common morphological, chemical and biochemical characteristics, with some morphological and chemical distinctions (Wachmuth et al., 2006).

First, the common characteristics pertain to all types of connective tissue (see 1.3). The predominance of the amount of extracellular matrix over the amount of cellular components is the most important common characteristic of all permanent types of cartilage tissue. This prevalence is so significant that quantitative biochemical data of tissue samples, with the exception of nucleic acid concentrations, actually reflect the composition of the matrix.

This pattern is illustrated in *Table 7.1*, which presents the results of a quantitative biochemical analysis of the most thoroughly studied type of hyaline cartilage –the articular cartilage (Pavlova et al., 1988).

Hydroxyproline is defined as a specific component of collagen. It accounts for at least 10% of the amino acid residues in fibrillar collagens. Therefore, the total content of collagenous proteins exceeds 60% of the total dry weight of the tissue. Compared to cartilage tissue, of all types of connective tissue, only the dense regular and irregular CT (tendons and dermis) contain more collagens.

Cartilage has the highest concentration of hexuronic acids (represented primarily by glucuronic acid) and hexosamines (glucosamine and galactosamine) within the connective tissue system. Hexuronic acids and hexosamines are monosaccharides, which form glycosaminoglycans – linear polysaccharide components of proteoglycan macromolecules. All cartilage matrix glycosaminoglycans (chondroitin sulfates and keratan sulfate), with the exception of hyaluronan, are sulfated, and, accordingly, cartilage tissue has a high sulfate sulfur content at around 1.3 g/100 g (McDevitt, 1973). The total concentration of glycosaminoglycans in the cartilage matrix reaches 10 g of a 100 g dry substance.

Hexosamines are found in the oligosaccharide groups of glycoprotein macromolecules, apart from being glycosaminoglycan components (and, therefore, proteoglycans). This explains why the hexosamine concentration is

Table 7.2

Biochemical composition of hyaline cartilage tissue

Components	g/100 g
Water	66–79*
Dry substance	21–34*
Collagenous proteins	48–62**
Non-collagenous proteins	8–15**
Glycosaminoglycans of proteoglycans	14–23**
Hyaluronan	< 1**
Other matrix components	< 3**

* g/100 g of fresh tissue.

** % of dry substance.

higher than the concentration of hexuronic acids. Cartilage matrix glycoproteins are numerous and, despite the low concentration of each individual protein, they play an important role in the supramolecular structure of the matrix (see section 7.2.1.2.4.1).

Data on the biochemical composition of the hyaline type of cartilage tissue is summarized in *Table 7.2*.

Second, all permanent cartilage is very rich in water. Water is the most abundant chemical component of cartilage tissue. In most cartilage, the content of dry residue does not exceed 20–30% of the fresh tissue mass. In this respect, hyperhydration is considered a normal state for cartilage tissue. Most of the water is not chemically bound to the structural matrix macromolecules and is actively exchanged.

Third, in addition to water, the basic components of the structural macromolecules of the extracellular matrix of all cartilages–both in terms of content and significance–are:

a) collagenous proteins (the main collagenous protein in hyaline cartilage is large type II fibrillar collagen, and

b) the large proteoglycan, aggrecan (see section 7.2.1.2.4.1), which forms large supramolecular aggregates with

hyaluronan (hyaluronic acid). The interaction between these two structural components and water plays a central role in determining the biomechanical properties of cartilage tissue.

The fibrous and elastic types of cartilage have special biomechanical functions; hence, the chemical composition of the extracellular matrix is supplemented with macromolecular components absent in hyaline cartilage. Thus, elastic (mainly extraskeletal) cartilages contain significant amounts of elastin and other components of elastic fibers. At the same time, the content of type II collagen is almost indistinguishable in elastic and hyaline cartilages. In fibrous cartilages (e.g. in articular meniscus), type II collagen is replaced, to a significant extent, by another large type I fibrillar collagen, typical for dense (fibrous) varieties of connective tissue. All three types of cartilage also show some quantitative differences in the amounts of the so-called "minor" collagen types V, VI, and X. There are also other differences in the chemical composition of hyaline, elastic and fibrous cartilages; however, type II collagen and aggrecan proteoglycans, the main components of the hyaline cartilage EM, are present in both elastic and fibrous types of cartilage, albeit at lower concentrations.

In addition to these radical differences between the three types of cartilage, there are also certain biochemical characteristics of the individual varieties of each type, as well as local (regional) features within each individual cartilage.

These peculiarities, extensively studied in human articular artilage, which is hyaline by nature, are manifested in the differences among the whole cartilage from various joints. Thus, considerable differences have been found in the content of the main structural macromolecules between the cartilage of human elbow and knee joints, functioning under unequal mechanical loads. Elbow joint cartilage has higher total proteoglycan content and lower water content compared to knee joint cartilage, which is indicative of lower matrix porosity and a correspondingly lower molecular transport efficiency (Fetter et al., 2006).

Biochemical differences, clearly detectable by histochemical (immunochemical) analysis, are also found between the layers and zones within an individual articular cartilage, and these differences are not just quantitative, but also of a qualitative nature (Poole et al., 2001).

The composition of type II collagen and the fibrillar collagen-associated small proteoglycans – decorin and biglycan – is higher in the extracellular matrix of the surface (tangential) layer, adjacent to synovia (synovial fluid), in comparison to deeper layers. In contrast, the total proteoglycan concentration in this layer is reduced, mainly at the expense of aggrecan, while the total concentration of proteoglycans rises relative to the increasing distance from the joint surface. The large proteoglycan, of surface zone, also known as proteoglycan-4 (PG 4), is present in the surface layer as well. This layer also contains other proteins that are absent in the deeper cartilage layers. These biochemical differences are indicative of the phenotypic peculiarities of the surface layer chondrocytes, the features of which are also manifested by differences in cell maturation dynamics (in integrin expression dynamics, for example) (Hidaka et al., 2006), and in the accumulation of matrix components induced by bone morphogenetic proteins (BMP) (Cheng, 2007).

The very thin, most superficial layer of articular cartilage has an entirely peculiar biochemical composition, similar to the composition of synovia. This layer is low in proteins and sulfated glycosaminoglycans compared to the most of the tissue, and is composed mainly of hyaluronan and phospholipids, with the phospholipids attached to the hydrophobic surface of the hyaluronan disaccharide residues (see section 3.2.1.2) (Crockett et al., 2007).

The deeper middle (intermediate) layer has a particularly high aggrecan concentration, while the type II collagen concentration is somewhat reduced, and type VI collagen is found. This layer contains a specific glycoprotein – cartilage intermediate layer protein (CILP).

Within the middle layer, there are also biochemical differences between the chondrocyte's pericellular microenvironment (PCME) and the rest of the extracellular matrix.

The pericellular (territorial) matrix – the matrix in a lacuna, which contains a chondrocyte (or more often, a small group of chondrocytes) – is different from the interterritorial matrix, which is located outside the **chondron**, the structural and functional unit of cartilage tissue. The main difference is that the chondron, particularly, the pericellular capsule that surrounds it, contains type VI collagen and decorin. The pericellular matrix is also distinguished by the presence of a protein related to WARP (von Willebrand factor A domain-related protein) (Allen et al., 2006), which participates in the chondron's assembly and maintains its stability.

Finally, the layer adjacent to bone tissue contains type X collagen, which is absent in all other layers, and appears only where chondrocyte hypertrophy and calcification proceeds.

The local and spatial heterogeneity in the biochemical composition of other cartilage species have not been studied in as much detail as in the case of articular cartilage. However, there is no reason to doubt that chemical composition varies along the length of other cartilage species, for example, massive rib cartilages, which represent another variety of hyaline cartilage.

The biochemical characteristics of the basic types of cartilage tissue will be thoroughly discussed in the subsequent sections of this chapter.

7.2. HYALINE CARTILAGE – CARTILAGE TISSUE

7.2.1. Hyaline articular cartilage

7.2.1.1. Cartilage cells differon

7.2.1.1.1. Morphology and histophysiology of chondroblast and chondrocyte

Articular cartilage is part of the articular ends of bones and ensures their optimal interaction inside the joint during movement. Cartilage is made of a special kind of connective tissue – cartilage tissue, which consists of cartilage cells and an extracellular matrix. The latter is the basic functional unit of the articular cartilage. Precisely its components – collagenous structures and an integrating buffer metabolic medium (ground substance) – provide the support, shape-maintenance and shock absorbing functions of cartilage, and are responsible for its tribological properties. The cellular constituents of cartilage synthesize and secrete the molecules of fibrous proteins and glycosaminoglycans into the extracellular space, as well as participating in their assembly into supramolecular aggregates: fibrous structures (collagen fibrils) and structured proteoglycans. This process occurs during cartilage formation during embryogenesis, and during its constant renewal throughout the postnatal period.

The cartilage cells differon arises in the process of cartilage tissue's formation from the mesenchyme. It includes:

connective tissue pluri potent stem cells; semi-stem (prechondroblasts), chondroblasts and chondrocytes. The distinction of prechondroblasts as committed chondroblast precursors is rather conditional, given that it is practically difficult to distinguish between the semi-stem cells of cartilage and those of bone, such semi-stem cells can generate either cartilage or bone differons depending on the composition of the environment. Chondroblasts are present predominantly in the inner layer of the perichondrium, in contact with the proper hyaline cartilage. The perichondrium is absent in mature articular cartilage, and, therefore, the majority of cartilage cells represent chondrocytes, which are fairly evenly distributed in the extracellular matrix. This is apparently related to the "responsibility" of each cell, or isogenic group of cells, to maintain local homeostasis in the territorial matrix and, in part, in the adjacent interterritorial matrix. In contrast to osteocytes, chondrocytes embedded in the intercellular matrix preserve their secretory activity and their capacity for cell division, including amitotic one. Another difference is the absence of structural connections among chondrocytes by means of cytoplasmic protrusions, even within isogenic groups (i.e. chondrocytes exist autonomously and do not form cell associations). The shape of cells and cell lacunae is determined by the extracellular matrix organization, which, in turn, depends on the shock absorbing function of cartilage. Obviously, the structural organization of chondrocytes is also influenced by mechanical load, and depends on the distance from food sources.

In addition, age dynamics impact on chondrocyte morphology. All the above-mentioned factors create an evident chondrocyte polymorphism, which is expressed, to a lesser or greater degree, in different regions and layers of articular cartilage.

In turn, the polymorphism is manifested by a number of features or characteristics, which comprise the chondrocyte morphotype (phenotype). These include cell shape, internal cell morphology, cytoskeletal organization, inclusions, synthetic activity, intracellular accumulation of synthetic products, and the composition of synthetic substances (glycosaminoglycans, collagen types, etc.).

There are several classifications of mature hyaline cartilage (more precisely–of articular cartilage) chondrocytes in the literature (Pavlova et al., 1988; Deduh & Pankov 2001; Gigante et al., 2006), which differ from each other, but combine both structural and functional characteristics. The articular cartilage chondrocyte characterization proposed here presents the most rational elements of existing classifications.

Morphotype I chondrocytes possess spindle or oval, elongated shapes (*Fig. 7.2*). An extended nucleus matches the shape of the chondrocyte, and euchromatin and heterochromatin distribution is clearly expressed. A thin rim of cytoplasm surrounds the nucleus. A small amount of general organelles are present in the cytoplasm at both poles of the nucleus. On the outside, cells are surrounded by a finely granular material, named pericellular aureole, or "halo". Beyond this layer is the extracellular matrix, represented by thin collagen fibrils (20–40 nm thick) made of type I collagen. The fibrils are densely packed and oriented, as are the cells, parallel to the articulating surface in the superficial zone of articular cartilage. This layer is composed mostly of collagen fibrils, made of type I collagen protein (A. Gigante et al., 2006). Such a structure of chondrocytes is indicative of their low metabolic activity. At the same time, this chondrocyte morphotype can be designated as fibroblastic on the basis of the aforementioned features. Even though the cells of this morphotype are not limited to the zone of collagen fibrils based ontype I collagen, a tight correlation is evident between the features of this morphotype and the expression of this collagen by these cells.

Chondrocytes of the morphotype II are small in size (3–6 micrometers), spherical, and have numerous short processes. A large part of the cell is occupied by a round nucleus with euchromatin and heterochromatin. Individual organelles are found in the cytoplasm. These cells are located mainly in the outer part of the middlezone. They are distributed individually (without isogenic groups) and directly contact with the EM without established lacunae (*Fig. 7.3*).

Obviously, this cell morphotype can be designated as chondroblastic, i.e. as cells with preserved proliferative ability.

Morphotype III chondrocytes are oval (egg-shaped) or round, with numerous pyramidal processes, an extensive GER in the cytoplasm, a lamellar Golgi complex, secretory vesicles, glycogen granules scattered throughout the cytoplasm, lipid droplets, round nucleus with euchromatin and heterochromatin, and a few mitochondria (*Fig. 7.4, 7.5*). These cells synthesize all EM components, including type II collagen protein. Two chondrocyte subtypes–physiologically active or inactive–can be distinguished within this morphotype on the basis of the degree of expression and the correlation of morphotype III features, and taking into account the structure of the cartilage EM.

Physiologically active chondrocytes have a well-developed synthetic apparatus and their activity can be manifested as either the synthesis or resorption of components of the EM. Chondrocytes involved in EM formation express its components and deliver them into the extracellular space. It should be noted that the number of

Fig. 7.2.
Morphotype I chondrocyte (1) in the superficial zone of articular cartilage.
Nucleus (2).
Cytoplasm (3).
Collagenous fibrils of EM (4).
"Halo" (5).
TEM-micrograph.
Contrasting of ultrathin sections with uranyl acetate and lead citrate.
x 10,000.

Fig. 7.3.
Morphotype II chondrocyte.
In the outer part of the middle zone of the articular cartilage.
Nucleus (1).
Cytoplasm (2).
Cellular processes (3).
Collagenous fibrils of EM (4).
TEM-micrograph.
Contrasting of ultrathin sections with uranyl acetate and lead citrate.
x 10,000.

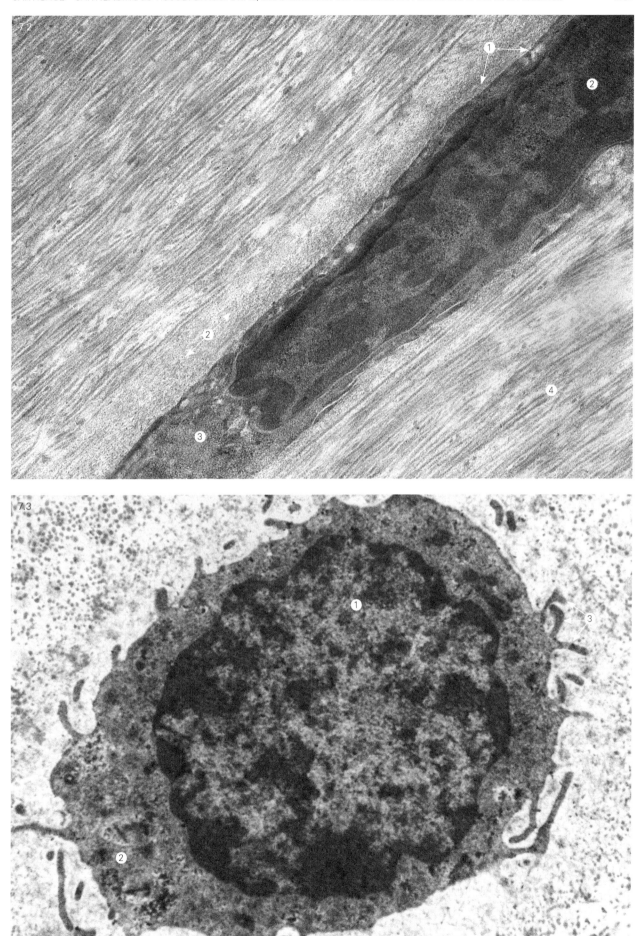

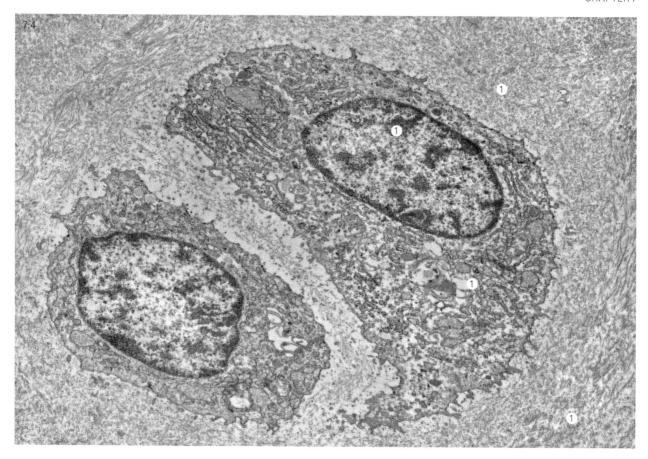

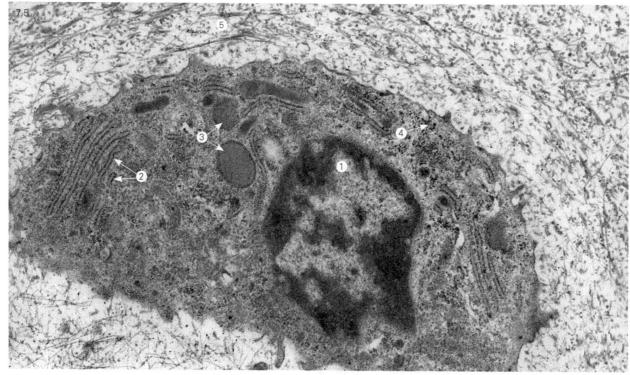

Fig. 7.4.
Morphotype III chondrocyte (active) from thecentral part of the middlezone of articular cartilage.
Nucleus (1).
Cytoplasm with developed GER (2).

Collagenous fibrils of the territorial EM (3).
Interterritorial EM (4).
TEM-micrograph.
Contrasting of ultrathin sections with uranyl acetate and lead citrate. x 5,000.

Fig. 7.5.
Morphotype III chondrocyte (inactive) from the central part of the middle zone of articular cartilage. Nucleus (1).
Cytoplasm with moderately developed GER (2).
Lipid droplets (3).

Collagen granules (4).
Collagenous fibrils of the territorial EM (5).
Interterritorial EM (6).
TEM-micrograph.
Contrasting of ultrathin sections with uranyl acetateand lead citrate. x 5,000.

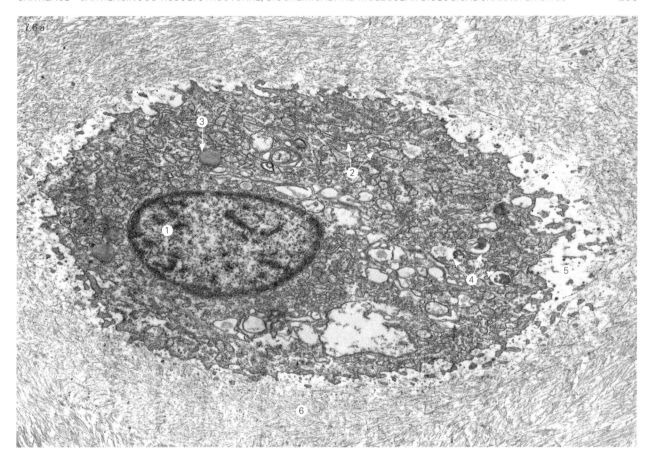

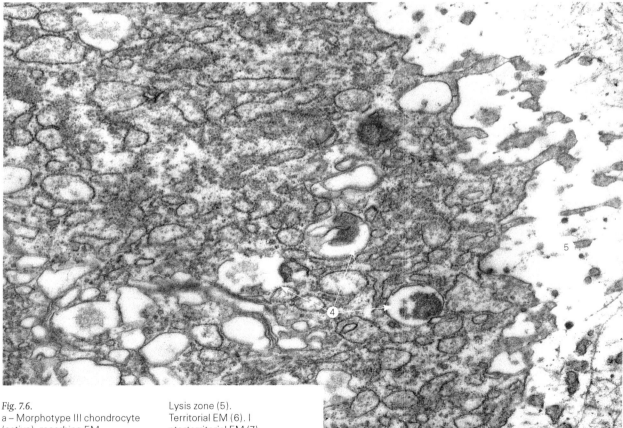

Fig. 7.6.
a – Morphotype III chondrocyte (active), resorbing EM.
b – a fragment of the chondrocyte. Nucleus (1). GER (2). Lipid droplets (3). Phagolysosome (4).

Lysis zone (5). Territorial EM (6). Interterritorial EM (7). TEM-micrograph. Contrasting of ultrathin sections with uranyl acetate and lead citrate. a – x 5,000, b – x 20,000.

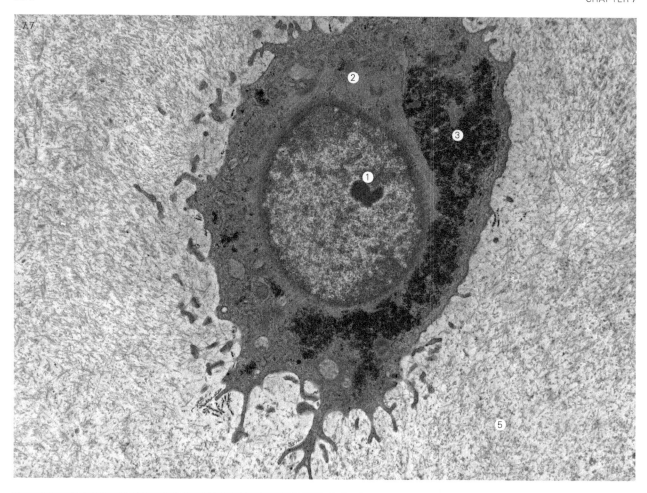

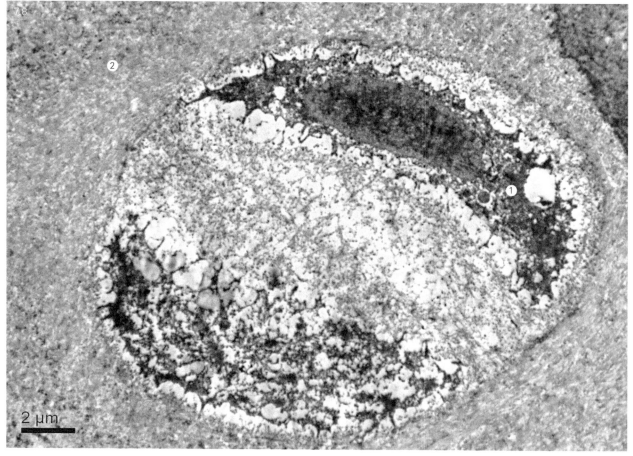

2 μm

organelles involved in the synthesis of EM components in these chondrocytes is much smaller than in the chondrocytes of embryonic tissues and growing cartilage. However, the amount of renewable cartilage EM cannot be compared to the matrix formation in embryonic chondrogenesis zones. The formation of the specific EM structure is also under cellular influence.

Chondrocytes that resorb the cartilage EM contain a large number of lysosomes in the cytoplasm, along with the synthetic machinery. The latter participate both in the extracellular lysis of EM, as indicated by the structureless zone surrounding individual active chondrocytes, and in engulfing macromolecular material from the extracellular space to digest it intracellularly in secondary lysosomes (phagolysosomes), as indicated by their presence in the chondrocyte cytoplasm. Part of the absorbed material is not fully destroyed and remains in the cytoplasm in the form of residual electron-dense bodies in the cytoplasm (Fig. 7.6).

Inactive chondrocytes have fewer organelles in the cytoplasm compared to the active subtype; GER is in the form of long, narrow cisternae; and the cytoplasm is denser, with detectable lipid droplets, glycogen granules and granule clusters of different sizes (Fig. 7.5).

It can be hypothesized that the described morphotype III chondrocyte subtypes represent cells in different functional states, with correspondingly variable amounts of organelles and cytoplasmic inclusions. Apparently, the life activity of this morphotype of chondrocytes is cyclical in nature. During periods of low activity, glycogen and lipids – energy substances necessary for active synthesis – accumulate in the cells.

For the regeneration of cartilage EM, the amount of organelles producing EM component-lysing enzymes in the cells increases. A free space (lysis zone) forms around the cell. Next, the organelle profile is altered towards the synthesis of EM components, the main one being the type II collagen protein. This protein, together with other (minor) collagens and proteoglycans, form the EM collagen fibrils. This step, in turn, is followed by an inactive period in the chondrocyte's life.

The functional state of cells can be appraised to a certain extent from the surrounding EM.

Collagen fibrils with a thickness of 30–80 nm, lying immediately adjacent to the cytoplasmic membrane of the chondrocyte, are indicative of its inactive state. A bright structureless area surrounding, as a rule, an active chondrocyte with resorbing characteristics, confirm the cata-

bolic orientation of its functions. A meshwork of thin filaments around an actively synthesizing cell confirms its building (matrix-forming) function.

Morphotype IV chondrocytes have lost the ability to synthesize EM components. They, too, can be divided into two subtypes: aging chondrocytes (i.e. a definitive form); and degenerating chondrocytes.

The amount of organelles in the cytoplasm of aging chondrocytes is markedly reduced. At the same time, the amount of lipid droplets and glycogen assembled into large aggregates, which occupy a significant portion of the cytoplasm, becomes greater (Fig. 7.7). The nuclear shape becomes lobular. Calcium phosphate crystals are detectable in some cells of the deep zone. Chondrocyte degradation represents the terminal stage of their existence.

Degenerating chondrocytes are wrinkled and have dark (dense) cytoplasm, fragmented nuclei with vague outlines, and swollen mitochondria with disorganized cristae. GER and the lamellar Golgi complex have dilated or vacuolated cisterns.

At the end of the degeneration process, the cells are degraded and their fragments remain in the lacunae (Fig. 7.8) (Palfrey & Davies, 1966).

Chondrocytes have various surface receptors responsible for EM adhesion and signaling. Examples include CD44, which binds hyaluronate (Knudson & Knudson, 2004) and bone morphogenetic proteins (Chen et al., 2004), and integrin family members (Loeser, 2002), which connect the cell with EM components (Svoboda, 1998).

Some of the articular cartilage chondrocytes possess a single cilium. This primary cilium shows the typical organization of a sensory cilium, including a ring of 9 microtubule doublets (9 × 2), which emerge from the basal body (9 x 3). The cilium core is immersed in the cell body through a cytoplasmic invagination, its base is anchored in the cytoplasm, and it associates with the additional centriole.

Another type of sensory cell organelles exists in the form of small (60 nm) flask-shaped dimples on the cell surface. These membrane invaginations are named caveolae, and have transport or sensory functions. Unlike the transport caveolae, sensory caveolae are abundant, permanent, and do not pinch off. They accumulate receptors involved in signal transduction. Their highest density in articular cartilage is on the flat side of the elongated cells from the superficial zone (Schwab et al., 1999). They also play a role in chondrogenesis (Rasmussen & Barrett, 1984).

In this way, chondrocytes actively interact with the surrounding extracellular matrix, which is necessary for its maintenance. Through the matrix adhesive proteins, the surface receptors and the cilia of chondrocytes receive information about the environment and adapt accordingly.

As functional cartilage cells, which create and maintain the specific structure of the cartilage EM, chondroblasts and chondrocytes do not fully correspond, from a termi-

Fig. 7.7.
Morphotype IV chondrocyte.
Definitive form. Nucleus (1).
Cytoplasm (2).
Granular aggregates
of glycogen (3).
Branching cell processes (4).
Extracellular matrix (5).
TEM-micrograph.
Contrasted with lead
citrate and uranyl acetate.
x 5,000.

Fig. 7.8.
Morphotype IV chondrocytes.
Degenerating forms (1)
in a double-chamber lacuna.
Territorial EM (2).
TEM-micrograph.
Contrasting of ultrathin
sections with uranyl acetate
and lead citrate.
x 5,000.

nology viewpoint, to fibrous connective tissue–the fibroblast/fibrocyte. A chondroblast is a cartilage cell, which actively synthesizes EM components and has retained its proliferative potency. Its activity results in cartilage EM formation during embryogenesis, and in the development and growing of cartilage during the early postnatal period of development and reparative chondrogenesis. Some chondroblasts die upon completion of the cartilage EM formation, whereas the rest differentiate into chondrocytes. The latter lose their proliferative ability, but retain their synthetic capacity for EM renewal during the life activities of the cartilage. Under these circumstances, the expression of EM components occurs at much lower levels compared to cartilage formation during embryogenesis and reparative chondrogenesis.

Under similar conditions, an actively synthesizing fibroblast of the fibrous connective tissue corresponds to a chondroblast.

A fibroblast in the physiological state of mature fibrous connective tissue corresponds to a morphotype III chondrocyte. A fibrocyte, being definitive, i.e. an aging form of the fibroblast, corresponds to a morphotype IV chondrocyte. These analogies are useful for to gain the proper understanding of literature terms denoting the cells of the fibrous connective tissue and cartilage tissue.

In vitro cultivation of chrondrocytes.

The isolation of chondrocytes from cartilage tissue and their subsequent cultivation in monolayer cultures provides an opportunity to study their behavior (proliferation, dedifferentiation and redifferentiation) outside the tissue, and the effects of different substances introduced in the culture medium, and also has significance in terms of practical applications. Harvested and expanded human chondrocytes can be used for reverse autotransplantation in restoring injured articular cartilage.

The extraction of chondrocytes from the extracellular matrix is performed by mechanical grinding of cartilage biopsies and subsequent enzymatic digestion for 12 hours. Cells released in this manner from their three-dimensional environment can grow in a monolayer in a culture medium containing calf serum.

Isolated chondrocytes round up when plated and passaged in a culture medium. The chondrocyte surface is quite uneven due to a few large, and numerous small, extrusions in the cell membrane. One feature of the previously presented structural and functional polymorphism of chondrocytes in cartilage tissue is their size variability (from 5–20 mm in diameter) immediately after their introduction in the culture medium. This size variability is further preserved in a monolayer culture.

Another polymorphic feature is the variability of time that cells spend in the culture medium (the stage of cell suspension) after the initial seeding (passage zero) or during reseeding (subsequent passages) until they are attached to the bottom of the flask. At the attachment stage, the cells retain their spherical or round shape, similar to the state of suspension, but do not change

their positions when the culture medium moves within the flask, or when it is replaced (*Fig. 7.9 a, b*).

The polymorphism is also manifested in the multitude of options for chondrocyte spreading on the bottom of the flasks (glass, plastic) and on the surface of various materials that can serve as carrier matrices for these cells. In the early stages of spreading on the bottom of the flask, some of the cells have a round shape, and already have a larger diameter. Other cells have an elongated or polygonal shape. At this stage in their cell cycle in the culture medium, and independent of their shape, the partition of the cytoplasm into endoplasm and ectoplasm occurs in the majority of cells. The endoplasm, which contains all cell organelles, including the nucleus, occupies almost the entire volume of the cell.

Small granules or larger globular structures can be present on the cell membrane surface over the endoplasmic region. The ectoplasm appears as a narrow peripheral rim with small processes (*Fig. 7.9 b, c*).

Depending on their positioning relative to each other during passaging, cells may touch or interact during spreading. Based on cell shape, two main groups of cells–elongated and polygonal–are established during spreading (*Fig. 7.9 d, e, f*). In the former group, a conditional aspect ratio–the shortest transverse and longest longitudinal measurements at the level of the nucleus–is 3 or more. In polygonal cells, this ratio does not exceed 2. All other cells fit in between. The elongated cells have few processes. As a rule, they are long, and are oriented mainly parallel to the longitudinal axis of the cell. The processes can branch. Polygonal cells have considerably more processes, which are short. The latter are part of the ectoplasm, which is more pronounced in polygonal cells.

The spreading of seeded cartilage cells is, in a way, an adaptation period, followed by the proliferation stage.

Fig. 7.9.
Chondrocytes in culture medium.
a – Stage of chondrocyte attachment (1) to the bottom surface of the flask.
b – Stage of attachment and initiation of chondrocyte spreading. Attached chondrocytes (1). Spreading chondrocytes (2).
c – Chondrocyte spreading stage. Spreading chondrocytes (1).
d, e, f – Chondrocyte spreading stage. Spreading (1) and spread (2) chondrocytes.
e, f – Chondrocyte spreading stage. Nucleus (1). Endoplasm (2). Ectoplasm (3).
g – Proliferation stage. Spread chondrocytes (1). Chondrocytes at various stages of division (2).
h, i – Stage of termination of

proliferation and formation of complete (confluent) monolayer. Nucleus (1). Endoplasm (2). Ectoplasm (3).
j – Stage of confluent monolayer. I phase. Chondrocytes (1) are immediately adjacent to each other. Chromatin clumps in the nuclei (2).
k – Stage of confluent monolayer. Phase II. Chondrocytes (1) are immediately adjacent to each other.
Small granules (2) and vacuoles (3) in the endoplasm.
LM-micrograph.
a–e; g–k–A light optic inverted microscope Ti Nikon (Japan) integrated with an incubator. Nomarsky (differential) interference contrast (DIC), f – azur-eosin staining, x 400.

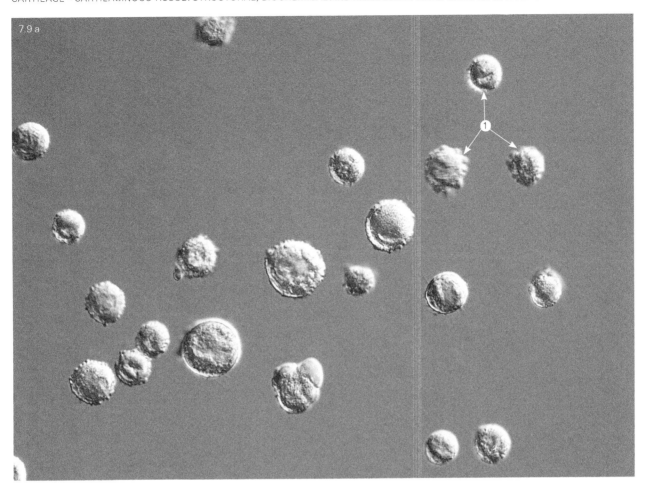

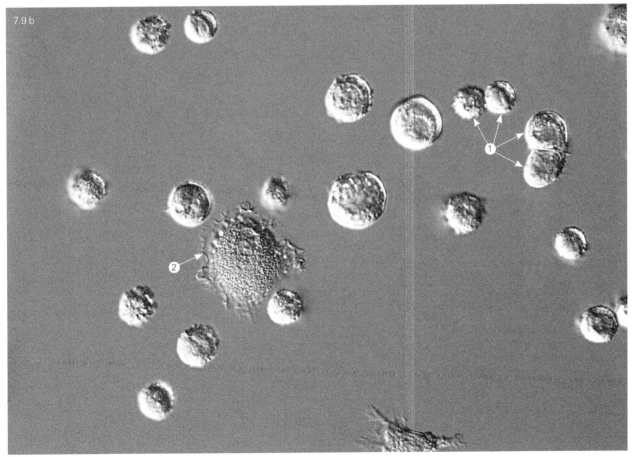

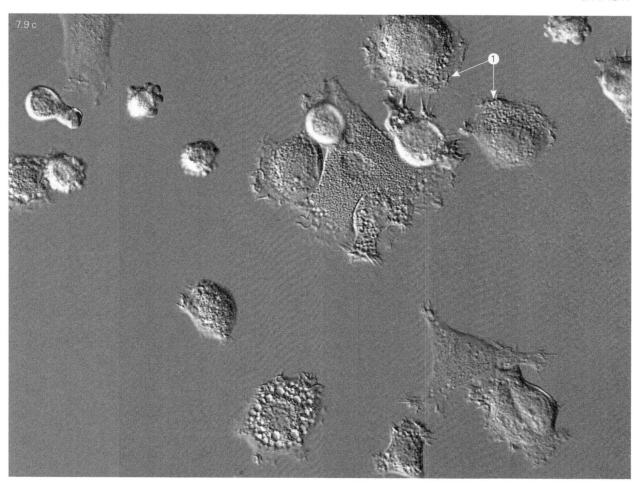

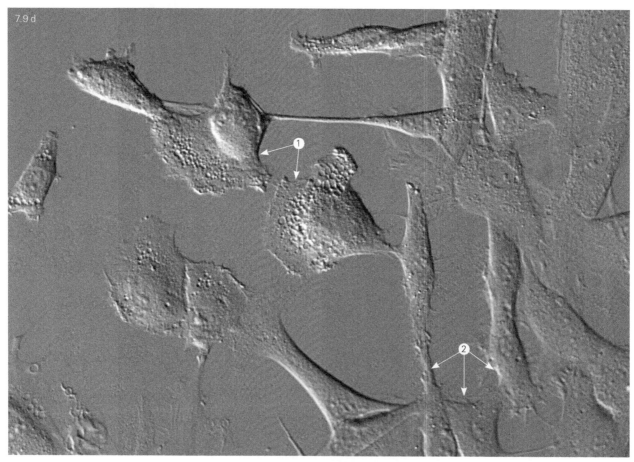

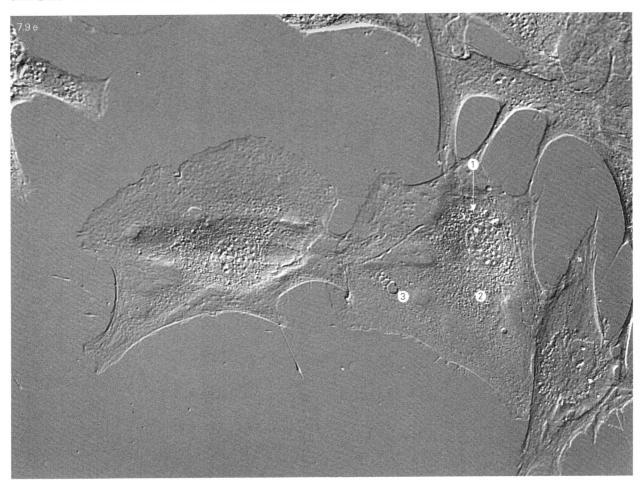

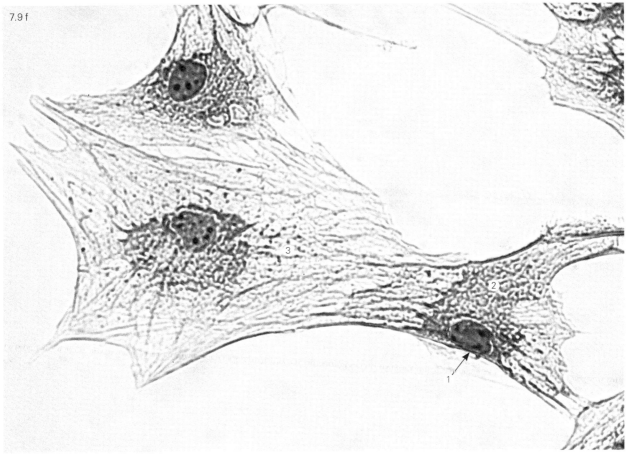

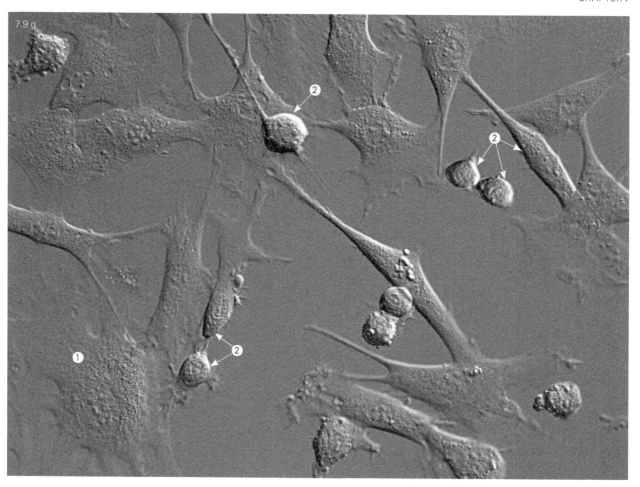

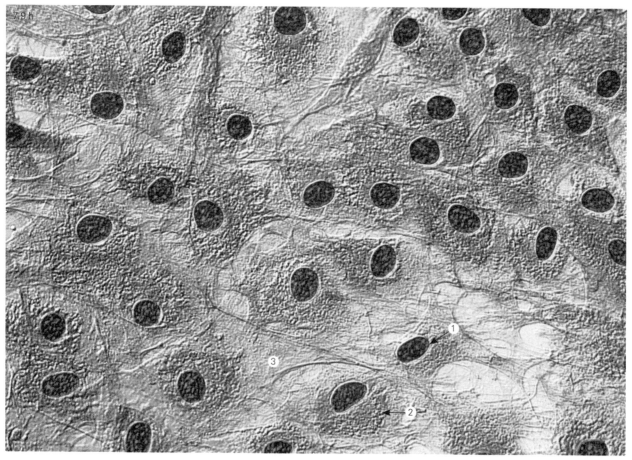

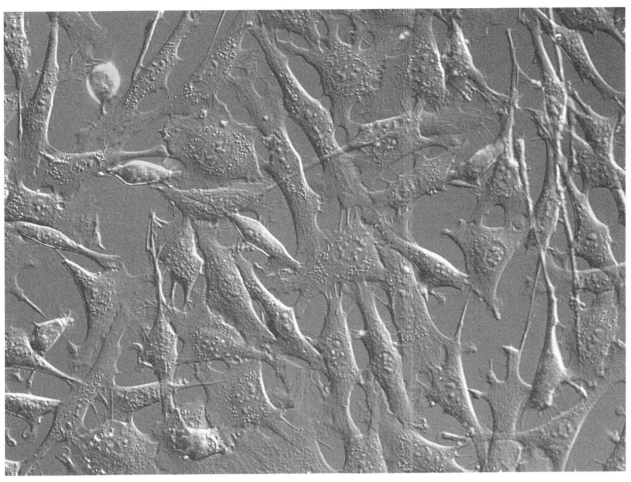

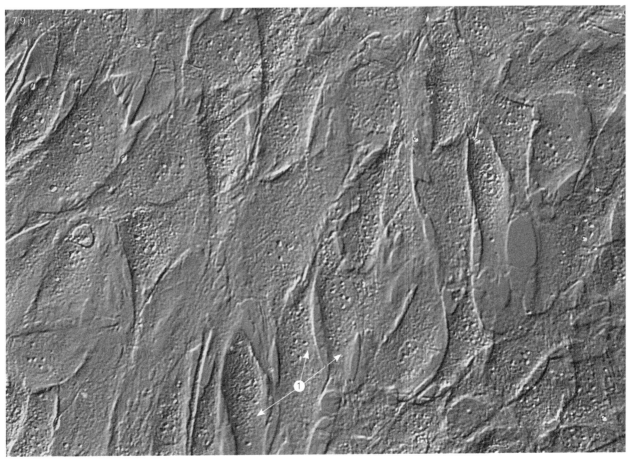

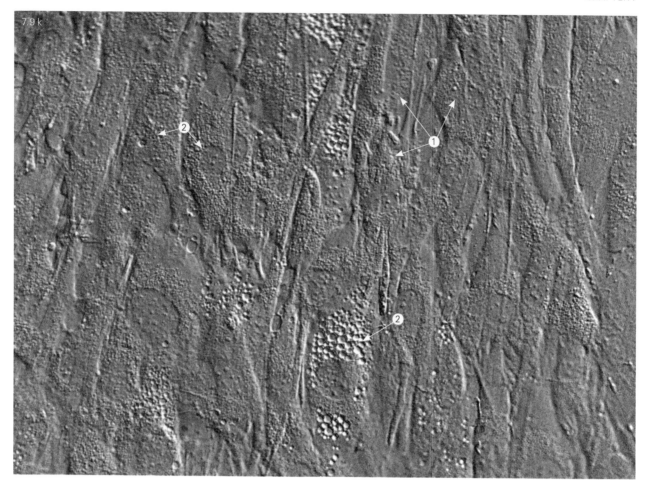

The mechanism of chondrocyte cell division is similar to that of fibroblasts (*Fig. 7.9 g*) (see section 2.2.1). The proliferation stage is accompanied by an increase in the number of cells and a corresponding decrease of the free space around them (*Fig. 7.9 h, i*). Cells affect each other mechanically and, thus, influence and change their own shape. However, the representation of the two main and the intermediate types described above, is preserved. The formation of a confluent monolayer, where the cells are adjacent to each other along nearly their entire lateral surfaces (*Fig. 7.9 j*), marks the termination of the proliferation stage. At this point, there is almost no free space left around the cells. A large part of the cells acquire intermediate shapes, which are slightly elongated. Their division ceases or slows down abruptly. Numerous vacuoles appear in the cytoplasm of some of the chondrocytes in the case of longer periods in a confluent monolayer (*Fig. 7.9 k, 7.10*). These vacuoles represent the dilated cisternae of endoplasmic reticulum with contents of moderate electron density (*Fig. 7.11*). Clearly, such chondrocytes have initiated the active synthesis of, probably, proteoglycans. This is indicated by the increase of hexuronic acids in the culture medium surrounding the cells.

There is an alternative method for isolating chondrocytes, in which mechanically ground cartilage biopsies are introduced into flasks, containing the culture medium. After about 10 days, the cells begin to migrate out of the cartilage pieces, attach, spread, and then proliferate in a monolayer, as already described above (*Fig. 7.12*).

The growth and multiplication of chondrocytes, and of other cells of the connective tissue differon, is possible not only on glass or plastic culture flasks. A collagen matrix, a specially demineralized bone matrix, containing a large amount of growth factors, is also favorable material for these cells. Currently in the field of tissue damage, this matrix is often used as a carrier (substrate) for transplanted CT cells to optimize the healing of injured tissues (*Fig. 7.13*).

The described staging of the life activities of chondrocytes in the monolayer culture is indicative of their entry in the cell cycle. This is accompanied by a gradual change in the morphological and molecular-biological characteristics of chondrocytes. This new state, acquired in cell culture, is termed dedifferentiation. Chondrocytes lose their round shape and acquire a flat, fibroblast-like appearance upon entry in the cell cycle *in vitro*.

The removal of chondrocytes from their natural (three-dimensional) environment triggers their dedifferentiation. This occurs due to loss of contact with the EM components, an increase in partial oxygen pressure, loss of mechanical stimuli and the ligands of surface receptors (Schlegel et al., 2006). Cultured chondrocytes continue to produce type II collagen for one week. The expression profile changes after one week. The synthesis of the car-

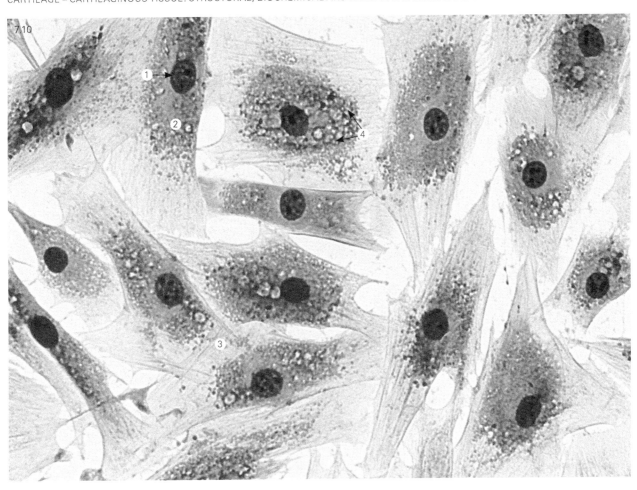

Fig. 7.10.
The confluent monolayer
stage of chondrocytes.
II phase.
Nucleus (1).
Endoplasm (2).
Ectoplasm (3).
Vacuoles (4).
LM-micrograph.
A light optic microscope
Ni Nikon (Japan).
Azur-eosin staining,
x 400.

tilage-specific type II collagen declines significantly, and the synthesis of type I collagen, not specific for cartilage, commences. The synthesis of type I collagen begins early in the dedifferentiation process, albeit at low concentrations. The regulation of the type I collagen synthesis occurs after three weeks of *in vitro* culture. At this very time, the synthesis of type II collagen nearly ceases. Nevertheless, production of type II collagen continues, albeit at a very low level. The collagen ratio for type I can be characteristic of dedifferentiated chondrocytes, and is maintained throughout the cultivation period in a monolayer. Later, the synthesis of other cartilage-specific proteins, such as aggrecan and type IX collagen, is also significantly reduced (Takahashi et al., 2007).

The proliferation of cartilage cells contributes to dedifferentiation. It has been shown that, during the repro-

duction of human chondrocytes, the degree of dedifferentiation correlates with the number of cell divisions, or passages. Thus, when investigating the possibility of the myogenic differentiation of chondrocytes, such did not occur when using early passage cells, whereas muscle-fiber derivatives were obtained using chondrocytes from later passages. This confirms that the multiplication of adult articular chondrocytes in vitro leads to a population of cells with progenitor properties (Dell Accio et al., 2003).

Redifferentiation of chondrocytes.

Chondrocytes can redifferentiate in monolayer cultures. The three-dimensional environment and suitable culture medium conditions are the main factors stimulating this process. The ability to redifferentiate is directly related to the number of cell divisions.

Three-dimensional structures appear to be one of the most important conditions for returning dedifferentiated chondrocytes to a phenotype, which most closely resembles the original chondrocyte phenotype. Some redifferentiation-supporting substrates have been developed.

One approach to get dedifferentiated chondrocytes to re-express the differentiated phenotype is by suspending culture in firm 0.5% agarose gels. In a three-dimensional agarose culture without attachment to the bottom of a flask, approximately 80% of the cells survive the transition

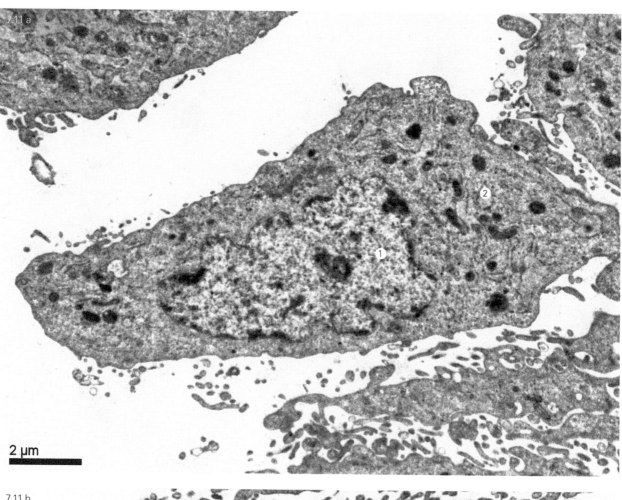

7.11 a

2 µm

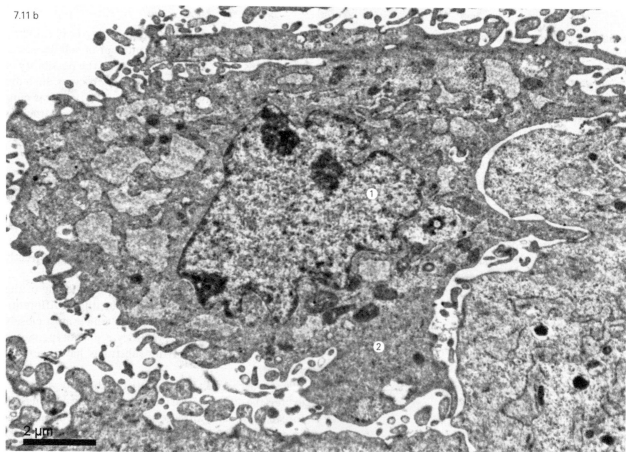

7.11 b

2 µm

from the flattened morphology of a spread-cell culture to the spherical shape of a monolayer culture, and then deposit a characteristic proteoglycan matrix. The ratio of proteoglycan and collagen synthesis reflects that of primary chondrocytes (Benya & Shaffer, 1982).

Another approach for the redifferentiation of dedifferentiated chondrocytes is through the use of alginate cultures. For this purpose, cells from a monolayer culture are transferred to a calcium chloride-containing gelatin solution, which forms three-dimensional beads.

This chondrocyte culture system allows the long-term maintenance of chondrocyte-specific phenotype (up to 180 days). Old chondrocyte cultures form structures resembling mature articular cartilage in morphology, ultrastructure, biosynthesis and genes expression (Yoon et al., 2002; Bonaventure et al., 1994; Reginato et al., 1994).

Growing chondrocyte cultures can be seeded in three-dimensional biological matrices, which create an environment similar to that of the cartilage extracellular matrix (Brodkin et al., 2004). The most common and promising biomaterials are composites of collagen biopolymer and hyaluronan derivatives. Studies show that chondrocytes exhibit variable growth and differentiation in different matrices (Marcacci et al., 2003; Cherubino et al., 2003; Chaipinyo et al., 2004). These differences can be monitored by using molecular biology techniques, such as PCR, Northern blotting, RT–PCR, or in situ hybridization.

7.2.1.1.2. Biochemical and molecular biological characteristics of chondroblast and chondrocyte

Given that there is just one cellular differon in cartilage tissue – the chondroblast/chondrocyte differon, only the cells from this differon (it actually comes down to two consecutive stages of differentiation of a single cell) carry out all biosynthetic and secretion processes of all structural components of the cartilage extracellular matrix. Therefore, the definition of chondroblasts/chondrocytes as "cartilage architects" is fully justified (Muir, 1995).

The formation of cartilage tissue occurs mainly during embryogenesis and terminates at a very young age. This means that the cartilage differon cells perform their basic function – extracellular matrix production – at the chondroblastic stage of differentiation. The rate of anabolic (biosynthetic) processes declines sharply in the cartilage of adult organisms, and the main function of the

cells' transitioning from chondroblasts to chondrocytes comes down to maintaining the matrix in a state of metabolic balance, ensuring its structural stability. Expression of type II collagen and the large aggregating proteoglycan, aggrecan, represent common and mandatory phenotypic markers of the chondroblasts/chondrocytes of all types of cartilage tissue. The pluripotent mesenchymal progenitor cell becomes (and is considered) a chondroblast from the onset of expression of both of these biopolymers, which, in terms of mass and functional significance, are the main specific components of the cartilage extracellular matrix. The chondroblast becomes a chondrocyte, losing the ability for mitotic division and proliferation, turning into a resident cell, and retaining its secretory phenotype, but with a significant decrease in biosynthetic activity (Archer & Francis-West, 2003).

The use of other expressed proteins as phenotypic markers of chondroblasts/chondrocytes has been proposed, in addition to using type II collagen and aggrecan. First is the minor type IX collagen. Cartilage homeoprotein 1 (**CART1**) (Iioka et al., 2003) and the serine protease inhibitor **Serpin A1**, whose onset of expression is especially closely correlated with the differentiation of the mesenchymal cell into a chondroblast, can also serve as cartilage cell markers (Boeuf et al., 2008). Expression of the gene ARG2, encoding the enzyme arginase II, is specific for the chondrocyte phenotype, too; in the process of chondroblast/ chondrocyte differentiation, expression of this enzyme begins together with the expression of type II collagen (Ko et al., 2006).

In cell cultures, **CEP–68** protein (chondrocyte expressed protein), secreted in the extracellular matrix (Steck et al., 2001), and CRTAC1 (glycosylated cartilage acidic protein 1) (Steck et al., 2007) represent specific markers that allow distinguishing human chondrocytes from mesenchymal progenitor cells.

The recently discovered growth factor **cartducin**, already produced by the chondrocyte differon progenitor cells at a very early stage of embryogenesis, is attracting much interest (Maeda et al., 2006). This signaling molecule contains 246 amino acid residues. It has a multidomain structure (one of the domains contains a collagen amino acid sequence) and is very similar to adiponectin, a hormone synthesized by adipocytes. Neither fibroblasts, nor osteoblasts express cartducin, which makes it a suitable chondrocyte-specific marker. Cartducin secretion is initiated almost simultaneously with the secretion of type II collagen, continues in the postnatal period, and is stimulated by insulin. Cartducin supports the growth of the chondrocyte differon progenitor cells, chondrogenesis and cartilage formation.

The chondroblast/ chondrocyte proteome is not well studied. Only a small part of it has been characterized: 127 proteins, 13 of which function in general and in energy metabolism processes; 5 – in protein biosynthesis; 26 – in protein processing, transport and degradation; 14 – as parts of the cytoskeleton and other cellular

Fig. 7.11.

Chondrocytes in a confluent monolayer.
a – I phase.
Nucleus (1).
Cytoplasm (2).
b – II phase.
Nucleus (1).
Cytoplasm (2).

Vacuoles – dilated cisternae of endoplasmic reticulum (3).
Cell processes (4).
TEM-micrograph.
Contrasting of ultrathin sections with uranyl acetate and lead citrate.
a, b – x 5,000.

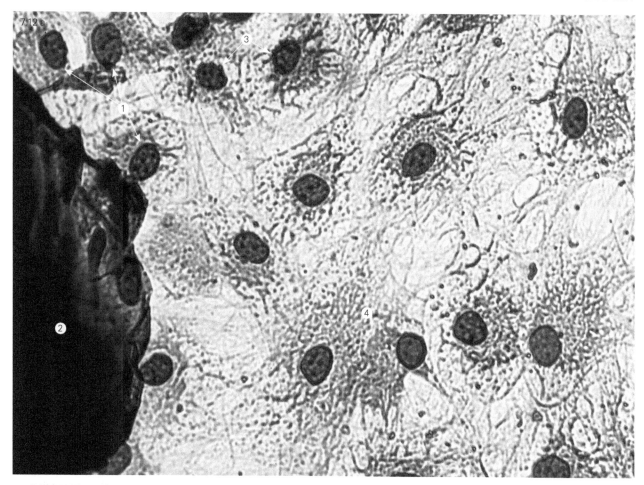

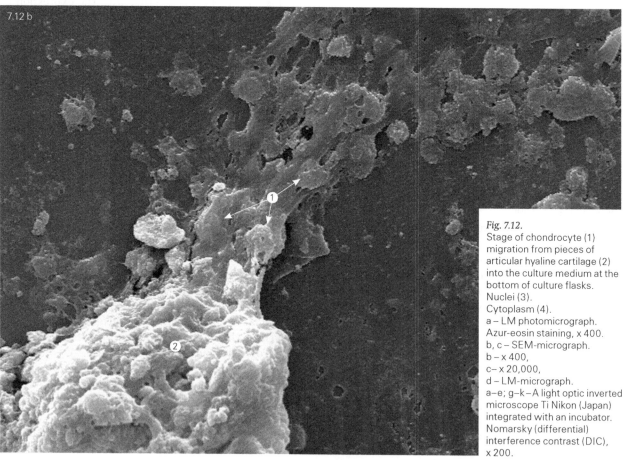

Fig. 7.12.
Stage of chondrocyte (1) migration from pieces of articular hyaline cartilage (2) into the culture medium at the bottom of culture flasks.
Nuclei (3).
Cytoplasm (4).
a – LM photomicrograph. Azur-eosin staining, x 400.
b, c – SEM-micrograph.
b – x 400,
c – x 20,000,
d – LM-micrograph.
a–e; g–k – A light optic inverted microscope Ti Nikon (Japan) integrated with an incubator. Nomarsky (differential) interference contrast (DIC), x 200.

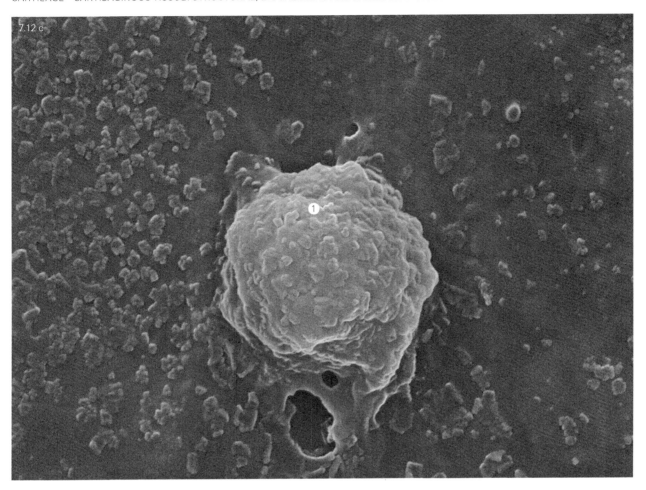

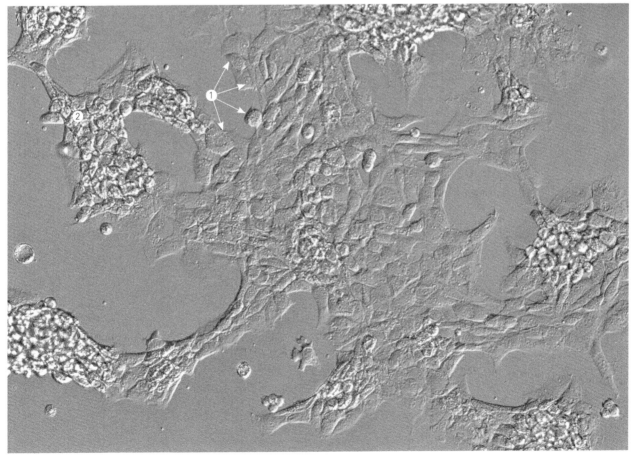

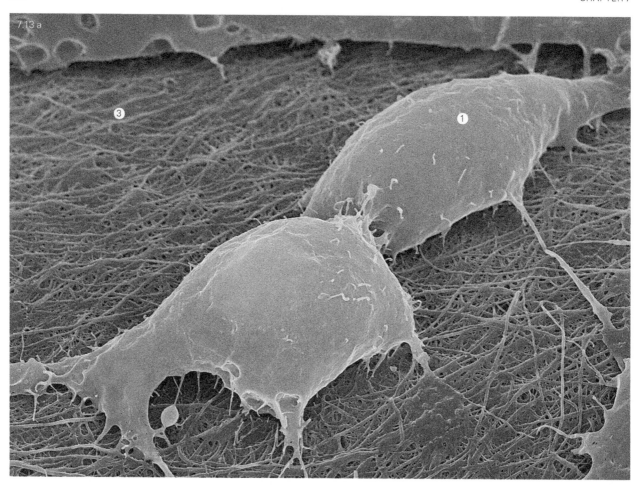

7.13 a

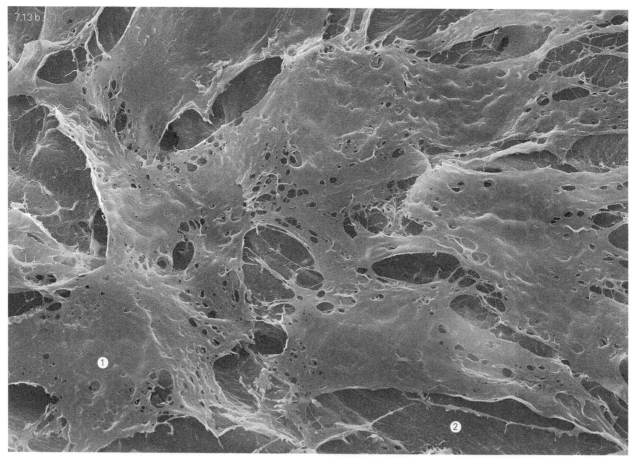

7.13 b

structures; 7–as cell defense factors; 15–in signaling pathways. 16 partially processed proteins of the extracellular matrix, 7 complement system factors, 22 blood plasma proteins (also present in synovial fluid), and 2 intracellular proteins with an unknown function (Vincourt et al., 2006) have also been isolated. The proteomes of normal chondrocytes and of mesenchymal progenitor cells show some quantitative differences: the content of proteins, such as annexin, vimentin, transgelin, destrin, cathepsin D, Hsp47, and mitochondrial superoxide dismutase is higher in chondrocyte cultures (Ruiz-Romero et al., 2005).

Two molecular biology methodologies have significantly added to the phenotypic characterization of chondroblasts/chondrocytes. The first one involves investigations of "DNA libraries"–a term for collections of genomic DNA fragments from cells or tissues, or of complementary DNA fragments obtained with the use of RNA-dependent DNA polymerase. These collections reflect the composition of the entire genome or a substantial part of it. One study used this methodology to analyze more than 13,000 cDNA fragments, derived from the cartilage tissue of human embryos, and identified 2,448 individual genes. Genes encoding proteins of the extracellular matrix quantitatively prevail among them; these are, in first place, genes for collagenous proteins, and, in second place, proteoglycan genes (aggrecan, decorin, glypican) (Zhang et al., 2003).

The second methodology involves determining the expression levels of individual genes from the transcription of messenger RNA (mRNA) and with the help of complementary DNA microarrays. The generation of such microarrays was made possible through the use of "DNA libraries".

This methodology also showed that the most highly expressed gene in cartilage tissue chondroblasts from an 18–20-week-old human embryo was, as expected, the gene COL2A1, encoding the polypeptide α-chain of type II collagen. Furthermore, 27 genes were found, which were previously known to give rise to skeletal deformities when mutated (Pogue et al., 2004). A similar study of human fetal articular cartilage identified 161 genes, whose expression levels were at least five times higher than their expression levels in all other tissues (a total of 34 tissues were analyzed). They were designated cartilage-selective genes and, undoubtedly, are important for defining the phenotypic characteristics of the cartilage tissue. A number of novel genes with unknown functions were found among these genes (Funari et al., 2007).

One of the phenotypic features of chondroblasts/ chondrocytes is the expression of proteoglycans containing sulfated glycosaminoglycans, primarily aggrecan, which is very rich in chondroitin sulfates and keratan sulfate. Intake of sulfate ions in the cell is required for this biosynthesis, and is mediated by three transmembrane proteins–anion transporters SLC4a2, SLC26a2 and SLC26a6 (Meredith et al., 2007), whose massive presence is a feature of the chondroblastic phenotype.

As the only cell type in cartilage tissue, the chondroblast/ chondrocyte phenotype includes pronounced biosynthetic activity, particularly significant at the chondroblastic differentiation stage. In this regard, chondroblasts resemble their prototypes–the fibroblasts, which build the extracellular matrix of soft types of connective tissue. This resemblance is manifested in the extensive development of intracellular systems for biosynthesis, transport and protein secretion in both cell types.

However, similar to fibroblasts, chondroblasts/ chondrocytes also demonstrate catabolic activity. They express all proteolytic enzymes functioning in the extracellular matrix (see section 3.7), in particular, metalloproteases that carry out the catabolism of collagens (Olsen et al., 2007) and proteoglycans (ADAMTS enzymes). The expression of catabolic enzymes by chondroblasts/chondrocytes is a cell function that is at least as important as the expression of the structural macromolecules of the matrix.

The cytoskeleton is of great importance for the formation and subsequent maintenance of the chondroblast/ chondrocyte phenotype. The chondroblast/chondrocyte cytoskeleton is built on the same principles, and consists of the same structural elements, as in other cell types, including fibroblasts: actin microfilaments, intermediate microfilaments, and microtubules. The cytoskeleton's particular importance for chondroblasts/chondrocytes is determined by the fact that these cells exist under conditions of constant hydrostatic compression due to the physical and mechanical properties of cartilage. In the absence of a certain degree of robustness of the cells, provided by the cytoskeleton, this would lead to their flattening. It has been established that changes in the chondroblast/chondrocyte shape due to cytoskeletonl defects lead to alterations of metabolic phenotype of cells (Vinall & Reddi, 2001).

Mutations that eliminate the expression of the Flnb gene, encoding the cytoplasmic protein **filamin B**, cause serious disruptions in chondrogenesis and skeletogenesis. These disruptions are associated with phenotypic changes in chondroblasts, namely, the disorganization of their actin cytoskeleton. This is because filamin B, which is not a structural component of the cytoskeleton, regulates the cross-linking of one of the main cytoskeleton components–the actin microfilaments–as well as the linking of the cytoskeleton to the cytoplasmic (cell) membrane, and the establishment of intracellular sign-

Fig. 7.13. Chondrocytes (1) of articular hyaline cartilage, grown in culture conditions: a – on a demineralized (collagen) bone matrix (2); b – on a collagen matrix, specially prepared from horse tendon (3). SEM-micrograph. a, b – x 4,000.

aling pathways (Lu et al., 2007). Disorganization of the intermediate filament vimentin cytoskeleton similarly leads to a serious disruption of the chondroblastic/chondrocytic phenotype (Blain et al., 2006).

Another phenotypic characteristic of chondroblasts/ chondrocytes is a unique set of transmembrane receptors, which provide two-way functional interactions between cells and the extracellular matrix.

The phenotypic features common to all chondroblasts/ chondrocytes are combined with the specific characteristics of chondrocytes from different types of cartilage (hyaline, fibrous, elastic) and their variants. Phenotypic features characteristic for the cells in the hyaline articular cartilage of different joints have been recognized. These characteristics are manifested *ex vivo*: human knee joint chondrocytes are less responsive to catabolic stimuli, and more sensitive to anabolic stimuli, compared with ankle joint chondrocytes (Eger et al., 2002). Chondrocytes isolated from different zones of the same articular cartilage also behave differently *ex vivo*: deep zone chondrocytes produce significantly more collagen and, in particular, proteoglycans (Hu & Athanasiou, 2006).

The phenotype of permanent chondrocytes acquired in the process of the differentiation of mesenchymal progenitor cells (see section 10.2), specifically in articular cartilage and nasal septal cartilage, is remarkably unstable compared to the phenotype of other connective tissue cells. This instability is preserved after chondrocytes reach full maturity (the unique dynamics of phenotypic changes in transient cartilage chondrocytes will be discussed in section 10.3.1.1).

The phenotypic instability is revealed when comparing chondrocyte gene expression *in vivo* and *in vitro*, showing the role that extracellular environmental signals play in the maintenance of a cell's phenotype. The transfer of chondrocytes from their natural environment into cell culture always results in similar changes in the expression of entire clusters of genes: the expression of several genes (matrix metalloproteases MMP-2 and MMP-13, bone morphogenetic protein BMP-2A, leukemia inhibitory factor LIF, etc.) increases, whereas the expression of other genes is suppressed (bone morphogenetic protein BMP-3B, some kinases, some transcription factors, ligands and receptors) (Zien et al., 2007).

The phenotypic instability of chondrocytes is manifested in their requirements for particular culture conditions *in vitro*. One prerequisite is a three-dimensional microenvironment. Pronounced phenotypic changes develop in monolayer (flat) cell cultures, which can be regarded as dedifferentiation. The cells' shape changes (from round to flattened) and their proliferative ability, which is lost during the differentiation of chondroblasts into chondrocytes, is restored. However, dedifferentiation does not cease upon returning from a chondrocyte to a chondroblast phenotype. Substantial changes in gene expression, with a defining impact on the chondrocyte phenotype, take place: aggrecan expression ceases,

and a switch in collagen expression, from cartilage-specific type II collagen to the fibroblast type I collagen, occurs. The expression of other genes active in chondroblasts/ chondrocytes is lost too and, conversely, the expression of genes that are active in fibroblasts and pluripotent mesenchymal progenitors of cartilage differon cells begins (Takahashi et al., 2007).

The small type IX collagen and the cartilage oligomeric matrix protein (COMP) (see section 7.2.1.2.4), whose expression ceases earlier (Zaucke et al., 2001), are even more sensitive markers of chondrocyte dedifferentiation than type II collagen and aggrecan. On the other hand, in the late stages of dedifferentiation, the expression of types III and IV collagen, which is normally absent in chondrocytes, is activated along with the expression of type I collagen, and the expression of the collagen-bound small proteoglycans–bi-glycan, fibromodulin and lumican–increases (Goessler et al., 2004). The expression of growth factors and cytokines also changes; for example, expression of the connective tissue growth factor (CTGF) increases. Overall, the expression levels of 62 genes have been found to change (in either direction) during the dedifferentiation of chondrocytes (Stokes et al., 2002). Among these changes, the decreased expression of the gene encoding the hypoxia-inducible transcription factor **HIF-1**α (hypoxia-induced factor 1α), essential for the metabolic homeostasis of chondrocytes in articular cartilage under conditions of anaerobiosis (hypoxia), which is physiologically relevant for this tissue, is of particular interest. It is probable that the transition from anaerobic to aerobic (in monolayer culture) type of metabolism itself is one of the basic mechanisms of chondrocyte dedifferentiation.

After a 10-day period in a monolayer culture, the dedifferentiation of chondrocytes from adult human articular cartilage is so advanced that they reacquire the phenotypic plasticity (i.e. the ability for de novo differentiation in different directions) characteristic of their predecessors, the pluripotent mesenchymal cells. When cultures are supplemented with certain growth factors, some clones of former chondrocytes can give rise to an osteogenic or adipogenic differon (Barbero et al., 2003).

However, the phenomenon of cell dedifferentiation is reversible, and most of these clones are capable, under certain conditions, to restore–to a greater or lesser extent–the chondrocytic phenotype. A major condition for redifferentiation is lowered ambient partial oxygen pressure, which is achieved experimentally by transferring the chondrocytes from monolayer to suspension culture (Malta et al., 2004). Here, the influence of local regulatory factors plays an important role: CTGF expression, elevated during dedifferentiation, is downregulated, and the expression of the cytokine IL-6 and factors involved in IL-6 signal transduction is upregulated (Haudenschild et al., 2001). The stimulating effect of bone morphogenetic proteins, especially BMP-7, on redifferentiation is also very significant. The main indication of chondrocyte redifferentiation is the resumption in the expression of genes regulating the early stages of chondroblastic differentiation (see stction 10.2.2) (Tallheden et al., 2004) and the biosynthesis of specific components of the cartilage extracellular matrix. However, the altered shape of chondrocytes, and the dedifferentiation-induced expression of macromolecules uncharacteristic of chondrocytes, namely, type I collagen, can both be partially preserved.

The impaired deacetylation of histones (nuclear proteins that bind DNA and affect the transcription process) is one of the important molecular mechanisms of chondrocyte dedifferentiation. Decreased activity of the enzyme histone deacetylase leads to inhibiting type II collagen expression. Expression of the morphogen Wnt-5a, which inhibits chondrogenesis, is simultaneously activated (Huh et al., 2007).

The phenomena of chondrocyte dedifferentiation and redifferentiation are observed not only under experimental conditions, but also during the development of pathological processes affecting cartilage tissue, in particular, osteoarthritis.

7.2.1.2. Extracellular matrix

7.2.1.2.1. Fibrillar components of cartilaginous tissue

7.2.1.2.1.1. Biochemical characteristics

Type II collagen predominates among the collagen proteins of cartilage tissue. In human articular cartilage, its mass represents 75% and over 90% of the total mass of collagens in embryos and adults, respectively, and about 50% of the mass of all cartilage proteins. Type II collagen is considered specific to cartilage tissue. Its expression is one of the most important phenotypic characteristics of chondrocytes. The appearance of type II collagen at the embryonic stage coincides" with the beginning of chondrogenesis. This same collagen appears in all cases of ectopic chondroid metaplasia.

Type II collagen expression was recently detected in rat ovarian tissue (Saha et al., 2007). This minor exception does not significantly diminish the value of type II collagen as a specific marker of cartilage tissue.

Type II collagen, a "large" fibrillar collagen is classified as a structural (interstitial) collagen, together with types I and III collagen. These three collagens are called "classical" (Kühn, 1987) because, following the completion of their intracellular and extracellular processing, they comprise a single continuous triple helical ("collagen") domain covering more than 97% of the macromolecule. The primary structure (amino acid sequence) of this domain contains all the necessary information for the assembly of the cross-striated collagen fibrils typical for fibrillar collagens.

The macromolecular structure of type II collagen is very similar to that of the other two large collagens, especially type I collagen. The "classical" collagens are grouped together primarily on the basis of the pronounced homology of the primary structure of their polypeptide α-chains. The degree of homology between the α-chains of types II and I collagen has been determined to be around 80% (Mayne & Mark, 1983). This results in similarly looking electron microscopic images of the cross-striated native fibrils and the SLS macromolecular aggregates of both collagens.

Nevertheless, the existing differences are sufficient to distinguish type II collagen as a specific isoform of collagen. The main difference from type I collagen is that type II collagen is a homotrimer. Its macromolecule is built from three identical polypeptide α-chains; accordingly, its molecular formula is $[\alpha 1(II)]3$.

According to Mayne & Mark, 1983. The number of amino acid residues per 1000 residues is indicated. The abundance of the remaining amino acid residues in all three polypeptide chains is virtually identical.

The most prominent features of the amino acid composition of the a1(II) chain, distinguishing it from the composition of the α1- and α2-chains of type I collagen, are shown in *Table. 7.3.*

The significance of the somewhat higher content of threonine and glutamic acid residues in type II collagen is unknown. The collective content of lysine and hydroxylysine residues in types I and II collagen is the same. However, the number of hydroxylysine residues is about three times higher in the type II collagen (Harst et al., 2004) at the expense of the number of lysine residues; this difference is clearly post-translational in nature. The elevated lysine hydroxylation probably provides the necessary conditions for interactions of collagen fibrils built of type II collagen with proteoglycans of the extracellular matrix. Furthermore, the presence of additional hydroxylysines enables the formation of intramolecular cross-links identified as hydroxylysino-5-oxonorleucine, characteristic of type II collagen.

The high hydroxylysine concentration is accompanied by an increase in glycosylation – an increase in the number of carbohydrates attached to this residue. The number of oligosaccharide groups in the type II collagen macromolecule is higher than in the macromolecules of types I and III collagen. There is a notable inverse correlation between the level of glycosylation and the diameter of collagen fibrils. This suggests that, during the process of fibrillogenesis, the numerous oligosaccharide groups of type II collagen are one of the factors limiting the growth in collagen fibrils' thickness.

The comparison between the structures of types I and II procollagen macromolecules, also reveals their close similarity. The only notable difference is that the N-terminal propeptide in the polypeptide chains of type II procollagen is slightly shorter and contains just one (not two) intrachain disulfide bond.

No matter how small the noted differences between the macromolecular structures of types I and II collagen, it can be assumed that the main information is contained in the primary structure of type II collagen.

Table 7.3

Peculiarities of the amino acid composition of type II collagen (number of amino acid residues per 1000 residues, according to Mayne & Mark, 1983)

Amino acids	α1(I)	α2(I)	α1(II)
Threonine	19	18	26
Glutamic acid	78	65	87
Lysine	30	24	13
Hydroxylysine	5	8	23

It determines the morphological features of cartilage collagen fibrils, in particular, their smaller diameter, branching, individual existence and the reticulate fibrillar structure of the fibrous framework. The role of all other factors that influence cartilage collagen fibrillogenesis (see below) is secondary to this primary information. This hypothesis is supported by the results from experiments with recombinant, i.e. free from any contamination procollagen type II. In vitro fibrillogenesis of this procollagen, which takes place after the cleavage of the amino- and carboxyterminal globular fragments of procollagen, concludes with the formation of the type of fibrils and supramolecular architectonics of the whole collagen network that are characteristic of cartilage tissue (Fertala et al., 1994).

It is namely the primary structure features of the collagen α1(II) polypeptide chain that are probably responsible for the high mechanical stability of type II collagen fibrils despite the fibers' smaller average diameter compared with type I collagen. The total surface of individual (not organized in fibers) fibrils is increased due to their lower thickness, which favors the efficient interaction of collagen fibrils with the glycoconjugates of the interfibrillar substance of the cartilage extracellular matrix. Given the relatively small thickness of the collagen fibrils built of type II collagen, tensile strength is achieved through additional intermolecular cross-links. These additional bonds are presumably formed with the participation of one of the minor (small) cartilage collagens, type IX collagen (see below) (Smith Jr. & Brandt, 1992). The low extractability of type II collagen from tissues is explained by these same additional triple-functional cross-links, which connect two polypeptide α-chains of type II collagen and one α-chain of type IX collagen.

Together with other components of the cartilage extracellular matrix, type II collagen controls and modulates chondrocytes' biosynthetic activity. Depending on the presence or absence of this collagen in the medium, the expression of proteoglycans and glycoproteins, specifically tenascin C, by chondrocytes cultured in vitro changes (Qi & Scully, 2003).

The mechanisms of type II collagen biosynthesis do not differ from those of collagen type I. The similarity of the primary structures of the α-chains of both collagens reflects the similarity of their genes, which consist of several discrete exons, each of which are 54 base pairs long. As a reminder (see section 3.1.1.1), each exon encodes six triplets Gly-Xxx-Yyy.

In humans, there are four known isoforms of type II collagen, encoded by a common gene **COL2A1**, and resulting from alternative splicing, which affects only one exon – exon 2 – of the messenger RNA (mRNA) (McAlinden et al., 2008). Differentiated chondroblasts express only collagen IIB, and this isoform, lacking exon 2, is the only one present in normal cartilage in the postnatal period. During embryogenesis, prechondroblasts express isoform IIA, encoded by a gene with completely preserved exon 2 and isoforms IIC and IID, partially lacking exon 2, which differ only slightly from isoform IIA. In chondroblasts, alternative splicing of the *Col2a1* gene, encoding type II collagen, is regulated by the splicing factor TASR-1, a serine- and arginine-rich phosphoprotein localized in the nucleus. The same factor regulates the alternative splicing of the minor collagen type XI, which plays a structural role in fibers formed by type II collagen (Matsushita et al., 2007).

The transcription factor Sox9A is central in the regulation of type II collagen expression (see section 10.2.2). It turns on the transcription of the *Col2a1* gene, acting on the enhancer element in its promoter. Promoter activity and therefore expression of this gene are also influenced by "zinc finger" transcription factors known as specificity proteins, Sp: Sp1 activates the promoter, while Sp3 suppresses it (Chadjichristos et al., 2003).

Table 7.4
Minor collagens of cartilage tissue

Collagen types, molecular formulas	Characteristics
Type IX, $\alpha1(IX)\alpha2(IX)\alpha3(IX)$	Located on the surface of type II collagen fibrils; promotes the binding of the fibrils to other components of the matrix and to each other; carries a glycosaminoglycan chain.
Type XI, $\alpha1(XI)\alpha2(XI)\alpha3(XI)$ or $\alpha1(XI)\alpha2(XI)\alpha1(II)$	Forms the core of the same fibrils. Regulates the formation and the diameter of the fibrils.
Type V, $[\alpha1(V)]2\alpha(V)$	Sometimes replaces the type XI collagen in cartilage; included in type I collagen fibrils in other tissues. Data on the composition and structure of the third a-chain are contradictory.
Type III, $[\alpha1(III)]_3$	Small amounts are covalently bound to type II collagen.
Type XII, $[\alpha1(XII)]_3$	Very small amounts are present on the surface of type II collagen.
Type XIV, $[\alpha1(XIV)]_3$	Very small amounts are present on the surface of type II collagen.
Type VI, $\alpha1(VI)\alpha2(VI)\alpha3(VI)$	As in other tissues, forms a network of microfibrils. Concentrated mainly in the pericellular areas, provides a connection between the chondrocytes and the matrix.
Type X, $[\alpha1(X)]_3$	Expressed only by hypertrophic chondrocytes in cartilage areas undergoing ossification.
Type XXVII, $[\alpha1(XXVII)]_3$	Expressed in cartilage tissue.

The cartilage extracellular matrix contains other collagens, apart from type II collagen. They are called minor (small) collagens, because their concentration is low in comparison with the concentration of type II collagen (in total, it does not exceed 10% of the overall amount of collagen proteins). A list of these collagens is provided in *Table. 7.4.*

Only two of the minor collagens, types IX and XI, are specific to cartilage (in all its varieties) to the same degree as type II collagen. The rest of the minor collagens are present in other tissues as well.

Type IX collagen accounts for up to 10% and about 1% of the total mass of collagen in embryonic and adult cartilage tissue, respectively. It is a heterotrimer: its macromolecule consists of three α-chains with molecular mass 84, 72 and 66 kDa (Ayad et al., 1989), and a molecular formula of $\alpha1(IX)\alpha2(IX)\alpha3(IX)$. Each chain is built of three typical collagenous (triple helical) and four non-collagenous (globular) domains (Diab, 1993). One of the globular domains has considerable flexibility, which makes it possible to bend the macromolecule.

Experiments with recombinant type IX collagen show that the assembly of heterotrimeric macromolecules is determined by the primary structure of the α-chains and does not require the participation of any additional factors (Pihlajamaa et al., 1999).

In approximately 70% of the molecules, a chondroitin sulfate chain is covalently attached to one of the globular domains of the $\alpha2(IX)$-chain. On this basis, type IX collagen is considered as a facultative proteoglycan.

Type IX collagen belongs to the family of FACIT collagens (see Table 3.1). It does not form separate supramolecular structures, but is associated with heterotypic collagen fibrils, whose main component is type II collagen. The association of type IX and II collagens is quite close – the affinity between them is weakened by certain point mutations (substitutions of single amino acid residues) in type II collagen (Steplewski et al., 2004). The existence of a covalent cross-link between lysine-930 in the helical domain of the $\alpha1(II)$ chain and one of the lysines in the NC1 domain of the $\alpha1(IX)$ chain has been established (Eyre et al., 2004).

The type IX collagen macromolecules are found on the surface of the large collagen fibrils, where they are arranged regularly in accordance with the D-periodic cross-striation of fibrils, and are oriented in an antiparallel fashion relative to the type II collagen molecules. The aminoterminal globular domain NC-4 of collagen IX protrudes above the surface of the fibrils (Bruckner & Rest, 1994).; this, as well as the presence of chondroitin sulfate, makes the surface of the fibers rough, which allows the to more strongly bind to other components of the extracellular matrix.

The surface location of type IX collagen probably contributes to limiting fibril lateral growth. In addition, it helps to improve fibril attachment to the cells: a specific site in the collagenous domain COL3 binds to the $\alpha2\beta1$ subunit of integrin $\alpha2$, an integrin typical of chondrocytes (Käpylä et al., 2004).

Knocking out the type IX collagen gene results in a disruption to the functional integrity of the cartilage matrix.

In particular, the expression of the glycoproteins COMP-3 and matrilin-3 is decreased; the integration of matrilin-3, produced by chondrocytes in cell culture, into the extracellular matrix is also disrupted (Budde et al., 2005). In the absence of type IX collagen, the healing of bone fractures is delayed due to the impaired maturation of the cartilage matrix of the developing bone callus (Opolka et al., 2007).

Type XI collagen, together with type V collagen, which resembles it very strongly in terms of the length of macromolecules, the primary and domain structure of the polypeptide chains, belong to the family of fiber-forming (fibrillar) collagens (Fichard et al., 1995). The heterotrimeric macromolecules of both of these collagens (they are classified as minor or small, because their abundance in tissues is much lower than the content of type I, II and III collagens) are built according to the same plan as macromolecules of the large fibrillar collagens: the majority of the molecule represents a continuous, triple-helical, "collagenous" domain. The molecular formula of collagen type XI is: $[\alpha1(XI)\alpha2(XI)\alpha3(XI)]$, where the polypeptide $\alpha3(XI)$-chain is probably encoded by the same gene COL2A1, as the $\alpha1(II)$-chain, but differs from the latter by the higher degree of glycosylation. *In vitro*, under appropriate conditions, types V and XI collagen macromolecules form typical SLS-aggregates with the same cross-

striation pattern as in the SLS-aggregates of the large collagens (Kadler, 2004).

In contrast to the large fibrillar collagens, the small fibrillar collagens do not form individual fibrils in vivo (or, more precisely, fibrils in which they would serve as the basic building material). The point is that the types V and XI collagens' polypeptide chains retain their aminoterminal propeptides during post-translational processing. These long (about 500 amino acid residues), nonhelical, structurally complex (Fallahi et al., 2005) terminal sections of the macromolecule impose substantial restrictions on the packing of the macromolecules in the fibrils and on their lateral growth. In this respect, the $\alpha1(XI)$-chain is especially important to ensure the optimal and uniform thickness of the fibrils (Fernandez et al., 2007).

Both of these collagens participate, usually in small amounts, in heterotypic collagen fibrils, i.e. made of several types of collagens. Within these fibrils they form a central core covered by a thick layer of the large collagen that defines their common name. Type V collagen participates in fibrils, called fibrils made of type I collagen. Type XI collagen is found predominantly in cartilage (in adults it represents about 3% of the total collagen mass), where it forms the core of collagen fibrils made of type II collagen (Bruckner & Rest, 1994). However, type XI collagen can be involved in the formation of fibrils made of type I collagen, following a slightly different model (Hansen & Bruckner, 2003). Similarly, collagen V (an isoform with a molecular formula $[\alpha1(V)]2\alpha(V)$ sometimes replaces collagen XI in the collagen fibrils of cartilage.

Type XI collagen, similarly to collagen IX, is covalently bound to the large type II collagen. Intermolecular pyridinoline-type covalent bonds are formed during the process of heterotypic fibrils' assembly, in which collagen II becomes involved prior to the aminoterminal propeptide's proteolytic cleavage from its macromolecules (Fernandes et al., 2003). Assembly defects due to mutations in the collagen XI encoding genes are manifested in mice as age-dependent accelerated denaturation of type II collagen within the collagen fibril network of articular cartilage (Rodriguez et al., 2004).

Thus, the collagen fibrils that determine the biomechanical properties of cartilage and can be designated more accurately as fibrils of the II/IX/XI type (Eyre et al., 2006) represent a heterotrimeric structure whose basic material is type II collagen. Participation of the minor collagens – type IX collagen macromolecules on the surface, and type XI macromolecules in the interior of the fibrils (collagen XI sometimes is replaced by collagen V in this location) – is essential for forming and maintaining the optimal properties of this structure. The minor components are covalently bound to type II collagen.

In human adult articular cartilage, type II/IX/XI collagen fibers contain a significant amount (at least 10% by weight) of type III collagen, whose macromolecules are covalently bound to type II collagen. It has been suggested that type III collagen, as an active participant in connective tissue repair reactions, is expressed by chondrocytes in response to microdamage. In addition to type IX collagen, a few easily extractable (without proteolysis) macromolecules of FACIT types XII and XIV collagens are located on the surface of fibrils (Eyre et al., 2006). One more FACIT collagen, type XVI collagen, is bound to very thin, type II and IX collagen-containing fibrils, which are localized inside the chondrons (Kassner et al., 2003). As a general rule reflecting the role of all type II collagen-bound minor collagens, the diameter of cartilage collagen fibrils is inversely proportional to the amount of minor collagens they contain. In other words, the minor collagens are necessary to ensure the optimum diameter of collagen fibrils (Bos et al., 2001).

Besides the network of heterotypic collagen fibrils formed by fibrillar collagens, cartilage contains another network built from type VI collagen microfibrillar aggregates.

The monomeric heterogeneous macromolecule of this collagen is constructed from three different polypeptide chains: two are almost identical–α1(VI) with a mass of 150 kDa, and α2(VI) with a mass of 140 kDa, and the much longer α3(VI) with a mass of 260 kDa.

The macromolecule consists of a short triple-helical domain and two globular terminal domains at both ends. The triple-helical domain contains at least 11 RGD-sequence repeats, giving it pronounced adhesive properties. The primary tetrameric (comprised of 4 molecules) structural units, linked by disulfide bonds, participate in noncovalent interactions and form microfibrils resembling beads on a string. The microfibrils, in turn, form a network that is present in many varieties of connective tissue, including cartilage. The formation of such networks *in vitro* occurs through the interaction of collagen VI with the small proteoglycan–biglycan. In cartilage, the cells of this network have a hexagonal form.

In cartilage tissue, type VI collagen is located almost exclusively inside chondrons, within the pericellular microenvironment of chondrocytes (Horikawa et al., 2004), and not only in the form of microfibrillar network, but also in the form of amorphous deposits. Type VI collagen plays a dual role in maintaining the structural integrity of the chondron. First, it stabilizes the collagen fibrils and proteoglycans in close proximity to the chondron. The connections between type VI collagen microfibrils, heterotypic collagen fibrils and aggrecan macromolecules are stabilized by complexes that consist of the glycoprotein matrilin-1 and small proteoglycans–biglycan or decorin (Wiberg et al., 2003). Second, type VI collagen binds to specialized receptors on the chondrocyte cell membrane, mediating not only the spatial attachment of chondrocytes, but also the transfer of information from the extracellular matrix to the cell nucleus.

Type VI collagen expression during the differentiation of chondroblasts/ chondrocytes coincides temporally with intensive biosynthesis of type II collagen.

Type X collagen is a minor collagen component of temporary cartilage undergoing ossification (see section 10.3.1.4). It is a mandatory participant in the process of mineralization during endochondral bone growth. It also appears in all locations where cartilage tissue is being replaced with bone tissue.

The recently discovered minor fibrillar type XXVII collagen is similar to type X collagen in the timing and location of its expression. Although these two collagens have completely different molecular structures, it can be can assumed that type XXVII collagen is also relevant to transforming cartilage into bone tissue (Hjorten et al., 2007).

The elastic cartilage tissue (auricle, larynx) is rich in elastin. Based on morphological data, of all types of skeletal cartilage, only the hyaline cartilage of nucleus pulposus of the intervertebral discs contains a significant amount of elastic fibers. Elastin is also found in the cartilaginous skeleton in buds of forming chicken limbs, where the elastic fibers form a temporary framework (Hurle et al., 1994). The molecular characteristics of cartilage tissue elastin are not known. There is also no quantitative biochemical data about the abundance of elastin in the elastic type of cartilage.

Chondrocytes are surrounded by fibrillin microfibrils in human adult joint and rib cartilage. They are built of fibrillin-1 and their characteristic feature is lateral cross-links between the macromolecules. The possible functions of these microfibrils are the inhibition of proliferation and differentiation of chondrocytes, and/or regulation of the cell traffic of TGF-b superfamily growth factors (Keene et al., 1997).

7.2.1.2.1.2. Morphological characteristics

The cartilage extracellular matrix represents an integrated complex of fibrous structures surrounded by ground substance (integrating a buffer metabolic medium). In terms of light microscopy, the cartilage EM structure appears homogeneous (*Fig. 7.14*). This is due to the fact that cartilage's fibrous foundation is built from individually (separately) existing collagen fibrils, i.e. but do not form collagen fibers–a more complex level of organization of collagen. Most collagen fibrils are less than 100 nm thick, making it impossible to distinguish them as separate entities under a light microscope. For the same reason, the cartilage intercellular matrix also appears homogeneous in SEM studies at low magnification (up to 1,000).

The outer part of the superficial zone of articular cartilage, directly bordering the joint cavity, is a thin "transparent" membrane called "*Lamina splendens*", which is structurally different from the rest of the cartilage (*Fig. 7.14 a, b*). When studied by SEM and TEM, the transparent membrane has an amorphous, finely granular structure, probably of proteoglycan nature (*Fig. 7.15, 7.16*). Its thickness varies from 4–7 mm. It does not contain any fibrillar elements. Another (inner) portion of the superficial zone of articular cartilage lies under this membrane. It contains collagen fibrils, ranging in size

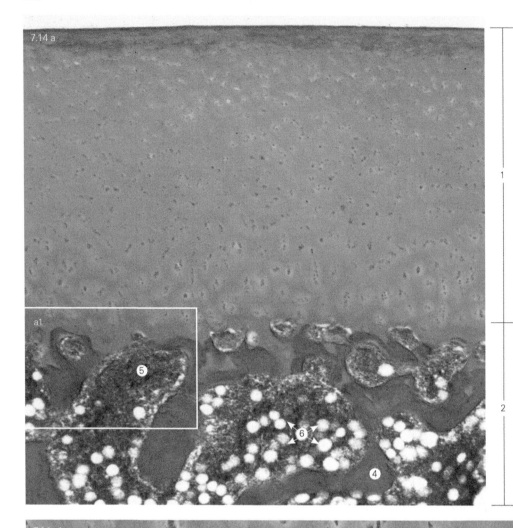

7.14 a

a1

Fig. 7.14 a.
Femoral head fragment.
Age 14 years.
Articular hyaline (non-
mineralized) cartilage (1).
Subchondral bone (2).
Chondrocytes (3).
Bone trabeculae (4).
Red bone marrow (5).
Fat cells (6).
Bone marrow and non-
mineralized cartilage
contact regions (7).
Histological section.
H-E staining.
LM-micrograph.
A light optic microscope
Ni Nikon (Japan).
a – x 32, a1 – x 100.
(see color insert)

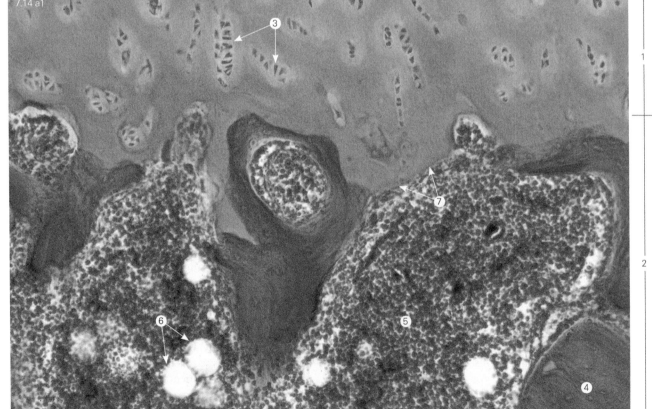

7.14 a1

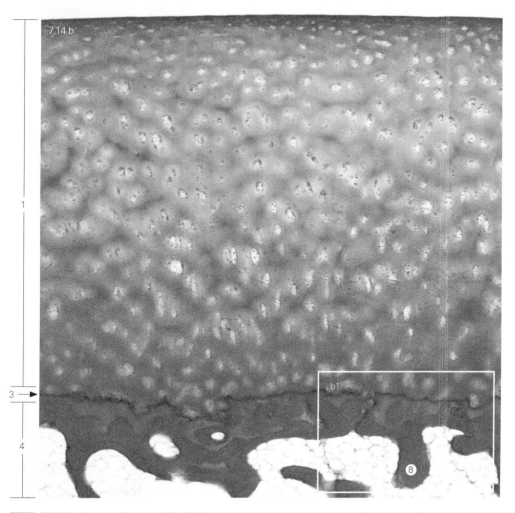

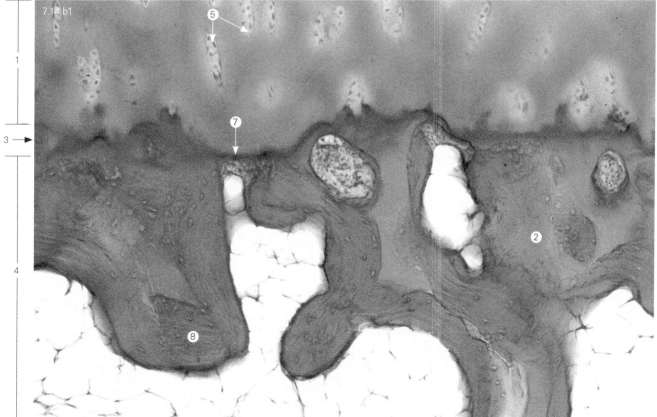

Fig. 7.14 b.
Femoral head fragment.
Age 40 years.
Articular hyaline (non-
mineralized) cartilage (1).
Mineralized cartilage (2).
Tide mark (3).
Subchondral bone (4).
Chondrocytes (5).
Yellow bone marrow (6).
Bone marrow and non-
mineralized cartilage
contact regions (7).
Bone trabeculae (8).
Histological section.
H-E staining.
LM-micrograph.
A light optic microscope
Ni Nikon (Japan).
b – x 32, b1 – x 100.
(see color insert)

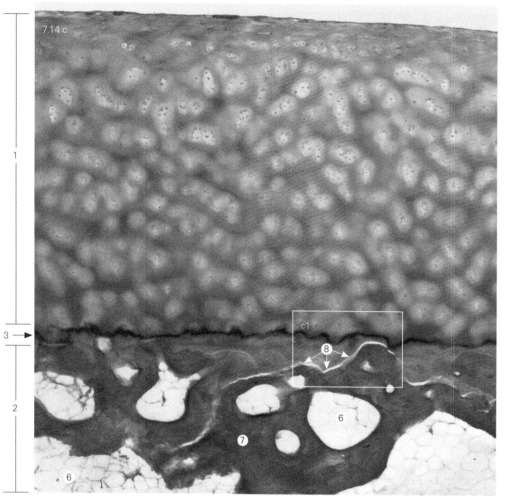

Fig. 7.14 c.
Femoral head fragment.
Age 80 years.
Articular hyaline (non-mineralized) cartilage (1).
Mineralized cartilage (2).
Tide mark (3).
Subchondral bone (4).
Chondrocytes (5).
Yellow bone marrow (6).
Bone trabeculae (7).
Separation of the mineralized cartilage from the subchondral bone (8).
Histological section.
H-E staining.
LM-micrograph.
A light optic microscope
Ni Nikon (Japan).
c – x 32,
c1 – x 250.

Fig. 7.15.
A region from the surface of femoral condylar articular cartilage.
"Transparent" membrane (Lamina splendens) (1).
The cartilage superficial zone without the membrane (2).
SEM-micrograph.
a – x 2,000;
b – x 10,000.
(see color insert)

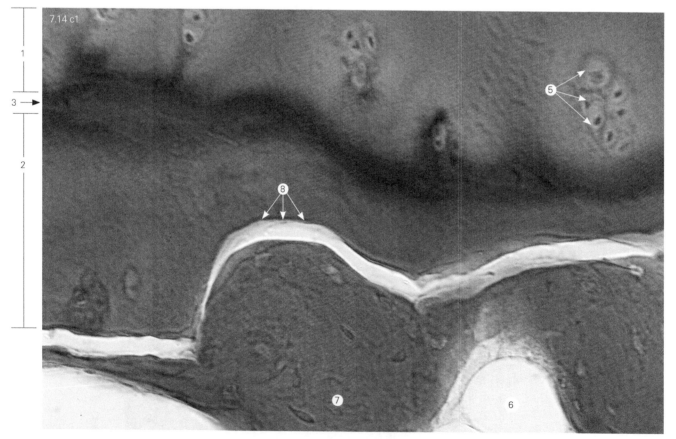

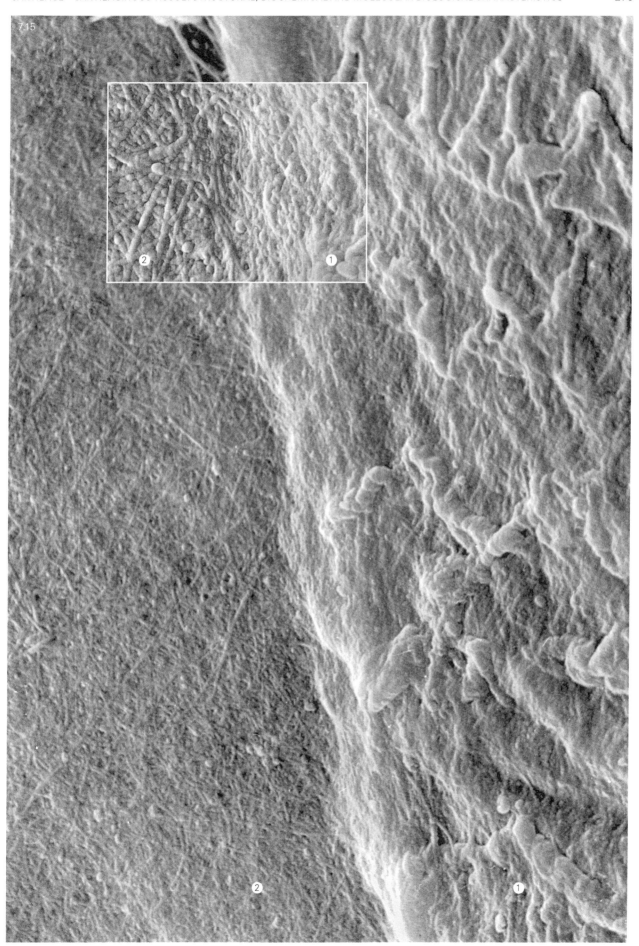

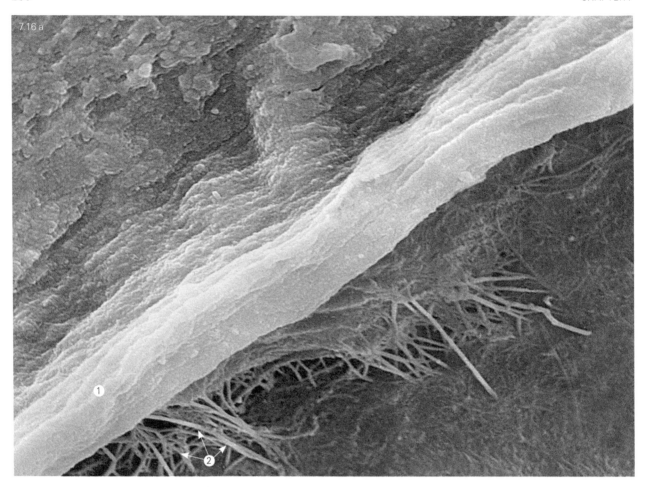

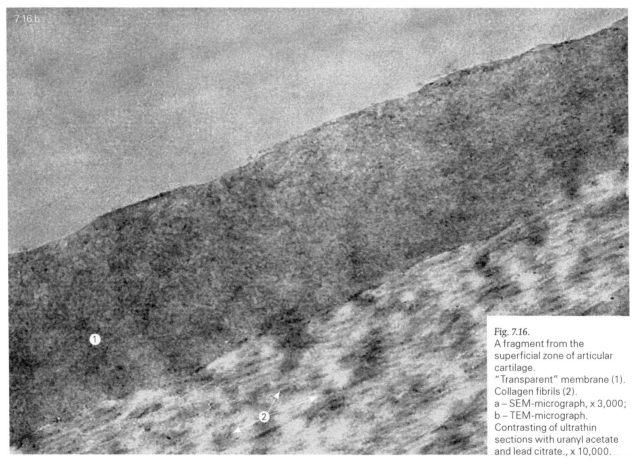

Fig. 7.16.
A fragment from the superficial zone of articular cartilage.
"Transparent" membrane (1).
Collagen fibrils (2).
a – SEM-micrograph, x 3,000;
b – TEM-micrograph.
Contrasting of ultrathin sections with uranyl acetate and lead citrate., x 10,000.

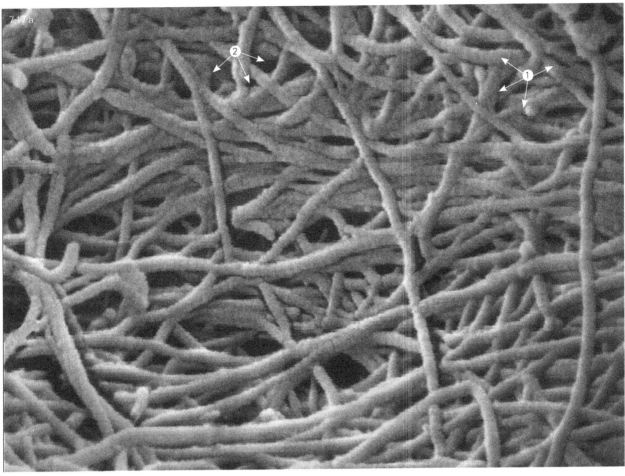

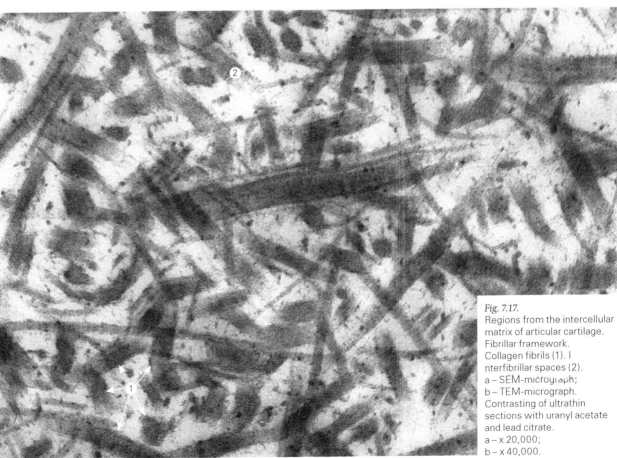

Fig. 7.17.
Regions from the intercellular matrix of articular cartilage. Fibrillar framework. Collagen fibrils (1). Interfibrillar spaces (2).
a – SEM-micrograph;
b – TEM-micrograph.
Contrasting of ultrathin sections with uranyl acetate and lead citrate.
a – x 20,000;
b – x 40,000.

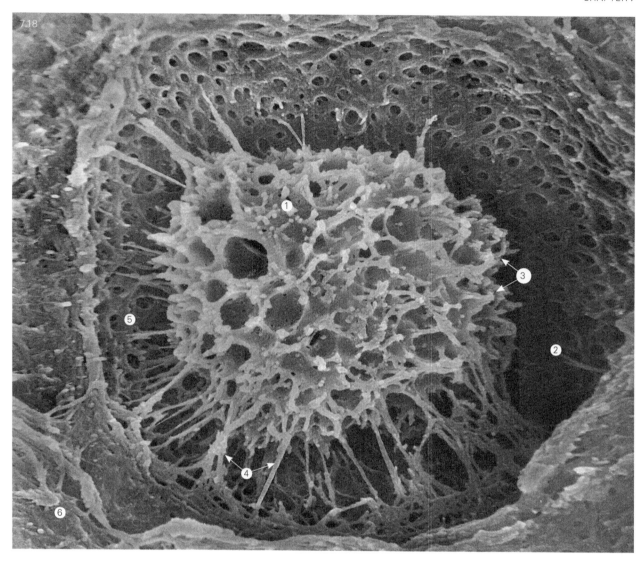

7.18

Fig. 7.18.
Articular cartilage
chondrocyte (1)
of morphotype III i
n a cell lacuna.
Pericellular space (2).
Cellular processes
of the chondrocyte (3).
Collagen fibrils (4)
connecting the
chondrocyte and the
walls of the lacuna (5).
Territorial EM (6).
SEM-micrograph,
x 5,000.

Fig. 7.19.
A fragment of articular cartilage.
Deep zone: non-mineralized (1)
and mineralized (2) cartilage.
Subchondral bone (3).
Fibrillar framework of the
cartilage (4) and of the
subchondral bone (5).
a – SEM-micrograph,
x 10,000.
b – TEM-micrograph.
Contrasting of ultrathin
sections with uranyl acetate
and lead citrate.
x 20,000.

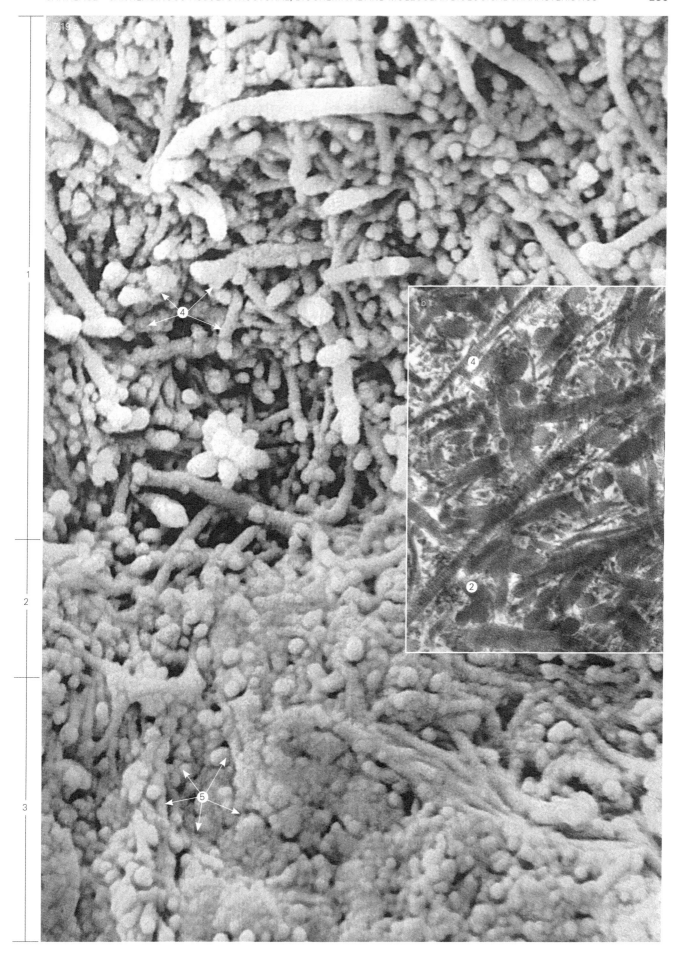

(as equivalent diameter) from 20–40 nm and with a periodicity of 60–70 nm. They are packed quite tightly, and for the most part, are oriented parallel to the articular surface with a 30% anisotropy coefficient (Omelyanenko, 1989; Omelyanenko et al., 1991). At the same time, their orientation within the plane parallel to the articular surface does not reveal any preferred direction, and has a anisotropy coefficient of 3%. Cartilage cells with a predominantly elongated or oval shape, whose long axis is parallel to the articular surface, reside among the fibrillar elements (*Fig. 7.2*). Most of the cells in this zone are arranged individually, whereas a few cells are found in isogenic groups. The abundance of organelles in the cytoplasm of chondrocytes varies considerably. With age, the number of cells in this layer decreases. The cells themselves are subject to degenerative changes. Dense eosinophilic "bodies", which are 10–30 mm long and with an elongated shape, can be found on the cartilage surface. Most often they occur after the age of 70 and therefore, are designated as "ageing bodies".

The superficial zone of articular cartilage forms its surface topography. It has three levels of structural organization: macro-, micro- and ultramicrorelief, generated by tuberosities and folds with sloping edges, and of various thicknesses and length. Folds of the I order have a thickness of 10–15 mm. Their organization does not exhibit a pronounced order. The thickness of folds and tuberosities of the II order is 2–4 mm. A parallel arrangement of the folds is noticeable only in some places. Particles (granules) with a round or oval shape and size of 0.4–0.1 mm are constituents of the transparent membrane of articular cartilage (*Fig. 7.15*), and define the topographic features of the III order (Omelyanenko et al., 2000, 2005).

The middle, most representative zone (70–80% of the overall thickness of cartilage) is dominated by branching fibrils with an equivalent diameter of 80–150 nm (*Fig. 7.17*). The collagen fibrils have a structural periodicity of 60–70 nm and a characteristic pattern of fine cross-striation lines in longitudinal ultrathin sections. The architectonics of this cartilage layer lack a preferred spatial orientation of collagen fibrils, i.e. they form a non-oriented, isotropic structure with an anisotropy coefficient of no more than 3% (*Fig. 7.17*) (Omelyanenko, 1989; Omelyanenko et al., 1991). Small regions of fibrillar structures with a rather high anisotropy coefficient of up to 25–30% are found within this zone. They are located in the area surrounding the cartilage cells (chondrocytes), where the fibrils form the walls of lacunae, or in the interterritorial zone. Despite the permanent presence of individual fragments with oriented structure, they cannot significantly affect the biomechanical properties of cartilage.

Chondrocytes of morphotype III are located in distinctive cavities – cellular lacunae (*Fig. 7.18*). They are distributed fairly evenly in the middle zone. In the outer part of this zone, they are distributed individually or as isogenic groups of two or three cells in coupled or multi-chamber lacunae. In the inner part, most of the isogenic groups are comprised of 2 to 5 cells, also located in lacunae. The cells are rounded, and have small processes or a relatively smooth surface. Pericellular space filled with ground substance is found between the walls of the lacunae and the chondrocytes. It has an ultrastructure comprised of fine granular material of intermediate electron density and thin fibrils with a thickness of 5–10 nm, which probably represent collagen fibrils in the early stages of extracellular aggregation. The walls of the lacunae are formed of tightly intertwined collagen fibrils (20–60 nm thick) arranged in parallel.

Such regions are called pericellular "baskets" or perilacunar zones. The density of fibrils becomes greater with increasing distance from the cell lacunae, but their preferred orientation around the lacunae is preserved. These areas are designated as territorial zones. The rest of the matrix is called interterritorial.

The middle zone transitions without a clear border into the deep zone, which is divided into non-mineralized and mineralized regions (*Fig. 7.19*). The transition from the middle into the deep zone is marked by an increase in the number of thicker collagen fibrils. The collagen fibrils forming the deep zone can be assigned into two groups of fibrils on the basis of prevailing equivalent diameters of 20–40 nm and 150–200 nm. Fibrils over 200 nm are found only in the deep zone and in the transitional zone between the cartilage and the subchondral bone. The cartilage fibrils transition directly into collagen fibrils of the bone trabeculae, where their thickness is 150–200 nm and they are "packed" more tightly than in the cartilage. In the interterritorial matrix, a significant fraction of the fibrils are oriented perpendicular or at a sharp angle to the subchondral bone (Omelyanenko, 2005). Part of the chondrocytes in this zone correspond to middle zone chondrocytes, but there are also chondrocytes of morphotype IV. In histological sections, the mineralized region of the deep zone is separated from the non-mineralized region by a basophilic line (Tide mark), which represents the border of the mineralization front, detectable by light microscopy in sections stained with H-E (*Fig. 7.14 b, c*). This boundary is not identifiable by electron microscopy. However, both cartilage and bone collagen fibrils transitioning into each other without interruption can be detected in the mineralized part of the deep zone. The fibrous framework, comprised of collagen fibrils made of collagen types I and II, is formed in this way. This region can be designated as bone-cartilaginous. Chondrocytes of morphotypes III and IV are also found in the lacunae of this matrix. Given the denser walls of the lacunae and the lack of long processes in the chondrocytes, which are capable of communicating with each other and penetrating into the mineralized bone-cartilage matrix, it must be assumed that the nutrient supply to these chondrocytes is limited, and, last but not least, that the excretion of metabolites outside of the cell lacunae is difficult. Electron-dense pyknotic nuclei, a small number of organelles, and the presence of glycogen and lipid inclusions, as well as osmiophilic particles have been discovered in chondrocytes of this zone. Chondrocytes with vacuolated cytoplasm can be encountered. In the age band over 60 years old, histological studies demonstrated the delamination of the mineralized cartilage (*Fig. 7.14 c*). Obviously, this is related to the degeneration and death of chondrocytes in the mineralized cartilage due to limited nutrition and therefore, loss of physiological regeneration capacity.

Endochondral ossification of the heads and condyles of joint-forming bones occurs from the first years of life. By 14–17 years of age, most of the cartilage of heads or condyles has been replaced by spongy bone substance. Thus, the bone trabeculae and red bone marrow are in direct contact with the remaining peripheral layer of hyaline cartilage, i.e. already articular cartilage (*Fig. 7.14 a*). The formation of the subchondral bone lamella as a border bone structure separating the spongy bone of the epiphysis (head or condyle) from the joint cartilage takes place by 18–20 years of age. Endochondral ossification ends by that time, concluding in cartilage resorption and its replacement by bone substance. The non-mineralized cartilage makes direct contact with the bone marrow in the interstitial space of the subchondral bone through open spaces remaining in the subchondral bone lamella (*Fig. 7.14 b*). These spots look like holes in the subchondral bone lamella. They obviously are involved in nourishing the cartilage and eliminating cellular metabolites. Furthermore, fluid flows through the holes upon compressive loading of the articular cartilage during movement in the joint, thus participating in the amortization func-

tion of cartilage. Observed changes with increasing age include a decrease in the reduction in the average diameter and the total quantity of holes per unit area of the subchondral bone lamella. By the age of 80, only a few holes are found in the entire femoral head (*Fig. 7.14 c*), which can result in the limitation or cessation of the above-mentioned processes.

Thus, the transition from the superficial through the middle and into the deep zone occurs without any sharp boundaries. The orientation, size range, degree of branching, and helicity of collagen fibrils, as well as their packing density, gradually change. The shape of chondrocytes and their lacunae, the number of cells in isogenic groups and their orientation relative to the surface of the articular cartilage change too. There are certain differences in chondrocytes' structure related to their zonal topography.

The integrated continuous structure (*Fig. 7.20*), which possesses intrinsic internal tension, is characteristic of the structural organization of the fibrous (fibrillary) framework of articular cartilage. This state is revealed in injured cartilage. When the superficial zone of articular cartilage is punctured with a needle, the round hole becomes stretched and takes the form of a crack. If the cartilage superficial zone is removed and the needle is stuck in the exposed middle zone, the hole formed after the puncture preserves its round shape. The injury was monitored with the help of ink. The study of the topography of internal tension in the superficial zone of femoral condyles is presented in the diagram (*Fig. 7.21*) (Meachim et al., 1974).

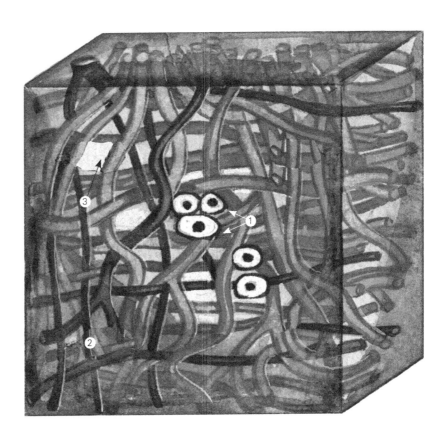

Fig. 7.20.
Diagram of the structural organization of hyaline articular cartilage.
Isogenic groups of chondrocytes (1).
Collagenous, fibrillar, non-oriented, fibrous framework (2).
Ground substance (3).
(According to Omelyanenko, 2005)

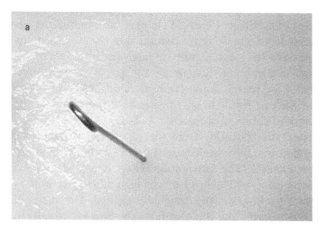

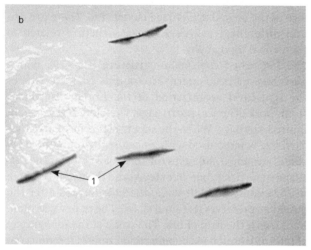

7.2.1.2.2. Structure of articular cartilage minerals

One of the characteristics of articular hyaline cartilage is the mineralization of part of its deep zone, which transitions into the subchondral bone. After removing the organic part of the cartilage and the deeper embedded organic components of the subchondral bone, the surface of the remaining cartilage mineral layer has a distinct multi-level relief, generated by: dips and tuberosities of various sizes; and holes or channels opening in the subchondral bone (Fig. 7.22 a). The surface of the mineral layer is mainly composed of round structures (microspherolytes) about 1 μm (0.5–2.0 μm) (7.22 b) in diameter. They form complexes separated by gaps (Fig. 7.23). The structure of microspherolytes is revealed by high resolution (magnification) SEM. They are built of nanocrystals with

a lamellar shape (Fig. 7.24). In whole (native) cartilage, the microspherolytes are connected to the collagen fibrils. However, the fibrils surrounding the microspherolytes are not mineralized (Fig. 7.25). These nanocrystalline plates are slightly curved and resemble the petals of mineral ("stone") flowers. Lamellar, or petalled, microspherolytes differ not only in size, but also in their internal structure. The small microspherolytes (about 0.5 μm) are built only of nanocrystalline plates, which are arranged inside them without a defined preferred orientation (Fig. 7.24; 7.25). In larger microspherolytes, the central part is represented by a denser mineral core ("nucleus", which lacks a defined structure (Fig. 7.25). Nanocrystalline plates pull out from the core. The thickness of the plates varies from 5 to 10 nm. The edges of the plates have "scalloped" or jagged contours. There are openings in the plates. The surface of the plates is textured, i.e. they are built of fine particles – granules (Fig. 7.24; 7.25). Obviously, the granules sized from 3–10 nm, as determined by both SEM and TEM, represent the primary nanocrystalline structures of calcium phosphate.

The structure of the mineral crystal aggregates changes with decreasing distance from the subchondral bone. The number of microspherolytes drops, and the lamellar nanocrystals are organized into more extensive aggregates ("fields"). Even closer, and transitioning into the subchondral bone lamella, the mineral aggregates comprise clusters of granular nanoparticles in the form of flattened, oval, elongated structures. There are fibrous mineral aggregates, which, obviously, represent the mineral matrices of collagen fibrils.

The above-mentioned aggregates proceed directly into the mineral framework of the subchondral bone. It consists of dense clusters of granular nanocrystals interspersed with mineral matrices of collagen fibrils arranged in bundles, and more rarely, arranged individually. This matches the structural organization of the fibrous framework of the subchondral bone: lamellae and trabeculae (Fig. 7.26).

It should be noted that cartilage mineralization does not have the same density as bones. The packing density of nanocrystals, microspherolytes and their aggregates in mineralized cartilage gradually increases from the non-mineralized cartilage towards the subchondral bone. The mineral matrices of individual collagen fibrils are found close to the subchondral bone, and possibly belong to bone collagen fibrils that turn (without interruption) into cartilage collagen fibrils.

Fig. 7.21.
Fragments of femoral condyles.
a – the surface of articular cartilage.
The needle is inserted in the cartilage.
b – cracks in the superficial zone of articular cartilage (1), formed after its piercing with a needle (marked with ink).

Fig. 7.22.
A fragment from the surface of sheep femoral condyle after removing the articular cartilage and the organic part of the subchondral bone with sodium hypochlorite (deorganification). Channels (holes) (1) connecting the interstitial space of the subchondral bone with the non-mineralized articular cartilage (removed in this preparation). Mineral matrix of mineralized cartilage. Mineral microspherolytes (2) and their complexes with the mineral matrix of mineralized cartilage.
SEM-micrograph.
a – x 800;
b – x10,000.

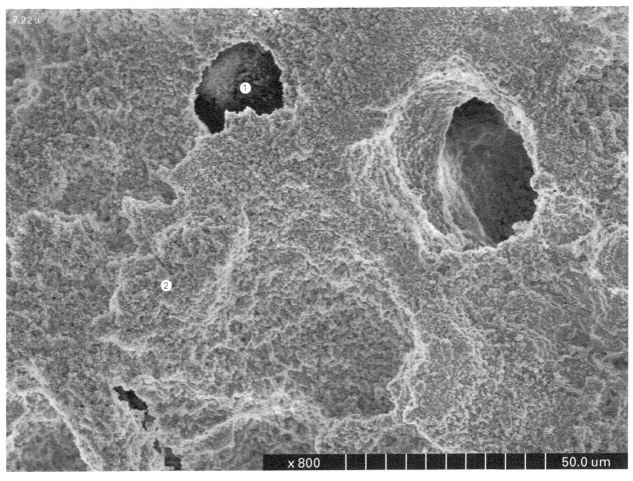

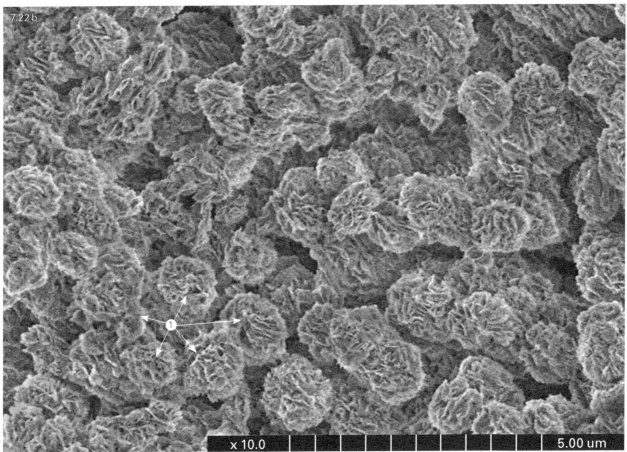

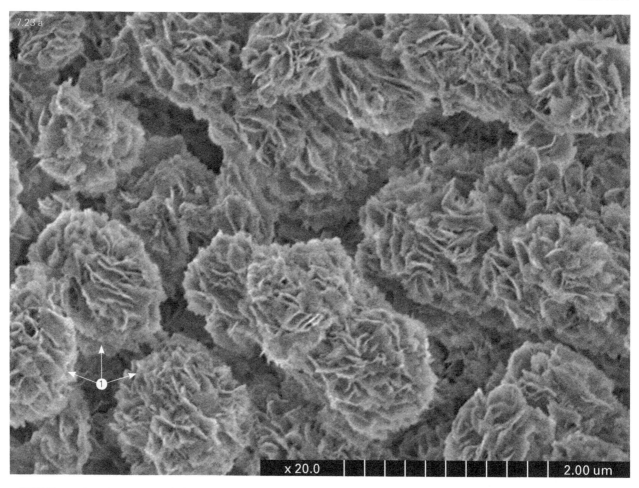

7.23 a

x 20.0   2.00 um

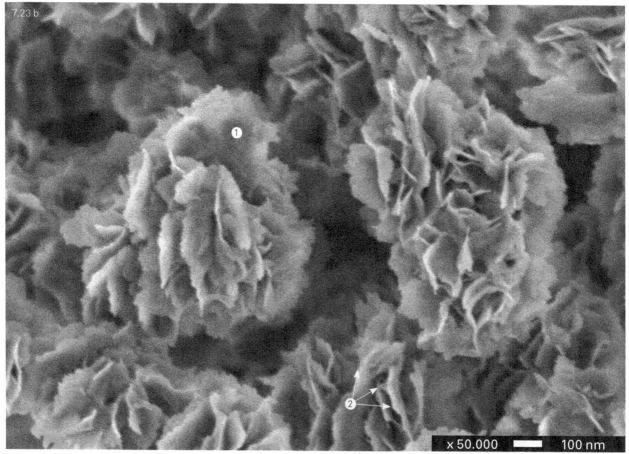

7.23 b

x 50.000   100 nm

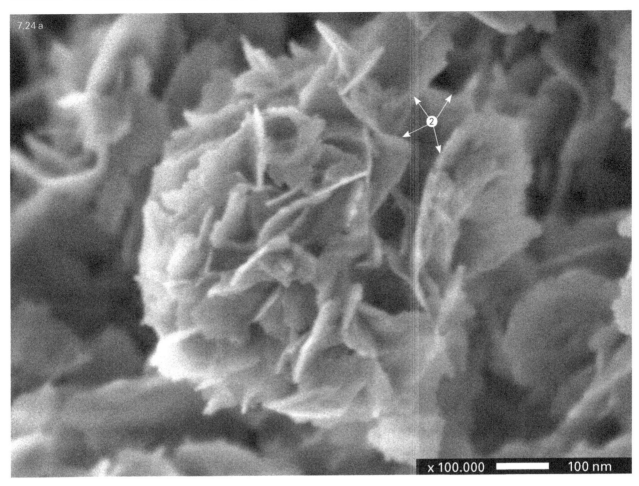

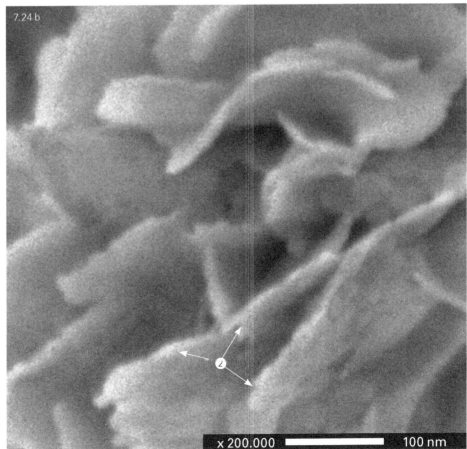

Fig. 7.23.
A fragment from the surface of sheep femoral condyle after removing the articular cartilage and the organic part of the subchondral bone with sodium hypochlorite (deorganification). Mineral microspherolytes (1) and their complexes with the mineral matrix of mineralized cartilage.
SEM-micrograph.
a – x 20,000;
b – x 50,000.

Fig. 7.24.
A fragment of sheep femoral condyle after removing the articular cartilage and the organic part of the subchondral bone with sodium hypochlorite (deorganification).
Mineral microspherolytes (1) and their complexes with the mineral matrix of mineralized cartilage.
Nanocrystalline plates (2).
SEM-micrograph.
a (1.0 kV) – x 100,000;
c (5 kV) – x 100,000;
b – x 200,000;
d – x 20,000.

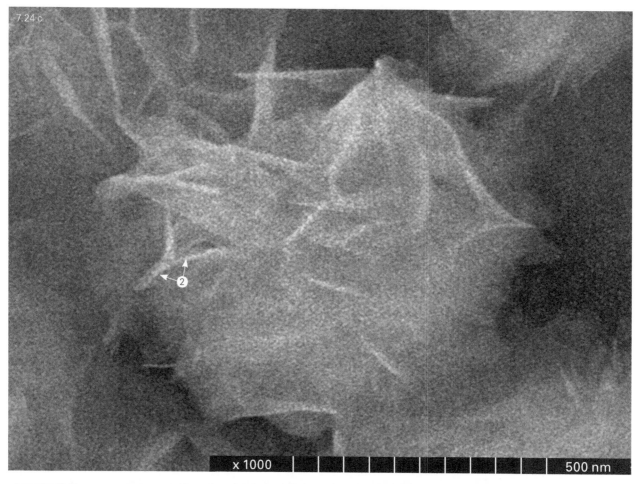

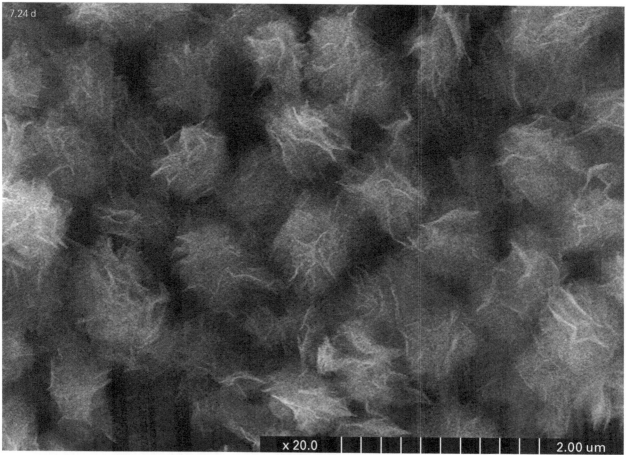

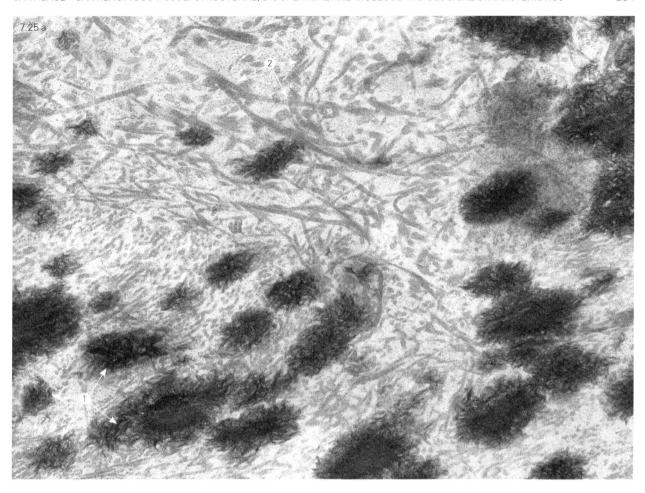

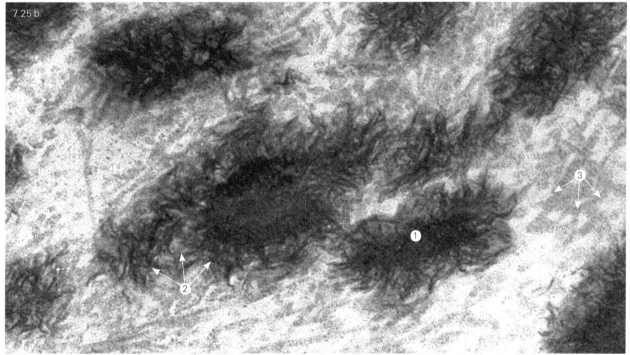

Fig. 7.25.
A fragment femoral condyle articular cartilage.
Mineral lamellar(1) and central "nucleus" microspherolytes (2) of the mineralized articular cartilage.

Collagen fibrils
(non- mineralized) (3).
TEM-micrograph.
Contrasting of ultrathin sections with uranyl acetate and lead citrate.
a – x 20,000; b –50,000.

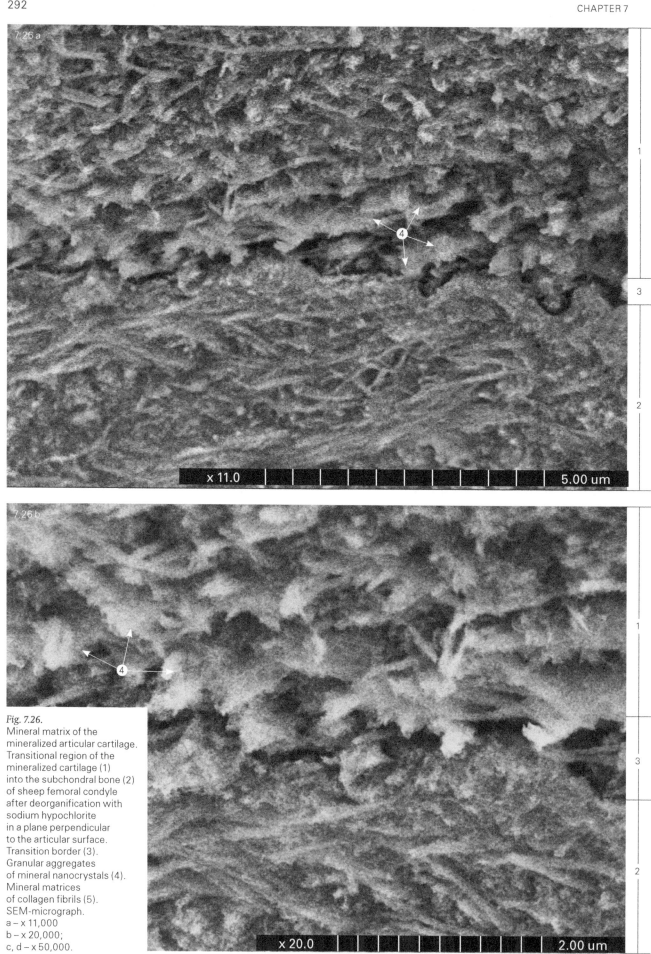

Fig. 7.26.
Mineral matrix of the
mineralized articular cartilage.
Transitional region of the
mineralized cartilage (1)
into the subchondral bone (2)
of sheep femoral condyle
after deorganification with
sodium hypochlorite
in a plane perpendicular
to the articular surface.
Transition border (3).
Granular aggregates
of mineral nanocrystals (4).
Mineral matrices
of collagen fibrils (5).
SEM-micrograph.
a – x 11,000
b – x 20,000;
c, d – x 50,000.

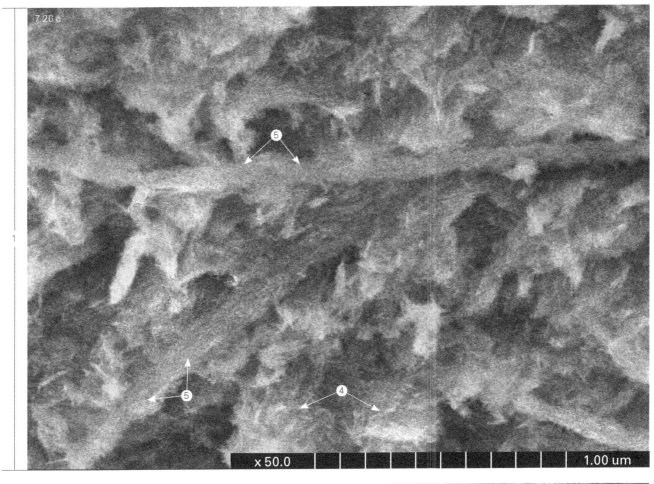

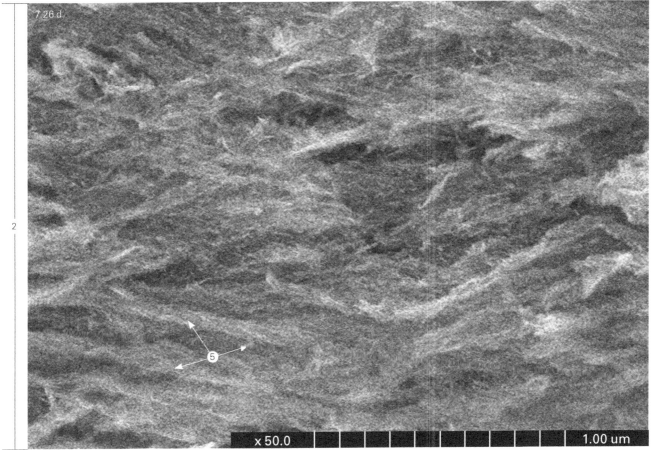

The different organization of the fibrous framework and the mineral matrix of articular cartilage and the subchondral bone may be a prerequisite for their separation at the bone-cartilage junction due to overload, especially in old age.

SEM X-ray microanalysis illustrates the chemical composition of the mineral component of mineralized articular cartilage and the subchondral bone (see *Fig. 7.27*).

7.2.1.2.3. Organization of articular cartilage interstitial space

The interstitial space (intercellular and interfibrillar) in articular cartilage is an integrated system of interstitial channels or tissue capillaries, the walls of which are formed by collagen fibrils. In this regard, their organization depends on the structural organization of the cartilage fibrillar framework. A SEM investigation of polymer replicas or micro-corrosion casts of interstitial space have shown that the interstitial channels form an integrated cellular system (Omelyanenko, 1990, 2005). The channels have different forms: tubes, cracks, circular cavities, and narrowings and widenings (sort of reservoirs) are encountered along their length. The equivalent diameters of the examined channels range from 100–800 nm. The channels are arranged in a disordered fashion in the middle zone of the cartilage. A certain preferential orientation is visually detectable in the superficial and deep zones, matching the organization of the fibrillar framework. The important quantitative parameters of the interfibrillar space are: its volume, the differential distribution of this volume, and the specific internal surface area of cartilage. It is these parameters that largely determine the metabolic activity of cartilage. The application of the mercury porosimetry technique has made it possible to obtain a quantitative characterization of the interstitial spaces of inertly dehydrated specimens of cartilage (Omelyanenko & Butyrin, 1994). Tissue structures occupy 63% of the total tissue volume, whereas interstitial space accounts for 37%. The total volume (V) of the interfibrillar space in articular cartilage is 0.96 cm³/g of dehydrated tissue. The differential distribution of this volume is as follows: spaces with an equivalent diameter of 300–150 nm amount to 11.2%; of 150–50 nm to 20.4%; of 50–30 nm to 20.5%; of 30–10 nm to 29.4%; and of 10–5 nm to 12.4%. I.e. channels that are in the range of equivalent diameters of 300 to 5 nm represent a total of 93.9%. The application of the gas adsorption method has shown that the specific surface area of 1 g of dehydrated articular cartilage is 23.8 m² (Omelyanenko, 2005). This huge surface suggests the potential that active exchange processes inside cartilage take place through the cartilage gel-like integrating buffer metabolic medium (ground substance) filling its entire system of channels.

7.2.1.2.4. Glycoconjugates of cartilaginous tissue

7.2.1.2.4.1. Biochemical characteristics of glycoproteins and proteoglycans

The cartilage extracellular matrix contains a large number (at least 40) of nonfibrillar proteins, commonly referred to as non-collagenous (Roughley, 2001). With very few exceptions, they belong to the glycoconjugates category, as their macromolecules contain carbohydrates attached to the polypeptide chains. We recall that glycoconjugates are subdivided into glycoproteins – molecules that carry oligosaccharide groups – and proteoglycans, which also contain glycosaminoglycans, as well as oligosaccharides.

The main nonfibrillar cartilage proteins that are not proteoglycans (mostly glycoproteins) are presented in *Table. 7.5*.

The nonfibrillar proteins of the cartilage extracellular matrix, mostly glycoproteins, represent:

1) structural macromolecules;
2) macromolecules with enzymatic activity (some proteins have both a structural role and an enzymatic function); and
3) signaling molecules involved in regulating metabolic processes (Neame et al., 1999).

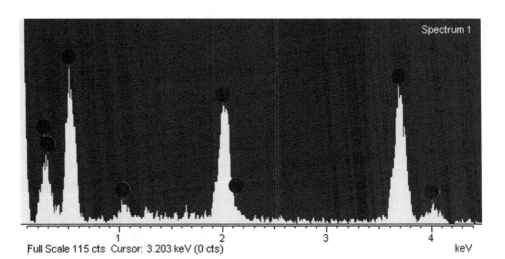

Fig. 7.27.
Diagram of the elemental composition of the mineral component of mineralized articular cartilage and the subchondral bone based on a SEM X-ray microanalysis.

Spectrum 1

Full Scale 115 cts Cursor: 3.203 keV (0 cts)

keV

Table 7.5

Main nonfibrillar proteins/glycoproteins of the cartilage extracellular matrix

Protein	Characteristics	Functions
Cartilage oligomeric matrix protein (COMP) (Thrombospondin-5)	Homopentamer with molecular mass ~ 430 kDa. Glycoprotein. Each monomer contains two N-linked oligosaccharides.	Maintains the connections between chondrocytes and the matrix with the help of integrins; stabilizes the structural organization of the matrix; participates in endochondral ossification; binds calcium; deposits hydrophobic molecules.
Matrilins: matrilin-1 (otherwise known as cartilage matrix protein, CMP) matrilin-2, matrilin-3, matrilin-4	Monomers with molecular mass of 53 to 107 kDa, form homo- and heteropolymers. Matrilins-1 and -2 contain one N-linked oligosaccharide, matrilin-4 – three N-linked oligosaccharides.	Binds to chondrocytes and structural macromolecules of the matrix, facilitating their interactions (adaptor function).
von Willebrand factor A-domain-related protein (WARP)	Multimeric protein; 415 amino acid residues-long monomers are linked by disulfide bonds. Located mostly inside chondrons.	Binds to perlecan inside chondrons and stabilizes the structure of the chondron. Involved in the formation of joints.
Chondrocalcin	Carboxy terminal propeptide of type II procollagen (amino acid residues 1,242–1,487). Homotrimer (molecular mass 105 kDa). Present in the transitory matrix surrounding hypertrophic chondrocytes.	Participates in endochondral ossification: binds hydroxyapatite and promotes mineralization.
Proline/arginine-rich protein (PARP)	A fragment (small part) of the large amino terminal propeptide of the a2-chain of type XI collagen (molecular mass 24 kDa). Present in the matrix of various cartilages.	Function is unknown.
Cartilage intermediate layer protein (CILP)	Monomeric glycoprotein. Consists of 1,163 amino acid residues. Contains 8 N-linked oligosaccharides. Present mainly in articular cartilage.	Component of the structural framework of cartilage tissue. Its content increases with age and in various arthropathies. Binds growth factors.
Chondroadherin	Based on the structure of the polypeptide component, it belongs to the family of small proteoglycans; however, instead of glycosamino-glycans, it contains one O-linked oligosaccharide. Contains 337 amino acid residues. Accumulates in the matrix of various cartilages.	Facilitates the attachment of chondrocytes to the matrix and to artificial substrates.

Prolargin (also known as PRELP, by the name of the coding gene)	Belongs to the family of small proteoglycans, but contains 4 N-linked oligosaccharides. Contains 362 amino acids. Accumulates in the matrix of various cartilages with age.	Binds to type II collagen and the proteoglycan perlecan.
Fibronectins (isoforms specific for cartilage tissue)	Large (molecular mass ~ 550 kDa) multidomain glycoproteins that contain up to 5% oligosaccharides. Possess adhesive, matricellular and regulatory properties. Present in various cartilages.	Stabilize the connections between chondrocytes and the matrix; stabilize the matrix structure by binding to COMP and decorin on the surface of collagen fibers. Interact with IGFBP-1.
Tenascin C (or Hexabrachion)	Hexameric glycoprotein expressed by chondrocytes in two isoforms – molecular mass of 220 and 320 kDa.	Activates extracellular matrix assembly.
Proteoglycan aggregate-binding protein (Link protein)	Located at sites of aggrecan macromolecules and hyaluronan chains.	Strengthens the binding between aggrecan and hyaluronan.
YKL-40 [cartilage glycoprotein 39 (gp39 or HC-gp39), chitinase-3-like protein 1]	Consists of 362 amino acid residues. Expressed by chondrocytes.	Involved in the differentiation and stabilization of the chondrocyte phenotype. May be involved in tissue adaptation to environmental changes and in tissue remodeling. Does not possess enzymatic activity.
YKL-39 (chondrocyte protein 39, chitinase-3-like protein 2)	Consists of 364 amino acid residues. Does not contain oligosaccharides. Expressed by chondrocytes.	Does not possess enzymatic activity. Binds to glycans. Expression is enhanced in osteoarthritis.
Matrix Gla-protein (MGP)	Consists of 77 amino acid residues, contains (in humans) 5 carboxylated glutaminyls. Expressed by chondrocytes.	One of the factors that prevent cartilage mineralization. Involved in the differentiation of chondrocytes.
Chondromodulin-I (Leukocyte Cell-Derived Chemotaxin 1)	Amino acid residues 215-334 of the *LECT1* gene product (humans). Contains 1 N-linked oligosaccharide. Found in the cytoplasm of chondroblasts and in the matrix of fetal cartilage.	A growth factor specific to cartilage tissues. Stimulates the growth of cartilage models of bones and exhibits antiangiogenic activity.
Chondromodulin-II (Leukocyte Cell-Derived Chemotaxin 2)	A product of the Lect2 gene (mice). Contains 133 amino acid residues. Present in the matrix of fetal epiphyseal cartilage.	Stimulates chondroblast proliferation.

Pleiotrophin (PTN)	A peptide with molecular mass of 15.3 kDa. Bound to the cytoplasmic membrane of fetal chondrocytes.	A growth factor present in various tissues and involved in many morphogenetic processes. Promotes chondrocyte proliferation; stimulates proteoglycan expression in mature cartilage.
Cartilage-derived morphogenetic proteins (CDMP) CDMP-1 (GDF-5, BMP-14) CDMP-2 (GDF-6, BMP-13) CDMP-3 (GDF-7, VMP-12)	Homodimeric glycoproteins. The subunits (monomers) consist of 120-129 amino acid residues. Expressed by chondrocytes; belong to the growth factor superfamily TGF-β1	Similar to the BMP, have osteoinductive and osteogenic activity. Stimulate chondrocyte proliferation and the growth of long bones.

The most important structural component is the **cartilage oligomeric matrix protein** (COMP), which belongs to the thrombospondin family (it is also called thrombospondin-5). This glycoprotein is a homopentamer: its macromolecule consists of five identical subunits. In humans, each subunit (monomer) consists of 737 amino acids and has a molecular mass of ~86 kDa; the entire macromolecule is 430 kDa. The subunits intertwine and are linked together by disulfide bonds at the junction of the helical amino terminal domains. The C-terminal part of each subunit ends with a globular domain.

COMP has pronounced acidity due to the high content of aspartic and glutamic acid residues, as well as the presence of negatively charged carbohydrate groups. Each monomer contains four amino acid repeat sequences similar to the sequence of the epithelial growth factor (EGF-like repeats). COMP also possesses calmodulin-like repeats (calmodulin is a calcium-binding protein), and the binding of calcium is required for the stability of the pentamer structure.

COMP, like all the other cartilage proteins, is expressed by chondrocytes. Although other cells can also produce COMP, and it is found in several other tissues, including tissues not related to the skeleton, its expression is particularly active in the cartilage. Therefore, it is considered to be a conditionally specific marker of the chondrocyte phenotype. In embryos, COMP is concentrated mainly in the pericellular matrix, whereas in adults, it is primarily in the interterritorial matrix.

Experimental data reveal a variety of COMP functions. Through its interactions with integrins, COMP supports two-way communication between chondrocytes and the extracellular matrix (Chen et al., 2005). COMP acts as a catalyst of type II collagen fibrillogenesis (Hallösz et al., 2007), binds to glycosaminoglycans in the aggrecan chains and to types II and IX collagen, which may be relevant to the organization of the matrix structure (Geng et al., 2008). Defects in this organization in articular cartilage, resulting from COMP deficiency, contribute to the early development of chronic arthritis (Chen et al., 2007; Geng et al., 2008).

The region of COMP monomer attachment is composed of five integrated helical domains and forms a cavity where small hydrophobic molecules can accumulate (including vitamins A and D, which are important for chondrogenesis and osteogenesis) (Özbek et al., 2002).

COMP is an abundant component of the metaphyseal cartilage matrix, suggesting its involvement in endochondral ossification (see section 10.3.1.1). This assumption is supported by its accumulation in the forming limb bones in human embryos (Koellig et al., 2006). It is also confirmed by the existence of at least 50 COMP mutations in humans, predominantly in the calcium-binding domain. These mutations cause chondrodysplasia with various degree of severity (Délot et al., 1999). In experiments on mice, COMP (thrombospondin-5) deficiency in the matrix of growth plates, combined with a deficit of thrombospondin-3 and type IX collagen, result in a serious disruption of skeletogenesis (growth is reduced by 20%) (Posey et al., 2008).

Finally, the importance of COMP for the functioning of cartilage tissue is confirmed by immunochemically detectable changes in COMP concentration in blood serum, urine, and synovial fluid in various pathological processes that affect cartilage, such as rheumatoid arthritis and osteoarthrosis. A rise in these parameters, which is due more to an increased expression of COMP, rather than to the destruction of cartilage tissue, has acquired diagnostic and prognostic value in clinical practice (Tseng et al., 2009). The enhanced expression of COMP in metaphyseal cartilage explains its elevated concentration in the blood serum of children in the pre-puberty stage following the introduction of pituitary growth hormone while treating growth retardation (Bjarnason et al., 2004).

Four proteins constituting the matrilin family, together with COMP, account for a significant proportion of the mass of structural nonfibrillar components of the cartilage extracellular matrix. Matrilin-1 and matrilin-3 are only present in cartilage, whereas matrilin-2 and matrilin-4 are also found in various types of fibrous (dense and loose) connective tissue (Mann et al., 2004).

Matrilin expression is characteristic of mature chondrocytes and appears relatively late in the chondrogenesis process, after the cessation of cell proliferation and following the onset of expression of the key chondrocyte phenotype markers–aggrecan and collagen II. However, the expression of matrilins continues in the final stages of metaphyseal cartilage chondrocyte differentiation prior to endochondral ossification (see 10.3.1.1), which indicates that matrilins participate in this process. Matrilin-2 and matrilin-4 are also expressed in the cartilage models of bones in areas of joint formation. Matrilins are present in the matrix of all types of cartilage tissue, being less abundant in articular cartilage than in epiphyseal and costal cartilage.

Even though each matrilin is encoded by a unique gene, the macromolecules of all four matrilins have a similar modular-type of structure: they consist of a von Willebrand factor A-domain-like (VWA-like) domain, an epithelial growth factor-like (EGF-like) domain, and a helical carboxy terminal domain. However, their molecular masses vary: 52.8 kDa for matrilin-3; 53.7 kDa for matrilin-1; 68.8 kDa for matrilin-4; and 106.8 kDa for matrilin-2. These differences are due to different numbers of EGF (from 4–10) and VWA (between 1–2) modules. The matrilins expressed by chondrocytes in cell culture often form homo- and heterooligomers whose carboxyterminal domains are linked by disulfide bonds. In the matrix, they tend to form filamentous structures that bind to types II and VI collagen microfibrils. Matrilins interact with other structural components of the matrix too, including COMP, hyaluronan, aggrecan, fibrillin-2, fibrinogen, and others (Piecha et al., 2002).

Furthermore, matrilins ensure a loose attachment of chondrocytes to the surrounding matrix without the involvement of integrins, which does not require the formation of adhesion loci (focal adhesions, see 3.8.3) or the restructuring of the actin cytoskeleton. It is possible that this attachment is mediated by glycosaminoglycans present on the cell surface (Mann et al., 2007).

This weak spatial fixation of chondrocytes, together with matrilins' numerous connections with the structural macromolecules of the matrix, make it possible to define the general function of matrilins as adaptive–enabling cartilage tissue to adapt to changing life conditions (Wagener et al., 2005). Thus, the expression of matrilin-3 in articular cartilage chondrocytes increases in joint dysfunction caused by osteoarthritis (Pullig et al., 2002).

The uniformity of the matrilin macromolecular structure is manifested in their at least partial interchangeability (capacity for biochemical compensation) and explains the results of knockout experiments in mice, in which the shutdown of one of the *Matn* genes caused no obvious phenotypic skeletal abnormalities (Nicolae et al., 2007).

If we were to turn off two matrilin genes, such as matrilin-1 (this matrilin, discovered before the others, was formerly called **cartilage matrix protein**, CMP) and matrilin-3, this would result in collagen fibrillogenesis abnormalities in cartilage tissue in the form of the fibrils'

thickening. A compensatory increase of matrilin-4 expression occurs at the same time, probably ensuring the lack of major changes in mouse skeletogenesis (Nicolae et al., 2007).

Despite these compensatory capabilities (matrilin interchangeability), mutations in the human *MATN3* gene, encoding matrilin-3, are accompanied by pathological alterations of the skeleton. There are three types of pathology: spondyloepiphyseal dysplasia, which affects cartilage structures of the spine; multiple epiphyseal dysplasia; and familial hand osteoarthritis.

The **cartilage intermediate layer protein** (CILP) is a large structural protein present in the middle (intermediate) zone of human articular cartilage (Lorenzo et al., 1998). It is not found in the superficial or deep zones of articular cartilage, but is present in the intervertebral discs and some other varieties of connective tissue (Mori et al., 2006). CILP is a monomeric glycoprotein, 1,163 amino acids in length, expressed by chondrocytes, and containing 8 N-linked oligosaccharides. It probably is one of the structural components of the cartilage framework. The content of CILP in the interterritorial matrix of articular cartilage, particularly in hip joint cartilage, progressively increases with age; the increase is especially abrupt at the initial stage of osteoarthritis.

Extracellular inorganic pyrophosphate content in cartilage rises in parallel with the upregulated CILP expression. The primary structure of the CILP carboxy-terminal domain bears some similarity to the enzyme nucleoside triphosphate pyrophosphohydrolase (NTPPPH), purified from pig cartilage. It has been suggested that CILP exhibits pyrophosphohydrolase enzymatic activity, and the combined name CILP/NTPPPH has been proposed for the entire macromolecule (Hirose et al., 2000). In line with this view, the accumulation of calcium pyrophosphate dihydrate (CPPD) crystals, produced by this enzyme, is the primary pathogenic factor causing the development of arthropathies. However, direct proof for CILP enzymatic activity has not been obtained, a catalytic domain has not been found, and the elevated CPPD levels in cartilage are evidently not of primary nature, but just one element of the pathological process. This may be related to the fact that CILP acts as an antagonist of the growth factor IGF-1; it is known that IGF-1 stimulates the chondrocyte function and decreases extracellular pyrophosphate levels (Johnson et al., 2003). It is also possible that the arthropathic phenomena caused by CILP are attributable to the presence of autoantigenic domains in its macromolecule and to its influence on the immune system (Yao et al., 2004).

The extracellular matrix of the superficial zone of articular cartilage contains specific proteins. First, **Del1** (developmental endothelial locus protein-1) is a protein with a molecular mass of 60 kDa, localized around chondrocytes, and strongly attached to them through the interaction of the "sticky" RGD-sequence with integrin avb3. It is believed that this attachment contributes to chondrocyte fixation in the superficial zone, compensating for the lack of chondrons therein; chondrons in the deeper cartilage layers provide optimal conditions for chondrocyte function (Pfister et al., 2001). Second, clusterin is a secreted multifunctional glycoprotein containing 427 amino acid residues and six N-linked oligosaccharides. Clusterin involved in the regulation of apoptosis is characteristically present near the "fluid–tissue" interface, in this case, the "articular cartilage–synovial fluid" interface (Khan et al., 2001).

Blood serum albumins, entering the cartilage tissue from the synovial fluid, are abundant in the most superficial layer of articular cartilage (Noyori et al., 1998).

The **von Willebrand factor A-domain-related protein (WARP)** represents the superfamily of connective tissue matrix proteins that contain this domain. On the basis of this feature it has certain similarity with a number of nonfibrillar collagens. It is possible that WARP is a descendant of one of the collagenous proteins that disappeared in the course of evolution.

WARP is a macromolecule that is 415 amino acid residues long and is found in developing articular cartilage tissue during embryogenesis. Its presence distinguishes this tissue from the adjacent epiphyseal cartilage tissue and it evidently participates in the formation of joints. In mature cartilage tissue, WARP is concentrated inside chondrons, where its association with the proteoglycan perlecan stabilizes the chondrons' structure (Allen et al., 2006).

On the basis of the primary structures of their polypeptide chains, chondroadherin and prolargin, two structural proteins of the cartilage extracellular matrix, belong in the same family of leucine-rich proteins as the small proteoglycans (SLRP). However, they do not contain glycosaminoglycans and, therefore, are not proteoglycans (Neame et al., 1999).

Chondroadherin consists of 337 amino acid residues and contains one O-linked oligosaccharide and two intramolecular disulfide bonds. In keeping with its name, chondroadherin attaches chondrocytes to artificial substrates in vitro, acting as a ligand of $\alpha2\beta1$ integrin; this attachment is accompanied by cell spreading. In vivo, the function of integrins is to strengthen the structural integrity of the "cell–extracellular matrix" system.

Prolargin (the name reflects the high content of proline and arginine, in addition to leucine), often called PRELP (for the name of the encoding gene), is a glycoprotein that is 362 amino acids long and contains four N-linked oligosaccharides. PRELP binds to type II collagen and to the proteoglycan perlecan present in articular cartilage. PRELP content in cartilage is low in embryos and newborns, but, similar to CILP, its content increases with age. Two structural components conserved in the extracellular matrix–**chondrocalcin** and PARP–represent products of the post-translational processing of collagens. Chondrocalcin is the carboxyterminal propeptide cleavable in its entirety from type II procollagen macromolecules already assembled in triple helices. The homotrim-

eric chondrocalcin molecule (mass of 105 kDa) consists of three monomers built from amino acid residues 1,242–1,487 of the a1(II) polypeptide chains. Chondrocalcin is present in the matrix of cartilage precursors of bones ready for endochondral ossification around hypertrophic chondrocytes. Its accumulation is indicative of active type II collagen biosynthesis. It facilitates mineralization thanks to its capacity to bind hydroxyapatite, and to associate simultaneously with the protein annexin V, a component of the membranous matrix vesicles (see section 8.3.2.3).

The **proline/arginine-rich protein** (PARP) is a fragment (the smaller part; mass of 24 kDa) of the large aminoterminal globular propeptide of the a2-chain of ctype XI collagen. It is present in the matrix of various cartilages, and especially abundant in epiphyseal cartilage. Its molecular structure is similar to propeptides of several other nonfibrillar collagens. Its function is unknown.

Cartilage tissue contains specific isoforms of the large multidomain glycoprotein, fibronectin, generated by alternative splicing (Parker et al., 2002). These isoforms are expressed by chondroblasts/ chondrocytes. Similar to all other isoforms of fibronectin, they are ubiquitous in the matrix of all varieties of connective tissue and combine the properties of adhesive and matricellular proteins (see section 3.3.1.1). Acting as ligands for integrins, fibronectins connect chondrocytes to the extracellular matrix. They impart additional stability to the matrix by binding to COMP and the small proteoglycan decorin, located on the surface of collagen fibrils. Fibronectins possess an additional regulatory function: they act together with one of the insulin-like growth factor-binding proteins, IGFBP-3, in regulating the IGF-1 effect on cartilage metabolism (Martin et al., 2002).

Fibronectin binds to tenascin C–another large glycoprotein expressed by cultured articular cartilage chondrocytes and embedded in the extracellular matrix (Savarese et al., 1996). This hexameric protein (also known as "hexabrachion", see section 3.3.1.1) is produced in two isoforms with: subunits of molecular mass 320 and 220 kDa. Most likely, both isoforms stimulate matrix assembly, but the smaller one is more active in this respect. The binding to fibronectins inhibits their adhesive activity.

The most important role in the structural organization of the extracellular matrix of all varieties of cartilage tissue is played by the proteoglycan binding protein–**link protein** (LP)–a glycoprotein that stabilizes the links between aggrecan and hyaluronan within the aggregates they form. LP will be further discussed below in regard to this function.

The cartilage extracellular matrix, similar to other types of connective tissue, contains a large number of different enzymes expressed by chondroblasts/ chondrocytes. These are:

a) enzymes acting in the final stages of anabolic processes–enzymes that complete the post-translational processing of structural macromolecules of the matrix (collagens, elastin, proteoglycans) after they exit the cells and following their assembly into supramolecular aggregates. In particular, chondrocalcin and PARP appear in the matrix thanks to the action of enzymes from this group. These enzymes' function will be discussed in more detail in the overview on the biosynthesis of the respective biopolymers;

b) enzymes that carry out the catabolism of structural macromolecules – metalloproteases (matrixins) and other proteolytic enzymes, hydrolases, etc. Information about these enzymes is presented in section 3.7, when we review the catabolic reactions taking place in the matrix.

Chondrocytes express, also *in vitro*, a small (molecular mass of 14.4 kDa) protein – lysozyme, which exhibits N-acetylmuramide glycanhydrolase activity towards mucopeptides and is known for its lytic action on a number of microorganisms. It is present in at least four isoforms in the extracellular matrix of articular and other cartilages (Moss et al., 1997). The significance of lysozyme enzymatic activity in normal cartilage tissue is unknown. This activity is determined by its cationic nature; the binding to the large anionic proteoglycan aggrecan suggests its involvement in the structural organization of the matrix.

Another two proteins expressed by chondroblasts/ chondrocytes and secreted in the matrix are very similar to each other in terms of primary structure and the size of molecules – YKL-40 and YKL-39 (these are trivial names – one-letter designations of the first three amino acid residues of the N-terminal domain: tyrosyl-lysyl-leucyl). They belong to glycosylhydrolase family 18 (GH18) and are similar to the enzyme chitinase-3, which is reflected in their official names. However, neither of them exhibits enzymatic activity, and they are essentially signaling molecules acting as regulatory factors. At the same time, there are significant differences between them.

Chitinase-3-like protein 1 (YKL-40, cartilage glycoprotein 39, gp39, or HC-gp39), is particularly actively expressed by chondrocytes, but is present in other tissues too. In human embryos, it is detectable (at the mRNA level) in the formation of cartilage, bone and muscle tissues in a very early stage of embryogenesis. Later, the active expression continues in those cells of the chondrogenic and osteogenic differons that are characterized by intense proliferation and differentiation and are involved in morphogenetic alterations (Johansen et al., 2007). YKL-40 influences the function of chondrocytes: it promotes the formation and the stabilization of their phenotype by regulating the functioning of signaling pathways, and by inducing the biosynthesis of the Sox9 factor and type II collagen (Jacques et al., 2007). The expression of YKL-40 is virtually absent in mature chondrocytes, but is activated when the cartilage needs to adapt to environmental changes, such as when it is necessary to inhibit the action of pro-inflammatory cytokines in rheumatoid arthritis. Expression is also activated in the course of tissue remodeling and during in vitro culture of chondrocytes. YKL-40 accounts for more than 30% of the proteins secreted by chondrocytes in the extracellular matrix.

Unlike YKL-40, chitinase-3-like protein 2 (YKL-39, chondrocyte protein 39) does not contain oligosaccharides and, therefore, is not a glycoprotein. In addition to chondrocytes, it is expressed, albeit in much smaller quantities, by synovial membrane cells. YKL-40 makes up about 4% of the proteins synthesized by chondrocytes in vitro. Similarly to YKL-40, YKL-39 does not have enzymatic activity. Its function in normal cartilage tissue is unknown, but it is noted that its expression in chondrocytes is upregulated in osteoarthrosis (Knorr et al., 2003).

The **matrix Gla protein** (MGP), expressed by chondrocytes, fulfills an important regulatory role. This small protein (its molecule consists of 77 amino acids in humans) contains five g-carboxylated (with the participation of vitamin K) glutamic acid residues. These residues are required for basic MGP functions – in preventing premature transitory cartilage mineralization in endochondral ossification (Newman et al., 2001), and participation in maintaining the non-mineralized status of the matrix in permanent cartilage (Neame et al., 1999). MGP is also involved in regulating chondrocyte differentiation and maintaining their viability. The effects of MGP explain its antagonism with the bone morphogenetic protein BMP-2.

Chondromodulins function as growth factors, which are actively expressed by chondrocytes in embryogenesis.

Chondromodulin-I, a cartilage tissue-specific glycoprotein, is composed of 100 amino acids (amino acid residues 215–314 of the protein encoded by the human gene *LECT1*) and contains an N-linked oligosaccharide. Chondromodulin-I is found in both chondrocytes and the extracellular matrix. Its expression is weak in mature chondrocytes. Chondromodulin-I supports chondrocyte proliferation and thus, stimulates the growth of the cartilage models of bones. By virtue of its anti-angiogenic activity, it prevents the vascularization of articular cartilage, especially during its formation (Kitahara et al., 2003).

Chondromodulin-II is not a glycoprotein and is not secreted into the matrix, but generally acts as an autocrine regulator. Like chondromodulin-I, this protein stimulates chondrocyte proliferation (Shukunami et al., 1999). Furthermore, it displays chemotactic activity toward neutrophils.

In fetal cartilage tissue, the intense expression of chondromodulin-I, monitored by the accumulation of mRNA, temporally coincides with at least equally intense expression by chondrocytes of another signaling molecule – pleiotrophin (PTN) (Azizan et al., 2000). Pleiotrophin [synonyms: osteoblast-stimulating factor-1 (OSF-1); heparin-binding growth factor (HB-GAM)] is a growth factor/cytokine involved in the growth and development processes of many tissues, and exhibits conditional activity in different directions. This small (136 amino acid residues, molecular mass of 15.3 kDa) peptide, secreted in the matrix, is abundant in cartilage during the fetal and early postnatal periods. It is bound to the chondrocyte cell membrane. Similarly to chondromodulin-I, the content of pleiotrophin in mature cartilage is sharply reduced. It increases again in pathological states, where anabolic reactions in cartilage are upregulated in the initial stages. An analysis of PTN receptor expression shows that, in situations of active morphogenesis, it stimulates, by autocrine mode, chondrocyte proliferation and the expression of matrixin inhibitors, whereas the expression of matrixins themselves (MMP-1 and MMP-13) is inhibited (Pufe et al., 2007). By contrast, PTN inhibits chondrocyte proliferation upon the completion of morphogenesis, but stimulates the biosynthesis of the proteoglycans aggrecan and biglycan in chondrocytes.

Proteoglycans in cartilage tissue. Large proteoglycans, aggrecan. Small proteoglycans (SLRP).

Proteoglycans are glycoconjugates that contain glycosaminoglycans, in addition to oligosaccharides (Roughley, 2006). In terms of mass, they are the dominant component of the interfibrillar substance of the cartilage matrix, and are of particular structural and functional (biomechanical) importance. A list of the major proteoglycans in the extracellular matrix of cartilage is presented in *Table. 7.6*.

The large cartilage proteoglycan, **aggrecan**, comprises up to 10% of the wet tissue. Its name reflects its ability to form supramolecular aggregates with the participation of hyaluronan.

The ability to bind to hyaluronan is also inherent to other large proteoglycans, which can be grouped on this basis in the hyalectan family.

The aggrecan protein core has a molecular mass of 210 kDa and is composed of multiple domains (Kiani et al., 2002). The polypeptide chain starts with the globular G1 domain, which is responsible for interaction between aggrecan and hyaluronan in the formation of aggregates.

The G1 domain contains two structural motifs. The amino terminal immunoglobulin (Ig) motif has a loop-like conformation. This loop is followed by two other loops, held together by disulfide bonds. These loop-shaped structures are called tandem proteoglycan repeat units (TPR), since the motif represents multiple reiterations (in tandem) of the same amino acid sequences. Domain G1 contains about 25% carbohydrates (some keratan sulfate and oligosaccharides).

The TPR-units of domain G1 represent the aggrecan region responsible for binding to hyaluronan and link protein, which was mentioned as being a cartilage glycoprotein (Knudson & Knudson, 2001). It is separated from the second globular domain (G2) by a short (21 nm in length, and 150 amino acid residues) linear peptide fragment, which carries a small portion of aggrecan's keratan sulfates. This interglobular domain (IGD) is the main point of proteolytic enzymes' activity on the aggrecan macromolecule (Hardingham & Fosang, 1995).

The second globular domain – G2 – is homologous in structure to the first globular domain, distinguished only by the absence of an immunoglobulin motif.

The linear region, called the keratan sulfate-binding domain, later follows. The structure of this domain is somewhat various in different species. In human aggrecan, the domain contains 11 repeats, each with six residues, which have almost the same, but not completely identical, amino acid sequences. Short keratan sulfate chains are attached via O-glycosidic bonds to a serine residue present within these sequences. More than 60% of all keratan sulfates aggrecan macromolecules are concentrated in this area.

The keratan sulfate attachment domain is followed by the most extended region of the protein core – the chondroitin sulfate-binding domain (domain CS), consisting of two sub-domains. In human aggrecan, the first subdomain (CS-1) consists of repeating 19-amino acid motifs. Chondroitin sulfate chains attach to paired serine-glycine residues within each of these repeats. The molecular mass of each chain is, on average, 20 kDa. The second, longer, subdomain (CS-2) consists of seven repeats of 100 amino acid residues each. Each repeat contains one segment of 30 amino acid residues, and seven repeating motifs of 10 residues. All of these regions contain at least one serine-glycine pair carrying bundled chondroitin sulfate chains, which, as in keratan, are attached to the protein core via O-glycosidic bonds. In total, there are 77 such dipeptides. About 40% of the total amount of keratan sulfate, and up to 90% of the chondroitin sulfate in proteoglycan macromolecules are concentrated in the chondroitin sulfate attachment domain (the remaining 10% of chondroitin sulfate are attached to the keratan sulfate-binding domain).

The human aggrecan gene exhibits size polymorphism in the exon encoding the CS domain (Doege et al., 1997). The total number of repeats, 26 on average, ranges from 13 to 33 in different individuals. This results in the variable length of the protein core and different amounts of attached chondroitin sulfates, leading to variations in the biomechanical characteristics of cartilage tissue.

The third globular domain (G3) resides at the carboxy terminus of the core protein, and it does not resemble the first two. One of the subdomains of this domain is homologous (in amino acid composition) to lectin C – a representative of the group of lectin proteins, which are distinguished for their ability to selectively bind to carbohydrate components of other proteins. The presence of a lectin-like subdomain, inherent also to the other large proteoglycans, warrants calling them lectins. This subdomain allows the attachment of aggrecan macromolecules to the cellular transmembrane proteins, since these proteins are usually glycoproteins. This fixation restricts the mobility of aggrecan macromolecules in the extracellular matrix. This same subdomain contains a module homologous to the epithelial growth factor. The second subdomain of the G3 domain is similar in primary structure to complement factor B.

The G3 domain contains 10 cysteine residues, which ensure the maintenance of globular conformation via disulfide bonds. It is nearly 100% conserved across species,

Table 7.6

Main proteoglycans of cartilage tissue extracellular matrix

Proteoglycan	Characteristics	Functions in cartilage tissue
Aggrecan (chondroitin sulfate proteoglycan-1, CSPG1)	A multidomain core protein, with a molecular mass of 210 kDa, carries more than 100 chondroitin sulfate and keratan sulfate chains. Expressed by chondrocytes.	Forms supramolecular aggregates with the participation of hyaluronan and the cartilage link protein; they protect the cartilage from compression.
Versican (large fibroblast proteoglycan; chondroitin sulfate proteoglycan-2, CSPG2; PG-M)	A multidomain core protein with molecular mass of 369 kDa, which carries only chondroitin sulfate chains. Expressed by mesenchymal cells and chondrocytes.	Forms supramolecular aggregates with the participation of hyaluronan and the cartilage link protein. Participates in the early stages of chondrogenesis. Possibly increases the resistance of articular cartilage to shear strain.
Lubricin (superficial zone protein, SZP; proteoglycan-4, PRG4)	Present in the superficial zone of articular cartilage.	Possibly important for imparting specific biomechanical properties to the superficial zone; enhances the lubrication function of synovial fluid.
Biglycan (DS-PG I)	See Table 3.5.	Function is the same as in other varieties of connective tissue.
Decorin (DS-PG II)	See Table 3.5.	Function is the same as in other varieties of connective tissue. In addition, imparts elasticity to collagen fibers.
Epiphican (DS-PG III)	Contained mainly in epiphyseal cartilage. Molecular mass of about 36 kDa.	Involved in the process of endochondral ossification.
PRELP (prolargin)	See Table 3.5.	Binds to perlecan and collagens.
Lumican	See Table 3.5.	Binds to laminin and collagens.
Perlecan	Large heparan sulfate proteoglycan (see 3.3.2 and Table 3.6). Contained mainly in the chondron.	Important for stabilizing the structure of the chondron. Involved in the regulation of growth factor activity.
Agrin	Large heparan sulfate proteoglycan. Contained in metaphyseal cartilage.	Involved in the process of endochondral ossification.

which points to its important functional role in biosynthesis and translocation (movement) in the process of glycosylation and the secretion of aggrecan macromolecules.

The core protein is a glycoprotein: it contains (in all domains, both linear and globular) 50–60 oligosaccharide groups attached to the polypeptide via O-glycosidic bonds and consisting of galactosamine, glucosamine, galactose and sialic acid in a molar ratio of 1:1:1:2. In addition, about 15 mannose-rich oligosaccharides attached to the polypeptide via N-glycosidic bonds have been found.

The organization of aggrecan macromolecules described above should be considered as generalized and idealized. Although aggrecan is the major proteoglycan in all varieties of cartilage tissue, notable differences in aggrecan composition have been found in different cartilages. Chondroitin-6-sulfate predominates in articular cartilage (and this predominance increases somewhat with age), whereas there is more chondroitin-4-sulfate in growth cartilage (in the metaphyseal plates of the bones). The majority of aggrecan macromolecules in the cartilage extracellular matrix are incorporated as subunits (monomers) into stable multimolecular aggregates with a molecular mass up to 100,000 kDa. Hyaluronan is the core component of these aggregates, with a single chain connecting numerous aggrecan macromolecules. A linear hyaluronan macromolecule with a mass of 1,000 kDa can carry up to 200 aggrecan subunits. Virtually all hyaluronan contained in the cartilage matrix (about 1% of the total tissue mass) is involved in the formation of aggregates. Thus, aggrecan, or rather, its core protein, acts as a hyaladherin in this interaction.

Aggregate formation can be observed in vitro, where it occurs spontaneously upon mixing aggrecan and hyaluronan solutions, even at very low hyaluronan concentrations of 0.01%. A sharp increase in the viscosity of the solution is an indicator of aggregation. Hyaluronan's role in this process is absolutely specific, and it cannot be substituted by any other polyanion. The minimum length of hyaluronan chains required for the binding of aggrecan is, theoretically, 10 disaccharide units; however in reality, this length is much greater, and the attachment points of two adjacent monomers are spaced at least 50–60 disaccharides apart.

As shown by in vitro studies (Mörgelin et al., 1995), during aggregate assembly, following the attachment of aggrecans or of link proteins alone, the hyaluronan chain length is reduced by about half compared with its length in a free state. This means that the spatial conformation of hyaluronan changes within aggregates.

Due to their size and mutual electrostatic repulsion, the aggrecan macromolecules can be oriented only perpendicularly to the hyaluronan chain. The resulting structure, which is compared to a "bottle-cleaning brush".

The attachment between aggrecan and hyaluronan within the aggregate is mediated by a globular G1 domain, whose structure (presence of PTR) is very similar to the transmembrane receptor CD44, the main hyaluronan receptor on the cell surface. This receptor has a single loop module, which, as in the G1 domain, is built from tandem repeats of amino acid residues. CD44 binds specifically to a hexasaccharide fragment of the hyaluronan chain. The G1 domain has two such modules and binds to a decasaccharide fragment.

Cartilage link protein (CLP), located directly at the point that aggrecan attaches to hyaluronan, further strengthens this bond. This small protein consists of 339 amino acid residues, has a molecular mass of about 45 kDa, and belongs to the hyaluronan and proteoglycan-binding link protein family (HAPLN). Cartilage link protein has two loop modules containing disulfide bonds and is generally very similar to the G1 domain; their genes are probably derived from a common ancestor (Spicer et al., 2003). The two-module structure of link protein allows it to attach simultaneously to hyaluronan and aggrecan; this binding makes hyaluronan more resistant to hyaluronidase action. The attachment to aggrecan and may be characterized as a cross-link of a carbohydrate nature formation.

Link protein does not carry glycosaminoglycans, but it contains N-linked oligosaccharides and is a glycoprotein. A study of mice with an inactivated link protein gene (Crtl1) indicates that this protein plays a rather significant role in the formation of cartilage tissue (Watanabe & Yamada, 1999). Most mice died shortly after birth due to respiratory failure caused by a deficiency of laryngeal and bronchial cartilage. The surviving mice developed dwarfism associated with the flattening of the vertebrae, limb shortening and skull deformation.

Density gradient centrifugation separates proteoglycan aggregates from articular cartilage into two populations, differing in length in terms of the hyaluronan chain (on average, 400 nm in one population, and 1,160 nm in the other) and the number of aggrecan macromolecules attached to it within an individual aggregate (on average, 15 and 44, respectively). Obviously, these two aggregate populations have different effects on the mechanical and metabolic stability of cartilage.

The main function of aggrecan is mechanical – it provides compressive resistance in cartilage tissue. Furthermore, in vitro experiments show that aggrecan protects cartilage collagen fibrils, composed predominantly of type II collagen, from degradation by metalloproteases. It has been proposed that aggrecan aggregates impede contact between enzymes and collagen (Pratta et al., 2003).

Data on the biosynthesis of proteoglycans, including aggrecan and hyaluronan, presented in section 3.2.1.2, must be supplemented by information pertaining specifically to the aggrecan of cartilage tissue.

The mouse gene encoding the core protein of cartilage tissue aggrecan has been characterized in detail (Watanabe et al., 1995) and contains 18 exons. Exon 2 contains the start (methionine) codon. The coding sequence, 6,545 base pairs in total, encodes a polypeptide chain of 2,132 amino acid residues. This includes the 18 amino acid residues that form the signal peptide. There is a complete correlation between the gene's exon structure and the domain structure of the polypeptide, indicating that the gene has a modular type of organization. This is also supported by the presence of aggrecan gene regions that are conserved in all investigated species. The domain that carries chondroitin sulfates is entirely encoded by a single exon that is 3,600 base pairs long. The promoter region contains segments that are structurally similar to the promoter of type II collagen, and other segments similar to the promoter of glucocorticoid hormone receptors.

The human aggrecan gene contains 7,137 base pairs, encoding a protein core polypeptide chain of 2,136 amino acid residues. The exon/intron structures of human and mouse genes are very similar; the bovine and chicken aggrecan genes also have similar structural patterns. The degree of homology between the amino acid sequences of the core proteins of human and mouse aggrecan is, on average, 75%, and approaches 100% in some domains. The intraspecies tissue specificity of aggrecans is determined by cis-elements in the gene controlled by transcription factors (Pirok et al., 2001).

Three isoforms of the human aggrecan protein are known, differing in the length of the polypeptide chains–the longest consists of 2,454 amino acid residues, and they are produced by alternative splicing.

After the completion of translation–the assembly of the polypeptide chain of the aggrecan core protein in polyribosomes on the cytoplasmic surface of the membranes of the rough endoplasmic reticulum–the macromolecule takes a path common to all secreted proteins: through the inner lumen of the endoplasmic reticulum and the cisternae of the Golgi system, to the plasma membrane, and finally to the extracellular matrix.

Along this path, the formation of spatial conformation of the globular domains is of particular importance (Luo et al., 2001). The folding of these domains proceeds through several intermediate stages and ends up in a state where the finished domains are completely hydrophobic on the outside and hydrophilic on the inside. These processes occur at a relatively slow rate. They must be precisely synchronized and properly carried out for all three globular domains–G1, G2, and G3. This order is achieved through the participation of molecular chaperones, acting at all stages of formation and the movement of the macromolecule. Chaperones do not catalyze folding, but prevent the hydrophobic groups from engaging in premature interactions between folding intermediates. They also control the correct addition of oligosaccharides and glycosaminoglycans to the polypeptide chain, which begins in the endoplasmic reticulum and continues in the Golgi cisternae. The proteins **calnexin** and **calreticulin** act as chaperones in the early stages of folding and glycosylation. The assembly of glycosaminoglycan chains attached to the linear domain of the protein core ends with their sulfation. Later, the chaperone hsp 27 selectively protects the G3 domain.

The completed formation of the G1 and G3 globular domains and the addition of glycosaminoglycans, modulating the secondary structure of the linear sections of the protein core, are essential for aggrecan secretion from the cell. The function of the G2 domain in aggrecan secretion remains unclear (Kiani et al., 2002).

Hyaluronan, essential for aggregates' formation, is produced by chondrocytes. In particular, the rate of hyaluronan synthesis in chondrocytes is high in the middle zone of articular cartilage. The expression of enzymes required for this synthesis–hyaluronan synthases (HAS-2, HAS-3) (Hiscock et al., 2000)–has been detected in chondrocytes. The assembly of proteoglycan aggregates occurs in the extracellular matrix (Asari et al., 1994). Aggrecan macromolecules secreted in the extracellular matrix interact with hyaluronan and become incorporated into an aggregate. Due to the huge size of aggregates, comparable to the size of chondrocytes, this interaction can only occur outside the cell.

The rate of the aggregation process slows down in the course of articular cartilage maturation: in adults, secreted aggrecan macromolecules remain longer (up to 18 hours) in the pericellular matrix, whereas, in immature cartilage, they immediately make their way to the interterritorial matrix and begin to be incorporated in aggregates. One limiting factor in the process of aggregation appears to be the maturation of the globular G1 domain. Another limiting factor is the age-related deceleration of link protein synthesis.

The cartilage link protein gene (CTRL1) has five exons and is similar in structure to the part of the aggrecan gene encoding the G1 domain. This is an indication of their evolutionary proximity. The non-translated region of the gene contains two cis-regulatory elements; the activity of one depends on the transcription factor Sox9, the main phenotype-determining factor of chondrocytes (see 10.2.2) (Kou & Ikegawa, 2004). Link protein expression in chondrocytes correlates with the expression of aggrecan, despite the fact that their genes are located on different chromosomes. The N-terminal peptide of link protein can act on chondrocytes as a growth factor stimulating aggrecan expression.

Alongside the aggregates formed by hyaluronan and aggrecan, the cartilage extracellular matrix contains aggregates, in which aggrecan is replaced by a similar large chondroitin sulfate glycoprotein, called **versican**.

Versican, a hyalectan, also known as PG-M and "large fibroblast proteoglycan", is expressed not only in embryongenesis by mesenchymal cells of prechondrogenic condensations, but also by chondroblasts/ chondrocytes after birth. In the postnatal period, the expression rate of versican, determined by the accumulation of mRNA, declines sharply (more than 10 times) and is much lower than the aggrecan expression rate. In mice aged 8 weeks, when the aggrecan concentration in cartilage is approximately 100 ng/mg, the concentration of versican does not exceed 20 ng/100 mg of wet tissue.

Like aggrecan, versican binds to hyaluronan and link protein CLP to form aggregates that are similar to aggrecan aggregates. In the postnatal period, versican incorporated in aggregates is present predominantly in the interterritorial matrix of articular cartilage. Due to the specific structure of the versican macromolecule (contains less glycosaminoglycans than aggrecan, has a lower degree of sulfation of chondroitin sulfate, and lower capability to bind to fibronectin and fibrillin-1), versican aggregates not only complement the anti-compression function of aggrecan aggregates, but also fulfill independent biomechanical functions. It has been proposed that versican aggregates increase the resistance of the superficial zone of articular cartilage to shear strain. Versican aggregates may be involved in the regulation of the effect of growth factors/cytokines on chondrocytes (Matsumoto et al., 2006).

Another characteristic large proteoglycan is present in the extracellular matrix of the superficial zone of articular cartilage, which differs from the deeper layers in the number of biochemical properties and phenotypic features of the chondrocytes (see section 7.2.1.1.2). This is proteoglycan-4 (PRG-4), or **superficial zone protein** (SZP). In vitro experiments have confirmed that SZP is expressed by chondrocytes in the superficial zone of articular cartilage (Blewis et al., 2007). The upregulated expression under the influence of dynamic shear strain and load is especially important for the superficial zone; such a change indicates the importance of SZP in maintaining the biomechanical properties of this zone (Nugent et al., 2006). SZP expression also increases under the influence of the bone morphogenetic protein BMP-7 and the growth factors FGF-2, IGF-1, PDGF, TGF-β1 (Khalafi et al., 2007). SZP expression is absent in the deeper cartilage layers, emphasizing the specific phenotype of chondrocytes in the superficial zone.

SZP is one of the proteins (i.e. one isoform) encoded by a gene known by the names PRG4, SZP and MSF. This gene contains 12 exons. The complete transcript of this gene represents an mRNA encoding a polypeptide with a mass of 400 kDa. The actual isoforms, expressed as a result of alternative splicing of this transcript in different cells, are encoded by different exons and have much smaller molecular size. The megakaryocyte-stimulating factor (MSF) was studied first, and represents a small molecule (with a molecular mass about 25 kDa), which appears to be a growth factor; this name is most often used when referring to the gene and the product of its complete translation.

The SZP (PRG-4) present in cartilage and the synovial fluid providing its lubricating properties, and lubricin (from the word lubricate) are two other isoforms encoded by the MSF gene, which are almost identical in terms of amino acid composition. Lubricin, a glycoprotein with a large amount of O-linked oligosaccharides and a molecular mass of about 227 kDa, is produced and secreted into the synovial fluid by synovial membrane cells. SZP (PRG-4) is expressed by chondrocytes in the superficial

zone, has a much higher (345 kDa) molecular mass and, besides oligosaccharides, contains glycosaminoglycans – chondroitin sulfate and keratan sulfate. These two homologous glycoproteins, encoded mostly by exons 6–9, the largest exons of the MSF gene, differ mainly by the specific features of their carbohydrate components (Jay et al., 2001).

In contrast to aggrecan and versican, SZP produced by chondrocytes does not form aggregates. Thus, it is not fixed in the matrix as firmly as hyalectans. Perhaps for this reason, chondrocytes respond, as previously mentioned, to dynamic mechanical stress by upregulating the expression of SZP, to prevent or limit possible disruptions of specific biomechanical properties of the superficial zone.

SZP, not being bound in aggregates, diffuses to the surface of articular cartilage and into the synovia. There is no direct evidence that the lubricating function of SZP complements the lubricating function of lubricin, and such can only be postulated on the basis of the close resemblance of the primary structures of the two macromolecules. However, it is known that SZP in synovial fluid, together with lubricin, protects the articular surface of cartilage from adhesion of proteins and cells, particularly polymorphonuclear leukocytes, and prevents the proliferation of synovial membrane cells (Rhee et al., 2005).

Large proteoglycans (hyalectans) make up the bulk of proteoglycans in the cartilage extracellular matrix, and they, especially aggrecan, play a defining role in establishing the biomechanical properties of cartilage. This function is mostly associated with the glycosaminoglycans, whose numerous long chains comprise 50% or more of their molecuar mass.

Alongside the large proteoglycans, a number of representatives of all subfamilies (classes) of the small leucine-rich proteoglycans (SLRP) family are present in the cartilage matrix (see Table 3.5.). Like the large proteoglycans, they are expressed by chondrocytes.

Class I SLRP is represented by decorin and biglycan in cartilage; in class II, by fibromodulin, lumican, osteoadherin and PRELP; and in class III, by epiphycan (Roughley, 2006).

Unlike the large proteoglycans, small proteoglycans contain only single, usually short chains of glycosaminoglycans. Accordingly, the functions of small proteoglycans depend on their protein components to an equal or even greater extent than on glycosaminoglycans.

These functions, common to all SLRP in various tissues, are determined by the ability of their core proteins to interact with many other proteins, in particular, with fibrillar collagens. During such interactions, SLRP bind to the surface of collagen fibrils (in cartilage – to fibrils built of type II collagen), thereby influencing the regulation of fibril diameter in the course of fibrillogenesis and interactions between the fibrils themselves. The ability to bind to collagen fibrils is most clearly expressed in decorin, fibromodulin and lumican. Similar interactions, which, according to some reports, require the participation of zinc ions, also occur between SLRP and non-fibrillar collagens. As a result, SLRP may protect collagens from the action of proteolytic enzymes. For example, it has been shown that the cleavage (at a specific site) of the macromolecule of cartilage type IX collagen by matrixin MMP-13 is facilitated by the simultaneous proteolysis of the fibromodulin associated with it (Danfelter et al., 2007).

SLRP interactions – not only with collagens, but also with other proteins – lead to the formation of stable complexes that stabilize the structural organization of the extracellular matrix, including the cartilage tissue matrix, and are necessary for the normal flow of the endochondral ossification process (Roughley, 2006).

Returning to fibromodulin, it should be noted that this keratan-sulfate small proteoglycan exhibits some other effects that are specific to articular cartilage. The content of fibromodulin and decorin – two SLRP that influence collagen (including type II collagen) fibrillogenesis more actively than the other SLRP – is higher in the superficial zone. Together with the presence of SZP, this represents another biochemical characteristic of the superficial zone. Perhaps due to this preferential localization of fibromodulin in mice with a null mutation of the *Fmod* gene, encoding fibromodulin, an increased frequency of spontaneous knee osteoarthritis has been observed (Gill et al., 2002).

Epiphycan (otherwise known as dermatan sulfate proteoglycan-3 is a small proteoglycan present mainly in the cartilage tissue of epiphyses, suggesting its involvement in endochondral osteogenesis. It may also participate in regulating the structural organization of the cartilage matrix. Epiphycan, whose protein core consists of 303 amino acid residues and contains seven leucine-rich repeats, carries one dermatan sulfate chain, three O-linked and two N-linked oligosaccharides (Knudson & Knudson, 2001).

Proteins that belong to the SLRP family but are not proteoglycans are present in cartilage tissue. Chondroadherin (or leucine-rich repeat protein, CRLP) contains 11 leucine-rich repeats, and has only one O-linked oligosaccharide. It forms complexes with type II collagen, which is concentrated in the pericellular matrix and contribute to strengthening the connections between collagen fibrils and chondrocytes (Månsson et al., 2001)

A unique protein from the SLRP family is present in large amounts in articular cartilage and menisci, which represent fibrous cartilage. It is structurally similar to the decorin and biglycan molecules, but, unlike decorin, it does not contain glycosaminoglycans and, therefore, is not a proteoglycan. This is **asporin**, a glycoprotein with molecular mass of about 43 kDa, which consists of 343 amino acids, and contains an O-linked and N-linked oligosaccharides. The most conspicuous feature of its primary structure is the high content of aspartic acid residues, as reflected in its name. Most of these residues are concentrated in the amino terminal section of the polypeptide chain, where there is a continuous sequence of D-residues (D is a one-letter code for aspartic acid) that contains 13–14 D.

In the cartilage tissue matrix, asporin binds to growth factors from the TGF-β superfamily, and inhibits their activity aimed at stimulating the expression of chondrocyte marker genes (Nakajima et al., 2007). This physiological function of asporin is characteristic of its more common isoform D13, which contains a sequence of 13 aspartic acid residues. In humans exhibiting a prevalence of the D14 isoform, in which this sequence contains an extra D residue, asporin's inhibitory function becomes excessive, the stability of the chondrocyte phenotype is disrupted, and the susceptibility to development of osteoarthritis increases dramatically (Kizawa et al., 2005). Asporin expression is elevated in patients with osteoarthritis.

Two members of the SLRP family – PRELP and lumican – known for their ability to bind to both collagens and structural components of basement membranes, are present in the cartilage extracellular matrix.

PRELP (or prolargin) is a proline- and arginine-rich protein that contains 12 leucine-rich repeats (LRR) among its 362 amino acid residues. It can carry two to three keratan sulfate chains but, for the most part, only contains four N-oligosaccharides. PRELP binds to the glycosaminoglycan chains of the large proteoglycan perlecan in basement membranes. These bonds, combined with the collagen links, enable PRELP to attach the basement membrane to the connective tissue matrix (Bengtsson et al., 2002).

Lumican, a protein with 12 LRR, is also a partial keratan sulfate proteoglycan of the cartilage matrix. During embryogenesis, when its concentration in the tissue is higher, it contains up to three to four keratan sulfate chains, but later it is present as a glycoprotein with four N-oligosaccharides. Lumican binds to laminin, the major glycoprotein of basement membranes, and its function may be similar to that of prolargin.

There is an explanation for the seemingly paradoxical presence of small, basement membrane-interacting proteoglycans (SLRP) in the cartilage extracellular matrix, which has no basement membranes as distinct morphological entities. All four major macromolecular components that form the basement membranes – type IV collagen, perlecan, laminin and nidogen – have been found in the territorial (pericellular) matrix of articular cartilage (Kvist et al., 2008). This means that PRELP and lumican can form the same intermolecular bonds they form at the interface of the connective tissue matrix with basement membranes.

Like all other connective tissue cells, cartilage cells are not isolated by the established basement membrane from the matrix they produce. Most structural macromolecules characteristic of basement membranes, and localized in the chondron in close proximity to the chondroblasts/chondrocytes plasma membrane, have recently been considered as the functional equivalent of the basement membrane. These macromolecules, together with the associated SLRP, probably reinforce chondron structure and contribute to the spatial fixation of chondrocytes in the matrix and to stabilizing their phenotype (Kvist et al., 2008).

In cartilage tissue, the functions of perlecan, the large, multidomain, heparan-sulfate proteoglycan (see section 3.3.2) are not limited to its involvement in the structural organization of the chondron, where perlecan binds to the WARP protein (see Table. 7.5) (Allen et al., 2006).

During embryogenesis, perlecan is diffusely distributed throughout the cartilage extracellular matrix, and it concentrates in the pericellular matrix only in the postnatal period. The changes in localization are not the only ones that take place during ontogenesis. The changes affect the size and structure of the protein core of the macromolecules; heparan sulfate can be replaced by chondroitin sulfate; and a complete loss of glycosaminoglycans can occur (Melrose et al., 2006). Depending on these changes, the links of perlecan with other molecules, and the related nature and direction of their effects, also change. Thus, the chondroitin-sulfate perlecan (perlecan in which heparan sulfate is replaced by chondroitin sulfate) is required for the normal formation of type II collagen fibrils. The absence of this perlecan isoform leads to the most severe, lethal form of chondrodysplasia, whose phenotypic pattern matches the pathological picture generated by null mutations in the type II collagen gene (Kvist et al., 2006).

Like other heparan-sulfate proteoglycans, perlecan binds to many signaling molecules in the matrix, thereby modulating the effects caused by these molecules. In particular, perlecan binds to the fibroblast growth factor FGF-2, which transmits impulses of mechanical origin to chondrocytes; in other words, perlecan regulates the mechanotransduction and tissue reaction to mechanical stress (Vincent et al., 2007).

During *in vitro* experiments, perlecan induces chondrogenic differentiation of embryonic mesenchymal cells, which suggests its possible role in the initial stages of chondrogenesis in vivo. At the same time, perlecan is actively expressed by chondrocytes undergoing hypertrophy during endochondral ossification; switching off the perlecan gene (*Pln*) at this stage of embryogenesis causes disruptions in the growth and shape of long bones (Gomes et al., 2004).

Growth plate (metaphyseal cartilage) chondrocytes actively express another large heparan-sulfate proteoglycan of the basement membranes – **agrin**. This proteoglycan is known mainly as a component of the basement membrane of the neuromuscular synapse. It consists of 2016 amino acid residues, its macromolecule contains 23 disulfide bonds, and it has two heparan sulfate chains. Turning off the agrin-encoding gene, *Agrn*, causes disruptions in the structure of the hypertrophic zone of growth cartilage and reduces the type II collagen and aggrecan content in this area. These disorders result in growth inhibition (Hauser et al., 2007).

7.2.1.2.4.2. Morphological characteristics of structured polysaccharide complex

In articular cartilage, as in other human connective tissues, the interstitial (interfibrillar and intercellular) space is filled with ground substance (integrating buffer metabolic medium). This medium is comprised of water, glycoconjugates, mineral salts, the molecular precursors of collagen, and plasma proteins. The properties of articular cartilage and its vital functions are strongly dependent on the qualitative and quantitative composition of this medium. Through the use of TEM, SEM and a proteoglycan-specific marker – the synthetic substance ruthenium red, several forms of structured proteoglycans have been found in articular cartilage: a fine granular amorphous substance, large granules, a meshwork structure, "shells" and crosslines of collagen fibrils (*Fig. 7.28*). All structures of a proteoglycan nature are interconnected and form an integrated system with the fibrous (collagen) core. Thus, there is a dense layer of spherical particles (globules), 20–60 nm in size, on the surface of collagen fibrils. The globules form an envelope for the fibrils by covering them. Similar structures occupy a significant part of the interfibrillar spaces. Here, the globules form aggregates, consisting of several spherical particles. Some of the gaps remain unfilled by ruthenium-positive structures. Such spaces have a round or oval shape and fuzzy contours with equivalent diameters of 20–150 nm. Evidently in native cartilage, the channels are filled with water, belonging to the fraction that is not firmly bound to proteoglycans, and, therefore, it moves relatively easily in the interfibrillar spaces during cartilage deformation, dampening the compressive mechanical load.

Thus, the main pathways for transporting metabolic products and for the movement of liquids are determined by the existence of two interacting, inseparable systems – microchannels of different diameters, interconnected with the chondrocyte lacunae and the joint cavity, and the integrating buffer metabolic medium, where water is also bound to a different extent. This is one of the mechanisms by which the organism regulates the life activity of articular cartilage and the execution of its biomechanical functions. The parameters of these systems constantly change during joint movement. This gives rise to the reversible deformation of cartilage fibrillar structures, which inevitably leads to an alteration in the balanced energy state of its fibrous core. The degree of orientation of contiguous collagen fibrils increases, i.e. they become organized. According to the literature, this should result in a reduction of the system's entropy, i.e. in an increase of its free energy. Furthermore, the deformation of the fibrils increases their internal energy due to changes in intermolecular distances. All of this creates the potential for restoring the structure of the fibrous core.

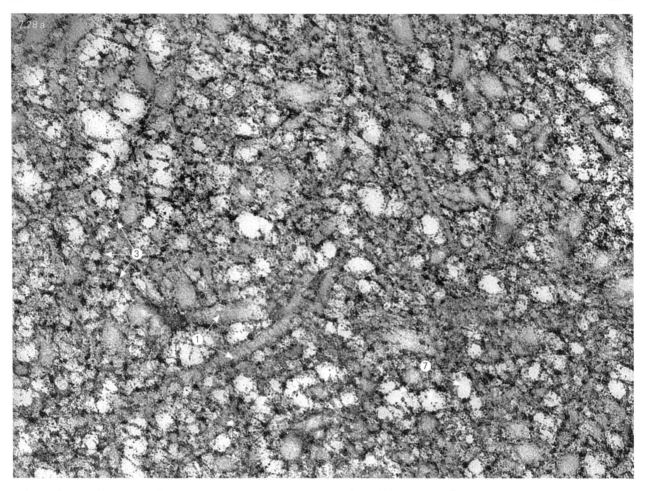

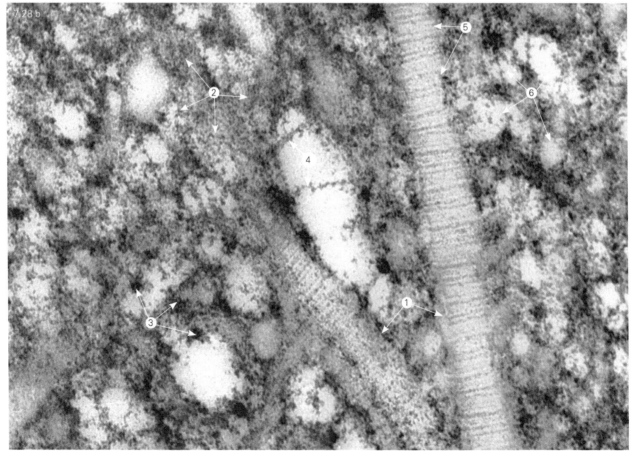

7.28 c

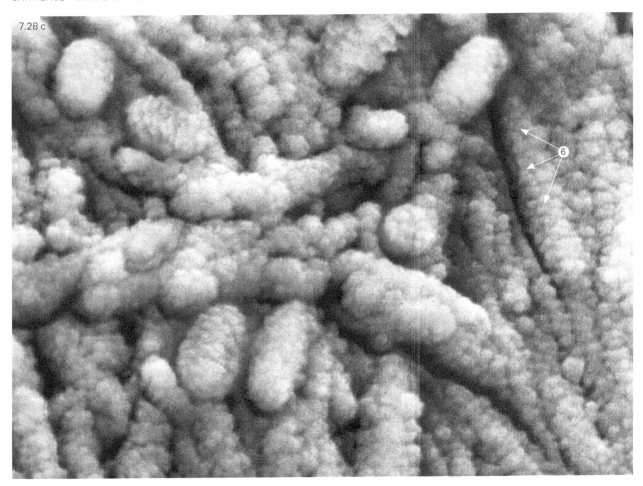

Fig. 7.28.
A fragment of articular
hyaline cartilage.
Collagen fibrils (1).
Ruthenium-positive structures
of proteoglycan nature: finely
granular amorphous
substance (2),
cluster "nodes" (3)
filaments (4),
cross-striation
of collagen fibrils (5)
Granules (6) on the surface
of collagen fibrils and in the
interfibrillar space.
Free Space (7).
a, b – TEM-micrograph.
Ruthenium red staining.
a – x 20,000;
b – x 40,000;
c – SEM-micrograph,
x 40,000.

When under pressure, fluid moves in different directions inside the cartilage. Part of this fluid can obviously go beyond the cartilage boundary into the joint cavity and mix with the synovia. Another part can exit into the interstitial space of the subchondral bone through holes in the mineralized cartilage and subchondral bone lamella (see section 7.2.1.2.1.2). The speed of this movement is limited by the porous structure of cartilage. Therefore, a burst of water bound into proteoglycan gel through "nozzles" (holes) can be observed. The above principle of damping the acting force is used in liquid shock absorbers. Therefore, the amortization function of cartilage depends on the fibrillar architectonics, channel diameter, the extent of water bound into the gel, i.e. the qualitative (chemical) composition of proteoglycans. Convergence of collagen fibrils increases the capillarity in the pressure area, whereas forcing the fluid out into adjacent areas, not subjected to the action of the load, shifts the osmotic balance of the tissue fluid. This is due to the fact that the concentration of proteoglycans, salts, and tissue proteins is higher in the load zone. Thus, the osmotic and capillary forces have to act in the same direction as forces generated in the fibrous framework, i.e. while gradually growing, they will resist the mechanical loading and will further participate in restoring the collagen fibrils' original architectonics once the load action on the cartilage ends. The described mechanism is presented in *Fig. 7.29*. Clearly, alterations in the shape of articular cartilage under load are associated with molecular rearrangement of its polymer network. The main forces resisting compression and regenerating the cartilage are the elasticity of the collagen network and the swelling pressure of the proteoglycan gel.

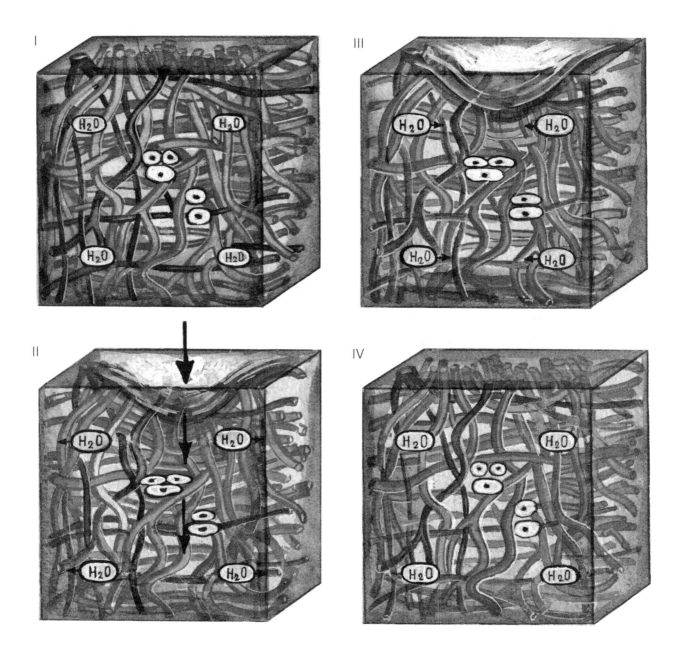

Fig. 7.29.
Schematic diagram of the hypothetical mechanism of articular cartilage's amortization function. (According to Omelyanenko) A cartilage fragment.

I. Intact state of the fibrous (fibrillar) core and the ground substance.
II. Load action (pressure) on the cartilage (I). Deformation of collagen fibrils, their convergence, and shrinking of interfibrillar spaces in the load area.

Water movement from the point of loading and deformation in the adjacent areas.
III. The deformed cartilage in the absence of load. Water returns to the area of load action. The shape of collagen fibrils is restored.

IV. The regenerated structure of cartilage.

7.2.1.3. Cartilaginous tissue as an integrated system (structural and functional unity of cells and matrix)

From a functional or biomechanical point of view, the cartilage extracellular matrix represents a three-phase composite material. Its main constituents are:

a) water;

b) collagenous fibrous elements; and

c) proteoglycan aggregates that fill the interfibrillar space of the matrix. The quantitative ratio of the masses of these three components varies among different types of cartilage and, for articular cartilage, can be expressed as 6.5 : 2.5 : 1. Water, which accounts for 2/3 of the matrix mass, is sometimes seen as a passive mobile phase that fills the pores between the supramolecular structures formed by the other two phases (Soulhat et al., 1999).

These supramolecular structures represent two interlocking frameworks or, in other words, two three-dimensional networks that regulate the content and movement of water in the matrix.

The first network is formed of collagen fibrils. The foundation of is collagen fibrils is collagenous proteins. Made primarily of type II collagen (often named incorrectly as type II collagen fibers), but also containing small fibrillar (V/XI types) and nonfibrillar (IX type) collagens linked by stable covalent bonds. Type VI collagen fibrils are associated with these heterotypic fibrils, and this association is secured by the macromolecules of the small proteoglycans–biglycan and decorin–as well as the glycoprotein matrilin-1 (Wiberg et al., 2003). Through these associations, the network of collagen fibrils in the matrix acquires reinforcing properties–strength and a certain toughness.

The second network is based on aggrecan aggregates, each containing aggrecan macromolecules linked by a hyaluronan chain. The aggrecan aggregates are stable supramolecular structures due to the covalent bonds between aggrecans, on the one hand, and hyaluronan, on the other. These connections are further strengthened by link protein.

Other matrix molecules are involved in building the proteoglycan network too–the non-collagenous cartilage matrix protein (CMP) and the cartilage oligomeric matrix protein (COMP/thrombospondin-5) (Chen et al., 2007), which bind to aggrecan. At the same time, some small matrix proteoglycans–decorin, biglycan, and fibromodulin–form bonds, possibly of a covalent nature, with the central part of the aggregates–hyaluronan (Roughley, 2006).

Thus, two three-dimensional networks (or two frameworks) coexist in the cartilage matrix: a collagenous network, and a slightly less rigid proteoglycan network. The existence of covalent bonds between the components of both networks has not been proven, and it is quite likely that the networks have some motility with respect to each other. The proteoglycan macromolecules forming the proteoglycan network are much more metabolically dynamic than collagens.

The function of both networks is primarily aimed at maintaining optimal, from a biomechanical point of view, water content in the tissue.

The aggrecan aggregates, by virtue of the polyanionic properties of their component, sulfated glycosaminoglycans, bind to a large number of electrically charged ions. The localization of these charges in the tissue is determined by local concentration and is fixed in accordance with the three-dimensional structure of the proteoglycan network. This creates a very important physicochemical property of the cartilage extracellular matrix, known as **fixed-charge density** (FCD). FCD is the main (albeit not the only) factor that imparts the ability to retain large amounts of water to the matrix (Chen et al., 2001). Such high water content is normal for cartilage tissue and is routinely assessed as hyperhydration.

Water retained in the tissue, as incompressible fluid that has the same volume at a constant temperature, provides resistance to compression (compressive strength) and endows the tissue with a certain degree of stiffness. At the same time, under compressive forces, water molecules can move in the pores among the structural macromolecular components of the cartilage matrix, as well as exit from and return to the cartilage. By virtue of the extent of deformability reached, mainly due to this water mobility, a uniform distribution of compressive stress is achieved in various regions of the articular cartilage move. The intrinsic deformability of some matrix macromolecules and the tighter overall packing of the matrix further contribute to cartilage deformability.

The collagenous framework acts in the opposite direction. By stabilizing the entire matrix as a whole, and reducing the mobility of its structural macromolecular components, it determines the spatial organization of aggrecan aggregates, compresses them, and limits the volume of space that aggregates occupy.

Due to the inability of the aggrecan protein core and the glycosaminoglycan chains to unfold completely, in the matrix this volume represents only about 15% of the volume occupied by the aggregates in an aqueous solution, given the absence of a collagen network. Such a restriction on the volume occupied by aggregates prevents the excessive accumulation of water in the tissue and helps to maintain the water content at a fairly stable level. Thus, the collagen framework prevents a transition from the normal state of hyperhydration to a pathological state, where excess water would lead to swelling of the tissue.

Furthermore, the collagen fibrils endow the tissue with resistance to stretching, or in other words, with tensile strength, whereby not just the amount of collagen in the cartilage, but also the extent of intermolecular crosslinking of the collagen fibrils is important (Williamson et al., 2003). At the same time, the compressive resistance of collagen fibrils is very low, and they cannot provide compressive strength (Myers & Mow, 1983).

The absence (or weakness) of covalent chemical bonds between the collagen fibrils network and the network of aggrecan aggregates is compensated by a set of mechanical bonds (mainly collagen fibrils' contacts with the keratan sulfate-rich region of aggrecan (Hedlund et al., 1999) and electrostatic bonds (interactions between negatively charged groups in glycosaminoglycan molecules and positively charged groups in collagen fibrils).

Both networks are dependent of each other for their structural organization and biomechanical functions. For example, experimental destruction of the cartilage tissue proteoglycan network by trypsin digestion enhances the disorganizing effect of mechanical stress on collagen fibrils' architecture (Saar et al., 2007). Disrupting aggrecan biosynthesis by inhibiting the incorporation of glycosaminoglycans into its macromolecules during cartilage extracellular matrix formation distorts the collagen network, leading to its disorganization and biomechanical deficiency (Bastiaansen-Jenniskens et al., 2009). Thus, the integrity of the cartilage extracellular matrix as a morphological and functional system is determined by the interaction of two organized supramolecular structures–the network of large collagen fibrils and the network of aggrecan aggregates. All other matrix components–numerous, but insignificant in terms of total mass, play very important roles that are complementary with respect to these main structures–they control their formation and modulate their properties.

Hyaluronan plays an especially important organizing role, by integrating the aggrecan macromolecules into aggregates and acting as a foundation for the proteoglycan network. Disruptions in the biosynthesis or depolymerization of hyaluronan cause serious pathological alterations in the cartilage tissue matrix (Bastow et al., 2007).

The morphological and functional integrity of the extracellular matrix is possible owing to the constant interaction between the matrix and chondrocytes. This interaction, which transforms the cartilage into an integrated system, is mediated by a number of proteins–chondrocyte plasma membrane receptors. The most significant of these receptors are the heterodimeric adhesion receptors- integrins.

Mature articular cartilage chondrocytes express at least nine types of integrins: α1β1, α2β1, α3β1, α5β1, α6β1, α10β1, α11β1, αvβ3, αvβ5. This set of integrins is sufficient for interactions with all ligands present in the extracellular matrix; integrin α10β1, in particular, is considered as specialized in the binding of type II collagen, α1β1–type VI collagen and matrilina-1; α11β1–type IX collagen and α5β1–fibronectins and thrombospondin-5. Ligand (matrix components)-bound integrins transmit into the cell signals, which regulate chondrocyte differentiation, its viability, matrix remodeling, and the reaction to the action of mechanical factors (Loeser, 2002).

Integrins containing the β1 subunit predominate among the chondrocyte integrins; these integrins are involved in regulating cell proliferation (the cell cycle) and chon-

drocyte motility in the chondrogenesis and endochondral ossification processes (Aszódi et al., 2003). β1 subunit deficiency in articular cartilage chondrocytes of the knee joint (in mice) is accompanied by the structural disorganization of cartilage, the accelerated terminal differentiation of chondrocytes, the destruction of their actin cytoskeleton, and a decline in their viability. These pathological changes occur in a paradoxical manner, in the absence of detectable disturbances in the metabolism of cartilage tissue (Raducanu et al., 2009).

The signals that influence gene expression of chondrocytes travel a complex route, which includes cell entry mediated by integrins, numerous proteins of focal adhesions, and the activation of several kinases [these include the focal adhesion kinases (FAK), proline-rich tyrosine kinase 2 (Pyk2) and mitogen-activated protein kinase (MAP)] (Loeser, 2002).

At the same time, the system of focal adhesion proteins transmits impulses from integrins to cytoskeleton components, in particular actin microfilaments, which brings about the restructuring of the cytoskeleton and the alteration of the entire structural organization of the cells (Lo, 2006).

Integrin gene knockouts, as well as integrin blocking through the introduction of specific antibodies or synthetic peptides containing the RGD-sequence into chondrocyte cultures (such peptides compete with natural ligands, since integrins use these same "sticky" sequences for binding with ligands) disrupt chondrocyte adhesion to the matrix and inhibit the stimulating effect on the biosynthetic activity of chondrocytes coming from the matrix (mainly from type II collagen). In this case there are also changes in the qualitative composition of the matrix expressed by chondrocytes (Qi & Scully, 2003).

Besides integrins, the transmembrane receptor, heparan sulfate glycoprotein CD44 (synonyms: epican, hyaluronate receptor) plays an important role in chondrocytes' interactions with the extracellular matrix. This glycoprotein is similar to the members of the syndecan family (see section 3.2.1.2). Its macromolecules gather in clusters in the plasma membrane, creating the possibility for the absorption (internalization) of hyaluronan by the cells. Internalization is the main path for the normal catabolism of this glycosaminoglycan. At the same time, CD44, which exists as several isoforms encoded by a single gene, is an adhesion receptor of the highest importance for the overall structure of cartilage tissue. It forms bonds that attach hyaluronan chains, the foundation of aggrecan aggregates, to the plasma membrane of chondrocytes (Knudson & Knudson, 2004).

The receptor role of CD44 is not limited to chondrocytes' adhesion to the matrix. Through interactions with ligands from the extracellular matrix (hyaluronan is the most significant, but not the only ligand of CD44), CD44 turns into a starting point of several intracellular signal transduction cascades for signals originating from the matrix. These signals affect both the cytoskeleton, and the metabolic functions of chondrocytes. Hence, CD44, together with integrins, can be considered to be among the signaling regulators of chondrocytes (Ponta et al., 2003). Inhibiting CD44 expression, or its blockage, which can be achieved using oligosaccharide fragments of hyaluronan, cause phenotypic changes to or even apoptosis of chondrocytes, as well as disturbances to the homeostasis of the cartilage matrix; chondrolysis (matrix destruction) is manifested as changes in the tinctorial properties of the matrix.

In contrast, stimulation of CD44 receptors, inducible in vitro by introducing polymeric hyaluronan into the chondrocyte culture, upregulates their biosynthetic activity, thus increasing the deposition of type II collagen and chondroitin sulfates into the matrix that they produce (Akmal et al., 2005).

In addition to CD44, chondrocytes express a number of other heparan sulfate proteoglycans in their plasma membrane. These are syndecans (see section 3.2.1.2) and glypican-3 – a proteoglycan, which is also a lipoprotein and whose molecule does not traverse the membrane, but is located entirely on the outer surface of the membrane and is covalently bound to it by means of glycosylphosphatidylinositol (Filmus, 2001). These proteoglycans function as co-receptors in the contacts of chondrocytes with signaling molecules, mainly growth factors, thereby modulating their interaction with the main receptors.

Chondrocytes express a representative of the large family of annexins, annexin V. Annexins, also known as lipocortins, are small proteins usually localized at the inner surface of the plasma membrane. They have the ability to bind phospholipids and calcium, and also possess anticoagulant activity. The molecules of all annexins contain four repetitive domains, with 60–80 amino acid residues in each of them. A sequence of 17 residues, which starts with lysine and ends with serine and arginine, is common to all these repeats. The carboxyl domain is markedly hydrophobic due to the predominance of hydrophobic residues therein (Mark & Mollenhauer, 1997).

Annexin V, found in cartilage tissue, is an exception. Similar to glypicans, it is located on the outer surface of the cell membrane. Its full name is cartilage annexin V, even though it is expressed by fibroblasts and osteoblasts too, and its amino acid composition is 100% homologous to annexin V, present intracellularly in other tissues. Human annexin V contains 319 amino acid residues. Its expression is high in the embryonic period, especially in the hypertrophic chondrocytes of growth plates. It is also found on the membrane surface of matrix vesicles, suggesting the possibility of its participation in mineralization (see section 8.2.2.1). During in vitro experiments, annexin V is highly selective for binding to native (but not denatured) type II collagen. The binding occurs via the macromolecule's aminoterminal telopeptide, whereas the carboxyterminal telopeptide and the triple-helical domain interact with integrins, but not with annexin V (Lucic et al., 2003).

The binding of annexin V to collagen fibrils of the cartilage matrix, consisting mainly of type II collagen, explains the other name for this receptor protein – anchorin CII. There is a lack of direct evidence of this binding in vivo, but there are sufficient grounds to consider annexin V (anchorin CII) as an important factor in the interactions between chondrocytes and the matrix, especially during morphogenesis. One of these reasons is its enhanced expression by chondrocytes in articular cartilage during the development of osteoarthrosis, when the compensatory reorganization of the tissue takes place (Mollenhauer et al., 1999). Annexin V, together with the $\beta5$ subunit of integrins, regulate the apoptosis of hypertrophic chondrocytes in the growth plate – an obligatory step of endochondral ossification (Wang & Kirsch, 2006).

A developed system of receptors in chondrocytes' plasma membrane ensures a constant flow of information between these cells and the extracellular matrix. Given that the small number of cells in mature cartilage tissue limits the possibilities for intercellular information-exchange contacts, the matrix plays the role of the principal information system, which regulates chondrocytes' metabolic functions.

First, chondrocytes perceive information about the very presence of the matrix in their environment, and about the concentrations in the matrix of its structural components. Experiments with cartilage tissue cultures have shown that the depletion of any structural component in the matrix, achieved by exposure of the culture to enzymes (collagenase, hyaluronidase, papain), entails (prior to the visible destructive changes in chondrocytes) the upregulation of biosynthetic processes directed at compensating for the deficit created around the cell. Dedifferentiation (loss of the chondrocyte phenotype) is a frequent consequence of the enzymatic destruction of the matrix, but the compensatory direction of the biosynthetic activity of chondrocytes is also preserved in this case; this activity is manifested as the expression of nonspecific macromolecules, for instance, the expression of type I collagen instead of type II collagen. Similar compensatory processes based on a feedback principle develop in vivo; for example, by intravenously administering the proteolytic enzyme papain to animals, causing the systemic destruction of the cartilage extracellular matrix.

Second, chondrocytes, mainly with the involvement of integrins, sense signals emanating directly from the macromolecular structural components of the matrix, and these signals have a positive impact on maintaining the phenotype of cultured chondrocytes. For example, supplementing a chondrocyte culture with exogenous native type II collagen enhances the TGFβ-1 growth factor-induced expression in chondrocytes of the two major structural components of the matrix – aggrecan and α1(II)-procollagen. A certain specificity of this effect is manifested in the inability of denatured type II collagen to provoke the same effect (Scully, 2001).

Third, hyaluronan, a macromolecular matrix component, has a positive effect on the chondrocyte phenotype. When cultured on artificial hybrid polymeric biomaterials, which have hyaluronan introduced in their composition, chondrocytes that have lost their phenotype under different culture conditions undergo redifferentiation. They resume the active expression of type II collagen and aggrecan, whereas the expression of type I collagen (not characteristic for chondrocytes) in chondrocytes is inhibited (Grigolo et al., 2002).

Macromolecular components of the matrix, particularly type II collagen and fibronectin, use integrins not only to transmit signals into chondrocytes. They can modulate the very expression of integrins by the cells, at least in vitro, making chondrocytes even more susceptible to influence from the matrix (Kim et al., 2003).

The functional activity of chondrocytes is rather strongly affected by components of the extracellular matrix concentrated in the chondron, i.e. in the territorial matrix in direct contact with the chondrocytes. Differences in the expression levels of 258 genes were found upon comparing (with the help of cDNA microarrays) the gene expression profiles of chondrocytes isolated from cartilage and cultured in cell culture conditions against chondrocytes cultured in cartilage fragments, where they reside inside intact chondrons (see section 7.2.1.1.1). These differences are indicative of the benefits of stabilizing the chondrocyte phenotype provided by the influence of the territorial matrix (Zhang et al., 2006).

Along with the direct information influence exerted on chondrocytes by structural macromolecular components of the extracellular matrix, another function of these components is at least as important–their involvement in the regulation of traffic in the matrix, and in modulating the activity of signaling molecules with system-wide (hormones, vitamins) and local (growth factors/cytokines, morphogens) actions. Several examples of this participation have already been presented when characterizing the functions of matrix components.

Complex interactions of several components play a role in performing these functions. For example, in chondrocytes, the anabolic factor, insulin-like growth factor IGF-1, which stimulates chondrogenic differentiation, is maintained in an inactive state in the territorial matrix of adult articular cartilage, where it is associated with a complex consisting of the insulin-like growth factor-binding protein 3 (IGFBP-3) and fibronectin. IGF-1 is released from this bond when it is necessary to stimulate chondrocytes' biosynthetic activity (Martin et al., 2002).

7.2.1.4 Metabolism of cartilaginous tissue

The peculiarity of metabolic processes in cartilage tissue lies in the fact that all of its varieties are deprived of blood vessels. The lack of vessels, inherent to both transitory and permanent cartilage, is determined by the common molecular mechanisms of their morphogenesis (Eames & Helms, 2004). The cartilage extracellular ma-trix contains components (chondromodulins and some others) that prevent angiogenesis.

In those cartilages (for example, rib cartilage), which are covered with a perichondrium, the lack of proper blood vessels is compensated by perichondrial blood vessels. Metabolite molecules from the latter diffuse into the interior of the extracellular matrix. Articular cartilages do not have a perichondrium and are separated by the tidemark from the subchondral bone, which is rich in vessels; chondrocytes can obtain the necessary materials for metabolic processes from the blood only after the prior diffusion through the synovia (synovial fluid), followed by movement through the matrix.

In aqueous solutions, diffusion dynamics depend on the diffusion coefficient–a parameter determined by the size and shape of the diffusing molecules. With respect to diffusion through a cartilage matrix filled with aggrecan aggregates and having the consistency of a dense gel, this ratio should be amended to account for the mechanical difficulty of molecular movement. The electric charges of aggrecan's glycosaminoglycans, which affect the movement of those molecules that also carry an electric charge, should be taken into account. In the case of articular cartilage, it is also necessary to make another correction regarding the mechanical difficulties of diffusion through the synovial fluid, which is a very viscous hyaluronan solution. These corrections are reflected in an additional parameter–the distribution coefficient, which is calculated by taking into account the ratio of the diffusion coefficient in the matrix to the diffusion coefficient in water. Such relative coefficients, characterizing the permeability of the cartilage matrix for different classes of molecules, are presented in *Table. 7.7.* As can be seen from the following table, the distribution coefficients of small nonpolar molecules (that do not carry an electric charge) is close to 1, suggesting that all or nearly all the water in the cartilage matrix is available for the penetration of small uncharged molecules.

Electrically charged molecules and ions behave differently. For monovalent cations (e.g. sodium), distribution coefficients are well above 1 and increase proportionally to the glycosaminoglycan content in the matrix. This illustrates the Donnan effect (Donnan law) caused by the fixed negative charges of glycosaminoglycan molecules. Due to the effect of this law, the distribution coefficients for divalent cations (e.g. calcium) are even higher, and this results in higher concentration of cations in the cartilage matrix than in the synovial fluid.

Similarly to other cations, the concentration of hydrogen ions in the cartilage extracellular matrix is also elevated, also proportionally to the glycosaminoglycan content. The matrix medium is more acidic than the synovial, with a difference of about 0.3 pH units.

For anions, the distribution coefficient between synovial fluid and cartilage matrix is less than 1 and, therefore, is considerably lower than is the case for the cations. The overall rate of penetration of electrolytes in the matrix is determined by the slowest ion, i.e. the anion, and there-

Table 7.7

Distribution coefficients and relative diffusion coefficients of various molecules in the cartilage extracellular matrix

Type of molecules	Examples	Molar distribution coefficient (mol/ml)	Ratio of the diffusion coefficient in the matrix to the diffusion coefficient in water
Small uncharged molecules	Water	1,0	0,40–0,45
	Urea, proline	1,0	0,40–0,45
	Glucose	1,0	0,40–0,45
	Saccharose	1,0	0,40–0,45
Small cations	Na^+	1,5	0,40
	Ca^{2+}	3,0	0,25
Small anions	Cl^-	0,75	0,40–0,45
	SO_4^{2-}	0,6	0,40–0,45
Globular proteins	Blood serum albumin	0,01	0,25
	Immunoglobulin IgG	0,01	0,20

fore the transport of electrolytes in cartilage tissues is slower than the transport of uncharged molecules. Thus, the diffusion of glucose is faster than the diffusion of sodium sulfate, even though the glucose molecule is larger in size.

Despite differences in the diffusion rates between polar and nonpolar molecules, the degree of diffusion of all low molecular mass substances in the matrix is quite sufficient to satisfy the metabolic requirements of chondrocytes throughout the entire thickness of articular cartilage, even in the most massive parts of human hip joint cartilage, where the thickness of the cartilage reaches 3.5–5 mm.

The only exception, particularly significant for articular cartilage, is oxygen, whose diffusion is additionally limited by its low concentration in synovial fluid. At the actual oxygen concentration in synovia ($3–10 \times 10-8$ mol/ml), the diffusion of oxygen only allows penetration to a depth of about 1.8 mm. Cells located in cartilage layers more remote from the articular surface experience a shortage of oxygen. If the partial pressure of oxygen in intercellular spaces of soft tissues is 15–20 mm Hg on average, in articular cartilage, it does not exceed 5–8 mm. Furthermore, it is about 10 times lower in the deep layers of cartilage than is the case on the surface (Archer & Francis-West, 2003).

As a consequence, the metabolic processes in chondrocytes from different layers of cartilage occur at different rates. This is another manifestation of the metabolic heterogeneity of articular cartilage.

The metabolic activity of cartilage chondrocytes that experience a shortage of oxygen is supported by energy generated by anaerobic glycolysis. This mode of energy supply is an adaptive mechanism, allowing the cartilage cells to function under conditions of very low oxygen concentrations. The lower the oxygen concentration in the cartilage matrix, the higher the rate of anaerobic glycolysis and, respectively, of lactic acid production in chondrocytes.

The phenotypic adaptation to anaerobic conditions (hypoxia), characteristic for chondrocytes, can be observed in in vitro experiments. With an increasing degree of hypoxia, not only are anabolic processes not inhibited, but are even activated (Rajpurohit et al., 1996). In particular, the efficiency of glucose utilization by the cells increases, enabling the more economical use of energy.

The decisive role in the molecular mechanism of this adaptation is ascribed to the transcription factor HIF-1α (hypoxia-inducible factor-1α), also known as MOP1. This phosphoprotein consists of 826 amino acid residues and has a molecular mass 93 kDa in humans. It is present in all body cells and is considered the main regulator of the adaptive response to hypoxia. HIF-1α is localized in the cytoplasm in normoxia (normal oxygen supply). In the case of oxygen deficiency, it translocates to the nucleus and binds to the so-called **hypoxia response element**

(HRE) in DNA, and activates the transcription of more than 40 genes by acting on their promoters. The proteins encoded by these genes (glucose transporters, glycolytic enzymes, vascular endothelial growth factor, erythropoietin, etc.) facilitate the metabolic adaptation to hypoxia.

These effects of the transcription factor HIF-1α are essential for the normal metabolism of chondrocytes, particularly for chondrocytes in the growth plate. In its absence, the biosynthesis of large matrix components – type II collagen and aggrecan – is reduced in chondrocytes cultured under hypoxia (Pfander et al., 2003). The effect of HIF-1α on the chondrocyte phenotype is most likely mediated by the HIF-1α-induced transcription of the Sox9 gene, which regulates the activity of chondrocyte-specific genes. The regulatory action of HIF-1α on Sox9 is required for chondroblast differentiation from its earliest stages, as well as to stabilize the phenotype and maintain the viability of chondroblasts/ chondrocytes (Amarillo et al., 2007).

According to some sources, another related transcription factor, HIF-2α (also known as EPAS-1), is even more important for the formation of hypoxia-adapted phenotype of chondrocytes in human articular cartilage. HIF-2α is a phosphoprotein containing 870 amino acid residues. It is localized in the nucleus, and its stimulating effect on the extracellular matrix biosynthesis is also associated with the activation of the SOX9 gene (Lafont et al., 2007).

Chondrocytes adapted to hypoxia exhibit a paradoxical reaction to the increasing partial pressure of oxygen: such an increase is accompanied by the inhibition of biosynthetic processes, in particular, a decrease in the biosynthesis of DNA, type II collagen and proteoglycans.

The predominantly anaerobic route of energy supply, in combination with the small number of cells, determines the relatively low overall level of metabolic rates in mature cartilage. The results of metabolic experiments using radioactive isotopes indicate that, in human adult articular cartilage, approximately 50% of all proteoglycan molecules are replaced per year, while other data (Maroudas et al., 1998) suggests that the half-life of aggrecan macromolecules is 3.4 years.

Collagenous proteins turn over much more slowly: at least 10 years are required to replace 50% of collagen molecules. This represents the minimum level of biosynthesis that is required to repair minor damage to articular cartilage, which will inevitably occur throughout a lifetime. The majority of collagen macromolecules deposited in the matrix during cartilage formation in embryogenesis is preserved throughout the entire ontogenesis. The catabolism of the macromolecular components of the articular cartilage extracellular matrix follows patterns common to the extracellular matrix of all connective tissues (see section 3.7), albeit with certain peculiarities.

Numerous proteolytic enzymes participate in the catabolism of the large cartilage proteoglycan aggrecan. The main site of their activity is the linear interglobular domain (IGD) of the protein core; this domain connects the globular G1 and G2 domains. In the IGD, there is a peptide bond DIPEN341-342FFGVG (single-letter code for amino acid residues, see the legend to Fig. 3.11), which is cleaved by neutral metalloproteases (matrixins) – collagenase, gelatinase, and stromelysin (see section 3.7.1). Besides this bond, collagenase-3 (MMP-13) also cleaves the bond VKP384-385VFE (Fosang et al., 1996). Different proteolytic enzymes – cathepsins (B and L), plasmin, elastase, urokinase, and matrilysin – cleave other peptide bonds in the IGD. The role of these proteases in the catabolism of aggrecan in vivo is unknown. The cleavage of any peptide bond in the IGD releases the majority (about 85% by mass) of aggrecan macromolecules from aggrecan aggregates, while only a small aminoterminal fragment containing the G1 domain remains attached to hyaluronan.

However, the leading role in the catabolism of aggrecan is played by aggrecanases – enzymes from the ADAMTS-family (ADAMTS-5 and ADAMTS-4) expressed by chondrocytes. One specific site of their proteolytic action in the core protein is the bond NVTEGE373-374ALGSW, located in the IGD. However, like the matrixins, they also cleave the N341-342F bond.

Furthermore, the aggrecanases cleave (perhaps not simultaneously, but sequentially) a number of bonds in the CS-2 subdomain of the chondroitin sulfate-binding domain of the aggrecan protein core. These bonds are: SSELE1279-1280GRGTI, FREEE1467-1468GLGSV, PTAQE1572-1573AGEGP and TVSQE1872-1873LGHGP, in addition to several others (Little et al., 2007).

The aggrecanases' proteolytic action on aggrecan precedes metalloproteases' activity. During the in vitro culture of articular cartilage explants, the aggrecanases trigger the start of releasing the bulk of glycosaminoglycan-bearing fragments from the core protein into the culture liquid.

The final stage of the aggrecan catabolism – the degradation of fragments of its macromolecule, generated by the action of aggrecanases and other proteases – is carried out by lysosomal glycosidases: hexosaminidases, β-galactosidase and glycoside sulfatases. These enzymes, which break down glycosaminoglycans (to monosaccharides), are expressed in the lysosomes of chondrocytes and are secreted into the extracellular matrix (Shikhman et al., 2000).

The large fibrillar cartilage collagen – type II collagen – is more stable than other fibrillar collagens owing to a more developed system of intra- and intermolecular cross-links. It is accessible for the proteolytic action of only a few selected collagenases from the MMP family. Collagenase-3 (MMP-13) is especially active on type II collagen: the activity of this enzyme, expressed by chondrocytes, towards type II collagen is 3 times higher than that of collagenase-1 (fibroblast collagenase-1; MMP-1). Within 15 minutes after injecting recombinant MMP-13 into a hamster joint cavity, fragments of type II collagen macromolecules appear in the synovial fluid (Otterness et al., 2000).

The small proteoglycans (SLRP) differ from aggrecan in their resistance to metalloproteases' action. This feature of the small proteoglycans, which stabilizes the network of collagen fibrils, likely protects collagen from degradation in the early stages of pathological processes. MMP-19 plays an important role in the catabolism of cartilage matrix oligomeric protein (COMP). This metalloprotease cleaves a large fragment with a molecular mass of 60 kDa (Stracke et al., 2000).

The tissue inhibitors of metalloproteases (TIMP) hold central place among catabolic process inhibitors in the cartilage matrix (see section 3.7.2). The activity of TIMP-1, TIMP-2 and TIMP-4 is aimed primarily at inhibiting the effect of collagenolytic metalloproteases, and they have only a negligible effect on the activity of aggrecanases. In contrast, TIMP-3 has a potent inhibitory effect on both major cartilage aggrecanases – aggrecanase-1 (ADAMTS-4) and aggrecanase-2 (ADAMTS-5). This activity is determined by certain peculiarities of the structure of its N-terminal domain, and it is already detectable in subnanomolar TIMP-3 concentrations (Kashiwagi et al., 2001).

7.2.1.5. Regulation of cartilaginous tissue metabolic functions

7.2.1.5.1. Systemic factors of regulation

Hormonal factors' influence on the metabolic functions of normal mature cartilage tissue is complicated by the same factor that complicates all metabolic processes in chondrocytes: as with all other molecules, hormones enter the cells exclusively by diffusion through the extracellular matrix. It should be kept in mind that most water-soluble hormones exhibit a polypeptide nature, i.e., they are large, poorly diffusing molecules. As for lipid hormones (steroid hormones in first order), these hydrophobic molecules can move through the hydrophilic matrix only when complexed with specific transport proteins (globulins). Such complexes are even bigger and, hence, particularly difficult to transport. Thus, it can be assumed that, under normal conditions and given physiological hormone concentrations in the body, their effects in vivo upon differentiated chondrocytes of permanent cartilage are very small, if any.

However, this does not mean that the chondroblastic differon cells do not need – at certain stages of differentiation and in particular physiological conditions – the active regulatory action of hormones. The first such occasion is in the chondrogenesis stage, which includes the condensation of mesenchymal cells, their proliferation and the acquisition of the chondroblastic phenotype by the cells (see section 10.2.2). The second occasion is in the final stages of chondrocytes' differentiation in provisory cartilage, specifically in metaphyseal cartilage (the growth plate). This stage includes the proliferation of chondrocytes, their hypertrophy and apoptosis, which ensure the normal flow of the endochondral osteogenesis process and growth of the organism

(see section 10.3.1.1). Hormones' influence on chondrocyte function is also clearly manifested in pathological processes that affect cartilage.

There is substantial direct evidence of hormones' effective influence on the metabolic functions of chondrocytes, based on studies performed on cultured cells in vitro, where conditions are created for the hormones' direct contact with the cells. The data obtained, naturally, should be interpreted with caution in regards to the processes occurring in vivo.

Chondrocytes' dependence on hormonal influences is suggested by the fact that they express hormone receptors – both plasma (cell) membrane receptors and nuclear receptors; steroid hormones serve as their ligands (Boyan et al., 2003). This is also indicated by chondrocytes' ability to synthesize their own hormones, acting as autocrine factors on chondrocytes.

For example, chondrocytes' ability to express mRNA for the entire set of specific enzymes catalyzing the local synthesis of sex steroids has been demonstrated (Takeuchi et al., 2007). The synthesis of **ghrelin** (growth hormone-releasing factor), a pituitary growth hormone-releasing peptide, has been detected in chondrocytes. Ghrelin is produced primarily by chondrocytes of the growth plate and has a local effect on chondrocytes, which possess two ghrelin receptors. In vitro ghrelin stimulates the production of cyclic adenosine monophosphate (cAMP) by chondrocytes and inhibits their overall metabolic activity (Caminos et al., 2005). Chondrocytes present in the developing bone tissue of growing rats express leptin, a peptide hormone known as one of the regulators of lipid metabolism.

Like other hormones, glucocorticoids' effect on chondrocytes is largely dependent on the dose. In cell culture experiments, glucocorticoids inhibit the biosynthetic activity of chondroblasts/chondrocytes. The expression of type II collagen and fibronectin isoforms typical of cartilage declines, and the biosynthesis of proteoglycans and hyaluronan is partially inhibited. These phenomena reveal phenotypic abnormalities (partial dedifferentiation) in cells under the influence of glucocorticoids; obviously, in vivo these effects are manifested as degenerative changes in cartilage tissue (Fubini et al., 2001).

Clinical practice shows that growth retardation due to impaired endochondral bone formation may be one of the consequences of the phenotypic changes induced by glucocorticoid drugs in chondrocytes during early postnatal ontogenesis. This effect is especially pronounced in terms of synthetic glucocorticoid drugs, the biological activity of which is considerably higher than that of natural hormones.

However, glucocorticoid steroids' effect on cartilage, in the natural concentrations occurring in the body, is considerably more complex. At a physiological concentration in the suspension cell culture medium, hydrocortisone – a synthetic analogue of the natural glucocorticoid cortisol – helped to maintain the optimum production of extracellular matrix components by chondrocytes of articular cartilage and reduced the catabolic processes (Wang et al., 2004). A similar result was obtained regarding the powerful synthetic glucocorticoid drugs dexamethasone, prednisolone and triamsinolon, which, in small doses, have inhibited the expression by chondrocytes of the catabolic metalloproteases–the matrixins MMP-1, MMP-3 and MMP-13, inducible by proinflammatory cytokines. Only high doses have caused an inhibition in the biosynthesis of type II collagen and aggrecan (Richardson & Dodge, 2003).

During in vitro experiments, dexamethasone, in proper doses, has a positive effect on the expression of genes involved in chondroblastic differentiation: it stimulates *Sox9* (the main regulator of this differentiation) (Sekiya et al., 2001b) and *IGFBP-1* (one of the proteins that bind insulin-like growth factors, which are anabolic for chondroblasts/chondrocytes (Nadra et al., 2003)), as well as genes encoding all the main structural components of the cartilage extracellular matrix (Derfoul et al., 2006). Furthermore, under the same conditions, dexamethasone inhibits the expression of genes relevant to angiogenesis and calcification, thus preventing premature ossification during endochondral osteogenesis.

Therefore, the regulatory influence of glucocorticoid hormones on cells of the cartilage differon is diversified and affects the expression of numerous genes (James et al., 2007).

Sex steroids (androgens and estrogens) are particularly active in provisional cartilage: cartilage models of future bones during embryogenesis, and cartilage of growth plates during puberty. This activity, together with the lifelong influence of sex steroids on bone cells, is a major determinant of sex differences in the morphological features of the skeleton (Vanderschueren et al., 2004) (see section 8.5.1 and 10.3.1.1). Both the direct effect of sex steroids on gene expression in provisional cartilage cells (Karperien et al., 2005), and their indirect effect mediated by the so-called "somatotropic axis", which includes the pituitary growth hormone, insulin-like growth factors IGF-1 and IGF-2 and their receptors (Parker et al., 2007), are important.

On the other hand, sex steroids are necessary for the normal functioning of chondrocytes in the homeostasis of permanent articular cartilage. Here, the effect of hormones (estrogen) is mostly anti-catabolic. It is known that postmenopausal estrogen deficiency in women causes the progressive degradation of articular cartilage, which often ends with the development of osteoarthrosis. Similar phenomena are reproduced in experimental animals by ovariectomy. The degradation is associated with the increased catabolism of type II collagen, with estrogen (17β-estradiol) successfully inhibiting this catabolism (Oestergaard et al., 2006). In vitro this estrogen has the same anti-catabolic effect on chondrocytes from osteoarthrosis-damaged articular cartilage: the expression of cell metalloproteases -1, -3 and -13 is inhibited, while that of the metalloprotease inhibitor TIMP-1 is stimulated (Lee et al., 2003).

17β-estradiol also exerts an anabolic effect when introduced into a culture of normal articular cartilage chondrocytes: it enhances the overall production of proteins, including the biosynthesis of type II collagen (Claassen et al., 2006). 17β-estradiol also accelerates the final stages of chondrocyte differentiation, as evidenced by the increased deposition of type X collagen in the extracellular matrix (Talwar et al., 2006).

Dehydroepiandrosterone, a steroid precursor of both androgens and estrogens, also exhibits anabolic effects. It not only inhibits the expression of metalloproteases, but also enhances the proliferation of cultured chondrocytes and the biosynthesis of the glycosaminoglycan component of proteoglycans (Sun et al., 2006).

The effect of calcitonin (a peptide hormone produced by the C cells of the thyroid gland) on articular cartilage tissue can be defined as chondroprotective–supporting normal tissue homeostasis (Karsdal et al., 2006). The chondroprotective effect of calcitonin, which supplements its anti-catabolic effect on bones (see 8.5.1), can be explained by its ability to limit the catabolism of type II collagen, and to inhibit the expression of matrix metalloproteases by chondrocytes, thereby reducing their activity in the matrix (Sondergaard et al., 2006).

Insulin has an expressly anabolic effect on cartilage tissue. According to data obtained during in vitro experiments with cultured chondrogenic ATDC-5 cells, insulin, together with the structurally similar insulin-like growth factor IGF-1, stimulate chondrogenesis. Unlike IGF-1, which enhances the proliferation of cartilage cells, insulin increases biosynthetic activity and promotes cell differentiation toward the chondroblastic phenotype by activating its receptors (Phornphutkul et al., 2006). Thus, insulin, along with estrogen, stimulates the expression of type II collagen in the cultured chondrocytes of articular cartilage (Claassen et al., 2006). The iodine-containing thyroid hormones of the thyroid gland–thyroxine (T4) and triiodothyronine (T3)–exhibit anabolic action on the cultured chondrocytes of articular cartilage, similar to the activity of insulin (and estrogen). They enhance the biosynthesis of the major matrix components, type II collagen and proteoglycans (Glade et al., 1994). Hypothyroidism causes many degenerative changes in cartilage *in vivo* (McLean & Podell, 1995). But the principal targets of thyroid hormones are provisional cartilage chondrocytes, primarily cartilage of bones' growth plates. T4 and T3 promote the proliferation and differentiation of chondrocytes in growth plates, acting through the thyroid hormone receptor β (Rabier et al., 2006). This thyroid hormone effect, whose mechanism includes the activation of transglutaminase and regulation of fibroblast growth factor (FGF-2 and FGF-18) receptors (Barnard et al., 2006), is required for normal endochondral osteogenesis and respectively for the organism to grow.

The peptide hormone parathyroidin (PTH), produced by the parathyroid glands, and the related small ubiquitous protein PTHrP (parathyroid hormone-related protein), whose basic functions are focused on regulating calcium metabolism by acting upon bone cells, are also involved in regulating the differentiation of proliferating chondrocytes in bones' growth plates. In these cells, PTHrP increases the expression of genes regulating intracellular signal transduction pathways (Hoogendam et al., 2006). In addition, PTHrP is involved in maintaining the homeostasis of articular cartilage, as indicated by its accumulation in cartilage in the case of osteoarthritis and the growth factor TGF-β-induced expression in chondrocytes. It is possible that PTHrP impedes the mineralization of articular cartilage, thus preventing the development of deep zone chondrocyte hypertrophy (Jiang et al., 2007).

From the vitamins family, vitamins D, C and A participate in the regulation of the chondrocyte's metabolic functions.

Vitamin D represents a group of biologically active steroid compounds, which are produced in the body (mainly in the skin under the influence of ultraviolet radiation) from low in activity fat-soluble precursors, thereby actually acting as hormones.

These compounds, collectively named the D-endocrine system (Bauman, 1989), induce various effects in the organism (strictly speaking, the name "vitamin D" must be used only for precursors (prohormones) found in food and, perhaps, for synthetic hormone pharmacological products). They play a particularly big role in the biology of bone tissue and in terms of calcium homeostasis (see section 8.5.1).

D-hormones have two modes of action for all cells. Like all steroid hormones, they freely diffuse through the cell membrane and, through interactions with nuclear (cytoplasmic) receptors (VDR, vitamin D receptor), they regulate the genome function. Besides this, they interact with specific receptors in the cell (plasma) membrane and influence the physical state (fluidity) of membrane lipids. This nongenomic signal transduction pathway creates the potential for the accelerated reaction to the action of vitamin D. In addition to these two, a third mode of action is active in cartilage: the active metabolites of vitamin D (together with other hydrophobic substances) are deposited inside the helical domain of COMP macromolecules; the chondrocyte receives additional signals from this peculiar depot (Özbek et al., 2002).

Articular cartilage chondrocytes express VDR in vitro. Furthermore, this expression is stronger and more frequently detectable in chondrocytes that have been isolated from the cartilage of patients with osteoarthrosis. Its localization, determined histochemically, overlaps with the sites of expression of metalloproteases, which demonstrates the role of vitamin D in regulating the catabolism of the articular cartilage extracellular matrix (Tetlow & Woolley, 2001).

However, the most important role of vitamin D lies in regulating the chondrocyte function in bones' growth plates. The most active natural metabolites of vitamin D (members of the D-endocrine system) – 1,25-(OH)$_2$D3 and 24.25-(OH)$_2$D3 – promote the chondrocytes' proliferation and differentiation.

Chondrocytes produce these metabolites (which exhibit autocrine effects) from the inactive precursor (prohormone) 25OHD, a process that is regulated by glucocorticoids and the TGF-β1 transforming growth factor (Schwartz et al., 1992). Vitamin D3 stimulates the production of the sex steroid 17β-estradiol in cultured chondrocytes from rib cartilage (which mediate the growth of the ribs) (Sylvia et al., 2002). The disrupted metabolism of D-system components leads to disruptions in endochondral osteogenesis and, along with other pathogenic mechanisms, in the development of rickets.

Like vitamin D, the molecular action mechanisms for vitamin A are similar to hormones (Reichrath et al., 2007). Its inactive precursors (retinyl esters contained in foods of animal origin, and carotenoids, contained in plant foods) enter the body. There, they acquire biological activity through the transformation of retinyl esters into retinol, and of carotenoids into retinal. Retinal can be oxidized to produce retinoic acid – particularly active and well known in several isomeric forms (see section 4.1).

These fat-soluble metabolites (retinoids) can freely diffuse through the membrane into the cytoplasm and further into the nucleus, where they interact with nuclear (cytoplasmic) receptors – transcription factors. This interaction is regulated by the binding of retinoids to specific proteins in the cytoplasm. One of these proteins, expressed almost exclusively by chondrocytes and known as cartilage-derived retinoic acid-sensitive protein (CD-RAP), is important for the formation of cartilage and for the subsequent maintenance of its stability (Yonekawa et al., 2002).

Hypovitaminosis A can be induced by insufficient amounts of inactive precursors in the diet, or by turning off the genes encoding the enzymes necessary for forming active metabolites from its precursors. Hypovitaminosis is accompanied by disruptions in the morphogenesis of connective tissue (including cartilage and bone) structures, during embryonic development. The origin of these disorders can be explained by in vitro experiments, which showed the catalytic role of retinoic acid in the chondrocyte differentiation at all stages, from the condensation of precursor cells, to hypertrophy and early mineralization (Kirimoto et al., 2005).

The stimulating effect of vitamin A on chondrogenesis occurs only within a narrow range of concentrations. Hypervitaminosis, especially the state of having excess retinoic acid, causes equally serious disruptions to chondrogenesis, even suppression (at the level of transcription) of the expression of Sox9 – the "master" gene of the chondroblastic differon (Sekiya et al., 2001). One of the early stages of chondroblast differentiation is also disrupted – the transition from the condensation of mesenchymal cells to establishing the chondroblast phenotype is delayed, accompanied by the continuous expression of N-cadherin (Cho et al., 2003) (see section 10.2.2).

Hypervitaminosis A condition, or more specifically–the unwanted activity of retinoic acid–arises not only as a result of the intake of excessive amounts of vitamins (or its inactive precursor), but mainly due to an imbalance in the finely tuned mechanisms regulating retinoic acid activity. This imbalance may be a consequence of the insufficient expression of retinoic acid-interacting proteins from the extracellular matrix and the cytoplasm (Dietz et al., 1996). It can also be due to a delayed repression of the genes encoding nuclear retinoic acid receptors (RAR). Under normal conditions, this repression, mediated by the large nuclear protein N-CoR1 (nuclear receptor co-repressor 1), is a prerequisite for the onset of *Sox9* expression (Weston et al., 2002).

Chondrocytes require vitamin C (ascorbic acid) for the synthesis of collagenous proteins, primarily type II collagen. The role of ascorbic acid in this synthesis is not only during the post-translational processing stage (as a cofactor in the enzymatic hydroxylation of proline and lysine residues, see section 3.1.1.1), but it also speeds up its initial stage–transcription. In articular cartilage explants, the expression of aggrecan and the hydroxylating enzyme prolyl-4-hydroxylase is enhanced under its influence (Clark et al., 2002). Significant amounts of ascorbic acid accumulate in cartilage tissue. With regard to ascorbic acid content (relative to cell mass), cartilage occupies an intermediate position between two tissues particularly rich in this vitamin–the liver and adrenal tissue (Stabler & Kraus, 2003). Chondrocytes are powerful concentrators of ascorbic acid–its concentration inside the cells is more than 900 times higher than the concentration in the environment. The sodium-dependent vitamin C transporter 2 (SVCT2) carried out the selective transport of only the biologically active stereospecific L-isoform of the ascorbate ion through the chondrocytes' cytoplasmic membrane (McNulty et al., 2005).

7.2.1.5.2. Local factors of regulation

Along with the systemic regulatory factors, signaling molecules that act locally (at a short-distance), such as growth factors, cytokines, and morphogens play an essential role in regulating differentiation (phenotype formation) and in the functional activity of chondroblasts/chondrocytes. Due to their small size, these protein molecules easily migrate through the cartilage extracellular matrix toward the cells. The results of studies of their effects in vitro (most of these studies are performed in cell culture) can be related reasonably well to the processes occurring *in vivo*.

Chondrocytes express receptors for short range signaling molecules. As ligands, these molecules act on the biosynthetic activity of the cells at all possible levels–gene expression (mRNA transcription), posttranscriptional processing and splicing of mRNA, translation, posttranslational modifications of biosynthetic products, intracellular transport, and secretion of proteins in the extracellular matrix.

Members of insulin-like growth factor (IGF) families, and the superfamily of transforming growth factor β (TGF-β), which includes the bone morphogenetic protein (BMP) family, act on chondrocytes as anabolic factors. The signals from these ligands are transmitted inside the cell and reach the nucleus with the help of Smad proteins. These molecules stimulate the expression of the Sox9 transcription factor, needed for chondrocyte phenotype establishment (Hashimoto et al., 2007).

The pro-inflammatory cytokines–tumor necrosis factor (TNF-α) and some interleukins (IL)–show mostly the opposite, catabolic, action on chondrocytes. These ligands act intracellularly via the nuclear factor ϰ B (NFkB) and the transcription factor AP1 (Hashimoto et al., 2006).

The activity of the signaling molecules from both groups–anabolic and catabolic–does not have a strictly defined direction, and some molecules cannot be assigned to either of these groups. Multi-directional activities are exhibited by various members of the fibroblast growth factor (FGF) family, or even by the same FGF, depending on the differentiation stage of chondroblasts/chondrocytes, or in experiments *in vitro*–depending on the age of the cell culture. They are also not the same toward cells of different types of cartilage (Bobick et al., 2007).

For example, the effect of FGF-2 (also known as basic fibroblast growth factor, bFGF), which uses the FGFR-1 receptor, on articular cartilage chondrocytes and intervertebral discs is predominantly catabolic (increased expression of metalloproteases, particularly MMP-13) and anti-anabolic (inhibiting proteoglycan biosynthesis) in nature. On the other hand, the action of FGF-18, carried out through the receptor FGF-3, in the chondrocytes of both these types of hyaline cartilage is stimulating and anabolic. It stimulates cell differentiation and the deposition of the extracellular matrix (Ellman et al., 2008).

The insulin-like growth factor IGF-1 is a particularly powerful anabolic factor (IGF-2 is somewhat less active) whose stimulating effect on the differentiation and especially the proliferation of chondrogenic cells through mitogenic signaling pathways greatly exceeds the analogous activity of insulin (Phornphutkul et al., 2006). Cultured chondrocytes increase the synthesis of proteoglycans and collagens under the influence of IGF-1. This results in a higher number of cross-links in collagens, i.e. in the improved biomechanical quality of the collagen network. In addition, IGF-1 prevents the apoptosis of chondrocytes in vitro.

The action of IGF-1 on chondrocytes is under the control of IGFBP-3–a member of the family of insulin-like growth factor binding proteins. Chondrocytes synthesize IGFBP-3 more actively than the cells of other tissues. Furthermore, IGFBP-3 regulates the binding of IGF-1 with the cytoplasmic membrane of chondrocytes (Evistar et al., 2003).

Members of the superfamily of transforming growth factor β (TGF-β), including the bone morphogenetic proteins (BMP) (see section 8.5.2), act on chondrocytes mostly in an anabolic direction. However, the multifunctional nature of these signaling molecules often makes their effects complex and diverse.

TGF-β1 plays a key role in initiating and maintaining chondrogenic differentiation *in vitro* (Goessler et al., 2005). It stimulates the growth of cartilage tissue in the process of its formation *in vivo*. It also contributes to maintaining a balance between the ability of the tissue to swell, which depends on the fixed charge density (FCD), i.e. the aggrecan concentration, and the rigidity of the collagen network, which limits swelling (Asanbaeva et al., 2007). TGF-β1 activates the specific kinase TAK1 in chondrocytes, and this activation stimulates the synthesis of type II collagen (Qiao et al., 2005).

In vivo the sensitivity of chondrocytes towards the action of TGF-β1 decreases with age. The expression levels of other TGF-β (2 and 3) and of the TGF-β-receptor in chondrocytes also drop (Blaney-Davidson et al., 2005).

All three isoforms of TGF-β with similar activities, together with IGF-1 and the platelet growth factor (PDGF), control the expression and accumulation of the articular cartilage superficial zone protein (proteoglycan-4, SZP) in chondrocytes. TGF-β is ascribed the primary stimulating role in this regulation (Niikura & Reddi, 2007).

BMP-7 (osteogenic protein-1, OP-1)–the member of the family of bone morphogenetic proteins that is most active toward chondrocytes, especially toward articular cartilage chondrocytes–makes its contribution to stimulating SZP expression (Chubinskaya et al., 2008). This BMP-7 action is just one of numerous effects that a number of BMPs have on chondrocytes.

The effects of the bone morphogenetic proteins, which act, like all members of the TGF-β superfamily, through the intracellular SMAD signaling system, are not just anabolic, but also anti-catabolic. IGF-1 synergizes with the anabolic effect of BMP (OP-1, BMP-2 and -9) and increases it (Chubinskaya et al., 2007a), whereas the anti-catabolic effect is manifested in the inhibition of catabolic enzyme expression (collagenases, aggrecanases) and the neutralization of the effect of other destructive factors, including of pro-inflammatory signaling molecules (Chubinskaya et al., 2007b).

OP-1 (BMP-7) and other BMP, in particular BMP-5, maintain the normal chondrocyte phenotype by stimulating the expression of a set of proteins making up the so-called focal adhesions (or adhesion loci) of cell membranes (see section 3.6.3), and play an important role in the exchange of information between cells and the extracellular matrix. BMPs stimulate the biosynthesis of type II collagen and aggrecan, characteristic of the chondrocyte phenotype, and they also activate chondrocyte proliferation (Mailhot et al., 2008).

Chondrocytes themselves produce three members of the BMP protein family. They have been isolated from cartilage tissue and described under the name of cartilage morphogenetic proteins, or **cartilage-derived morphogenetic proteins** (CDMP). They are also known as growth and differentiation factors (GDF). The directionality of the functional activity of these signaling molecules does not differ from the activity of most bone morphogenetic proteins, such as, OP-1 or BMP-6, for example (Yeh et al., 2005). In the modern nomenclature, GDFs are referred to as BMP-12, BMP-13 and BMP-14 (see section 8.5.2, *Table. 8.6*).

The structure of CDMP molecules does not differ from the molecular structure of the bone morphogenetic proteins (BMP), as discussed in detail in section 8.5.2. Like BMP, they are homodimers whose subunits are connected by a disulfide bond in the carboxy terminal domains. Each subunit is a glycoprotein, 120–129 amino acid residues in length, containing one or two N-linked oligosaccharides and 7 obligatory (conservative) cysteine residues, one of which participates in the creation of the just-mentioned disulfide bond between the subunits, while the other six form three intramolecular disulfide bonds (within a single polypeptide chain).

The biosynthetic processes of CDMP and BMP are also identical: the primary transcripts of either protein encode a propeptide, which is almost three times longer than the one included in the subunits of the homodimer, and is removed during the post-translational processing. As signaling molecules, CDMPs act on cells using the same receptors (BMPRs), and, accordingly, the same intracellular signal transduction pathways (SMAD protein system) as the BMPs (Mazerbourg et al., 2005).

All three CDMPs possess osteoinductive and osteogenic activity, characteristic of the BMPs too, albeit manifested in different fashions. In cultured cells of mesenchymal origin–CDMP-1 (GDF-5, BMP-14) and CDMP-3 (GDF-7, BMP-12), but not CDMP-2 (GDF-6, BMP-13)–direct differentiation toward the osteoblastic pathway by stimulating the expression of osteogenic markers–alkaline phosphatase, osteocalcin, bone sialoprotein (BSP) and type I collagen (Yeh et al., 2005).

CDMP-1 exhibits particularly high osteogenic activity comparable to, and even higher than, the activity of the osteogenic protein OP-1 (BMP-7). Moreover, CDMP-1 has an important role in the morphogenesis of articular cartilage (Thomas et al., 2006). CDMP-2 induces chondrogenic differentiation of mesenchymal cells (Nochi et al., 2004). CDMP-1 and CDMP-2 (CDMP-2 expression is especially pronounced in endochondral ossification) also stimulate chondrogenesis and actively participate in the growth of long bones and in the healing of fractures.

In vivo CDMP-3 induces the ectopic formation of tissue, which is similar to tendon tissue. However, in vitro this CDMP also exerts an osteogenic effect, for example, stimulating the proliferation of cultured cells of the osteoblastic differon, and the increased activity of alkaline phosphatase in these cells (Furuya et al., 1999).

The connective tissue growth factor CTGF/CCN2, also known as CCN family 2 factor and hypertrophic chondrocyte-specific gene product 24 (HCS24), exerts a distinct anabolic effect on chondrocytes. This molecule, secreted by endothelial cells, stimulates the proliferation and differentiation of chondrocytes. CTGF/CCN2 also has a positive influence on the production of cartilage extracellular matrix components by chondrocytes, and the expression of integrins, especially of the integrin α5 subunit, as well as the activity of the integrin-associated kinases FAK and ERK1/2, which are necessary for signal transduction from integrin receptors (Nishida et al., 2007). CTGF/CCN2 stimulates the proliferation and differentiation of chondrocytes in the elastic cartilage of the ear (Fujisawa et al., 2008).

The importance of CTGF/CCN2 for chondrocyte differentiation is underscored by the activity of a peculiar mechanism for regulating its expression in chondrocytes. This mechanism is associated with the activity of a cofactor – the phosphoprotein nucleophosmin (synonyms – nuclear protein B23 and numatrin), which is present in the nucleus (more precisely, in the nucleolus) and contributes to maintaining the posttranslational stability of mRNA in the biosynthesis of CTGF/CCN2 (Mukudai et al., 2008).

CTGF/CCN2 interacts with BMP-2, one of the most active bone morphogenetic proteins, in chondrocytes to form stable complexes. The anabolic effect of these complexes is different from the BMP-2 effect itself: it is weaker with respect to stimulating the growth and proliferation of chondrocytes, but stronger in stimulating the expression of chondrocyte phenotype markers and extracellular matrix proteoglycans. Thus, CCN2 acts as a modulator of BMP-2 (Maeda et al., 2009).

It is interesting that the anabolic effect of CCN2 is opposed by the catabolic action of another representative of the same family, CCN3. This counteraction, which contributes to the accuracy in regulating chondrocyte differentiation, is particularly strong in its late stage (Kawaki et al., 2008).

The anabolic factors are counterbalanced by another group of factors acting on chondrocytes by inhibiting the anabolic and stimulating the catabolic processes. This group consists of pro-inflammatory cytokines.

Such activity is especially conspicuous in interleukin IL-1β. The effect of this interleukin is versatile. While the powerful anabolic factor BMP-7 (OP-1) modulates the expression of 36 of 3400 tested genes in human articular cartilage chondrocytes, IL-1β simultaneously modulates the expression of more than 900 genes, exerting both anti-anabolic and catabolic effects on chondrocytes. The repression of anabolic genes is manifested by the inhibited expression of structural components of the extracellular matrix – collagen, aggrecan and SZP. The catabolic action represents the enhanced expression of the genes encoding catabolic factors. The expression of matrixins (MMP-1, MMP-3, MMP-13), which carry out collagen proteolysis, and aggrecanases (ADAMTS-4, ADAMTS-5), which degrade aggrecan, increases. Incidentally, the activating effect of IL-1β on the expression of aggrecanases in chondrocytes is synergistic with the activity of retinoic acid observed in hypervitaminosis A. Such a widespread effect is possible due to the fact that IL-1β utilizes multiple signal transduction pathways at the same time (JNK kinases, p38, Erk) (Saas et al., 2006).

The direct effect of IL-1β on chondrocyte metabolic functions is supplemented by the influence on other proinflammatory cytokines – IL-6 and IL-18, whose expression is induced by IL-1β. IL-6 exerts the same effects as IL-1β; however, its anti-anabolic effect on the synthesis of proteoglycans is somewhat weaker. IL-18 impedes the accumulation of type II collagen in the matrix, disrupts the expression of the β subunit of integrins and of one of the focal adhesion proteins – vinculin. High concentrations of IL-18 stimulate chondrocyte apoptosis (John et al., 2007).

The action of IL-1β is markedly synergistic with the action of another cytokine – interferon-γ (IFN-γ), which also induces the expression of IL-6, together with all the effects of this interleukin. IFN-γ exerts a catabolic effect in yet another way – by inducing the expression of nitrogen oxide synthase (iNOS), an enzyme that catalyzes the formation of NO. This free radical gas causes the apoptosis of the cells (Henrotin et al., 2000).

The expression of nitric oxide synthase also represents the main mechanism of the catabolic activity of tumor necrosis factor α (TNF-α) (Hashimoto et al., 2007). At the same time, TNFα influences the function of enzymes involved in the glycosylation of glycoproteins of the extracellular matrix; this leads to changes in the structure of the oligosaccharides contained in the glycoprotein macromolecules (see section 3.2.1.2) (Yang et al., 2007).

The proinflammatory cytokines affect chondrocyte function in complex interactions with prostaglandins, another group of chemical mediators. Amongst them, PGE2 is particularly active in these interactions. PGE2 stimulates the production of cytokines, and cytokines induce the production of this prostaglandin by chondrocytes, which, depending on the activity of other regulatory factors, can alter the overall effect (Goldring & Berenbaum, 2004).

Neuropeptides are relevant to the development of catabolic and anti-anabolic effects caused by pro-inflammatory cytokines. Fibroblast growth factor 2 (FGF-2 or bFGF), which was mentioned above for its catabolic and anti-anabolic effects on chondrocytes of articular cartilage, uses a neuroendocrine signaling pathway. It induces the expression by chondrocytes and synovial membrane cells (synoviocytes) of a small, only 11 amino acids-long neuropeptide, known as substance P, as well as the expression of the receptor of this peptide (NK1-R) by chondrocytes. Acting through this receptor, substance P stimulates the production of metalloproteases and inhibits the accumulation of proteoglycans in the cartilage. This mechanism is important in the pathogenesis of osteoarthrosis (Im et al., 2008).

The Wnt family morphogens, whose nature and molecular mechanisms of action are discussed in section 10.1, have diverse regulatory influences on the chondrocytic differon. The role of Wnt is especially significant in embryogenesis. In particular, they control the main stages of chondroblast differentiation, whereby the activities of individual Wnt family members have different directions, both stimulating and repressing (see section 10.2.2). Wnt are involved in controlling the final stage of chondrocyte differentiation in a process that takes place during postnatal growth via endochondral ossification, as well as in the lifelong chondroblastic differentiation of bone marrow stromal mesenchymal stem cells (Yates et al., 2005).

Wnt influence on cartilage tissue persists in mature cartilage (Chun et al., 2008). This is evidenced by the expression of several Wnt (5b, 7a, 10b, 2b/13, 9a/14), their receptors, antagonists and intracellular components of signaling pathways of mature articular cartilage chondrocytes and the changes in this expression during the development of pathological processes that affect cartilage (Yates et al., 2005). Mechanical trauma of articular cartilage activates the canonical Wnt signal transduction pathway, which leads to the stimulation of regenerative and anabolic processes (Dell'Accio et al., 2006).

The signaling molecules with local action, anabolic and catabolic, acting on chondrocytes use numerous intracellular signal transduction pathways. Upon reaching the cell nucleus, the signals induce, activate or inhibit gene expression with the help of transcription factors and cofactors. In particular, transcription factors from the NFκB family (including factor RelA) play a significant role in influencing genes (Raymond et al., 2007). The activator protein AP-1 is involved in the process too. But the central point of application of all signals in chondrocytes at this level of incoming signals activity is the Sox9 transcription factor, the master coordinator of the function of genes involved in the formation and maintenance of the phenotype of the chondrocytic differon cellular elements (see section 10.2.2).

Intracellular signal transduction pathways form an integrated, functionally organized network, which ensures the maintenance of homeostasis (metabolic equilibrium) of mature cartilage. Imbalances between the activities of anabolic and catabolic factors in this network serve as triggers for the development of many pathological processes, including osteoarthrosis (Aigner et al., 2006).

7.2.1.6. Biomechanical (mechanochemical) aspects of articular cartilage

The main function of cartilage tissue – mechano-supporting – is best manifested and studied in most detail in articular cartilage. It should be considered in two aspects.

First, articular cartilage exists under conditions of high mechanical loads throughout life. These loads have both static (especially in the joints of the lower extremities in humans) and dynamic (due to the motion of the cartilage-covered joint surfaces of the bones relative to each other) natures. Therefore, the biomechanical properties of articular cartilage must match up these conditions and be adapted to both these loads. In other words, the material must possess the necessary strength and durability.

Second, the kinematic (motor) function of joints demands articular cartilage's adaptability to the constant motion of the bone surfaces relative to one another. A major role in the kinematic joint function is played by the joint lubricant – the synovia (synovial fluid). Obviously, the role of the surface quality of articular cartilage and its deformation properties is of no less importance. The cartilage surface must be sufficiently smooth and slick and the deformability of the tissue must not only alleviate the effect of mechanical loads, but also facilitate the maintenance of maximum compatibility between the shapes of the articular ends of bones. In addition, tissue deformability must create conditions for the optimal interaction of cartilage with the synovial fluid, and for the flow of synovial fluid during joint movements.

The biomechanical characteristics of articular cartilage that are necessary and sufficient to perform these functions are defined, on the one hand, by its morphology and, on the other hand, by the biochemical composition and supramolecular architectonics of the extracellular matrix.

The role played by main articular cartilage extracellular matrix components in providing the biomechanical functions of the tissue has been already discussed in section 7.2.1.3.

The main biomechanical properties of articular cartilage are listed in *Table. 7.8.*

The zonal (layered) morphology of articular cartilage, manifested, in particular, in the qualitative and quantitative variations of the macromolecular composition of the matrix and the characteristics of the spatial orientation of collagen fibrils in the different zones, determine the biomechanical inhomogeneity (heterogeneity) of articular cartilage as a material.

The different spatial orientation of collagen fibrils is also a major factor affecting the anisotropy of the biomechanical properties of cartilage. Anisotropy – the differential behavior of the material in response to stress in different directions – is a common property of all biological tissues that have a fibrous framework. The spatial orientation of the glycosaminoglycan chains participating in the proteoglycan aggregates is another significant determinant of the biomechanical anisotropy of cartilage tissue. The glycosaminogly-can meshwork impedes the flow of fluids, thus leading to uneven hydraulic permeability – the uneven distribution of tissue fluids under compression (Quinn et al., 2001). This uneven deformation facilitates the sliding of the articular cartilages in the joint. (Mow et al., 1992).

The nonlinear mechanical behavior of cartilage, manifested both during compression and tension.

Changes in the macrostructure and the spatial orientation of the collagen fibrils are the basis of the nonlinear tensile response of the tissue, (Mow et al., 1992).

The nonlinearity of the biomechanical parameters is observed in all zones of articular cartilage However, the specific numerical values of these parameters are very

Table 7.8

Basic biomechanical properties of articular cartilage

Inhomogeneity (heterogeneity)

Zonal differences in tensile strength (layer-specific differences in the structural organization of collagen fibrils and the amount of collagen).

Zonal differences in terms of the ability to swell (layer-specific differences in the amount of proteoglycans).

Regional differences in both of these properties (local variations in collagen and proteoglycan content in the extracellular matrix).

Anisotropy

Orthotropic mechanical properties.

Orthotropic swelling capacity.

Nonlinearity

Tension-compression.

Exponential behavior during tension-compression (stress-strain).

Dependence of permeability on compression.

Dependence of the deformation on the magnitude of the impact (large deformation).

different in different zones (layers) and in different regions. These differences are especially pronounced in the cartilage of large joints, such as the hip and knee (Treppo et al., 2000; Laasanen et al., 2003). *Table 7.9* shows the values of Young's modulus for different directions of strain stress in the cartilage zones.

The origin of the nonlinearity of cartilage deformation under compression is different from the origin of nonlinearity under strain. Under compression, the main biome-

chanical role lies in the flow of interstitial fluid (water), not the collagen fibrils, whose compressive resistance is insignificant. The extracellular matrix is a microporous material, whose pores are filled with water and whose surface is permeable to water molecules. Compression causes the exudation (extrusion) of water and thus, the compacting of the solid–macromolecular–phase of the matrix. Two additional factors are at play here: reduced permeability and higher friction between the macromolecules due to increased density. Water outflow from the tissue slows down as permeability decreases and friction increases, (Mow et al., 1992), indicative of the non-linear proceeding of this process.

The flow of interstitial fluid (water) under pressure does not come down to exudation alone. Water also moves from articular cartilage regions, subjected to stronger compression, toward the less compressed ones. The exudation of water is also enhanced under compression, and the geometric shape of cartilage changes to accommodate the conditions for the movement of the articular ends of the bones.

Under the influence of pressure, which represents the predominant mechanical load on articular cartilage, deformations related to the flow of water are accompanied by deformations caused by changes in the macromolecular organization of the extracellular matrix. From a biomechanical point of view, cartilage is considered a two-phase composite material (Soulhat et al., 1999): the proteoglycan aggregates occupying the bulk of the matrix represent the first phase, and the reinforcing framework of collagen fibrils represents the second phase. Water in this case represents a third, extremely significant, but passive phase.

As a rule, such reinforced biphasic macromolecular materials combine the properties of elasticity and plasticity. This combination is called viscoelasticity. The intrinsic nonlinear viscoelasticity of concentrated aggrecan solutions is increased manifold by the viscoelasticity resulting from the biphasic state (Meechai et al., 2001). The viscoelasticity of articular cartilage is manifested as shear strain under the dynamic compression caused by movement, and is characterized by the shear modulus. The shear modulus of cartilage is low (0.2–0.4 mPa, micropascals), indicative of low stiffness. Thus, in addition to the intratissual displacement of water, viscoelasticity contributes to the ability of articular cartilage to acquire fairly easily various geometric shapes in order to adapt to the changing loads during movement without altering its volume.

The tension in the diagonally oriented collagen fibrils gains high importance under such shear strains, (Mow et al., 1992).

The elastic component of articular cartilage's deformability is the predominant one during short-term stresses arising from movements in the joint. During long-term stresses, such as a prolonged period of staying in an upright position, the elastic deformation is accompanied by viscous deformation, caused mainly by water outflow

Table 7.9

Direction of strain	Cartilage zone	Young's modulus E (MPa)
Parallel to the long axis of collagen fibrils	Superficial (tangential) zone	42,2
	Middle zone	13,0
	Deep zone	2,6
Perpendicular to the long axis of collagen fibrils	Superficial (tangential) zone	15,6
	Middle zone	4,7
	Deep zone	1,1

According to Mow et al. (1992).

from cartilage tissue. This phenomenon is defined as creep. The recovery of the cartilage shape after a viscous deformation requires a longer time than recovering from elastic deformation. The combination of elasticity and viscosity makes it possible for articular cartilage to effectively reduce the stress transmitted under static and dynamic loads on the relatively fragile articular ends of the bones. In this respect, the function of articular cartilage is comparable to the function of the shock absorbers used in various technical devices.

All of the above-mentioned information about the patterns of articular cartilage's biomechanical function demonstrates a direct causal relationship between the biochemical composition and supramolecular organization of the extracellular matrix, on the one hand, and the biomechanical properties, on the other. Normal biomechanical properties can be maintained only for as long as the normal structural organization of the matrix is preserved–an organization that is constantly maintained by chondrocytes' metabolic activity.

The chondrocyte is a cell, which constantly exists under conditions involving some compression (Urban, 1994). Mechanical load is the key regulator of articular cartilage chondrocytes' function. In these circumstances, the pericellular (territorial) matrix (PTM), localized in the so-called chondron, is a direct transducer (transmitter) of the cell's mechanical signals. This matrix, which is the microenvironment of one or more chondrocytes, differs from the rest of the extracellular matrix by the presence of type VI collagen. Type VI collagen microfibrils impart special mechanical properties on the PTM that affect the perception of mechanical impulses by the cells (Guilak et al., 2006).

Changes in the magnitude, amplitude and frequency of stresses in the cartilage influence the expression of structural matrix macromolecules and the agents regulating anabolic processes, such as growth factors and cytokines. As previously noted, the composition of the extracellular matrix reflects the preferential distribution of loads; for example, proteoglycan concentration is higher in areas, subjected to stronger compression in the normally functioning joint. It has been suggested that the differences in mechanical loads pressing on different parts of articular cartilage and especially on cartilage of different joints is the reason for the postnatal phenotypic modulation of chondrocytes and for the selection of those cell clones providing the necessary biomechanical properties to the tissue through their biosynthetic activity (Little & Ghosh, 1997). Under these circumstances, it is very important that the biomechanical properties of different cartilages are well adapted to the stress values prevailing in a particular cartilage under physiological conditions. For example, a two-fold difference has been found in the values of the compression modulus (similar to Young's modulus) for cartilage in human elbow and knee joints (Yao & Seedhom, 1993).

The general inhibition of protein biosynthesis and, in particular, the inhibition of aggrecan biosynthesis was revealed in experiments where cultured fragments of articular cartilage had been subjected to excessive (damaging) stress through compression (Kurz et al., 2001). The intensity of these biochemical changes amplified in parallel with the rate at which compression increased. At very high rates, part of the chondrocytes died, while the cells that preserved their viability lost the ability to adequately respond to even a small stress. Together with metabolic changes, other biomechanical parameters, such as compressive and shear resistance, also deteriorated.

In contrast, low magnitude, short compression triggers a temporary increase in aggrecan mRNA expression in articular cartilage explants cultured in vitro (Valhmu et al., 1998). This phenomenon is regarded as a mechanical modulation of aggrecan gene expression.

In other experiments performed in vivo on guinea pigs (Wei et al., 2001), increased compression on some regions of articular cartilage, induced by the surgical disruption of the joint configuration, resulted in the accumulation of excess water in the tissue and a reduction in proteoglycan and collagen concentrations.

Similar biochemical disorders (e.g. increased water content, decreased aggrecan and collagen content) were observed in some parts of the articular cartilage of knee joints in dogs undergoing intense running training. These disorders resemble the beginning of degenerative cartilage changes in osteoarthrosis (Säämänen et al., 1994). In addition, elevated decorin concentration has been registered during very high dynamic loads (Visser et al., 1998).

The mechanotransduction (transmission of mechanical impulses to the cell) occurring in all these experiments is mediated by physical factors. Thus, the altered shape of chondrocytes under the influence of compression changes the configuration of ion channels (potassium ion channels in particular) in the plasma membrane, and affects their function. These are caused by the modulation of activity in terms of intracellular metabolic processes. The movement of ions present in interstitial water is altered under the influence of compression, accompanied by changes in the electrical potential acting on chondrocytes and by the hyperpolarization of the cell.

Mechanotransduction is also associated with molecular interactions between chondrocytes and the extracellular matrix. Integrin $\alpha V\beta 5$, which possesses mechanosensory properties, participates in these interactions. Under moderate intermittent compression not exceeding the physiological loads, this integrin activates the expression of interleukin-4 by chondrocytes (IL-4), which affects cell polarization through the paracrine and autocrine pathways (Millward-Sadler et al., 1999).

Under these conditions, IL-4 stimulates the biosynthesis of aggrecan by chondrocytes and inhibits the biosynthesis of metalloprotease MMP-3, as confirmed by corresponding changes in the mRNA levels of these macromolecules. Furthermore, this anabolic and, essentially chondrogenic response to the IL-4-mediated mechanical force (compression) involves the inhibition of catabolic factors –the proinflammatory cytokine IL-1β and the tumor necrosis factor TNF-α. It is characteristic for normal chondrocytes, but is absent in chondrocytes from osteoarthrosis-affected cartilage (Millward-Sadler et al., 2000).

Stronger compressive stresses exceeding the physiological limits cause a catabolic anti-chondrogenic effect.

This is manifested by the elevated expression of IL-1β and matrix metalloproteases, and the inhibition of their tissue inhibitors (TIMP). Additionally, extremely high mechanical overloads induce the expression of the vascular endothelial growth factor (VEGF), not typical for the avascular cartilage tissue, and the inhibition of its antagonist–endostatin, a fragment of the type XVIII collagen macromolecule. Penetration of capillaries into articular cartilage tissue results in its destruction (Pufe et al., 2005).

The family of the transcriptional activator, nuclear factor NF-κB (see section 10.2.4), is considered to be the endpoint of the intracellular molecular signaling pathways (both chondrogenic and anti-chondrogenic), generated by the biomechanical impact on chondrocytes (Knobloch et al., 2008).

Thus, an analysis of the biomechanical properties of articular cartilage illustrates the concept of the extracellular matrix of connective tissue as a mechano-chemical, as well as mechano-biochemical structure (see section 1.3).

7.2.2. Hyaline non-articular cartilage–cartilage tissue

7.2.2.1. Morphological characteristics

The presence of two types of connective tissue–dense fibrous and cartilage–is characteristic of the organization of hyaline non-articular cartilage (airways, ribs). The former forms the basis of the perichondrium, which is penetrated by nerves and blood vessels providing nutrients to the cartilage and carrying away its metabolites. The fibrous structures of the perichondrium (collagen and elastic fibers and fibrils) directly proceed into the hyaline cartilage tissue, the basis of the hyaline cartilage itself. Chondrocytes of variable shapes and degree of maturity represent its cellular elements. They are located in the extracellular matrix, either individually or in isogenic groups of cells in the lacunae.

The fibrous framework of non-articular hyaline true cartilage is fibrillar (the same as articular cartilage). In other words, it is constructed of individual collagen fibrils. Their characteristic feature is the presence of only two layers or zones: peripheral and central (as opposed to the three zones in articular cartilage). In the peripheral zone, collagen fibrils, although not incorporated into fibers, retain a predominant orientation parallel to the perichondrium, as well as a round shape in cross sections and a diameter of 50–80 nm. The fibrils do not branch. The preferential orientation of collagen fibrils in the fibrillar framework of proper cartilage is lost with increasing distance from the perichondrium. The organization of the framework in the central zone is isotropic. Fibrils in this zone branch into thinner fibrils or subfibrils (Omelyanenko, 1984) (*Fig. 7.30*). This phenomenon is especially pronounced in the collagen fibrils of the central layer of rib cartilage. In cross sections, the fibrils have irregular shapes, fuzzy outlines and lighter regions in the structure (*Fig. 7.31*). Clearly, the branching of the fibrils reaches the level of microfibrils (Omelyanenko, 1981). Nevertheless, the 60–70 nm periodicity in the structure of these fibrils is preserved. The equivalent diameter of the fibrils in all hyaline cartilages is in the range of 20–200 nm.

There are also fibrils with an equivalent diameter of up to 1,000 nm. Many authors refer to them as "asbestos" or "amianthoid" fibers (Hough et al., 1973; Hukins & Knight, 1976; Ghadially et al., 1979). Significant differences in the thickness of the fibrils do not affect their periodicity. At the interface of the perichondrium and the proper cartilage, elastic perichondrium fibrils thin out to the size of collagen fibrils, and ramify into even thinner branches, which probably proceed into the proper cartilage, where they are indistinguishable from the thin collagen fibrils. This data suggests the presence of either very thin elastic fibrils, or their individual components–fibrillin (glycoprotein) microfibrils–in proper cartilage.

The organization of structured proteoglycans into several types is similar to that of hyaline articular cartilage, with some minor differences related to the structural features of the fibrous components of hyaline non-articular cartilage.

The cartilage end-plate (CEP), part of the intervertebral disc, represents one type of non-articular hyaline cartilage. Similarly to articular cartilage, CEP are in direct contact with the underlying (subchondral) vertebral cancellous bone. On the opposite side, the hyaline cartilage tissue of the plate transitions into nucleus pulposus, i.e. it is not bathed by the synovial fluid as articular cartilage, and also has no perichondrium characteristic of the above-mentioned non-articular cartilages. Therefore, CEP feeding takes place only from the side of the subchondral bone, which affects the structure of CEP. Nevertheless, the general principles of hyaline cartilage's organization and its individual components (cellular and fibrous elements, and the integrating buffer metabolic medium) are conserved in CEP. The prevalence of "amianthoid" fibers in the composition of CEP is notable. These unique collagen fibrils, with a thickness of 200–1,500 nm, are present in the end-plates of people of all age groups and, like regular fibrils, undergo degenerative changes with age (see *Fig. 7.32 a, b*).

7.3. ELASTIC CARTILAGE – CARTILAGINOUS TISSUE

7.3.1. Morphological characteristic

Elastic cartilage is included in the composition of the human ear auricle, larynx and epiglottis, giving these anatomical structures elastic properties. The auricular elastic cartilage is the most informative in terms of structure and properties. It consists of two parts: the perichondrium and the proper elastic cartilage

(*Fig. 7.33 a, b*). The perichondrium has protective, trophic and plastic functions with regard to the true cartilage: it limits unnecessary strain, provides nutrients, removes metabolites through the vessels passing through it, and contains cartilage progenitor cells in the inner layer. In turn, external (larger) and internal (smaller) parts are distinguished in the perichondrium; the latter proceeds directly into the proper cartilage. The external layer of the perichondrium is made of dense fibrous regular connective tissue, and the internal part is formed of dense and loose irregular connective tissue. The fibrous framework of the perichondrium is fibro-fibrillar. Collagen fibrils, incorporated in fibers or found individually, are of fairly uniform thickness (50–80 nm) and rarely branch. They have a characteristic periodicity (a period is 60–70 nm).

The elastic fibers are another fibrous constituent of the perichondrium fibrous framework. The elastic fibers are arranged in the same way as the collagen fibers in the external layer of the perichondrium–parallel to the surface of the cartilage plate. They ramify into finer branches in the internal layer of the perichondrium. All of the fibrous constituents of the perichondrium directly proceed into the fibrous framework of the proper elastic cartilage.

In LM studies, the homogeneity of the extracellular matrix of the proper elastic cartilage in hematoxylin-eosin-stained sections is associated with the very compact arrangement of the fibrous constituents (Omelyanenko, 1983). Individual collagen fibrils are the basic collagen structures here. Thin bundles of collagen fibrils and the collagen fibers they form are found in some areas. The majority of fibrous constituents are oriented parallel to the cartilage plate in the peripheral regions of proper cartilage. The elongated chondrocytes are oriented the same way. Chondrocytes become rounded in the transition to the central layer. Thicker elastic fibrils and fibers appear. Collagen fibrils represent the majority of collagen structures (*Fig. 7.34 a*). The constituents of the fibrous framework do not have a preferential orientation (*Fig. 7.35*). Chondrocytes are found in 1–4-chamber lacunae (*Fig. 7.33 a, b*). The walls of the lacunae are made of collagen and elastic fibrils. Collagen fibrils have the same characteristics as in the perichondrium. The structure of elastic fibrils (*Fig. 7.34 b b*) is identical to the elastic fibrils described earlier (see section 3.1.2). Structured proteoglycans of the granular ground substance fill the interfibrillar space, and surround both the collagen and elastic fibrils, combining them into an integrated "monolithic" structure (*Fig. 7.36*).

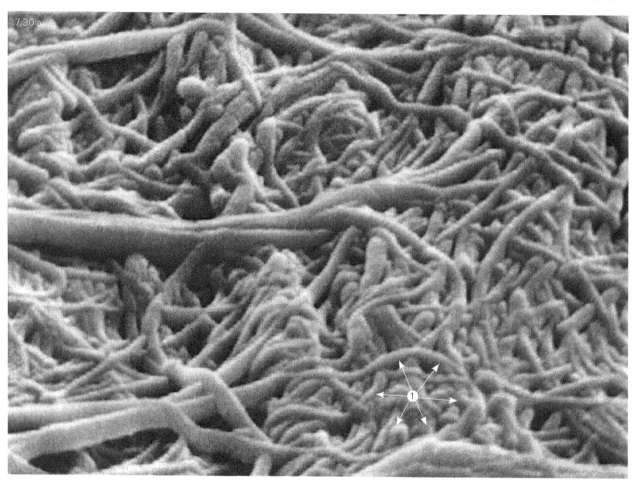

7.30 a

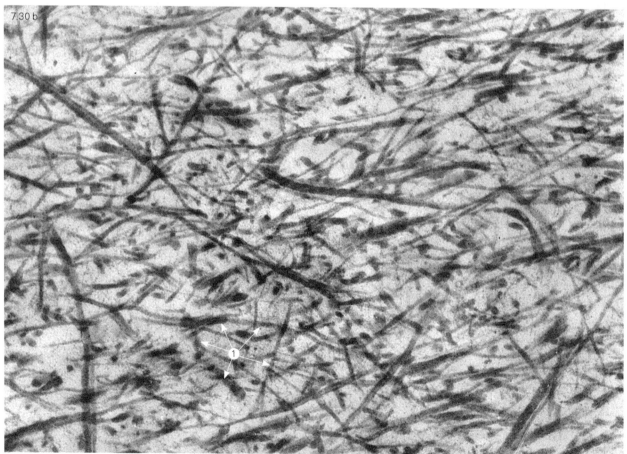

7.30 b

7.31

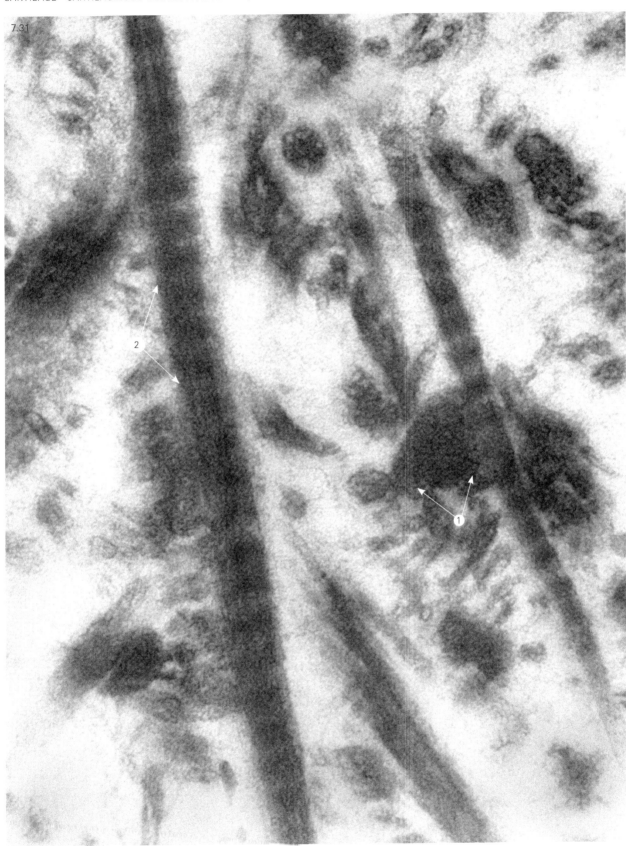

Fig. 7.30.
A fragment of the central part
of the hyaline cartilage of nasal
septum.
Fibrillar framework.
Collagen fibrils (1).
a – SEM-micrograph.

x 20,000.
b – TEM-micrograph.
Contrasting of ultrathin
sections with uranyl acetate
and lead citrate.
x 20,000.

Fig. 7.31.
A fragment of rib hyaline
cartilage.
Collagen fibrils in a cross
section (1)
and in a longitudinal section (2).
TEM-micrograph.

Contrasting of ultrathin
sections with uranyl acetate
and lead citrate.
x 50,000.

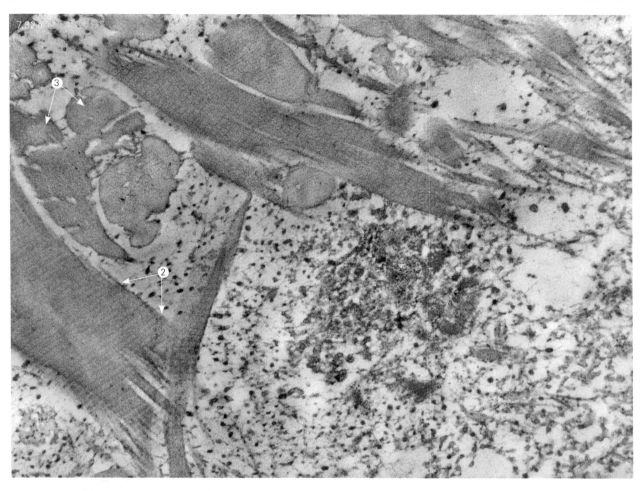

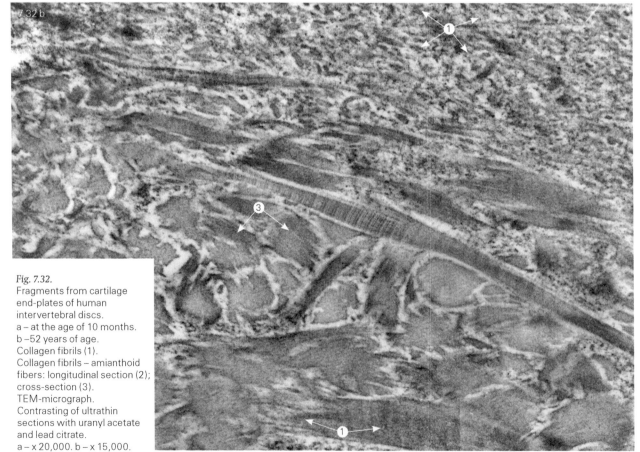

Fig. 7.32.
Fragments from cartilage
end-plates of human
intervertebral discs.
a – at the age of 10 months.
b – 52 years of age.
Collagen fibrils (1).
Collagen fibrils – amianthoid
fibers: longitudinal section (2);
cross-section (3).
TEM-micrograph.
Contrasting of ultrathin
sections with uranyl acetate
and lead citrate.
a – x 20,000. b – x 15,000.

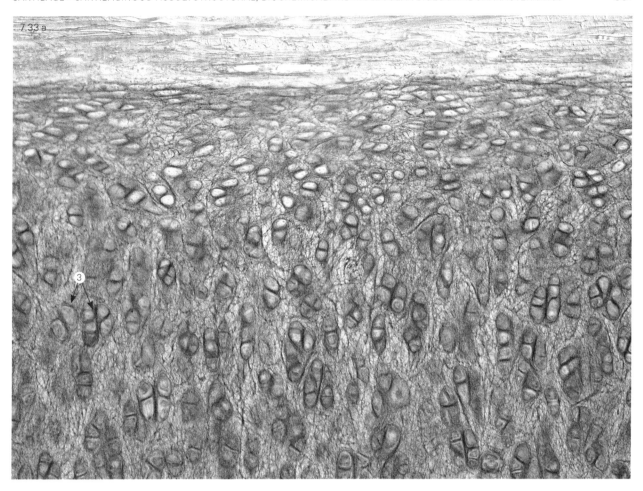

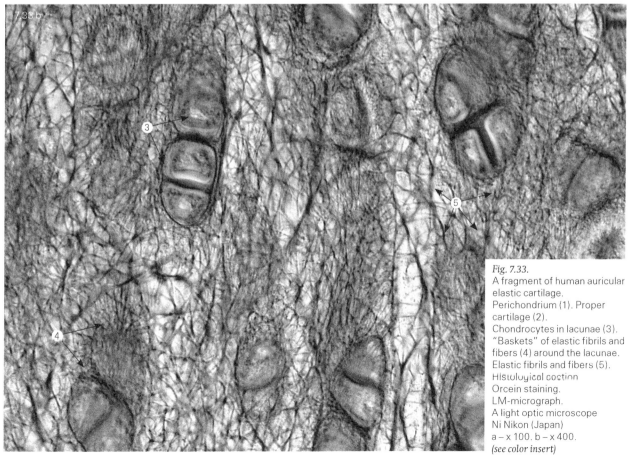

Fig. 7.33.
A fragment of human auricular elastic cartilage.
Perichondrium (1). Proper cartilage (2).
Chondrocytes in lacunae (3).
"Baskets" of elastic fibrils and fibers (4) around the lacunae.
Elastic fibrils and fibers (5).
Histological section
Orcein staining.
LM-micrograph.
A light optic microscope
Ni Nikon (Japan)
a – x 100. b – x 400.
(see color insert)

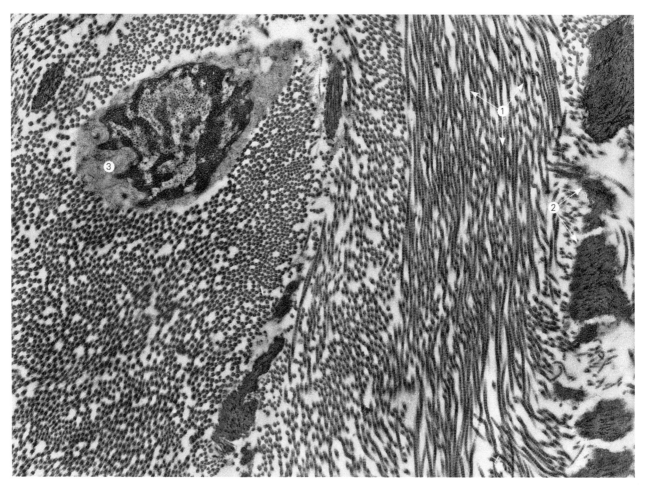

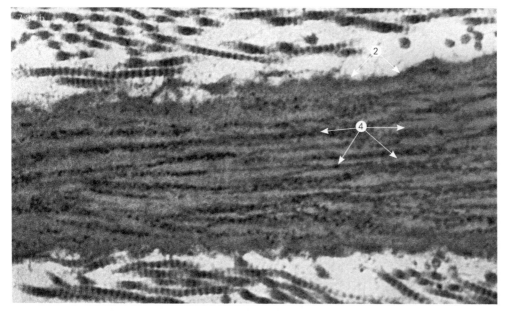

Fig. 7.34.
A fragment of human auricular
elastic cartilage. Collagen (1)
and elastic (2) fibrils and fibers.
Chondrocyte (3).
Framework microfibrils (4).
Amorphous substance (5).
TEM-micrograph.
Contrasting of ultrathin
sections with uranyl acetate
and lead citrate.
a – x 10,000. b – x 30,000.

Fig. 7.35.
A fragment of human
auricular elastic cartilage.
Collagen (1) and elastic (2)
fibrils and fibers.
SEM-micrograph.
 x 3,000.

Fig. 7.36.
A fragment of human auricular
elastic cartilage.
Collagen (1) and elastic (2)
fibrils and fibers, surrounded
by electron-dense, ruthenium-
positive amorphous substance
of proteoglycan nature.
TEM-micrograph.
Ruthenium red staining.
x 10,000.

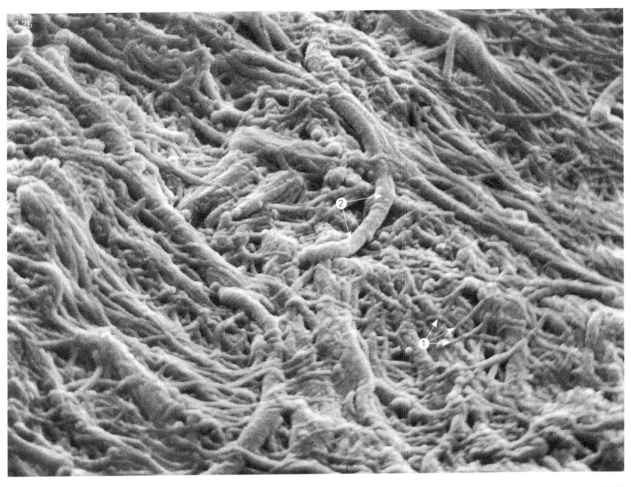

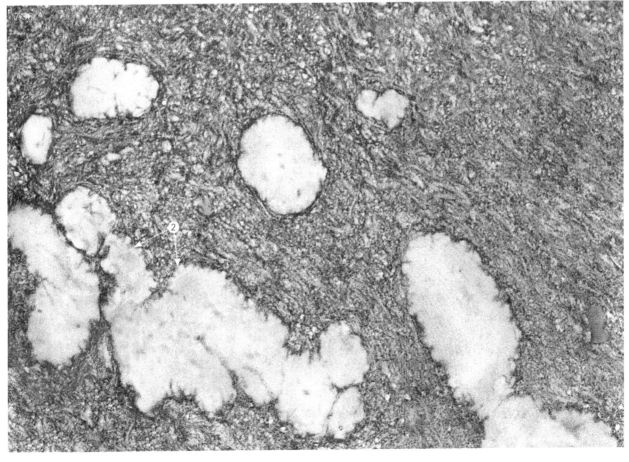

7.4. FIBROUS CARTILAGE–CARTILAGINOUS TISSUE

7.4.1. Morphological characteristic

The fibrous cartilage–cartilage tissue–is defined, according to the international histological classification, as a type of skeletal connective tissue.

Despite the official approval of this notion, a number of investigators do not consider it appropriate to assign the fibrous cartilage–cartilage tissue to the proper cartilage category. Obviously, this view is based on the morphology of this cartilage species.

The structure of fibrous cartilage is discerned in the transition regions from tendons into hyaline cartilage and further into bones. In these areas, the fibrous framework corresponds to the dense fibrous regular connective tissue. The cells are round and elongated in shape, and are arranged in single chains between the longitudinally oriented collagen and elastic fibers. The collagen fibrils forming the collagen fibers are made up of both type I (the majority) and type II (the minority) collagen protein. The cellular constituents occupy an intermediate position between fibroblasts and chondrocytes.

The features of hyaline cartilage tissue become more pronounced when approaching the cartilage; the features of dense fibrous regular connective tissue, (i.e. a tendon) emerge in the opposite direction.

The designation of this transitional region as a separate individual species of cartilage tissue and, even more so, designating the cartilage as a separate anatomical structure, lacks foundation.

The fibrous ring of an intervertebral disk is the most frequently cited example of fibrous cartilage (as an anatomical structure). However, the bulk of it (the larger part)–the outer and middle thirds–represents fibrous dense regular connective tissue, in terms of its structure, and a typical tendon, in terms of its fibrillar composition. There are two predominant groups of fibrils therein, with diameters of 30–50 nm and 120–150 nm. The fibrils of the latter group branch out constantly. The thin fibrils merge together. The basic structural units of the intercellular substance of the fibrous ring are collagen fibers with a flat shape, located between the cartilage end-plates at an angle of 30–40° to their planes (*Fig. 7.37*). The fibers is are 0.5–0.8 mm thick. Adjacent fibers are oriented in the opposite direction with regard to the arrangement of collagen fibrils. The angle of inclination to the plane of end-plates is preserved (Omelyanenko, 1984). Upon approaching the nucleus pulposus, the fibers become looser and less oriented.

The fibrous ring and other parts of the intervertebral disc, contains elastic fibers; the structure is presented in detail in section 3.1.2.

The differential distribution of interstructural spaces shows that 41% of the total volume of spaces have equivalent diameters ranging from 150 to 5 nm. Interfiber spaces represent 28% (15,000–1,500 nm). Spaces, occupying an intermediate position, represent 31% (1,500–150 nm). The volume of the interstitial spaces is equal to 0.91 cm^3/g of dehydrated tissue (Omelyanenko, 1991).

While, on the one hand, all of the data provided above does not fit the structure of hyaline cartilage, on the other hand, it is close enough to the structure of the dense fibrous regular connective tissue (e.g. a tendon).

Apparently, the reason that the fibrous ring is considered as fibrous cartilage is the structure of the areas where it transitions into the hyaline end-plate (analogous to the transition of a tendon into cartilage) and into the nucleus pulposus.

From a functional point of view, the fibrous cartilage mediates the transmission of stress-strain during spine loading and the compression of the nucleus pulposus on the fibrous ring. By their nature, such loads are characteristic for the tendons. Other types of cartilage perform a damping or amortization function owing to their elastic properties.

Thus, without conflicting with the existing classification, the conditional nature of the fibrous cartilage–cartilage tissue must be considered when using this term, and its structure and function should be presented with care.

Another type of connective tissue structure is the nucleus pulposus–part of the intervertebral disc. Its gel-like consistency, i.e. high water content, is a peculiar structural feature, which allows nucleus pulposus to perform an amortization function in the spinal intervertebral disc. During spine loading, the nucleus pulposus moves into the interfibrillar and interfiber space of the inner and middle parts of the fibrous ring, and returns to the central part of the intervertebral disc after relaxation (i.e. once the load is removed).

Toward the center of the intervertebral disc, the fibrous, oriented structure of the inner part of the fibrous ring becomes fibrillar and non-oriented. Furthermore, the density of the fibrous framework decreases. Cellular constituents are less common than in hyaline cartilage, and some of them are structurally similar to chondrocytes (*Fig. 7.38*), whereas others resemble fibroblasts.

In young individuals, the central part of nucleus pulposus contains only individual, widely spaced collagen fibrils made of type II collagen protein and with a diameter of 20–70 nm. They do not have a defined preferred orientation with respect to the relatively large interfibrillar spaces (Omelyanenko, 1991) (*Fig. 7.39*).

Fig. 7.37.
Fibrous foundation of the fibrous ring of a human intervertebral disc. Outer part. Alternating differently oriented collagen fibers (1). Collagen fibrils (2) incorporated in fibers.
a – SEM-micrograph.
x 1,000.
b – TEM-micrograph.
Contrasting of ultrathin sections with uranyl acetate and lead citrate.
x 10,000.

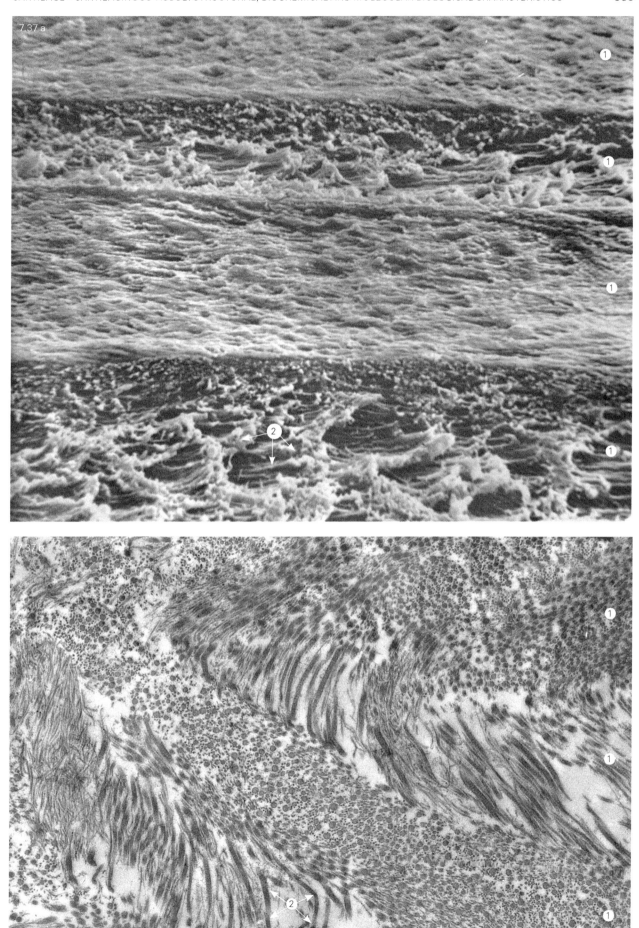

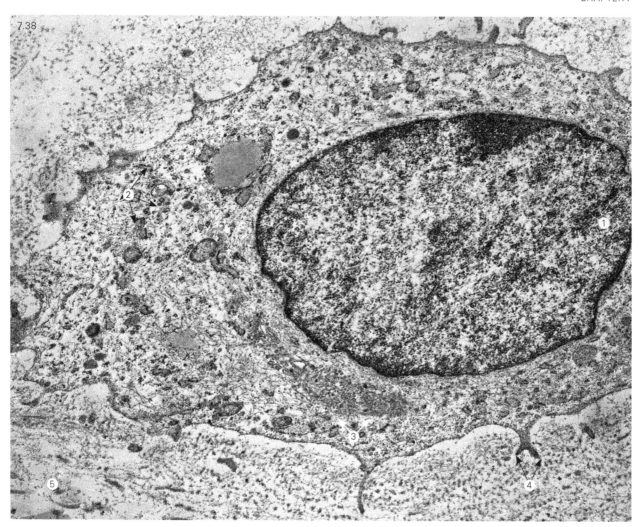

Besides these major collagen fibrils, various other (less representative) fibrous structures can be found in the nucleus pulposus, but the role played by most of them has not been defined.

Thin filaments with a thickness of 3–5 nm, similar to the microfibrils of collagen fibrils, stand out among these structures. A significant portion of the filaments exist individually, forming a network that lacks a defined preferred orientation. Another portion of the filaments are arranged in parallel and form aggregates, within which they can interact with each other or be separated by spaces of up to 10 nm. This determines the "loose" structure of the aggregates. The thickness of the aggregates depends on the number of filaments that they contain. This could be 2–5 filaments or several hundred, corresponding to a thickness of 10–250 nm (Fig. 7.40 a).

The aggregates have a periodic (repeating) structural organization. Each period has a length of about 120 nm and consists of two regions. In the more rarefied region, the filaments have low interaction density, which makes it possible to visualize them well. The length of these regions (lighter in the TEM-micrograph) is about 65 nm. Apparently there is high density of cross-links (i.e. active groups) between the filaments in the other part of the

period. This results in higher concentrations and density of the contrasting agents (lead citrate and uranyl acetate) in these regions (darker in the TEM-micrograph). Their length is 55 nm (Fig. 7.40 b). The approximate nature of the length of the periods is related to the roughness of their contours. Due to the presence of such dense (dark) regions within the periods, the aggregates are called striated. Type VI collagen is the basic component of the filaments.

The thickness of the filamentous aggregates varies along their length due to their branching or the merging of fine aggregates.

Some supergiants can be found, the thickness of which

Fig. 7.38.
A chondrocyte cell from the nucleus pulposus of a human intervertebral disc.
Cell nucleus (1).
GER (2).
Lamellar complex (3).
Cellular processes (4).
Extracellular matrix (5).
TEM-micrograph.
Contrasting of ultrathin sections with uranyl acetate and lead citrate.
x 10,000.

Fig. 7.39.
A region of nucleus pulposus from a human intervertebral disc.
Collagen fibrils (1) of the fibrous framework.
a – TEM-micrograph.
Contrasting of ultrathin sections with uranyl acetateand lead citrate.
x 20,000.
b – SEM-micrograph,
x 10,000.

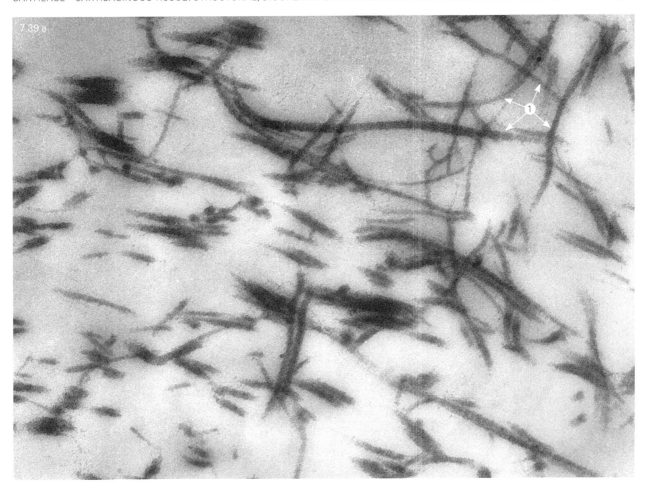

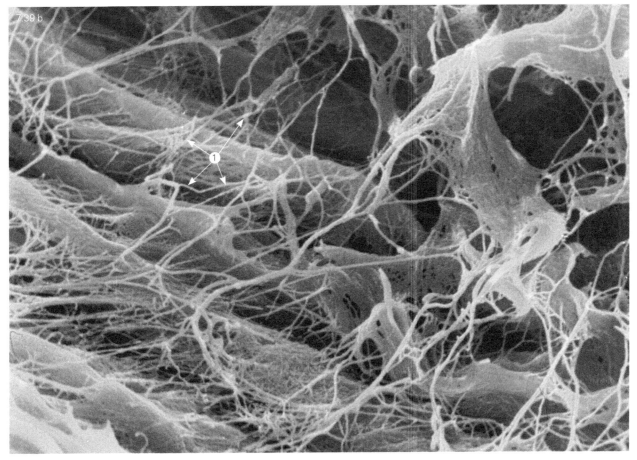

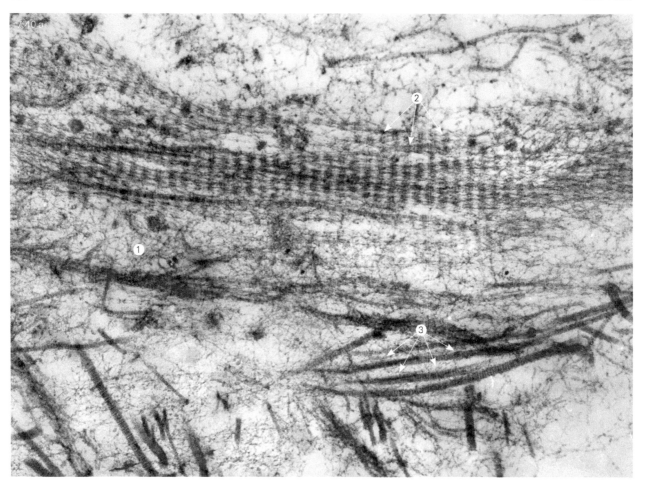

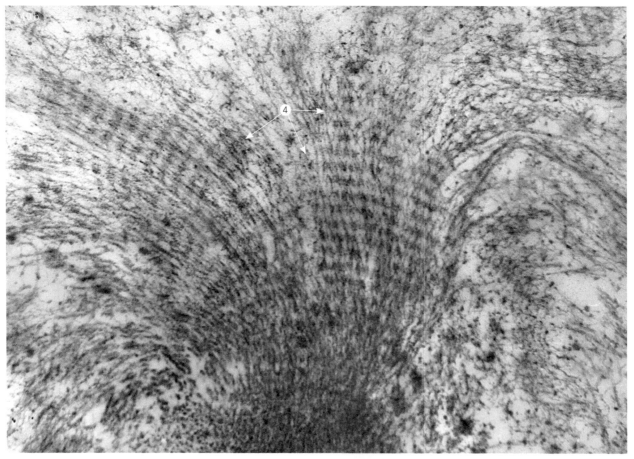

7.40 c

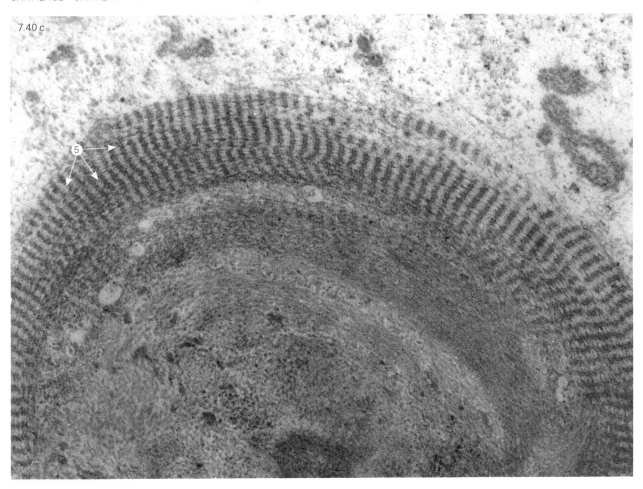

can reach 2,000–3,000 nm. Some of these aggregates have a fan-like appearance, with fine fillamentous aggregates heading in different directions away from the dense core (*Fig. 7.40 b*). Other superaggregates have a circular structure. Their dense core, composed of protein granules or fibrils closely adjacent to each other, is surrounded by filamentous aggregates or superaggregates in the form of a ring (*Fig. 7.40 c*).

Fig. 7.40.
A region of nucleus pulposus from a human intervertebral disc. Network of individual filaments (1). Longitudinally striated filamentous aggregates (2). Collagen fibrils (3). Filamentous striated superaggregates of the "fan" type (4) and "circular" type (5). TEM-micrograph. Contrasting of ultrathin sections with uranyl acetate and lead citrate.
a – x 20,000.
b, c – x 15,000.

The low density of fibrils in nucleus pulposus is reflected in the size distribution of interstructural spaces. Sixty-three percent of them represent spaces with equivalent diameters from 15,000 to 500 nm. The total volume of the interstitial spaces is 2.13 cm^3/g dehydrated tissue.

The cellular constituents of nucleus pulposus, to a large extent, resemble the chondrocytes of hyaline cartilage.

The intercellular and interfibrillar spaces are filled with various types of structured proteoglycans. The most abundant among them are thin filaments (made of individual granules), which form a meshwork where the free cells apparently are filled with water in the native tissue. It should be noted that the structure of nucleus pulposus is characterized by the uneven distribution of its components. Obviously, this is reflected in its biomechanical properties and, most importantly, in the distribution of loads generated in the spine.

With age, the structure of nucleus pulposus changes significantly. The fibrous framework becomes denser. There are collagen fibers among the increased number of collagen fibrils. The number of degenerative forms of cells increases.

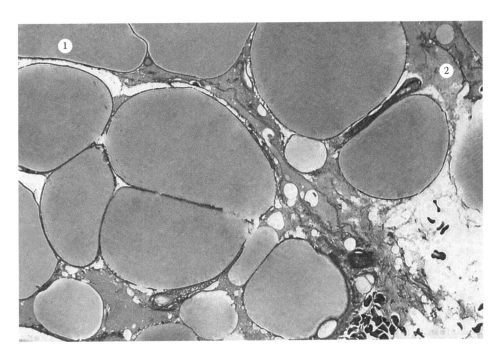

Fig. 2.13 b
White adipocytes (1) of the subcutaneous adipose tissue. The loose fibrous irregular connective tissue between adipocytes (2). b – LM-micrograph.
A light optic microscope Ni Nikon (Japan). Contrasting with an OsO4 solution in fragments and staining of the section with methylene blue + azure II, counterstaining with basic fuchsine, × 700.

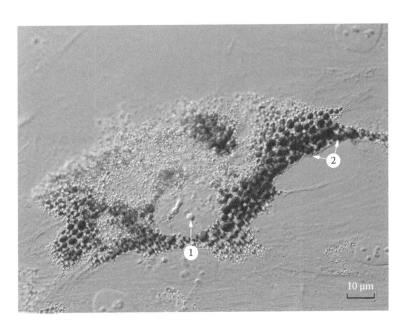

Fig. 2.14 c
Multicameral adipocyte (lipocyte) of the subcutaneous fat in culturing with large, medium and small lipid droplets. LM-micrograph. A light optic microscope Ni Nikon (Japan). Cultured cells after fixation and staining with Oil Red. × 600.

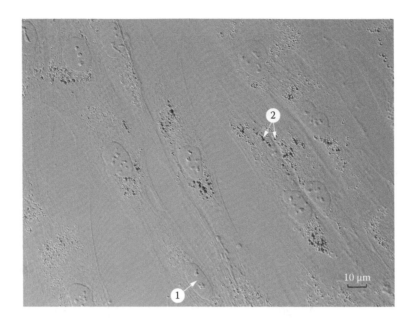

Fig. 2.14 d
Fibroblast-like cells containing small lipid droplets. A nucleus with nucleoli (1). Lipid droplets (2).LM-micrograph. A light optic microscope Ni Nikon (Japan). Cultured cells after fixation and staining with Oil Red. × 600.

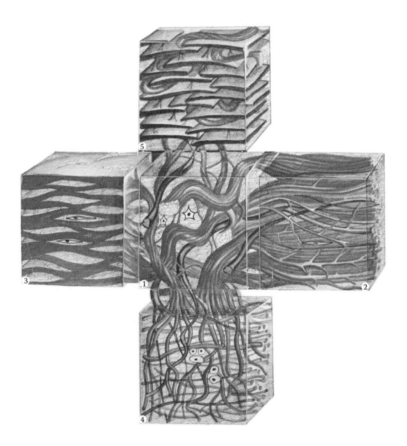

Fig. 3.31
A summary image of the structural organization of different connective tissue types, their relationship, and the constructive transformation of the fibrous elements and frameworks in transitioning from one type to another.(according to Omelyanenko,1984).
1 – fibrous loose irregular CT, collagen-elastic, fiberfibrillar, non-oriented type of a fibrous framework.
2 – fibrous dense regular CT, the collagen-elastic, fibrillar, oriented type of a fibrous framework (tendon).
3 – fibrous dense regular CT, the collagen, fibrillar, combined in orientation type of a fibrous framework (cornea).
4 – hyaline cartilaginous tissue. The collagen, fibrillar nonoriented type of a fibrous framework (hyaline cartilage).
5 – the elastic-collagen, fibrillar combined type of a fibrous framework (the aorta middle layer).

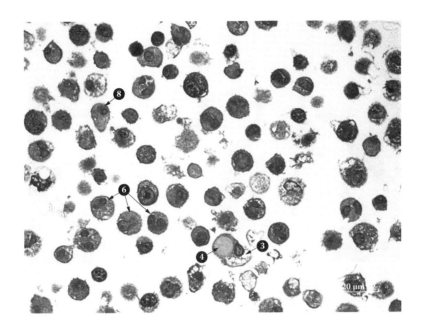

Fig. 6.12 b
Human bone marrow cells immediately upon isolation. Semi-thine sectione. A lipocyte (3). A drop fat(4). White blood cells (6). Cells changing their form (8). LM-micrograph. A light optic microscope Ni Nikon (Japan). Semi-thine sectione. Azur-eozin. × 800.

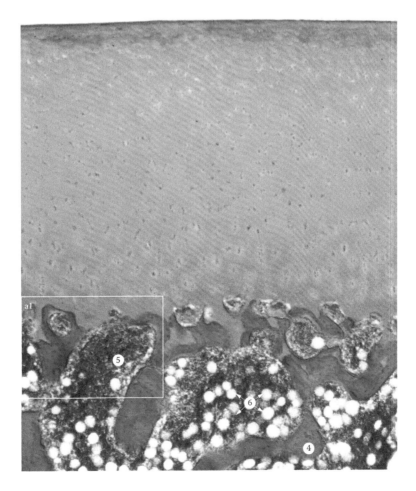

Fig. 7.14 a
Femoral head fragment. Age 14 years. Articular hyaline (nonmineralized) cartilage (1). Subchondral bone (2). Chondrocytes (3). Bone trabeculae (4). Red bone marrow (5). Fat cells (6). Bone marrow and nonmineralized cartilage contact regions (7). A light optic microscope Ni Nikon (Japan). Histological section. H-E staining. LM-micrograph. × 32.

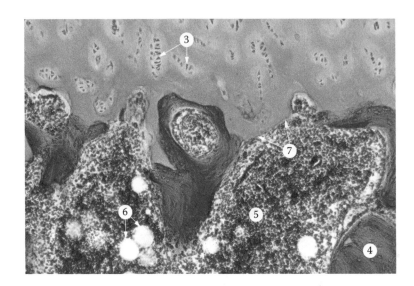

Fig. 7.14 a1.
Femoral head fragment. Age 14 years. Articular hyaline (nonmineralized) cartilage (1). Subchondral bone (2). Chondrocytes (3). Bone trabeculae (4). Red bone marrow (5). Fat cells (6). Bone marrow and nonmineralized cartilage contact regions (7). A light optic microscope Ni Nikon (Japan). Histological section. H-E staining. LM-micrograph. × 100.

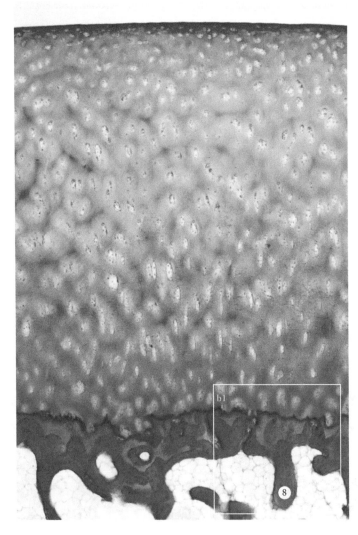

Fig. 7.14 b
Femoral head fragment. Age 40 years. Articular hyaline (nonmineralized) cartilage (1). Mineralized cartilage (2). Tide mark (3). Subchondral bone (4). Chondrocytes (5). Yellow bone marrow (6). Bone marrow and nonmineralized cartilage contact regions (7). Bone trabeculae (8). LM-micrograph. A light optic microscope Ni Nikon (Japan). Histological section. H-E staining. × 32.

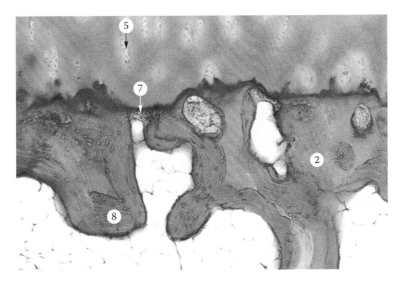

Fig. 7.14 b1
Femoral head fragment. Age 40 years. Articular hyaline (nonmineralized) cartilage (1). Mineralized cartilage (2). Tide mark (3). Subchondral bone (4). Chondrocytes (5). Yellow bone marrow (6). Bone marrow and nonmineralized cartilage contact regions (7). Bone trabeculae (8). LM-micrograph. A light optic microscope Ni Nikon (Japan). Histological section. H-E staining. × 100.

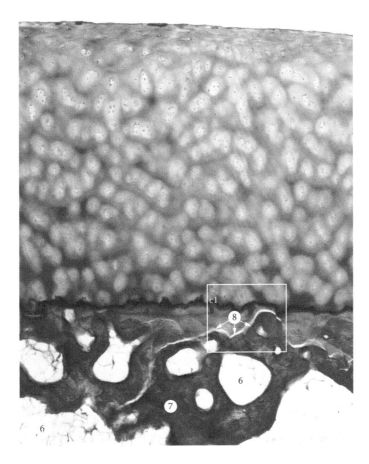

Fig. 7.14 c
Femoral head fragment. Age 80 years. Articular hyaline (nonmineralized) cartilage (1). Mineralized cartilage (2). Tide mark (3). Subchondral bone (4). Chondrocytes (5). Yellow bone marrow (6). Bone trabeculae (7). Separation of the mineralized cartilage from the subchondral bone (8). LM-micrograph. A light optic microscope Ni Nikon (Japan). Histological section. H-E staining. × 32.

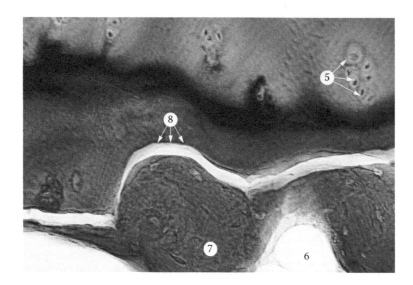

Fig. 7.14 c1

Femoral head fragment. Age 80 years. Articular hyaline (nonmineralized) cartilage (1). Mineralized cartilage (2). Tide mark (3). Subchondral bone (4). Chondrocytes (5). Yellow bone marrow (6). Bone trabeculae (7). Separation of the mineralized cartilage from the subchondral bone (8). LM-micrograph. A light optic microscope Ni Nikon (Japan). Histological section. H-E staining. × 250.

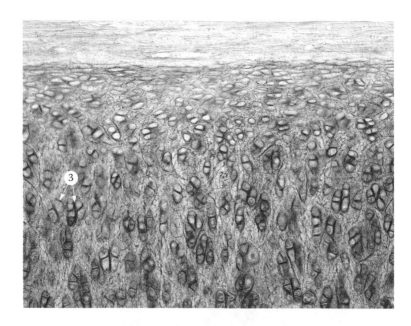

Fig. 7.33 a

A fragment of human auricular elastic cartilage. Perichondrium (1). Proper cartilage (2). Chondrocytes in lacunae (3). "Baskets" of elastic fibrils and fibers (4) around the lacunae. Elastic fibrils and fibers (5). LM-micrograph. A light optic microscope Ni Nikon (Japan). Histological section. Orcein staining. × 100. b – x 400.

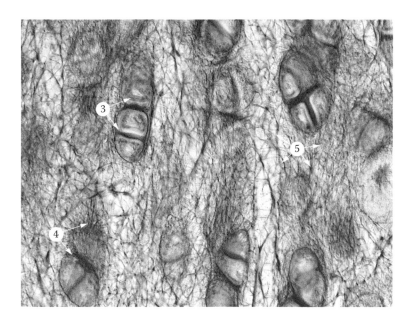

Fig. 7.33 b
A fragment of human auricular elastic cartilage. Perichondrium (1). Proper cartilage (2). Chondrocytes in lacunae (3). "Baskets" of elastic fibrils and fibers (4) around the lacunae. Elastic fibrils and fibers (5). LM-micrograph. A light optic microscope Ni Nikon (Japan). Histological section. Orcein staining. × 400.

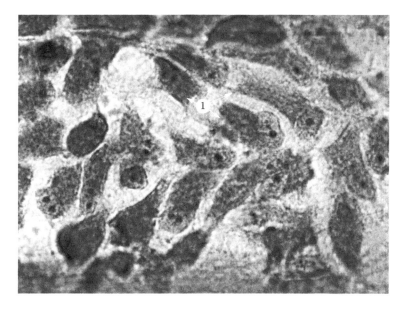

Fig. 8.4 a
Primary osteoblasts in a regenerated bone (1). a - LM-micrograph A light optic microscope Ni Nikon (Japan). Histologic section. Hematoxylin and eosin stain. (Japan). × 1000.

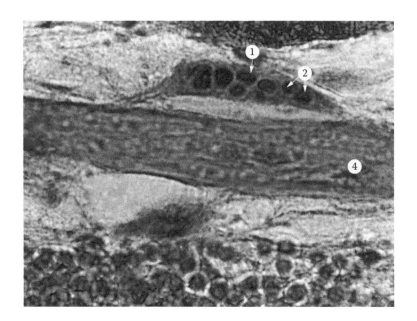

Fig. 8.10a
Osteoclasts in a regenerated bone (1). Nuclei (2). A primary trabecule (4). LM micrograph. A light optic microscope Ni Nikon (Japan). Histologic section. Hematoxylin and eosin stain. × 1,000.

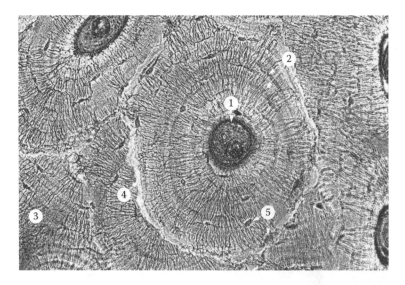

Fig. 8.14a
Osteons of the cortical part of the tibial diaphysis. Central canal (1). Osteonic bone lamellae (2). Intermediate bone lamellae (3). Cement lines (4). Osteocytes with processes in the bone canaliculi (5). Cross section. LM-micrograph. A light optic microscope Ni Nikon (Japan). Histologic sections. Schmorl staining. × 400.

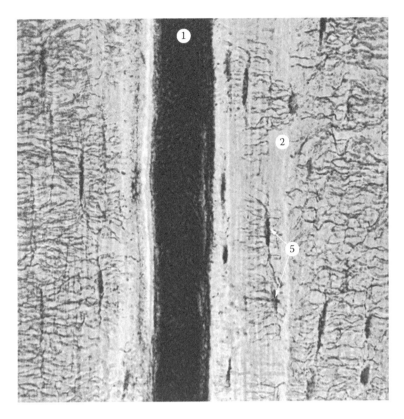

Fig. 8.14b
Osteons of the cortical part of the tibial diaphysis. Central canal (1). Osteonic bone lamellae (2). Osteocytes with processes in the bone canaliculi (5). longitudinal section. LM-micrograph. A light optic microscope Ni Nikon (Japan). Histologic sections. Schmorl staining. × 400.

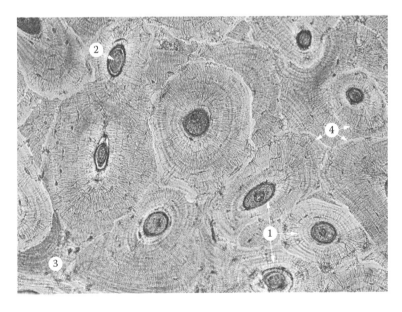

Fig. 8.17a
Fragment of the cortical part of the tibial diaphysis. Compact bone tissue. Osteons on a cross-section (1). Central canals of osteons (2). Intermediate lamellae (3). Cement lines (4). LM -micrograph. A light optic microscope Ni Nikon (Japan). Histologic section. Schmorl staining. × 200.

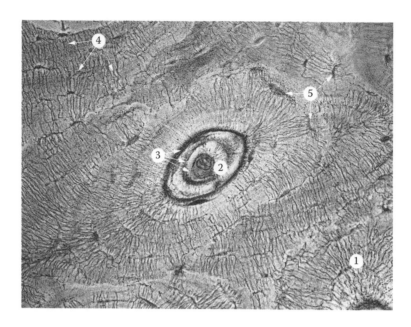

Fig. 8.35
A fragment of lamellar compact bone tissue. Osteons (1) in a cross-section. Central canal (2). Circular (collector) canaliculi (3). Canaliculi (4). Lacunae (5). LM-micrograph. A light optic microscope Ni Nikon (Japan). Histological section. Schmorl staining. × 200.

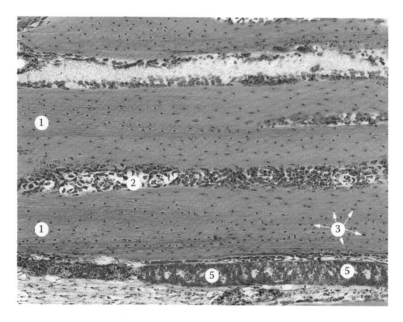

Fig. 8.40a
A fragment of 21-day-old dog distraction bone regenerate. Zone of primary (reticulofibrous) osteogenesis. Primary bone trabecula (1). Primary osteoblasts (2) and osteocytes (3). Sinusoidal capillary (5). LM-micrograph. A light optic microscope Ni Nikon (Japan). Histological sections. Hematoxylin-eosin staining. × 200.

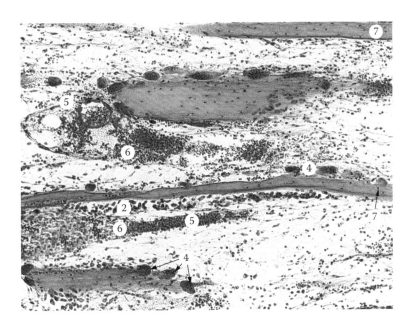

Fig. 8.40b
A fragment of 21-day-old dog distraction bone regenerate. Bone resorption zone. Primary osteoblasts (2). Osteoclasts (4). Sinusoidal capillary (5). Erythrocytes (6). Resorbing bone trabecula (7). LM-micrograph. A light optic microscope Ni Nikon (Japan). Histological sections. Hematoxylin-eosin staining. × 200.

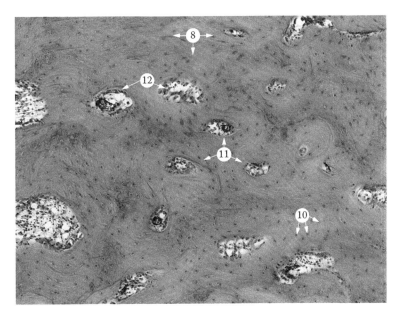

Fig. 8.40c
A fragment of 21-day-old dog distraction bone regenerate A cross-section. Zone of secondary (lamellar) osteogenesis. Primary bone lamellae (8). Secondary osteoblasts (9) and osteocytes (10). Forming primary osteons (11) and central canals (12). LM-micrograph. A light optic microscope Ni Nikon (Japan). Histological sections. Hematoxylin-eosin staining. × 200.

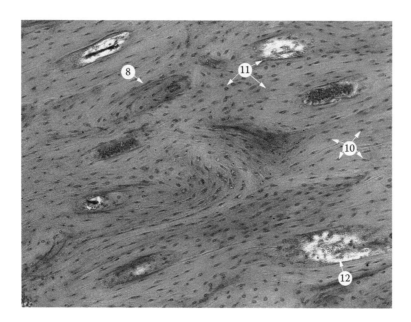

Fig. 8.40d
A fragment of 21-day-old dog distraction bone regenerate. A tangential section Zone of secondary (lamellar) osteogenesis. Primary bone lamellae (8). Osteocytes (10). Forming primary osteons (11). Central canals (12). LM-micrograph. A light optic microscope Ni Nikon (Japan). Histological sections. Hematoxylin-eosin staining. × 200.

Chapter 8

BONE TISSUE:
THE STRUCTURAL-
FUNCTIONAL,
BIOCHEMICAL
AND BIOMOLECULAR
CHARACTERISTICS
OF ITS COMPONENTS

8.1. GENERAL OVERVIEW OF BONE TISSUE STRUCTURE AND COMPOSITION

8.1.1. The structure of bone tissue

Bone tissue is dense, mineralized and well-shaped connective tissue characterized by an organized association of specialized cellular elements, an arranged fibrous base, and an extracellular fluid space comprised of a complex multilevel system of interconnecting canals.

All bone tissue components are interconnected in a specific manner and are quantitatively balanced. Its cellular elements are mesenchymal derivatives. Within the body, this type of tissue performs biomechanical (support and protection) functions and constitutes the basis of the bone, an organ of the locomotor system and a link in the functional system regulating the circulation of calcium levels in humans and animals. Three main types of bone tissue – reticulofibrous, rough fibrous and lamellar – may be distinguished, depending on the respective degree of maturity and the structural properties of fibrous matrix elements (*Fig. 8.1*).

The formation and the further structural maintenance (renewal) of bone tissue involve two types of differons (histogenetic series of cells). The first one is the osteal differon, with the majority of its cells constantly present in the bone tissue. Another cellular differon related to the bone tissue (that is associated with it) is that of mononuclear phagocytes (the osteoclastic differon).

Fibrous structures of bone tissue, similarly to those of other types of connective tissue, are comprised of a complex multilevel hierarchy system involving molecular and supramolecular levels (see Fig. 3.3). The basic component of these structures – type 1 collagenous protein – makes up about 95% of the organic part of the bone matrix. Mature bone tissue mainly consists of flat and flattened collagen fibers; in a mineralized state, their complexes are referred to as bone lamellae. Because morphological studies of bone tissue are mostly performed on demineralized samples, the terms "bone lamella" and "flat collagen fiber" convey the same meaning. It is due to the presence of lamellae in the bone tissue that it is known as "lamellar". The lamellar bone tissue was previously referred to as "fine-fibrous"

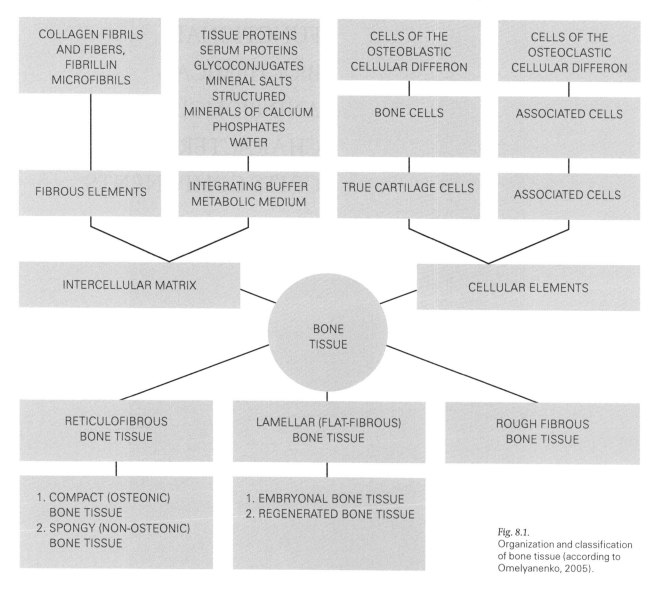

Fig. 8.1.
Organization and classification of bone tissue (according to Omelyanenko, 2005).

or "flat-fibrous". Obviously, the term "fiber-lamellar" would offer a more precise description for the architecture of lamellar bone tissue, constituting 97–98% in an adult body and comprising the basic element of osteonic and non-osteonic lamellar complexes, which, in turn, form the basis of spongy and compact bone tissue. All bones in the body are made up of a varying ratio of these types of tissue.

Rough fibrous and reticulofibrous bone tissues are treated as one type in the literature. However, the comparative morphological analysis of these tissues shows considerable variability in their structural organization. Thus, embryonic or regenerated bone tissue has a reticulofibrous structure that is, in the early stages of its formation, similar to the structure of spongy bone tissue. This justifies the use of the term "primary bone rods" ("trabeculas"). The latter are collagen fibers (non-flat) or bundles thereof. The basic structural element of these fibers is type 3 collagenous protein. In the remodeling process, the reticulofibrous bone tissue undergoes resorption in order to be replaced with a newly formed lamellar bone tissue, whose collagen fibers are flat in shape and basically made up of type 1 collagenous protein. The mineral phase is comprised by crystalline hydroxyapatite.

Classical sources have claimed that rough fibrous bone tissue does not have a lamellar arrangement. It is found at the tendon to bone insertions, i.e. regions of transition from tendons' collagen fibers to those of a bone (lamellae). The considerable thickness and dense concentration of mineralized collagen fibers (non-flat in shape) in these areas suggests a formal reason to recognize a rough fibrous bone tissue as a separate type, while it would be incorrect to equate it with the reticulofibrous type. No rough fibrous bone tissue is found in the area of cranial sutures (another site reported in the literature).

Bone tissue of the cranial bones, including the region of the sutures, has a lamellar arrangement (osteonic in particular). The structural elements of bone lamellae (collagen fibrils or fibers) do not pass from the lamellae of one cranial bone into another. The edges of the jointing bones have protrusions and indentations in them, which interact to form a bone suture. The tightness of fit between the scull bones is ensured by the presence of a thin layer of fibrous connective tissue directly attached to both bones.

The strength of the suture depends entirely on the mineral components maintaining the shapes of the aforementioned formations. In a demineralized skull, the bones detach from each other easily enough without changing their structure. It is only the fibrous layer, apparently a remainder of the mineralized periosteum, which comes loose. Such a structure cannot justifiably be referred to as reticulofibrous bone tissue. It is evident that further morphological and biochemical analysis will support the appropriateness of classifying rough fibrous and reticulofibrous bone tissues into two separate types.

A complex consisting of mineralized collagen structures and a ground substance is the main functional link in terms of compact bone tissue, which performs the support function and thus, requires constant renewal. Within the bone tissue, plastic material access and the elimination of breakdown products occur via interstitial space, a widely developed multilevel network of interconnecting canals. These canals differ in size, direction and function, while belonging to a single system.

Unlike most tissues of the body, bone is a multiphase material and, as such, is equally extensively studied using both morphological and physicochemical methods. In terms of the latter, the interstitial spaces (canals) are a kind of pores, making the bone a porous material. This arrangement determines bones' high mechanical strength properties.

Therefore, physicochemical research methods considerably widen opportunities in terms of understanding the nature of the interstitial, or pore, space of the bone tissue and filling the gaps in our knowledge thereof.

In the above diagram of the organization and classification of bone tissue (*Fig. 8.1*), the concepts of compact and spongy bone substances used in the Nomina Histologica are replaced by "compact and spongy bone tissues". The rationale for such a replacement is evident. The term "substance" designates a certain matter (bone matter, in this case), but we are dealing with two types of bone tissue. Therefore, they should be identified accordingly. Besides, the categorization of bone tissue as lamellar compact and spongy bone tissues conforms to the classification of connective tissue (fibrous dense and loose connective tissues).

8.1.2. Chemical composition of bone tissue

Biochemically (and morphologically), the key feature of bone tissue is the presence of a considerable amount of mineral (inorganic) component in its extracellular matrix. As shown in *Fig. 8.2*, generalizing the chemical composition of bone tissue, the mineral phase accounts for about 70% of its overall mass.

Since the weight of cellular elements in the bone tissue (as well as in cartilaginous tissue) is very small compared to the extracellular matrix, the numerical data shown in *Table 8.2* actually refers to the matrix.

To gain a fuller understanding of the proportion between bone tissue components, the weight parameters shown in *Table 8.3* should be supplemented with volumetric data. A comparison of the weight and volumetric data shown in *Table 8.1* makes it discernible that, despite the impression one might get from the weight parameters, the organic component prevails over the mineral one in the overall volume of bone tissue. This apparent paradox is due to the differences in specific gravities (densities) of the components, the specific gravity of mineral component exceeding that of the organic one more than two-fold. The volumetric data is essential to under-

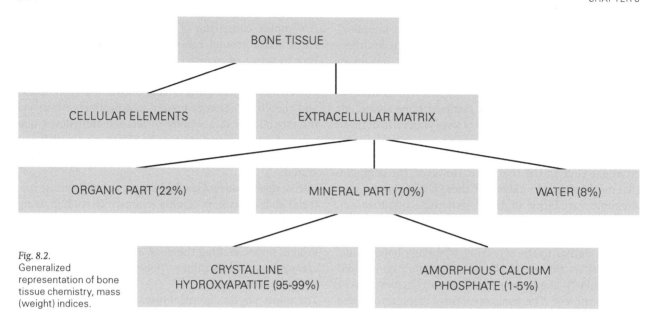

Fig. 8.2.
Generalized representation of bone tissue chemistry, mass (weight) indices.

Table 8.1

Weight and volumetric composition of compact bone tissue

Components	Density (g/ml)	Weight (%%)	Volume (%)
Cells + liquid	1,05	10	16
Organic componnt	1,41	30	45
Mineral component	3,15	60	40

Table 8.2

Chemical composition of compact bone tissue

Components	g/100 g
Inorganic (mineral) components	68–73
Collagenous proteins	20–23
Non-collagenous proteins	12–15
Lipids	0,7–0,8
Water	7,0–10,0

Table 8.3

Basic quantitative biochemical characteristics of compact and spongy bone tissue in the distal femoral epiphysis in humans

Parameters	Compact bone tissue	Spongy bone tissue
	g/100 g fried defattedc tissue, M±m, p<0.05	
Calcium, total	26,6±0,4	21,4±1,5
Nitrogen,total	5,3±1,4	5,6±0,5
Collagenous proteins	21,4±0,9	19,6±1,6
Non-collagenous proteins	5,8±1,1	6,5±1,6
Hexosamines	0,11±0,03	0,18±0,01
Hexuronic acids	0,09±0,03	0,13±0,03
Deoxyribonucleic acid	0,21±0,05	0,24±0,11
Ribonucleic acid	0,14±0,04	0,18±0,05

standing the functions of the bone tissue (including the biomechanical function).

The overall average density of compact bone substance is 2.10 g/ml or 0.48 ml/g, reaching 2.33 g/ml in completely mineralized compact bone tissue (Mbuyi-Muamba et al., 1989).

The mineral component here is conventionally considered to consist purely of hydroxyapatite Ca10(PO4)6(OH)2 (see section 8.3.2.1).

Table 8.2. shows the bulk/integral chemical composition of fresh (non-dehydrated) compact and spongy bone tissue.

Our data in *Table 8.3* gives a general quantitative concept of the basic biochemical parameters of bone tissue.

Research has been conducted both on tissues received from surgical interventions and cadaveric tissues that were preserved by freezing.

Total calcium reflects the content of the mineral component, while total nitrogen serves as a net measure for the level of proteins.

As suggested by the data presented, the mineral component (inorganic phase) constitutes about 70% of the overall mass of compact bone tissue. Higher concentrations of mineral substances occur only in tooth dentine, but

most of the minerals in the body are contained in the bone tissue due to the greater total weight of the latter.

An adult human body contains about 1 kg of calcium. Apart from its structural and mechanical role, this defines another major function of the bone tissue as the main depot of mineral substances in the body.

Because of the complex structure of bone tissue (both at the macroscopic and microscopic levels), the results of the quantitative biochemical analysis of tissue samples are typically averaged ones.

Quite considerable quantitative variations in the chemical composition of bone tissue are observed between different age groups, different bones of the same body, or even – within the limits of compact substance – between different areas of the same cross-section of a bone. This was demonstrated in our research, using the human tibial bone as an example (Saulgozis et al., 1973)

A segment of human tibia was dissected along a plane perpendicular to the long axis of the bone and divided into six zones (two anterior, two posterior and two lateral). From each of these, 1,0--1,5-ml³ samples were withdrawn.

Differences in the concentrations of collagenous proteins in the samples, as determined according to hydroxyproline content, reached as much as 18.9% of the average for this bone. Approximately the same results were seen in terms of the differences in mineral component levels which, in this experiment, were measured based on inorganic phosphate content. For non-collagenous glycoconjugates (whose levels were reflected by hexosamines content), the sample to sample differences reached 47%.

Collagenous proteins are quantitatively dominant among extracellular organic components of bone tissue, forming the basis of the supramolecular structure of the extracellular matrix (see section 8.3.1.1). Their mass exceeds 20% of the total mass of the bone, but their volume is comparable to that occupied by mineral substances.

The quantitative ratios of mineral and organic constituents in human bone tissue do not remain constant throughout life. The total content of non-collagenous proteins in the compact bone tissue of the tibia in healthy adult humans (determined based on tyrosine levels) was shown to progressively increase with age. In the youngest age group (19–44), the tyrosine content averaged at 0.23 ± 0.04 g per 100 g of dry, defatted bone tissue, whereas, in the oldest age group (75–89), it reached 0.92 ± 0.35 g/100 g. In middle-age groups (45–74), tyrosine levels rise as the collagen content increases, measured by hydroxyproline content, and this allows considering the accumulation of non-collagenous proteins to not only be relative but also absolute (Slutsky & Pfafrod, 1980).

On the contrary, a study of spongy bone tissue in humans between 18–96 years of age (also with no evidence of any systemic changes in bone tissue), showed a gradual drop in collagen levels, accompanied by a similarly gradual increase in the degree of mineralization. These changes occur in parallel with a decrease in the total mass of the skeleton (Bailey and Knott, 1999).

8.2. DIFFERONS OF BONE CELLS

8.2.1. Osteogenic cells (osteoblasts and osteocytes) and their progenitors

8.2.1.1. Morphology of preosteoblasts and osteoblasts

The osteal differon, with the majority of its cells always present in the bone tissue^, includes the following types of cells:

1) multipotent stromal stem cells of the connective tissue, found in the bone marrow;
2) semi-stem, or committed progenitors of osteogenic cells (preosteoblasts);
3) osteoblasts; and
4) osteocytes.

Multipotent stromal stem cells of the connective tissue derived from the marrow are mesenchymal derivatives retaining the potencies of mesenchymal cells. They con-

stitute an element in the hematopoietic cells' microenvironment and may become the descendants of bone cells' differon. Pericytes and adventitious cells may probably possess similar capacities. A characteristic feature of connective tissue stem cells is their functional purpose of maintaining the population of several connective tissue differons of the body (including osteal) through intermittent division, during which one group of cells remains maternal while another starts differentiation and gradually loses the ability to divide in the process of acquiring a specialized function. Stem cells are capable of indefinite self-maintenance and remain in a condition of physiological rest during the body's physiological functioning. The specialized function of CT cells lies in the production of components of the intercellular matrix of an organ's connective-tissue framework and the subsequent maintenance of its homeostasis.

Preosteoblasts (committed* cambial** osteogenic cells) are derivatives of multipotent connective-tissue stromal stem cells of the bone marrow (apparently, pericytes or adventicytes). Preosteoblasts are characterized by retaining proliferation potencies, along with the acquired ability to produce the bone matrix components, as evidenced by elements of the GER and Golgi apparatus, as well as the corresponding nuclear-cytoplasmic ratio. Pre-osteoblasts are found in the inner layer of the periosteum, adjacent to the osteoid layer on the outer surface of the bone (periosteal cells) and within the endosteum (endosteal cells) that lines medullary spaces, haversian (central) and Volkmann's (perforating) canals, and also covers the trabeculae in spongy bone. Depending on their degree of differentiation, functional activity and location (surface of a growing bone, areas of remodeling, sites of reparative regeneration, or intact mature bone), these cells differ in shape (they can be flattened, spindle-shaped, oval, etc.) and they have varying nuclear-cytoplasmic ratios, and differ in the amount and variety of cytoplasmatic organelles (Fig. 8.3) (Ross et al., 1995).

In growing bones, a single layer of preosteoblasts lines the outer and inner surfaces of the bones, alternating with osteoblasts. Pre-osteoblasts have short processes, enabling them to establish gap junctional intercellular communication with each other or with neighboring osteoblasts.

In mature adult bone, where remodeling is relatively rare, the outer and inner surfaces of bones contain flat-

Fig. 8.3.
Pre-osteoblasts in a regenerated bone (1).
A fragment of primary trabecula (2).
Nucleus (3),
GER (4),
mitochondria (5).
a – SEM-micrograph;
b – TEM-micrograph.
Contrast of ultrathin sections enhanced with uranyl acetate and lead citrate.
a, b x 10,000.

* Cell commitment – limitation of the possible ways of differentiation.
** Cambiality – a cell's ability to replenish the pool/population/supply of differentiating cells by division (proliferation)

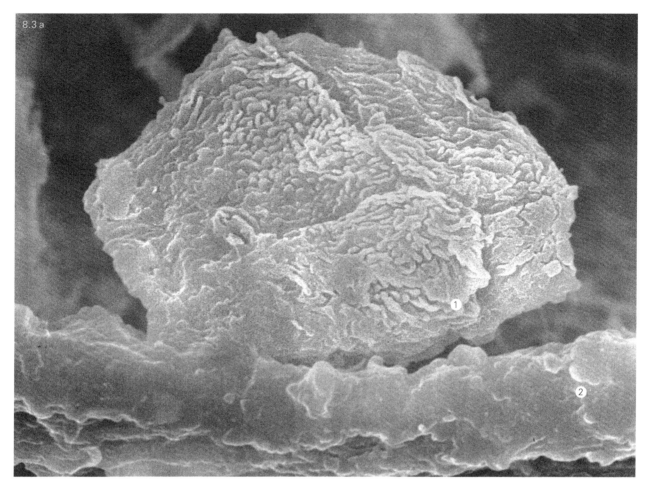

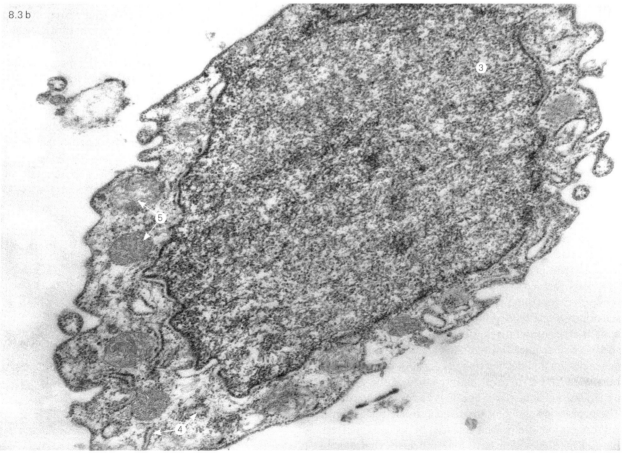

tened pre-osteoblasts with a rarefied cytoplasm depleted of "multi-purpose" organelles, localized mainly around the perinuclear area. These cells do not form a continuous cellular lining on the bone surface, interacting only at the sites of gap junctional communication of cell processes. Some longer processes extend into the osteoid (the non-calcified part of the formed bone matrix) and penetrate into bone canaliculi, interacting (communicating) with the osteocyte processes via gap junctions. Apparently, this is the way in which pre-osteoblasts participate in maintaining the trophism of osteocytes embedded in the bone matrix. Based on morphological data, such pre-osteoblasts exist in a more quiescent state than cells localized at the sites of active osteogenesis. The basic role of these cambial cells (found mostly in the G_0-period of the cell cycle) lies in maintaining the population of osteogenic cells as the need arises (physiological regeneration, including renewal, remodeling and reparative regeneration).

Numerous factors lead to a transformation of these cells into osteoblasts: the differentiation of pre-osteoblasts, morphologically evident by the formation and accumulation of GER, components of the Golgi complex and other multipurpose organelles, along with an increase in the cell volume, nuclear polarization, and a reduction in the nuclear-cytoplasmic ratio.

Osteoblasts are differentiated osteoblastic cells that produce and release components of the bone matrix that are involved in its formation and physiological regeneration (renewal), i.e. in maintaining the structure of bone tissue in its normal functional state. These cells are justifiably regarded as the "architectural managers" of bone tissue (Mackie, 2003). They retain the ability to divide. Due to their synthesis potencies, osteoblasts possess all of the necessary (essential) components, including a well-developed GER, a Golgi apparatus and mitochondria. Depending on their functional activity, osteoblasts may be resting or active. The latter typically localize in the areas of intensive osteogenesis (a growing bone, a bone in the process of reparative regeneration or remodeling) (Fig. 8.4). Active osteoblasts may also be subdivided into two groups. Primary osteoblasts take part in the formation of reticulofibrous bone tissue during embryogenesis or reparative regeneration. In this process, they become embedded, or "immured", into the primary trabeculae created by them (Fig. 8.5), transforming into flattened-shaped primary osteocytes with numerous short processes that do not penetrate into trabeculae. This prevents them from interacting and forming ordered associations (Fig. 8.6). An important fact is that, once the bone matrix mineralizes, the diffusion of nutrients to these cells becomes limited. This leads to their gradual degeneration and destruction. As a result, the process of formation and structural maintenance of the primary (regenerating) bone tissue becomes disrupted and ceases. The neoformed reticulofibrous bone tissue undergoes a full resorption and is then replaced by secondary osteoblasts (Fig. 8.7), which have long processes that enable

their interaction. The result of this cell activity is the lamellar bone tissue, while the cells themselves, embedded into the organic bone matrix, turn into secondary mature osteocytes, which form organized associations, wherein their communication via long cellular processes is retained. Osteocytes are located in the lacunae, with their processes extending into the canaliculi interconnected with the central and Volkmann's (communicating) canals (Fig. 8.8). Resting osteoblasts reside in the periosteum or endosteum of the mature bone (see Fig. 8.9) and do not form a continuous layer, while being capable of interacting with each other and the osteocytes of the underlying bone tissue via their cell processes. Communications between them are apparently established in the earlier stages in the same way as with neighboring osteoblasts and are retained after being embedded into the bone matrix. The cells embedded in the bone matrix and their processes are surrounded by free spaces that, in turn, form a system of bone canals – the lacuna-canalicular system – filled with interstitial fluid, the circulation of which provides for the metabolism of bone cells. Components of the intercellular bone matrix – fibrous (collagenous) proteins, glycosaminoglycans, polypeptide chains of proteoglycans, and enzymes (alkaline and acid phosphatase) – are accumulated and transported within the cytoplasm of osteoblasts as a result of their synthesis on GER in the vesicles of the Golgi apparatus.

Young osteoblasts, functionally active mature osteoblasts and hypertrophic osteoblasts, which may be considered "depot cells" for secretions, are distinguished based on the intensity of their osteogenic function and the degree of development of their synthetic and secretory apparatus (Rodionova, 1989).

Upon the completion of osteogenesis, the mature osteoblasts remaining on the bone surface are left with a partially reduced GER and Golgi apparatus, while, in young ones, the synthetic apparatus' development slows down as they turn into inactive forms of osteoblasts.

Inactive osteoblasts are flat cells with a poorly developed synthetic apparatus. Together with pre-osteoblasts, they cover about 70–80% of the bone surface in an adult human skeleton without the underlying osteoid (4–8% with the underlying osteoid).

Fig. 8.4.
Primary osteoblasts
in a regenerated bone (1).
Nucleus (2). GER (3).
a – LM-micrograph.
Histologic section.
Hematoxylin and eosin stain.
A light optic microscope
Ni Nikon (Japan) x 1000.
(see color insert)
b, c – SEM-micrograph.
b – x 1,500;
c – x 11,000.
d – TEM-micrograph.
Contrast of ultrathin sections,
enhanced with uranyl acetate
and lead citrate.
x 10,000.

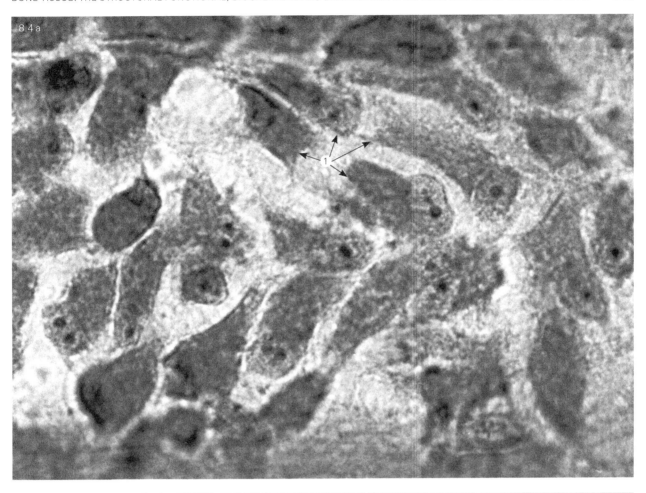

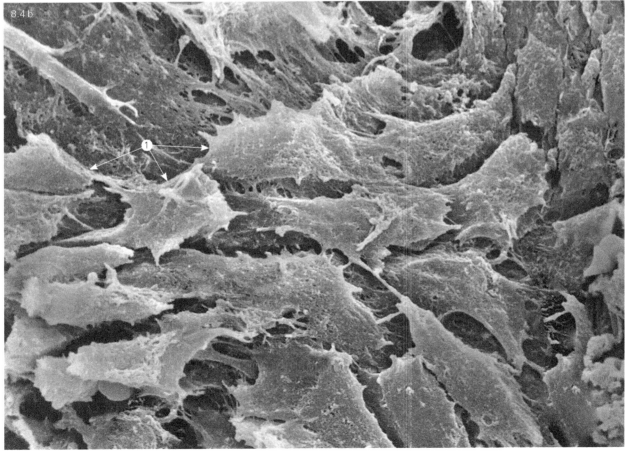

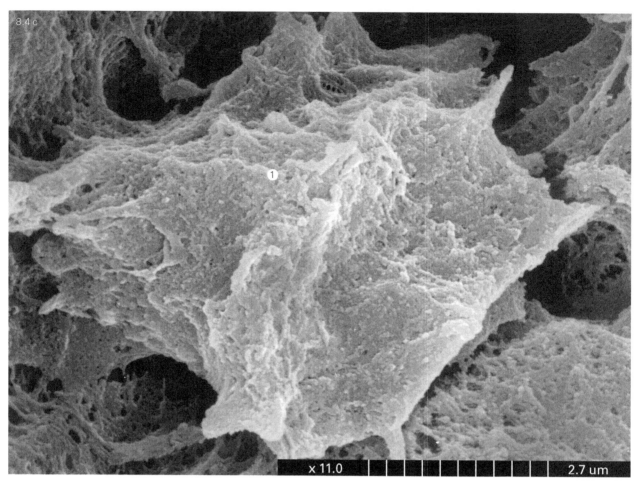

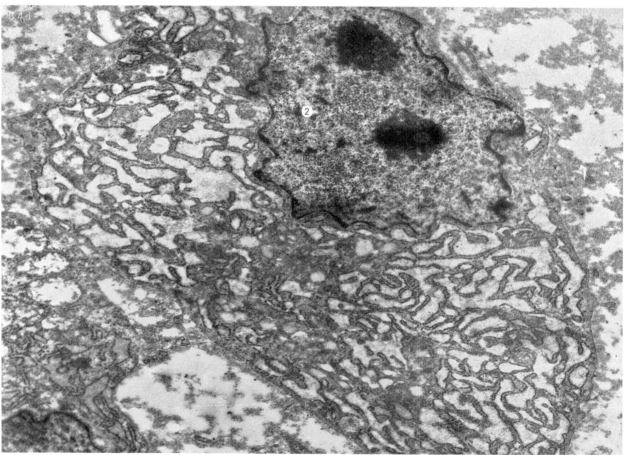

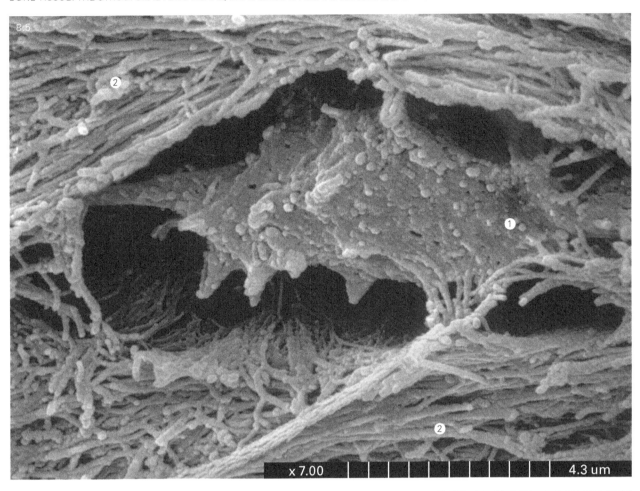

x 7.00   4.3 um

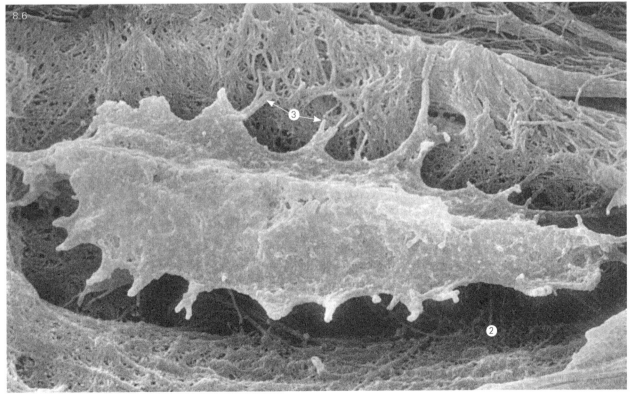

Fig. 8.5.
A primary osteoblast (1)
in a regenerated bone
surrounded by collagenous
fibers and fibrils (2) that make
up the major part of the
intercellular matrix.
SEM-micrograph. x 7,000.

Fig. 8.6.
A primary osteocyte (1)
in a lacuna (2).
Processes of an osteocyte (3).
SEM-micrograph.
x 4,000.

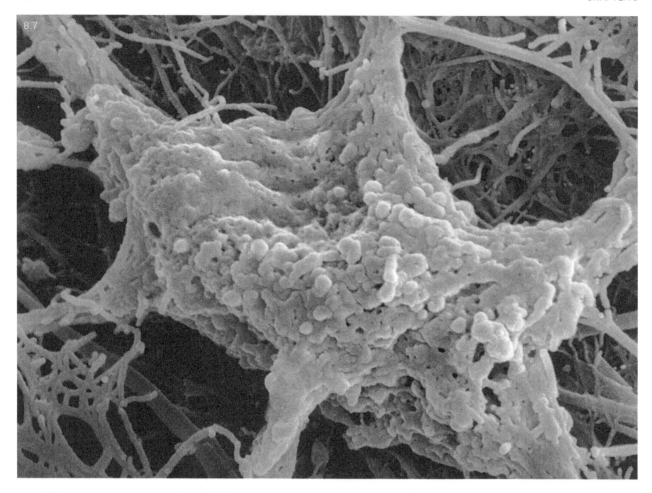

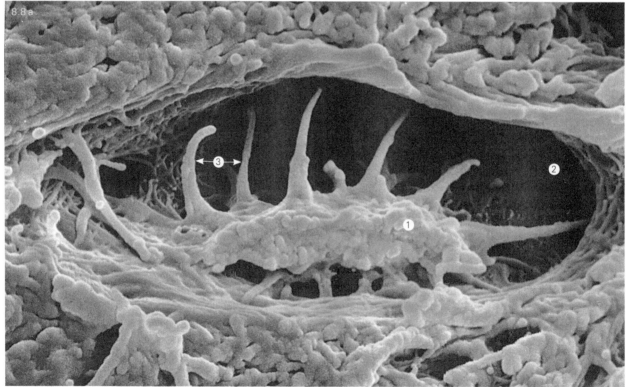

Fig. 8.7.
A secondary osteoblast on the surface of a neoformed lamellar bone after remodeling of the primary (reticulofibrous) regenerated bone. SEM-micrograph. x 5,000.

Fig. 8.8.
Osteocytes (1) in lacunae (2). Cellular processes (3). Nucleus (4). Lamellar bone tissue (5).

a, b – SEM-micrograph.
c – TEM-micrograph.
Contrast of ultrathin sections enhanced with uranyl acetate and lead citrate. a, b, c – x 5,000.

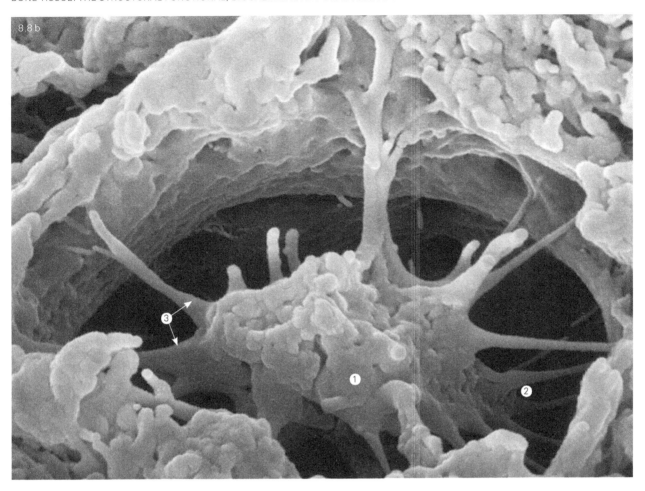

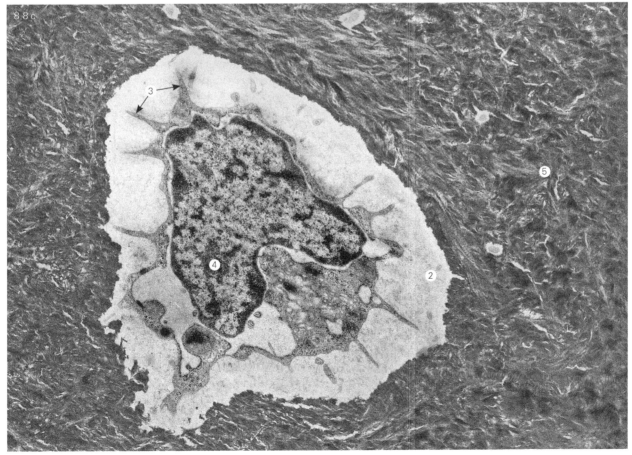

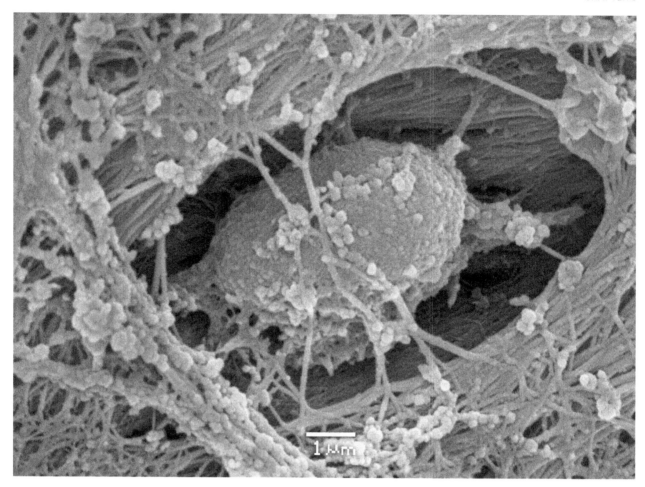

8.2.1.2. Molecular biological and biochemical characteristics of osteoblasts

The main function of the osteoblast is the active secretion of structural components for the extracellular matrix of bone tissue and the mineralization. This function is fulfilled at a certain stage of its differentiation from a multipotent connective tissue (mesenchymal) cell into an osteocyte. It is this stage of differentiation (the mature osteoblast stage) where the biochemical and biomolecular phenotypes of the osteoblast become similar in terms of the main characteristics to an active fibroblast (see section 2.2.1 and 2.2.2). During this stage, an osteoblast that has lost its capacity for mitotic division (typical to the previous stages), becomes focused, very much like a fibroblast, on the production and secretion of the macromolecular components of the extracellular matrix.

The similarity between the osteoblast and active fibroblast is clearly evident at the molecular level. In a comparative study of the expression of 7,500 genes by human osteoblasts and fibroblasts cultivated in vitro (Han et al., 2002), significant differences (more than three times higher) in the levels of expression were detected for just 120 genes: in 64 cases, a higher expression was seen in osteoblasts over fibroblasts, and in 56 cases, the opposite held true.

However, despite the apparent similarity between the osteoblast and the fibroblast, there are a number of important differences in their biochemical and biomolecular characteristics, which suggest the unique nature of the osteoblast's functional phenotype and justify the description of this cell as a "more complex" or "sophisticated" fibroblast (Ducy et al., 2000). This "sophistication" is related to major changes in the cell proteome and transcriptome. Thus, the osteoblast is characterized by a peculiar phenotype (Blonder et al., 2006).

The first and most pronounced group of differences affects the osteoblast's secretory function. Like the fibroblast, the osteoblast produces all the basic macromolecular components of the extracellular matrix. Nevertheless, osteoblast secretions have their own peculiarities and are, to a greater or lesser degree, specific to the organic matrix of the bone tissue, defining the features that are prerequisites for mineralization. Accordingly, the osteoblast is characterized by the active expression

Fig. 8.9.
A fragment of the endosteum
with pre-osteoblasts/
osteoblasts (1)
on the surface of the osteoid.
SEM-micrograph.
x 5,000.

of genes encoding these structural components of the matrix. There is also an active expression of enzymes and other proteins involved in the mechanisms of production, transport and the posttranslational processing of these components.

Most of the proteins expressed by the osteoblast do not exhibit absolute specificity in terms of the markers of the osteoblastic phenotype. Two structural non-collagenous proteins – bone sialomucoprotein and osteocalcin (and, to a lesser degree, the alkaline phosphatase enzyme) – are regarded as the most specific. The other molecules used as markers, secreted into the matrix in osteoblast studies, are type I collagen, which somewhat differs in the bone tissue from those found in other types of connective tissue (see section 8.3.1.1.1), and proteoglycan lumican (Raouf et al., 2002). The presence of this proteoglycan indicates the transition from a pre-osteoblast, capable of proliferating to an osteoblast that has lost this ability. The intensive expression of osteocalcin, a noncollagenous protein that binds the ion of calcium and plays a role in regulating matrix mineralization, is indicative of the complete differentiation (maturing) of the osteoblast. Osteocalcin is the most commonly used marker for a mature osteoblast and a pre-osteocyte.

The second group of differences is related to osteoblasts' intracellular proteins: cytosolic proteins and those of cellular organelles; the latter include cytoskeletal proteins (Billiard et al., 2003).

The third group of osteoblasts' distinguishing features is determined by the properties of proteins bound to their cellular (cytoplasmic) membrane and participating in osteoblasts' interactions with each other, with other cells (including osteocytes), and with the extracellular matrix.

The cytoplasmic membranes of osteoblasts possess a unique set of integrins, including $\alpha v \beta 3$, $\alpha v \beta 5$, $\alpha 5 \beta 6$, $\alpha v \beta 8$, $\alpha 2 \beta 1$, $\alpha 3 \beta 1$ and $\alpha 5 \beta 1$. This peculiarity is defined by a prevalence of $\alpha v \beta$ integrins, which bind osteoblasts to non-collagenous proteins of the extracellular bone matrix (v designates the α-subunit of integrins, whose specific ligand is vitronectin; the subunit αv also interacts with fibronectins) (Siebers et al., 2005). The $\alpha v \beta$ integrins (containing different β-subunits) are required for the osteoblast differentiation, induced by bone morphogenetic proteins in a relevant experiment (see 8.5.2) (Lai and Cheng, 2005). The $\alpha 2 \beta 1$ integrin binds osteoblasts to type I collagen, the main structural protein of the matrix. The $\beta 1$-subunit of integrins is essential for mature osteoblasts. In the absence of the external domain of this macromolecule, which protrudes into the matrix, osteoblast differentiation proceeds normally before osteocalcin expression commences, which indicates the osteoblasts' maturity. However, a functional impairment takes place as of this moment, reflected by a considerable reduction in the bone tissue mass in growing animals to 45% (Zimmerman et al., 2000). The $\beta 1$-subunit also plays a critical role in the activation of kinases, stimulating the expression of those genes in the osteoblasts that are most important for its specific biosynthetic functions. This role of the $\beta 1$-subunit is determined by its sensitivity to mechanical stimuli, generated by the movements of interstitial fluid (Lee D.Y. et al., 2008). The inhibition of the integrin function by specific antibodies leads to the suppression of mineralization: the use of the anti-$\alpha v \beta 3$-integrin antibody causes a 65% reduction in the degree of mineralization, while adding the anti-$\alpha 2 \beta 1$-integrin antibody reduces it by nearly 95% (Schneider et al., 2001).

The OF45 protein, expressed by osteoblasts and containing a "sticky" RGD sequence, participates, together with integrins, in interacting between cells and the extracellular matrix. The expression of OF45 (also known as MEPE) is more pronounced in osteocytes.

The fourth distinctive feature of the osteoblastic phenotype is the active expression of a large number of local (short-distance) signaling molecules, which play a role in regulating osteoblasts' and osteoblast-interacting cells' functions. The most important of these molecules are those involved in regulating osteoclastic resorption and the remodeling of bone tissue – RANKL and osteoprotegerin. These molecules also include the parathyroid hormone-related protein (PTHrP), exerting an anabolic effect in bones (Miao et al., 2005).

A number of molecules expressed by osteoblasts (osteopontin, Jag1, angiopoietin Ang-1, cadherins, etc.) take on a signal role and take part in regulating the differentiation of haematopoietic (stem) progenitor cells that contact the osteoblasts in the bone marrow stroma (Haylock & Nilsson, 2006; Yin & Li, 2006).

Some of the signaling molecules expressed by osteoblasts and larger molecules with a similar action mechanism play important roles in the processes of osteoblastogenesis and the formation of bone tissue.

Thus, in cultivated osteoblasts and in human osteoblasts *in vivo* at the time of the intensive deposition of bone matrix, as well as in young osteocytes, a protein called osteocrin (abbreviated as Ostn) is expressed and secreted into the matrix (Thomas et al., 2003; Bord et al., 2005). In humans, this is a short protein containing 54 amino-acid residues after removing a signal peptide and a propeptide. Its primary structure bears a certain similarity to that of peptide hormones. Osteocrin is also expressed by the myocytes of skeletal muscles (alternatively known as musclin) and actively influences the carbohydrate metabolism in muscle tissue. Therefore, in a strict sense, **osteocrin** is not a specific marker for the osteoblastic differon. However, its expression in osteoblasts shows a number of intriguing patterns. In cultivated osteoblasts, this expression coincides in time with the intensive formation of the extracellular matrix and is suppressed by vitamin D3; *in vivo*, its maximum occurs immediately after birth. The addition of osteocrin to an osteoblast culture leads to a delay in the final stage of differentiation (Thomas et al., 2003). All this data demonstrates the importance of osteocrin in the metabolism of osteoblasts (Moffatt and Thomas, 2009).

It is rather probable that this importance stems from the fact that osteocrin is a ligand for the C-type natriuretic peptide receptor (NPR-C) and, as such, competes with the natriuretic peptides themselves (Moffatt et al., 2007), while these peptides, particularly CNP, stimulate osteoblast differentiation.

Osteoblasts also express a protein that was initially referred to as osteoblast-specific factor 2 (OSF2) but was subsequently renamed **periostin** (Horiuchi et al., 1999), as the abbreviation OSF-2 became relatively common as an alternative name for an isoform of the transcription factor Cbfa1/Runx2, discussed later in this chapter. This glycoprotein, which is secreted into the extracellular matrix and has an average length of about 800 amino-acid residues and a molecular mass of 86–93 kDa, contains up to 20 y-carboxyglutamic acid (Gla) residues. This enables it to bind calcium, which promotes the mineralization of the matrix. The active expression of periostin is typical for intramembranous ossification, but is absent in endochondral ossification (Kashima et al., 2009).

Several isoforms of periostin are known, with differences between them concentrated in the C-terminal domain. The expression of periostin isoforms is stimulated by TGF-β growth factors (Litvin et al., 2004). Periostin is not only actively expressed in osteoblasts; considerable importance is also attached to it in heart morphogenesis. More specific to osteoblasts, especially those located on the surface of bone trabeculae, is the periostin-like factor (**PLF**), which is regarded to as one of the periostin isoforms. The hyperexpression of PLF stimulates the proliferation and differentiation of osteoblasts and amplifies bone tissue development in the medullary cavity (Zhu et al., 2009).

The glycoprotein osteoactivin, whose cDNA was originally isolated in an osteoblast study, has a variety of functions (Safadi et al., 2001). **Osteoactivin** exists as two isoforms, one of which is transmembranous and the other secreted into the extracellular matrix. The transmembrane isoform contains a greater number (up to 13) of N-linked oligosacharide groups; the mass of the osteoactivin macromolecule, consisting of 372 amino-acid residues, is 115 kDa given the highest level of glycosylation.

Osteoactivin expression in osteoblasts is induced and regulated by a bone morphogenetic protein (BMP-2) with the participation of Smad-1 protein (see section 8.5.2). At the same time, osteoactivin (its cytoplasmatic domain) acts as an intracellular mediator in terms of BMP-2's effect on osteoblasts' differentiation and function. The cytoplasmic domain also participates in regulating the movement of osteoblast-produced matrix components towards the cell membrane. The level of expression of the secreted osteoactivin correlates with the activity of alkaline phosphatase, which indicates its anabolic role in the final stage of bone matrix formation and mineralization (Abdelmagid et al., 2007; 2008).

A bioinformatical (mathematical) analysis of the structure of an osteoactivin macromolecule, which consists of two spiral domains divided by a double β-plate and contains a large number of various motifs, has shown that the range of its conformations, its function and action mechanisms may be more diverse than is currently thought. Osteoactivin is capable of playing the roles of a ligand, a receptor or an enzyme (Selim, 2009).

Osteoactivin is not a specific marker for the osteoblastic phenotype. Besides the osteoblasts, within the bone tissue, it is actively expressed by osteoclasts. In other tissues, it is expressed by various cells, particularly by fibroblasts.

Finally, the fifth group of proteins expressed by osteoblasts are the transcription factors, which play a crucial and direct role in the formation of the osteoblast phenotype. Their action determines the transcriptional profile and, consequently, the proteome of the osteoblasts.

Runx2 plays the key role among all these transcription factors (Komori, 2008; Franceshi et al., 2009). It is regarded as a "master regulator" of gene transcription in osteoblasts, with its gene known as a "master gene" (Schroeder et al., 2005). Its role in osteoblast differentiation is similar to that of the Sox9 factor in the differentiation of chondroblasts (Karsenty, 2008).

The main functional role of Runx2/Cbfa1 becomes obvious in the early stages of osteoblastogenesis, ranging from determining an osteoblastic direction in the differentiation of the multipotent connective-tissue (mesenchymal) cell to reaching the stage of a pre-osteoblast. In all of these stages, Runx2/Cbfa1 has a stimulating effect.

Runx2/Cbfa1 is also essential to mature osteoblasts, and is involved in maintaining their phenotype. It slows down their differentiation into osteocytes, which prolongs their biosynthetic activity (Karsenty, 2001).

In mature osteoblasts, Runx2/Cbfa1 serves as a target for mechanical stimuli. A careful stretching of a layer of cultivated osteoblasts leads to an increase in the expression of Runx2/Cbfa1, accompanied by the activation of intracellular signaling systems (Ziros et al., 2002). In vivo experiments in heterozygotic mice carrying a zero mutation in the Runx2/Cbfa1 gene (in these animals, the expression of Runx2/Cbfa1 in osteoblasts is reduced by 50%), involving a mechanical unloading of the skeleton (tail suspension), showed a two-fold reduction (compared to control mice) in the rate of bone matrix formation and mineralization. This confirms that the Runx2/Cbfa1 protein is essential in maintaining the functional activity of a mature osteoblast (Salingcarnboriboon et al., 2006).

The function of Runx2/Cbfa1 becomes redundant in postnatal mature osteoblasts in the case of mutations, switching off the gene encoding the **Shn3** (Schnurri-3) protein. This adapter protein, which promotes the formation of protein complexes and contains zinc fingers, limits the activity of Runx2/Cbfa1, inducing its proteosome-dependent degradation and thus, regulates the bone tissue's mass gain (Jones et al., 2007).

The activity of Runx2/Cbfa1, which acts within the cell nucleus, drops in the context of a deficiency of lamin A/C, a phospholipoprotein with a molecular mass of

70 kDa forming a fibrous layer on the nucleoplasmic side of the inner nuclear membrane. This fact is apparently associated with the age-related decline in osteoblast differentiation and bone loss (Akter et al., 2008).

The function of Runx2/Cbfa1 is associated with the Sp7 transcription factor (the official term for this protein in humans is specificity protein 7), which is more commonly known by its alternative name osterix, proposed for this factor in mice (Nakashima et al, 2002).

Like Runx2/Cbfa1, osterix, which is required for the osteoblast differentiation during embryogenesis, retains its coordinating role in osteoblasts in postnatal life. For example, this has proven to be the central target for signals generated by mechanical stress, which activate a number of kinases in the cells of the ligamentum flavum in the human backbone. A subsequent increase in the expression of osterix leads to an abnormal ossification of the ligament (Fan et al., 2007). Postnatal inactivation of the *Osx* gene, encoding osterix in mice causes the animals to develop osteopenia due to the insufficient anabolic function of osteoblasts that have not reached maturity, while the osteoclasts retained their normal resorbing activity (Baek et al., 2009).

Besides Cbfa1/Runx2 and osterix, the normal biosynthetic activity of a mature osteoblast requires the protein encoded by the protooncogene *c-Src*, as well as a transcription factor known as the microphthalmia factor, coded by the gene *Mitf* and containing a so-called leucine zipper (a domain containing at least 7 leucine residues) (Boyce et al., 1999). The protein FHL2, which is rich in "zinc fingers" (see section 10.2.3), supports the viability of osteoblasts and prevents the reduction in the overall bone tissue mass and its mineralization in ovariectomized female mice (Govoni et al., 2006). A transmembrane protein known as the "progressing ankylosis protein homolog"(abbreviated as ANK), which transports inorganic pyrophosphate from within the cell to the extracellular matrix, promotes the formation of a mature osteoblast phenotype, its mineralization, and the expression of its markers. The role of ANK is more distinctly expressed in osteoblasts of craniofacial skeleton bones than in those of long bones of the extremities (Kirsch et al., 2009).

The main function of osteoblasts, which is producing all the basic components of the extracellular matrix (both in the embryonic morphogenesis of bone tissue and in its remodeling throughout life), is collectively performed by cells. This process is coordinated, firstly, by adhesive interactions between osteoblasts and secondly, by two types of junctions (contacts)–adhesive junctions and communicative gap junctions (nexi) (Stains and Civitelli, 2005).

Adhesive junctions (AJ), adherens junctions) are protein complexes mainly comprised of cadherins. Osteoblasts express N-cadherin, 11-cadherin (also known as osteoblastic (OB) cadherin), and small amounts of 4-cadherin (Cheng et al., 1998). In the presence of calcium ions, the cadherin homodimers of one cell bind to the respective homodimers in a neighboring cell, and the intracellular domains of the cadherins are connected to the cytoskeleton.

While AJs are especially important in the course of osteoblast differentiation, gap junctions (GJs) play a key role in communications among mature osteoblasts and osteocytes (Civitelli, 2008).

Transcellular gap junction contacts (intercellular canaliculi) are formed by the connections of two connexons belonging to the contacting cells. Each connexon consists of six connexin subunits (structurally-related transmembrane protein molecules). Gap contacts establish communications between osteoblasts, or between them and osteocytes' processes. A connexon not connected to a connexon in another cell is a hemichannel opening into the extracellular space. Besides adhesive and gap junctions, osteoblasts are interconnected by tight junctions (TJs) and express the whole complex of proteins required for their arrangement. Among them, the most important ones are four-pass transmembrane proteins (claudins and occludins) (Wongdee et al., 2008). TJs almost completely isolate cells from each other, while fixing them in an oriented position. Tight junctions are essential for osteoblasts in two ways. First, they turn the layer of osteoblasts located on the bone surface into a barrier separating the intraosseous fluid circulating in the lacunae and canaliculi from the blood serum; such a separation is important for metabolic processes in the bone tissue. Secondly, by fixing the position of cells and being closely connected with the cytoskeleton, TJs maintain the polarization typical to osteoblasts consisting of a unidirectional movement (towards the apical portion of the membrane) and the subsequent unidirectional secretion of extracellular matrix components produced by the osteoblasts. This promotes the formation of the required (such as osteonic) matrix structure (Prêle et al., 2003). Proteins required for such organization of intracellular movement (rsce 6, NSF, VAMP1, syntaxin 4) accumulate at the same cell pole. At the opposite ("rear") side of the osteoblast, the extracellular matrix is deposited by the next layer of osteoblasts.

Osteoblasts maintain their biosynthetic activity when cultivated in vitro. They continue to express all basic macromolecular components of the extracellular matrix but the levels of expression of individual components largely depend on the cultivation conditions–in particular, the chemical nature and structure of the surface of the substrate being used, such as a synthetic polymer (El-Amin et al., 2003). This data is of interest in relation to the development of biomaterials for bone surgery.

After the formation of the extracellular bone matrix and mineralization (ossification) thereof, the main (secretory) function of osteoblasts is fulfilled. The molecular mechanisms underlying the choice between the three possible scenarios of their subsequent fate remain obscure. These scenarios are as follows:

1) entering into an inactive state in the surface layer of the bone, characterized by lowered biosynthetic activity,

2) apoptosis, or

3) transforming into osteocytes.

For the majority of osteogenic differon cells, the osteoblastic stage of their differentiation ends up in apoptosis, a naturally programmed cell death (Hock et. al, 2001). Mature osteoblasts are characterized by active genes for proteins, which take part in the apoptosis process, whose development mainly depends on the ratio between proapoptotic (Bax) and antiapoptotic (Bcl-2) factors (Bax/Bcl-2 ratio) (Wiren et al., 2006), and on caspase enzymes. The apoptosis of osteoblasts is stimulated by androgenic hormones and changes in the extracellular matrix due to its natural resorption: a rise in the concentration of free ions of calcium and inorganic phosphate and the appearance of peptide fragments of structural proteins rich in RGD-sequences (Adams and Shapiro, 2003). Osteoblast apoptosis is inhibited by systemic and local signaling factors of an anabolic nature, including insulin and IGF-1. They use intracellular pathways, starting from the receptors to which the multifunctional serine/threonine protein kinase (Akt1) is associated (Kawamura et al., 2007).

The cell population resulting from the osteoblast differentiation is not homogeneous. Some of the osteoblasts–those located on bones' outer or inner surface–retain their osteoblastic phenotype characterized, in particular, by a marked expression of the *Cbfa1/ Runx2* gene. These cells possess the ability to actively produce the extracellular matrix, which enables the normal remodeling of bone tissue (and thus, the maintenance of the metabolic balance of calcium in the body) throughout life.

Another group of osteoblasts become immured in the lacunae within the mineralized matrix. These osteoblasts undergo a further final differentiation, acquiring the phenotype of a controller bone cell, the osteocyte.

8.2.1.3. Morphology of osteocytes

Osteocytes are differentiated bone cells with a characteristic phenotype ensuring the efficient structural and functional status of bone tissue through remodeling mechanisms (resorption and plastic ones, including their own), which regulate the functions of other bone cells and are involved in mineral metabolism. These cells are unable to divide or undergo a reverse transformation (dedifferentiation). They make up 90% of the cell population of mature, completely mineralized bone tissue. They are slightly less in size than osteoblasts and have a flattened polygonal shape with numerous long processes (*Fig. 8.8*), which link them to each other via gap contacts, thus forming a fairly ordered cellular association unique to bone tissue. The nuclei of osteocytes have a round or oval shape with invaginations, occupying considerable space within the cytoplasm, which accounts for a high nuclear-cytoplasmic ratio. Their cytoplasm contains multi-purpose organelles, including a relatively small amount of GER, a Golgi complex, mitochondria

and lysosomes. Based on the shape and condition of cells, their processes and cytoplasm, the structure and number of organelles and the structure of the lacunae, four different types of osteocytes may be distinguished:

1) matrix-forming

2) matrix-resorbing

3) resting, and

4) degenerating (Ross et al., 1995; Rodionova, 1989). The first type of osteocytes may be also subdivided into two groups. The first of them, matrix-forming osteocytes, are found in areas of osteogenesis. They are similar in structure to actively producing osteoblasts (primary or secondary osteocytes). Apparently, their isolation from the newly-formed bone matrix and the resulting limited access to nutrients have not been happening for so long as to affect their structure. At the same time, they continue to participate in the formation of the bone matrix. The second group are secondary osteocytes. These are involved in the formation of lamellar bone tissue in the final stage of reparative regeneration and the subsequent remodeling that occurs with increased bone-loading, and also form the bone matrix in a mature bone during its natural (physiological) renewal. These cells contain a much smaller number of organelles, particularly GER and Golgi complex components, but then the volume of the renewed bone matrix is incomparable to that formed in the areas of active osteogenesis. The second type of osteocytes (matrix-resorbing) contain a larger number of lysosomes within their cytoplasm. These cells resorb the bone matrix in the walls of the lacunae and, probably, in the canalicular walls as well. Resting (type 3) osteocytes contain the least number of cell organelles, apparently required to maintain the cell's viability. It is quite logical to assume that the first three types of osteocytes are actually the same cells with a varying number of organelles, depending on the required functional condition. Such osteocytes may be referred to as "areal", i.e. responsible for the condition of an area in the bone matrix to which the processes of the osteocyte extend. Degenerating (type 4) osteocytes have practically no organelles, a wrinkled, electron dense nucleus and a cytoplasm reduced to a narrow band. Such osteocytes are typically found in intermediate lamellae and at the periphery of osteons.

8.2.1.4. Biochemical and molecular biological characteristics of osteocytes

Phenotypically, the osteocytes differ dramatically from their precursors, the osteoblasts, and not only in a morphological way (which is mainly due the development of numerous long processes). They also differ in terms of the peculiarities of their biochemical phenotype (Franz-Odendaal et al., 2006).

"Immured" in the mineralized matrix, the osteocytes are adjusted to low oxygen partial pressure. This adjustment occurs, in particular, through a raised expression of the ORP150 protein, which differentiates osteocytes from osteoblasts. ORP150 (oxygen-regulated protein) is a glycoprotein with a molecular mass of 150 kDa, one of the proteins that protect cells from stress. It promotes the differentiation of osteoblasts into osteocytes (Hirao et al., 2007).

Long processes typical to osteocytes are located in the bone canals communicating with bone cells' lacunae to form networks that permeate the mineralized extracellular bone matrix. An important role in the formation of the canaliculi is played by the matrix metalloproteinase MMP-2, expressed by differentiating osteocytes. Inactivation of the gene encoding this enzyme leads to osteocyte death and a decrease in the mineral density of the bone tissue (Inoue et al., 2006).

The osteoblast-to-osteocyte differentiation is accompanied by a complete rearrangement of its cytoskeleton. There is a sharp rise in the level of actin, the basic protein of the cytoskeleton, with major amounts concentrating in the processes. According to cytochemical research, the spatial distribution of actin-binding proteins within the cell is also significantly changed. **Fimbrin** and α-actinin mostly accompany actin in processes, while villin accumulates in the cytoplasm of the cell body and filamin is found mainly at the base of the processes. **Spectrin**, which, in osteoblasts, appears as punctate dots in the cytoplasm, acquires a filamentous structure in osteocytes. Such a rearrangement is inevitably accompanied by functional changes in the cytoskeleton (Kamioka et al., 2004).

Unlike osteoblasts, the osteocyte does not express **vigilin** (from the Latin *vigilo*—"to stay awake; be vigilant"). This protein, binding to mRNA and controlling the balance between the rate of its synthesis in the nucleus and degradation in the cytoplasm, is specific to cells with a high biosynthetic activity. Its absence in osteocytes indicates a decrease in their biosynthetic potential in comparison to osteoblasts (Dodson and Shapiro, 2002).

Other important changes in the proteome during the osteoblast-to-osteocyte transformation correspond to those in the orientation and level of secretory activity. Although the expression of structural components of the extracellular matrix (osteocalcin, bone sialoprotein, osteopontin, osteonectin, fibronectin, vitronectin, type 1 collagen) does not cease altogether, it becomes much less intensive than in osteoblasts (Franz-Odendaal et al., 2006). It recedes to the background in comparison to a number of signaling molecules and those that modulate the functions of osteoblasts and osteoclasts and are involved in calcium and phosphate homeostasis.

These molecules include members of transforming growth factor-β (TGF-β) superfamily, in particular the bone morphogenetic proteins BMP-2 and BMP-4 (Heino et al., 2002), which suppress bones' osteoclastic resorption.

This group of molecules also includes **sclerostin**, a small secreted glycoprotein (containing 213 amino-acid residues in humans) encoded by the *SOST* gene (Bezooijen et al., 2004). Inactivation of this gene results in the amplified formation of bone tissue and increased bone mass (when occurring in humans, this disorder is called sclerosteosis). The role of sclerostin is to inhibit osteoblasts' activity (and thus, bone growth). In this respect, the effect of sclerostin is antagonistic to that of bone morphogenetic proteins (BMPs), which stimulate osteoblastic activity. However, the mechanism of sclerostin's action is different. Since it is not a direct extracellular competitor of BMPs, it blocks the receptors for Wnt morphogens, interrupting one of the signal pathways used by BMPs in their osteoblastogenesis-stimulating action. In the absence of sclerostin, this stimulation becomes excessive (Bezooijen et al. 2007; Dijke et al., 2008; Veverka et al., 2009).

The expression of the above-mentioned phosphoglycoprotein, osteoblast/osteocyte factor-45 (OF45), is more active in osteocytes than in osteoblasts. Its name reflects its molecular mass of 45 kDa, but it is also known as **MEPE** (matrix extracellular phosphoglycoprotein) (Gowen et al., 2003; Nampei et al., 2004). This protein, consisting of 525 amino acid residues and containing a "sticky" RGD-sequence of amino acid residues, belongs to the SIBLING family. The "sticky" sequence promotes the binding of cells to the extracellular matrix. In addition, MEPE is involved in the regulation of phosphate homeostasis. ASARM peptides (also known as **minhibins**), which are rich in serine and asparaginic acid and control mineralization by binding to hydroxyapatite, are cleaved from MEPE with the participation of PHEX endopeptidase (Addison et al., 2008).

Another phosphoglycoprotein that is more actively expressed by osteocytes relative to osteoblasts is dentin matrix protein-1 (DMP-1), which is mainly secreted into the matrix, but is also found within the cell. It is essential for osteoblast-to-osteocyte differentiation and plays a role in regulating mineralization (Qin et al., 2007).

Mutations in the genes encoding MEPE and DMP-1 and in the proteins interacting with them lead to the development of osteomalacia and hypophosphatemic rickets. This indicates the participation of these molecules in regulating phosphate homeostasis in the body (Feng et al., 2006). The fibroblast growth factor-23 (FGF-23), expressed by osteocytes and viewed as a hormone influencing the renal function, is also involved in this regulation, which permits speaking of the "endocrine" function of osteocytes (Quarles, 2008). At the same time, FGF-23 plays a local (paracrine) role, aimed at controlling osteoblast differentiation and the mineralization of the matrix (Wang H. et al., 2008).

Osteocytes have receptors for systemic hormones (such as the parathyroid hormone, androgen and estrogen hormones), which determine their ability to respond to hormonal impulses (Riggs et al., 2002). The presence of receptors for parathyroid hormone (PTHR), along with one for calcium ions (CaSR), supports the suggestion that osteocytes are involved in maintaining calcium homeostasis. PTHR in osteocytes controls the overall mass of bone tissue, beneficially affecting the support and protection function of the bones (O'Brien et al., 2007). This involvement is not limited to the remodeling mechanism, which is relatively slow, taking days or weeks. Some evidence suggests the existence of an additional fast-acting mechanism, the osteocytic osteolysis of the mineralized bone matrix. Apparently, this mechanism involves the alkaline phosphatase expressed by osteocytes (Teti and Zallone, 2009).

The gap junction contacts connecting osteocytes with each other and with osteoblasts are represented by groups of **connexons**. Each connexon is comprised of six molecules of transmembrane proteins, or connexins; the one most commonly found in humans is **connexin 43**, with its name reflecting its molecular mass. Following a change in the conformation of connexin molecules, a hemichannel in the connexon connected to an identical hemichannel in the next cell opens to form a canaliculus, through which cells exchange signaling molecules that carry information. The information that is thereby transmitted is vital for osteocytes (Plotkin et al., 2002). Osteocytes have abundant connexons, which are assembled together to form hemichannels in the cytoplasmic membrane remaining open. Through these hemichannels, the signaling molecules enter the periosteocytic fluid circulating in the lacunae and canaliculi. Osteocytes have receptors for these molecules, which makes information exchange between osteocytes even more efficient (Jiang et al., 2007).

Besides their contacts with other cells, osteocyte processes also have points of contact with the walls of the canaliculi in which they are located. At these points, there is contact with the collagenic fibers of the extracellular matrix. This contact, mediated by $\alpha v \beta 3$ integrin, enables information exchange between osteocytes and the matrix (McNamara et al., 2009).

Thus, in having contact amongst themselves, with osteoblasts and with the matrix, the osteocytes form an integrated information system – an osteocytic network – basically similar to that of neurons in the central nervous system (Turner et al., 2002). This network involves the same signaling molecules as the one in the CNS (glutamic acid, prostaglandins, nitrogen oxide), as well as calcium ions.

The main function of the osteocytic network is to respond to mechanical impulses that constantly influence the bone tissue. Within this network, osteocytes play a sensory role (Bonewald, 2006). Bone micro-deformations resulting from mechanical stress cause deformations in the cell membranes of osteocytes, which brings about changes in conformation of the transmembrane receptors. The changes affect many receptors, including integrins and connexons.

Special importance in the perception of mechanical stimuli is attributed to the α-receptor for estrogens (Zaman et al., 2006). Membrane stretch brings about a change in the activity of transmembrane channels and increases the entry of potassium and calcium ions into the cells. Changes occur in the configuration of the membrane itself, which promotes changes in the conformations of the cytoskeletal proteins adjoining it and, consequently, in the entire cytoskeleton (Rubin et al., 2006). It is exactly here, at the cytoplasmic membrane, where mechanical energy is converted into chemical energy (Silver and Siperko, 2003), and mechanical signals into biochemical ones, and where the propagation of biochemical signals through the osteocytes network begins, called mechanochemical transduction or mechanotransduction (Yang et al., 2004).

The process of mechanotransduction involves a number of intracellular kinases – protein-phosphorylating and protein-activating enzymes – (FAK, MAPK, PKC, JNK, ERK1/2). Other enzymes, including phospholipase C and cyclo-oxygenase-2, are also switched on. Cytoplasmic and cytoskeletal proteins altered by these enzymes enter the cell nucleus, probably as a complex called **mechanosome** (Pavalko et al., 2003). The nuclear matrix transcription phosphoprotein 4 (NMP4, also known as zinc finger protein 384) seems to be the main probable candidate as the integrator of all mechanochemical signals (Liedert et al., 2006). The genes *c-fos* and *c-jun*, encoding the proteins that belong to the family of activator transcription factors AP-1, are activated under its influence.

Factors of the AP-1 complex, in their turn, activate a variety of mechanosensory genes, whose promoter regions contain elements sensitive to mechanical stress. These genes include those of growth factors such as the insulin-like growth factors IGF-I and IGF-II, the vascular endothelium growth factor VEGF, the transforming growth factor TGF-β1 family, and the bone morphogenetic proteins BMP-2 and BMP-4. The autocrine and paracrine actions of these and some other factors stimulate the expression of signaling molecules, which regulate the differentiation, proliferation and functions of both the osteoblasts that produce bone tissue and the osteoclasts responsible for its resorption (Liedert et al., 2006). The signaling system, WNT/β-katenin, which stimulates the osteoblastogenesis, becomes activated (Robinson et al, 2006). In other words, this starts the mechanism of bone tissue remodeling that enables its renewal and maintaining its biomechanical properties.

Another protein associated with the mechanosensory function of the osteocytes is the osteocyte-expressed HB-GAM protein (heparin-binding growth-associated molecule, also called **pleiotrophin**). The expression of this molecule, consisting of 163 amino-acid residues, is stimulated by mechanical loading, which is evidenced *in vivo* by a reduction in the mass of load-carrying bones following the inactivation of the pleiotrophin-encoding gene (Imai et al., 2009).

Mechanical influences cause osteocytes to exert not only a sensory, but also an effector function. Within them, there is an increase in the level of cyclic adenosine monophosphate (cAMP) stimulating the kinases activity, and in the expression of a number of genes, such as those encoding the glutamate/aspartate transporter (GLAST)–an enzyme required for the formation of glutamic acid–and two other enzymes: nitric oxide synthetase (NOS) and prostaglandin G/H synthetase (PGHS-2). The biosynthetic activity of osteocytes increases accordingly (Nomura &Takano-Yamamoto, 2000). In particular, the enhanced expression of tenascin C, one of the extracellular matrix glycoproteins, is observed (Webb et al., 1997). In this respect, it may be noted that tenascin C biosynthesis is also intensified in other connective tissue cells (such as fibroblasts or chondrocytes) under the influence of mechanical factors. The enhanced expression of tenascin in response to mechanical stress is regarded as one of the early manifestations of bone tissue rearrangement and a developing osteogenic reaction (enhanced bone formation).

There is one more mechanotransduction pathway to activate the osteocyte response to mechanical stimulation (Cowin, 2002). Tissue microdeformations accompanying the mechanical loading applied to a bone induce the movement of periosteocytic fluid, which fills the lacunae and canaliculi. The fluid flow is perceived by receptors in the cytoplasmic membrane of the osteocytes, mainly by integrins (Wang Y. et al., 2007), which leads to an increase in the expression of the mRNA of prostaglandin synthase enzyme. The synthesized prostaglandin $PGE2_2$, transported through the canaliculi to the bone surface where the bone-forming cells reside, activates the transformation of osteoprogenitor cells into osteoblasts and the proliferation and secretory functions of osteoblasts and osteoclasts. A local activation of osteoclasts leads to the formation of a bone tissue remodeling unit (BMU) where needed, which ensures the maintenance of the bone's biomechanical properties.

The formation of BMU, where it is required due to local biomechanical damage to bone tissue properties (especially as microcracks arise), is facilitated by the apoptosis of osteocytes (Cardoso et al., 2008). At the apoptosis site, there is an increased expression of proapoptotic molecules promoting its expansion, including the protein encoded by the *Bax* gene. At the same time, osteocytes undergoing apoptosis release HMGB1 cytokine, activating the neighboring cells, HMGB1, thereby functioning as an "alarmin" (Bidwell et al., 2008).

Around the apoptosis site, in the neighboring osteocytes, there is an increased expression of genes that beneficially influence the cells and are known as "survival" (antiapoptotic) genes, such as *Bcl-2*. Cell survival is promoted by weak mechanical impulses at the periphery of the damage zone, which have a stimulating effect on the osteocytes; its mechanism involves integrins and kinases of the Src and ERK families (Plotkin et al., 2005). A kind of protective shield of metabolically active osteocytes is formed. Through their processes, these transmit a signal to osteoblasts, which are the main source of signaling molecules controlling the osteoclastogenesis process and osteoclasts' functional activity. Under the effect of these molecules, a group of active osteoclasts accumu-

lates at a certain location on the bone surface; a BMU arises, which restores the bone's biomechanical properties. This effect is weakened by a reduction in the population of osteocytes that progresses with age, which suppresses osteoclastogenesis and bone tissue remodeling and increases bones' brittleness (Gu et al., 2005).

Thus, the mechanical impacts on the bone are converted, in a variety of ways, into a series of biochemical reactions. The osteocyte not only performs a large part of these reactions by itself, but is also the center in terms of detecting reactions occurring in other cells. It directs and coordinates molecular/ biochemical processes in the osteoblasts and osteoclasts, the cells that are responsible, respectively, for the building and destruction of bone tissue. In other words, it regulates the functions of these opposite-acting cells, which puts the osteocyte in a role of a "mechanostat" (Taylor et al., 2007). It is namely the osteocyte that determines the bone structure by controlling the adaptation of the micro- and macro-architectonics of bone tissue to the effects of mechanical factors (Klein-Nulend et al., 2003; Noble, 2008). Such is today's understanding of the molecular mechanism for the classical Wolff's law (describing the relationship between the bone's structure and function) triggered by the osteocyte (Huiskes, 2003).

8.2.2. Osteoclasts. Osteoclastic resorption of bone tissue

8.2.2.1. The morphology of osteoclasts

Another cell differon related to bone tissue is that of mononuclear phagocytes. This includes:
1) multipotent hemopoietic stem cells of red bone marrow;
2) multipotent committed myeloid progenitor cells of the red bone marrow;
3) oligopotent committed myeloid progenitor cells;
4) unipotent precursors of monocytes;
5) monoblasts;
6) promonocytes;
7) monocytes;
8) macrophages/osteoclasts.

Osteoclasts are specialized bone resorbing cells. The biological importance of their function, catabolic in its nature, is twofold:
a) enabling, by way of remodeling, constant renewal and thus, maintenance of the mechanical properties of bone tissue and control of its mass, and
b) maintenance of calcium homeostasis in the body. Osteoclasts have a characteristic structural organization enabling them to dispose of components of bone tissue and mineralized cartilage. These cells may have a round, spherical, spheroid or ellipsoid shape with a flattened base, which are located on the tissue to be resorbed and constitutes its main working part. The central part of the osteoclast contains the nuclei,

whose number may range from one to several dozens. The cisternae of the Golgi complex are located close to the nuclei, but its vesicles are dispersed throughout the cytoplasm. There is a well developed GER, and a considerable number of middle-sized and small mitochondria. Some authors describe the entire complex of the above-mentioned cell organelles as the basal part of the cell, which is responsible for the regulation of its vital activity, synthesis and secretion, and energy supply(Fig. 8.10). However, only the narrow somewhat ring-shaped peripheral immediately adjoins the bone surface, thus isolating the resorption zone and limiting the possible passage of formed acid and released enzymes to the rest of the bone surface. The intracellular base of the ring is formed by an actin cytoskeleton. The actin filaments in its structure are parallel to the surface of the underlying substrate. Besides, the ring contains dot-like local structures consisting of actin filaments, oriented perpendicularly to the substrate plane, which are called podosomes. The latter occur only in cells of monocytic origin (osteoclasts and monocytes) (Marchisio et al., 1987). In addition to bundles of actin filaments, the podosomes contain proteins involved in cell-cell and cell-matrix interactions (Teti et al., 1991). Among those, the following have been found: fimbrin, α-actinin and gelsolin, which are closely bound with actin filaments in the core of the podosome, as well as vinculin and talin, which form "rosettes" around the core of the podosome (Teti et al., 1991). There are certain differences between the structures of the actin cytoskeleton of the ring-shaped base and podosomes in a moving osteoclast and in an osteoclast fixed at the site of would-be resorption (Lakkakorpi et al., 1989).

The transmembrane proteins of the adhesive molecules family mediate cell-matrix interactions within the space between the osteoclast and the bone. Integrins are heterodimeric molecular assemblies of alpha and beta subunits with a specific receptor-like sequence to bind the matrix via the Arg-Gly-Asp (RGD) (Horton and Davies, 1989). Osteoclasts express many integrins, some of which are involved in the osteoclast's adhesion to the bone matrix (Nesbit et al., 1993). Remarkably, the osteoclasts independently synthesize and secrete such proteins as osteopontin and bone sialoprotein, which are involved in integrating the organic part of the bone matrix. A TEM study has shown that the actin cytoskeleton of the peripheric area of the osteoclast is surrounded by a fine-granular substance. This part of cytoplasm contains no organelles. Due to this fact, this area is referred to as the clear zone. All structures within this area, along with the adhesive proteins, represent a specialized complex aimed at fixing the osteoclast to the bone surface at the resorption site.

The cytolemma adjoining the bone surface and limited by the clear zone has numerous, rather deep foldings and crypts. In the literature, this area of the osteoclast is termed a ruffled border. Its dimensions (extent) or percentage of cell perimeter are variable enough, apparently reflecting the functional activity of the osteoclast. A ruffled border may be completely absent in some osteoclasts. From the periphery towards the center of the cell, the ruffled border is followed by a vesicular region. This area of the cytoplasm contains a multitude of various-sized membrane-enclosed "bubbles" or vesicles. These structures may be terminal regions of crypts in the cytoplasm or may be detached from them to become endocytotic vacuoles (phagosomes) with bone matrix resorption products, or secretory vesicles budded from the Golgi cisternae (Fig. 8.11). The ruffled border and the vesicular region constitute a specialized part of the cell that is directly involved in the bone matrix resorption. This is where some of the synthesized classes of enzymes are carried to (Baron, 1995).

8.2.2.2. Functions of osteoclasts and biochemical mechanisms of osteoclastic bone tissue resorption

The biochemical phenotype of a multinuclear mature osteoclast is formed in the course of osteoclastic differentiation (osteoclastogenesis), during which the osteoclast arises through the fusion of its precursors (monocytes or macrophages). The resulting phenotype reflects the osteoclast's function (the resorption of bone tissue) in both of the aspects described above and significantly differs from that of its precursors.

The osteoclastic phenotype is characterized by much higher activity on the part of enzymes involved in the resorptive function than in macrophages, in particular, by the high activity of proteolytic enzymes, primarily cathepsins and other hydrolases acting in lysosomes and endosomes. As a phenotypic marker of the osteoclast, histochemical studies employ the unusually high activity of the tartrate-resistant (resistant to the action of tartaric salts) acid phosphatase 5 (TRACP5, more commonly known by its shortened name TRAP); this enzyme will be discussed in more detail later in this chapter. The osteoclastic phenotype is also characterized by the intensive expression of proteins acting as transmembrane ionic channels, through which the flow of ions takes place in the process of bone tissue destruction (Teitelbaum, 2000). Besides, the osteoclast phenotype has a special set of other transmembrane receptors, including those for calcitonin and vitronectin (see section 8.5.1), as well as specialized integrins not found in other cells such as osteoblasts (Teitelbaum, 2006). Of these special integrins, integrin αvβ plays an important role in the resorptive function of osteoclasts. The αv-subunit is required for binding to mineralized bone surface (v stands for vitronectin). The resorptive activity largely depends on the cytoplasmic (intracellular) domain of the β3-subunit activating signaling pathways with the participation of Src and Syk protein tyrosine kinases and several signaling pathways bound to Pyk2 and c-Cbl molecules and gp130 glycoprotein (Nakamura et al., 2007). In addition, β3 affects the cytoskeletal proteins through the participation of guanosine triphosphatases of the Rac family and the guanine nucleotide exchange factor VAV3, which activates these enzymes. Inactivation of the gene encoding β3 results in cytoskeleton defects and interferes with osteoclasts' attachment to the bone surface; their ability to resorb the bone tissue becomes limited (Faccio et al., 2003). Besides, β3 deficiency deprives osteoclasts of the beneficial influence of the vascular endothelial growth factor (VEGF), which, with the participation of theVEG-FR2 receptor present in the osteoclast membranes, supports their viability and stimulates their resorbing activity (Yang et al., 2008).

Characteristic of osteoclasts are also integrins α9β1(Rao et al., 2006) and αvβ5 (Lane et al., 2005). The former is associated with the regulation of the cytoskeleton: in its absence, the actin ring locking the lacuna, where the resorbing factors of osteoclasts act, is not formed. The latter or, more precisely, the β5-subunit is involved in regulating the osteoclast differentiation rate.

β1 and β3 integrin subunits assemble into heteromeric complexes with the transmembrane glycoprotein osteoactivin expressed by osteoclasts (formerly, osteoactivin was known to be found only in osteoblasts) being one of the players in the process of endocytosis (absorption) of bone tissue degradation products by the osteoclast (Sheng et al., 2008).

Due to their important role in homeostasis, osteoclasts also possess a considerable number of sensory receptors for ionized calcium and others for signaling molecules that regulate the functions of cells involved in calcium metabolism.

The transmembrane RANK receptor, the receptor activator of nuclear factor kappa B (NF-κB), holds a special place in osteoclast biology. This receptor provides a starting point for signaling systems, which end with transcription factors of the NF-κB family. The latter hold a central place in regulating osteoclast phenotype formation and retain this place in regulating the vital activity of mature osteoclasts.

RANK, also called TNFR11A, belongs to the tumor necrosis factor (TNF) receptor family (see section 4.2). RANK is activated by a special ligand expressed by osteoblasts (RANKL) and is a member of TNF-superfamily; factors of this superfamily are involved in many aspects of regulating the vital activity of osteoclasts, such as apoptosis (Feng, 2005a).

Just as the other receptors for TNFR-family, RANK does not exhibit its own kinase activity. It uses intracellular pathways for the transmission of signals, starting from factors associated with it, such as adaptor proteins TRAF and TSG-6. RANK also interacts with the Vav3 protein (the guanine nucleotide exchange factor for guanosine triphosphatases of the Rho-family), as well as with the protein Cdc42 involved in cell cycle regulation, and with Rac1 kinase.

Another factor, osteoprotegerin (OPG), also known as OCIF (osteoclastogenesis inhibitory factor), is a critical component of the RANKL/RANK signaling system (axis). This dimeric glycoprotein, containing sialic acid, consists of 380 amino-acid residues (after the removal of the signal peptide) and is homologous to RANK. Like RANK, osteoprotegerin belongs to the tumor necrosis factor receptor family, hence, its alternative name TNFR11B (or TR11B). Osteoprotegerin is expressed by many tissue cells; in bone tissue, it is expressed by osteoblasts. Unlike RANK that is bound to the cytoplasmic membranes of osteoclasts and their progenitors, osteoprotegerin is secreted into the extracellular matrix (Simonet et al., 1997). Osteoprotegerin acts as a false (competing rather effectively with RANK) receptor for RANKL, which is a ligand for it. By binding RANKL, osteoprotegerin reduces the intensity of RANKL's activating effect on RANK, interrupting the RANK/RANKL axis. This leads to the suppression of osteoclastogenesis and a reduction in the number of active osteoclasts. The ratio between the expressed amounts of RANKL and OPG thus appears to be the major determinant of the rate of bone modeling and remodeling and thus, of bone tissue mass (Boyce and Xing, 2008; Kearns et al., 2008).

It should be noted that this ratio is defined by osteoblasts. Thus, the deficiency in OPG expression by osteoblasts, caused by the absence of the homeotic protein Dlx5 (leading to the suppression of osteoblasts' biosynthetic activity), increases the RANKL/OPG ratio and induces the acceleration of osteoclastogenesis and the intensification of bone resorption (Samee et al., 2008). On the contrary, morphogens of the Wnt family, which stimulate OPG expression in osteoblasts and accordingly lower the RANKL/OPG ratio, block osteoclastogenesis (Kubota et al., 2009). This effect of Wnt in differentiated osteoblasts is mediated by the main component of the intracellular pathway for the transduction of Wnt signals (Glass II et al., 2005).

NF-κB (nuclear factor-κB) is a member of a small family of pleiotropic (regulating the expression of multiple genes) transcription factors. Its effect is evident through the consecutive activation of c-fos protooncogene (a component of the AP-1 transcriptional activator complex) and the nuclear factor of activated T-cells 1 (NFATc1) (Yamashita et al., 2007). In osteoclasts, NFATc1 takes on a role comparable to that of Sox9 in chondroblasts/ chondrocytes or of Cbfa1/Runx2 (as well as that of Osterix) in osteoblasts. It is the role of a central regulator and coordinator ("master") of the expression of the entire set of genes determining the osteoclastic phenotype (Kobayashi et al., 2009). This role remains extremely important in the postnatal period as osteoclastogenesis continues throughout life due to the constant remodeling of bone tissue.

The blockage of NF-κB stops the resorption activity in osteoclasts that have completed their differentiation. Their migration is thus broken, the activity of TRAP decreases and the disorganization of the cytoskeleton takes place (Soysa et al., 2009). The blockage of RANK also leads to ruptures in the actin cytoskeleton of mature osteo-

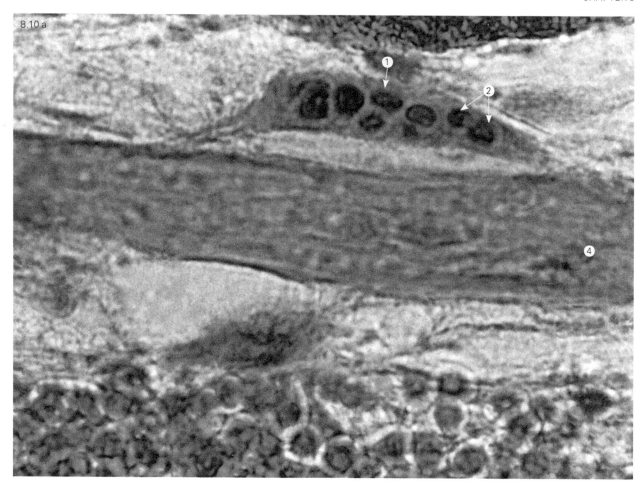

8.10 a

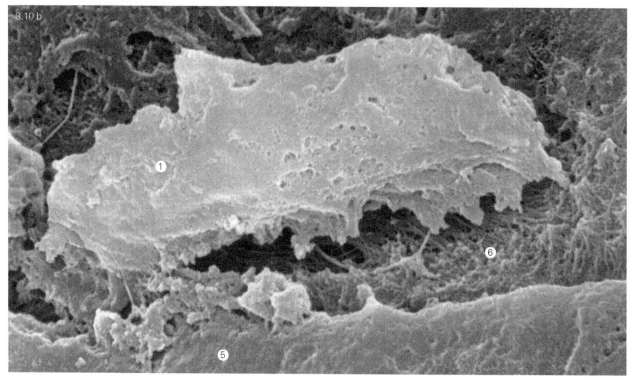

8.10 b

Fig. 8.10.
Osteoclasts in a regenerated bone (1).
Nuclei (2). Mitochondria (3).
A primary trabecule (4).
Bone matrix, mineralized (5)

and demineralized (6).
Lysis zone (7).
Foldings of the ruffled border (8).
Cytoplasm (9).
a – LM micrograph.

A light optic microscope Ni Nikon (Japan). Histologic section. Hematoxylin and eosin stain x 1,000.
(see color insert)
b,c – SEM-micrograph.

b – x 5,000. c – x 7,000.
d – TEM-micrograph.
Contrast of ultrathin sections, enhanced with uranyl acetate and lead citrate.
x 15,000.

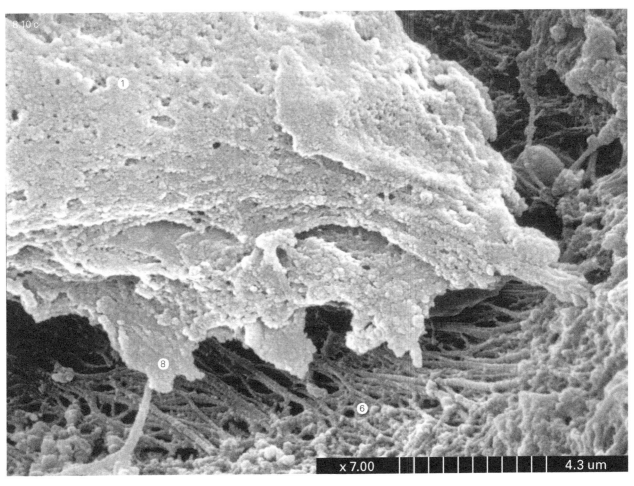

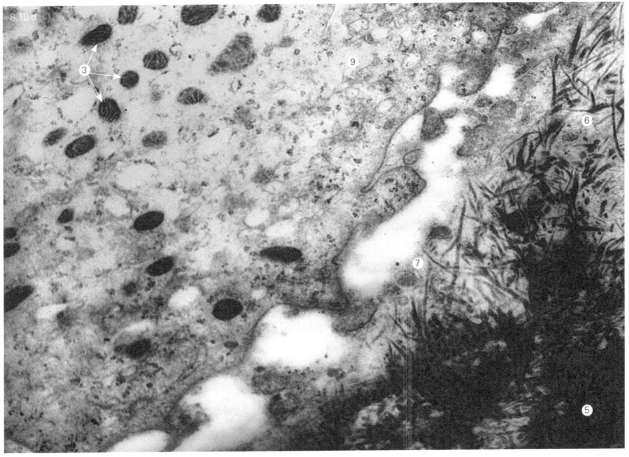

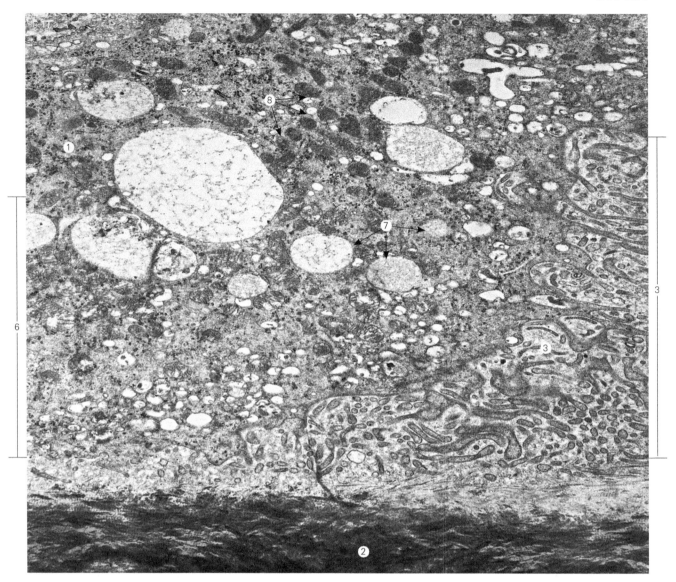

Fig. 8.11.
An osteoclast fragment (1)
touching the resorbing bone
surface with its cytolemma (2).
Ruffled border (3).
Foldings (4) and crypts (5)
of the ruffled border.
Vesicular region (6).
Vesicles (7).
Mitochondria (8).
Dissolving bone mineral (9).
Lysis zone (10).
ТЭМ micrograph.
Contrast of ultrathin sections,
enhanced with uranyl acetate
and lead citrate.
a – x 15,000;
b – x 30,000.

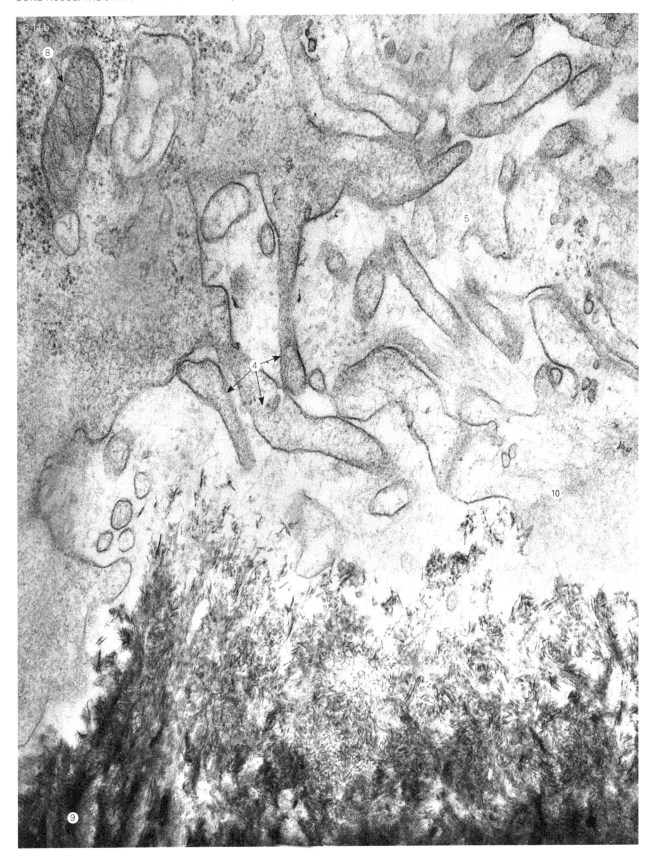

clasts and inhibits the destruction of bone tissue (Kim et al., 2009).

For an osteoclast to resorb bone tissue, it is critical that it appear in the right location on the bone surface. This is achieved through the migratory ability of osteoclast precursors. Their attraction is enabled by the chemotactic effect of the lipid factor (mediator) sphingosine 1-phosphate (S1P); osteoclast progenitors have receptors for this factor (Ishii et al., 2009).

Other prerequisites are the attachment (adhesion) of the cell to the bone surface and the formation of a special environment at the contact site. The latter is created by isolating this area from the surrounding extracellular space (lacuna) resulting from the formation of podosomes within the cell. Podosomes are adhesive structures found in many mobile cells and are similar to focal adhesions in regard to their functions and molecular structure. The main part of a podosome is formed by the F-actin core. Numerous podosomes of the osteoclast, upon contacting each other, form a continuous isolating barrier that tightly attaches to the bone surface and becomes fixed in this position. This affixing becomes possible due to the rearrangement of the actin cytoskeleton forming a tight actin ring. The actin dynamics during this rearrangement are positively regulated by the protein tyrosine kinase activity of s-Src protooncogene; inhibiting that activity impairs the formation of podosomes (Destaing et al., 2008). Inversely, the Wrch1 enzyme, one of the small guanosine triphosphatases of the Rho family, negatively affects podosome formation, as well as the migration and adhesion of osteoclast precursors (Brazier et al., 2009). Regulation of osteoclast actin cytoskeleton dynamics also involves the high-molecular tropomyosin, expressed by the osteoclast controlling actin's interactions with other cytoskeletal proteins (Kotadiya et al., 2008).

As the osteoclast affixes to the bone surface, the cellular membrane in the lacunar zone adjoining the bone surface acquires a corrugated (villous) structure. Carbonic anhydrase II (carbon dioxide anhydrase), catalyzing the formation of protons (H_+) and HCO_3, becomes activated. A distinct polarization of the cell takes place, manifested, in particular, by the increasing number of canals in the lacunar area of the membrane, which are formed by the vacuolar (functioning within the vacuoles) adenosine triphosphatase (V-ATPase). Through these canals, (H+) protons are actively transported to the lacuna. This is also where the number of ClC-7 ion exchangers increases; these transport chlorine ions (Cl-) to the lacuna. An excess of chlorine ions inside the cell (as well as maintaining the intracellular pH at a normal level) is made possible by the activity of Cl-/HCO3−(Ae2) anion exchangers concentrated in the membrane of the opposite cell surface (Teitelbaum, 2007).

Interaction between H+ and Cl- makes the hydrochloric acid, acidifying the environment to pH in the range of 4.5–4.8, accumulate in the lacuna. The hydrochloric acid dissolves the mineral component of the bone matrix and makes the organic components of the matrix, including the collagen structures, susceptible to the destructive effect of non-specific proteases, mainly cathepsins. This effect, which is apparently central in osteoclastic bone resorption, makes the lacuna similar to lysosomes, where hydrolytic enzymes exhibit optimum activity in an acidic environment (Teitelbaum, 2006). Inactivation of the gene encoding Ae2 leads to the impairment of the osteoclasts' resorptive function and the development of osteopetrosis (an excessive accumulation of bone tissue) (Josephson et al., 2009).

A complex of cathepsins (cathepsins C, D, B, E, G, and L) is involved in the osteoclastic resorption of the demineralized bone matrix. The highest proteolytic activity against type 1 collagen, which prevails in the matrix, is exhibited by cathepsin K in endochondrally-formed bones. This activity is regulated by fragments generated from the type I collagen molecule. Cathepsin K is also associated with the formation of the actin ring locking the resorption lacuna. Its activity, like that of other cysteine proteases, is regulated by cystatin C, an endogenous inhibitor produced by osteo-clasts (Goto et al., 2003; Wilson et al., 2009). Cathepsin L is more active in the degradation of proteins in skull bones formed via intramembranous ossification (see section 10.3.1.3) (Everts et al., 2006). The absorption of calcium ions released from the bone matrix is promoted by calmodulin, which accumulates in the villi of the resorptive membrane (Seales et al., 2006).

The products of bone tissue destruction move from the lacuna to the osteoclast by way of endocytosis, which involves osteoactivin (as described above). Further on, they are transported via a system of phagosomes (intracellular vesicles), characterized by a complex dynamic protein structure, to the free, anti-resorptive region of the cytoplasmic membrane (Sakai et al., 2001). Within this pathway, called transcytosis, the degradation of bone substance fragments absorbed by the osteoclast continues. Cathepsin D acts along with cathepsin K in phagosomes, where the basic cytochemical marker of osteoclasts, the aforementioned tartrate-resistant acid phosphatase (TRAP or TRACP), is also concentrated. The biological role of this enzyme is not fully understood but it has been established that, in addition to its phosphatase function, it is capable of generating the so-called reactive forms of oxygen (ROS). ROS actively destroy a vast variety of biological macromolecules, thereby supplementing cathepsins' action (Vaaraniemi et al., 2004).

The process of bone substance degradation, beginning in the lacuna and occurring in the transcytotic vesicles of osteoclasts, ends up in small fragments of macromolecules and ions entering the bloodstream. It should again be stressed that the passage of calcium ions (Ca^{2+}), released from bone mineral, into the bloodstream constitutes the basic mechanism for maintaining calcium homeostasis in the body.

Amino acids released by the proteolysis of the organic matrix are reutilized for the biosynthesis of new proteins. However, the bone type I collagen-specific domains, containing the cross-links formed during the posttranslational stage of fibrillogenesis, are protease resistant. They are excreted with urine, the numerical parameters of their excretion reflecting the overall rate of bone tissue metabolism.

The acid phosphatase (TRACP) or, more precisely, its TRACP5b isoform, which differs from the macrophage- and dendritic cell-derived TRACP5a, also enters the bloodstream from the functioning osteoclasts. The increased activity of the TRACP5b acid phosphatase in the blood serum is a specific and sensitive clinico-biochemical indicator of abnormally increased osteoclastic bone tissue resorption (Halleen et al., 2006).

Osteoclastic bone tissue resorption occurs within the so-called basic metabolic units (BMU), in which they act in a functional coupling with osteoblasts. While the leading role in osteoclast differentiation, as well as in the initiation and stimulation of their resorptive activity, is played by the osteoblast-expressed molecular signals, the "initiative" in this coupling is transferred to osteoclasts. Osteoclasts are a source of molecular signals that attract osteoblasts into BMU and activate their anabolic activity to replace the resorbed bone matrix. Therefore, the resorptive (catabolic) function of osteoclasts within BMUs cannot be regarded as their only one, as it is also combined with an anabolic role (Karsdal et al., 2007).

Osteoclasts' anabolic function is not just the other side of their resorptive function. A reduction in the population of osteoclasts, caused by mutations of genes involved in osteoclastogenesis, such as *Csf* or *c-fos*, is accompanied by abnormalities in bone formation. Such abnormalities are explained by the insufficient osteoclastic expression of anabolic signaling molecules of the TGF-β and IGF families, expressed by osteoclasts irrespective of their resorptive activity (Karsdal et al., 2007). Equally irrespective of their resorptive activity, the osteoclasts secrete the cardiotrophin-1 (CT-1) cytokine, which promotes the proliferation and biosynthetic activity of osteoblasts, as well as stimulating bone growth. This cytokine belongs to the interleukin IL-6 family and is known for its ability to cause myocardial hypertrophy (Walker et al., 2008). Hence, osteoclasts' biological role is not limited to bone tissue resorption; they also actively control its formation (Segovia-Silvestre et al., 2009).

Another distinguishing feature of osteoclasts' biochemical phenotype is the presence of a number of active signaling systems that support the viability of cells and inhibit apoptosis. Typically, these intracellular systems include receptors for growth factors of TGF-β superfamily. The signal from these receptors directly activates TAK1 kinase, which calls the signaling pathways activated by other kinases, such as MEK, AKT, NIK, or IKK, into action. This is followed by the activation of transcription factors NF-κB (whose role in the osteoclast function has been discussed above), as well as I-κB. This support of osteoclasts' viability is unrelated to the Smad protein system usually employed by TGF-β in its other effects (Gingery et al., 2008).

In addition to its effect, mediated by RANK and RANK-controlled signaling pathways, RANKL is used as a receptor for another member of the TRAF family, is Fas, the key stimulator of apoptosis. RANKL enhances the expression of Fas in osteoclast progenitors, thereby reducing the osteoclast population. In mature osteoclasts, RANKL inhibits Fas expression, acting as a factor that raises the viability of osteoclasts and enhances bone tissue resorption (Wu et al., 2005).

One of the major local regulators of osteoclastogenesis, the macrophage colony-stimulating factor, or M-CSF (see section 10.2.4), continues to influence mature osteoclasts' function with the participation of αvβ3 integrin. This influence affects the cytoskeletal development and the activity of a number of cytoplasmic kinases (Ross and Teitelbaum, 2005). M-CSF stimulates the expression of Mitf (microphthalmia-associated transcription factor), which, in turn, controls the expression of such executory proteins of the osteoclast as cathepsin K, TRAP acid phosphatase, and chloride channel protein 7 (OC-7) (Sims & Gooi, 2008). In addition, with the participation of PAK1 kinase, M-CSF detains the osteoclast apoptosis by stimulating the expression of the apoptotic inhibitor survivin (Bradley et al., 2008).

Osteopontin, a non-collagenous protein (a phosphorylated sialoglycoprotein) of the organic bone tissue matrix plays an especially important role in terms of the osteoclast function. It is alternatively known as bone sialoprotein I (BSPI), secreted phosphoprotein 1, and uropontin. In humans, its molecule consists of 314 amino-acid residues. Osteopontin is produced by many cells in a variety of tissues, and is especially actively expressed in osteoblasts. Zero mutations of the osteopontin-encoding gene (*Opn*) lead to a decrease in the size of the corrugated (villous) surface of the osteoclast's cell membrane, which indicates a decrease in its resorptive activity. These mutations prevent the development of osteoporosis in mice (Franzen et al., 2008).

Osteopontin is a ligand for αvβ integrin, a typical osteoclastic integrin that apparently mediates the osteopontin's influence on the osteoclast. Studies involving the inactivation of the osteopontin gene in mice (Chellaiah et al., 2003) have shown that osteopontin deficiency causes a rearrangement of the osteoclastic cytoskeleton, accompanied by a retardation of cell mobility and a suppression of the expression of the cytoplasmic transmembrane receptor CD44, which is required for the osteoclast to attach to the bone surface. Thus, the effect of osteopontin on the osteoclast differs in its mechanism from that of osteoprotegerin, the former suppressing the differentiation and the resorptive function of osteoclasts and the latter acting as a decoy receptor (a competitor of RANK). In addition, osteopontin stimulates the apoptosis of osteoclasts.

8.3. EXTRACELLULAR MATRIX OF BONE TISSUE

8.3.1. Organic component of the bone matrix

8.3.1.1. Biochemical characteristics of bone matrix organic component

8.3.1.1.1. Collagenous components of matrix: fibrillin

Collagenous proteins are the major component of the organic extracellular matrix of bone tissue in terms of their mass. They make up about 85–90% of the overall mass of the matrix.

The quantitatively dominating collagen of bone tissue is type I collagen, comprising at least 90% of the overall mass of collagenous proteins in the bone. Like other "major" fibril-forming collagens (type II and III collagens), this collagen forms strong, structurally stable fibrils and fibers; it is these fibrils and fibers that endow the bone tissue with such a biomechanical property as tensile/rupture strength.

Type I collagen of the bone tissue has certain peculiarities of posttranslational origin. Unlike type I collagen of the dermis, bone collagen has hydroxylated lysine residues in the position 16C (in the carboxyterminal telopeptide) and in the position 87 (in the triple-helical domain of the molecule) of the α1(I) chain. Additional hydroxylysyls may be used for the formation of additional intramolecular cross-links, increasing the stability of collagen structures.

It was also shown that type I collagen of the bone tissue contains additional specific (lysyl pyridinoline and lysylpyrrolic) cross-links located at the lysine (rather than hydroxylysine) residues (Knott and Bailey, 1998). These cross-links are so highly specific to bone tissue collagen that the low-molecular peptide fragments of collagen fibrils (formed during the catabolism and excreted with urine) maintaining these links can serve as markers for the catabolism of bone tissue.

The properties of the type I collagen of bone tissue also depend on pentosidine cross-links forming with age due to the non-enzymatic addition of reducing sugars (see Chapter 5). More pentosidine cross-links occur in those parts of bone tissue characterized by a higher level of mineralization, which is indicated by higher bone mineral density (BMD), which is however, accompanied by a worsening of the tissue's biomechanical parameters (Saito et al., 2006).

While it is the quantitatively prevailing type I collagen that plays a critical role in the structure and functions of the extracellular matrix of bone tissue, the latter also contains a number of other collagens.

Thus, type V collagen plays an important role in terms of matrix formation. This collagen, with a heterotrimeric macromolecule described by the formula α1(V)α2(V)α3(V), is, similar to type XI collagen, a minor fibrillar collagen. It is very similar to the fibril-forming type I, II and III collagens in the continuous triple-helical structure of its macromolecule and its ability to form cross-striated fibrils.

Type V collagen does not form any independent structures in the bone tissue. All type V collagen detected in the bone extracellular matrix is found to be central (axial) cores of collagen fibrils, mainly consisting of type I collagen (Birk, 2001), the collagen fibrils and bone tissue fibers thus being heterotypic.

Such localization of type V collagen indicates its possible involvement in the formation of fibrils from type I collagen. One notable peculiarity of the type V collagen macromolecule in this respect is that its polypeptide chains retain their N-terminal propeptide during posttranslational processing; this propeptide projects into the gap zone between the type I collagen macromolecules. This adds to the strength of the supramolecular organization of collagen fibrils and fibers forming the framework of the organic matrix of bone tissue.

The stability of the collagenous framework is additionally contributed by the presence of type XII collagen of the FACIT group (see section 3.1.1.1). Collagens of this group have macromolecules that are located on the surface of collagen fibrils, composed predominantly of type I collagen. This limits the fibrils' diameter growth while, at the same time, binding them to each other.

Type III collagen forms independent small bundles of fibrils in the bone's cortical layer, especially noticeable on the surfaces of the haversian canals walls and on the border between the bone and the periosteum. Fibrils built of type III collagen have been found in human bones of all ages, ranging from the 30th week of embryonic development to 80 years of age (Keene et al., 1991), but their levels are the highest in the embryonic period, during the formation of the primary buds of bones.

Short filaments of type VI collagen are found within the bone, in particular, at the insertions of tendons and joint capsules, in the periosteum and endosteum. Their function consists of strengthening connections between cells, collagen fibrils and fibers. After 7 years of age, these filaments are found almost solely in contact with cells (Keene et al., 1991).

There are reports of finding small amounts of type VIII collagen in the bone (within the periosteum), as well as of transmembrane type XIII collagen (during the embryonic period). No data explaining the functional roles of these non-fibrillar collagens in the bone tissue is available.

In the earliest stages of osteogenesis in a mouse embryo, a considerable osteoblast expression of type XXIV collagen has been detected at the sites of bone tissue formation (Koch et al., 2003; Matsuo et al., 2006) (see section 3.1.1.1). This expression is regarded as a specific (in no lesser degree than osteocalcin) marker for osteoblastic differentiation and the beginning of osteogenesis (Matsuo et al., 2008).

Type XV collagen belonging to multiplexins (collagens with multiple interruptions of the triple-helical domain) are also expressed and secreted into the matrix by osteoblasts. This expression arises during osteoblastic differentiation in the mesenchymal progenitor cells and is further observed in mature bone-forming osteoblasts (Lisgnoli et al., 2009).

Bone tissue contains no elastic fibers. However, it contains one of the two structural components of elastic fibers–microfibrils composed of fibrillin–and the third (beside collagens and elastin) fibrillar component of connective tissue's extracellular matrix, and of glycoproteins bound to it.

The structural-functional importance of the presence of fibrillin in bone tissue has been indisputable since the Marfan's syndrome, a serious systemic skeletal disorder manifested by pronounced bone deformations, was proven to be caused by a mutation in the *FBN1* gene responsible for the synthesis of fibrillin-1, which is an isoform of fibrillin (Plantin et al., 2000).

According to Keene et al. (1991), the localization of fibrillin microfibrils in the bones of a human embryo is similar to that of fibrils built of type III collagen (in particular, at the insertions of tendons), but after 7 years of age, discrete fibrillin fibers remain almost solely on the surface of the cortical part of bones, in the areas of pronounced osteoblastic activity.

It has been shown, both in molecular-biological studies in vivo and in experiments on cell cultures (Kitahama et. al., 2000), that osteoblasts express mRNAs encoding fibrillin-1 and fibrillin-2, along with MAGP-1, MAGP-2 and MP78/70 glycoproteins associated with microfibrils, and the high-molecular (260310 kDa) protein LTBP-2. Within the bone tissue, fibrillin-1 is concentrated on the endosteal surface and inside the lacunae, where osteocytes reside. The fibrillins and MAGP-2 promote the fixation of osteoblasts in the tissue with the involvement of $\alpha v\beta 3$ integrin. Loss of fibrillin-2 expression (due to a zero mutation in the *Fbn2* gene) in mice leads to a contraction of the tubular phalangeal bones in the fore and hind limbs. (Boregowda et al., 2008). All these facts suggest that proteins of the fibrillin microfibrils serve not only a structural but also a regulatory role in the bone tissue. The latter is apparently associated with microfibrils' ability to bind signaling molecules of the TGF-β superfamily, including BMPs, and to control the dynamics of their interactions with cells (Ramirez and Sakai, 2009).

8.3.1.1.2. Non-collagenous components of bone matrix

Table 8.4 provides an overview of the basic non-collagenous proteins in the extracellular matrix of bone tissue. Among non-fibrillar non-collagenous proteins, the one found in bone tissue in relatively high amounts is the glycoprotein osteonectin (SPARC). Its molecule is not large. In humans it contains 286 amino acid residues and its mass is 32 kDa after the removal of the 17-residue signal propeptide (43 kDa together with the attached oligosaccharide groups). The molecule consists of three major domains. All these domains bind calcium ions but the degree of affinity for calcium is especially high in the so-called EF-hand structural motifs with a characteristic "helix-loop-helix" structure. Calcium ions considerably affect the secondary structure, or molecular conformation, of osteonectin.

The first, the N-terminal domain (residues 1–52) has an acidic character due to considerable levels of aspartic and glutamic acids. This domain has a high affinity to hydroxyapatite and is apparently involved in the mineralization process. The second domain (residues 53–137) is rich in cysteine, with all its cysteine residues involved in the formation of intramolecular disulfide bonds. A mannose-rich N-oligosaccharide is attached to the Asn99 residue. The second domain participates in interactions with other extracellular matrix proteins, particularly with collagens, and with cells. The third domain (residues 138–286) has an α-helix conformation and is characterized by an especially high affinity for calcium; it also binds to collagens and cell membranes (Yan and Sage, 1999).

Just after its discovery, osteonectin found in bone tissue was believed to function solely as an adhesive protein. Its adhesive properties manifest in vitro by the ability to bind both collagens and hydroxyapatite. It has been shown that osteonectin binds with the amino acid sequence PSGPRGQOGVMGFOGPKGNDGAO (where O stands for 4-hydroxyproline) common for the α-polypeptide chains of large fibrillar collagens (types I, II and III) (Giudici et al., 2008). These adhesive properties were thought to account for the impairment of bone tissue properties arising with osteonectin deficiency in a disorder called osteogenesis imperfecta, or in some forms of hereditary fragility of bone in animals. Further research has shown that, in its role of a matricellular protein in bone tissue, the functions of osteonectin are much more complex and diverse, going far beyond its adhesiveness (Sodek et al., 2002). Osteonectin has been shown to be capable of regulating the proliferation of bone and endothelium cells, angiogenesis and the expression of matrix metalloproteases. Induction of MMPs is a property of the small domain, located between the amino-acid residues 154 to 173. The osteonectin expression is the highest in the bone remodeling units, located on the outer surface (see section 8.6.2). Studies in mice, with a deletion of exon 4 of the osteonectin gene, have shown decreased bone remodeling activity, leading to osteopenia due to a negative balance between resorption and formation. Such a disbalance results from a derangement in the process of differentiation and maturing, as well as a decrease in osteoblasts' viability (Delany et al., 2003).

Osteoadherin (Wendel et al., 1998), or osteomodulin, is a proteoglycan of the leucine-rich proteoglycans family (PRELP), expressed only in bone tissue and found around mature osteoblasts on the surface of bone trabeculae.

Table 8.4

Structural peculiarities and functional characteristics of the key non-collagenous proteins of the bone matrix

Protein (synonyms)	Structural features	Basic functions
Osteonectin (SPARC, BM-40, 43- kDa protein)	Contains EF-hand structural motifs and mannose-rich oligosaccharides; N-terminal domain markedly acidic	Binds calcium ions and hydroxyapatite; promotes the proliferation and differentiation of osteoblasts; stimulates angiogenesis and matrixin expression
Osteoadherin (osteomodulin)	Proteoglycan. Contains keratan sulfate, 11 repeats of leucine-rich sequences, and a large, markedly acidic C-terminal Ensures the adhesion (attachment) of cells	hydroxyapatite; promotes the domain
Fibromodulin	Proteoglycan. Contains keratan sulfate, 11 repeats of leucine-rich sequences; 4 tyrosine residues may be attached near the N-terminal domain	Involved in the processes of enchondral and intramembranous ossification
Osteopontin (2ar, 44 kDa phosphoprotein, SPP, bone sialoprotein I, BSP-I)	Phosphorylated; contains a RGD-sequence	Attachment of cells, in particular of osteoclasts to the bone surface; involved in the osteoclastogenesis; binds hyaluronan
Bone sialoprotein II (BSP-II)	Contains a RGD-sequence and sulfated tyrosine residues	Attachment of cells, initiation of mineralization
Acidic bone protein (glycoprotein) (BAG-75)	Polyasparagine acid	Mineralization?
Biglycan (PG-I)	Proteoglycan. Contains leucine-rich repeats and two GAG-chains near the NH2-terminal	Interaction of cells among themselves and with proteins
Decorin (PG-II, PG-40)	Proteoglycan. Contains leucine-rich repeats and one GAG-chain near the NH2-terminal	Binding of collagen; regulation of the fibrillogenesis
Bone Gla-protein (osteocalcin, BGP)	Contains γ-carboxy glutamate	Binds calcium and hydroxyapatite
Matrix Gla-protein	Contains γ-carboxy glutamate	Detains osteogenesis?
TSP-1, TSP-2, TSP-3 and TSP-4 thrombospondins	TSP-1 and TSP-2: homotrimers TSP-3 and TSP-4: homopentamers. Contain a RGD-sequence	Exert multifaceted effects of matricellular proteins. Affect the attachment of cells, mineralization and angiogenesis
Dermatopontin (22 kDa matrix protein)	Proteoglycan. Contains dermatan sulfate	Stimulates the cell adhesion. Regulates the activity of BMPs

It contains keratan sulfate, and the main peculiarity of the central domain of its polypeptide chain is the presence of 11 leucine-rich repeats of amino acid sequences, each of which is 20–30 residues long. Osteoadherin is distinguished by a large, markedly acidic C-terminal domain. Osteoadherin promotes the adhesion (affixing) of cells, which is mediated by αvβ integrin. Mature osteoblasts actively express osteoadherin in vitro, and this stimulates mineralization in the culture (Rehn et al., 2008).

Another keratan sulfate proteoglycan is fibromodulin, which also belongs to the PRELP family. The expression of fibromodulin has been detected in osteoblasts (as well as in chondroblasts) in the course of endochondral and intramembranous ossification in mouse embryos (Gori et al., 2001b). As implied by its name, fibromodulin also affects the process of collagen fibril and fiber formation. Two other small proteoglycans of the SLRP family–biglycan and decorin–are expressed at different stages of bone tissue formation with their macromolecules containing different glycosaminoglycans. This was shown in osteo-blast cultivation experiments (Waddington et al., 2003). The expression of biglycan, which contains dermatan sulfate, is active at the proliferation stage. It decreases during the deposition of the extracellular matrix (osteoid) and reactivates with the beginning of matrix mineralization, but, at this stage, biglycan contains chondroitin sulfate. Decorin expression occurs somewhat later than that of biglycan; likewise, the prevalence of dermatan sulfate in decorin at the stage of matrix formation is followed by the dominance of chondroitin sulfate during mineralization.

Three non-collagenous proteins of bone tissue–osteopontin (also known as BSP-I), bone sialoprotein (BSP-II or simply BSP) and acidic bone glycoprotein (BAG-75)–occur in detectable amounts only in mineralized tissues and are usually isolated from the bone tissue, together with the mineral component. All these proteins share two basic peculiarities: they are phosphorylated (thus belonging to phosphoproteins) and are markedly acidic (Gorski, 1992). Their acidity is caused by large repeats of acidic amino-acid residues, aspartic (D) and glutamic (E) acids. Thus, the region located between residues 77 and 84 in human bone sialoprotein has an EEEEEEEE structure, while the structure of the region between residues 151–160 is DEEEEEEEE; the region between residues 70 and 78 in the rat osteopontin contains only D. In all three proteins, additional acidity is due to the residues of sialic acid and phosphate groups. This anionic primary structure implies that one of the functions of bone matrix phosphoproteins (in particular, of the bone sialoprotein BSP-II) is binding calcium cations and, probably, in the nucleation of hydroxyapatite crystals.

Phosphorylated glycoproteins of the bone and dental tissues are classified as a family of proteins called **SIBLINGs** (small integrin-binding ligand, N-linked glycoproteins), similar in structure and the chromosomal localization of the encoding genes (Fisher and Fedarko, 2003; Young, 2003). This family also includes the dentine matrix protein, dentine sialophosphoprotein and the osteocyte-expressed MPE (matrix extracellular phosphoglycoprotein). All these proteins contain a RGD-sequence, defining their ability to bind with integrins. Two phosphoglycoproteins of the SIBLING family that contain sialic acid–osteopontin and BSP–are involved in regulating the osteoclastogenesis and osteoclastic functions through a variety of mechanisms. Due to this involvement, they affect the remodeling of bone tissue and its mechanical properties (Malavia et al., 2008)

Cultivated osteoblasts actively express fibronectin; considerable amounts of fibronectin are also found in the extracellular bone matrix in vivo. It is therefore assumed that fibronectin is required for the formation of the matrix's structural arrangement (Young, 2003). By binding with bone morphogenetic protein 1 (BMP-1), fibronectin raises its proteolytic activity. This effect of fibronectin activates the posttranslational processing of the secreted structural components occurring in the extracellular matrix (Huang et al., 2009).

About 2% of the overall mass of the matrix proteins are comprised of two proteins, distinguished by the presence of γ-carboxylated residues of glutamic acid. One of them is bone Gla-protein (BGP), or osteocalcin, which is synthesized only in osteoblasts and osteocytes and has a small molecule of 49 amino acid residues, including one hydro-xyproline residue uncharacteristic to non-collagenous proteins, and three γ-carboxy-glutamyl residues. Osteocalcin is specific to bone tissue and serves as a credible marker for the completion of the differentiation (phenotypic maturity) of the osteoblast. Blood levels of osteocalcin are used as an indicator for the activity of osteogenesis. The γ-carboxy-glutamate residues make it possible for osteocalcin to bind to calcium ions and hydroxyapatite. Mutant mice with the inactivated osteocalcin gene show excess bone mass and density in postnatal life, which indicates the regulatory (or optimizing) effect of osteocalcin on bone tissue formation (Ferland, 1998).

The second protein, which contains four γ-carboxy-glutamate residues, matrix Gla protein (MGP), has the ability to control and restrain mineralization. This protein is found not only in bone tissue; its function is especially distinctly seen in cartilaginous tissue and in vessel walls, i.e. in tissues that normally do not undergo mineralization.

The carboxylation of glutamate residues in Gla-proteins requires the involvement of vitamin K. Besides, the synthesis of these proteins is stimulated by vitamin D.

Four members of the thrombospondin family are present in the bone extracellular matrix: TSP-1, TSP-2, TSP-3, and TSP-4. All four exert multifaceted activity typical to matricellular proteins affecting angiogenesis, the proliferation and adhesion of cells and the mineralization. In other words, thrombospondins modulate the development, remodeling and regeneration of bone tissue (Alford and Hankenson, 2006). In the bone matrix, the most abundant is thrombospondin 2, which detains osteogenesis. This action's mechanism differs from that underlying the action of Gla-proteins: thrombospondin 2 regulates the size of the osteoblast population by affecting the marrow stromal cells, precursors of osteoblasts. The inactivation of the gene encoding this protein leads to thickening of the cortical bone layer and an abnormal increase of bone density in response to mechanical load (Hankenson et al., 2006).

A demineralized extracellular bone matrix contains a significant amount of dermatopontin, a proteoglycan in which dermatan sulfate is a glycosaminoglycan component of its small (22 kDa) macromolecule. Dermatopontin suppresses bone morphogenetic proteins' stimulating effect on the formation of the osteoblastic phenotype in osteogenic precursor cells, in particular, on alkaline phosphatase expression (Behnam et al., 2006). Besides, dermatopontin promotes cell adhesion.

Non-collagenous proteins of the bone matrix have intra- and intermolecular covalent cross-links. In terms of their chemical nature, these links are similar to fibrillins' cross-links: they are formed under the effect of the osteoblast-expressed transglutaminases and belong to γ-(glutamyl)-ε-lysyls. The cross-linking pertains to macromolecules of fibronectin, osteopontin and bone sialoprotein, resulting in homo- and heterotypical polymeric protein complexes that are more stable than individual molecules. Similar links bind these complexes to macromolecules of type I collagen. Such an interconnection of fibrillar and non-fibrillar components of the bone matrix improves its biomechanical properties. The interaction of these complexes with the integrin receptors of osteoblasts is also possible, improving the adhesion between cells and the extracellular matrix. Two members of the transglutaminase family are involved in the formation of cross-links: TG2 and the coagulation factor XIIIA enzymatic subunit (Nurminskaya and Kaartinen, 2006). The suppression of transglutaminases in the early stage of osteoblast differentiation, which disrupts the formation of the entire cross-linking system in the matrix, blocks the further production of the matrix components and its mineralization.

8.3.1.1.3. Matrix non-specific components

In addition to the above-mentioned components of the extracellular organic matrix forming its supramolecular structure, it also contains some other constituents.

Like all biological tissues, bone tissue contains water, which accounts for up to 10% of its mass. Water makes up the basis of the interstitial fluid infiltrating the matrix. An electrophoretic analysis of this fluid indicates the presence of a number of blood plasma proteins: albumin, apolipoprotein A-I, transferrin, α2-HS-glycoprotein, and the immunoglobulins IgG and IgM.

The prevailing protein in the interstitial fluid of bone tissue is albumin. The albumin clearance from plasma to the interstitial fluid in bone tissue is more intensive than in the skin or muscle tissue and is comparable to that in the intestine. Besides, albumin that does not differ from blood plasma albumin in terms of its amino-acid structure and molecular mass is expressed by osteoblasts (Yamaguchi et al., 2003). However, interstitial fluid contains only about 30% of the total albumin detected in bone tissue. This is due to the fact that crystalline hydroxyapatite is an excellent adsorbent and, as such, is capable of actively accumulating many proteins. Therefore, the major part of albumin is bound to the mineral phase of bone tissue.

Due to hydroxyapatite's adsorptive properties, bone tissue can accumulate plasma proteins so that the levels of some of them in the bone exceed their concentrations in plasma. This is true not only for albumin, but also for α2-HS-glycoprotein and the immunoglobulins.

The accumulation of immunoglobulins increases bone tissue's inherent resistance to infection. The antimicrobial peptides present in the matrix – osteoblast-produced **β-defensins** (hBD-1,-2,-3) – act in the same direction (Warnke et al., 2006).

In immunohistochemical studies on a mineralized bone, these blood plasma proteins are localized together with the typical bone tissue glycoproteins, osteopontin and osteocalcin (McKee et al., 1993). This gives reason to assume that those amounts of plasma proteins not adsorbed on hydroxyapatite interact with structural proteins of the matrix, playing a functional role in the matrix, which remains to be clarified.

Peptide signaling molecules (growth factors/cytokines) have accumulated within the organic matrix of the bone. Thus, levels of the transforming growth factors of the TGF-β superfamily in the bone matrix are dozens of times higher than their counterparts in other tissues of the body; some of these factors (bone morphogenetic proteins) have actually been initially isolated from a demineralized bone matrix. Such a high level of signaling molecules is obviously beyond the requirements of local regulation, indicating that bone tissue is a depot for these factors.

Bone tissue contains lipids. Their total content (triglycerides, fatty acids, free and esterified cholesterol) makes up about 12% of the dehydrated tissue mass (Boskey et al., 1983). Lipids are detected in the organic matrix, making up 1% to 3% of its mass (or even more, according to some sources), as well as in the mineral phase.

The demineralized bone matrix contains all the above-mentioned lipid fractions, more than 40% of which are comprised by fatty acids. A considerable percentage of matrix lipids are extracted from the non-collagenous fraction, together with bone morphogenetic proteins (Urist et al., 1997). The physical nature of interactions between non-polar (water insoluble) lipids and proteins is still not entirely clear. The formation of lipoproteins (complex macromolecules consisting of lipid and protein components) may likely take place. The origin of the matrix lipids is most apparently associated with osteoblasts, which are genetically close to fat cells (adipocytes). This relatedness becomes evident in some pathological conditions, where changes in the functional condition of osteoblasts are accompanied by changes in the spectrum of matrix-contained fatty acids (Plumb and Aspden, 2004).

Despite the fact that their quantitative proportion is less than that of non-polar lipids, phospholipids are of great importance in bone tissue biology. Glycosphingolipids such as lactosyl ceramide are required for normal osteo-clastogenesis (Fukumoto et al., 2006). Phospholipids, at least some of them, originate from matrix vesicle membranes disintegrated in the course of mineralization and, according to some reports, are involved in the mineralization process per se. Some phospholipids are extracted from bone tissue only along with the mineral phase.

Atomic force microscopy, in combination with immunochemical methods, have shown that, within the compact bone tissue, spherical particles about 145 nm in diameter are located between the surfaces of collagen fibrils and fibers and the mineral crystals deposited on them. As evidenced by their solubility in organic solvents, these spheres have a lipid or lipoprotein nature. Apparently, the layer of lipid particles mediates the binding between mineral crystals and collagens (Xu and Yu, 2006).

8.3.1.2. Morphological characteristic of organic component of bone matrix

The majority of the molecular elements of the bone matrix organic component described above are part of the structure of the fibrous base of bone tissue which, like in other types of connective tissue, is represented by a complex, multi-level hierarchical system that includes collagenous molecules, microfibrils, fibrils, fibers and fiber complexes.

The major part of the mature bone tissue is comprised by bone lamellae consisting of flat and flattened collagenous fibers. It should be kept in mind that morphological studies of bone tissue are usually conducted on demineralized samples. For this reason, the concept of a "bone lamella" is equated with its organic (demineralized fibrous) base. Depending on the area occupied by bone lamellae within the compact or spongy bone tissue, they are termed as outer and inner peripheric general, osteonic (haversian), intermediate (interstitial, transition, fragmentary), or trabecular bone lamellae. All lamellae share a common structure pattern (Fig. 8.12). Their thickness varies from 2–5 μm on average. They are arranged parallel to each other and along the long axis of structures formed by them (the cortical part of the diaphysis or a trabecula). The width and length of bone lamellae vary from several dozens to hundreds of microns. Bone lamella's structure can include from several hundreds to several thousands of collagen fibrils (Fig. 8.13) (N.P.Omeliyanenko, 1990). Collagen fibrils are finely cross-striated, which can be well detected on their longitudinal sections by contrasting them with uranyl acetate and phosphotungstic acid. Narrow longitudinal crevices (the apparent locations of crystalline hydroxyapatite, which are removed during demineralization) are seen in the structure of most fibrils. These crevices also are clearly visible on cross-sections of round-shaped collagen fibrils. The structure of collagen fibrils in the lamellae exhibits a number of peculiarities. A computerized morphological orientation analysis made it possible to provide quantitative characteristics for the architectonics of the fibrillar base of bone lamellae (Omelyanenko, 1990; N.P.Omeliyanenko, 1992). In their central parts, collagen fibrils have a predominantly longitudinal orientation with an anisotropy factor of 25%. This orientation of collagen fibrils coincides with the long axis of the osteon. In the periphery of the lamella, the fibrils have tangential and transverse orientations in addition to longitudinal ones. Here, the tangential orientation predominates. The anisotropy factor is 23%. Flat collagen fibers forming the bases of bone lamellae become split (branched), i.e. a redistribution of their fibrillar structure occurs without the fibrils being interrupted in any place. This ensures the integrity of the entire fibrous base of the bone. Besides, flat fibers of bone lamellae are permeated and divided into kind of segments by thin collagen filaments and individual fibrils running perpendicular to the plane of the bone lamellae from the cylindrical and flattened collagen fibers, which are located in the intermediate layers on either side of the bone lamella.

Such fibers have a predominantly circular-transverse orientation. Apparently, they perform an integrating function within the fibrous framework (Omelyanenko, 1990). Together with them, the bone lamellae form lamellar complexes, whose structure includes two or more lamellae arranged both in line and in parallel. Bone tissue contains three types of lamellar complexes: flat, cylindrical and semi-cylindrical. Cylindrical lamellar complexes form the fibrous base of the osteon (haversian system), a cylindrical formation consisting of "tubes" "inserted" one into another (telescopic structure). Accordingly, the diameter of individual "tubes" built of cylindrical bone lamellae decreases toward the center of the osteon, where the central (haversian) canal is located (Fig. 8.14; 8.15). It should be noted that the term "cylinder" is used only conventionally here since, in a strict geometrical sense, osteons are not cylinders. On longitudinal sections, their diameter does not remain constant. Its equivalent diameter varies from 120–160 microns. These variations depend, first, on the number of bone lamellae in the osteon's structure; secondly, on the thickness of lamellae themselves that varies largely, thirdly, on the osteon being located in the surface (peribone), medial or deep (endbone) areas of the "cortical". The central canal does not usually run through the geometrical center of the osteon but is shifted sideways. The diameters of central canals are also variable (30–40 μm). Besides, central canals may be filled with loose unshaped connective tissue surrounding one or more vessels passing through the central canal, or partially so, or missing some of the inner structures. The currently available morphological data set has led to the proposal for a new, more ideal model for the osteon fibrous base (*Fig. 8.16*) (Omelyanenko, 1990, Omelyanenko et al., 1997). Its basic difference from earlier models offered since 1901 (Gebhardt, 1901) or those currently existing (Cooper et al., 1966) lies in the following:

1. The orientation of collagen fibrils in the bone lamellae is characterized by two major directions relative to the central canal of the osteon: tangential (at the periphery of the lamellae) and longitudinal (in the central part of the lamellae).
2. The orientation of fibrils is similar in different bone lamellae (including adjoining ones).
3. Within the bone lamellae, there is a system of ligament fibers running transversely to the orientation of the lamellae.
4. Bone lamellae located in parallel are separated by spaces filled with cylinder-shaped (round) or flattened-shaped collagen fibers and are generally situated circularly relative to the central canal.

It should be noted that osteons might occasionally have two haversian canals, one located closer to the osteon's center and the other to its periphery. An important feature of the lamellar bone tissue's structural arrangement is the system of canals penetrating the entire bone matrix. Its detailed characteristic is provided in Section 8.4 below. Here it should be noted that the distribution of canals and canaliculi is irregular both in the osteons and within the entire compact bone tissue. On osteon cross-sections (mainly at their periphery) there are visible sites with no detectable canaliculi. In addition, almost all osteons are bounded by a limbus–a relatively homogeneous bone lamella containing no bone canaliculi or lacunae. In the literature, this lamella is termed (not quite accurately) the "cement line". The thickness of lines varies from one to several microns. These variations can be associated with the orientation of the section plane. The lines have a wavy contour. In some locations, this lamella is absent so that one osteon is in direct contact with the other, which includes interaction between the canalicular systems.

Some osteons may intrude into neighboring osteons, thus altering their ordered structural arrangement.

Semi-cylindrical lamellar complexes, built of intermediate bone lamellae, are located between the osteons and in close association with them (*Fig. 8.17*). Osteons and semi-cylindrical lamellar complexes (intermediate bone lamellae) make up most of the compact bone tissue. At the periphery, both outer and inner parts of the bone "cortical" are composed of flat lamellar complexes consisting of several common bone lamellae. All types of lamellar complexes are interrelated and form a composite mass of compact bone tissue (see *Fig. 8.17*). The aforementioned "cement lines", encircling the complexes around their periphery, serve as boundaries between them. In some locations between osteons, stretches of homogeneous bone matrix with no canaliculus (only with cell lacunae) occur instead of intermediate lamellae. These are probably areas of degenerating bone matrix.

Flat lamellar complexes form bone trabeculae (rods). Trabecular lamellar complexes are built of bone lamellae that somewhat differ from those in osteons, both in their structure and in their tighter packing within the trabeculae. Intermediate layers between the lamellae are absent (*Fig. 8.18*). When the diameter of the trabeculae exceeds 250–300 μm, osteons and semi-cylindrical complexes appear in their structure. The spongy bone tissue characterized by a cancellous arrangement (*Fig. 8.19*) is, in turn, built of trabeculae. The shape of trabeculae varies from cylindrical to flat (lamellar). Accordingly, the structure of spongy bone tissue also varies from cancellous to multi-chamber or honeycomb-like. All bones contain both types of bone tissue, one of which dominates depending on the specific nature of the biomechanical function of the bone.

8.3.2. Mineral component of bone matrix

8.3.2.1. Chemical characteristic of mineral component

The mineral component, or inorganic phase, of the bone tissue basically consists of calcium/phosphorus salts. Ninety-nine percent of the total calcium and 85% of the total phosphorus content in the body are found in the bone tissue.

The mineral component of the bone tissue results from the mineralization process, i.e. the deposition of calcium/phosphate salts in a crystalline form in the bone tissue organic matrix (a similar process occurs in dental tissue). So far as a living tissue's function is concerned, a more accurate term for this process would be biomineralization. It should not be equated with the concepts of the calcification or ossification. Calcification is a term designating any deposition of various (generally calcium) salts in a variety of tissues, which is sometimes abnormal. As to ossification, this term covers the entire process of bone tissue formation through the differentiation of mesenchyma that precedes it in the development or replacement of the cartilaginous tissue; this process includes mineralization as its final stage.

At least 95% of the bone mineral component mass is accounted for by crystalline hydroxyapatite. The chemical composition of hydroxyapatite crystals is described by the following formula:

$Ca_{10}[PO_4]_6[OH_2]_2$.

So far, the detailed crystallographic structure of hydroxyapatite contained in the bone tissue cannot be considered fully ascertained, and the information related to it remains controversial. The matter is that crystals of bone hydroxyapatite are never fully terminated. They re-

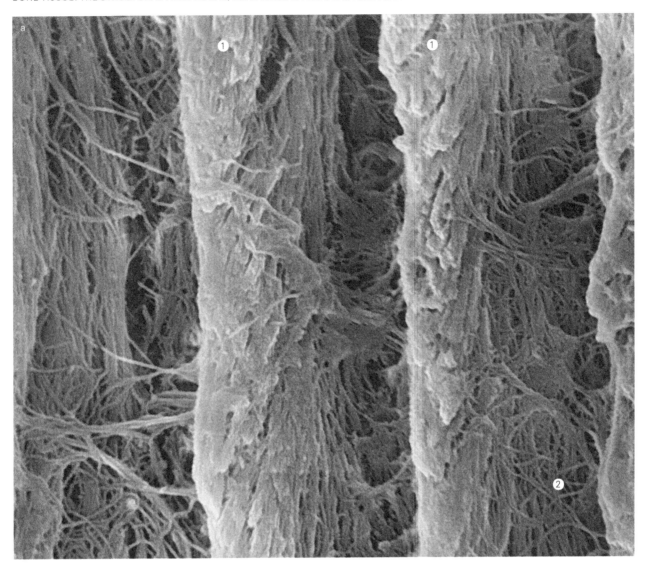

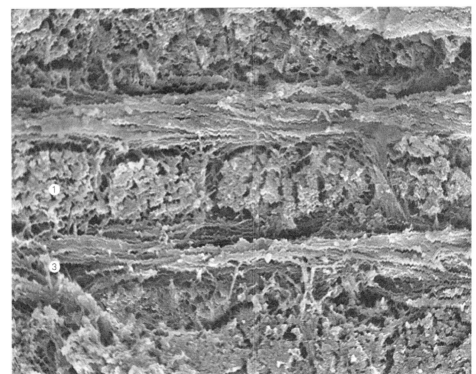

Fig. 8.12.
Bone lamellae (1) in the
compact bone tissue.
Collagen fibers and fibrils (2).
Intermediate layers of circularly
oriented collagen fibers (3).
a – longitudinal section;
b – cross section.
SEM-micrograph.
a, b – x 5,000.

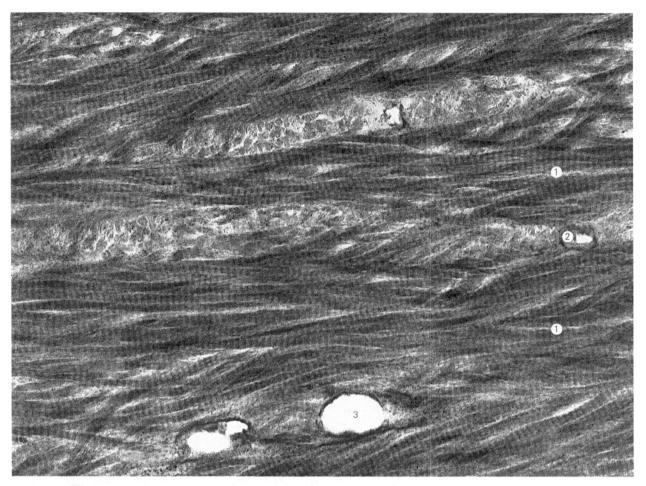

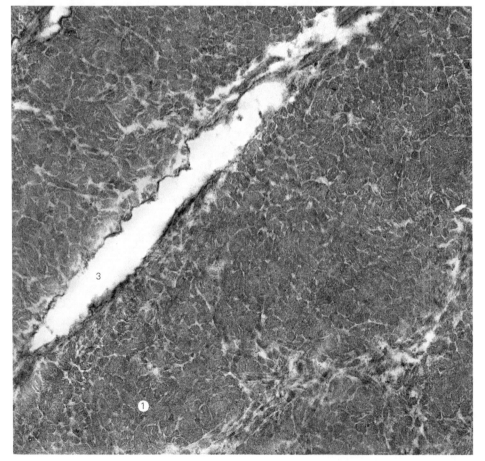

Fig. 8.13.
Bone lamellae (1) in the
compact bone tissue.
Intermediate layers of collagen
fibers and fibrils (2).
Bone canaliculi (3):
a – longitudinal section;
b – cross section.
TEM-micrograph.
Ultrathin sections contrasted
with uranyl acetate and lead
citrate.
a, b – x 30,000.

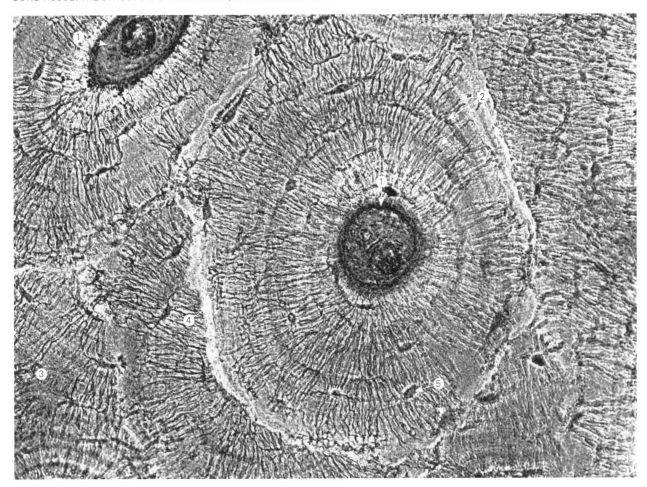

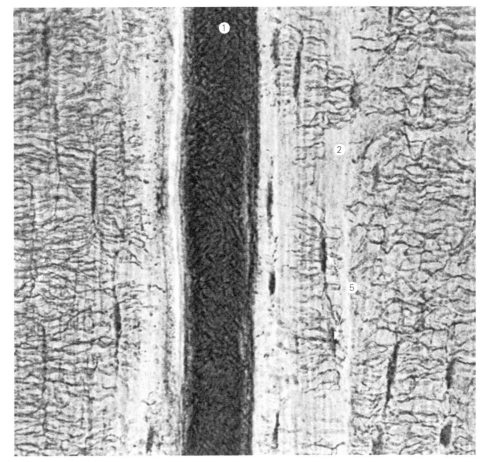

Fig. 8.14.
Osteons of the cortical part
of the tibial diaphysis.
Central canal (1).
Osteonic bone lamellae (2).
Intermediate bone lamellae (3).
Cement lines (4).
Osteocytes with processes in
the bone canaliculi (5).
a – cross section;
b – longitudinal section.
LM-micrograph.
Histologic sections.
Schmorl staining.
x 400. *(see color insert)*

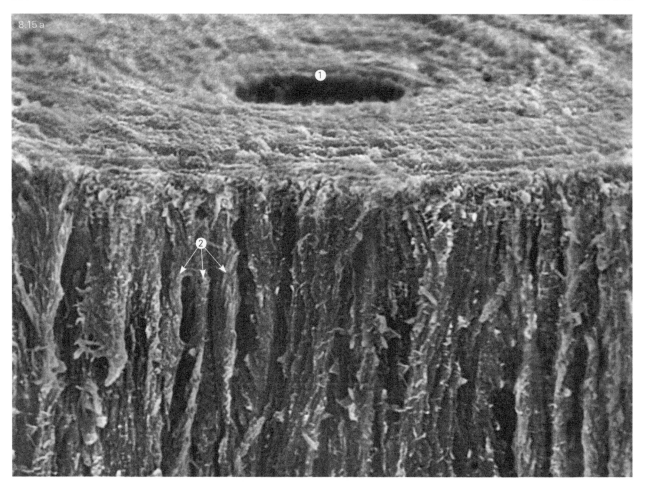

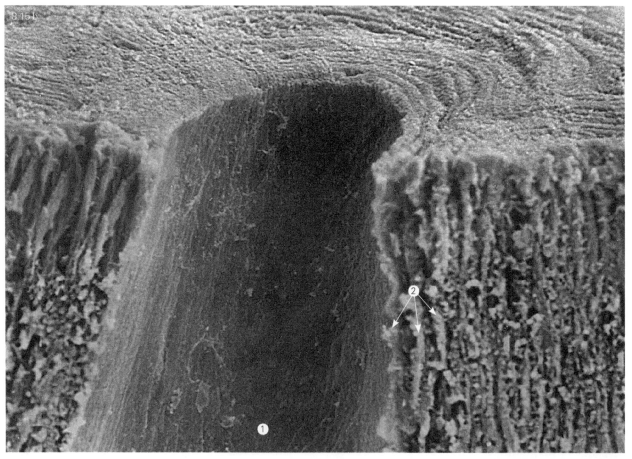

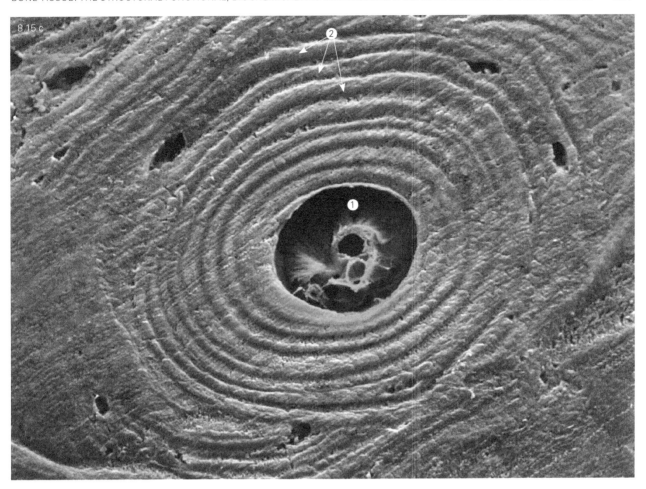

8.15 c

Fig. 8.15.

Fragments of osteons in various geometrical sections.
Central canal (1).
Bone lamellae (2).
Lacunae of bone cells (3).

a – lateral-longitudinal section;
b – section of an osteon along the central canal;
c – osteon cross section. SEM-micrograph. x 500.

main in a constant state of exchange and dynamic equilibrium with their environment. The phosphate ions $(PO_4)^3$ therein are partly replaced with $(HPO_4)^{2-2}$ acid phosphate and $(CO_3)^2$ carbonate ions. The levels of these ions may change with the aging of crystals (Buckwalter et al., 1995). The presence of OH groups in the crystals is being disputed; should these doubts be confirmed, it would be more correct to speak of apatite rather than hydroxyapatite. Despite these reservations, we will henceforth follow the established tradition of referring to the bone tissue mineral component as hydroxyapatite. During the 1970s and 1980s, a commonly accepted point of view (Posner, 1985) was that in crystallographic studies, the crystal structure of hydroxyapatite in bone tissue is masked by the presence of considerable amounts (up to 30% of the entire mineral component) of amorphous forms of calcium/phosphate salts. However, it was proven that the content of amorphous salts does not exceed 1–5%. The ambiguity of crystallographic data is explained not by the presence of the amorphous mineral, but by the peculiarities of bone hydroxyapatite, in which the calcium level is somewhat lower than would be expected according to stoichiometric patterns. Basically, calcium ions in the crystals are partly replaced by other ions. Accordingly, the crystal structure of hydroxyapatite formed in the course of biomineralization does not reach the perfection characteristic to crystals grown *in vitro* or those found in geological formations (Boskey, 1997).

Ions present on the surface of hydroxyapatite crystals remain in a hydrated condition, i.e. they retain water molecules. At the same time, superficial ions adsorb free ions from the interstitial fluid, which, in turn, undergo hydration, whereby another layer of water molecules is formed. Thus, each crystal becomes surrounded with a kind of hydration "coating". Complementary (in relation to hydroxyapatite) ions – sodium, magnesium, hydrocarbonate HCO_3, citrate and others – become inserted in significant amounts, mainly into these surface regions of crystals. The bone mineral consists of about 40% sodium, 60% magnesium and 90% citrate (Vlasov, 1987), in terms of the percentage of these ions total content in the body.

Due to their surface location, these additional ions are easily exchanged. Sodium, hydrocarbonate and citrate ions become involved in the acid-base equilibrium maintenance (Lemann et al., 2003).

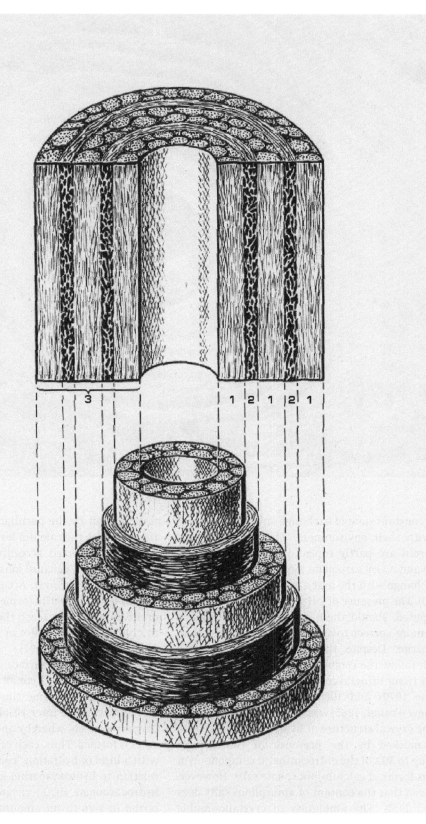

Fig. 8.16.
Structural arrangement of the
fibrous base of the osteon.
Bone lamellae (1).
Intermediate layer (2).
Lamellar complex (3).
(according to Omelyanenko,
2005).

Fig. 8.17.
Fragment of the cortical part
of the tibial diaphysis.
Compact bone tissue.
Osteons on a cross-section (1).
Central canals of osteons (2).
Intermediate lamellae (3).
Cement lines (4).

a – LM-micrograph.
A light optic microscope
Ni Nikon (Japan).
Histologic section.
Schmorl staining.
x 200 (see color insert);
b – SEM-micrograph.
x 200.

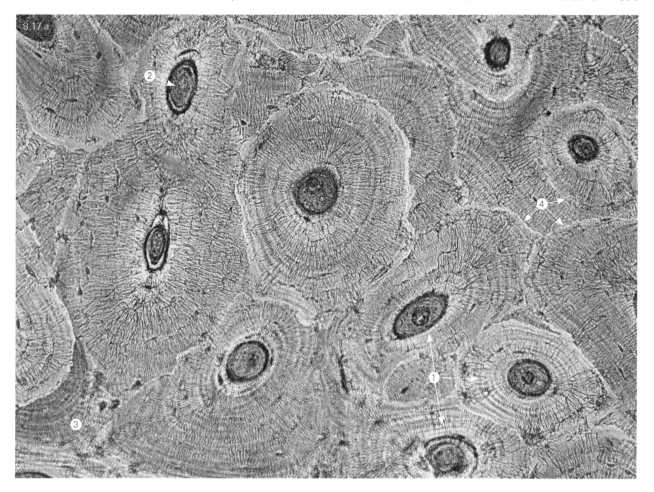

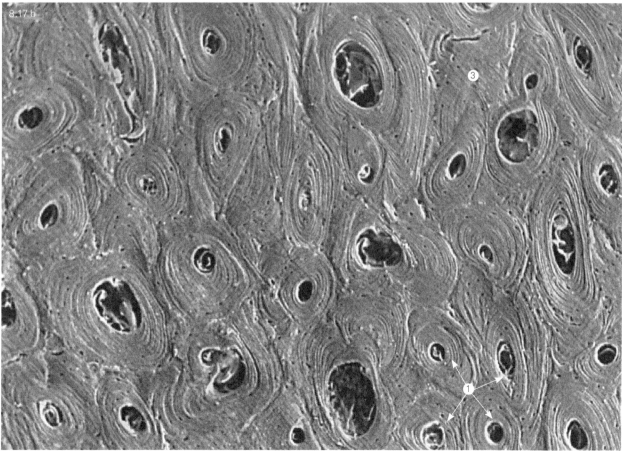

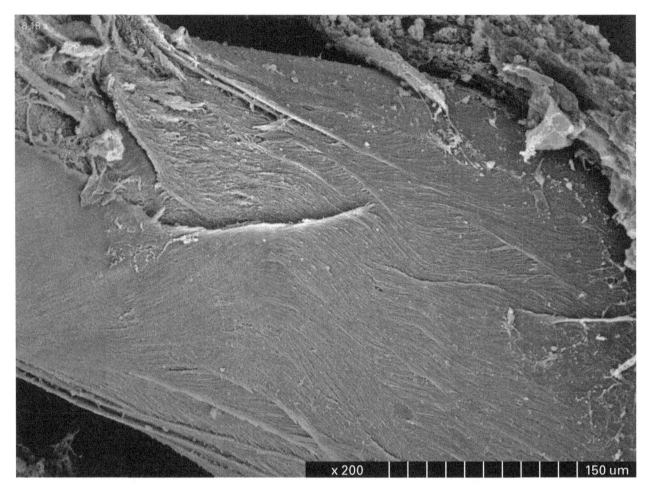

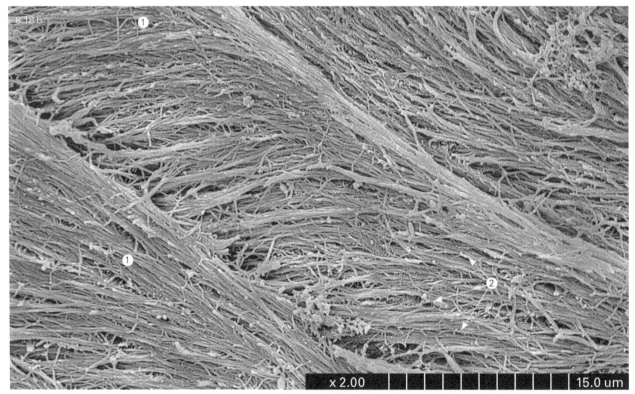

Fig. 8.18.
Fragment of a bone rod (trabecula) of the spongy bone tissue.
Bone lamellae (1).

Collagen fibrils within a bone lamella (2).
SEM-micrograph.
x 2,000.

Fig. 8.19.
Fragments of a vertebral body. Spongy bone tissue.
a – cylinder-shaped bone trabeculae (1);

b – lamellar-shaped bone trabeculae (1).
Intertrabecular spaces (2).
SEM-micrograph. a, b – x 100.

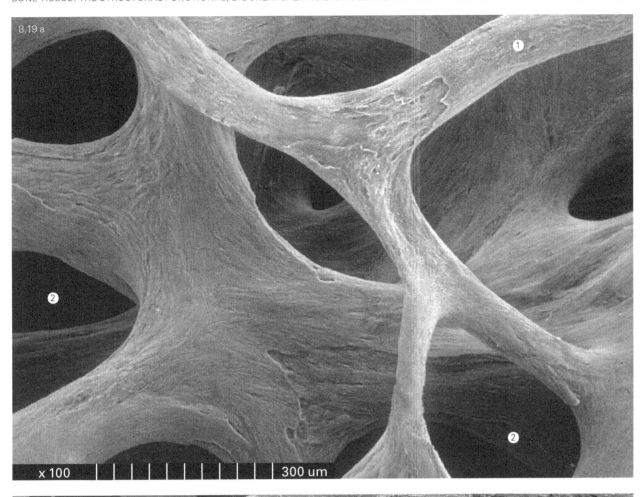

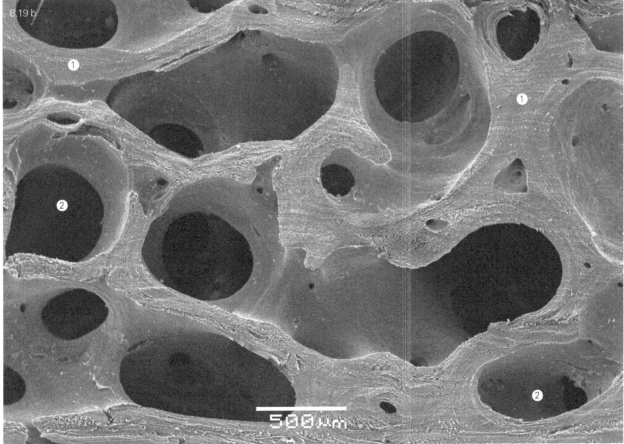

The calcium ion in hydroxyapatite found in bone tissue may easily be replaced with ions of other alkaline-earth elements such as barium, radium or strontium. From an ecological point of view, the replacement of calcium with strontium is of particular interest, since the radio-active long-lived isotopes of this element (Sr89 and Sr90), released into the atmosphere during nuclear explosions, become strongly fixed within bones' inorganic phase upon entering the body. The mineral component of bone tissue can also strongly absorb ions of actinides and tran-suranium elements, which has been shown by the examples of plutonium and americium (Guilmette et al., 2003).

8.3.2.2. Morphological (structural) arrangement of mineral component

The available data on the structural organization of the mineral component of bone and other mineral-contain-ing tissues is rather varied and sometimes controversial. This apparently reflects the results of studying the struc-tured "biominerals" using a variety of methods. Howev-er, with a whole variety of methods being used, the shapes and sizes of individual crystals, as well as their more complicated hierarchical arrangement within mineral aggregates, are based on indirect methods of visualization of elementary crystal units, or nanocrys-tals. Small-angle x-ray scattering (SAXS) and transmis-sion electron microscopy (TEM), in combination with to-mography, have been used to infer the size and geometry of bone and dentine crystals (Fratzl et al., 1997; Paris et al., 2000; Tesch et al., 2001; Landis, et al., 1993; Landis, 1995; Landis and Hodgens, 1996).

Mineral crystals were platelet-shaped, 3 nm thick and up to 100 nm long. In enamel, these values were 15–20 nm and up to 1000 nm, respectively (Warshawsky, 1989). In nacre, the thickness of mineral platelets is 200–500 nm and their length is 5–8 µm (Wang et al., 2001; Kamat et al., 2000). The size and geometry of mineral crystals are believed to play an important role in the mechanical properties of mineralized biomaterials.

The orientation and arrangement of mineral crystals in the protein matrix of bone and dentine were studied by Fratzl and co-workers (Fratzl et al., 1992, 1996 a, b, 1997; Rinnerthaler et al., 1999; Paris et al., 2000; Tesch et al., 2001) using SAXS, and by Landis and his colleagues (Lan-dis et al., 1993; Landis, 1995; Landis and Hodgens, 1996) using TEM tomography.

Mineral crystals in the bone microstructure are known to have a preferred orientation inside the fibril parallel to the longitudinal axis of the bone (Bundy, 1985).

Non-hydrostatic thermodynamics indicate that crystal growth is parallel to the principal stress directions and suggests that mineral orientations in biological tissues may depend on functional loading (Williams, 1989).

Based on their research of biominerals using the above-mentioned methods, Kager and Fratzl (2000) and Landis (1995) proposed a model for crystals' arrangement in the protein matrix in a tile-shaped pattern. The tile-shaped

organization of mineral platelets is consistent with the arrangement of collagen molecules in a collagen fibril (Hodge and Petruska, 1963).

Denisov-Nikolsky and his colleagues (2002) have shown the probability of the coplanar orientation of prismatic aggregates of bone mineral crystals.

Calculations were made to show that, due to the small size of an individual crystal, the total surface area of hy-droxyapatite crystals in the bones of an adult human, with a body weight of 70 kg, amounts to 40 hectares; the total surface area of crystals in 1 g of bone tissue reaches 200 m². Such an area offers exceptional opportunities for ion exchange between crystals and the environment and constitutes a prerequisite for bone tissue's functioning as the main depot ensuring calcium homeostasis in ver-tebrates.

The possibilities of modern high-resolution scanning electron microscopy has made it possible to obtain a di-rect image of the mineral structure in mineral-contain-ing tissues after the selective removal (dissolution) of their organic part (Omelyanenko, 2009–data not previ-ously published), whereby the mineral phase remained intact. The finest non-discrete (under SEM) mineral structures formed a polymorphic group, which included nanocrystals of the following shapes:

1) granular;

2) needle-like or rod-like;

3) platelet-like.

A significant part of bone tissue's mineral component is comprised of granular nanocrystals, ranging in size from 3 to 10 nm. These crystals make up the major part of the mineral base of mineralized collagen fibrils and interfi-brillar spaces (*Fig. 8.20*). They are distributed diffusely or in chains aligned along the long axes of fibrils. In some regions of the mineral matrix of collagen fibrils, perio-dicity is observed, the length of which correlated with the periodicity of collagen fibrils. A period, i.e. the repeti-tiveness of the structure along the long axis, consists of dark (less dense) and light (more dense) zones. In a dark zone, mineral nanocrystals and their chains are distrib-uted more sparsely and hence, are more clearly detecta-ble. In light zones, nanocrystals are arranged more dense-ly, making their visual separation more difficult. The pe-riod's length varies from 60–70 nm, which is only dis-tinctly traceable in individual locations. The mineraliza-tion degree of collagen fibrils, as estimated visually (un-der SEM) by the density of their mineral matrices, varies considerably, which makes the matrix' contour irregular; in some locations, matrices are rarefied and completely disappear. Interfibrillar spaces contain assemblies (aggre-gates) of granular nanocrystals. There are also free spaces throughout the entire mineral part, which indicates the incomplete and irregular mineralization of bone tissue.

Needle-like or rod-like nanocrystals also occur in lamel-lar bone tissue (*Fig. 8.21*). The crystals are 7–10 nm thick and 50–150 nm long. They may be distributed loosely or densely, forming bundles with a preferred orientation (anisotropic bundles) or without it (isotropic bundles).

Platelet-shaped nanocrystals occur in the lamellar bone tissue. Mineral platelets have a round shape with an equivalent diameter of about 50 nm and are 7–10 nm thick (*Fig. 8.22*). Nanocrystal platelets contact each other with their end faces or become layered over one another, thereby forming platelet aggregates, which may have a preferred orientation, apparently correlating to that of the fibrous structures they were part of.

Platelets and their aggregates form mineral complexes that basically have a "porous" structure (*Fig. 8.22*). Pores are spaces remaining after the removal of collagen fibrils. In addition, there occur areas characterized by the dense distribution of nanocrystals. Apparently, in such areas, fibrils had been absent or the space had been filled with micro- or subfibrils instead. It is known that the mineralization of the bone matrix with calcium nanocrystals, as described above, requires the presence of collagen structures. The deposition of minerals in biological tissues is also possible without the presence of collagen structures, but the shape of mineral crystals and their aggregates will be different.

The distribution of various shaped nanocrystals in the bone tissue may exhibit a mosaic pattern. In some locations, the prevalence of the same shapes may be observed, while in others, the tissue's mineral matrix may combine several types of nanocrystals. This is apparently determined by peculiarities in the structural arrangement of fibrous elements within the lamellar bone tissue, age and functional loading.

The identification of the elements present in the studied mineral matrices is reflected by SEM/X-Ray microanalysis charts (*Fig. 8.23*), which make it clear that the reliably detected dominant elements are calcium, phosphorus, oxygen and, in some instances, carbon, sodium, and magnesium. This corresponds, to some extent, with the chemical composition of the bone tissue's mineral component as determined by chemical methods.

The mineralization degree of the organic (principally collagenous) matrix or the distribution of minerals within it varies significantly and may be determined using SEM in back-scattered electron mode. This method confirms and essentially supplements the classical X-ray micrography. Interosteonic lamellae are much more mineralized than osteons (*Fig. 8.23*). This is apparently due to the fact that they are older that osteons. The mineralization degree also varies within the osteon, being more pronounced in the osteon lamellae than in interlamellar interfaces, although the boundary of this interface has a diffuse nature. In some locations, bone lamellae are not separated by a lower-mineralized area. The mineral matrix of bone lamellae is not a monolithic structure. It has numerous visible canals, canaliculi and microcanals. This is consistent with the porometric studies of the interstitial space of the bone tissue, in which the dimensions of these canals have been determined (see section 8.3.2.2). Around the periphery, almost all osteons are encircled by a thin, strongly mineralized limbus, which is about 1 μm thick.

The elements present in the studied samples of the lamellar compact bone tissue are shown in the SEM/X-Ray microanalysis charts (*Fig. 8.25*), indicating that the reliably detected dominant elements are calcium, phosphorus, oxygen and carbon, as well as small amounts of sodium and magnesium. The presented ratios of elements in native bone tissue somewhat differ (especially in carbon and oxygen contents) from the composition of the pure mineral matrix.

The above data imply that the mineral component of bone tissue consists of a multi-level hierarchical structural arrangement including:
1) a molecular level comprised by molecules of calcium-phosphate and other accompanying minerals;
2) a supramolecular level comprised by various shaped hydroxyapatite nanocrystals;
3) a tissue components level comprised by various order nanocrystal aggregates: mineral matrices of collagen fibrils, interfibrous and intercellular (interstitial) mineral matrices;
4) a tissue level comprised by the whole mineral matrix of the bone tissue.

The granular nature of the mineral component is observed in tooth enamel. Non-discrete granules are between 7 and 10 nm in size. However, they are detected only as part of various sized mineral aggregates (20–200 nm). Such aggregates may be distributed relatively loosely. In such locations, the contours (borders) of each of them are clearly detectable. In other places, aggregates merge to form a kind of dense conglomerate, in which only small aggregates remain detectable. On the surface of a tooth (i.e. its enamel), regions of loosely and densely distributed mineral aggregates occur in an alternating pattern. Such arrangement of the surface layer of enamel is probably not physiologic; further, more extensive studies will provide data to supplement this knowledge.

8.3.2.3. Dynamics and biochemical mechanisms of structuring (mineralization) of bone minerals

The formation of insoluble crystals from a solution (crystallization) is not a chemical reaction. It is a phase transformation of a substance – its transition from one state into another. A typical example of phase transition is the conversion of water into ice.

The initial stage of crystallization is called nucleation, i.e. the formation of a critical nucleus of a crystal from molecules moving chaotically in the solution and gathering into the smallest organized assemblies, which gain stability only after they reach a certain size. In many cases, the onset of crystallization is crucially determined by the presence of any foreign molecules or particles acting as heterogeneous nuclei. Crystal-forming molecules attach to these nuclei, which gives a specific orientation to the crystal growth. This process is called epitaxy, and crystallization that occurs on heterogeneous nuclei is referred to as heterogeneous.

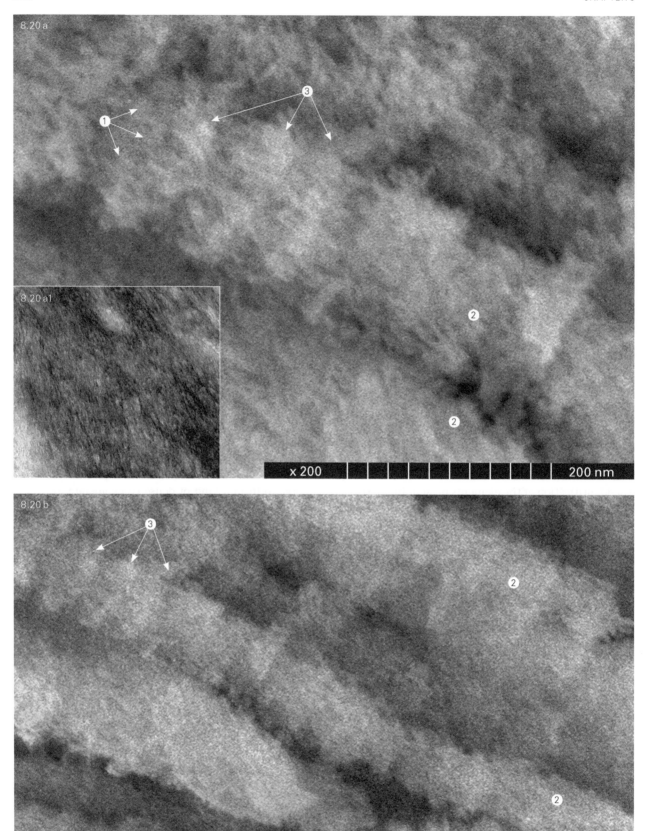

8.20 a1

x 200   200 nm

8.20 b

x 100   500 nm

Fig. 8.20.
Fragments of lamellar bone
tissue:
a, b, c, d – deorganified
(mineral matrix),
e – native bone tissue.

Granular structure of the mineral
component (matrix) (1).
Mineral matrix of collagen
fibrils (2).
Periodic structure of the
mineral in mineral matrix

of a collagen fibril (3).
Mineral matrix of collagen
fibers (bone lamellae) (4).
Needle-like nanocrystals (5).
a, b, c, d – SEM-micrographs.
a – x 200,000, b – x 100,000,

c – x 50,000,
d – x 10,000.
a1, e – TEM-micrograph.
Ultrathin sections,
a1 – x 200,000;
e – x 50,000.

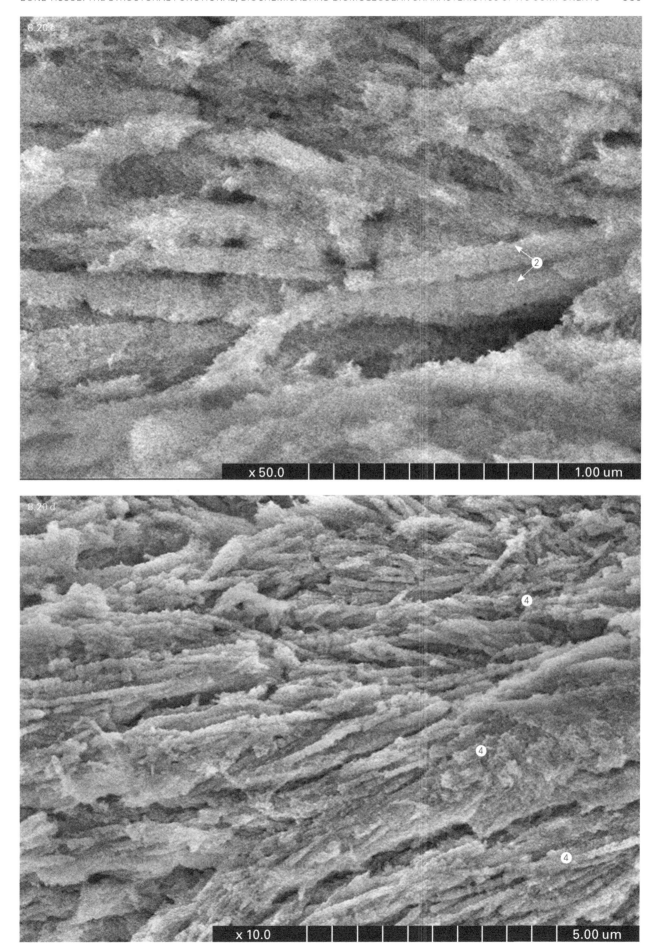

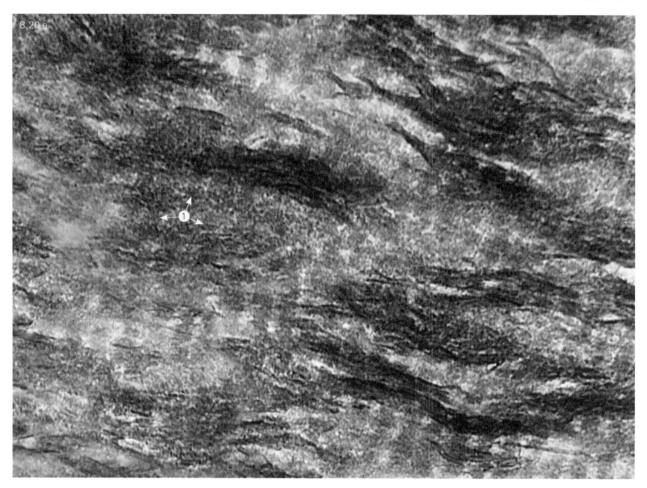

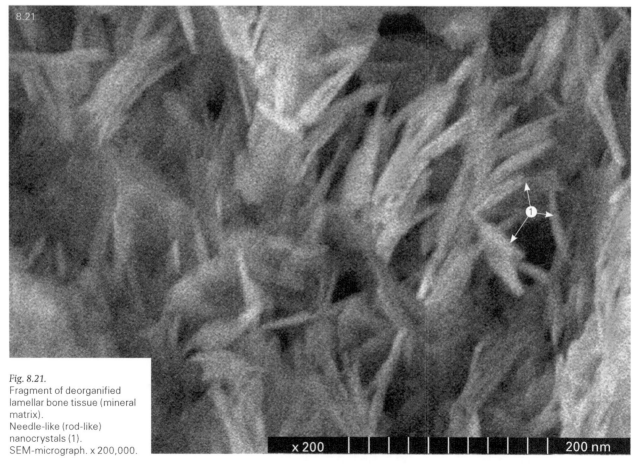

Fig. 8.21.
Fragment of deorganified
lamellar bone tissue (mineral
matrix).
Needle-like (rod-like)
nanocrystals (1).
SEM-micrograph. x 200,000.

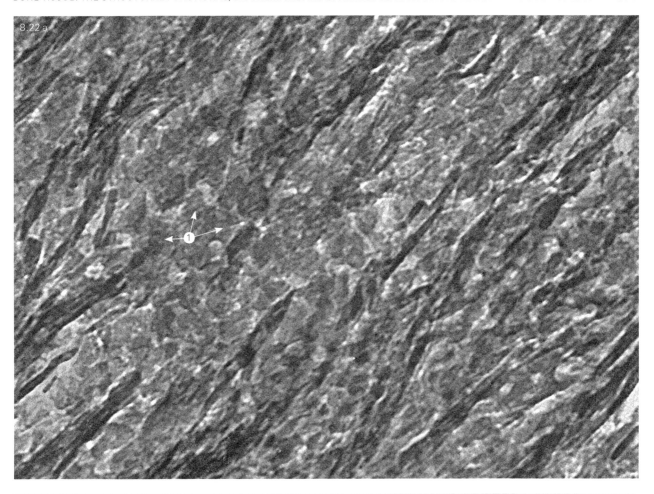

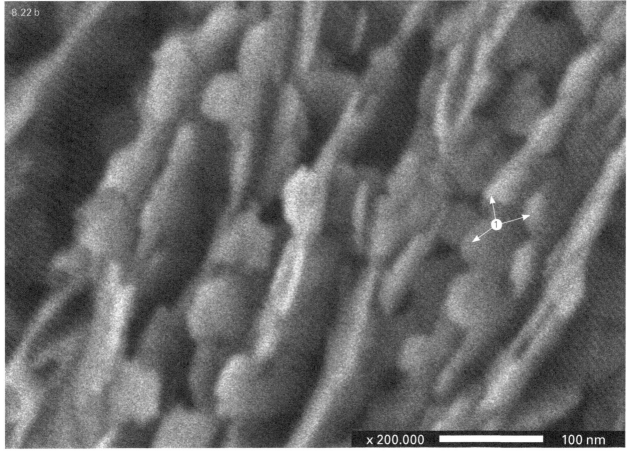

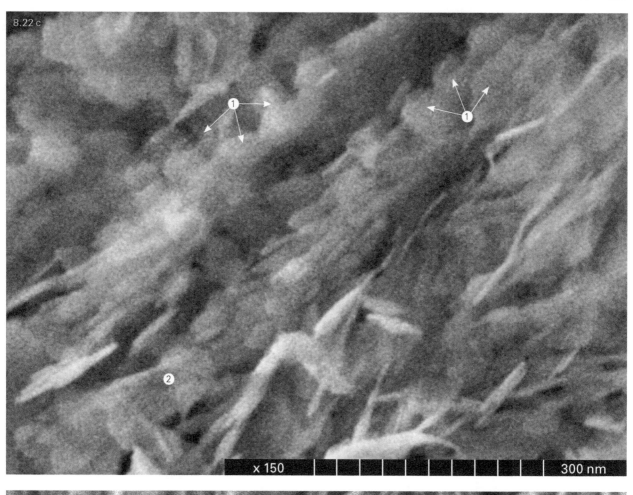

8.22 c

x 150   300 nm

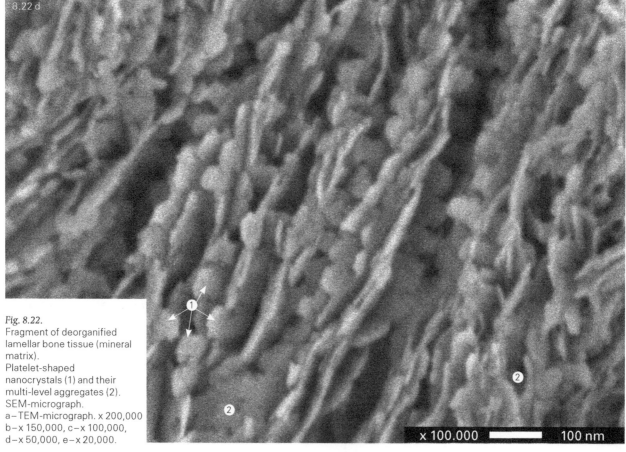

8.22 d

Fig. 8.22.
Fragment of deorganified
lamellar bone tissue (mineral
matrix).
Platelet-shaped
nanocrystals (1) and their
multi-level aggregates (2).
SEM-micrograph.
a−TEM-micrograph. x 200,000
b−x 150,000, c−x 100,000,
d−x 50,000, e−x 20,000.

x 100.000   100 nm

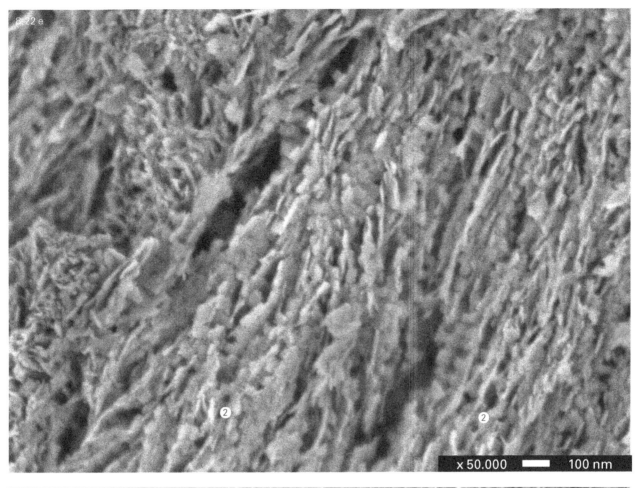

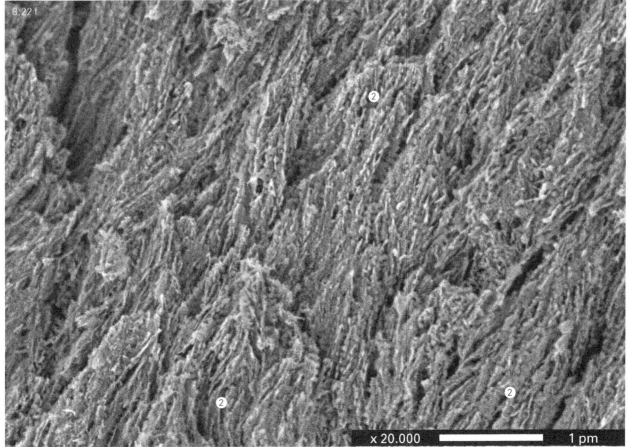

An example of heterogeneous crystallization is the hydroxyapatite crystallization underlying the mineralization of the organic matrix of bone tissue (as well as of the cartilaginous matrix in the course of bones' endochondral formation (see section 10.3.1.1). In this instance, heterogeneous nuclei may be comprised by various anionic (acidic) macromolecules of the matrix, whose chemical nature and structural conformations (particularly the β-sheet conformation) make them capable of binding calcium ions or calcium-containing molecules.

Such diversity of potential crystallization nuclei makes it impossible to trace the processes involved in the mineralization of various biological substrates, including that of bone tissue, to a single molecular mechanism. There are reasons to believe that this process may occur in various ways and that there exists a certain redundancy of mineralization mechanisms that supplement or, at least, do not theoretically exclude each other.

The currently dominating concept of hard tissue mineralization in vertebrates defines it as a two-stage process, in which the nucleation of crystals and their subsequent growth are spatially separated (Wiesmann et al., 2005).

The first stage (stage I), involving the accumulation of a sufficient concentration of hydroxyapatite and nucleation of crystals, occurs in the so-called matrix vesicles (MV), which are found in the foci of the beginning calcification (mineralization). They develop by outpouching from areas of plasma membranes of the cells responsible for calcification. The cytoplasm of the resulting outpouchings contains a cytoskeleton, which rearranges so that they detach from cells and become independent blebs. This process is believed to play a role among the phenomena making up the apoptosis process. The production of matrix vesicles is found in a variety of cells, such as hypertrophic chondrocytes of the bone growth plates, which are responsible for the mineralization of provisional cartilage during endochondral ossification, and osteoblasts that mineralize the bone tissue in all other instances of ossification, and odontoblasts (dental tissue cells homologous to osteoblasts). This gives reason to believe that the formation of MVs is a universal stage in the mineralization of skeletal tissues in vertebrates (Anderson et al., 2005).

Matrix vesicles are complicated structures. Since the vesicle's wall is a fragment of a cytoplasmic cell membrane, its basic components are the same lipids as in the parent membrane (cholesterol, sphingomyelin and other phospholipids), only with an increased content of acidic phospholipids (phosphatidylserine and phosphatidic acid). Acidic phospholipids may act as traps for calcium not requiring energy consumption (Anderson, 1995). The vesicle is located between two cross-striated collagen fibrils. Type X collagen, linking aggrecan proteoglycan protein and hyaluronan become linked to the vesicle's membrane from the outside. Phosphatases occupy a transmembrane position. Annexin V (anchorin CII), carbonic anhydrase, calpactin and actin are found inside the vesicle, contacting the inner surface of the membrane. Molecules of lactate dehydrogenase, calbindin and various proteinases move freely within the vesicle's cavity.

Matrix vesicles are characterized by a complex and peculiar protein composition. The proteome of osteoblasts' matrix vesicles have been shown to contain 133 proteins (Xiao et al., 2007). A matrix vesicle proteome differs in its structure and quantitative ratio of proteins from any cell organelles, both in terms of cells (osteoblasts) and of the bone tissue extracellular matrix as a whole. This means that MVs are specialized, dynamic independent structures used by cells to create favorable conditions for the onset of crystallization and tissue mineralization.

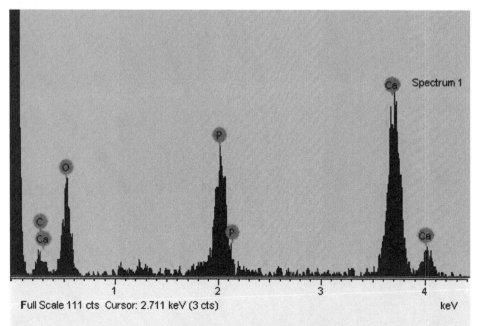

Full Scale 111 cts Cursor: 2.711 keV (3 cts)   keV

Fig. 8.23.
A diagram showing the elemental composition of the mineral matrix of the lamellar bone tissue.

Fig. 8.24.
Fragment of the cortical part of tibial diaphysis. Compact bone tissue. Osteons on a cross-section (1). Central canals of osteons (2). Intermediate lamellae (3). Lines of increased mineralization (4). Bone lamellae (5). Lacunae of osteocytes (6). SEM-micrograph taken in back-scattered electron

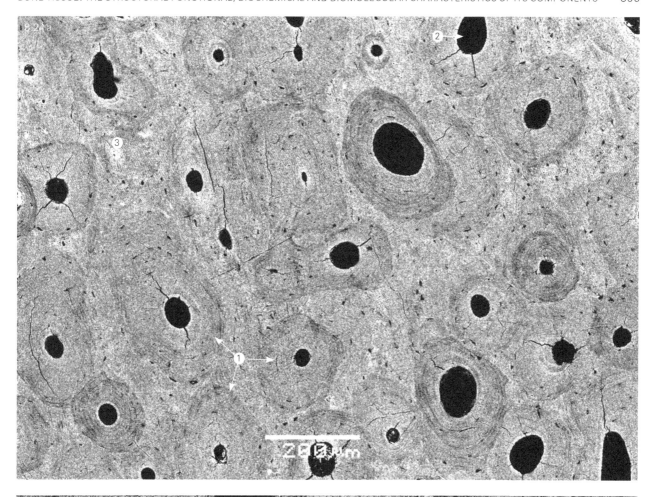

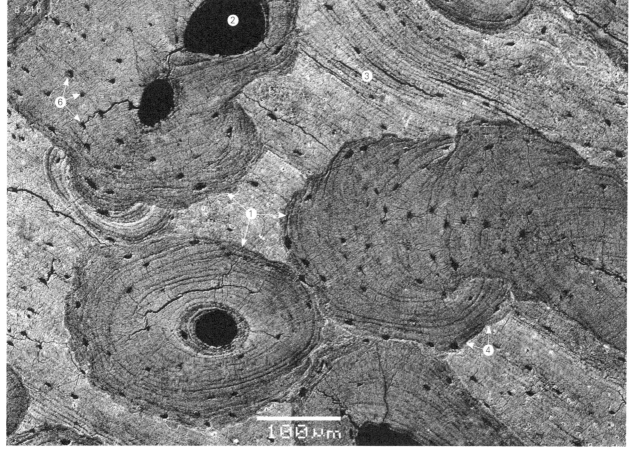

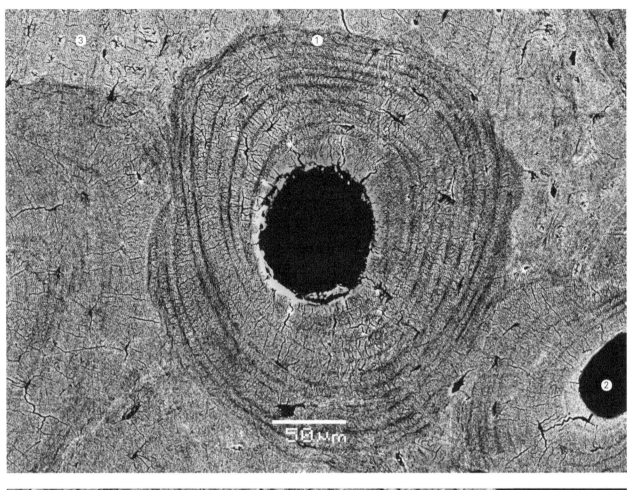

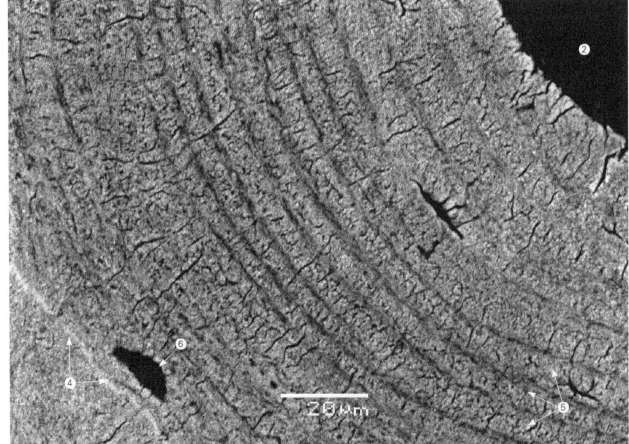

The following proteins have been found in MVs' structure:

a) cytoskeletal proteins forming an outpouching that subsequently turns into a vesicle;

b) plasma membrane proteins, including receptors and ion channel proteins;

c) structural proteins, including those that actively bind calcium (bone sialoprotein, osteonectin and osteocalcin), as well as extracellular matrix enzymes;

d) proteins involved in intracellular signaling;

e) proteins involved in the intracellular transport of secreted molecules; and

f) numerous enzymes. The factors most directly related to the mineralization process are proteins of two classes: specific proteins regulating the calcium metabolism and phosphatase-type enzymes that ensure the required concentration of phosphatic (or, more specifically, orthophosphate) ions. The functions of a number of proteins recently detected in the vesicle proteome remain obscure.

The specific proteins regulating the calcium metabolism within MVs include **annexins**, involved in the transmembrane transport of calcium ions and, at the same time, affecting membrane configuration dynamics (Gerke et al., 2005). Annexin A1 (calpactin) and annexin A11 (calcyclin) actively bind calcium ions and promote calcium's accumulation in vesicles. The accumulation of calcium ions is also promoted by other calcium-binding proteins, such as calbindin, calnexin, calpain and S100.

The accumulation of the second component of hydroxyapatite, the phosphate ion, within the vesicles involves several phosphatases, contacting the inner surface of the cytoplasmic membrane. These are: alkaline phosphatase, 5-adenosine monophosphatase, calcium adenosine triphosphatase, inorganic pyrophosphatase (PPi), and nucleoside triphosphate pyrophosphohydrolase (NTPPase). The role of the tissue-non-specific alkaline phosphatase isoenzyme is especially important: inactivation of the gene encoding this enzyme impairs mineralization. The basic substrate for these phosphatases (the source of free orthophosphate ions) is adenosine monophosphate (AMP).

The function of another phosphatase known as PHOSPHO1 is probably particularly important in accumulating the orthophosphate ions required for mineralization. This assumption is based on the extremely high selective expression of this enzyme (phosphoethanolamine/phospholine phosphatase) in vivo in those regions of the cartilaginous tissue (during endochondral ossification) and bone tissue where the matrix undergoes active mineralization. *In vitro*, PHOSPHO1 is expressed by SaOS-2 osteoblasts that deposit the mineralized matrix, but never by MG-53 osteoblasts whose cultures do not undergo mineralization (Houston et al., 2004).

Reaching the required concentration of hydroxyapatite (formed through a chemical reaction between calcium and orthophosphate ions) in the cytosol of matrix vesicles triggers the nucleation of crystals. The role of nuclei

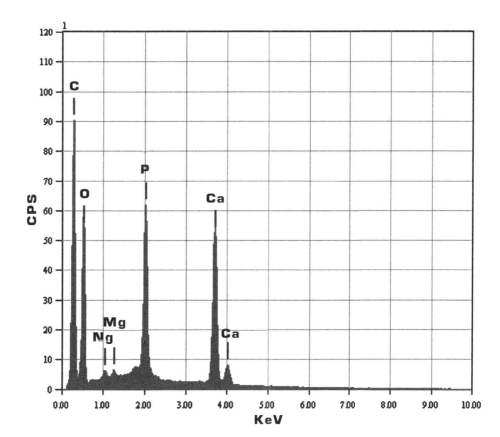

Fig. 8.25.
A diagram showing the elemental composition of the lamellar compact bone tissue.

for heterogeneous crystallization in the vesicles is played by anionic phospholipids such as phosphatidylserine. Nucleation occurs near the inner surface of the vesicle membranes consisting of phospholipids. This process is influenced by the composition of the vesicles'environment. Thus, the mineralization of bones' growth plates during endochondral ossification requires that the macromolecules of types II and X collagens contact the vesicles (Kirsch et al., 1994).

In the subsequent development of the mineralization process, matrix vesicles become unnecessary. The second stage of mineralization starts after the tiniest primary crystals of hydroxyapatite are released from the rupturing matrix vesicles, coming into contact with the tissue (interstitial) fluid and assuming the role of nuclei in the subsequent crystallization. The levels of Ca^{2+} + and PO_4^{3-} ions in the interstitial fluid are sufficient to maintain the high concentration of hydroxyapatite and ensure the subsequent appositional crystal growth. The appositional growth involves the successive joining of new hydroxyapatite molecules and their ordered deposition on the surface of primary crystals.

The matrix mineralization is actually the mineralization of collagen fibrils and fibers formed of type I collagen; moreover, hydroxyapatite crystals locate in spaces between α-chains previously filled with water (Wiesmann et al., 2005). Therefore, to be packed within these spaces, primary nanocrystals should not exceed the size of molecules with a molecular mass of 40 kDa. Hence, a mechanism to restrict the growth of crystals should exist. Such inhibition of their excessive growth is assumed to be ensured by a protein called **fetuin** (also known as α2-HS-glycoprotein), which transports primary crystals. The fetuin level in the interstitial fluid is high during the embryonal period (Price et al., 2009).

The subsequent appositional growth of hydroxyapatite nanocrystals is presumed to initially occur within the holes between the ends of collagen macromolecules in the fibrils (gap zones) (see section 3.1.1.2). However, there is not enough space within these intervals, so the process of crystal growth within the collagen fibrils spreads along the macromolecules, also covering those areas where free spaces are absent (overlap zones). This forces apart the collagen macromolecules within fibrils. Yet, the resulting space is still insufficient, so crystals growth proceeds between fibrils and, subsequently, between fibers. This process is characterized by an ordered packing of crystals, both within fibrils and fibers and between them: like collagen macromolecules, they are oriented along the length of fibers and have shifted lengthwise relative to each other. Such a spatial organization of crystalline substance ensures the optimization of the biomechanical properties of bone tissue (Jäger and Fratzl, 2005).

The specificity of the crystals' locations in relation to collagen fibrils depends on the non-uniformity of hydrophilic and hydrophobic amino-acid residues along the length of a collagen macromolecule. Crystals generally bind to the hydrophilic segments of a macromolecule, with special importance of amino-acid residues containing electrically charged side groups (glutamic or aspartic acid, lysine, arginine and histidine residues), their localization and combinations in all three α-chains of the macromolecule (Landis and Silver, 2009). It should be noted that the proposed concept is largely hypothetical in nature and, in many respects, there is no direct evidence to support it.

An alternative model of tissue biomineralization in vertebrates does not imply the involvement of matrix vesicles. It suggests that matrix vesicles are an obligatory component only in the mineralization of the provisional cartilage during endochondral ossification. According to this concept, the nucleation of crystals and their subsequent growth are not locationally separated; both stages of mineralization take place directly where the crystals are deposited, that is, within collagen fibrils or in their close environment (Glimcher, 2006).

This concept contemplates two possible ways of crystal nucleation. In the first, selected sites on the surface of type I collagen macromolecules play the role of nuclei. These sites are characterized by the chemical features and electrical charge of side groups of amino-acid residues; in other words, these are the same sites that are regarded as loci of affixion and appositional growth of already nucleated crystals. The active participation of collagen in nucleation is believed to be associated, in particular, with the phosphorylated γ-glutamic acid residues found in some samples of bone-derived type I collagen.

The primary role of collagen fibrils in crystal nucleation is supported by the results of genetic studies showing that optimum conditions for mineralization require a unique bone tissue combined osteoblastic expression of:

1) the above-mentioned tissue-nonspecific alkaline phosphatase (TNAP), and

2) type I collagen, characterized in bone tissue by a number of peculiarities in terms of its molecular and supramolecular architecture. TNAP ensures the accumulation of sufficient amounts of free orthophosphate ions around the collagen fibrils. This occurs due to the hydrolysis of pyrophosphate, which detains the crystallization of hydroxyapatite (see below). The collagen fibrils possessing a normal cross-linking system typical to bone tissue-specific type I collagen create the conditions for nucleation (Murshed et al., 2005).

Non-collagenous proteins of the bone tissue play a certain role in the formation of the collagen fibrils' properties required for mineralization, in particular biglycan and decorin, small proteoglycans of the PRELP family. Biglycan improves the conditions for crystal growth, restricting the lateral growth of collagen fibrils and thus, reserving space for crystals between them. Inactivation of the gene encoding biglycan leads to the suppression of bone tissue mineralization (Boskey et al., 2005). Decorin modulates the assembly of the collagenous matrix in a similar way, and the inactivation of *Dcn* gene encoding decorin results in the suppression of mineralization (Mochida et al., 2009). At the same time, small proteoglycans of the PRELP family can actively bind hydroxyapatite molecules, limiting their incorporation into the growing crystals.

Another known version of the alternative concept of biomineralization (mineralization without the participation of matrix vesicles) assigns the primary role in nucleation and the subsequent formation of hydroxyapatite crystals not to type I collagen itself but to non-collagenous protein components of the bone tissue matrix, which are bound to this collagen and interact with it. This is influenced by the transglutaminase-catalyzed intra- and intermolecular cross-linking of non-collagenous proteins among themselves and with collagens.

Thus, some of the phosphorylated non-collagenous proteins (in particular, those containing phosphorylated serine residues) are considered very probable candidates for the role of nuclei for the heterogeneous nucleation of hydroxyapatite crystals. Such activity is established in phosphoseryl-rich phosphophoryn (George & Hao, 2005). In addition, phosphorylated proteins of the matrix promote the stabilization of mineral crystals binding to collagen fibrils.

A crystallization nucleator function has also been found in bone sialoprotein II (BSPII), which acts jointly with the bone acidic glycoprotein-75 (BAG-75). BAG-75 molecules capable of self-association form spherical structures at a very early stage of the extracellular matrix formation in mineralizing cultures of MC3T3-E1 osteoblasts. These structures, referred to as primary foci of biomineralization (biomineralization foci, BMF), are enclosed spaces; this is viewed as a functional similarity between BMFs and matrix vesicles. Bone sialoprotein II and alkaline phosphatase accumulate within BMFs. Upon introducing a substrate for phosphatase into the culture (an organic source of orthophosphate ions), sialoprotein II linked to BAG-75 binds a considerable amount of calcium ions inside the BMFs, followed by the formation of primary nanocrystals of hydroxyapatite (Midura et al., 2004). BMFs consisting of BAG-75 and sialoprotein II have been found in vivo in the course of intramembranous ossification (Gorski et al., 2004).

Some non-collagenous proteins containing considerable amounts of acidic amino-acid residues (aspartate, glutamate, and carboxyglutamate) have the opposite (suppressing) effect on the mineralization process, especially when grouped into clusters. They bind hydroxyapatite molecules, thereby interfering with their ability to attach onto the growing crystals. This effect is exerted by bone Gla-protein (osteocalcin) and matrix Gla-protein. A similar mineralization-detaining effect is shown by osteopontin (BSP I). The blood serum proteins present in the interstitial fluid of the matrix also interfere with mineralization.

Both concepts of mineralization do not exclude, but rather supplement each other. New hydroxyapatite nanocrystals, forming within collagen fibrils and between them through the action of the second nucleation mechanism,

can attach to those entering the collagen fibrils from matrix vesicles. The functions of both nucleation mechanisms thus appear synergistic.

Not much time is required for the completion of mineralization: it occurs in a matter of several hours from the onset of crystallization.

Some artificial materials may become involved in the mineralization process. In the in vivo implantation of ceramics (or synthetic polymers) containing the Si-OH, Ti-OH, Zr-OH, Nb-OH, and Ta-OH functional groups into the bone tissue, a layer of hydroxyapatite crystals is deposited on the implant surface, allowing a direct (without an intermediate layer of a granulation-fibrous tissue) bond between these materials and the surrounding bone tissue. In in vitro studies, the formation of hydroxyapatite crystals on the surface of the same materials occurs when they are placed in a cell-free fluid that is similar in composition to blood plasma, but without the proteins. Hence, these materials not only ensure the growth of crystals, but may also serve as heterogeneous nuclei in crystal nucleation. This data is of great importance in the development of artificial bone tissue substitutes (Kokubo, 2005).

Of the amorphous phosphate compounds that, as previously mentioned, are found in trace amounts in the bone tissue, inorganic pyrophosphate (PPi) containing two phosphate residues is of special importance. (Terkeltaub, 2001).

The phosphate ions combining to form pyrophosphate are released from nucleoside triphosphates. This occurs in osteoblasts under the effect of the enzyme phosphodiesterase 1 (full name: nucleotide pyrophosphatase phosphodiesterase 1 or NPP-1; alternative name: plasma cell membrane glycoprotein-1 or PC 1). Phosphate ions are excreted into the extracellular matrix via channels formed by another transmembrane glycoprotein, ANK. Impairment in the expression of each of these proteins (through the inactivation of their respective genes), especially with the simultaneous inactivation of the osteopontin gene, results in hypermineralization. Hypermineralization is also caused by the inactivation of *Akp2* gene encoding alkaline phosphatase (TNAP), the above-mentioned enzyme catalyzing the hydrolysis of excess PPi (Harmey et al., 2004). The maintenance of an optimum PPi level in tissues is ensured by a coordinated interaction of a number of systemic and local regulatory factors. The formation of PPi occurs in the extracellular matrix. For this purpose, two free ions of inorganic phosphate (Pi) are spent for each PPi molecule and, therefore, cannot be subsequently used for the growth of hydroxyapatite crystals; the growth of crystals is thereby inhibited. Inorganic pyrophosphate thus proves to be antagonistic to factors that stimulate the mineralization.

This antagonistic effect of pyrophosphate is especially distinct in tissues that do not normally undergo mineralization, such as articular cartilages and tendons. PPi prevents mineralization in these tissues, its deficiency leading to such abnormalities as the calcification of articular cartilages in osteoarthrosis, or of longitudinal ligament of the spine in ankylosing spondylitis (Terkeltaub, 2001).

The inhibiting (competitive) effect of inorganic pyrophosphate on mineralization acts directly on the process of formation and especially the growth of hydroxyapatite crystals. However, as has been shown, pyrophosphate affects already-formed hydroxyapatite crystals in an opposite manner, reducing the solubility and thus increasing the stability of crystals.

This effect of pyrophosphate has substantiated the use of synthetic analogs of pyrophosphate, bisphosphonates (often also referred to as diphosphonates) as pharmacological agents for the prevention or delay of the abnormally enhanced destruction of the bone tissue mineral component. Such enhanced destruction occurs in osteoporosis of various geneses. It has been subsequently established that the therapeutic effect of bisphosphonates in osteoporosis is due not only to the physicochemical mechanisms of their interaction with crystalline hydroxyapatite, but also to their suppressing influence on the functional state and resorptive activity of osteoclasts (Fleisch, 2002).

8.3.2.4. Structuring of bone minerals in reparative bone regeneration

The morphological dynamics of bone tissue mineralization are seen clearly enough in the course of reparative bone regeneration. After the formation of primary collagen fibrils and fibers, areas with an elevated concentration of calcium ions (detected by means of topographic TEM-elemental microanalysis via electron energy-loss spectrometry) arise in the intercellular matrix (Omelyanenko et al., 1995). Further on, these areas extend so that the bulk of the neoformed fibrous structures is found in regions with an increased concentration of calcium and phosphate ions. A routine TEM study (without a spectrometer) does not detect a local increase in calcium ions.

The smallest mineral structures detected by TEM as mineralization loci are aggregates (primary aggregates), 7 to 10 nm in size and consisting of calcium phosphate pellets (nanocrystals) ranging 3 to 5 nm in size. These aggregates are combined into larger (secondary) aggregates, the size of which may reach several microns. Primary aggregates may be evenly distributed within secondary ones or form chains that sometimes look like needle-like crystals in a TEM image (*Fig. 8.26*). The formation of mineral aggregates has a multifocal nature, but it does not occur per saltum. Therefore, at the initial stages of mineralization, various-sized mineral aggregates can be found in the mineralization zones. They usually appear close to the actively synthesizing primary bone cells (osteoblasts), which indicates their role in the mineralization process (*Fig. 8.27*). A loose distribution of fibrous structures (collagen fibrils) is observed at the sites of beginning mineralization. The mineralization subse-

quently spreads to the interfibrillar spaces, where collagen fibrils are also distributed relatively loosely. The size, density and number of mineral aggregates around primary osteoblasts and, subsequently, around primary collagen fibers (primary bone rods), gradually increase. This growth proceeds until they merge with the neighboring aggregates and a more extensive mineral matrix (mineral complex) is formed around both cells and fibers. The dynamics of this process is shown in *Fig. 8.27*. Collagen fibers (round-shaped on cross-sections) are mineralized basically at the periphery. Some fibers are mineralized to a greater degree; however, unmineralized areas also occur within them. Fuller mineralization of the primary (reticulofibrous) bone tissue, identical to a mature bone tissue, does not occur because of the short-lived existence of primary fibrous and cell structures of the reparative bone "regenerates".

The increase in their concentration around and within the fibrous collagenous structures can be explained by their structural arrangement and biochemical composition, one peculiarity of which is the presence of the BMP family, sialoprotein II (BSPII), glycoprotein 75 (BAG-75) and other non-collagenous components of collagen fibrils defining their affinity to minerals (see section 8.3.1.1.1). Another probable factor of the local increase in the concentration of calcium salts initiating crystal formation may be fluid movement in these sites during the secretion of various intercellular matrix components by cells (osteoblasts). The remodeling of primary reparative bone "regenerates" (fibrous structures and cell elements) is accompanied by their resorption. During subsequent bone formation, the mineralization process recurs. In a mature tissue-specific bone "regenerate", hydroxyapatite nanocrystals are comprised by the three above-mentioned shapes, their aggregates characterized by a more pronounced integration with the organic (basically collagenous) bone matrix and, in many respects, repeating the structure of the collagenous fibrous base of the bone matrix and filling its major part.

The appearance of primary nanocrystals, in association with any certain locations of collagen fibrils, such as gap zones of collagenous microfibrils, should be considered hypothetical since the TEM resolution limit does not permit visualizing it. Collagen fibrils may be tightly "filled" with fine pellets, while retaining their periodic pattern, i.e. the presence of a recurrent structure consisting of dark (more electron-dense) and light (rarefied) regions (*Fig. 8.20*). This indicates that the deposition of hydroxyapatite, i.e. the formation of the mineral "skeleton" of a fibril is, to a certain degree, directed by fibrils' own molecular organization. This process also does not proceed per saltum.

a

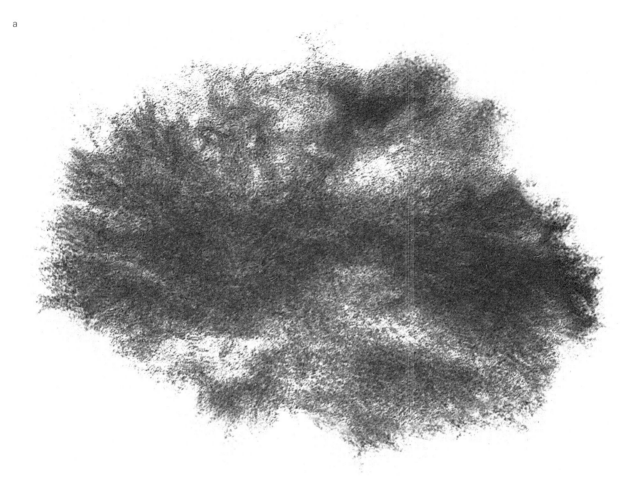

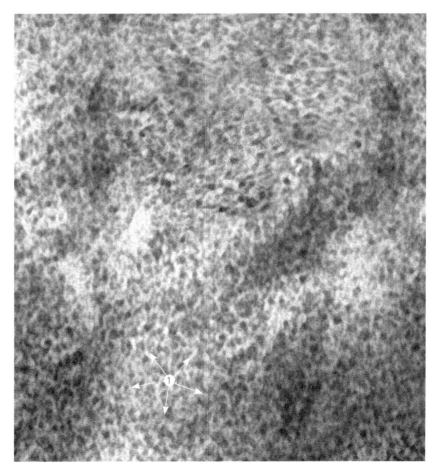

Fig. 8.26.
A secondary mineral aggregate
in a regenerating bone.
Primary mineral aggregates (1).
TEM-micrograph.
a – x 140,000,
b – x 250,000,281.

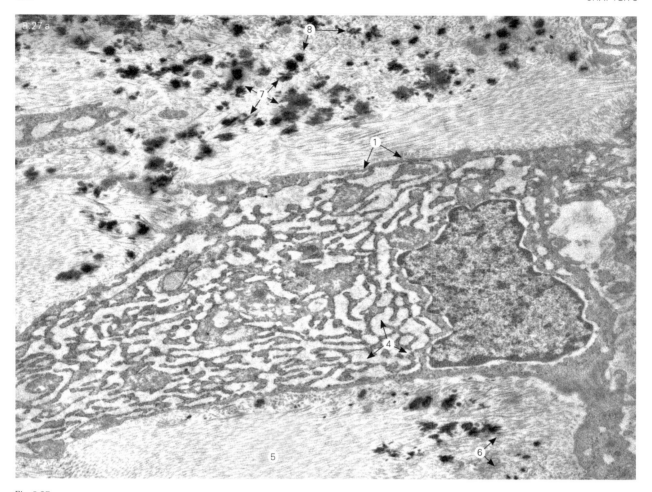

Fig. 8.27.
Fragments of regenerating
bone at different stages
(maturity) of the intercellular
matrix mineralization.
Primary osteoblast (1).
Primary osteocyte (2).
Nucleus (3). GER (4).
Collagen fibers (5). Collagen
fibrils not bundled into fibers (6).
Mineral aggregates (7).
Mineral complexes (8).
Non-mineralized areas
of collagen fibers (9).
TEM-micrograph. Ultrathin
sections contrasted with uranyl
acetate and lead citrate.
a – beginning of the intercellular
matrix mineralization near a
primary osteoblast. Separately
located mineral aggregates.
b – increased number of small
and large mineral aggregates.
Merging of some aggregates.
c – "loose" mineral matrix
(mineral complex) forming
around a primary osteoblast.
d – "dense" mineral matrix
(mineral complex) formed
around a primary osteoblast
(osteocyte).
e – mineral aggregates in interfiber spaces, around collagen
fibers (primary bone rods).
f – fragment of a mineralized
primary bone rod.
a, b, c, d – x 10,000,
e – x 5,000, f – x 20,000.

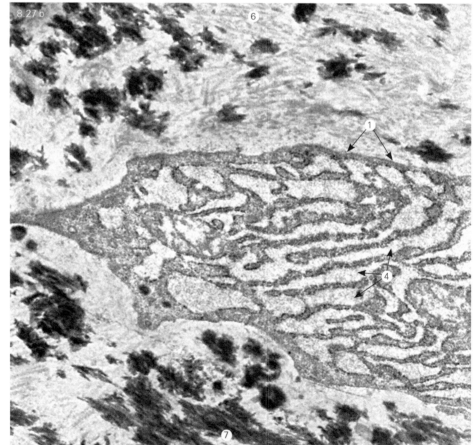

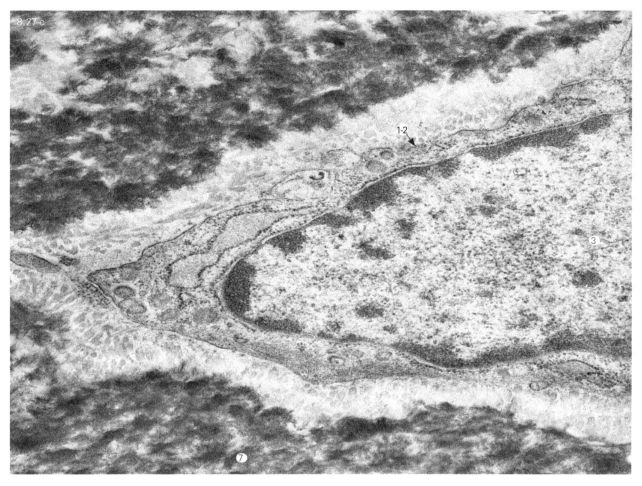

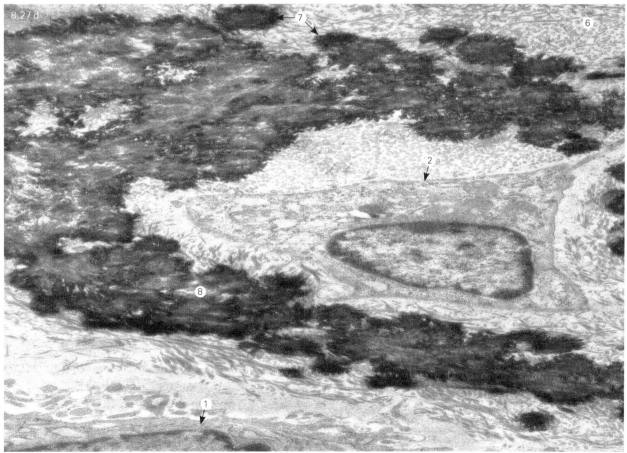

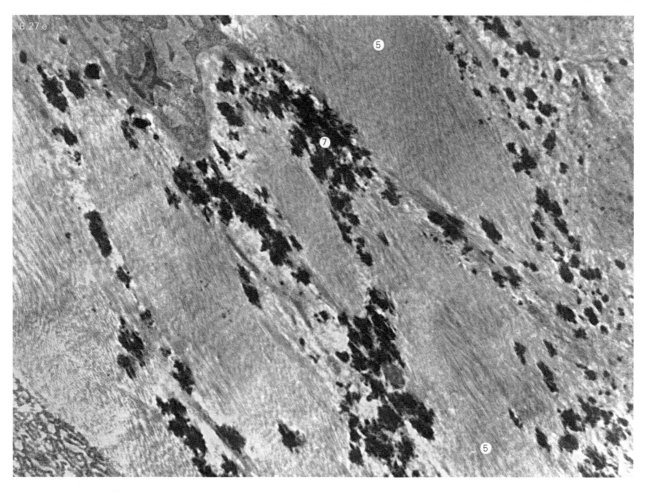

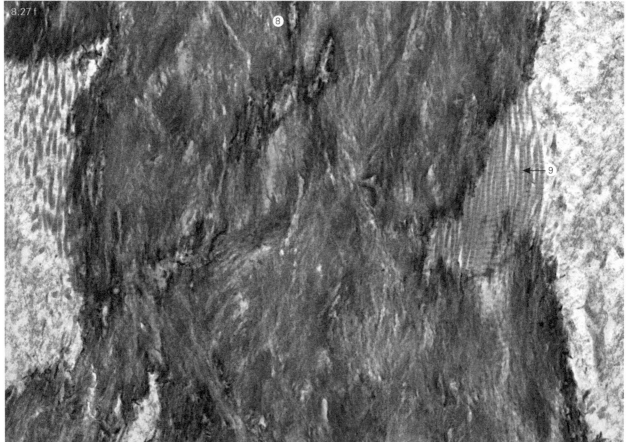

8.3.2.5. Demineralization of bone matrix *in vitro* and subsequent structuring (crystallization) of bone minerals dissolved on its surface

Demineralization of the bone matrix using hydrochloric and other acids is widely known and employed in scientific studies of bone tissue, as well as in the production of demineralized or partially demineralized bone matrix (DBM, PDBM) for use in traumatology and orthopedics, as well as in stomatology as dental implants, in gelatin production in the food industry, etc. The demineralization process consists of the dissolution of mineral salts through the chemical reactions discussed below (*Fig. 8.28*). With the constant replacement of hydrochloric acid, the demineralization proceeds continuously up to full dissolution of the bone mineral and its release from the bone matrix into the solution.

The structural specificity of bone tissue (the presence of a great number of interconnecting canals of various diameters, and internal spaces) affects the rate and uniformity of demineralization, which, in turn, influences the properties of DBMs implanted in bone defects. The contact between a demineralizing (most commonly, hydrochloric) acid and the outer surfaces of bone tissue fragments leads to the fairly rapid dissolution of the calcium-phosphate crystals contained therein. However, with advancing of the demineralization front deeper inside the bone sample, this process slows down due to the less favorable conditions for the quick exchange of the acid (saturated with, and partially neutralized by the calcium-phosphate dissolved therein) through the increasing DBM layer. Therefore, after the full completion of the demineralization of the collagen matrix from DBM, its different areas (peripheric or deeper) will have been exposed to hydrochloric acid for varied lengths of time and hence, will be hydrolyzed to a different degree depending on the thickness of DBM. This should be borne in mind in the production of DBM implants. At the same time, a slower demineralization also proceeds from within the bone sample since the acid penetrates the sample via numerous bone canals and spaces.

Using a limited amount of hydrochloric acid or its neutralization through interaction with minerals of the bone matrix leads to the oversaturation of the solution surrounding the bone sample, causing the demineralization process to slow down or stop. The resultant non-equilibrium state leads to the crystallization of the released mineral salts into a multi-level hierarchical mineral structure on the surface of the demineralized bone matrix. These structures have a form of radial monomineral aggregates (spherulites). The terms have been borrowed from mineralogy (Betekhtin, 2008). The size of spherulites reaches 500 µm (*Fig. 8.29*). The central part (nucleus) of a spherulite has a granular structure. Radial rays in the form of prismatic-shaped crystals grow away from the nucleus (*Fig. 8.29 a, b*). Their shapes somewhat vary in length, the number and sizes of planes (3–5), and the peak shape (pointed, flat, pyramidal, or occasionally cylindrical). The length and width of radial crystals vary from 3–5 to 120 µm and from 3–5 to 50 µm, respectively (*Fig. 8.29 c, d*). The structure of these crystal aggregates is discrete and consists of bundles (40–200 nm in equivalent diameter) of needle-like- or rod-like aggregates, which are 5–10 nm thick and 40 to 100 nm long (*Fig. 8.29 e, f, g, h*). These bundles are anisotropic formations since the bulk of the aggregates of which they are formed is oriented parallel to each other and perpendicular to the surface of the radial crystal aggregate. Bundles may be in contact with each other or be separated by spaces comparable to their own size. Needle-like crystal aggregates, in their turn, are chains of granules or grains 5–10 nm in diameter (*Fig. 8.29 g, h*). If the latter are to be considered the smallest (primary) morphological structures (as detected by SEM), then the recrystallized mineral has a five-level organization:

Level 1 – primary nanocrystals (granules sized 5–10 nm);

Level 2 – secondary needle-like nanocrystals (primary mineral aggregates; monochains of granules);

Level 3 – bundles of needle-like nanocrystals (secondary mineral aggregates);

Level 4 – radial crystals (tertiary crystal aggregates);

Level 5 – crystalline spherulites (quaternary crystal aggregates).

On the lateral surfaces of the radial crystals of spherulites, there are numerous "embryos" or already-formed lateral processes perpendicular to radial crystals. These processes exhibit the same crystalline structure (*Fig. 8.30*).

The above-stated data suggests that the formation of granules, needle-like aggregates and their bundles does

Fig. 8.28.
Chemical equations for calcium phosphate and carbonate reactions occurring during the demineralization of bone tissue.

1. $Ca_3(PO4)_2 + 4HCL = Ca(H2PO_4)_2 + 2CaCL_2$

2. $Ca_3(PO_4)_2 + 6HCL = 2H_3PO_4 + 3CaCL_2$

3. $Ca_3(PO4)_2 + 4H_3PO_4 = 3Ca(H2PO_4)_2$

4. $CaCO_3 + 2HCL = CaCL_2 + H_2O + CO_2$

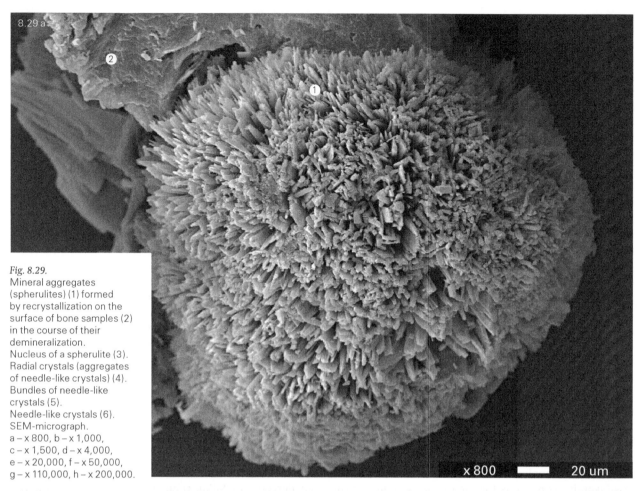

8.29 a

Fig. 8.29.
Mineral aggregates
(spherulites) (1) formed
by recrystallization on the
surface of bone samples (2)
in the course of their
demineralization.
Nucleus of a spherulite (3).
Radial crystals (aggregates
of needle-like crystals) (4).
Bundles of needle-like
crystals (5).
Needle-like crystals (6).
SEM-micrograph.
a – x 800, b – x 1,000,
c – x 1,500, d – x 4,000,
e – x 20,000, f – x 50,000,
g – x 110,000, h – x 200,000.

x 800   20 um

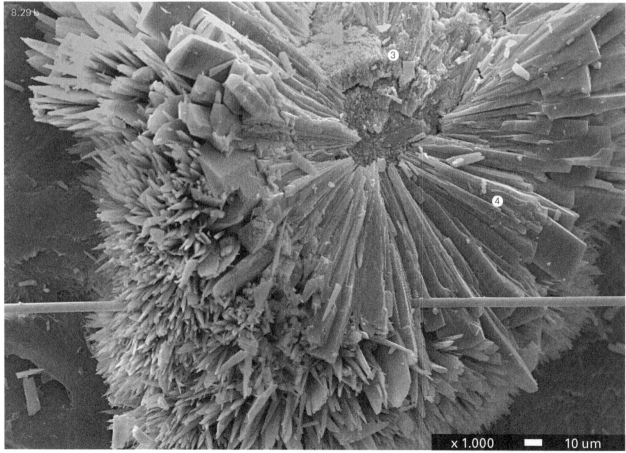

8.29 b

x 1.000   10 um

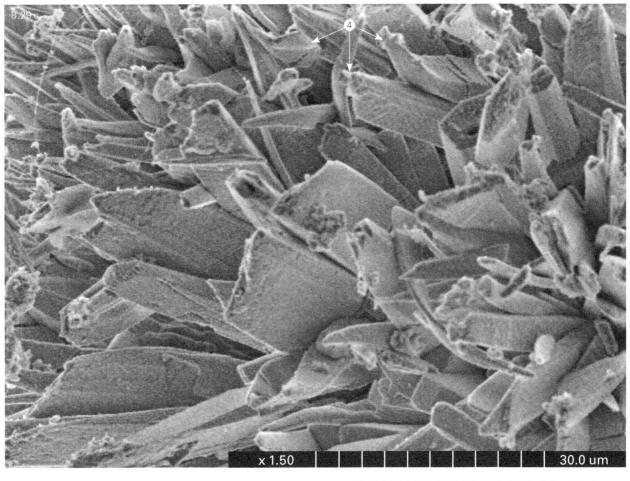

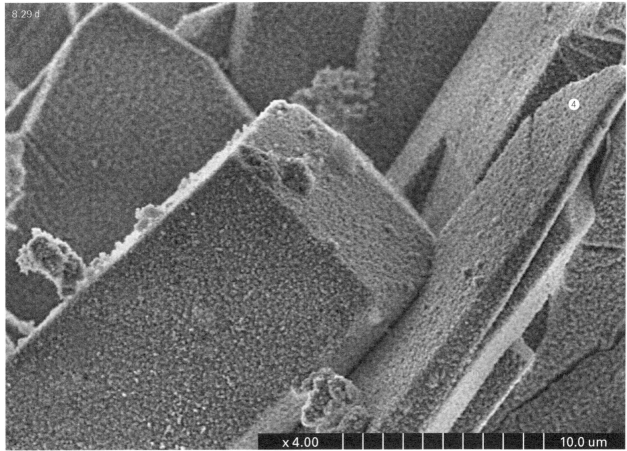

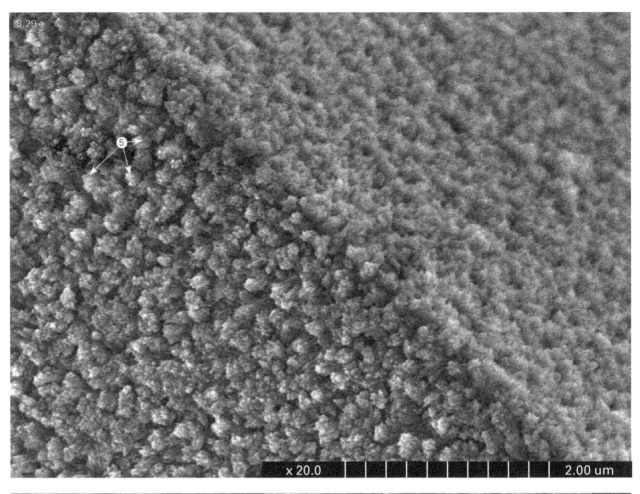

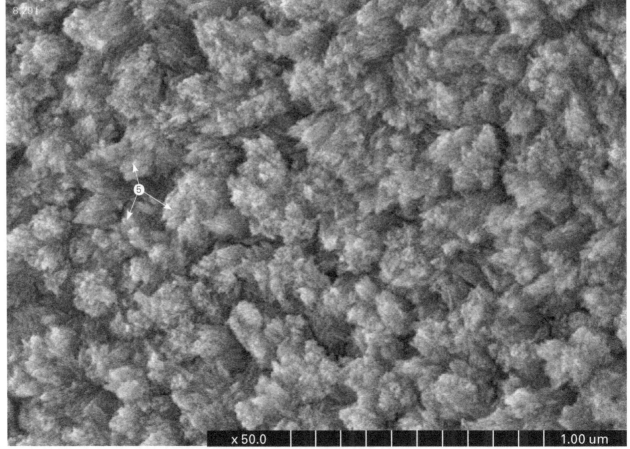

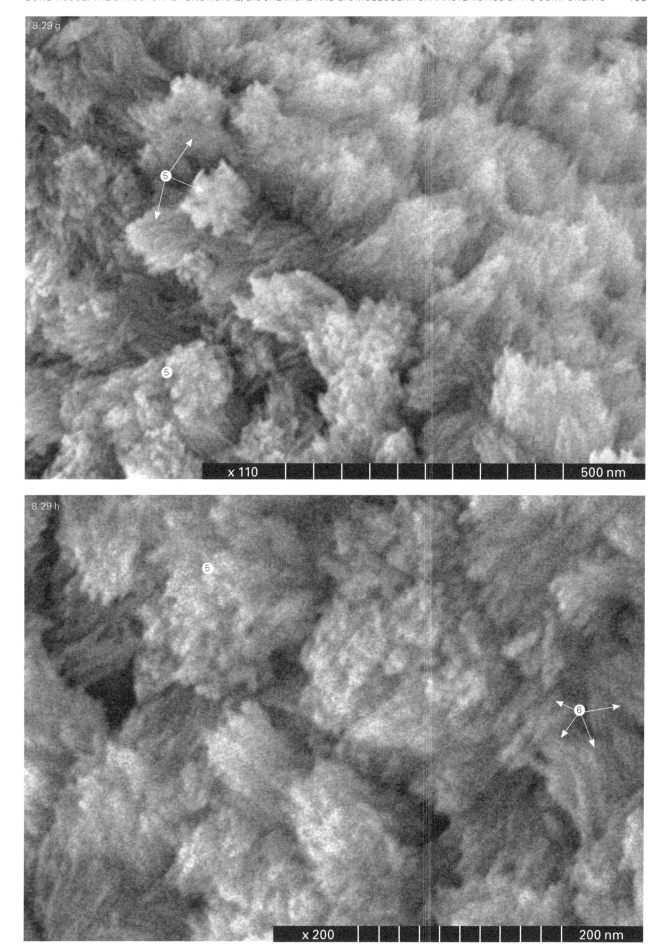

not require the presence of collagen structures. The pre-requisite for crystal formation is the oversaturation of the solution with calcium, phosphorus, magnesium, carbonate and other ions, as well as a certain temperature (room temperature in this instance). Apparently, the same condition is also required for the mineralization of fibrous (collagen) structures during bone tissue formation. Fibrous structures (collagen fibrils or, more specifically, collagen molecules present in their structure) that presumably have an affinity to the above-mentioned minerals, are involved (along with other mechanisms) in the mechanism of their attraction to the site of their formation and the subsequent tissue-specific structurization, i.e. forming a single mineral matrix as part of the intercellular bone matrix.

8.3.2.6. Structure of coral skeleton

The possibility of the formation of multi-level mineral aggregates without a fibrous matrix is illustrated by the formation of a coral skeleton (corallite) in certain kinds of sea polyps. In this instance, the primary units of the structured mineral (basically, calcium carbonate), as detected by SEM, are elongated oval-shaped crystals whose equivalent diameter varies from 50–500 nm. Their ends exhibit a rounded or conical shape. They form pronounced anisotropic structures in the form of bundles (a secondary structure with an equivalent diameter of 5–20 μm), containing several thousands of primary crystals. The latter are packed tightly enough against each other, with only narrow spaces left between them. The bundles form groups with the same orientation. The latter, together with the less structured mineral aggregates, form the third level of the mineral organization and, subsequently, the fourth and the fifth. All above-listed structural organization levels for the coral mineral are shown in *Fig. 8.31,* presenting a series of SEM-micrographs from the nanolevel through the ultra-micro-, micro- and macrolevels.

8.3.2.7. Structure of sea-shell mineral

Sea shells have a similar pattern of mineral structures in the nano- and ultra-micro level; aragonite, one of calcite forms ($CaCO_3$), comprises their base. Rectangular or oval elongated crystals detected by SEM (*Fig. 8.32 a, b*) are a primary morphological unit of its structure. A thickness of these crystals ranges from 100–500 nm, at the same time the same fluctuations in thickness can be observed along the entire length of one crystal. A surface of crystals can be smooth or they can have an imbricate relief. The crystals are arranged in parallel in the aforementioned levels i.e. their superstructure is evidently anisotropic. The adjacent crystals contact closely by their side surfaces or fuse with each other forming thin bridges. Sometimes the crystals can wedge between adjacent crystals. In the micro-level parallel-oriented crystals are presented by flattened aggregates with a thickness of

about 5–10 μm, which interchange with other (adjacent) flattened aggregates which are tangentially oriented (*Fig. 8.32 c, e*). They closely adjoin to each other without a distinct gap. This aggregate complex being a unity is penetrated by canals with a diameter of 7–10 μm. A canal bed is formed by rod-like crystals with a diameter of 100–200 nm which are located in parallel and bound into complexes (*Fig. 8.32 d*).

8.3.2.8. Role of mineral component in bone biomechanical properties

Natural biomaterials such as bone, tooth, nacre, coral, etc. containing proteins and minerals are high-strength nanocomposites.

Stiffness and hardness are the most important properties for the support and protection function of bone-like biocomposites. This is apparently ensured both by their structure (protein and mineral) and by the nature of their interactions within the structural arrangement of endo- and exoskeletons.

Despite the fact that the protein component is softer than the mineral approximately by a factor of 10^3 (Ji & Gao, 2004), biocomposites' stiffness is not significantly decreased through the presence of protein. Actually, Young's modulus of biocomposites approaches the upper limit (0.45) defined by the Voigt model. For mineral-protein hybrid systems, the range between the upper (Voigt model) and lower (0.002 for bone, as defined by the Reuss model) limits of stiffness may be very large due to the considerable difference in stiffness between mineral and protein. Protein, as the organic component of biomaterials, plays an essential role in achieving and maintaining the high strength of mineralized tissues. The protein matrix apparently acts to protect the mineral structures from the peak stresses created by external influences by dissipating them within the composites.

The fact that the endoskeleton in mammals contains much more protein than in sea-shells is significant. Thus, the volume fraction of protein accounts for approximately 50% in bone (Jäger and Fratzl, 2000) and only 5% in nacre (Jackson et al., 1988). This difference may be caused by the fact that the animal endoskeleton is exposed to more severe dynamic deformations during its lifetime than that of seashells, for instance. In addition, protein can help dissipate the dynamic fracture energy more effectively due to its viscoelastic properties (Lakes, 2001; Sasaki et al., 1993) and hierarchical structural organization (Smith, et al., 1999; Thompson, et al., 2001). The latter is ideally suited for the dispersion and dissipation of fracture energy (Smith et al., 1999). Acting as a template for the formation of crystallization centers and the deposition of mineral crystals in the course of mineralization, the protein matrix organizes the size and assembly of mineral crystals at several levels of mineralization.

From the mechanical point of view, proteins endow biocomposites with special characteristics that distinguish them from conventional composites, such as Young' modulus ratio between the hard and soft phases, as well as well-developed microstructures and effective viscoelastic properties that help in dissipating the fracture energy within the biocomposite under dynamic loads (Ji & Gao, 2004).

The mechanism of high strength of mineralized biocomposites is being explained from various points of view, including their multi-level hierarchical macro- and microstructures (Menig et al., 2000, 2001; Kamat et al., 2000; Kessler et al., 1996), the mechanical properties of proteins in terms of dissipating fracture energy (Smith et al., 1999), protein-mineral interface roughness (Wang et al., 2001), and the reduction of stress concentration at cracks (Okumura and de Gennes, 2001). The organized arrangement of mineral platelets makes biocomposites anisotropic to environmental conditions during their lifetime. Bone can reach an anisotropic ratio of 1.7–2.1 in two normal directions (Hasegawa et al., 1994; Turner and Burr, 1997; Turner et al., 1995; Pidaparti et al., 1996).

At the same time, not enough attention is paid to the relationship between strength mechanisms and other mechanical properties and the nanostructural organization of mineralized biocomposites. It is obvious that the properties of the latter depend on their structural arrangement at all levels of hierarchy (Ji & Gao, 2004).

Within the bone tissue, five levels of the collagen fiber structures' architecture have been distinguished (Omelyanenko, 2005), as well as (in a certain conformity with the latter) four levels of mineral structures organization (see section 8.3.2.2).

At a molecular level, calcium ions cross-link negatively charged peptides, forming relatively stable bonds with a strength up to 30% of the covalent bonds of the peptide backbone. These protective bonds bind functional groups along different segments of protein and along the protein-mineral interface, increasing the effective stress in protein and creating a high threshold for fracture energy (Thompson et al., 2001).

Another mechanism for fracture energy dissipation may be the viscoelastic properties of the protein (collagen) forming the organic basis of the bone tissue.

At the level of individual mineralized collagen fibrils, their mechanical properties will probably depend on the exact arrangement of mineral crystals within the fibrils (Weiner and Wagner, 1998; Rho et al., 1998; Jäger and Fratzl, 2000; Landis, et al., 1993; Landis, 1995; Landis and Hodgens, 1996). It should be kept in mind that the distribution of various-shaped nanocrystals is irregular along fibrils' length.

The packing (distribution) of mineral within the interfibrillar and interfiber spaces is also irregular, having a systemic patterned nature in some locations while, in others, varying according to the topography and the tissular peculiarities of the structure. Apparently, such mineral distribution in the bone tissue contributes to its biomechanical properties, enabling the collagen fibrils

to shift in relation to each other within fibers and bone lamellae, as well as the latter to shift in relation to each other.

The nanometric size of the mineral crystals in the mineralized biocomposites endows them with optimum fracture strength and maximum crack resistance (Gao et al., 2003).

8.4. INTERSTITIAL SPACE OF BONE TISSUE

8.4.1. Morphological characteristics of bone canals

The complex of collagen structures and mineralized ground substance represents the main functional unit of compact bone tissue, which has a support function and therefore, requires constant renewal. Accessing nutrients and the removal of metabolic products in bones take place through interstitial spaces, which represent a widely developed network of interconnected channels. Despite being parts of an integrated system, they differ in shape, size, direction and destination. Each group of channels has a specific name in the literature: central (Haversian) canals (HC); Volkmann's (perforating) (VC) canals; interconnecting, radial canals (IC) (anastomoses); canaliculi; lacunae (cellular and noncellular); interstructural (interfibrillar and intercrystalline) spaces (Bogonatov & Gonchar-Zaikin, 1976; Omelyanenko & Butyrin, 1990).

The central (Haversian) canals are located in the center of the osteon – bone's structural unit (*Fig. 8.14, 8.15, 8.17*). The walls of the canals consist of bony plates (lamellae). The surface relief is formed by mineralized collagen fibrils, which are part of the bony plates.

The system of bone canals is most clearly revealed by microcorrosion casts. To this end, dehydrated bone samples are impregnated with epoxy resins (usually methacrylate or ethacryl), which penetrate even small pore spaces well. Following the polymerization of the epoxy resin, the mineral part of the bone is removed with acid (usually hydrochloric acid), and the organic part is removed with sodium hypochlorite. The remaining polymer replica – microcorrosion cast – is studied by SEM.

The central canals typically run along the long axis of the bone, although some of them have tangential and even transverse orientation. They branch out, but their orientation does not change significantly after the branching (*Fig. 8.33*). The central canals are 30–150 mm in diameter. All of the other types of channels listed above open into their lumen. Volkmann's canals run transversely from the periosteal bone surface to its long axis and open into the central canals. Their diameters are somewhat smaller – 30–60 µm. The Haversian canals communicate with the outer surface of the bone or, more precisely, with the bone environment through these canals. The interconnecting canals (anastomoses) between the central canals exhibit the same size and orientation (Omelyanenko & Butyrin, 1990).

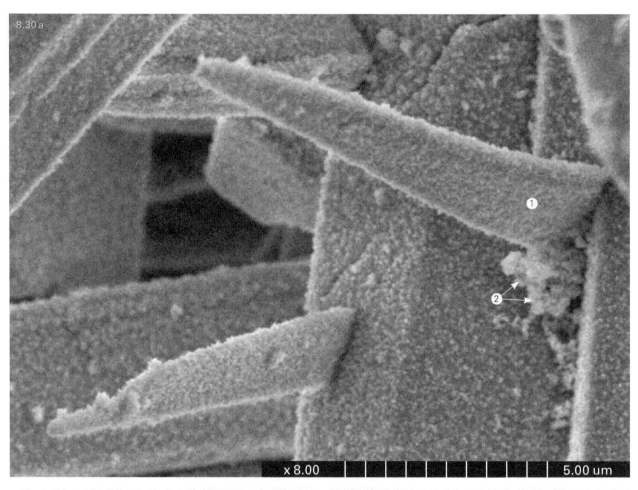

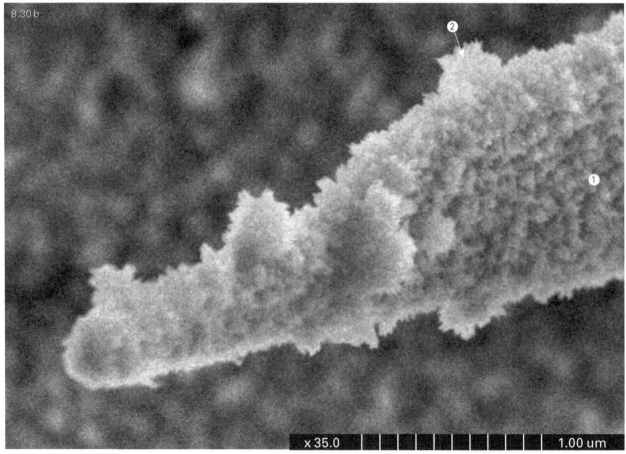

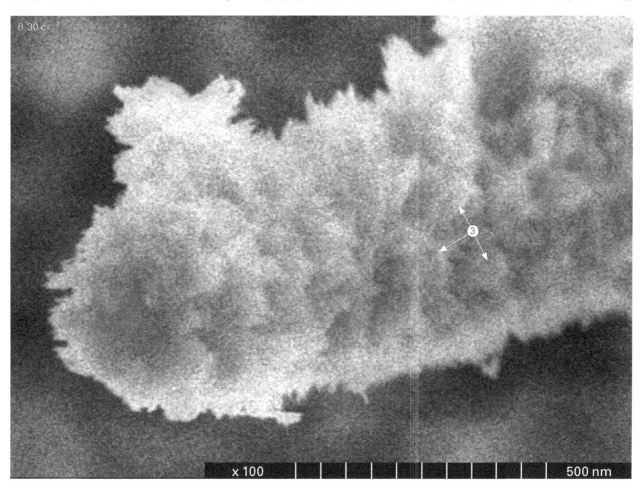

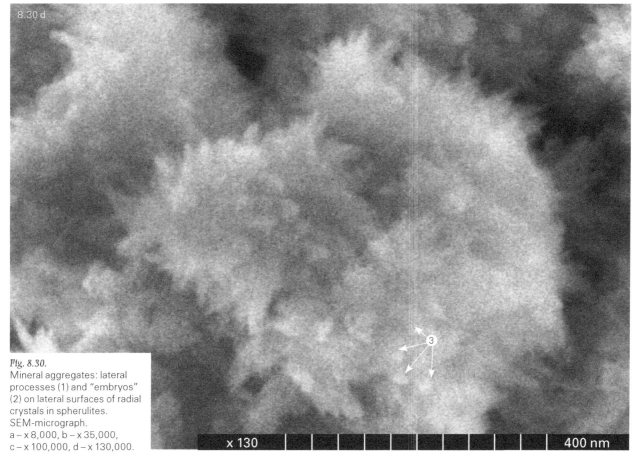

Fig. 8.30.
Mineral aggregates: lateral processes (1) and "embryos" (2) on lateral surfaces of radial crystals in spherulites. SEM-micrograph.
a – x 8,000, b – x 35,000,
c – x 100,000, d – x 130,000.

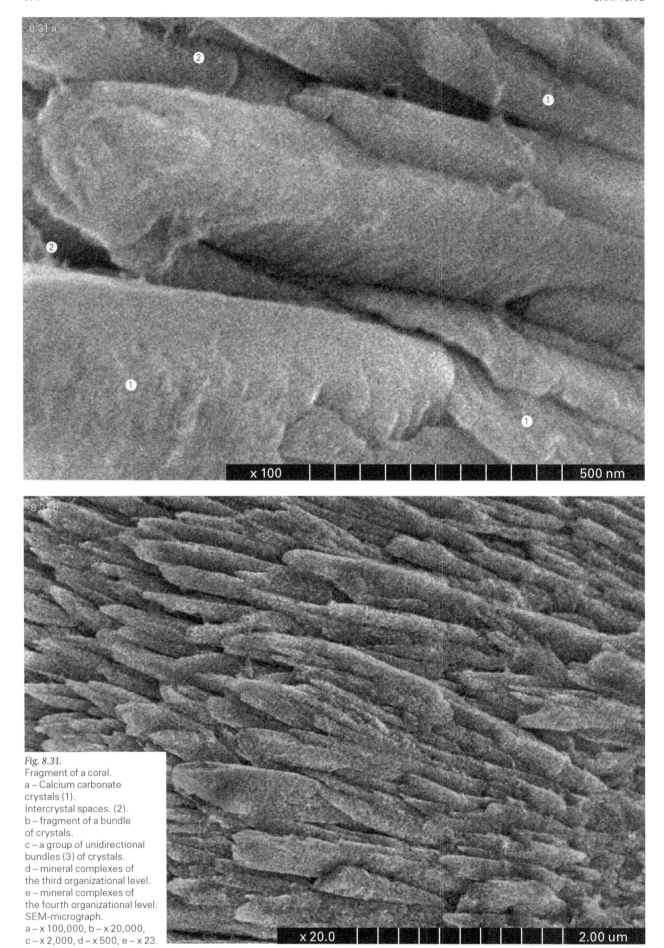

Fig. 8.31.
Fragment of a coral.
a – Calcium carbonate
crystals (1).
Intercrystal spaces. (2).
b – fragment of a bundle
of crystals.
c – a group of unidirectional
bundles (3) of crystals.
d – mineral complexes of
the third organizational level.
e – mineral complexes of
the fourth organizational level.
SEM-micrograph.
a – x 100,000, b – x 20,000,
c – x 2,000, d – x 500, e – x 23.

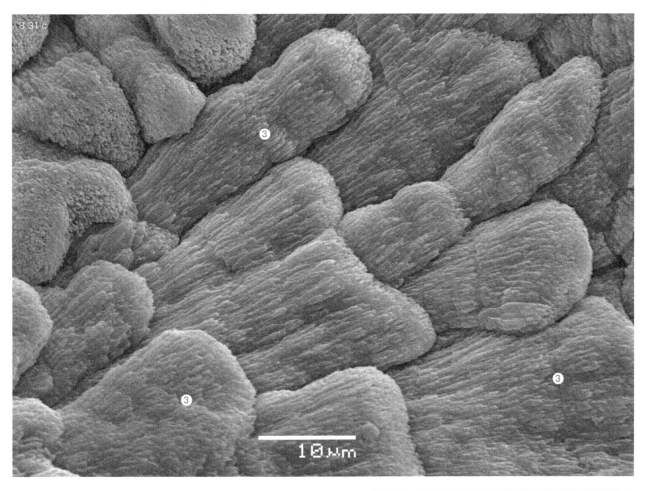

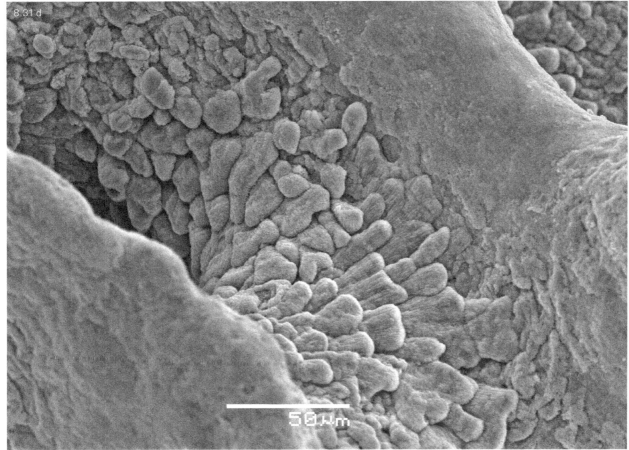

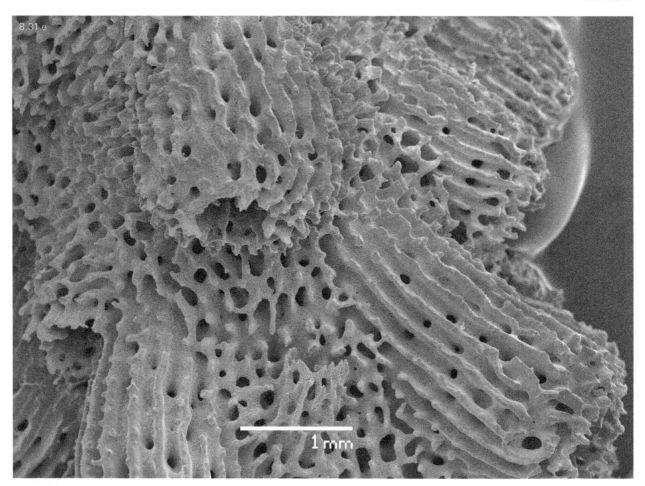

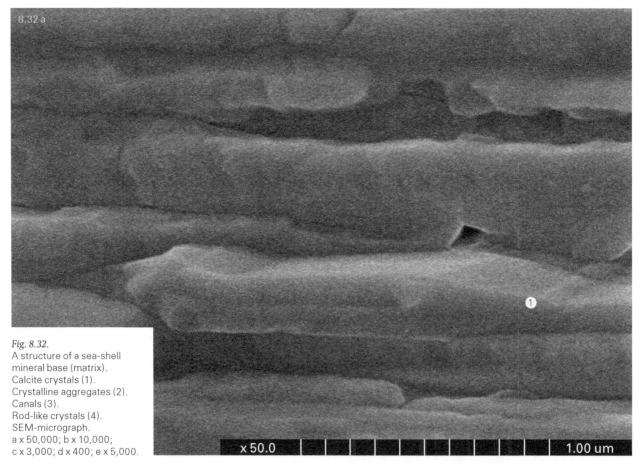

Fig. 8.32.
A structure of a sea-shell mineral base (matrix).
Calcite crystals (1).
Crystalline aggregates (2).
Canals (3).
Rod-like crystals (4).
SEM-micrograph.
a x 50,000; b x 10,000;
c x 3,000; d x 400; e x 5,000.

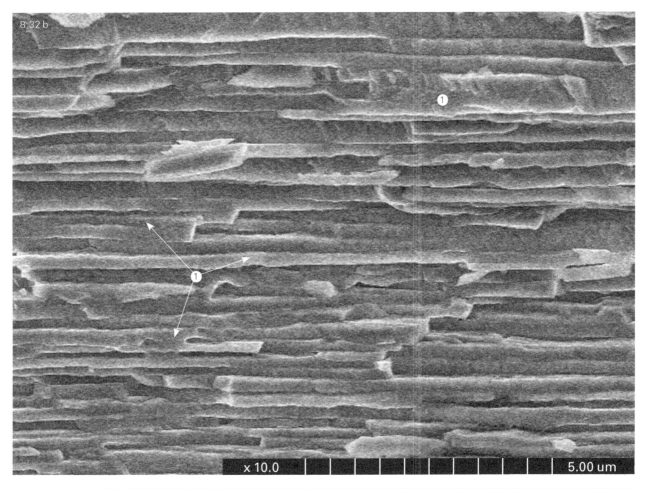

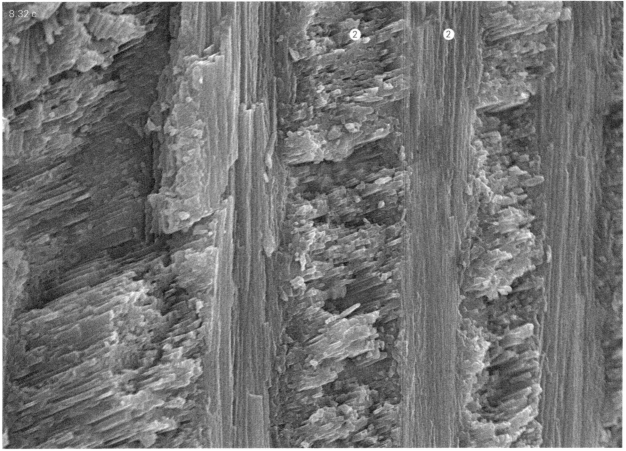

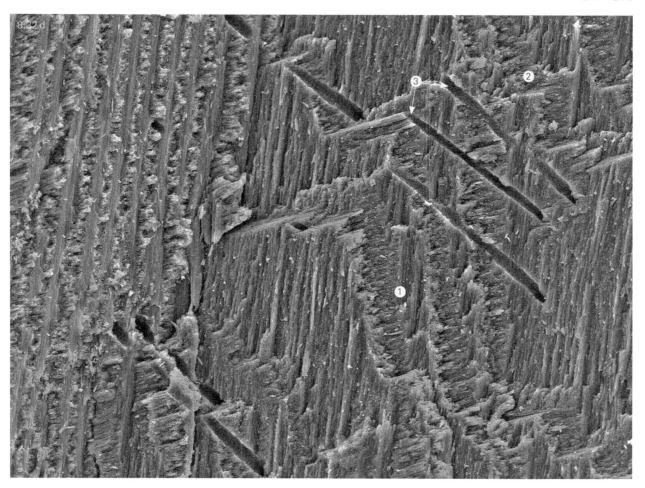

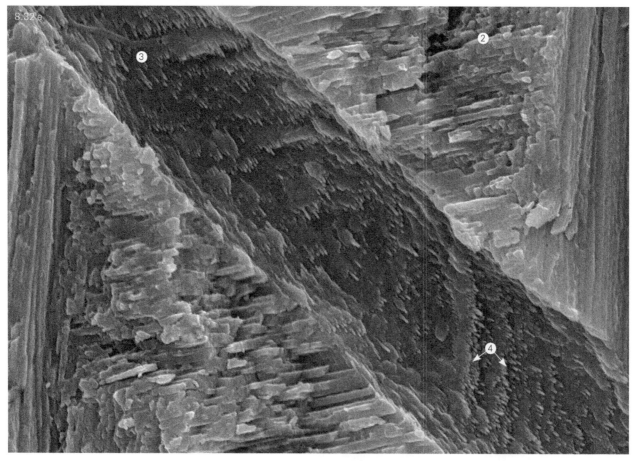

The next sector of the bone channel system are comprised of canaliculi and lacunae. Canaliculi are units of the bone's microcirculatory system. In compact bone osteons, they connect the lacunae between themselves and with the central canals (*Fig. 8.17, 8.34*). Canaliculi exhibit various orientations. A quantitative evaluation of the degree of orientation, produced by a computer orientation analysis in different parts of the cortical layer of compact bone tissue of long bones performed on methacrylate replicas, revealed the presence of three preferred orientation directions with respect to the central canal:

1) along the central canal;

2) radial; and

3) circular. Canaliculi branch out, merge and anastomose. The length of the straight part of canaliculi can be 5–25 μm. Canaliculi range from 1.5–0.1 μm in diameter. Some canaliculi are obliterated. The number of canaliculi per unit area, i.e. their density, varies markedly. Some canaliculi open into the central canals, while others open into the lacunae. In some osteons, particularly in the compact bone tissue of the cortical layer of flat bones, there are circular (collector) canaliculi that, to some extent, reproduce the circular structure of the osteon fibrous framework (*Fig. 8.35, 8.36*). These canaliculi are formed like slits positioned on the outer and inner sides of the bony plate and, therefore, their replicas have lamellar shapes.

Canaliculi are connected to lacunae either directly, or through a "stalk" common to 2–3 canaliculi (*Fig. 8.34 d*). Two types of lacunae – cellular and non-cellular – are distinguished in compact bone tissue or in the trabeculae of the spongy bone substance. Cells reside in the cellular lacunae (*Fig. 8.34 d*). The latter are 8–15 μm wide and 25–35 μm long. One cellular lacuna can be connected to 20–40 canaliculi. There are "spike-like" formations on the surface replicas of the microcorrosion casts of cellular lacunae, which are apparently the remnants of obliterated canaliculi. The cellular lacunae can be divided into two groups:

1) lacunae located in close proximity to the central canals and connected to them through own canaliculi; and

2) lacunae located inside lamellae and connected with the central canals, either directly via long bony canaliculi or by means of canaliculi through other bony lacunae. Based on the replica forms, lacunae in the first group have various shapes: flat stellate, spindle-like, spherical and intermediate. Non-cellular lacunae have flattened, spherical and cylindrical shapes. Their size range is much wider. Interstructural spaces are 0–5 nm or less in size. Morphologically, they are identified only by TEM (Omelyanenko & Butyrin, 1990).

The trabeculae of spongy bone lack Haversian, Volkmann's and connecting canals. The organization of canaliculi and lacunae is determined by the structure of the bony plates forming the trabeculae's foundation. Canaliculi connect the microcirculatory system of the bone beams with the interstitial space (*Fig. 8.37*).

8.4.2. Physico-chemical characteristics of interstitial space of bone tissue

Unlike most body tissues, bone is a multiphase material. Hence, it is studied extensively through equal use of both morphological and physico-chemical methods. From a physico-chemical perspective, the interstitial spaces resemble pores, making bone a porous material. Such a structure determines the high strength properties of bone. In this regard, the physico-chemical methods of research greatly expand our ability to study the interstitial or pore space of bone tissue. It has been established that the total amount of open (accessible) porosity (OP) of the compact bone substance of the cortical layer of the diaphysis of long bones is 11–13%, while the rest of the bone is represented by organic and mineral components. At the same time, the apparent density (AD) of dehydrated bone samples varies from 1.79–1.84, whereas the pycnometric density (D_{pycno}), using isooctane, is from 2.057–2.074, and, when using helium, it ranges from 2.10–2.25 g/cm^3. The specific volume of open (accessible) pores (V) varies between 0.055 and 0.077 cm^3/g, and the specific surface area (S_{sp}) ranges from 0.44–1.95 m^2/g.

Integral curves (*Fig. 8.38*) built from mercury porosimetric data (*Table 8.5*) show the distribution of the pore (interstitial) space of native dehydrated and demineralized dehydrated bone tissue. An analysis of the distribution curves of V values versus equivalent pore diameter (D_{ekv}) values for the compact bone tissue samples studied indicates the presence of three prevailing groups in bone porous structure, with D_{ekv} values in the order of 20, 0.12 and 0.006 mm. These groups account for 20–36, 6–14 and 17–27% of the open porosity, respectively. The presence of bone canals with such dimensions is confirmed by morphological (TEM and SEM) data.

After selective removal of the mineral phase from bone tissue, the total open porosity makes up about 45% of the total tissue volume, and the specific volume (V_{sp}) is 0.2–0.3 cm^3/g, which is several times more than similar parameters for native dehydrated bone tissue. The specific internal surface (S_{sp}) is also increased to 4.6–62.2 m^2/g. The apparent density (AD) values – 0.96–1.17 – are lower.

An analysis of integral distribution curves of total interstitial space for demineralized bone tissue indicates the presence of four groups of pores in the porous structure of the organic bone substance, with dimensions D_{ekv} in the order of 12–28, 0.4, 0.08 and 0.006 μm, accounting for 25–29%, 12–17%, 9–11%, and 4–9% respectively of the total open porosity of the bone tissue samples studied. The appearance of pores with $D_{ekv} = 0.4$ μm in this series apparently is determined by the predominant size of structural elements, which form the dissolved mineral component of bone. When the organic component is removed from bone tissue samples (after the preliminary filling

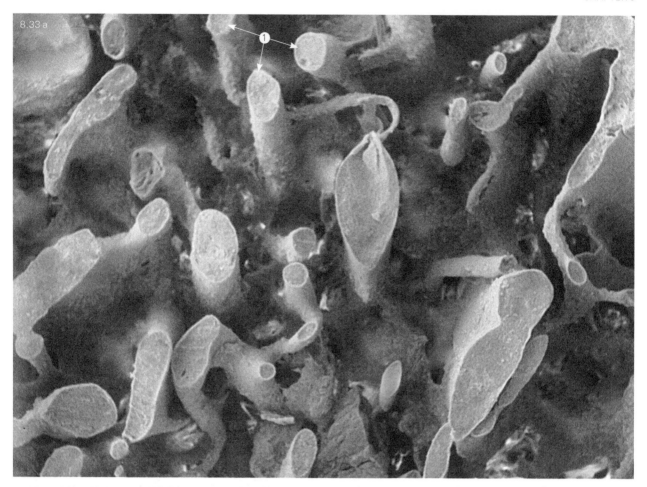

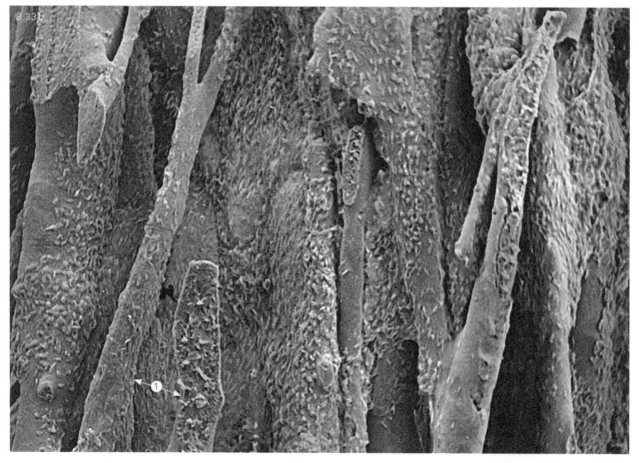

of the open porosity of the original sample with methacrylate), the value of the newly formed open porosity (i.e. the space that used to be occupied by the organic part) is 41.2%, its specific volume is 0.2 cm^3/g, and its specific internal surface (S$_{sp}$) is about 100 m^2. Such a huge inner surface apparently derives from the microcrystalline structure of the mineral component of bone, whose surface is concealed (occupied) by the organic matrix. The volume (expressed as a percentage) occupied by different sectors of the interstitial channel system of compact bone tissue is determined by comparing the equivalent pore diameters presented in Table. 8.5 with the diameters of the bone canals and canaliculi measured in TEM and SEM-micrographs. The central and perforating canals and their anastomoses, ranging in diameter from 150 to 30 μm, account for 13.5% of the total interstitial (pore) space.

The anastomoses and perforating canals, 30–1.5 μm in diameter, account for 10%, and lacunar spaces with a diameter of 15–1.5 μm account for 24.4%. Canaliculi, which are 1.5–0.1 μm in size, occupy 19.3% of the total interstitial space. Interfibrillar and intercrystalline spaces, with equivalent diameters up to 50–5 nm, account for 35.5%. This data confirms the existence of microchannels with diameters of 20–150 nm in compact bone (N.P.Omeliyanenko, 1990).

The whole set of data on the interstitial space of bone tissue, obtained using morphological (LM, TEM, SEM) and physico-chemical (mercury porosimetry, gas adsorption, pycnometry) methods, enabled simultaneously building a schematic model of the system of bone canals (Fig. 8.39) and providing a quantitative characterization of the various parts of this system.

Despite the fact that the interstitial channels are parts of an integrated system, they can be divided into two groups:

1) lined with endosteum (HC, VC, IC); and
2) free of bone-lining cells (canaliculi, lacunae, interstructural gaps). In addition, the volume of the latter group of channels (77%) is almost three times larger than the former (23%) and, most importantly, the internal specific surface area of the small channels (pores) is several times bigger. It is possible that the first group of channels exhibits mainly a transport function, whereas metabolism takes place along with transport in the second group.

It is obvious that the volume of the interstitial (pore) space constantly changes. In other words, it is in a dynamic state, since there is a continuous solubilization and aggregation of bone mineral in connection with one

Fig. 8.33.
A polymor replica
of the central canals (1)
of lamellar compact
bone tissue osteons.
Microcorrosion cast.
a – Cross section.
b – Longitudinal section.
SEM-micrograph, x 100.

of its functions – a calcium depot. A similar process called resorption occurs with fibrous structures in connection to their constant renewal. A comparison of the differential distribution of interstitial spaces in bone tissue with that in cartilage, tendon and skin showed the marked specificity of this parameter for each of these tissues. Hence, in certain cases, it can be used as their identifying attribute.

8.5. REGULATION MECHANISMS OF BONE TISSUE METABOLISM AND FUNCTIONS

8.5.1. Systemic factors and regulation mechanisms (hormones, neuroendocrine factors, vitamins)

Hormonal factors are the main systemic factors regulating bone tissue's morphogenesis and function. Based on their chemical nature, they are divided into two groups distinguished by the mechanism of their interaction with the cell: water-soluble protein (peptide) hormones and fat-soluble, mostly steroid, hormones. The action of protein hormones is mediated by transmembrane receptors, located in the cell (cytoplasmic) membrane. The action of fat-soluble hormones, which can diffuse freely through the membrane into the cell, is mediated by a principally different kind of receptors – so-called nuclear receptors, located in the nuclear envelope (nucleolema). Ligands (hormones) form complexes with these receptors, and are translocated into the nucleus, whereby they act as transcription factors on the genetic apparatus of the cell (on the promoter regions of the corresponding genes in the DNA).

Among the peptide hormones, the growth hormone (GH; also known as somatropin or somatotropin) plays a particularly important role in the morphogenesis of bone tissue (Ohlsson et al., 1998). It is secreted into the bloodstream by cells of the anterior pituitary gland and circulates in a complex with a specific binding protein (growth hormone binding protein, GHBP). It is the chief factor determining the total mass of bone tissue in the body and the longitudinal growth of human long bones. GH has a single polypeptide chain consisting of 191 amino acid residues and a molecular mass of about 22 kDa. It affects osteoblasts in two ways. The first one is a direct independent action through a specific receptor in the osteoblast plasma membrane – GHR. The second way is apparently a lot more significant and is mediated by the insulin-like growth factor 1 (IGF-1). IGF-1 acts on cells through the IGFR receptor, for which it is the primary ligand, and via the insulin receptor IR.

Together, GH and IGF-1 are recognized as an integrated functional system ("axis"). This system also includes the above-mentioned receptors and six IGF-binding proteins (IGFBP). IGFBPs not only regulate (modulate) IGF-1 activity, but they themselves exhibit some biological activity. IGF-1 (also known as somatomedin C) is also a polypeptide (70 amino acid residues, molecular mass about

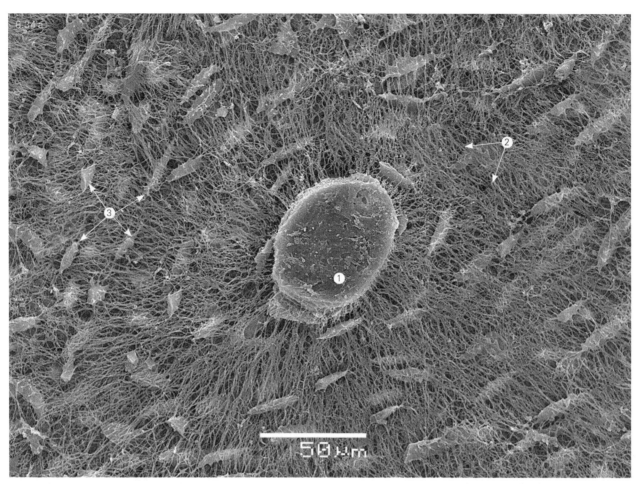

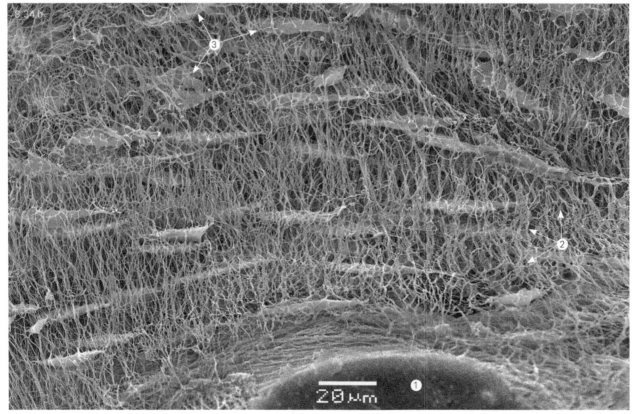

Fig. 8.34.
Polymer replicas of the central canals (1) and lacuno-canalicular system of lamellar compact bone tissue osteons. Canaliculi (2). Lacunae (3). Microcorrosion cast. SEM-micrograph. a – x 400, b – x 600, c – x 1,400, d – x 5,000.

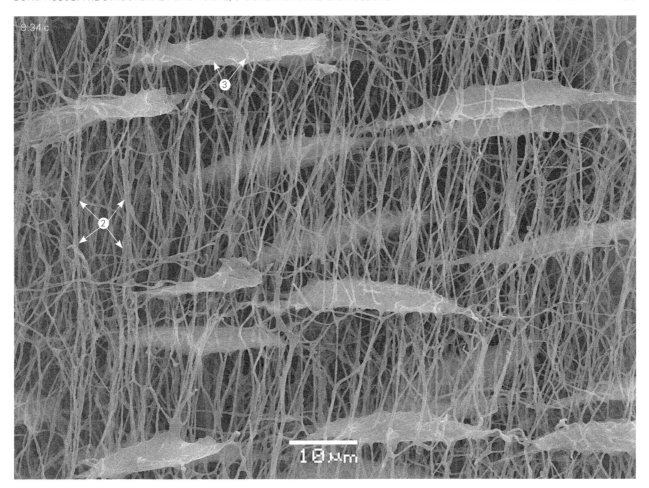

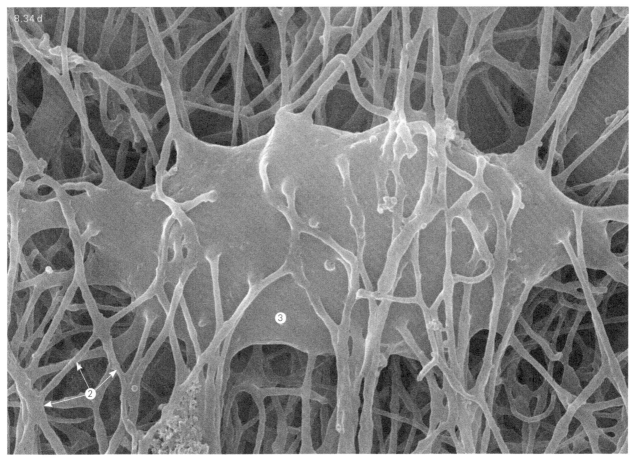

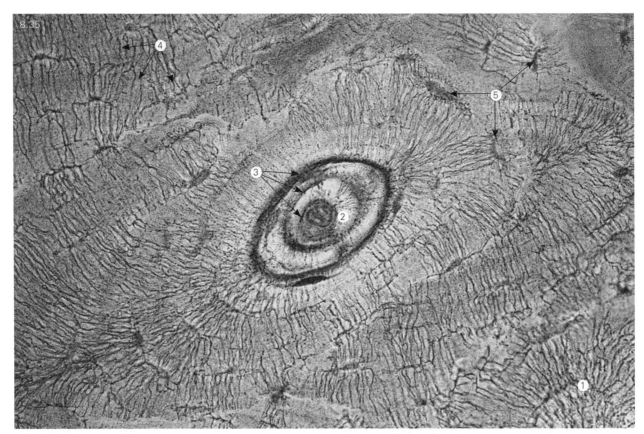

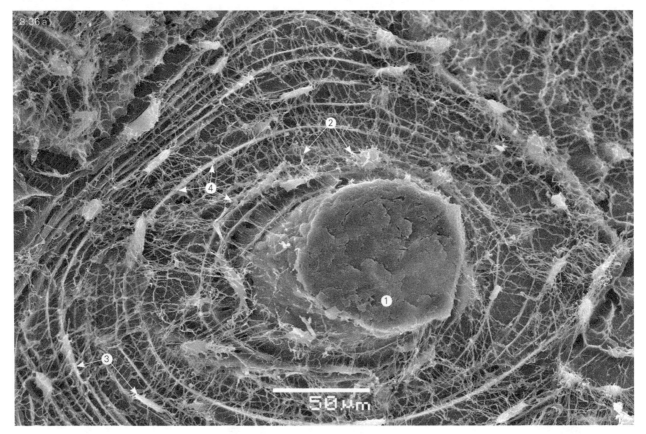

Fig. 8.35.
A fragment of lamellar compact
bone tissue.
Osteons (1) in a cross-section.
Central canal (2).
Circular (collector) canaliculi (3).

Canaliculi (4). Lacunae (5).
LM-micrograph. A light optic
microscope Nikon (Japan).
Histological section.
Schmorl staining.
x 200. *(see color insert)*

Fig. 8.36.
Polymer replicas of lamellar
compact bone tissue channel
system.
Osteon central canals (1).
Canaliculi (2).

Lacunae (3).
Circular (collector) canaliculi (4).
Microcorrosion cast.
SEM-micrograph.
a – x 400; b – x 1,100; c – x 1,700.

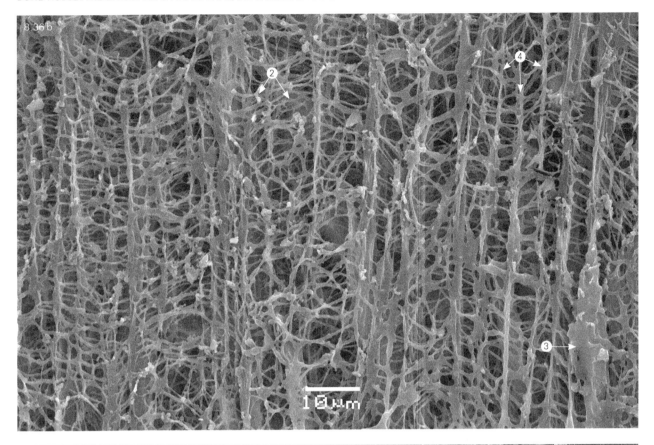

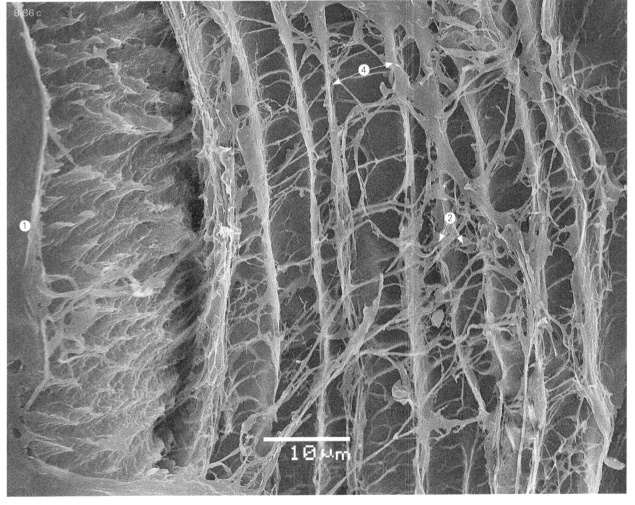

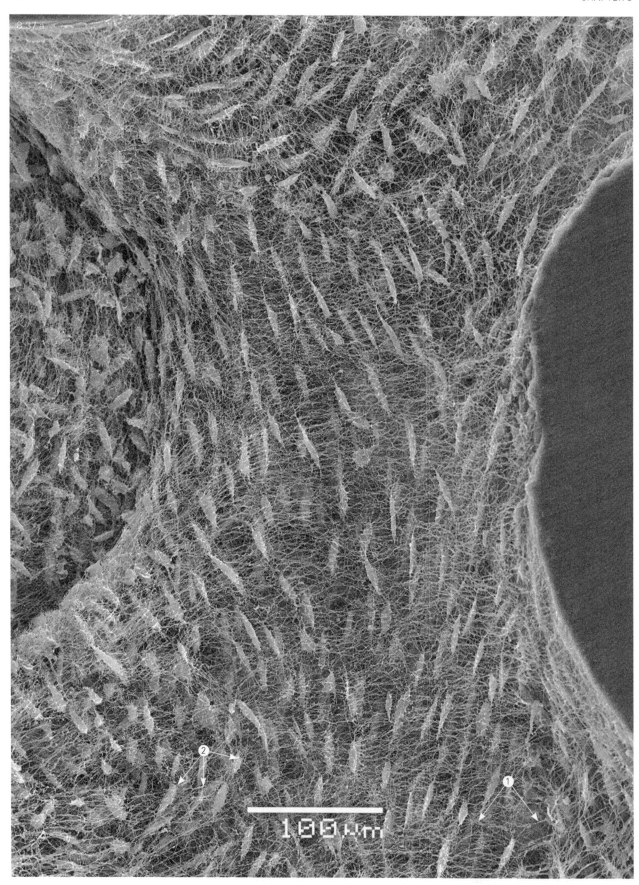

8.37 a

Fig. 8.37.
A fragment of lamellar spongy
bone tissue trabecula.
Canaliculi (1). Lacunae (2).

a, c, e, f – Polymer replicas of
the lacuno-canalicular system.
Microcorrosion casts.

SEM-micrograph.
a – x 200, c – x 300,
e – x 1,200, f – x 3,500.

b, d – Histological section.
Schmorl staining.
LM-micrograph.
b – x 200, d – x 300.

8.37 b

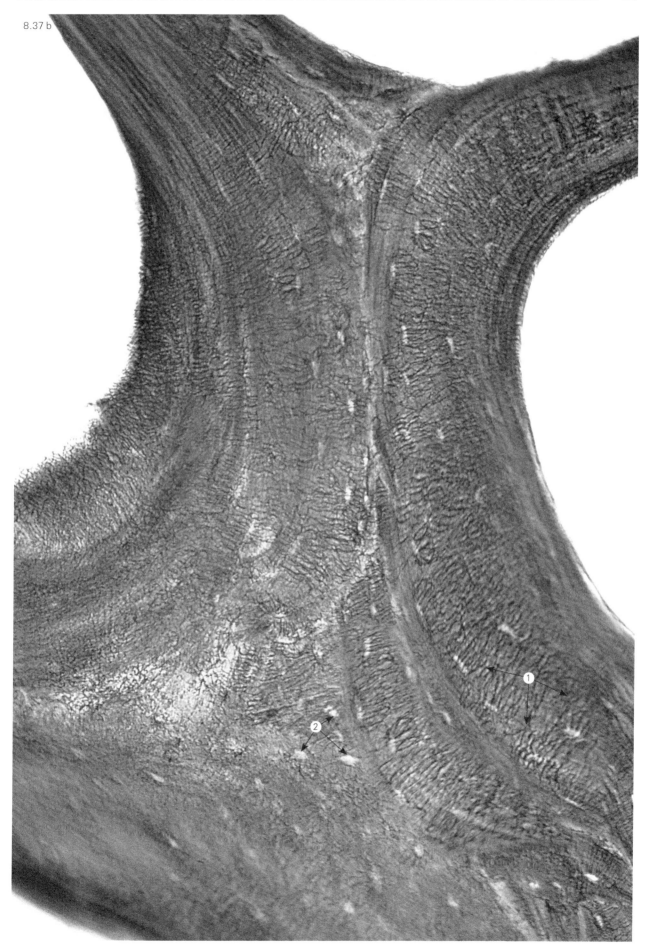

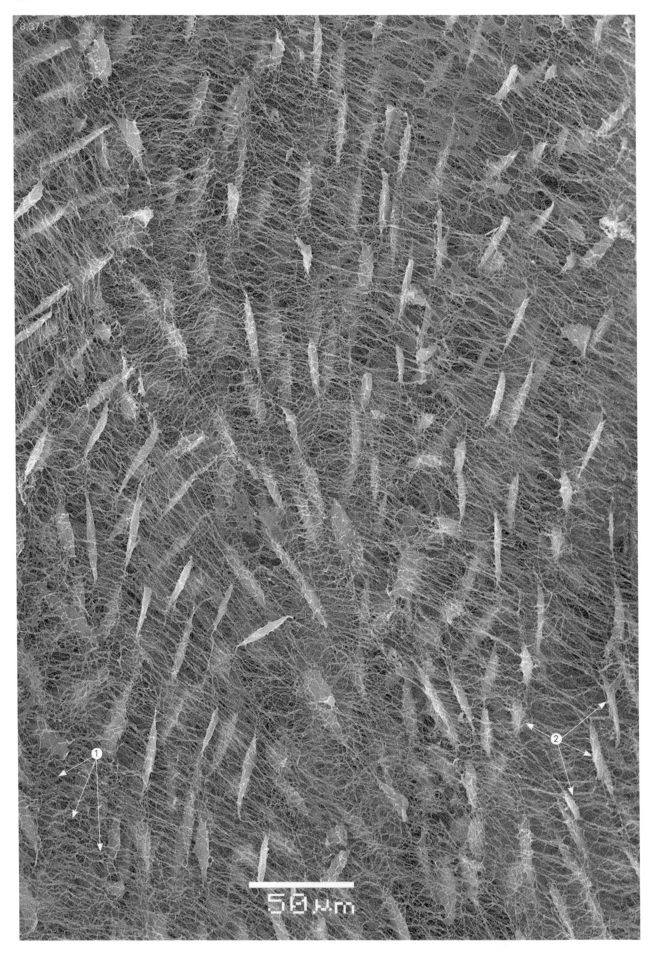

50 μm

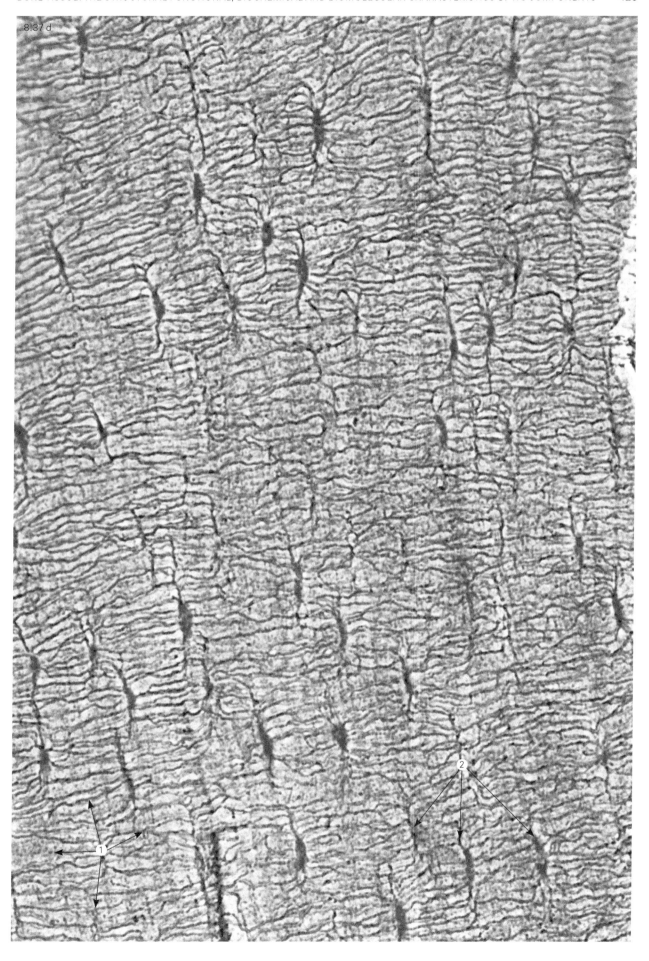

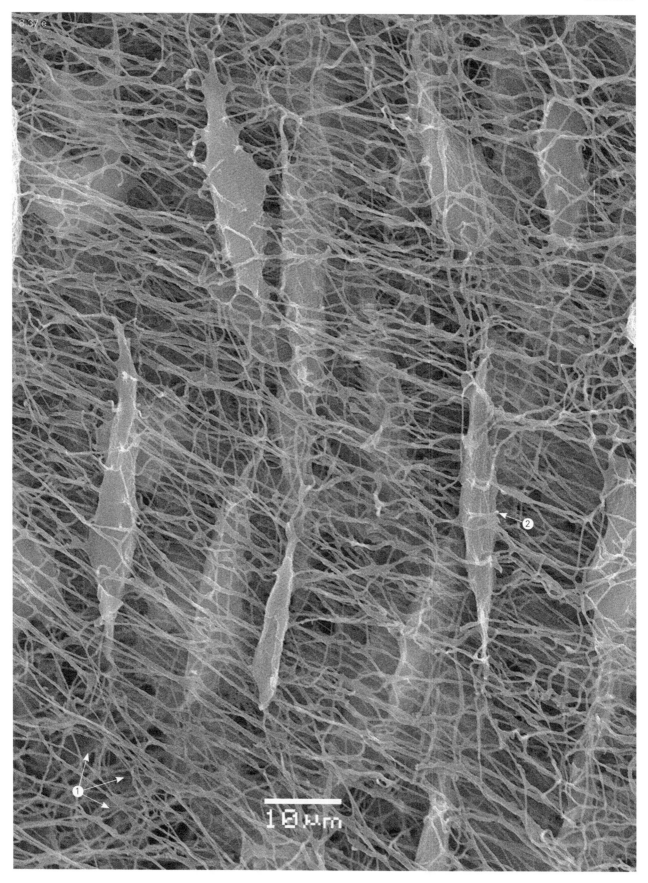

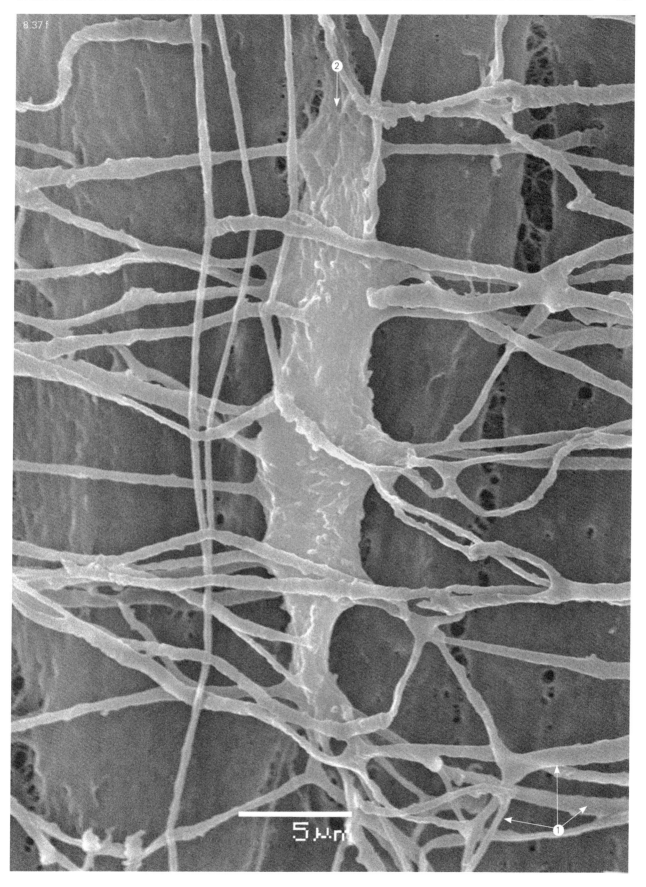

Table 8.5

Results of the mercury porosimetry of compact bone fragments of human tibial diaphysis

Size of the equivalent diameters, nm	Specific pore volume (V) share for the samples studied, %				
	1	2	3	4	Average value
113,636	5,2	3,7	1,9	1,8	3,15
37,974	9,7	8,9	3,8	7,2	7,4
28,517	2,9	3,7	1,0	3,6	2,8
22,796	4,0	3,7	1,9	3,6	3,3
19,011	2,9	4,7	1,4	4,2	3,3
15,000	4,0	3,7	1,9	4,2	3,5
6,000	8,6	4,7	12,5	9,3	8,8
3,000	5,7	10,5	9,1	7,5	8,2
1,500	6,9	5,2	7,2	6,6	6,5
750	4,0	3,7	2,4	3,0	3,3
500	1,2	3,1	1,0	1,2	1,6
300	1,2	0,5	0,7	0,9	0,8
214,2	0,6	0,8	0,7	0,9	0,8
150	1,2	1,0	1,0	0,6	0,95
50	12,0	12,6	11,1	11,4	11,8
30	1,7	2,0	2,9	2,4	2,3
21,4	1,7	2,1	2,4	1,8	2,0
15	1,7	1,6	1,9	1,8	1,8
10	3,4	2,6	3,4	3,0	3,1
7,6	2,9	3,1	4,3	3,0	3,3
6	4,0	3,1	4,8	4,2	4,0
5	4,0	4,2	6,7	6,0	5,2
<5	10,3	13,1	15,4	12,0	12,8

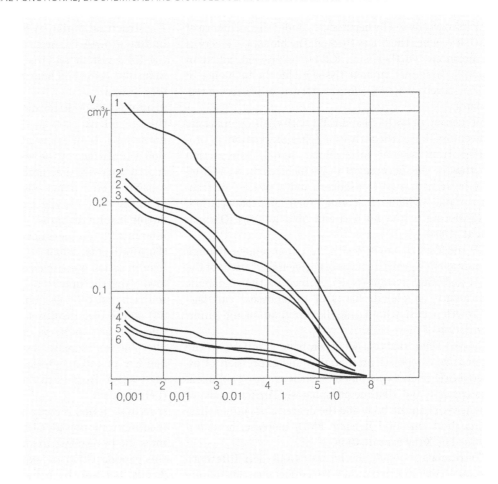

Fig. 8.38.
Integral distribution curves
of the specific volume
of the interstitial space
of the compact bone
of human tibial diaphysis
versus equivalent
diameter values.
4, 4*, 5, 6 – native bone
samples;
1, 2*, 2, 3 – demineralized
bone samples.
According to Omelyanenko,
2005.

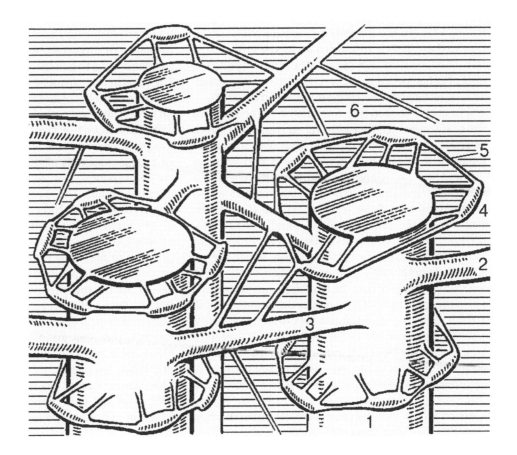

Fig. 8.39.
Schematic representation
of the organization
of the interstitial channels
of compact lamellar bone
tissue.
Central canals (1).
Volkmann's canals (2).
Interconnecting canals (3).
Lacunae (4).
Canaliculi (5).
Interstructural space (6).
According to Omelyanenko,
2005.

7.7 kDa) expressed by hepatocytes under the influence of GH. It reaches the bones through the blood, i.e. it acts as a hormone. Furthermore, IGF-1 is expressed, albeit in smaller amounts, in bone tissue under the influence of GH, whereby it acts as a local autocrine or paracrine regulator.

Interaction of both GH and IGF-1 with their cytoplasmic receptors causes the activation (phosphorylation) of proteins from several intracellular signal transduction pathways. One of these pathways includes the STAT family proteins (signal transducers and activators of transcription), which, following their phosphorylation, translocate to the nucleus and bind to DNA (Ohlsson et al., 1998).

GH and IGF-1 act anabolically. The enhancement of longitudinal bone growth – the most pronounced effect of the GH and IGF-1 system – is determined by their anabolic influence on chondroblasts of metaphyseal cartilage (growth plates), stimulating the proliferation and differentiation of these cells.

GH and IGF-1 anabolic action on bone manifests in the intensive osteoblast proliferation and expression of osteoblastic phenotypic markers, such as type I collagen, osteocalcin and alkaline phosphatase. The total mass of bone tissue in the body and the degree of its mineralization (bone mineral density, BMD) increase, as determined by X-ray examination.

The osteoclast population increases and their differentiation accelerates in parallel. This effect depends mainly on IGF-1 and interleukin IL-6, whose expression is also controlled by GH. As a result, the number of basic metabolic units (BMU) engaged in bone tissue remodeling increases, whereby the biosynthetic activity of the osteoblasts in these BMU is stimulated under the influence of IGF-1. Bone renewal is accelerated. In this respect, the effect of GH is indeed anabolic, rather than anti-catabolic, i.e. limiting bone resorption (Riggs & Parfitt, 2005).

Growth hormone secretion is regulated by the so-called releasing factors or, alternatively, secretagogues (from the Greek agogos – cause, reveal). The most important among these is ghrelin, whose name is derived from "GH" and "release". Ghrelin is a hormone known to be a factor that stimulates the appetite. It is a small (28 amino acid residues) peptide secreted by cells in the mucous membrane of the stomach fundus. Ghrelin and its analogs, synthetic secretagogues (GHS) used in clinical practice, act through specific GHSR receptors, which are enriched in hypothalamic cells (van der Lely et al., 2004). Therefore, it is likely that the hypothalamus is involved in ghrelin's effect on GH secretion by the pituitary gland. At the same time, ghrelin also acts directly on osteoblasts that possess one of the isoforms of its receptor (GHS-1a). In osteoblast cell cultures, ghrelin stimulates cell proliferation and the expression of key markers of the osteoblastic phenotype – Runx2, type I collagen, alkaline phosphatase, and osteocalcin. In in vivo experiments on rats, it increases the degree of mineralization of bone tissue (Fukushima et al., 2005).

The structural similarity between the molecules of insulin-like growth factor 1, the main active factor of the GH–IGF-1 system, and insulin determines the similarity in insulin's effect on bone tissue with that of this regulatory system.

Insulin is a peptide hormone produced by the β-cells of the Langerhans islets in the pancreas. Like the growth hormone, it is an essential anabolic factor. This conclusion is confirmed by the severe growth disorders and disrupted microarchitectonics, as well as the regenerative capacity of bone tissue, observed during insulin deficiency in the body in type 1 diabetes mellitus (T1DM) and during insulin resistance caused by the deficiency of cellular insulin receptors in type 2 diabetes mellitus (T2DM) (Thrailkill et al., 2005).

Insulin action is complex and cannot be reduced to only mediating the uptake of glucose as a primary energy source by the cells. Osteoblasts possess insulin receptors (IR) and in vitro insulin stimulates osteoblast proliferation and the expression of type I collagen and alkaline phosphatase, increases osteoblasts' sensitivity to IGF-1, and has an anti-apoptotic effect on osteoblasts by sending a signal from IR to the BAD factor, thus increasing their survival.

Insulin secretion is controlled by the glucose-dependent insulinotropic peptide GIP, produced by cells of the small intestine in response to glucose intake. The receptors of this peptide (GIPR) are expressed not only by pancreatic β-cells, but also by bone cells – osteoblasts and osteoclasts. The interaction between the osteoclast GIPRs with the ligand leads to the inhibition of bone resorption (Zhong et al., 2007). This means that the increase of insulin secretion during glucose uptake in the body is accompanied by an anti-catabolic effect in the bone tissue, thus supplementing the anabolic effect of insulin.

The parathyroid hormone and calcitonin – two oppositely acting peptide hormones, have a powerful regulatory influence on bone tissue, particularly on its metabolic and homeostatic functions.

The parathyroid hormone (parathormone, PTH), secreted by the chief cells of the parathyroid gland, is a single-chain polypeptide containing 84 amino acid residues in humans. The specific biological activity of PTH is determined by its N-terminal domain, which consists of 34 amino acid residues. This fragment of the PTH molecule (teriparatide) elicits the full range of effects inherent to the whole PTH molecule; hence the alternative name of teriparatide – PTH(1-34), whereas the suggested name for the native hormone is PTH(1-84) (Poole & Reeve, 2005).

The physiological effect of the parathyroid hormone is to increase the concentration of ionized calcium in the blood and other body fluids, mainly through the release of calcium deposited in the mineral component of bones. This release occurs via osteoclastic resorption. Thus, PTH plays the most important role in regulating the function of bone tissue as a calcium depot (Blair et al., 2002).

However, PTH is unable to affect osteoclasts directly, because these cells do not express PTH receptors (PTHR). Only osteoblasts have PTHR receptors in bone tissue. With the help of the PTHR1 receptor, PTH controls transcription factors in the osteoblast nucleus, in particular, the Runx2/Cbfa1 transcription factor involved in regulating osteoblasts' metabolic activity, as well as other transcription factors. Furthermore, PTH causes an increase in the cAMP (cyclic adenosine monophosphate) content in osteoblasts. In addition, PTH is capable of delaying apoptosis in osteoblasts. Thus, the hormone stimulates the biosynthetic activity of osteoblasts and increases their viability.

This anabolic effect of PTH on osteoblasts enhances the production of RANKL by osteoblasts–a ligand, which stimulates osteoclastogenesis and the resorptive function of osteoclasts. By acting on osteoblasts, PTH simultaneously influences osteoclasts, thus intensifying bone tissue remodeling. The outcome of such complex action is the elevated concentration of ionized calcium in the blood, observed in patients with parathyroid gland hyperfunction.

The dual nature of the PTH influence on bone tissue explains a seemingly paradoxical phenomenon observed during the clinical application of the hormone (or of teriparatide). In agreement with its physiological function, the long-term continuous administration of the hormone indeed causes enhanced osteoclastic bone resorption. However, the predominant effect is anabolic during the intermittent introduction of PTH, even in large doses. This allows use of PTH (or, recently, teriparatide) as an effective pharmacological means for treating osteoporosis (Potts, 2005).

The carboxy terminal fragments of the hormone, starting from the Tyr35 residue or even shorter, have a varied influence on bone tissue, varying from the activity of the intact PTH molecule and its amino terminal domain (Murray et al., 2005). These PTH fragments act as ligands for specific receptors (CPTHR) that are expressed, in particular, by the hypertrophic chondrocytes in the growth plate during endochondral ossification. The carboxy terminal fragments have an anti-apoptotic effect on osteocytes, which are particularly rich in CPTHR receptors. Other effects of these fragments include the elevated expression of alkaline phosphatase by cultured osteoblasts and the enhanced intake of ionized calcium by osteoblasts and chondrocytes.

Hypercalcemia, caused by osteoclastic bone resorption, often develops in various malignancies. It is caused by excessive osteoclastic resorption, particularly intense in tumor metastasis to bone tissue. However, in these cases it is not PTH that acts on bone cells, but the PTH-related protein (PTHrP, parathyroid hormone-related protein), also known as osteostatin, which is expressed by tumor cells (Liao & McCauley, 2006).

PTHrP is expressed by many other cell types in the body, including those of bone tissue itself. It is considered that PTHrP and PTH form the family of parathyroid hormones (Guerreiro et al., 2007). PTHrP circulates in the blood and acts both as a hormone and a signaling molecule with a local (paracrine) action.

The PTHrP molecules are similar to PTH in the N-terminal domain (8 of the first 13 amino acid residues in this domain are identical) and do not need their own cell surface receptors. PTHrP uses the same receptors (PTHR) as PTH; therefore, it is more accurate to call these receptors PTHR/PTHrPR. Accordingly, the intracellular effects of PTHrP are similar to the effects caused by PTH.

However, the biological role of PTHrP is not limited to these effects observed in osteoclastic bone destruction caused by metastatic cancers. This protein exists in several isoforms and can serve as a ligand for other receptors, different from PTHR/PTHrPR. It is an active participant in many physiological and, during embryogenesis, morphogenetic processes such as growth, proliferation, differentiation and apoptosis (Strewler, 2000).

The multifunctionality of PTHrP is explained, to some extent, by the fact that its molecules can be present inside the cell nucleus, and even within the nucleolus. They are either internalized into the cytoplasm in a complex with the receptor, or are retained in the cytoplasm of the cells that produce them. In the latter case, the effect exercised by a molecule, which then translocates into the nucleus, is called intracrine. Inside the nucleus, PTHrP interacts directly with the genetic apparatus of cells (with both DNA and RNA) (Lam et al., 2000). The importance of these PTHrP interactions is supported by the fact that switching off the gene that encodes the protein is lethal.

PTHrP activity affects developmental processes in many tissues and organs; PTHrP involvement in regulating the development of metaphyseal cartilage (growth plate) in the process of long bones' formation and growth is especially important for skeletal biology.

Calcitonin is a peptide hormone of 32 amino acid residues secreted by the C-cells of the thyroid gland. Its effect–a decrease in the concentration of ionized calcium in the blood–is opposite to the effect of the PTH family of factors. This effect is mainly due to the direct inhibitory effect on the proliferation and resorptive activity of osteoclasts. Such anti-catabolic action is possible due to the presence of a corresponding receptor (CTR) in osteoclasts, which belongs to the type II family of G-protein-coupled receptors (Findlay & Sexton, 2004). According to some data, calcitonin also exhibits anti-anabolic activity, having an inhibitory effect on bone formation (Lerner, 2006).

Calcitonin is a member of the calcitonin family of homologous peptides expressed in various cells. This family also includes amylin, adrenomedullin and the calcitonin gene-related peptide (CGRT, see below). Members of this family share a common feature in their molecular structure: the first 7 amino acid residues at the N-terminus form a ring, sealed with a disulphide bridge between cysteine residues at positions 1 and 7, whereas the last residue in the COOH-terminus (prolyl) is amidated. Despite this similarity, their biological activities are different.

Amylin resembles calcitonin in its mode of action on calcium metabolism. This peptide consists of 37 amino acids and is produced (together with insulin) by the β-cells–of pancreatic islets. Amylin lowers the blood calcium concentration, thereby inhibiting, similarly to calcitonin, osteoclastic bone resorption. Furthermore, amylin is an osteoblast mitogen, stimulating their proliferation. Such combination of effects allows recommending amylin (and its synthetic analogues) for treating osteoporosis (Bronsky et al., 2006).

Adrenomedullin–a product of the adrenal medulla, known mainly as a vasodilator peptide (52 amino acids)–does not cause significant changes in blood calcium concentration. It has a mitogenic effect on osteoblasts and actively stimulates their biosynthetic activity.

Osteoblasts, but not osteoclasts, express adrenomedullin receptors, and intracellular signal transduction from these receptors occurs via the same pathways that transmit IGF-1 signals (Cornish et al., 2004). Therefore, despite its structural similarity to calcitonin, adrenomedullin can be considered a signaling molecule with an anabolic, rather than anti-catabolic effect on bone tissue.

In addition to the aforementioned peptide factors, **stanniocalcin** participates in controlling mineral homeostasis, carried out with the participation of bone tissue. It was initially discovered in teleosts (bony fishes), whereby it is secreted by the corpuscles of Stannius attached to the kidneys. Its hormonal function in fish is to prevent an excessive increase of blood calcium. Stanniocalcin 1 (STC1), a peptide homologous to stanniocalcin, is produced by osteoblasts in mammals and man. In humans its molecule consists of 247 amino acid residues, and the homology of STC1 and the fish stanniocalcin reaches 73%. STC-1 stimulates the differentiation of osteoblasts in vitro and in vivo in the process of skeletal development, acting as a local factor in an autocrine-paracrine mode. This increases the consumption of calcium and phosphate by the cells (Yoshiko et al., 2003).

Steroid hormones are highly important for the regulation of bone tissue metabolism.

The bulk of information about the effect of glucocorticosteroids (glucocorticoid hormones) on bone tissue has been collected in studies of synthetic pharmaceutical drugs with glucocorticoid hormonal activity used in clinical practice. The effect of these drugs on bone tissue is destructive: they cause the development of osteoporosis and avascular necrosis. These phenomena are often accompanied by bone fractures.

Glucocorticoid drugs act on osteoclasts and this effect, as shown by experiments with knockout mutation of the glucocorticoid receptor gene in osteoclasts, is the basis of glucocorticoid osteoporosis (Kim et al., 2006). Osteoblasts' expression of factors contributing to osteoclastogenesis, in particular, RANKL and M-CSF, is stimulated in the early stages of glucocorticoid use, leading to increased bone resorption (Canalis, 2005). Next the direct effect of glucocorticoids on osteoclasts becomes dominant, resulting in an increase of their lifespan (Jia et al., 2006). At the same time, the osteoblast apoptosis increases and, consequently, the renewal of the bone matrix in remodeling foci (BMU) is inhibited (O'Brien et al., 2004).

These data are very important for the use of glucocorticosteroid drugs in clinical practice, but they provide little information about the physiological role of endogenous glucocorticoids secreted by the adrenal cortex. The fact is, the hormonal activity of synthetic drugs significantly exceeds the activity of the main endogenous glucocorticoid, cortisol (also known as hydrocortisone) and the applied pharmacological doses of these drugs are generally high in comparison with the natural concentration of the hormones.

Osteoblasts (but not osteoclasts) express glucocorticoid receptors (GR), which belong to the superfamily of cytoplasmic (nuclear) receptors. The presence of GRs in osteoblasts indicates that these cells are sensitive to the cortisol concentrations observed *in vivo*.

Studies of cortisol's effect on bone metabolism are complicated by the fact that the shutdown of the genes encoding enzymes, which carry out the synthesis of cortisol, is lethal due to the necessity for this hormone by other tissues and organs. A detailed investigation was made possible after ascertaining the role of the enzyme 11β-hydroxysteroid dehydrogenase (11-βHSD), expressed by osteoblasts. 11-βHSD inactivates the hormone inside the osteoblasts, thus disrupting its interaction with GRs. *11-βHSD* gene knockout experiments have shown that the cessation of cortisol action in osteoblasts by the selective interruption of its intracellular signaling pathway disrupts osteoblast differentiation and the growth of cortical bone material, as well as the mineralization of the bone matrix (Sher et al., 2006). This established the targets of endogenous glucocorticoid action in the process of bone tissue formation and the subsequent maintenance of its normal life activity.

The role of sex steroid hormones (sex steroids)–estrogens and androgens–in regulating the metabolic functions of bone tissue is even more significant. Both estrogens (estradiol, which is prevalent in the body before menopause, estriol and estrone, which persists after menopause) and androgens (the main one is testosterone) are produced by the gonads and the adrenal cortex. Both estrogens and androgens are present, albeit in different amounts, and function in the bodies of both sexes. Furthermore, some androgens are converted to estrogens (testosterone–to estradiol, androstenedione–to estrone) in the metabolism process by a special enzyme, aromatase, which is active in bone cells (Gennari et al., 2004). With respect to the bone tissue, sex steroids actually represent a complex integrated regulatory system, despite the fact that each of its components is of individual importance.

In ontogenesis, estrogens and androgens act independently or, in other words, carry out their characteristic activities before the end of puberty. They exert a powerful influence on bone morphogenesis, determining the development of sexual dimorphism (gender differences) in the structure of the skeleton, and, at this stage, their effects can be viewed primarily as parallel.

Steroids participate in maintaining biochemical homeostasis and the biomechanical stability of bone tissue in adults. At this stage, estrogens and androgens act unidirectionally on bone tissue: they slow down the remodeling process. This effect is achieved by acting on the BMUs – temporary units consisting of joint "teams" of osteoclasts and osteoblasts, which carry out this task (see section 8.5.2).

The slowdown of remodeling results from:

a) the inhibition of the formation of new BMUs by both female and male hormones, which leads to a reduction in their numbers; and

b) the inhibition of the destructive, osteoclastic component of BMU activity. The positive component of the remodeling process, associated with the biosynthetic function of osteoblasts, is not affected significantly at this stage, thus maintaining the stability of bone mass and structure (Syed & Khosla, 2005). This activity of sex steroids can be described as anti-osteoporotic.

The situation changes radically in women after menopause, when estrogen secretion by the gonads ceases and the inhibitory effect of estrogens on the destructive (osteoclastic) component of the remodeling process is eliminated (or greatly reduced). This is not accompanied by osteoblast activation, which could compensate for the intensive resorption of bone tissue, leading to the development of progressive osteoporosis and increased risk of bone fractures. The male skeleton undergoes similar, but much less pronounced changes. The importance of aromatase increases at this stage. By converting androgens into estrogens, it maintains a minimum concentration of estrogen in the body. In the absence of aromatase, caused by a mutation of the gene encoding the enzyme, osteoporotic events are more dramatic in men and women, as well as animals of both sexes used in experiments, and the therapeutic use of testosterone by men is ineffective in these cases.

This general picture of the influence of sex steroids on bone tissue, indicating the dominant role of estrogens in the regulation of metabolic processes in the bone tissue of both sexes, has been quantified. A clinical study (Falahati-Nini et al., 2000) found that estrogen regulates 70% of bone tissue resorption in older men, and only 30% of the regulatory effect is accounted for by testosterone.

Indirect support for this is provided by the fact that bone cells possess only one androgen receptor (AR), whereas they have three estrogen receptors: the so-called estrogen-related receptor α (ERRα), actively operating in osteoblasts, was recently added to the two previously known receptors ERα and ERβ (Bonnelye & Aubin, 2005).

The cytoplasmic (nuclear) receptor-mediated interaction of sex steroids, mainly estrogens, with the DNA of bone cells regulates osteoblasts' expression of components of the RANKL/ RANK/osteoprotegerin system.

The expression of RANKL – the leading osteoclastogenesis stimulator – is suppressed, while the expression of other factors (M-CSF, CFU-GM) with similarly targeted activity in hematopoietic bone marrow cells and cells of the immune system are simultaneously inhibited. Furthermore, sex steroids decrease the expression of pro-resorptive (contributing to bone resorption), cytokines, in particular, IL-6 and its receptor IL-6α, and accelerate osteoclast apoptosis. The majority of these factors are not expressed by osteoclasts, but by other cells, primarily osteoblasts. Thus, the effect of sex steroids on osteoclasts is mostly indirect, rather than direct, and is mediated by their effect on osteoblasts, since the latter contain significantly more ER and AR receptors than osteoclasts. Sex steroids deficiency activates the expression of all the mentioned factors, leading to the stimulation of osteoclastogenesis and increased bone resorption (Syed & Khosla, 2005).

Unlike estrogens, whose action is primarily anti-catabolic, androgen activity has a clear anabolic component. They enhance the expression of the anti-resorptive (bone resorption-inhibiting) interleukin IL-1, delay the apoptosis of osteoblasts and osteocytes, and increase their functional activity. Androgens' anabolic effect is particularly pronounced in the cortical bone substance (Vanderschueren et al., 2004).

Sex steroids and their receptors represent a higher regulatory system of bone remodeling than local factors regulating this process, i.e. it controls the action of local factors and co-ordinates their functions.

In addition to the steroid (glucocorticoid and sex) hormones previously discussed, a set of isomeric steroid compounds, grouped under the name vitamin D, is a powerful hormonal factor regulating the metabolic functions of bone tissue.

This name is inaccurate, since the biologically active factors in this group are produced by mammals, including humans, and act as systemic hormones. The term D-endocrine system is gaining increasing popularity (V.K. Bauman, 1989; Dusso et al., 2005). The name "vitamin D" can be reserved for the group of fat-soluble inactive precursors of these hormones (prohormones), ingested with food and perhaps, for the pharmacological derivatives of active hormones applied during hormone D deficiency in the body. Some of these analogues are much more active than the na-tural D-hormones (Ke et al., 2005). Besides malnutrition, the main reason for D-hormone deficiency is a deficiency of sunlight.

Hormones of the D-system are very similar to other steroid hormones in terms of their chemical nature. They belong to the so-called secosteroids – a group of steroids with open six-atom rings (from the Latin word seco – to cut). In most mammals, including humans, cholecalciferol ($1\alpha,25(OH)_2$-dihydroxyvitamin D3 or D-calcitriol) is the most active. It is produced in the kidneys from less active precursors and will henceforth be referred to as D3. 25(OH)-hydroxyvitamin D2 (ergocalciferol or D-calcidiol) is also active.

D-system hormones circulate in the blood, complexed with the vitamin D-binding protein (VDBP), and, after release from this complex, act on cells through the vitamin D receptor (VDR). This receptor, together with the glucocorticoid and sex steroid receptors, belongs to the steroid and thyroid hormone receptor superfamily. Like other members of this superfamily, VDR is localized intracellularly (according to some data within the nucleus). Its complex with the (D3) ligand, also bound by the retinoid X receptor (RXR), interacts as a transcription factor with a hormone-sensitive DNA element. Unlike other steroid receptors, VDR is also present in the cell (cytoplasmic) membrane, in the so-called caveolae–membrane invaginations containing a unique set of lipid and protein molecules. Instead of acting on the cellular genetic apparatus, D3 (probably in a specific molecular conformation) activates through the cell membrane-specific form of VDR, the intracellular signal transduction pathways associated with the function of certain kinases. Owing to this, it becomes possible to significantly accelerate cellular responses (Norman, 2006).

The discovery of D3 effects occurring in cells without the participation of VDR has led to the proposal of local D3 production from its precursors (Dusso et al., 2005). This suggestion has been further supported by the discovery of the enzyme 25-hydroxyvitamin D-1α-hydroxylase (CYP27B1) in osteoblasts, which converts inactive precursors into D-calcitriol. Therefore, bone tissue represents an intracrine organ (Anderson & Atkins, 2008).

The functional effects of D-hormones in the body are diverse, and their role in the vital activity of bone tissue is complex.

First, D-hormones regulate blood calcium and phosphorus levels. They stimulate calcium absorption in the intestine, and enhance the expression of the calcium-binding protein calbindin-D28k (the letter D emphasizes the protein's dependence on D-hormones) by the epithelial cell lining. They also contribute to calcium reabsorption (reuptake) in the kidney tubules. Furthermore, they inhibit the secretion of parathyroid hormone (PTH). In parallel, D-hormones stimulate the absorption of phosphorus in the small intestine. The calcium and phosphorus concentrations in the blood decline, and alkaline phosphatase activity increases in response to D-hormone deficiency (traditionally referred to as D-avitaminose). There is a deficit of ions needed to form the mineral component of bone tissue, and the mineralization process is disrupted. These disorders, leading to the biomechanical inferiority of bones, are especially dangerous during the organism's growth and are accompanied by the development of rickets in children, manifested as bone deformities. A similar disease, called osteomalacia (softening of the bones), is observed in adults.

Second, D-hormones, especially D3, exert an anabolic effect in osteoblasts by stimulating the expression of TGF-β family growth factors and their receptors. They also stimulate the expression of anabolic growth factor IGF-I and IGF-II receptors, and of specialized proteins binding to the IGF receptors (Blair et al., 2002). The modulating effect of D3 on the synthesis and activity of some cytokines (activation of IL-1α and IL-6, and inhibition of IL-8) contributes to its anabolic effect (Gurlek et al., 2002).

Third, D-hormones have direct effects on bone tissue. Osteoblasts and their progenitors express the vitamin D receptor (VDR). In *in vitro* experiments, D3 – the most active D-hormone – stimulates the differentiation of osteoblasts and the formation of their phenotype.

Similar to other cells, the D-hormone induces calbindin-D28k expression in osteoblasts and osteocytes; calbindin-D28k exerts an anti-apoptotic action and thus, prolongs the duration of osteoblast anabolic activity (Liu et al., 2004).

Furthermore, D3 affects osteoclastogenesis and osteoclast function. This effect is mediated by osteoblasts and can have a different directionality depending on the action of other systemic factors and osteoblast maturity. Thus, D3 prevents the parathyroid hormone (PTH)-induced increase in osteoblasts' expression of the main osteoclastogenesis stimulator – RANKL, as well as the expression of cathepsin K by osteoclasts (Suda et al., 2003), i.e. it shows an anabolic effect. On the other hand, D3 induces the expression of semaphorin 3B – a member of the semaphorin family of proteins that direct axonal growth – by osteoblasts. Semaphorin 3B enhances RANKL expression by young osteoblasts and, therefore, intensifies osteoclastogenesis, which leads to increased bone resorption and osteopenia (catabolic effect) (Sutton et al., 2008).

Vitamin D deficiency often occurs in older people, whose blood shows higher values for the parameters (markers) indicative of enhanced bone resorption (Need, 2006). In this respect, maintaining optimal D3 levels in the organism nowadays is considered a way to prevent osteoporosis and reduce the risk of bone fractures.

The cell interaction mechanism of thyroid hormones (hormones of the thyroid gland) is similar to that of steroid hormones. This interaction occurs through receptors (TR), which belong to the nuclear receptor superfamily; complexed with ligands (hormones), they bind to hormone-sensitive DNA elements (TRE), thus serving as transcription factors.

The variety of thyroid hormone receptors (their four isoforms – α1, α2, β1, β2 – have been characterized) indicates the complexity of the physiological effects of these hormones. Functional TRα and TRβ receptors are expressed by osteoblastic progenitors located in bone marrow stroma and by differentiated osteoblasts, TRα receptors being the predominant isoform.

The amino acid tyrosine is used for the synthesis of two thyroid hormones: thyroxine (T_4), which has four iodine atoms in its molecule, and the more active triiodothyronine (T_3), whose molecule contains three iodine atoms. Only a small portion of these hormones is present in a free state in the blood, and only this portion is active.

T3 and its receptors are required for normal skeletal development during ontogenesis. It also participates in regulating the remodeling and mineralization of bone tissue in adults. Growth retardation and delayed ossification are observed in mutant mice lacking TRα receptors and these animals are, therefore, resistant to the action of the hormone (TRβ can replace TRα only to a small extent). These phenotypic changes experimentally reproduce the symptoms observed in children with hypothyroidism (Murphy & Williams, 2004). However, thyrotoxicosis phenomena caused by an excess of the hormone in the body (hyperthyroidism) have been discovered in people with mutations that disrupt the function of the TR3β receptors, and in animals with similar mutations. At the same time, alterations in the skeleton show the opposite trend: accelerated ossification, premature bone aging and early osteoporosis have been observed (O'Shea et al., 2003). Hence the need for a coordinated effect of thyroid hormones and their receptors in bone formation and the metabolic functions of bone tissue becomes obvious.

Besides enhancing the secretion of thyroid hormones by the thyroid gland, thyrotropin (thyroid-stimulating hormone, TSH) exerts its own effect on bone tissue. TSH is a hormone of peptide, rather, glycoprotein nature, which, like all peptide hormones, acts through a transmembrane receptor (TSHR); this receptor is present in osteoblasts and osteoclasts. Experiments involving mutant animals resistant to thyroid hormone have shown that TSH inhibits osteo-clast differentiation and activity by weakening their response to RANKL. On the other hand, TSH inhibits the differentiation of osteoblasts in BMU and their expression of type I collagen, and this effect is not associated with Runx2 and Osterix factors. Thus, TSH is a negative regulator of bone remodeling (Galliford et al., 2005).

Leptin is one of the hormonal factors involved in the control of bone tissue. The peptide hormone leptin is a small peptide with a molecular mass of about 16 kDa; after cleavage of the signal peptide, it contains 146 amino acid residues. Adipocytes (fat cells containing all triglycerides – the organism's energy reserves) are the main source of leptin (see section 2.4.2). Adipocytes scattered throughout the adipose tissue are regarded as an integrated endocrine organ, which produces leptin and other biologically active peptides (adiponectin, resistin). It is known that adiponectin stimulates the proliferation and differentiation of osteoblasts, which possess a specific receptor, AdipoR, for interactions with this ligand. The amount of leptin and adiponectin in the blood is directly proportional to the mass of triglycerides accumulated in the body, or, in other words, to the total number of adipocytes.

It should be recalled that adipocytes and osteoblasts have a common origin; their common progenitor is the mesenchymal multipotent stem cell of the bone marrow stroma, which can differentiate into both an adipocyte and an osteoblast. Therefore, bone and adipose tissues are genetically similar. Progenitor stem cells – potential osteoblasts or adipocytes – are the main target of leptin circulating in the blood; it controls which one of these differentiation pathways will be selected.

The expression of the intracellular protein peroxisome proliferator-activated receptor γ (PPARγ) is necessary for the differentiation of progenitor stem cells into adipocytes. Some pharmacological agents for the treatment of diabetes are known peroxisome proliferators. PPARγ deficiency makes adipocyte differentiation impossible or limited (Akune et al., 2004).

PPARγ is a nuclear/cytoplasmic receptor that functions similarly to the steroid and thyroid hormone receptors. In the absence of ligands, this protein shuttles between the nucleus and the cytoplasm and is not available for interaction with leptin. To be able to connect with PPARγ, leptin, like all other peptide (water-soluble) hormones, must first enter the cell using its own transmembrane receptor. This receptor exists in multiple isoforms and is called OB-R.

Leptin forms a heterodimeric complex with OB-R, which relocates from the cell membrane to the cytoplasm and associates with a kinase from the JAK family. The JAK kinase activates (phosphorylates) proteins of the STAT (signal transducers and activators of transcription) signal transduction system. Activated STAT penetrates into the nucleus and interact with DNA sensor elements, thus modulating the expression of the PPARγ encoding gene (Gordeladze et al., 2001).

It is not entirely clear whether PPARγ itself is included in this signaling pathway as a nuclear receptor transforming into a transcription factor after binding to the ligand (leptin), possibly with the participation of fatty acids (Rosen & Spiegelman, 2001). If so, then leptin appears to be the only hormone that needs two different types of receptors (transmembrane and nuclear) for its action on the cell. It is more probable, however, that in this case, PPARγ acts as a transcription product rather than as a receptor. This viewpoint is supported by data showing reduced PPARγ mRNA expression under the influence of leptin.

The inhibition of PPARγ expression is not the only effect of leptin's direct action on stem cells. Switching progenitor cells from adipocytic to osteoblastic differentiation is a complex process that involves many intracellular factors (Gimble et al., 2006). Particularly notable is the activated expression of factors required for osteoblastic differentiation, such as Runx2/Cbfa1 and Osterix. This activation takes place with the participation of the transcriptional modulator TAZ (Hong et al., 2005).

The activation of osteoblastogenesis by inhibiting adipocytogenesis is not the only effect of leptin's direct action on bone tissue (also known as peripheral). In vitro leptin stimulates the proliferation of cultured osteoblasts, type I collagen synthesis and the mineralization of the matrix, as well as delaying osteoblast apoptosis and increasing the expression of osteoprotegerin, which delays osteoclastogenesis (Gordeladze et al., 2002). Similar positive effects are also observed in vivo when high doses of leptin are administered in the blood. This results in an increase of the total mass of the skeleton (Thomas, 2004). This result agrees with clinical observations showing that, in obesity, when the number of adipocytes in the body is increased and blood leptin concentration is therefore elevated, the development of osteoporosis is delayed or halted, and the risk of bone fractures is reduced.

These OB-R transmembrane receptor-mediated effects of leptin, whereby it acts as a regulator of the osteoblastic differon and bone remodeling, represent only one aspect of the broader action of this hormone on the whole organism.

Osteoblasts and their progenitors are not the only cells that possess OB-R receptors for leptin. These receptors are present in a variety of cells and, together with the JAK/STAT signaling system, they activate several other equally functionally important intracellular signal transduction pathways. This enables various peripheral effects of leptin, which affect angiogenesis, immune processes, wound healing, and the functions of the cardiovascular system (Frübeck, 2006).

However, the major effects of leptin on the organism are not peripheral, but of a central character – they are mediated by the central nervous system, more specifically by the hypothalamus.

There are spontaneously arising mouse strains lacking either the *ob* gene (these mice do not produce leptin) or the *db* gene encoding the leptin receptor (these mice are resistant to peripheral leptin activity). In the absence of leptin activity, bone mass in mice of both strains is increased, and this effect is associated with heightened activity of osteoblasts. In other words, leptin does not stimulate, but inhibits bone formation.

This conclusion has been confirmed in experiments on mice (and later on sheep) by introducing very small doses (insufficient to enter the blood) of leptin into the ventricles of the brain (intraventricularly). Introduced in this way, leptin acts on the cells of the so-called arcuate zone of the hypothalamus. Endogenous leptin, produced by hypothalamic cells after transfection of the leptin-encoding *ob* gene, acts similarly (Iwaniec et al., 2007). Through its action on the hypothalamus, leptin inhibits bone formation and increases osteoclastic bone resorption. These effects are manifested in mutant animals that lack OB-R receptors in the bone tissue, and, therefore, transmit the signal to the bone cells in some other way.

A number of experiments have proven that changes in the tone of the sympathetic nervous system serve as a mechanism for transforming changes in hypothalamic neuron function into a regulating effect on bone tissue (Karsenty, 2006). The sympathetic nervous system transmits its impulses to osteoblasts through the β2AR adrenergic receptor available in osteoblasts. The sympathetic neurotransmitter noradrenaline serves as a ligand for β2AR. Turning off the *Adrβ2* gene, which encodes β2AR, is accompanied by the stimulation of osteoblasts and a sharp increase in bone mass, indicative of an interruption in leptin's inhibitory effect on osteogenesis. The intraventricular administration of leptin in mice carrying such a mutation does not inhibit osteogenesis.

The β2AR-mediated activation of osteoblasts increases their cyclic adenosine monophosphate (cAMP) levels; ATF4, a protein from the CREB family, becomes phosphorylated, in turn activating the osteoblastic expression of RANKL, the main osteoclastogenesis stimulating factor. Thus, the sympathetic β2AR receptor regulates not only bone formation, but also osteoclastic bone resorption.

In this regard, it should be noted that pharmacological β-blockers impede bone resorption and osteoporosis, which is manifested in increased roentgenologic bone density (bone mineral density, BMD) (Turker et al., 2006), and also reduce the risk of bone fractures (especially of the hip) in humans.

Thus, data accumulated over the past years suggest that the specific effect of leptin on bone tissue is anti-osteogenic, even destructive, and this effect is mediated by the hypothalamic brain regions. As is well known, the hypothalamus is the center that coordinates all basic vegetative reactions. The hypothalamus-mediated leptin activity coordinating the anti-osteogenic effect is secondary in comparison with other leptin effects that are more important from an evolutionary and biological point of view. The principal of these effects is the regulation of energy intake by the organism (in lay terms – the regulation of appetite) and its utilization, in other words, the energy homeostasis. This major leptin effect is accompanied by hypothalamus-coordinated changes in the activity of many hormonal factors relevant to energy homeostasis: insulin and insulin-like growth factors; glucagon; thyroid hormones; adrenal hormones; and hormones that regulate the reproductive system (Karsenty, 2006).

Incidentally, it is exactly the wide range of effects caused by leptin that is the main reason for its assignment to the group of systemic hormones, despite the structural similarity between the leptin molecule and cytokines, the similarity of its receptors and cytokine receptors, and its autocrine and paracrine activities typical of cytokines and growth factors.

In agreement with modern views, it is more accurate to call leptin a "signal of starvation" (the name "leptin" is derived from the Greek word leptos – lean, thin, and the name of the leptin-encoding gene *ob* – from the English word obesity; leptin's alias is obesity hormone).

By secreting leptin, adipocytes signal about the organism's state of fat (energy) reserves via the central nervous system, and this signaling is the main function of leptin's hormonal activity. Leptin deficiency (reduced numbers of adipocytes) turns on all neuroendocrine mechanisms for adaptation to an energy deficit. This adaptation is an essential condition for the survival of most wild animals. The same process has been active throughout the evolution of mankind. In order to survive in conditions of acute malnutrition, the organism must limit the functions of all systems that are not directly involved in efforts to obtain food. These restrictions, in particular, affect bone formation and remodeling. Small doses of leptin acting on the hypothalamus indeed induce this specific reaction.

Understanding the adaptive function of leptin explains the seemingly paradoxical stimulatory effect of high leptin concentrations on bone tissue–a positive balance between its remodeling and the increase in its total mass. High leptin concentrations occur during the intake of sufficient energy sources and intensive adipocytogenesis. The organism takes advantage of the emergent possibilities to eliminate the effects of malnutrition and to restore the energy (fat) reserves. The peripheral (including osteogenic) effects of leptin take priority and resistance to its principal activity develops; it is possible that the dynamics of leptin's entry into the cerebrospinal fluid changes, and its influence on the hypothalamus decreases. The appetite, improved during the period of low-level leptin production, persists, and the functions and structures affected by starvation are restored; in particular, the total bone mass is restored (Khosla, 2002).

Leptin's mechanism of action is an example of the regulatory role of the central nervous system in the functioning of bone tissue, particularly in its remodeling. Studies of this mechanism make a great contribution to a developing new scientific field called neuroskeletal biology (Patel & Elefteriou, 2007).

Sensory and sympathetic nerve fibers are present not only in the bone marrow, periosteum and endosteum, but also in the mineralized, trabecular and cortical bone substance, and nerve endings make direct contact with bone cells. Such innervation must have functional significance, and experimental data and clinical observations show a disruption in the remodeling process and the development of osteoporosis during bone denervation.

The regulating influence of the nervous system on organs and tissues, including bone tissue, occurs with the participation of neuromediators–substances produced by neurons. Neuromediators represent:

1) neurotransmitters–low molecular mass compounds that enhance, modulate and transmit electrical nerve impulses from a neuron to another cell; and

2) neuropeptides–diverse biologically active peptides (around 100 are known), synthesized by different populations of neurons. Neuropeptides exert their activity, regulating metabolic processes in the neurons themselves and influencing other cells via specialized receptors. In the latter case, neuropeptides act either directly on the cells, similarly to hormones, or use neurotransmitters and other substances for transmitting signals. Such a coordinated interaction of nerve impulses and biochemical signals makes it possible to speak about a special system of neuroendocrine factors involved in the regulation of bone metabolism, which represent the central subject of neuro-skeletal biology (Spencer et al., 2004).

In most studied cases, the role of neuroendocrine factors completing the transfer of information from the central nervous system and transmit regulatory signals to the cells, are considered low molecular mass (referred to as "traditional") neurotransmitters–monoamines, acetylcholine, glutamic and γ-aminobutyric acid, derivatives of some fatty acids, purines.

Thus, leptin injection into the brain's ventricles acts on the hypothalamus, altering the expression of several neuropeptides, particularly neuropeptide Y, by the neurons in this part of the brain. The expression of neuropeptide Y receptors also changes, affecting the exchange of information between neurons. Experimental mutations, which selectively switch off the expression of these receptors, are accompanied by changes in the osteoblastic stage of bone remodeling, which significantly resemble the changes caused by intraventricular leptin injection; the bone mass decreases (Allison et al., 2007). However, the signal about processes occurring in the hypothalamus is not transmitted via humoral pathways: upon joining the blood circulatory systems of two mice (parabiosis), the emergent changes affect only the bone tissue of the mouse that has received mass. Therefore, neither neuropeptide Y nor its receptor gets into the circulating blood. Information about the changing hypothalamus function is transformed into nerve impulses in the sympathetic nervous system, and, as mentioned above, the final signal is transmitted to osteoblasts by a monoamine neurotransmitter, noradrenalin, through its receptor β2AR.

Osteoblasts have receptors and channels for penetration through the cell membrane of other low molecular mass neurotransmitters: the monoamine 5-hydroxytryptamine (5-HT or serotonin), acetylcholine (neurotransmitter of the parasympathetic nervous system), glutamic acid, and γ-aminobutyric acid (GABA). All of these neurotransmitters influence the functional activity of osteoblasts. Glutamic acid (a neuromediator for glutamatergic nerves, and the most important factor in neurons' interactions in the central nervous system) is necessary for the functioning of the integrated network of osteocytes and osteoblasts in the reception of mechanical impulses acting on bone tissue (see section 8.2.1.4) (Spencer et al., 2004).

Oxytocin (OT) has a pronounced systemic anabolic action on bone tissue. This 9-amino-acid neuropeptide (its primary structure is described by the formula CYIQNCPLG) is known primarily as a neurohypophyseal hormone that affects the function of the female reproductive system. Turning off the oxytocin Oxtr receptors induces osteoporosis in mice. OT stimulates osteoblast differentiation by increasing the expression of BMP-2, which activates Osterix, ATF4, and other factors controlling osteoblastogenesis, whereby this stimulation takes place against the background of intense remodeling (Tamma et al., 2009).

All bone cells–osteoblasts, osteocytes and osteoclasts–express CB2 receptors for endogenous cannabinoids–derivatives of arachidonic acid produced by the organism, and analogs of the plant terpenophenols in hemp. Endogenous cannabinoids belong to the family of N-acetazolamides and are considered as low molecular mass lipid neurotransmitters. The CB2 receptor-mediated effect of cannabinoids manifests as elevated numbers and increased activity of osteoblasts in the cortical bone layer, and restricted osteoclastogenes in trabecular bone (Ofek et al., 2006).

The possibility of larger neuropeptide molecules' direct activity on bone cells should not be completely excluded. Information about the expression of neuropeptide receptors by bone cells is still controversial, but immunocytochemical data confirms the presence of several neuropeptides, particularly neuropeptide Y, in nerve fibers in bone tissue. Neuropeptide VIP receptors have been found in osteoblasts, and neuropeptide SP receptors found in osteoclasts (Spencer et al., 2004).

The effect of hypothalamic neuropeptides such as the cocaine- and amphetamine-regulated transcript (CART) and melanocortin (MC), a ligand for the receptor MC4r, on bone tissue is transmitted to effector cells by a yet unclarified pathway, different from the signaling pathway of the Y4 neuropeptide. The role of the sympathetic nervous system as a possible pathway for the signals of these neuropeptides has not been established. CART and melanocortin act on the remodeling process. Both of these peptides inhibit osteoclastic bone resorption in vivo, and knockout mice for the Cart and Mc4r receptor-encoding genes exhibit lower bone mass. It can therefore be assumed that these neuropeptides have a direct effect on bone cells (Patel & Elefteriou, 2007).

A peptide from the calcitonin family–α-calcitonin gene-related peptide (αCGRP), encoded through alternative splicing by the same Calca gene as calcitonin–is present in the nerve fibers in trabecular bone tissue. This neuropeptide acts on osteoblasts via a calcitonin receptor-like receptor (CRLR), which binds to αCGRP after dimerization with the transmembrane protein receptor activity-modifying protein (RAMP). αCGRP stimulates the biosynthetic activity of osteoblasts (Lerner, 2006).

Coordinated primarily by the hypothalamus, the neuroendocrine regulation of bone tissue function is controlled by the higher central nervous system. This control is revealed by clinical studies on the development of osteoporosis in people with severe mental depression. The influence of depression on bone tissue is confirmed by experiments on mice exposed for 4–5 weeks to various stress treatments affecting the cerebral cortex (for example, exposure to bright light and noise around the clock). There is an observable decrease in the total bone mass and density of the trabecular substance in these animals. These disorders are prevented by pharmacological blockade of β-adrenergic receptors, indicative of the sympathetic nervous system's involvement in the observed reaction of bone tissue to stress (Yirmiya et al., 2006).

Prostaglandins are among the systemic regulatory factors that actively influence bone tissue. These are products of the enzymatic modification of 20-carbon atom-long fatty acids belonging to the class of eicosanoids. Prostaglandins' mechanism of action is similar to hormones. Despite their hydrophobic nature, prostaglan-

dins need receptors (PE) to penetrate into cells. Prostaglandin PGE2 from the group of exogenous prostaglandins exhibits a peculiar activity. This prostaglandin stimulates bone resorption by accelerating osteoclast proliferation and differentiation, but simultaneously exhibits an anabolic effect by stimulating osteoblast function; the latter results in accelerated bone remodeling and may even intensify its formation (Vrotsos et al., 2003). Prostaglandins are also involved in the mechanosensory function of osteocytes.

Dietary factors, including vitamins, represent a separate group of systemic factors relevant to the regulation of the metabolic functions of bone tissue (Palacios, 2006).

Vitamins D, A, C and K are most important for bone tissue. The biologically active factors grouped under the name vitamin D are similar to hormones and their effects are discussed above, together with other hormones. Vitamin A is also similar to hormones in terms of the molecular mechanisms of its action (Reichrath et al., 2007). Its metabolites produced in the organism have biological activity; retinoic acid and retinoids are the most important. Osteoblasts and osteoclasts possess nuclear (cytoplasmic) receptors for retinoic acid (RAR) and retinoids (RXR). This fact suggests that retinoic acid and retinoids are involved in the regulation of bone remodeling (Palacios, 2006). Vitamin A deficiency leads to a thickening of the cortical bone substance, whereas its excess increases the risk of bone fractures.

Vitamin C (ascorbic acid or, more precisely, ascorbate ion) is a cofactor of enzymes involved in the post-translational processing of collagen–peptidyl prolyl and peptidyl lysyl hydroxylases. These enzymes carry out the hydroxylation of proline and lysine residues already incorporated in procollagens' polypeptide chains, transforming them into hydroxyproline and hydroxylysine, respectively. Hydroxyprolines and hydroxylysines are necessary for the formation and stabilization of collagen macromolecules and the supramolecular organization of collagen structures (see section 3.1.1.3), which play a major role in the bones' mineralization and biomechanical properties. Accordingly, ascorbate deficiency during the process of bone tissue formation inevitably affects its properties and functions.

The dependence of the bone tissue's forming collagen structures on ascorbate is clearly manifested in the process of reparative osteogenesis: the healing of experimental fractures in rats is greatly accelerated by the inclusion of additional amounts of vitamin C in the diet, despite the fact that rats, unlike humans and guinea pigs, are capable of synthesizing ascorbate.

There is a mouse strain, sfx, in which the Gulo gene, encoding the enzyme gulonolactone oxidase, is turned off. This enzyme is necessary for the biosynthesis of ascorbic acid in the organism, and its activity makes normal mice independent of the intake of vitamin C with food. Animals of this strain exhibit reduced bone mass and unusual frequency of spontaneous bone fractures at a very early age (Mohan et al., 2005).

Besides its universal, system-wide role in the post-translational processing of collagens in connective tissue, ascorbate exhibits some effects specific to bone tissue. Accelerating the proliferation and differentiation (especially the early stages of differentiation) of osteoblasts is one such effect, which can be explained by ascorbate's ability to induce expression of the transcription factor Osterix (see section 10.2.3), required for the formation of osteoblastic phenotype (Xing et al., 2007). Ascorbate also inhibits RANKL-induced osteoclastogenesis *in vitro* (Xiao et al., 2005).

Vitamin K plays a significant role in the metabolism of bone tissue. Its main function is as a cofactor of the enzyme γ-carboxylase. By adding a carboxyl group, this enzyme converts some glutamic acid residues (glutamyls), incorporated in the polypeptide chain, to γ-carboxyglutamic acid residues; these residues are called Gla.

Several molecules whose structure is based on a methylated naphthoquinone ring are grouped under the name of vitamin K. A side chain of 4 isoprenoid residues is attached to this ring in vitamin K1 (phylloquinone), which enters the body through vegetarian food. Vitamin K2 represents a group of menaquinones produced by the bacterial flora of the colon, which differ from each other by the variable length of the isoprenoid side chain.

The process of γ-carboxylation of glutamic acid residues affects the biosynthesis of 14 proteins in the human body called vitamin K-dependent Gla-proteins (Ferland, 1998). Most of them are produced by the liver, and some are part of the blood coagulation system. Two of the vitamin K-dependent Gla-proteins are expressed and secreted in the extracellular matrix by osteoblasts. Vitamins K1 and K2 are found in bone tissue, and osteoblasts have a receptor (LRP1) that mediates the internalization of these lipophilic vitamins by the cells (endocytosis) (Niemeier et al., 2005).

Proteins containing γ-carboxyglutamyl, whose biosynthesis by osteoblasts is disrupted in vitamin K deficiency, control and optimize the formation and mineralization of bone tissue. They include osteocalcin (bone Gla-Protein, BGP), which contains three Gla, and matrix Gla-protein (MGP), containing five Gla (Vermeer et al., 1995). Osteocalcin and MGP, with an insufficient amount of γ-carboxylated glutamyls, are expressed in vitamin K deficiency, and such defective proteins cannot perform their functions. Furthermore, a vitamin K deficit enhances osteoblasts' expression of the RANKL factor required for osteoclast differentiation, and prevents osteoclast apoptosis.

According to some reports (Vermeer et al., 1995), besides these two proteins, in vitro osteoblasts secrete another vitamin K dependent Gla-protein in the extracellular matrix – protein S, also found in human bone tissue. This protein, synthesized by the liver, previously known as one of the anticoagulant components of the blood clotting system, contains 11 Gla-residues in its molecule. The function of protein S in bone tissue is not clear. The only known fact is that it serves as a ligand for the Axl (UFO)

family of receptors, which exhibit protein kinase activity and are found in osteoclasts, whereby they regulate the osteoclast osteoresorptive activity and apoptosis (Hafizi & Dahlbäck, 2006).

The development of osteoporosis caused by metabolic abnormalities in hypovitaminosis K can be prevented or slowed down through the administration of vitamin K (Iwamoto et al., 2004).

Lactoferrin (lactotransferrin) is a pleiotropic protein with anabolic activity in regards to bone tissue, known primarily as an iron transporter (Naot et al., 2005). The highest concentrations of lactoferrin are found in colostrum and milk, hence its particularly big role in the early stages of postnatal development in mammals. Lactoferrin molecules are absorbed from an infant's gut and they act on the cell through the LRP1 protein, a member of the low density lipoprotein receptor-related protein family. Together with this protein, lactoferrin enters the cell by endocytosis, stimulates the differentiation and proliferation of osteoblasts, delays osteoblast apoptosis, and inhibits osteoclastogenesis.

8.5.2. Local (short distance) regulation factors of bone tissue metabolic functions

Local (short-distance) regulators of a polypeptide nature are growth factors/cytokines, comprising up to 0.1% of the total mass of bone tissue organic components. Such a high concentration of molecules, which perform only signaling functions, is explained: first, by their intensive expression by bone cells; and, second, signaling molecules binding with the organic matrix and their absorption from the blood plasma by the mineral component of bone tissue. Bone tissue can be regarded not only as a depot of minerals, but also of signaling molecules. Furthermore, the high content of signaling molecules indicates their active participation in the vital activity of bone tissue.

Representatives of all major families of signaling molecules with local action affecting the connective tissue play substantial roles in the regulation of bone cells function (see Table. 4.1). Their influence primarily targets the cells function in the formation and development of bone tissue. Another direction in the activity of local regulatory factors is the regulation of cell function in bone remodeling (Simpson et al., 2006).

In quantitative terms, members of the transforming growth factor-β (TGF-β) superfamily, including bone morphogenetic protein (BMP) superfamily members, predominate among short-distance signaling molecules in bone tissue.

Transforming growth factors-β (TGF-β) are the prototypes of a very large (containing at least 100 members) superfamily of structurally similar dimeric growth factors/cytokines.

Three isoforms of TGF-β are known. They are encoded by the related genes *TGF-β1, TGF-β2 and TGF-β3*. The presence of a cluster of cysteine residues ("cysteine knot"), linked by intramolecular disulfide bonds, is a structural feature of their molecules common to all functionally different members of the superfamily, and preserved during evolution from lower invertebrates to higher mammals. The C-terminal domain of the TGF-β molecule contains 9 cysteines; 8 of these are linked by intramolecular sulfhydryl bonds, whereas the ninth is used to form a sulfhydryl bond with a similar molecule in the formation of homodimers. Another feature common to the entire TGF-β superfamily is the post-translational processing that occurs in the extracellular matrix. Besides the N-terminal signal peptide (20–30 amino acids long), the secreted molecules contain a large domain, which comprises more than 60% of the original length of the molecule. The name of this domain is latency-associated peptide (LAP), and, after cleavage of the signal peptide, the whole molecule is regarded as a small latent complex (SLC). In addition, in many tissues TGF-β latency is achieved through the formation of complexes consisting of SLC and the large molecules of one of the four latent TGF-β-binding proteins (LTBP). These complexes are called large latent complexes (LLC) (Rifkin, 2004). The dimeric TGF-β molecules acquire signaling activity only after their liberation from this complex, following the cleavage of LAP. The active dimeric molecule consists only of the cysteine-containing knots of the C-terminal domains of the secreted precursors.

Despite the pronounced homology of their primary structures, each of the three TGF-β isoforms has a different function. This is demonstrated by the different phenotypic disorders of their gene knock-outs (Janssens et al., 2005).

The active molecules from the TGF-β superfamily interact with cells with the help of a transmembrane receptor system, consisting of two receptors–TβRI and TβRII; both receptors are serine/threonine kinases. Further transmission of the signal can be carried out via two pathways.

The first pathway consists of the intracellular signaling molecules of the SMAD system. TGF-β action on the receptors activates the SMAD2 and SMAD3 proteins, which form a trimeric complex with the SMAD4 protein. This complex translocates to the nucleus, where it modulates the transcription of genes sensitive to it. The second TGF-β signal transduction pathway consists of the so-called adapter proteins of the DAXX system. This pathway leads to switching on the genes that activate apoptosis.

All three isoforms of TGF-β have been detected in bone tissue, but transforming growth factor-β1 (TGF-β1), the most common isoform prevalent in other tissues, significantly predominates. Its concentration in bone tissue (200 mg/kg) is much higher than in other tissues; by this parameter, bone tissue is second only to platelets.

In bone tissue, TGF-β1 is secreted by osteoblasts, osteocytes, and periosteum cells, and it accumulates in the organic matrix. Unlike other tissues, the small (SLC), not the large (LLC), latent complex accumulates preferentially, making TGF-β1 in bone tissue more available for inclusion in the acting network of signaling systems. Active TGF-β1 is produced by proteases activity, including proteases released by osteoclasts. The completed monomeric TGF-β1 is a short-lived (a half-life of about 2 min.) peptide consisting of 112 amino acid residues.

The regulatory activity of TGF-β1 in bone tissue is diverse. It is different at different stages of osteogenesis *in vivo* in the embryonic period and during osteoblast differentiation in cell cultures in vitro, on the one hand, and in the normal postnatal development of the skeleton and the subsequent bone remodeling in adult organisms (Janssens et al., 2005; Kanaan & Kanaan, 2006).

TGF-β1 interacts with other systemic and local regulatory factors. With regard to interactions with systemic factors, it reduces immature osteoblasts' sensitivity to the parathyroid hormone (PTH) and the parathyroid hormone-related protein (PTHrP), inhibiting the expression of the PTHR/PTHrPR receptor common for both of these hormonal factors. In contrast, the TGF-β1-influenced expression of the vitamin D receptor (VDR) by mature osteoblasts increases, while the active forms of vitamin D stimulate the secretion of TGF-β1 by osteoblasts. The stimulating effect of TGF-β1 on osteoblast proliferation is mediated by the same enzymatic mechanism used by the PGE$_2$ prostaglandin. TGF-β1 enhances the production of prostaglandins by osteoblasts.

The interactions of TGF-β1 with other local regulators of bone metabolism are numerous (Janssens et al., 2005). TGF-β1 in osteoblasts enhances the expression of the basic fibroblast growth factor (bFGF), increases the expression and activity of the macrophage colony-stimulating factor (M-CSF), enhances expression of interleukins IL-6 and IL-11, as well as the secretion of the insulin-like growth factor IGF-I. The connective tissue growth factor (CTGF/CCN2) is a TGF-β1 effector, mediating its stimulatory effect on osteoblasts' production of extracellular matrix components (Arnott et al., 2007).

TGF-β1 interacts with members of the other family within the TGF-β superfamily–the bone morphogenetic proteins (BMP), specifically, with the most active of these–BMP-2.

Bone morphogenetic proteins (BMP) have been discovered in the extracellular matrix of bone tissue. The implantation of demineralized matrix in rodent muscle tissue induces the ectopic formation of bone structures, which indicates the presence of growth factors called bone morphogenetic proteins in the matrix. Further studies have shown that these factors form a family of molecules with different functions (see section 10.1).

Cartilage cells produce molecules that are very similar in chemical nature to BMP. These proteins are called cartilage-derived morphogenetic proteins (CDMP), or growth and differentiation factors (GDF). These proteins belong to the unified BMP/GDF family (Katoh & Katoh, 2006; Bessa et al., 2008).

The total number of molecules that can be assigned to BMP, based on the homology of amino acid composition,

Table 8.6.

Main families of morphogenetic proteins in mammalian bone and cartilage

BMP family	Original name	Current name
BMP-2/4	BMP-2A BMP-2B	BMP-2 BMP-4
BMP-3	Osteogenin Growth and differentiation factor 10 (GDF-10)	BMP-3 BMP-3D
OP-1/BMP-7	BMP-5 Vegetal related 1 (Vgr-1) Osteogenic protein 1 (OP-1) Osteogenic protein 2 (OP-2) Osteogenic protein 3 (OP-3)	BMP-5 BMP-6 BMP-7 BMP-8 BMP-8B
Various BMP	Growth and differentiation factor 2 (GDF-2) BMP-10 Growth and differentiation factor 11 (GDF-11)	BMP-9 BMP-10 BMP-11
Cartilage-derived morphogenetic proteins/growth and differentiation factors (CDMP/GDF)	Cartilage-derived morphogenetic protein-3 (CDMP-3) or growth and differentiation factor 7 (GDF-7) Cartilage-derived morphogenetic protein-2 (CDMP-2) or growth and differentiation factor 6 (GDF-6) Cartilage-derived morphogenetic protein-1 (CDMP-1) or growth and differentiation factor 5 (GDF-5)	BMP-12 BMP-13 BMP-14
Other BMP	BMP-15 BMP-16	BMP-15 BMP-16

is 47 (Chubinskaya & Kuettner, 2003). They are divided into families according to the extent of homology, which ranges from 20–92% in these proteins. Thus, a BMP/GDF superfamily can be recognized within the more extensive TGF-β superfamily.

A list of the main families within this superfamily, studied in higher vertebrates, is provided in *Table. 8.6*, together with nomenclature variants. This list remains controversial and cannot be considered definitive; this remark applies specifically to the BMP-3 family.

It is not by accident that BMP-1 is missing from the table. This was the first protein identified in the demineralized bone matrix exhibiting osteoinductive activity. However, as it turned out later, it does not exhibit osteoinductive activity and differs significantly from other BMPs in size and molecular structure; hence it cannot be included in their group. This glycoprotein macromole-

cule possesses proteolytic activity. It belongs to the M12A family of peptidases, which are Zn-containing metalloproteases with an astacin domain. It is also similar to tolloids, a group of proteolytic enzymes in invertebrates. There are seven known isoforms of BMP-1. They function as C-proteinases in the process of large collagen fibrillogenesis, cleaving the carboxyl propeptide from types I, II and III procollagen macromolecules. Knockout of the BMP-1-encoding gene leads to a lethal phenotype caused by the impaired formation of the collagen structures of the abdominal wall (Gazzerro & Canalis, 2006). Lacking its own osteoinductive activity, BMP-1 activates other–osteoinductive–BMPs and signaling molecules of the TGF-β superfamily (Hopkins et al., 2007).

BMP molecules exhibit all the features common to members of the TGF-β superfamily. These are small dimeric molecules with two oppositely oriented identical polypeptide chains held together by a disulfide bond. As with other TGF-β, BMPs' polypeptide chains are synthesized as precursor molecules, containing from 396 (BMP-2) to 513 (BMP-6) amino acid residues. Each chain starts with a signal peptide, while the main part of the molecule represents the cleavable propeptide.

The posttranslational processing of the synthesized monomeric polypeptide chains, which involves a subtilisin-like proprotein convertase, begins in the granular endoplasmic reticulum, whereby the 30-amino acid-long signal peptide is removed. N-glycosylation, formation of the secondary structure (folding) and dimerization with the formation of a disulfide bond between the monomers occur after molecules' entry in the lamellar complex (Golgi). The processing ends with the removal of the large propeptide. The completed monomers contain a total of 114 (BMP-2) to 139 (BMP-7) amino acid residues. Seven obligatory cysteine residues form a cluster–a "cysteine knot" typical for all TGF-β–and they are called "canonical" cysteines. One of them participates in the formation of the already mentioned disulfide bond between monomers; the other six cysteine residues form three intrachain disulfide bonds. The molecular mass of the mature BMP dimer is nearly 25 kDa.

This pattern, common to all BMPs, varies only in the length of the individual domains. Seven cysteine residues (C) are present in the monomer chain, which is 114 to 139 amino acids (AA) long (highlighted in black), after the cleavage of the signal peptide and propeptide. The 32 AA-long amino terminal domain is basic in nature.

The specific activity of BMPs is a function of their C-terminal domains. It is mediated by two types of transmembrane serine/threonine kinase receptors. BMPR-IA and BMPR-IB are type I receptors. Receptors of this type are somewhat different in various cells and are specialized for binding to specific BMP ligands. Type II receptors (BMPR-II) are less specific and participate in binding to most BMPs. Furthermore, some BMPs can use ActR-II and ActR-IIB receptors, which act simultaneously as activin receptors (Wan & Cao, 2005). Activins are growth factors, which, like BMP, belong to the TGF-β superfamily, and regulate cell proliferation, differentiation and apoptosis (Chen et al., 2006). BMPs initially bind to type II receptors, which then form heterodimeric complexes with type I receptors. Preformed heterooligomeric BMPR complexes participate in the binding of BMP ligands, and are joined by co-receptors/coactivators in the process of binding (Gazzerro & Canalis, 2006).

The so-called RGM (repulsive guidance molecules), which repel conductive molecules, are especially important among the co-receptors. RGMs are a small family of glycoproteins with three members, which are anchored to the outer side of the cell (cytoplasmic) membrane by a glycosylphosphatidylinositol. The mechanism of RGM involvement in interactions with BMP remains unclear; however, it has been determined that only the presence of RGM makes the cells sensitive to the action of BMP. This detail significantly distinguishes BMP from other members of the TGF-β superfamily, which use the same receptors as BMP (Halbrooks et al., 2007).

Furthermore, receptor colocalization with integrins containing an αv-subunit is important for binding BMPs to their receptors. BMPs stimulate the expression of these integrins by osteoblasts, and the normal function of these integrins is necessary for the manifestation of the BMP effects (Lai & Cheng, 2005). It is possible that the intracellular signal transduction begins with the endocytosis of the ligand-activated receptor complexes (Hartung et al., 2006).

Activated receptor complexes phosphorylate molecules from the intracellular signaling pathways via the receptors' own serine/threonine kinase activity, or through the activation of several other kinases: MAPK, ERK, c-JUN (JNK), TAK1, and others (Nohe et al., 2004). Phosphorylation turns on several signaling pathways, the most important of which are the SMAD signaling protein molecules (phosphoproteins). The same happens during the propagation of signals from all TGF-β.

There are eight known SMAD proteins, divided into receptor-regulated SMAD (R-SMAD) (which include SMAD-1, SMAD-2, SMAD-3, SMAD-5, SMAD-8) and inhibitor SMAD (I-SMAD), which include SMAD-6 and SMAD-7. Unlike other TGF-β (and activins), which activate SMAD-2 and SMAD-3 (these proteins are referred to as AR-SMAD), the signals from BMP are transmitted through SMAD-1, SMAD-5 and SMAD-8, called BR -SMAD (Zwijsen et al., 2003). The formation of a complex between R-SMAD and a specific SMAD, SMAD-4, is very important for transmitting signals to the cell nucleus. The inhibitory effect of I-SMAD results from competition for SMAD-4. R-SMAD complexes with SMAD-4 enter the cell nucleus and influence transcription directly by binding to DNA. The complexity of the SMAD signaling system is not limited to this. Along the signaling pathway, BR-SMAD interact with numerous adapter proteins, nuclear membrane proteins and nuclear transcription factors (Zwijsen et al., 2003; Nohe et al., 2004). In addition, they interact with specific transcription factors, particularly the Runx2/Cbfa1 factor, required for chondrogenic and osteogenic differentiation. Along with the SMAD system, other kinase-activated signaling cascades, which use the AP-1 transcription factor, join in regulating transcription by BMP receptor signals (Canalis et al., 2003).

The signaling cascades triggered by BMP intersect with the signal transduction pathways originating from morphogens of the Wnt and Hh families (see 10.1). BMP molecules have direct contact with the molecules of these morphogens, as well as with intracellular molecules that transmit their signals (β-catenin, calmodulin, etc.) (Bubnoff & Cho, 2001).

The discovery of osteoinductive activity in the organic bone matrix marked the beginning of the isolation and study of bone morphogenetic proteins; this activity is most pronounced in BMP-2. Subcutaneous or intramuscular injection of 0.5 mg rhBMP-2 (recombinant human BMP-2) in rats induces the almost immediate accumulation and proliferation of undifferentiated (progenitor) mesenchymal cells. These cells differentiate into chondroblasts, secreting components of the cartilage extracellular matrix, specifically the large proteoglycan aggrecan and the cartilage oligomeric matrix protein (COMP). The formed cartilaginous matrix becomes mineralized against the background of chondroblast hypertrophy and apoptosis, with the simultaneous invasion of blood vessels into the provisional cartilage. Osteoblasts and osteoclasts appear at this stage and specific bone matrix macromolecules are expressed. The provisional cartilage is completely replaced by bone tissue. The latter undergoes remodeling, a tiny bone is revealed at the site of BMP injection, and bone marrow develops therein; this testifies to BMP's ability to stimulate the proliferation and differentiation of hematopoietic cells. The rate and intensity of the process of bone formation are BMP-2 dose-dependent; at a dose of 30 mg, bone formation is already observed at day 7 post injection. Thus, a single BMP injection can recapitulate the *de novo* formation (by an endochondral type of ossification, see section 10.3.1.1) of a complete bone in an arbitrarily chosen location. This phenomenon is called osteoinduction.

The induction of bone formation indeed represents the specific effect of BMP. It is based on influencing the genetic system of multipotent mesenchymal cells to switch on the expression of the genes determining the formation of osteoblastic phenotype, such as *Runx2/Cbfa1, Osx, Dlx5, Msx2* (see section 10.2.3) (Ryoo et al., 2006). Induction equals quality selection of a cell phenotype, and in this, it is fundamentally different from stimulation, which is an intensification, i.e. quantitative change of rate and intensity of the cell differentiation and proliferation processes that were already initiated under the influence of other stimuli. For example, factors such as platelet-derived growth factors (PDGF) and the numerous representatives of the transforming growth factor superfamily (TGF-β), which are not BMP, induce cell division, thereby increasing cell numbers, and enhance the production of secreted proteins without altering the cells' phenotypic characteristics.

Osteoinductive activity (this term denotes solely the ability to induce ectopic, i.e. extraskeletal, bone formation) is characteristic only of certain BMPs and is reproducible, to emphasize this again, only in experiments on rodents (rats and mice). This represents just a small part of the strong osteogenic activity (both initiating and stimulating osteoblastogenesis) (see section 10.2.3) inherent to a wider range of BMPs.

The osteogenic activity of different BMPs varies not just in quantitative, but also in qualitative terms. Experiments investigating the effect in cell cultures of 13 recombinant BMPs (BMP-2 to BMP-to 15, except for BMP-13) (Cheng et al., 2003) have shown that only BMP-2, BMP-6 and BMP-9 have an intrinsic osteoinductive effect on multipotent mesenchymal cells. At the same time, BMP-2, -4, -7, -9, stimulate the osteoblastic differentiation of cells at an early, osteoprogenitor, stage. All tested BMPs,

except BMP-3, stimulate the final stage of differentiation – the transition from osteoblast to osteocyte.

BMP-3, known in two isoforms (BMP-3 and BMP-3b, or by the other nomenclature – BMP-3A and BMP-3B) and quantitatively predominant in the demineralized bone matrix, represents an exception in the BMP superfamily. Recombinant BMP-3A is not only devoid of osteoinductive activity, even though the structure of its molecules does not differ fundamentally from the structure of other BMPs but, in contrast, shows antagonism to osteoinductive BMPs, such as BMP-2. This is explained by competition for the use of receptors and intracellular signaling pathways. BMP-3A lowers the total bone mass and its roentgenologic density, i.e. it delays mineralization (Bahamonde & Lyons, 2001).

BMP-13 is another exception; it inhibits the osteoblastic differentiation of mesenchymal progenitor bone marrow stromal cells in vitro. The inhibition is manifested as suppression of alkaline phosphatase expression and mineralization (Shen et al., 2009).

The functions of osteogenic BMPs are necessary not only in bone tissue formation, but also in the regulation of its subsequent vital activity. Obviously, the main function of BMP in normal bone tissue is to maintain the optimal proceeding of remodeling (Abe, 2006). As shown in experiments *in vitro*, BMP is also required for the maintenance of the osteoblastic phenotype and for osteoblast biosynthetic activity, in particular, for their ability to carry out matrix mineralization (Martinovic et al., 2006). This ability is associated with BMP stimulation of osteoactivin expression.

Thus, the osteogenic activity of the bone morphogenetic proteins is supplemented by osteostimulating activity. This combination of properties has prompted the testing of BMPs as therapeutic agents to stimulate orthotopic bone formation – in reparative bone tissue regeneration disorders, and possibly to reduce the healing time of uncomplicated fractures. Another area of potential BMP application is the surgical treatment of various skeletal defects, such as spinal fusion surgery to correct abnormal mobility of the vertebrae.

Mesenchymal cell commitment to chondroblastic differentiation (in healing fractures of bones of endochondral origin) or to osteoblastic differentiation (fractures of bones of endesmal and endochondral origin) is a prerequisite for the successful proceeding of reparative bone regeneration, recapitulating the basic patterns of embryonic bone formation. Intense BMP-4 mRNA expression is noted already at the initial stage of healing in undifferentiated cells in the region of the future callus (in the periosteum, marrow cavity, and surrounding soft tissue). The enhanced expression of BMP-2, -4 and -7, as well as molecules involved in the propagation of the BMP signal – BMPRIA, BMPRIB, BMPRII, Shh – occurs a little later in the cells of the developing callus. Such expression is found not only in animal experiments, but also in human studies, including in distraction osteogenesis (Nakase & Yoshikawa, 2006).

Clinical trials, conducted initially in the form of the implantation of demineralized bone matrix as a carrier of BMPs, has been met with particular interest after the generation of recombinant human BMP. Two of the most studied proteins, rhBMP-2 and rhBMP-7, have manifested undeniable efficiency in clinical use (Termaat et al., 2005). However, gene therapy has proven to be even more effective, at least in in vivo experiments on animals, increasing BMP expression by an organism's own cells by means of transfection of the appropriate DNA. In a comparative trial of adenoviral constructs (vectors), each of which carries one of the 14 BMP (*BMP-2–BMP-15*) genes, it has been shown that the osteogenic activity of individual BMPs is different. Judging by the expression of alkaline phosphatase in the area of vector injection, only five BMPs–namely (in ascending order) BMP-4, BMP-7, BMP-2, BMP-6 and BMP-9–clearly express osteogenic activity. The fact that BMP-9 has the highest activity is particularly interesting, because this BMP is resistant to the antagonistic effect of BMP-3 (Kang et al., 2004), as well as to the action of another extracellular BMP antagonist (see section 10.1)–noggin (Rosen, 2006).

The overall biological significance of BMPs is much wider than their roles in regulating bone formation and bone tissue function. Other effects of these pleiotropic growth factors (their expression begins very early in embryogenesis, prior to the formation of bone tissue), and the control mechanisms over their activity will be discussed in section 10.1.

Connective tissue growth factor (CTGF; synonyms CCN2, HCS24), which is part of the CCN family, as well as other members of this family, represent an intermediate target for BMP action and all growth factors of the TGF-β superfamily in osteoblasts. The CCN family consists of relatively large (molecular mass over 300 kDa) glycoprotein molecules, particularly rich in cysteine. They are found in the extracellular matrix and combine signaling activity with the properties of matricellular proteins (see section 3.2.1), playing the role of adapter molecules mediating and modulating the effect that other signaling factors have on the cells (Leask & Abraham, 2006). Among factors that require adapters, besides TGF-β and BMP, are morphogens from the Wnt family, involved in regulating osteoblastogenesis and being assigned a key role in determining bone mass (Baron et al., 2006; Krishnan et al., 2006).

CCN act on the cells using signal transduction pathways from BMP and the Notch protein signaling system (Minamizato et al., 2007). CCN have a broad spectrum of activity, they affect cell differentiation, proliferation, migration, adhesion and apoptosis.

Of the six known CCN family glycoproteins, five (CTGF, CYR61, NOV, WISP1, WISP2) are expressed by osteoblasts along with many other cell types, and BMPs, specifically BMP-2, are among their transcriptional regulators in osteoblasts (Parisi et al., 2006). This expression, whose intensity varies at different stages of differentiation, is a direct indication of their role in osteoblastogenesis. This

role is particularly important in the growth and reparative regeneration of bone tissue, and recombinant CTGF (rCTGF) is regarded as a potential means to accelerate the healing of fractures (Kubota & Takigawa, 2007).

Fibroblast growth factors (FGF) are small peptides (molecular mass of 17–34 kDa), which are quite conservative in the structure of their coding genes and amino acid composition. They play an important regulatory role in bone tissue biology, and this role is especially big during the embryonic period.

The FGF action on cells is mediated by specific, high affinity (though different for different ligands) FGFR receptors. Only four types of FGFR (FGFR1–FGFR4) are known, each being able to bind to several FGF ligands. The intracellular FGFR domains represent receptor tyrosine kinases (RTK), which exist in a latent state before binding a ligand. Ligand binding causes dimerization of the monomeric FGFR and activates their enzymatic activity, resulting in the phosphorylation of specific tyrosine residues in the receptor molecule. This phosphorylation leads to the binding of a special adapter protein, and further induces activation of several intracellular kinases, whose action turns on several signal transduction pathways to the cell nucleus. Thus, the JAK kinase activates proteins belonging to the family of signal transducers and activators of transcription (STAT)–latent transcription activators, which, following phosphorylation, transmit a signal to the cell nucleus. STAT1 regulates the controlling (restrictive) effect of some FGFs, specifically FGF-18, on endochondral bone formation in postnatal osteogenesis (Xiao et al., 2004). Another pathway for the propagation of signals originating from FGF leads to the induction of the Sox2 transcription factor, which is highly important in regulating chondroblast differentiation (Mansukhani et al., 2005). Using these signaling pathways, FGFs exert a modulating effect on virtually all major intracellular events, including cell commitment, and cell proliferation, differentiation, migration, and apoptosis (Chen & Deng, 2005).

Bone cells express three of the four known types of FGFR receptors: FGFR1, -2 and -3 receptors. In clinical studies, it has been noted that spontaneous point mutations in the genes encoding these receptors cause 14 forms of skeleton lesions. These genetic diseases are divided into two groups–chondrodisplasia syndromes and craniosynostoses. Chondrodisplasias affect skeletal elements formed by endochondral ossification. These syndromes manifest as dwarfism and a shortening of the limbs. Craniosynostoses affect bones formed via the endesmal (intramembranous) pathway. The premature closure of craniofacial sutures occurs in these pathologies.

Since several different FGFs serve as ligands for each of the three mutated receptors, these clinical observations do not make it possible to distinguish the exact FGF signal, whose interruption is responsible for the individual observed syndromes. However, these observations are sufficient to establish that FGF signals are needed for normal skeletogenesis (Chen & Deng, 2005).

The directionality of fibroblast growth factors' activity in bone tissue is diverse. It varies among different members of this large family and, within an experiment, is largely dependent on the applied dosage and receptors' function. The most acceptable general conclusion about the role of FGF signals in bone tissue biology should be considered the definition of their role in controlling osteoblast differentiation (Marie, 2003).

Insulin-like growth factors (IGF) act on bone tissue mostly within the pituitary growth hormone (GH/IGF) "axis", which, in addition to the two ligands (IGF-1, IGF-2), includes two receptors (IGF1R, IGF2R) and six binding proteins (IGFBP1-IGFBP6). Within this axis, both IGFs, but mostly IGF-1, mediate the growth hormone's stimulatory effect on bone growth and the anabolic effects on osteoblast activity.

The regulatory effect of insulin growth factors on the cell is controlled by binding proteins. Among the latter, IGFBP-4 and IGFBP-5 are quantitatively predominant in bone tissue; according to some reports, IGFBP-5 induces the expression of IGF-1 by osteoblasts (Mukherjee & Rotwein, 2007). The appearance of osteocytes expressing IGFBP-2 mRNA in compact bone tissue following mechanical impact (compression and bending) on the bone (Reijnders et al., 2007) indicates the participation of the IGFBP-2 protein in the bone mechanosensory function (see section 8.2.1.2).

Stimulation of the expression of genes encoding factors required for osteoclastogenesis has been noted as one of IGF-1's effects. The mRNA levels of the M-CSF, RANKL and RANK factors are decreased by more than half in the bone tissue of *Igf1* gene knockout mice (Wang Y. et al., 2006a); in other words, the remodeling process maintaining optimal properties of the bone substance is disorganized.

Osteoclastogenesis is the main target of the activity of signaling molecules from the tumor necrosis factor (TNF) superfamily in bone tissue. A member of this superfamily – TNF-11 or TRANCE, recently often referred to as RANKL – is a necessary participant in this process, thereby maintaining the functional well-being of bone tissue through constant remodeling.

TNF-α, another ligand from the TNF superfamily, acts independently from the RANKL-RANK axis and stimulates osteoclasts' differentiation and functional activity. TNF-α is important mainly in the pathogenesis of osteoclastic bone destruction (osteolysis) during inflammatory processes, for example in rheumatoid arthritis (Teitelbaum, 2007). TNF-α is also involved in the intensification of ongoing bone resorption by osteoclasts during the development of postmenopausal osteoporosis.

TNF-α exerts a catabolic (pro-resorptive) effect on bone tissue not just by stimulating osteoclastogenesis. It also inhibits osteoblast differentiation induced by bone morphogenetic proteins. This inhibition involves two mechanisms. First, TNF-α controls the expression of the BMPR-IA, BMPR-IB and BMPR-II receptors by osteoblasts; the effectiveness of BMP's action on osteoblasts depends on this expression (Singhatanadgit et al., 2006). Second, TNF-α disrupts BMP-triggered intracellular signal transduction pathways by interfering with the activity of certain kinases, including SAPK/JNK (Mukai et al., 2007).

Besides growth factors/ cytokines, some small (no bigger than 30–40 kDa) signaling molecules, classified as cytokines on the basis of their structural features and representing the numerous families of interleukins and chemokines, as well as some interferons, exert intensive, multidirectional regulatory influence on bone cells *in vitro*.

The action of individual interleukins in bone tissue is controversial, and their separation into osteotropic and anti-osteotropic (pro-resorptive, in most cases also showing proinflammatory activity) is largely arbitrary. The directionality of the action depends on many factors, but the interactions between interleukins themselves and with other signaling molecules should be emphasized, as well as the general condition of the organism, and the influence of systemic, more specifically – immune pathological processes.

For example, in rheumatoid arthritis, activated T lymphocytes express pro-inflammatory interleukins IL-1 and IL-17, which enhance RANKL expression by osteoblasts, thereby stimulating osteoclastogenesis. This causes the intense osteoclastic destruction of bone tissue (Udagawa et al., 2002). Many other interleukins of the IL-1 family and the genetically related IL-33 family exhibit a proinflammatory and accordingly, pro-resorptive action, on bone. However, IL-10 – a member of the same family – as well as IL-19 and IL-21 exhibit anti-inflammatory activity and inhibit osteoclastic bone resorption. IL-7, IL-12 and IL-18 inhibit osteoclastogenesis. IL-32 induces the expression of the TNF-α factor with the resulting consequences for bone tissue.

The osteotropic effect – the stimulation of osteoblast proliferation and differentiation – has been discovered in IL-6 (Franchimont et al., 2005) and IL-11. The expression of one of the interleukin-11 receptors, IL-11Rα, is necessary for normal bone remodeling (Sims et al., 2005).

Among interferons, a type II interferon – interferon-γ (IFN-γ) – is the most important in terms of the regulation of bone tissue. It can stimulate the formation of osteoclasts through the activation of RANKL-producing immunocompetent T-cells, but can also have the opposite effect by competing with RANKL for binding to its receptor RANK (Gao et al., 2007).

Among the local regulatory factors, morphogens from the Wnt signaling system play a key role in controlling bone cell function; we have already encountered them in the description of cartilage tissue, and their nature and mechanism of action will be presented in detail in section 10.1. The expression of some Wnt-ligands (Wnt5a, Wnt7b) and other molecules that belong to this system is most active in differentiating osteoblasts in vivo during the embryonic period, and *in vitro* in cultures of mesenchymal progenitor cells derived from young animals. However, the expression of other Wnt (1, 9b), on the contrary, increases with age (Rauner et al., 2008). Wnt support cell viability (block apoptosis) in mature osteoblasts. In the postnatal period, β-catenin, a Wnt effector, restricts osteoclastogenesis, thus contributing to an increase in bone mass (Holmen et al., 2005). Enhanced Wnt expression, characteristic of the embryonic period, resumes during reparative bone regeneration (Issack et al., 2008; Chen & Alman, 2009; Kubota et al., 2009).

8.6. REMODELING OF BONE TISSUE

8.6.1. Definition, classification, general characteristics

Bone tissue remodeling (rebuilding) is the replacement of some of its bone structures with other, newly formed structures, leading to the recovery (creation) of tissue organization in accordance with the specific functions.

The general remodeling mechanism consists of two stages: I–resorption, and II–*de novo* formation of bone structures. Each of these stages has substages.

Stage I.

Resorption. First substage–the gradual disintegration of a mineral's multilayered, tissue-specific structure to nanoparticles (2–3 nm in diameter), the subsequent dissolution of the latter into molecules, and release of the fibrous structures (collagen fibrils and fibers); Second substage–the disintegration of collagen fibrils to subfibrils, microfibrils and protofibrils. The fragmentation of protofibrils to macromolecules, polypeptides and fragments thereof, and the utilization of the latter. Three variations of this process have been described:

1) lysis of collagen peptides to amino acids by osteoclast-secreted enzymes, including collagenase, near the osteoclast surface; and

2) the formation of phagolysosomes inside osteoclasts, the digestion of the fragmented fibrils and collagen molecules to amino acids, and discharge of the latter into the extracellular medium;

3) the internalization of fragmented fibrils and collagen molecules by osteoclasts with the formation of vesicles.

Stage II.

Formation of new bone structures. First substage–collagen protein synthesis, formation of collagen supramolecular structures (microfibrils, fibrils, fibers, fibrous aggregates: osteons, trabeculae, etc.); second substage is integration with the remaining bone structures; third substage is mineralization of the newly-formed fibrous structures in accordance with their multilevel organization.

Three variations of the mechanism of bone resorption have been described in the literature:

1) osteoclastic;

2) osteocytic;

3) non-cellular ("chemical") or "smooth". The first two variations postulate the involvement of cellular elements. The visible participation of cells has not been established in non-cellular resorption. This variation is observed as perivascular lysis of newly formed bone regenerates.

With regard to the condition of the human or animal organism, bone remodeling can be classified as:

1) physiological;

2) reparative; and

3) pathological.

1. a). The physiological remodeling of mature bone tissue enables the gradual local replacement of "worn-out" mature bone tissue (i.e. microdamage) without disturbing the hosting bone function. Microdamage does not reach a critical volume capable of affecting bone function.

b). The physiological multistage remodeling of immature bone tissue leads to the formation and "maturation" of bone tissue. The primary (reticulofibrous) bone tissue formed during embryonic development is completely resorbed by osteoclasts in accordance with the genetic algorithm, and lamellar bone tissue forms in its place, which is also subjected to remodeling under the influence of biomechanical factors, as well as the growth and development of the whole organism.

2. Reparative remodeling occurs during the formation of bone regenerates and consists of two stages. The complete resorption of the (primary) reticulofibrous bone tissue, formed following the genetic algorithm as in embryonic development, occurs in the first stage. The considerable amount of simultaneously resorbing bone tissue does not allow the damaged bones to carry out their specific functions at this stage (*Fig. 8.40*).

In the second–adaptive–stage, lamellar bone tissue formed in the place of the reticulofibrous bone tissue also undergoes remodeling under the influence of biomechanical factors, which increase gradually in the process of loading the healed bone. The simultaneous remodeling occurs on a smaller scale, allowing the restored bone to partially fulfill its function.

3. The replacement of normal bone tissue with abnormal occurs in pathological bone remodeling. The further remodeling of the pathologically altered bone structures into similar structures is possible. Given the small amount of abnormal bone tissue in the bone, the function of the latter is not impaired. In the case of gradual expansion of the area of pathological remodeling, the amount of altered bone tissue increases, which can lead to an impairment of bone function.

8.6.2. Molecular and biochemical mechanisms of bone tissue remodeling

About 10% of the skeletal mass is renewed in a human adult each year owing to bone remodeling. This indicates a high metabolic activity. Such activity distinguishes bone tissue from the metabolically inert cartilage tissue in adult organisms. This activity is determined by the aerobic nature of the metabolism of bone cells, which requires a sufficient supply of oxygen to the cells, and is supported by a well-developed system of blood supply system to the bone.

Remodeling has a dual biological significance. First, remodeling maintains the optimal physico-mechanical state of bone tissue, preventing it from wear, thus ensuring the fulfillment of the supporting and protective functions of the skeleton. During growth and skeletal formation, remodeling is the mechanism that, in accordance with the classical law of biomechanics–Wolf's law, ensures the adaptation of bones' form, macro- and micro-architectonics to the realization of these functions.

Second, the inorganic components are released from the resorbing bone tissue during the remodeling process. They enter the blood, other body fluids, and ultimately the cells of other tissues. Their content in the mineralized bone tissue is so high that it makes the skeleton the main depot of inorganic substances in the body, whereas ongoing remodeling makes this depot metabolically active. It has been estimated that about 2 million clusters of osteoclasts and osteoblasts, named basic metabolic/multicellular units (BMU), operate simultaneously in the bones of a human adult. Each BMU operates in a confined space (bone remodeling compartment, BRC), isolated from the bone marrow by a layer of osteoblast-like cells (Kaunitz & Yamaguchi, 2008). It performs the complete remodeling cycle in a coordinated fashion, which includes local bone resorption and the replacement of the resorbed tissue with newly formed tissue (Sims & Gooi, 2008). On average, a new BMU appears in the body every 10 seconds.

The activity of the remodeling process is particularly important for calcium metabolism. Its total amount in a human adult is about 1 kg. Ninety-nine percent of the calcium in the body is found in bone tissue. Owing to the remodeling, the bone tissue releases 500 mmol (0.7–0.8 g) of calcium into the body fluids daily, and it is important that osteoclasts release calcium into the blood serum in an ionized, biologically active form (Ca^{2+}) (Li Z. et al., 2006). Under normal conditions, such an amount of calcium is used for the mineralization of the organic bone matrix generated by osteoblasts working within BMUs.

Thus, the bone tissue, together with the kidneys and intestines, is a member of the triad of organs stabilizing the calcium balance in the organism.

The calcium ion participates in metabolic processes, and also acts as their regulator in all living cells. Maintaining stable calcium ion concentration in the body fluids is an essential requirement for the normal vital activities of the organism. The concentration of ionized calcium in the blood serum cannot go beyond the 1.1–1.4 mmol/liter range (4.5–5.7 mg%) without serious consequences for the functions of the heart, neuromuscular and endocrine systems. It can be argued that, from a general biological point of view, the role of bone tissue in maintaining calcium homeostasis via the remodeling process is no less crucial than the support and mechanical func-

tions of the skeleton.

Both major functional tasks of the main metabolic unit (BMU) in the bone remodeling process–optimizing the skeleton's biomechanical properties and maintaining calcium homeostasis–determine the origin and the essence of the molecular mechanisms controlling this process.

The emergence of BMU as a means of fulfilling the first of these tasks–changing bones' biomechanical properties–is related to the action of mechanical stress on bone tissue and the inevitable microcracks caused by the loading. Osteocytes sense local mechanical stress and part of their population undergoes apoptosis. Osteocyte apoptosis is considered to be the primary element in stimulating osteoclastogenesis (Noble, 2003). The expression of apoptosis-promoting (proapoptotic) molecules, including proteins encoded by the Bax gene, increases in the immediate apoptotic region. However, the expression of genes with a positive effect on the cells, known as "survival genes" (anti-apoptotic)–the Bcl-2 gene in particular–in nearby osteocytes surrounding the apoptotic region is enhanced (Verborgt et al., 2002). The surviving metabolically active osteocytes form a kind of a protection. These osteocytes transmit the signal through their processes to the osteoblasts, which, in turn, become activated (Wang X. et al., 2006). As already noted, osteoblasts are the primary source of signaling molecules (M-CSF, RANKL, TNF, c-fos, IGF-I, IL-1, prostaglandins, etc.), controlling the process of osteoclastogenesis and the functional activity of osteoclasts. Under the influence of these molecules, a group of active osteoclasts accumulates in a specific location on the bone surface to initiate bone resorption.

The aging of bone tissue, more specifically, of its collagen components, contributes to this accumulation. The "preference" for aged bones shown by osteoclasts has been confirmed in experiments whereby the age-related isomerization (altered arrangement of certain functional groups) of the type I collagen macromolecule served as a sign of aging (Henriksen et al., 2007).

Changes in the calcium concentration in the body fluids serve to signal the initiation of bone remodeling and the fulfillment of the second task–maintaining calcium homeostasis. More precisely, the concentration of ionized calcium itself, either reduced or elevated, represents a signal for the appearance or suppression of BMUs, respectively. First, this signal turns on systemic (hormo-

>
Fig. 8.40.
A fragment of 21-day-old dog distraction bone regenerate.
a,a1 – zone of primary (reticulofibrous) osteogenesis;
b – bone resorption zone;
o, d – zone of secondary (lamellar) osteogenesis.
Primary bone trabecula (1).
Primary osteoblasts (2) and osteocytes (3).
Osteoclasts (4).
Sinusoidal capillary (5).
Erythrocytes (6).

Resorbing bone beams (7).
Primary bone lamellae (8).
Secondary osteoblasts (9) and osteocytes (10).
Forming primary osteons (11) and central canals (12).
LM-micrograph.
A light optic microscope
Ni Nikon (Japan).
Histological sections.
Hematoxylin-eosin staining
(see color insert).
x 200.
a1 – SEM-micrograph.

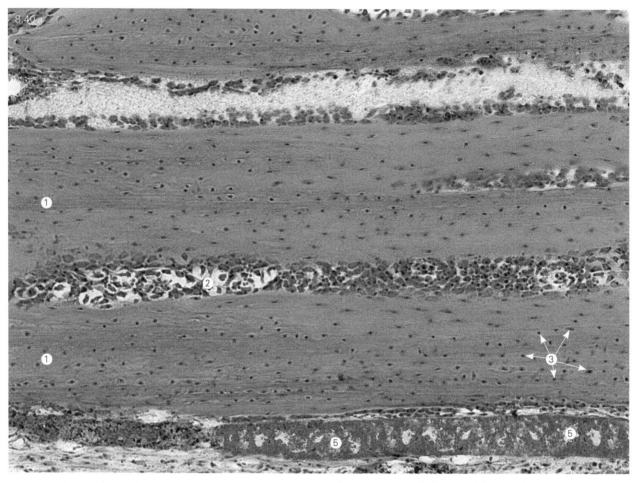

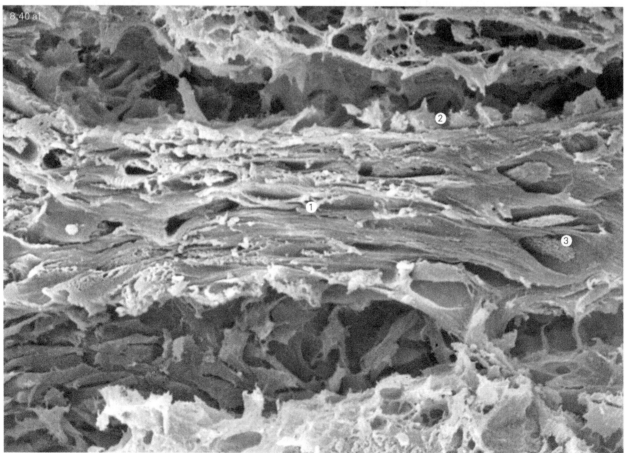

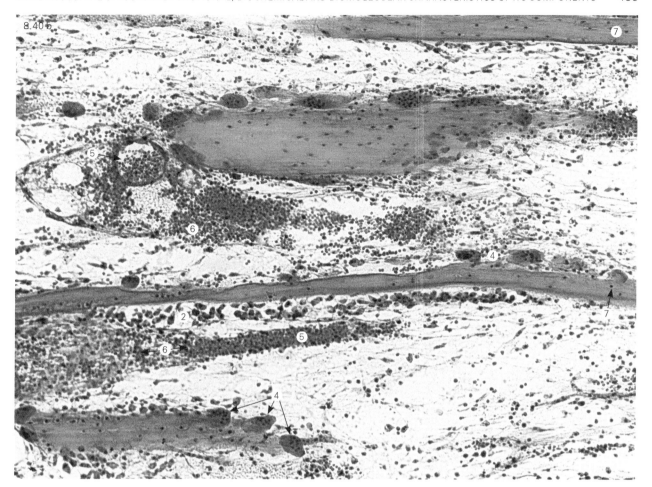

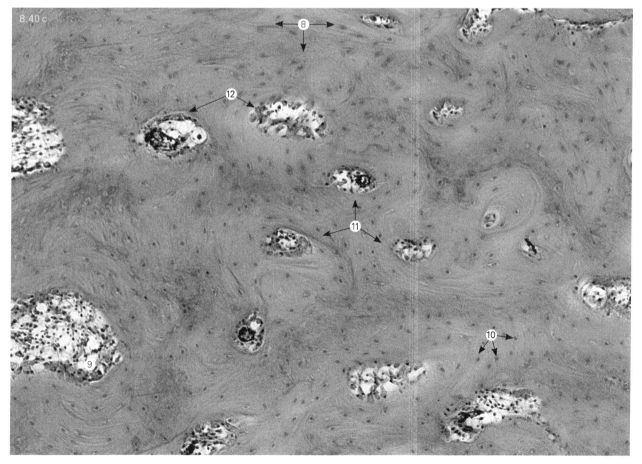

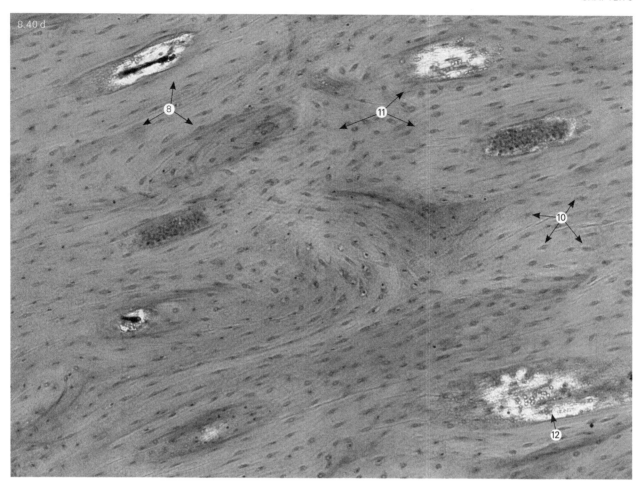

nal) regulatory factors. The cells of endocrine organs producing these factors possess the respective receptors. In turn, bone cells possess a developed system of receptors (CTR, CLR) and modulators of receptor activity (RAMPs), whose ligands are these systemic factors, particularly calcitonin and peptides, which belong to the calcitonin family (see section 8.5.1) (Davey et al., 2008; Naot & Cornish, 2008).

Bone cells, both osteoblasts and osteoclasts, also have receptors enabling them to respond directly to changes in calcium ions' concentration in the cellular environment; this ability is clearly manifested in vitro (Purroy & Spurr, 2002). The calcium receptor of bone cells is probably the same CaSR receptor (Calcium Sensing Receptor, otherwise known as CaR), which operates in cells of the parathyroid gland and other organs responsible for calcium homeostasis (Chang & Shoback, 2004; Dvorak & Riccardi, 2004). Calcyclin (S100A6), a representative of the S100 protein family, contributes to this receptor's sensitivity in bone cells (Tu et al., 2003).

CaSR belongs to a large group of so-called metabotropic transmembrane receptors; the propagation of their signals within the cell is mediated by the G-protein. This receptor-coupled G-protein (the name G-protein derives from its ability to bind guanine nucleotides) activates the enzyme phospholipase C and a number of kinases, whose action is aimed at opening and closing the transmembrane calcium channel (Tfelt-Hansen & Brown, 2005).

The most important biological role of osteoclasts in maintaining calcium homeostasis in the organism is manifested in their biochemical phenotype by the intense expression of calcium ions sensory receptors and transmembrane channels for their transport. The ryanodine receptor 2 (RYR2), a giant macromolecule consisting of 4965 amino acid residues, combines both of these functions – the function of a sensor and that of a channel (Zaidi et al., 2004).

By acting on bone cells via the CaSR receptor, a decline in extracellular calcium ion concentration ([Ca2+]e) initiates osteoclast resorptive activity in the BMU. However, the excessive local increase in the concentration of [Ca2+]e on the osteoclast villous surface, resulting from this activity, does not stop the ongoing resorption process. The fine regulation of the resorptive activity, including its complete inhibition, is associated with the dynamics of intracellular calcium ion concentration ([Ca2+]i); the intracellular distribution (compartmentalization) of [Ca2+]i is important herewith (Li Z. et al., 2005).

The osteoclasts that carried out the resorption are immediately replaced by osteoblasts, which actively produce and deposit the new extracellular organic matrix and regulate its mineralization. The mechanisms of the onset of the first stage of remodeling – osteoclastic bone resorption – are explained by the reviewed factors initiating the process of remodeling (BMU formation). These are the mechanical fatigue of the tissue sensed by osteocytes and the accompanying apoptosis, and the changes in ionized calcium concentration in the body fluids sensed by osteoclasts. However, these factors are not sufficient to understand the mechanisms that activate osteoblasts' differentiation, proliferation, involvement in BMU, and biosynthetic function, enabling the recreation of new complete tissue in the remodeling focus. The above-mentioned signals, expressed by osteocytes and propagated through the network of osteocyte processes, which come into contact with osteoblasts and quiescent progenitor multipotent cells on the bone surface, may form the basis of one of these mechanisms.

However, osteoclast activity plays a more significant role in the formation of the osteoblastic (anabolic in essence) component of remodeling (Martin & Sims, 2005). First, by resorbing the bone matrix, osteoclasts release large amounts of growth factors contained in the matrix, which stimulate osteoblastogenesis, particularly insulin-like growth factors (IGF-I and IGF-II) and members of the TGF-β transforming growth factor superfamily. Second, osteoclasts express signaling molecules that enable the coupling of bone resorption with its formation through osteoblast activation. This impact is provided by cytokines, particularly interleukin IL-6, which use different receptors and signaling pathways mediated by the transmembrane glycoprotein gp130 in the capacity of a co-receptor. This co-receptor, required for the further transmission of the signal within the cell, is important for regulating bone metabolism and bone growth (Sims et al., 2004).

Other molecular factors, expressed by osteoclasts, participate in coupling the osteoclast and osteoblast functions in the remodeling process. These are sphingosine-1-phosphate (S1P), mentioned in section 8.2.2.2, the mim1 protein, and the hepatocyte growth factor (HGF). These also include the Wnt10b morphogen and BMP-6 (Pedersen et al., 2008). The signaling system of the Eph family of transmembrane receptors and their ligands, as well as the transmembrane proteins of the ephrin family, is probably of great importance for the coupling. This concerns, first of all, the EphB4 receptor expressed by osteoblasts and the ephrin-B2 ligand expressed by osteoclasts. The ligand-activated osteoblast EphB4 uses numerous intracellular signaling pathways to activate a variety of anabolic functions (Edwards & Mundy, 2008). In contrast, the interaction of the EphA2 receptor and the ephrin-A2 ligand inhibits osteoblastogenesis and stimulates osteoclast differentiation, thereby activating the catabolic aspect of remodeling (Irie et al., 2009).

The ability of osteoclasts to stimulate osteoblasts' expression of the keratan sulfate proteoglycan osteomodulin (osteoadherin) (see section 8.2.1.2), one of the osteoblast maturity markers facilitating mineralization, is also important for the coupling of osteoclast and osteoblast functions (Ninomiya et al., 2007).

Osteoblasts' anabolic function in the BMU is stimulated by the bone morphogenetic proteins BMP-2, -4, -6 and -7,

expressed by osteoclasts (Garimella et al., 2008). An interruption of the main intracellular BMP signaling pathway (and those of other TGF-β superfamily members), caused by mutations in the Smad4-encoding gene, results in skeletal growth disorders during the postnatal period in mice (Tan et al., 2007).

The paracrine action of the osteoclast-secreted glutamic acid is of relevance to the exchange of information between osteoclasts and osteoblasts, required for coupling their functions in the remodeling process (Skerry, 2008). This action is analogous to the role played by glutamic acid in the mechanosensory function of osteocytes.

The zinc finger transcription factor Snail1 is one of the main factors controlling the influence of remodeling on the bone mass. The molecular mechanism of its action involves the repression of Runx2 and vitamin D receptor (VDR) transcription in differentiating osteoblasts (Frutos et al., 2009).

The above information does not exhaust the complexity of the set of factors with local action regulating the process of remodeling bone tissue and, accordingly, bone mass (Lai SF et al., 2009). The entire set is under the control of systemic (hormonal) factors, among which the most important roles are played by calcitonin, the parathyroid hormone, estrogens, and hormones from the vitamin D group.

Molecules relevant to the central (hypothalamic) and peripheral (sympathetic) nervous systems' functions – neuropeptide Y, neuromedin U, dopamine, serotonin, endocannabinoids and others, as well as their receptors – undoubtedly participate in the regulation of remodeling. The mechanisms of this participation are poorly understood. They are probably similar to the action mechanism of leptin and other neurohormones on bone metabolism (Elefteriou, 2008).

As has already been noted several times above, kinases (phosphotransferases) – enzymes that carry out the activation of proteins by phosphorylation (addition of phosphate groups) of specific amino acid residues – are the intracellular effectors of the signals for both the local and systemic factors regulating osteoclastogenesis and osteo-clasts' function. Many receptors exhibit kinase activity, as well as proteins that directly interact with receptors and proteins affecting intracellular signal transduction pathways. Tyrosine and serine/threonine residues are the most frequent phosphorylation targets. This role of protein kinases is common to all cells.

In addition, cells possess an enzymatic mechanism, which limits the results of the kinase activity of protein phosphorylation in the cell and ensures optimal levels therein. This restriction is achieved in osteoclasts through protein tyrosine phosphatases (PTP) – enzymes that cleave the phosphate group from tyrosine residues in proteins. In the osteoclast, there are four active PTP, three of which (Cyt-PTP-ε, PTP-PEST and PTP-oc) are positive regulators of osteoclastic bone resorption, while the fourth (SHP-1) has a negative effect on the resorptive function (Sheng & Lau, 2009).

Coupling or, in other words, attaining a positive outcome of remodeling, requires the presence of osteoprotegerin in the remodeling focus. Turning off the osteoprotegerin gene disrupts the coupling of osteoclast and osteoblast functions, and the resorbing bone is not replaced with new one (Nakamura et al., 2003).

Short-distance signaling molecules – RANKL, growth factors and cytokines – evidently represent direct regulators of the remodeling process. For this reason, one of the essential conditions for effective coupling of bone resorption and formation is close contact of interacting cells inside BMU. Connexons provide this contact (Stains & Civitelli, 2005).

The participation of Wnt-morphogens in the regulation of bone remodeling is associated with mechanobiological processes. Mechanical stress causes the rapid accumulation in osteoblasts of β-catenin, the central element of the canonical Wnt signal pathway (see section 8.5.2). The expression of genes affected by Wnt intensifies in osteoblasts (Case et al., 2008). Furthermore, mechanical stress decreases the expression by osteocytes of sclerostin, an inhibitor of Wnt signals. Owing to this, Wnt successfully exert their stimulating activity on the anabolic stage of remodeling (Turner et al., 2009).

Signals about the dynamics of the intracellular calcium ion concentration are transmitted from cell to cell in the bone tissue, in particular, in BMUs, through more complex pathways. Besides calcium ions, small molecules affecting the opening and closing of calcium channels of the cytoplasmic membrane can pass into neighboring cells through gap junctions. Calcium level fluctuations in osteoblasts caused by mechanical stimuli are accompanied by the secretion of nucleotides (probably adenosine triphosphate), which act as ligands for the P2Y2 transmembrane receptor of neighboring osteoblasts. The signal transmitted by this receptor enhances the production of inositol-3-phosphate (IP3), releasing the calcium ion from its links within the cell. A similar paracrine effect of adenosine triphosphate, expressed by osteoblasts, also extends to nearby osteoclasts, stimulating their resorptive activity. The effect on osteoclasts is mediated by another, very similar, transmembrane receptor – P2X7 (Jorgensen, 2005).

The molecular mechanisms of regulating osteoclastic resorption in bone remodeling are connected to the molecular mechanisms of the immune system's functioning. The fact is that osteoclasts and cells of the immune system – phagocytes (macrophages) and dendritic antigen-presenting cells – are descendents of a common progenitor – the hematopoietic stem cells in bone marrow. The same signaling molecules participate in regulating the differentiation of osteoclasts and these immunocompetent cells. The receptors sensing these signals are similar in nature, including the so-called Toll-like receptors, represented both in osteoclasts and in different cells of the immune system – not just in macrophages, but also T cells, B cells and NK (natural killer) cells (Takayanagi, 2005).

The connections between bone tissue and the immune system are not limited to the common origin of immune cells and osteoclasts. These relationships are also determined by osteoclasts' and immune cells' common reaction to the action of numerous regulatory factors – a number of interleukins and other cytokines, interferons and growth factors (Lee DH et al., 2008). The common reaction results from the participation of the same transcription factors therein. Among these factors, the transcription factor (phosphorylated nuclear protein) c-Fos (Matsuo & Ray, 2005) and representatives of the RANK and nuclear factor of activated T-cells (NFAT) families, specifically NFATc1, are particularly important (Takayanagi, 2007).

For this reason, the ongoing processes in the immune system inevitably affect the dynamics of osteoclastogenesis and osteoclast functional activity in normal remodeling and, even more so, in pathological states, particularly by inflammatory and infectious conditions (Wu et al., 2008).

Through constant contact and information exchange between osteoclasts and cells of the osteoblastic differon, the latter also become involved in interaction with the immune system. Regulatory factors functioning in the immune system (e.g. NFAT) participate, with the intermediation of osteoclasts, not only in bone resorption, but also in the formation of bone tissue (Koga et al., 2005; Winslow et al., 2006).

Furthermore, cytokines and other signaling molecules with short-distance activity, expressed by cells of the immune system, directly influence the differentiation and function of cells of the osteoblastic differon. This direct effect is especially pronounced in the bone marrow, where it occurs via physical contact between the cells of both systems (Lorenzo et al., 2008).

The widely developed network of systemic regulatory factors and local (short-distance) factors make the skeleton a stable metabolic system, whose functions are controlled according to a feedback principle (Harada & Rodan, 2003). The influence of various signals entering the cells of both differons – osteogenic and osteoclastic – and regulating the mechanisms of apoptosis is of principal importance. These signals ensure the necessary and sufficient viability of bone cells (Xing et al., 2005).

Under normal conditions, this entire system preserves its stability by solving two opposing tasks:

1) maintaining the optimal calcium concentration in the body fluids and, therefore, in the cells; and

2) maintaining the strength and other biomechanical properties of bones. The stability of the total bone mass is the main indicator of the system's stability (Civitelli, 2008. Harada & Rodan, 2003).

8.7. TOOTH CONNECTIVE TISSUE

8.7.1. Structural Organization

Human and animal teeth are specific bone formations mainly involved in food processing (primary mechanical processing–disintegration). This function of the teeth is provided by their structure, form and properties. Like any other bone formations a tooth base is comprised of dense regular and irregular mineralized and non-mineralized connective tissue as well as structured mineral in the form of calcium phosphate (hydroxylapatite). This connective tissue borders (surrounds) a cavity, which is filled in with loose irregular connective tissue directly passing into non-mineralized connective tissue. Loose irregular connective tissue performs all the functions specific for connective tissue. Four basic components of teeth–the dentin, enamel, cementum and the pulp are made of the aforementioned types of connective tissue.

8.7.1.1. Pulp is made of loose irregular connective tissue (*Fig.8.41*) which comprises an intercellular matrix made up by loosely arranged collagen fibrils without particular preferred orientation (I and III type collagen) which exist independently or form fine collagen fibers or membranes where the fibrils are located as a non-oriented network; elastic fibers, an integrating buffer metabolic medium (glycoconjugates, mineral salts, tissue proteins and water). Fibrous structures form special meshes inside which a glycoconjugated gel is located. There are cellular elements (cells of fibroblastic and odontoblastic differons, lymphocytes, macrophages, dendritic cells, mast cells and plasmatic cells as well as blood vessels and nerves) inside the intercellular matrix.

8.7.1.2. Dentin is the main functional part of a tooth, which base is composed of a connective tissue mineralized to a variable degree. Mature dentin contains about 70% of inorganic substances (hydroxylapatite crystals predominantly), about 20% of organic substances (type I collagen mainly) and 10% of water. There are no cellular elements in the dentin.

Morphologic characteristics of dentin organic component

Dentin contains dense regular and irregular mineralized and non-mineralized connective tissue (*Fig.8.42*). As in a bone tissue the dentin intercellular matrix has numerous tubules radiating outward where odontoblast processes are located (*Fig. 8.42*). The tubules can be seen in tissue cross- and longitudinal sections or studied in micro-corrosion specimens (*Fig.8.43*). Unlike a bone the odontoblasts are only in the pulp mainly near or on a dentin inner surface faced towards the pulp chamber or a tooth root canal. The dentin comprising the tooth main part has no cells. There are anastomoses between the tubules in which odontoblast process branches are located. An organic component of the tooth intercellular matrix is comprised of individual collagen fibrils mainly composed by type I collagen and having a specific periodic structure of 64–70 nm (*Fig. 8.42*). The fibrils have a diameter of 40–50 nm, are located relatively dense and without particular preferred orientation around dentin tubules. Individual collagen fibrils fix the spatial position of odontoblast processes in a dentin tubule. In some regions the fibrils form fibers, which may also have an ordered or non-ordered orientation. Along the border between the pulp and the dentin mineralized connective tissue there is a thin layer of non-mineralized intercellular matrix, which is an analogue to osteoid in a bone.

Characteristics of mineral component structure

A mineral matrix is one of two main tooth intercellular components as in bone. Its base is composed by calcium phosphate in the form of crystalline hydroxylapatite. Its crystal organization has a prominent polymorphism, which specificity differs from that of a bone. The crystal form depends on a part of the tooth where it is present, the tooth topography, the degree of its maturation, a person's age, the chemical composition of the food he/she takes and so on. A selective removal of a tooth organic part by dissolving it in sodium hypochlorite allows isolating and retaining a tooth mineral matrix and its further examination with SEM as in a bone.

The dentin structural organization has the pattern of formation of a bone tissue. Several forms of crystalline hydroxylapatite (*Fig. 8.44*) make up a native (free of organic materials) dentin mineral matrix. A layer of the mineral directed particularly into a lumen of the dentin tubule is the most variable in structure. It can be presented by:

1) rectangular-shaped (including square-shaped) lamellar crystals with a thickness of 5–10 nm with side sizes ranging from 30 to 100 nm (the largest part has a size of 50–70 nm);
2) rod-like or needle-shaped crystals with a width of 10–20 nm, contacting with each other and forming a 3D network inside which lamellar crystals can be located;
3) a granular substance consisting of 3–7 nm-sized mineral granules diffusely located or forming chains from which a meshed structure can be made up (*Fig. 8.44*).

A mineral matrix located between the tubules comprises crystals which differ in form. These can be loosely arranged crystal conglomerates, lamellar crystals with a width of 5–10 nm without definite borders as they are part of a crystal complex looking like a peculiar "monolith", rod-like or needle-shaped crystals with a width of 10–20 nm and a length of up to 100 nm (*Fig. 8.44*). The mineral main mass surrounding the tubules consists of all types of the aforementioned hydroxylapatite crystals which can be arranged with a varying degree of density i.e. calcification or mineralization of the given part of the tooth dentin. Polymorphism of crystals is obviously due to a constant physiologic (non-physiologic in particular cases) dynamic structuring and rearrangement (re-crystallization). This is associated with meta-

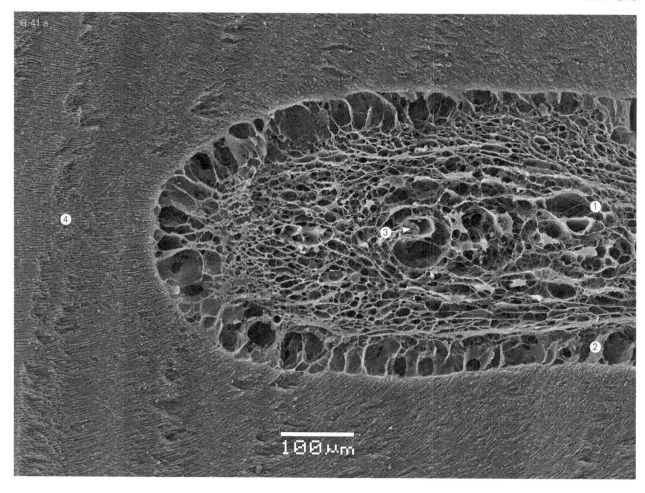

8.41 a

100 μm

Fig. 8.41.
An organic (fibrous) part
of a tooth intercellular matrix.
A surface of a tooth cut
parallel to its long axis.
The pulp–central (1)
and peripheral (2) parts.
Blood vessels (3).
Dentin (4).
Dentinal tubules (5).
Fine collagen fibers
and fibrils(6).
Flat collagen
fibers(membranes) (7).
SEM-micrograph.
a–x 150;
b–x 300;
c–x 600;
d–x 3,000;
e–x 5,500.

>
Fig.8.42.
An organic (fibrous) part
of a tooth dentin.
A surface of a tooth cut parallel
(a, b) and perpendicular (c, d)
to its long axis.
Dentinal tubules (1).
Collagen fibrous(2) fibrils(3)
of the extracellular matrix.
An odontoblast process
in a dentin tubule (4).
SEM-micrograph.
a, c–x 3,000;
b, d–x 10,000.

>
Fig. 8.43.
A polymer replica (impression)
of tooth dentinal tubules (1).
Anastomoses (2).
SEM-micrograph.
a – x 500;
b – x 2,000.

>
Fig. 8.44.
A tooth mineral base (matrix).
Tooth dentin.
a, b, c, d, e – a sample surface
of split parallel to the
arrangement (radiation) of tooth
dentinal tubules.
f, g, h, i – a sample surface
of split tangential to the
arrangement (radiation) of tooth
dentinal tubules.
Dentinal tubules (1).
Intratubular mineral matrix (2).
Lamellar crystals in the form
of rectangule (3).
Rod-like or needle-shaped
crystals (4).
Granular substance (5).
Granule chains (a meshed
structure) (6).
Lamellar crystals in the form of
scales (7).
SEM-micrograph.
e, i – x 5,000;
d, h – x 20,000;
c – x 50,000;
a, b, g, f – x 100,000.

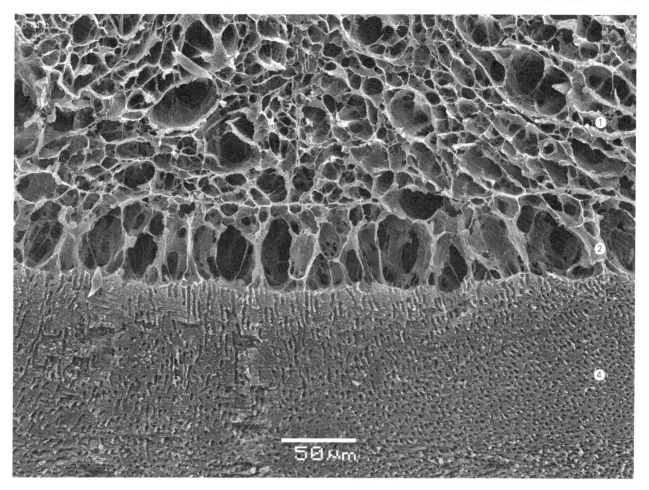

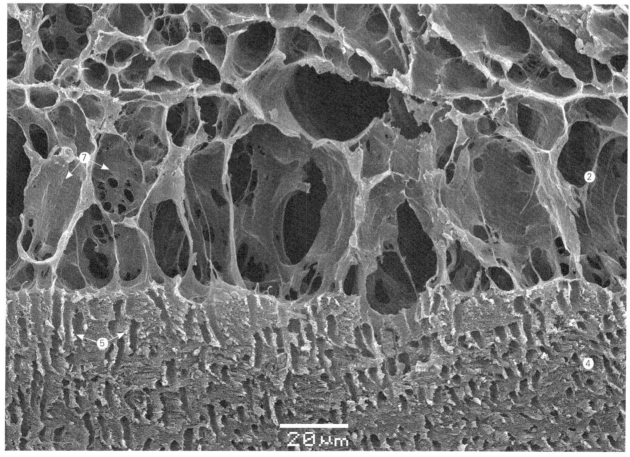

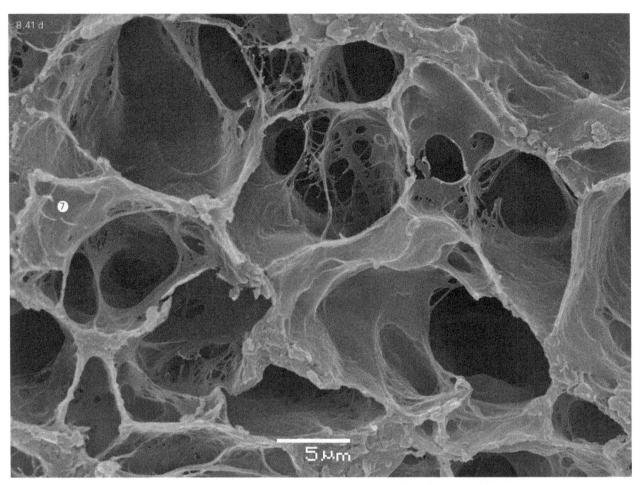

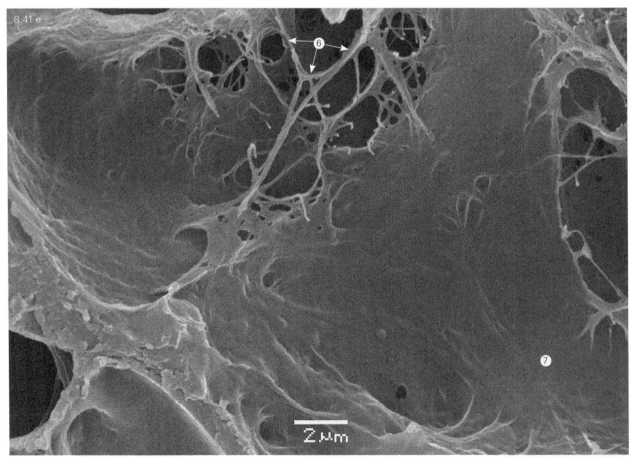

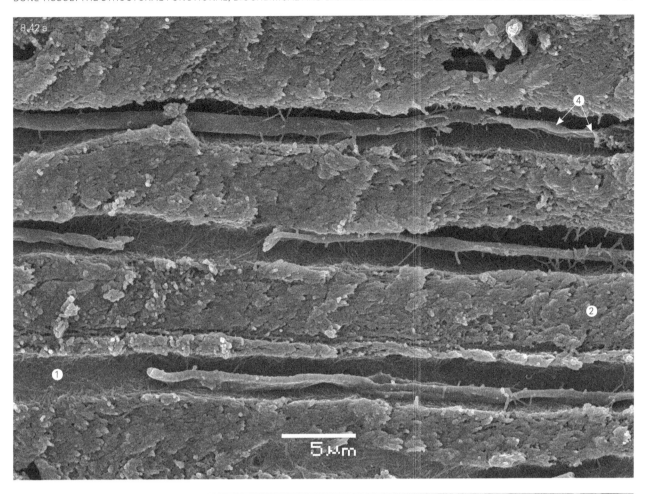

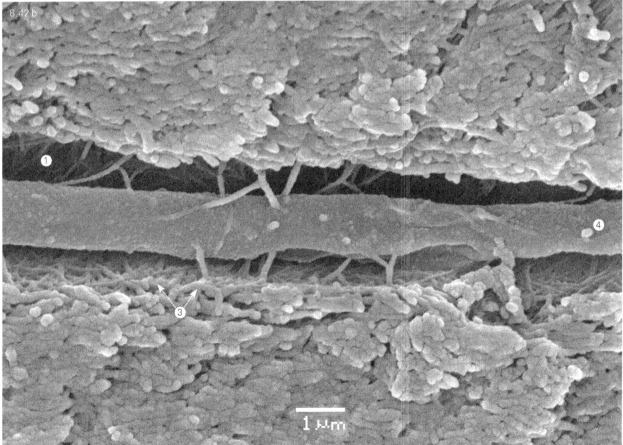

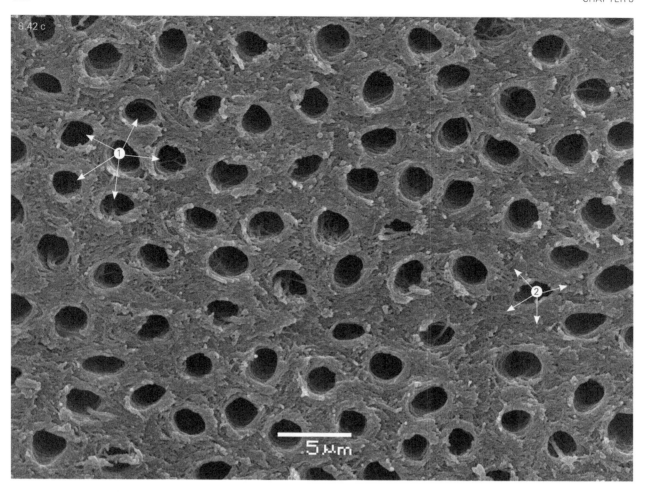

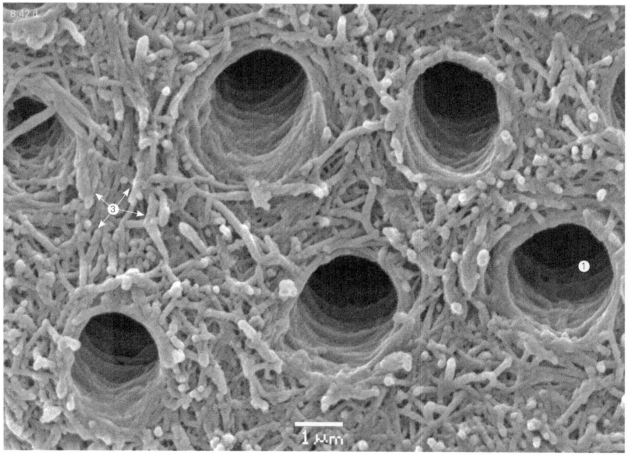

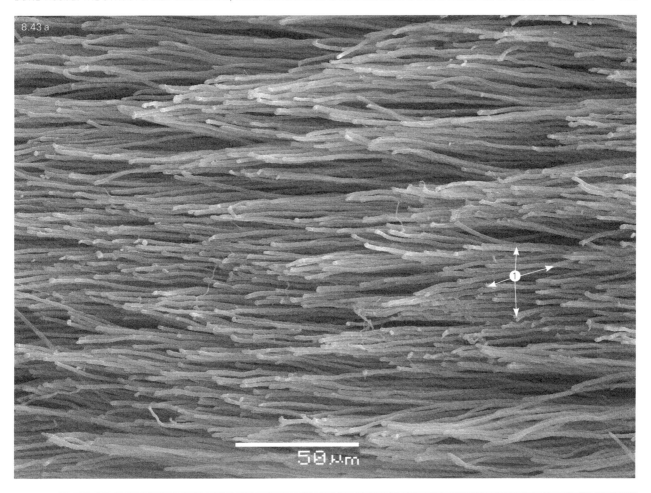

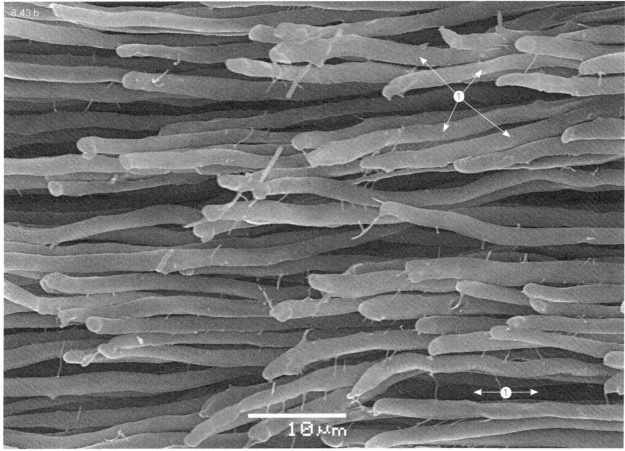

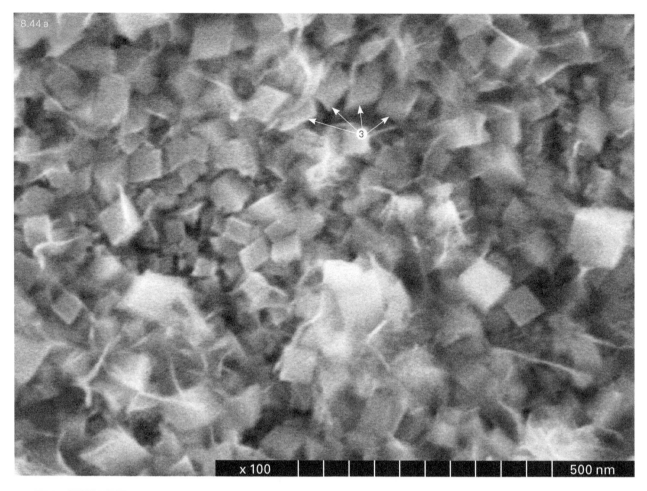

8.44 a

x 100   500 nm

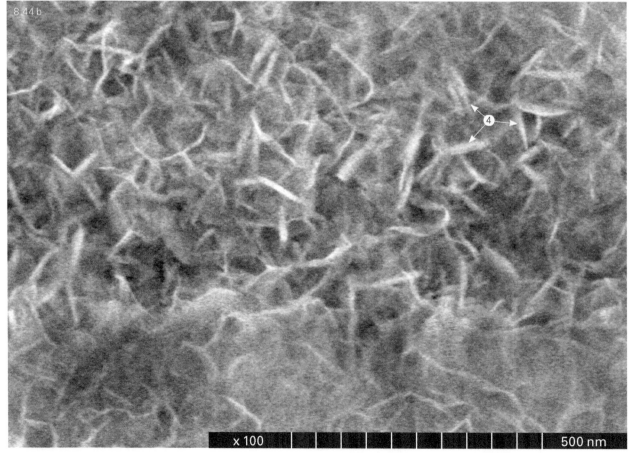

8.44 b

x 100   500 nm

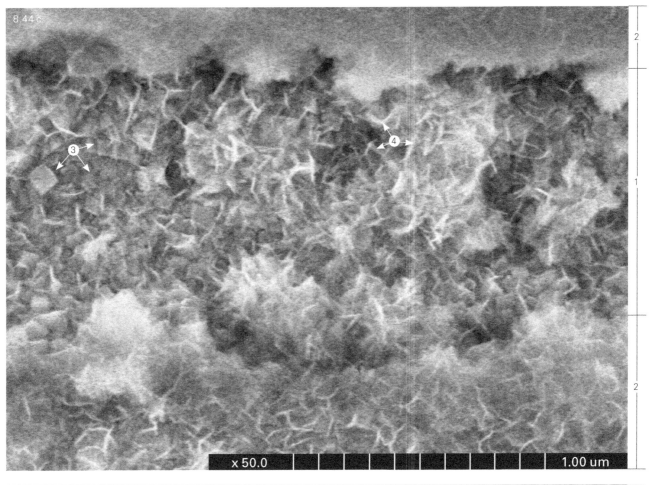

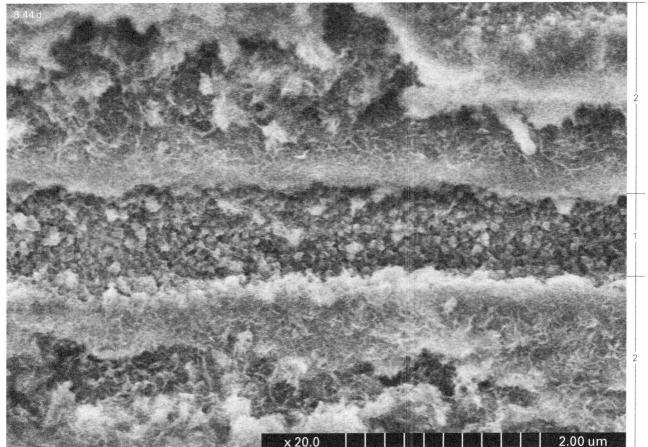

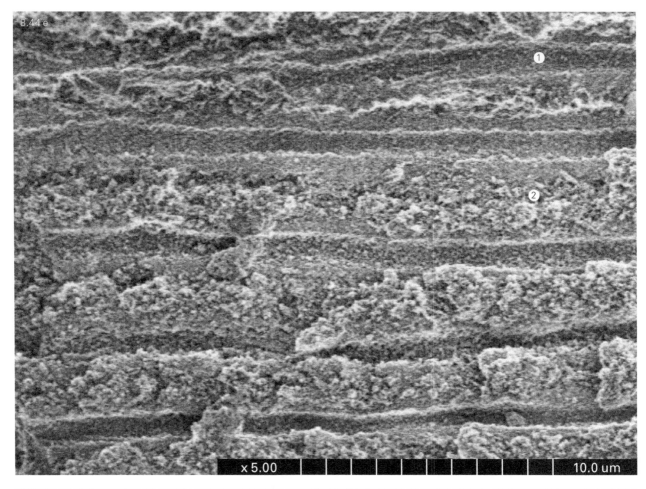

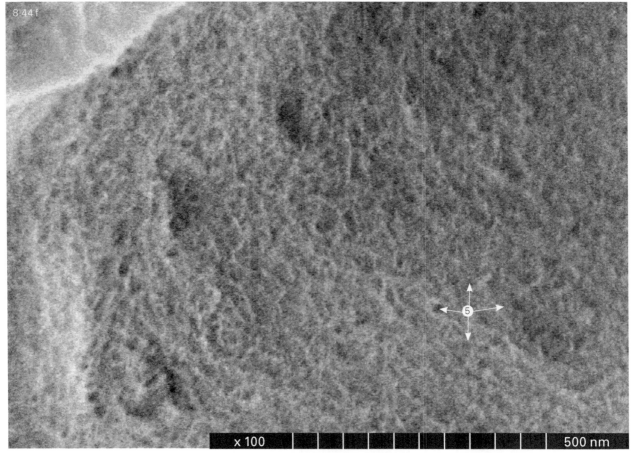

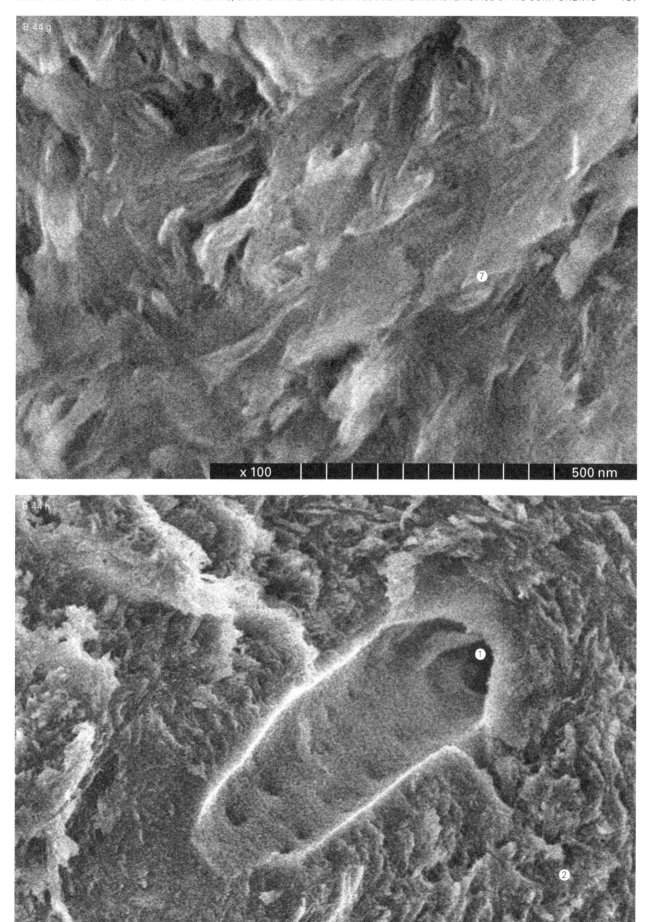

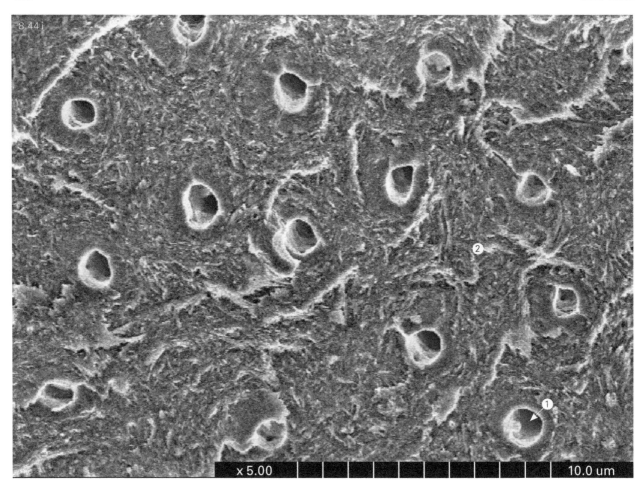

8.44 i

x 5.00   10.0 um

bolic processes ongoing in tooth tissues, their physiologic renewal and possibly reparative regeneration. Dentin directly passes into enamel, which covers it. But collagen fibrils of dentin do not pass into enamel.

8.7.1.3. Enamel

An inorganic fraction comprises 97% of a tooth enamel dry weight. 98% of this fraction consists of hydroxylapatite, carbonate apatite, fluor apatite, while 2% being non-apatite crystals. Enamel has a high hardness and is comparable to some sorts of steel by this parameter. It is rather brittle and could be cracked under significant mechanical loading, but it does not occur owing to a layer of more resilient dentin underlying it. Enamel contains no cells therefore it is not capable to regeneration. Nevertheless there is ion exchange in it; these ions enter it from both the dentin and saliva. Enamel de-mineralization and remineralization take place. Enamel is made up by enamel rods, an interrod substance and rod-free enamel and is covered by a cuticle. Enamel rods are its main structural and functional units. Their form significantly varies. They pass in bundles tangentially from the surface to a dentin-enamel border.

An enamel superficial (cuticle-free) layer consists of granular (granules of 3–5 nm in diameter) nanoaggregates (20–100 nm), which are distributed with a varying density in this layer (Fig. 8.45). In dense flattened regions

the aggregates are separated between each other by narrow (5–7 nm) tortuous furrows. In other regions there are crypts where the aggregates are located more loosely. Such a structure is obviously due to the peculiarities of a mechanical effect on teeth. In deeper layers (when studying splits perpendicular to a tooth surface) hydroxylapatite crystals are lamellas with a thickness of 5–7 nm, a width of 20–100 nm and an undetermined length that are located parallel to each other and perpendicular or tangentially to a tooth surface (Fig. 8.45). The lamellas are densely adjacent to each other, forming complexes in which they have a particular preferred orientation. The complexes can be located angled to each other as part of an integrated mineral matrix (Fig. 8.45).

>
Fig. 8.45.
A tooth mineral base (matrix).
Tooth enamel.
a – a natural surface of tooth enamel.
b, c, d, e, f – a surface of an enamel split perpendicular to the tooth surface.
Granular nanoaggregates (1).
Crypts (2).
Intraaggregate furrows (3).
Lamellar long rectangular

crystals of hydroxylapatite (4).
Lamellar crystalline complexes (5).
Enamel prisms (6)
Intraprismatic crystalline aggregates (7).
SEM-micrograph.
a, b – x 100,000;
c – x 50, 000;
d, e – x 20,000;
f – x 10,000.

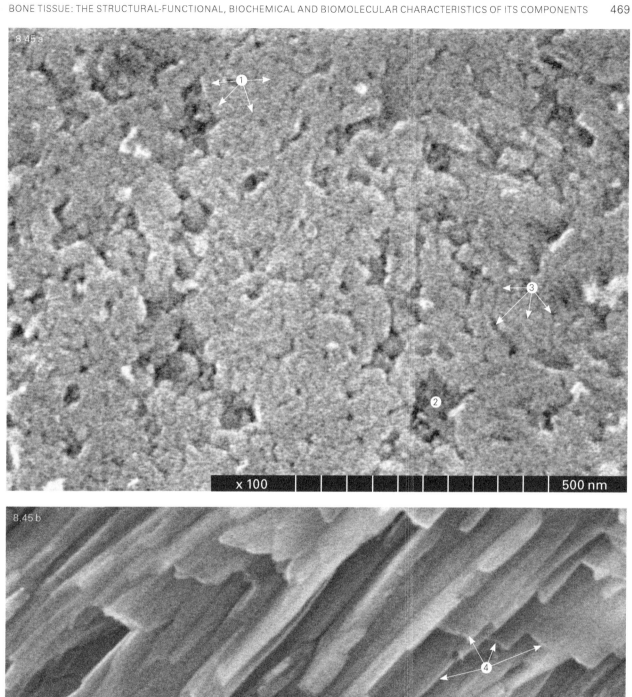

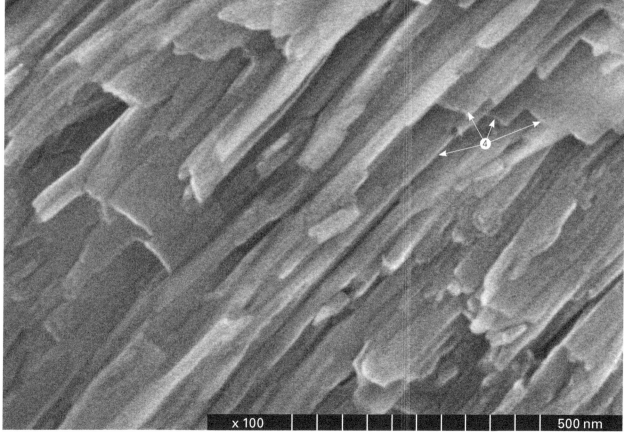

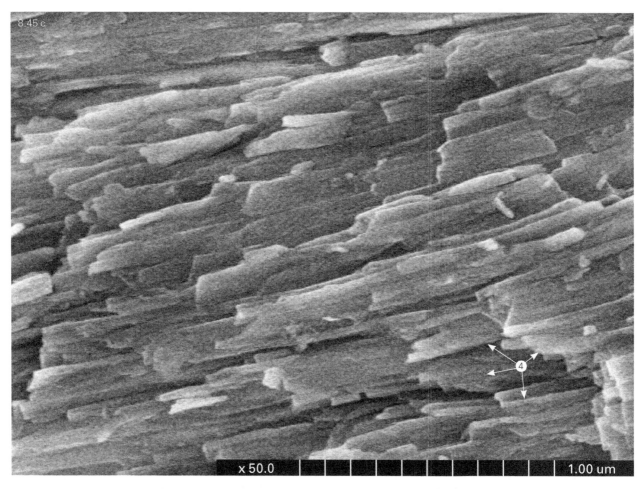

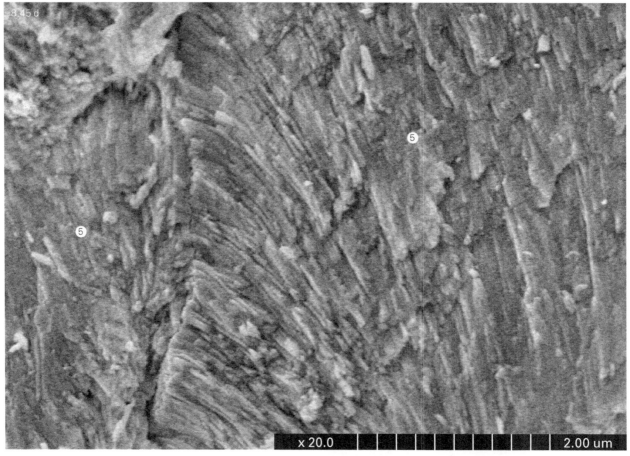

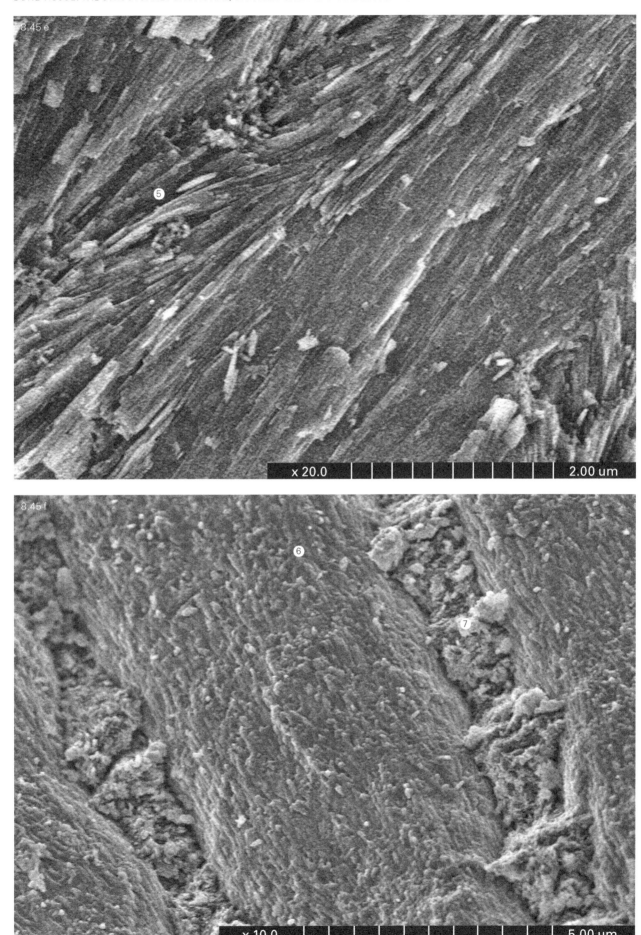

Chapter 9

BIOCHEMICAL
CHARACTERISTICS
OF SYNOVIAL
MEMBRANE
AND SYNOVIA

9.1. SYNOVIAL MEMBRANE

Diarthrosis, a synovial joint, which provides a flexible unification of the skeleton bone elements, comprise four structural components:
1) articular cartilages;
2) a joint capsule and intra-articular ligaments;
3) a synovial membrane; and 4) synovia (synovial fluid).
The biochemical and molecular biological characteristics of articular cartilages, which are typically hyaline cartilaginous tissue, were already described in Chapter 7. The peculiarities of the special subtypes of intra-articular ligaments in some joints, meniscs and disks, composed of fibrous cartilaginous tissue, have also been discussed therein.

The joint capsule and intra-articular (and periarticular) ligaments uniting bones to other bones are made of dense formatted fibrous connective tissue, the biochemical and molecular biological features of which are outlined in section 3.5.3.

The synovial membrane (synovial coat)–the fine inner layer of the joint capsule composed of loose non-shaped fibrous connective tissue–borders the joint cavity on one side, and, on the other, turns into dense fibrous connective tissue of the outer, thicker layer of the capsule. There is no synovial membrane on the uncovered intraarticular surfaces of the inner articular cartilages. It is of significance that, from the side of the joint cavity, neither the synovial membrane nor the articular cartilages have any special border-line coating.

The synovial membrane is one of varieties of connective tissue where the cell elements quantitatively predominate the extracellular matrix, particularly due to the surface layer. The specialized (covering) cells of the membrane are referred to as synoviocytes, with two known types: type A synoviocytes and type B synoviocytes. These cells do not constitute a continuous layer and there are areas of uncovered extracellular matrix between them. Besides synoviocytes, the membrane contains an insignificant number of histiocytes, plasma cells, mast cells (heparinocytes), lymphocytes and blood macrophages.

Type A synoviocytes are mobile and are capable of actively phagocyting cell wastes from the synovia. They express antibodies and some cytokines (interleukins). The type A cells originate from blood mononuclear cells and are considered as tissue (resident) macrophages, unlike blood macrophages. They are also referred to as macrophage-like synoviocytes.

The type B synoviocytes are characterized by an intensive development of the granular endoplasmic reticulum and the presence of branching processes that form a network on an inner (inward to the joint cavity) membrane surface. Having significant biosynthetic activity, these cells produce the main macromolecular components of the synovia (in particular, hyaluronan) and the synovial membrane extracellular matrix. Type B synoviocytes are a specialized kind of fibroblast in terms of their morphological and functional characteristics (Iwanaga et al., 2000). Sometimes they are called synovial fibroblasts (SF).

The synovial membrane has no clear-cut outer boundary and its fineness can account for the practical inability to its precise preparative separation. This also makes it difficult to carry out a biochemical study of the membrane. Therefore, a significant part of the findings on the biochemical characteristics of the membrane has been obtained by means of various histochemical and cytochemical methods, and this data are not quantitative. The advantage of this data is that it makes it possible to evaluate the distribution of the components revealed according to the membrane layers–an inner layer, directly adjoining the synovia (intimal), and a deeper (subintimal, collagen-elastic) layer. At the same time, this data is also significantly contradictory; this divergence might be due to the differences between membrane layers, which were not always taken into account when studying the entire membrane, as well as interspecific differences inherent to the synovial membrane (Revell et al., 1995).

The collagen-elastic layer is comprised of a network of fine collagen fibers, characterized by argyrophily (impregnated with silver), which indicates a deposition of glycoproteins on the surface of these fibers, predominately consisting of type III collagen. These fibers are defined as reticular (Ushiki, 2002).

Data on collagen components of the synovial membrane are rather inconsistent. On the one hand, there are reports that the synovial membrane of rabbits contains type III, V and VI collagen, with the quantitative prevalence of type III collagen forming the above-mentioned network of reticulin fibers. According to these data, type III collagen makes up more than 50% of the total collagen mass, which significantly exceeds this collagen content in other connective tissue varieties in adults.

The formation of a network of microfibrils (with a diameter of about 9 nm) have also been described (in rabbits as well). This network is located within the intimal layer at a depth of 2–3 μm from the surface i.e. it can be referred to a surface collagen-elastic complex (Levick & McDonald, 1990). The ultrastructural characteristics of these microfibrils correspond to the properties of type VI collagen; they are not like fibrillin microfibrils. The expression of type VI collagen by cultured synovial membrane cells has also been detected (Wolf & Carsons, 1991). Both *in vivo* and in an extracellular matrix produced by the culture, type VI collagen is found in the surface (intimal) layer, together with fibronectin, which generally indicates its expression by synoviocytes located nearer to the surface and a certain functional relationship between these macromolecular components. Type VI collagen is also found in the walls of synovial membrane blood vessels.

Other immunohistochemical investigations of the human synovial membrane intima (Revell et al., 1995) have confirmed the presence of only type V and IV collagens in this layer (the latter shall be discussed separately). It may be supposed that type III collagen is concentrated in a deep collagen-elastic layer, and whether it is present in the intima of the human synovial membrane remains unclear.

One of the specific peculiarities of synovial membrane collagens is the presence of a glucosylgalactosylpyridinoline non-reducib-le cross-link (Glc-Gal-PYD) (Garnero et al., 2001). Bone and cartilage collagens have no such cross-link; the appearance of peptides containing this link in urine in joint disorders might be considered as an indicator of the destruction of synovial membrane collagens and of its involvement in a pathological process.

Together with collagen fibers, the collagen-elastic layer contains the fibers stained with orcein–a staining substance specific for elastic fibers. There is a lack of any information about the biochemical properties of the synovial membrane elastin.

The presence of hyaluronan in significant amounts within the surface layer is the most essential peculiarity of the in- terfibrillar matrix of the synovial membrane (Worrall et al., 1991), which is absolutely natural in terms of the immediate contiguity of the membrane and the synovial f luid. It is the synovia where the hyaluro- nan concentration is especially high. In a healthy human, synovial membrane hyaluronan is mainly found around synoviocytes in the surface layer, with lower concentration in deeper layers.

Proteoglycans, containing chondroitin 4-sulfate, chondroitin 6-sulfate, keratan sulfate and heparin sulfate as glycosaminoglycan components, have been shown to be present in the synovial membrane. According to research findings in rabbits whose synovial membranes contained the corresponding core proteins, chondroitin sulfate was found to be present in biglycan and decorin macromolecules, while keratan sulfate was found in fibromodulin (Coleman et al., 1998).

According to immunohistochemical findings, there is a very thin layer of fibronectin macromolecules in the most superficial layer of a mouse's synovial membrane (Linck et al., 1983). This suggests that fibronectin plays an important functional role in the vital activities of the synovial mem- brane. This suggestion is confirmed by a biosynthesis of fibronectin by the cultured sections of a normal human membrane (Lavietes et al., 1985). Upon being synthesized in such a culture, fibronectin was not only secreted into the cultural medium but also embedded into a resulting matrix. It is probable that both type A and type B synoviocytes take part in fibronectin production. It may be assumed that interacting with a network of collagen fibers and proteoglycan components of the extracellular matrix fibronectin forms a special layer on the border between the synovial membrane and synovial f luid. This layer controls the exchange of substances between these two media. One of tenascins, tenascin-X, appears to be an obligatory component of the normal synovial membrane (Li et al.,2000). It is also found in a synovial pseudomembrane, developed around loosening joint prostheses, and it is of probable impor-

tance for stabilizing the supramolecular structural organization of the membrane extracellular matrix.

Macromolecules known as basement membrane components (the above-mentioned type IV collagen and laminins) have been detected in synovial membrane tissue, particularly around blood vessels, using immunohistochemical methods. This is of particular interest in connection with the lack of morphologically structured basement membranes within the synovial membrane. There are basement membranes neither inside nor outside the membrane, neither between the membrane layers, nor around blood vessels (Revell et al., 1995).

Type IV collagen is represented by a limited set of isoforms, mainly, α1(IV) and α2(IV) polypeptide chains, together with a few α5(IV) and α6(IV) chains within the synovial membrane. This is the difference between the synovial membrane and the tissues, with formed basement membranes containing all of the six known isoforms. The mRNA of type IV collagen isoforms of the membrane has been found in synovial fibroblasts (type B synoviocytes). It is assumed that components of the basement membrane in the synovial membrane play a certain organizing role in the extracellular matrix structure. The fact that the abrupt decrease in type IV collagen observed in rheumatoid arthritis is accompanied by the increased permeability of the synovial membrane for white blood cells favors this hypothesis (Poduval et al., 2007).

As in other types of connective tissue, all the structural components of the extracellular matrix in the synovial membrane are expressed and secreted by fibroblasts and, in the given case, by specialized synovial fibroblasts (type B synoviocytes, SF). The same cells are producers of macromolecular components, enabling interaction between the synovial membrane cells. These components are the adhesive molecules of cell membranes (VCAM-1, ICAM-1) and desmosome proteins, as well as two cadherins–cadherin 11 and N-cadherin–specific for mesenchymal cells (see section 3.6.3). Each of these cadherins acts as a part of separate supramolecular complexes within the synovial membrane (Agarwal et al., 2008).

Type B synoviocytes produce not only components of the synovial membrane extracellular matrix but also specific components of the synovial fluid–proteins that differ from blood plasma proteins–as well as hyaluronan. In vitro studies demonstrate that the synthesis of hyaluronan is controlled by pro- and anti-inflammatory cytokines (Hyc et al., 2009).

Along with the structural components, the synovial fibroblasts express enzymes that participate in metabolic processes within the synovial membrane, synovia and articular cartilages. Metalloproteases of the ADAMTS family (see section 3.7.1) are among these enzymes. ADAMTS-enzymes, particularly ADAMTS-5, which is responsible for the catabolism of aggrecan, a large proteoglycan of cartilaginous tissue, enters articular cartilage through the synovia (Vankemmelbeke et al., 2001). Cathepsin K, expressed by synovial fibroblasts, is engaged in the destruction of the collagens of articular cartilages during pathological processes (Hou et el., 2001).

Apart from the biosynthesis of the macromolecular components of its own extracellular matrix and specific components of synovia, and the opposite processes of the catabolism and resorption of the synovia, the synovial membrane serves the function of controlling substance exchange (diffusion) between blood plasma and the synovia. This exchange depends on two factors.

The first factor is constituted by the physical and chemical features of the synovia (synovial fluid) itself due to the high concentration of high-polymeric glycosaminoglycan, hyaluronan, therein. This factor, conditioning the high viscosity of the synovial fluid, creates special circumstances for the bilateral diffusion of molecules through the synovial membrane. In vitro experiments demonstrate that the greater the hyaluronan's molecular mass (and respectively the longer its macromolecules are), the more significant impact that this polymer will have on the physical and chemical conditions of molecule diffusion (Coleman et al., 2000). With a molecular mass of 530 kDa and more, hyaluronan becomes a buffer, restraining the fluid release from the synovia into the interstitial spaces of the synovial membrane.

The second factor is the structure of the synovial membrane. As previously mentioned, it lacks structured basement membranes, as a result of which there are no other barriers except for the capillary endothelium, not tightly adjoining cells of the synovial membrane (synoviocytes), and the extracellular matrix that is located between the circulating blood and the synovia. This means that there is actually no barrier for low-molecular substances to penetrate the synovial fluid from the blood plasma and back. In fact, under normal conditions, the concentrations of electrolytes, glucose, uric acid, low-molecular antibiotics and other small molecules in the synovial fluid differ only a little from their concentrations in blood.

However, a detailed investigation into the kinetics of this balance have shown that this process cannot be reduced to only the physical diffusion of molecules through a membrane permeable for them. In fact, the transsynovial exchange of a number of the molecules studied appeared to be different from that which was expected based on their molecular mass. For instance, the rate for the transsynovial exchange of water, studied in a normal human knee joint using tritium marking, is significantly lower in comparison with the ideal rate for diffusing molecules of this size. It appears that a molecule's traffic through the synovial membrane is subject to more complicated regularities in relation to metabolic processes taking place in the membrane and synovia.

9.2. SYNOVIA (SYNOVIAL FLUID)

9.2.1. General general characteristics of synovia. Protein components

The synovia (synovial fluid) is found inside synovial joints (diarthroses), in an enclosed space (a cavity) that is bounded by cartilage-covered bone ends and a joint fibrous capsule, lined with the synovial membrane.

The synovia is often considered as a biologic fluid, enabling the free movement of bones connected to each other and facilitating movement conditions thanks to the synovia's inherent lubricating properties. At the same time, the synovia is considered as a blood plasma dialysate, formed mainly by diffusing molecules from plasma. The synovia is distinguished from other body fluids by its pronounced viscosity. As for synovia that just resulted from puncturing a joint, the term tenacity would be appropriate. In storage, even in the short-term, at room temperature and especially when kept in a fridge, the viscosity increases so much that the fluid becomes a gel that cannot be poured from a tube. In more precise physics terms, these characteristics of the synovia are described as a property of non-Newtonian fluid and a property of thixotropy. A non-Newtonian fluid is a fluid, the viscosity of which depends on changes in its flow rate (the dependence is not linear). Thixotropy (*Greek thix-* is – act of touching, *tropé* – alteration) is the dependence of fluid viscosity on mechanical impact. The viscosity of a thixotropic fluid increases gradually at a constant temperature over time when under continuous exposure, for instance, at the same flow rate. At the same time, a thixotropic fluid is able to gradually restore the original structure (viscosity) that has been mechanically destroyed.

These properties are due to the presence of a significant amount of high-polymeric hyaluronan interacting with numerous protein components in the synovia. At the same time, the concentration of most low-molecular organic components and electrolytes differs a little from that of these components concentrations in blood plasma (*Table 9.1*).

The synovia, like blood plasma, is slightly alkaline – its pH in human ranges between 7.2 to 7.8, more often being around 7.4 (blood plasma pH is 7.35 – 7.45).

But the definition of the synovia as "a blood plasma dialysate plus hyaluronan" is not precise. A number of facts showing to the existence of some other differences between the synovia and blood plasma/serum, besides the presence of hyaluronan in the synovia, do not agree with the definition given. Even the small differences that attract our attention in *Table 9.1* (in the urea and glucose concentrations) do not fit with the presentation of the synovia as a plasma dialysate. Moreover, differences (both an increase and decrease) in the concentration of a number of microelements, such as aluminum, nickel, cobalt and cadmium, have been detected between plasma and the synovia. The normal synovia is hyperosmo-

Table 9.1.

Concentrations of some low-molecular components in synovia of the knee joint and human blood plasma (mmol/100 g)

Component	Synovia	Blood plasma
Sodium	136	135–155
Potassium	4	4–6
Calcium	2,4	2,2–2,75
Uric acid	2,35	1,8–2,9
Urea	3	3,4–7,5
Glucose	4	4,2–5,5

lar relative to blood serum: the synovia osmolality is 400 mM/kg on average, while the serum osmolality is 300 mM/kg.

These factors are enough to draw the conclusion that the inflow of its components into the synovia from circulating blood is not confined to the phenomenon of dialysis and is not limited to diffusion. The process of forming the synovia composition is more complicated.

One of the factors complicating diffusion is the size and shape of the molecules diffusing through the synovial membrane. The role this factor plays becomes distinctly clarified upon studying the protein composition of the synovia. While, as shown in *Table 9.1*, the concentrations of non-organic salts and ions, urea, uric acid, glucose in the synovia hardly differ from those of the low-molecular substances in blood plasma, the concentration of macromolecular protein components differ significantly in blood plasma and the synovia.

The total content of proteins in knee synovia (nearly all studies have been carried out on this object) is 1.3–2.0 g/100ml. This concentration is 3–4 times lower than the total concentration of proteins in blood plasma (6.0–8.0 g/100ml), which provides evidence of the limited diffusion of protein macromolecules through the synovial membrane. Other more prominent element of support for the significance of the macromolecule size involved in this process is the complete lack of fibrinogen (the largest protein macromolecule in blood plasma) in the sinovia. In the absence of fibrinogen, the synovia protein set is similar to that of blood serum in terms of its composition, with the majority of proteins detected in the synovia identical to those found in blood serum by immunochemical parameters.

However, the mechanism of forming the quantitative and qualitative protein composition of the synovia cannot be reduced to the diffusion of protein molecules from serum into the synovia, and the macromolecules' size is not the only factor determining the intensity of the diffusion. This concept contradicts the fact that the differences in the relative concentrations of some globulins in the synovia and in blood serum are not very significant – even less than the difference in concentrations of albumin, the smallest macromolecule among all blood serum proteins (*Table 9.2*). In particular, this refers to some immunoglobulins. For example, the concentration of albumin in the synovia is about one-third the amount of its concentration in plasma, while the concentration of immunoglobulins IgM and IgA amounts to 70–90% the level found in the synovia although their molecular mass greatly exceeds that of albumin.

One of explanations for this seemingly paradoxical fact might be related to the dynamic state of the synovia (Simkin, 1995). The quantitative biochemical parameters of the synovia reflect the balance of the import or inflow of molecules diffused from the blood to the synovia, and the export or outflow of molecules from the synovia, preferably to the lymph. Therefore, the relatively high concentration of immunoglobulins (and other globulins) in the synovia might depend upon a slower

Table 9.2

Comparison of the concentration (mg/100 ml) of some proteins in the synovia and blood serum

Proteins	Synovia	Serum	Synovia/ Serum
Albumin	1,400 ± 200	3,800 ± 350	0,37 ± 0,00
α1-acid globulin	65 ± 3	135 ±15	0,48 ± 0,20
Ceruloplasmin	19 ± 4	36 ± 6	0,53 ± 0,09
IgA	120 ± 70	150 ± 100	0,90 ± 0,40
IgM	93 ± 40	145 ± 55	0,71 ± 0,30
IgG	500 ± 110	1,030 ± 190	0,49 ± 0,57

rate of the outflow from a joint in comparison with albumin.

There might be active selective permeability of the synovial membrane in response to certain immunoglobulins that promote the maintenance of their concentration at the required level within a joint. Moreover, the maintenance of this level may be enabled by the local synthesis of immunoglobulins by the immunocompetent cells of synovial membrane classified as type A synoviocytes (see section 9.1.1).

All these qualitative peculiarities of the synovia protein composition are in complete contradiction with the definition of the synovia as a blood plasma dialysate.

The evidence that there are qualitative differences in the protein composition of the synovia and blood serum, such as the presence in healthy synovial and appearance in pathologically altered synovia of a number of proteins that are absent in the serum, runs counter to this definition even more.

Thus, normal synovia contains chondroitin sulfate proteoglycans (about 150 nM/ml of chondroitin sulfates), which are present only in blood cells but not in plasma and, therefore, cannot penetrate the synovia by diffusing from plasma, i.e. they have a local (synovial) origin (Nakayama et al., 2000).

Proteoglycan 4 encoded by a *PG4* gene is such a proteoglycan containing chondroitin sulfate and keratan sulfate. Several homologous proteins are the result of alternative splicing and post-translational modifications of this gene transcript. One of them, known as lubricin,

takes part in fulfilling the lubricating function of the synovia (Schmidt et al., 2009).

The use of modern highly sensitive methods of proteomic analysis to study synovia proteins showed the number of proteins found in the synovia to be significantly higher than was previously thought. One such study (Gobezie et al., 2007) of knee joint synovia in normal people and patients with osteoarthrosis identified the total 135 proteins. The expression intensity of 18 of them was statistically reliably different between the groups of normal subjects and the patients. The concentration of three proteins whose function in the synovia is to be studied, was higher in the normal synovia. They are

1) aggrecan, a large proteoglycan of articular tissue expressed by chondrocytes;
2) cystatin A (or stefin-A), an inhibitor of thiol (cystein) proteases;
3) dermcidin (DCD-1), a small protein with an antibacterial activity previously studied in the secret of sweat glands. The two latter proteins are expressed by synovial fibroblasts.

It is pertinent to note that puncturing normal joints is rare and is only performed in special studies with volunteers. The most interesting are the findings on the activity of synovial fibroblasts (type B synoviocytes) in different pathological conditions, as these findings allow to evaluate the functional potential of these cells and their role in the formation of the synovia macromolecular structure.

The biosynthetic potential of synovial fibroblasts is especially obvious in inflammatory pathological processes involving joints, particularly in the case of rheumatic arthritis. One of the products of this activity is c190rf10 protein (anti-inflammatory cytokine) secreted into the synovia, which is also known as UPF0556 or interleukin 25, consisting of 142 amino acid residues after a signal peptide removal (Weiler et al., 2007).

In rheumatoid arthritis there is also hyperexpression by synovial fibroblasts and secretion into the synovia of fibronectin, semaphorine 7a epidermal growth factor receptorbound protein 7 (GRB7), galectin-1 and several other proteins (Kim C.W. et al., 2006). Synoviolin, a transmembrane phosphoprotein of the endoplasmic reticulum membrane, expressed by synovial fibroblasts, is very important in preventing their apoptosis and maintaining homeostasis within a joint. This protein exhibits enzymatic activity of the ubiquitin-protein ligase, which enables it to discard protein molecules with impaired (malfolded) conformation. The need in such a molecule 'controller' in the synovia is justified as the amount of defect molecules synthesized in rheumatic arthritis reaches 30% (Yagishita et al., 2008).

Using methods of proteomic analysis, 501 peptides of an endogenous origin have been identified in the normal synovia and in that of patients with osteoarthrosis (in the absence of inflammation symptoms). These peptide fragments are the metabolic products of 40 proteins, expressed by the synovial fibroblasts and chondrocytes in articular cartilage. These include six proteins whose presence in the synovia is typical for osteoarthrosis (type II collagen, proteoglycan 4, tubulin, vimentin, matrix Gla-protein, serum amyloid A protein–SAA) (Kamphorst et al., 2007).

Type B synoviocytes secrete fibronectin, a structural adhesive glycoprotein of the extracellular matrix of all types of connective tissue, into the synovia (Iwanaga et al., 2000). Its normal concentration in the synovia is, on average, 170 µg/ml (Belousov et al., 1987). Synovial fibronectin cannot penetrate into the synovia by diffusing from plasma. Firstly, the molecular mass of fibronectin is high enough for it to be identified as proteins unable to diffuse through the synovial membrane; a prolate form of a fibronectin macromolecule also prevents its diffusion. Secondly, in some pathologies, the fibronectin concentration in the synovia significantly exceeds that in plasma. Thirdly, peculiarities of the fibronectin macromolecule structure in the synovia give evidence that this fibronectin isoform differs from that in plasma. One of fragments of this isoform, released in rheumatic arthritis, with a molecular mass of 45 kDa (Fn-f45), induces an expression of matrix metalloprotease MMP-13 (collagenase-3) by chondrocytes of articluar cartilages and stimulates the activity of aggrecanases, proteases that destroy the proteoglycans of cartilaginous tissue (Stanton et al., 2002).

In this context, it must be noted that the proteolytic enzymes (MMP and ADAMTS) acting in the synovia play a significant role in the pathogenesis of arthropathies, although their activity controlled by tissue inhibitors is not high under normal conditions (Jones et al., 2008). The functions of the synovia proteases, generated by the surrounding tissues, are not limited to the destruction of the macromolecular components of these tissues and the synovia itself. Proteases also regulate the activity of numerous signal molecules (growth factors, cytokines) in the synovia and thus, enable the maintenance of homeostasis in a joint (Punzi et al., 2002).

The synovia is also a medium where protein-arginine deiminases act. Protein-arginine deiminases are the enzymes performing the so-called citrullination of some arginine residues in the macromolecules of several proteins, particularly in fibronectin. Citrullination (the trasnformation of arginine into citrulline) deprives a protein of its electric charge and changes the macromolecule conformation, which converts it into an autoantigen. This process is deemed as rather important in the pathogenesis of rheumatic and other inflammatory arthritides (Kinloch et al., 2008).

All these data characterize the complexity of the synovia protein composition and the metabolic processes therein. They comprise a set of arguments that demands abandoning the conception, according to which the synovia is considered as a just blood plasma dialysate with the addition of hyaluronan.

At the same time, these findings support another, more general point of view, according to which the synovia is a distint highly specialized type of a connective tissue extracellular matrix.

There are three types of bone connection synarthrosis (this type combines syndesmosis, synchondrosis and synostosis), amphiarthrosis and diarthrosis. (Gay & Miller, 1978).

All three types of joints evolve from the same mesenchyme tissue areas where primary cartilaginous buds (limb buds) are formed. The first two types–synarthroses and amphiarthroses–are strong but do not provide mobility of connected bones or enable it insufficiently.

As for kinds of synarthroses, synostosis (the joining of the cranial bones in an adult) absolutely lacks any mobility, where the mesenchymal (intermediate) interlayer is replaced by bone tissue so that there is no gap between the bones. Syndesmosis is characterized by a very limited flexibility, persisting between the bones in very small children, when a dense fibrous tissue develops between bones and is gradually displaced right until the complete fusion of bones is achieved. Synchondrosis is almost immovable as it is a joint that consists of hyaline cartilage between the epiphysial and diaphysial regions of long bones in embryonal and early postnatal development (growth plates). As the growth ceases, the hyaline cartilage therein is also displaced by bone tissue.

Some more flexibility persists in amphiarthrosis throughout the entire life, an example being the joint uniting the two pubic bones. In this joint, the space between the bones is filled with fibrous cartilage, which is rich in type II collagen and is elastic and extensible to some extent. Similar joints also develop between vertebral bodies.

Thus, both in synarthrosis and in amphiarthrosis, bones are united with various types of connective tissue, originated in primary mesenchyma. Diarthroses, joints providing extremity bones with the maximal motility required for the normal existence of the vertebrate, are of the same origin. On the one hand, the evolvement of diarthroses required the origination of special structures fastening a joint (a joint capsule, intra-articular and capsular ligaments) and, on the other hand, it required the differentiation of a specialized extracellular matrix–the synovia. This peculiar matrix, unifying tissues that comprise a joint, does not prevent but rather facilitates movements of bone ends.

The definition of the synovia as a type of extracellular matrix is confirmed by the anatomy of diathroidal joints. The joint cavity, filled with the synovia, differs from other fluid-containing cavities of the body (serous–abdominal and pleural) by the absence of a continuous cell sheet separating the joint content from the surrounding tissue. The walls of serous cavities are lined with a continuous layer of mesothelial cells, which is a distinct border between the fluid and the tissues, with nothing separating the joint cavity from surrounding tissues, i.e. articular cartilages and the synovial membrane. The synovia directly washes against the superficial cells of these tissues in the same way as the extracellular matrix contacts a cytoplasmic membrane of the cells of other connective tissue types. Herein the cells that the synovia adjoins are type B synoviocytes (synovial fibroblasts), which are cells of connective tissue with typical functions, the biosynthetic function being the main one. Synoviocytes secrete macromolecules directly into the synovia and, like in other types of connective tissue, cells synthesize extracellular matrix (this can be seen in fibroblasts, osteoblasts, and chondroblasts/chondrocytes). The most active biosynthesis made by synoviocytes B, the biosynthesis of hyaluronan, is indigenous to other connective tissue cells; this glycosaminoglycan is present in the extracellular matrix of many varieties of connective tissue, although its concentration there is not so high as in synovia. Along with hyaluronan, synoviocytes secrete other macromolecules, which can be considered as its structural components, as well as enzymes and biologically active peptide factors (growth factors, cytokines) into the synovia. Synoviocytes A also contribute to the composition of the synovial fluid, being in a direct contact with it.

The synovia also adjoins directly to the articular cartilages–there are no separating structures here, and the continuous cross-diffusion of molecules occurs between the synovia, which is a means of providing cartilaginous cells with basic substances for metabolism, and the extracellular cartilage matrix. The regularities of this diffusion are not determined by the functioning of any specialized barriers but preferably by the physical and chemical and structural properties of the contacting cartilaginous matrix and synovial media.

Regarding the synovia as a special kind of the extracellular matrix unifying various types of connective tissue present in a diarthroidal joint increases the importance of the synovia (synovial fluid) as an object for investigations in terms of clinical practice. Widening the scope and improving the methods and control systems for these investigations are important issues for consideration in the field of present-day arthrology (Swann et al., 2002).

9.2.2. Synovial hyaluronan

The most prominent peculiarity of the synovia is an extraordinarily high concentration of hyaluronan. The concentration of hyaluronan (hyaluronic acid) is significantly higher in the synovia than that in any other tissue with the exception of the eye vitreous body; this concentration is not less than two orders higher than the level of hyaluronan concentrations in other biologic fluids.

Some differences in hyaluronan concentrations are ascertained to be in various joints. This conclusion is based on the results of investigations carried out on animals, since, as a rule, only synovia of the knee and, sometimes, temporomandibular joints are studied in humans. It has been determined that changes in the hyaluronan concentration in the synovia of a human knee joint are dependent on age: an increaing during growth and subsequently decreasing as of 29 years of age. None of these differences and changes are very large.

Hyaluronan (hyaluronic acid) is present as a sodium salt in the synovia, which is why it is not hyaluronan but hyaluronate that is often spoken about. This is of specific significance, as cation bound to hyaluronan greatly affects the conformation of its molecules. The conformation of hyaluronan is especially actively changed by divalent cations, calcium and magnesium, changing the location of intramolecular cross-links in a spiralized macromolecule.

The physical properties of hyaluronan solutions (viscosity, sedimentation, light scattering and light refraction) form the basis for the idea that its macromolecule at a salt concentration close to the physiologic one, particularly in synovial fluid, has a conformation of a chaotic tangle. The radius of this tangle is very large in the molecular scale–about 150–400 nm. Thus, the macromolecule occupies a volume in a solution that is 1,000–10,000 times more as its own volume. Although the molecular mass of hyaluronan is truly gigantic, sometimes being 10,000 kDa, the density of a resulting macromolecular tangle does not exceed 0.003 g/ml. In other words, one milliliter of a normal synovial fluid contains not more than 3 mg of hyaluronan.

Such a behaviour of a hyaluronan molecule accounts for some properties of the synovia. The first of these properties is the so-called sieve or filter effect (Laurent et al.,

1995). This effect is that other molecules entering a hyaluronan-containing solution diffuse slower than they otherwise would do in the absence of hyaluronan. This slowing down occurs in the sedimentation of molecules by centrifugation as well, and is more strongly expressed the larger the diffusing molecules are. Therefore, it concerns high molecular substances much more. Also, the movement of smaller molecules up to free ions is altered to some extent under the influence of a sieve formed by hyaluronan tangles.

The sieve effect in the synovia due to a high concentration of hyaluronan is one of the factors determining the above-mentioned specific quantitative characteristics of the synovia biochemical composition, distinguishing it from the blood serum dialysate, together with the peculiarities of the synovial membrane permeability.

The sieve effect in itself is close to another property of the synovial fluid–the so-called excluded volume effect (Laurent et al., 1995). It is that other molecules cannot penetrate a space occupied in fluid by a hyaluronan tangle despite this tangle looseness. This space appears to be unavailable and excluded for other molecules. The value of an excluded volume is not the same for different molecules; this value depends on molecules' size, and is higher for larger molecules.

The consequence of the excluded volume effect, in combination with the sieve effect, is a peculiar phenomenon that can be referred to as the phenomenon of the uneven distribution of molecules. It can be explained in the following example.

If two spaces (we designate them A and B) are separated by a membrane with pores that are 100–200 nanometers in size (such pores are sufficient for the passing of macromolecules of serum albumin and globulins, but are too small for hyaluronan macromolecules), then both spaces are filled with a buffer solution, and hyaluronan is put only in space A. After adding, for example, albumin in an equal concentration to both spaces, equilibrium is achieved as a result of the diffusion of protein macromolecules when the albumin concentration in space A, containing hyaluronan (C_A), will be lower than the concentration in space B (C_B). In other words, the equilibrium constant K-value $= C_B/C_A$ will exceed a unit at any initial concentration of albumin.

Given the concentrations of hyaluronan attributable to the normal synovia, the volume excluded for serum albumin macromolecules is calculated as approximately one-third of the total volume of synovial fluid. This result corresponds to the actual difference in the concentration of albumin in blood serum and that in synovia. It also corresponds to the difference in values of the albumin-globulin ratio in the synovia and serum, which can be explained by the fact that, when increasing the size of diffusing molecules, the excluded volume for them increases. Thus, the excluded volume for globulins is larger than that for albumin. For low molecular substances such as glucose, for example, the excluded volume effect in the synovia is so small that it can be neglected.

A theoretical background for the sieve effect and excluded volume effect is based on the concept of the chaotic character of hyaluronan tangles conformation. However, there are findings that lead to seeing this concept as simplified. Some molecules diffuse in the synovial fluid not only quicker than should otherwise be expected according to the sieve effect but even more rapidly than occurs in a pure solvent (for instance, in water), even when some part of the non-excluded volume has already been occupied by macromolecules of the proteins impeding the free diffusion.

This effect can be explained by the origination of an interaction between diffusing molecules, on one side, and an organized supramolecular structure of hyaluronan, on the other. The main factor determining the origination of this structure is hyaluronan macromolecules' ability to form supramolecular aggregates through self-assembly. It seems probable that the synovia protein components acting as hyaladherins participate in organizing the supramolecular structure. The bond of hyaluronan and hyaladherins is not covalent; the hypothesis on the existence of a special proteoglycan, hyaluronate-protein, has not been confirmed. But this non-covalent bond is so strong that hyaluronan preparations absolutely free of a slight admixture of proteins cannot be obtained by using any methods of extracting and purifying hyaluronan from the synovia.

Albumin appeared to be one of hyaladherins in the synovia (Scott & Heatley, 1999). Hyaluronan's ability to bind and restrain fluid within a joint appeared to decrease by 20% in the absence of albumin (when replacing a natural synovia in a joint with an artificial hyaluronan solution free of other components).

The presence of organized tertiary and quaternary structures of hyaluronan (involving protein components) confirmed by nucleic magnetic resonance as well as electron microscopic and X-ray results, provides a network of hyaluronan macromolecules in the synovia with a certain rigidity. "Corridors" or "tunnels" appear where accelerated diffusion takes place.

As hyaluronan is the quantitatively prevailing component of the synovia (the synovia can be considered as a concentrated solution of hyaluronan), it is hyaluronan–a structural organization of its solution–that determines the specific biomechanical and rheological behavior of the, synovia which, while not identical to the properties of a hyaluronan solution without impurities, is essentially similar. These peculiarities combine two properties: elasticity and viscosity (a property that is opposite to flow ability) (Fam et al., 2007).

This is because the network structure formed by very long convoluted hyaluronan macromolecules in a solution is connected by numerous intra–and intermolecular bonds. Given a rapid but short-term flow of fluid, these bonds are retained; the synovia (hyaluronan network) behaves as an elastic material in such settings (for example, in the case of a fast movement in a joint). Given a slow, prolonged flow of a solvent (for example, in the case that a bending angle in a joint is altered for some time), the bonds are broken, the hyaluronan threads are straightened, and the fluid proceeds between them, submitting to viscosity laws. Shift deformations peculiar to viscous materials occur, improving the biomechanical conditions of interaction of articular cartilage surfaces. Thus, it is possible to say that hyaluronan performs the same function in the synovia as it does in other types of connecting tissue – the function of organizing an extracellular matrix structure. This conclusion is additional support of the view that synovia is one of the extracellular matrix types, adapted to the motor function of diarthrodial joints during their evolution.

9.2.3. Molecular mechanisms of synovia lubricating function

Apart from transporting nutrients for biosynthetic (anabolic) reactions to chondrocytes in articular cartilages (which blood vessels do not reach) and the reverse transport of catabolism products, synovia solves a number of tasks of great importance for joints' biomechanical functions. These include the amortization of load on jointed bones; synovia bolsters the shock-absorbing function of articular cartilage and enlarges the conglutination of articular surfaces. But the main function of the synovia is to maintain the diarthrodial joints' basic function i.e. mobility of jointed bone elements of the skeleton. Mobility demands "lubrication" between the moving opposed articular surfaces of bones. The lack of "lubrication" in a joint would inevitably lead to a rapid process of wearing jointed surfaces, owing to friction caused by movement. The synovia provides such necessary lubrication.

The synovia's lubricating activity is determined by three co-operating molecular factors entailed therein:
1) the basic macromolecular component of the synovia, hyaluronan;
2) a special "lubricating" protein, lubricin;
3) surface-active phospholipids. The presence of all three factors is considered as an indispensable condition for the functional completeness of the synovia (Meng & Long, 2008).

The decreasing effects of **hyaluronan** solutions and the synovia on the friction coefficient between glass and rubber surfaces has been proven in an experiment. This effect is in a direct ratio to viscosity which, in turn, is directly proportional to the hyaluronan concentration and polymerization degree. However, despite the high concentration of hyaluronan, causing the expressed lubricity of the synovia, hyaluronan's own lubricating effect in joints is insignificant. This was already established a long time ago through the depolymerization of the synovia hyaluronan in an experiment involving incubation with hyaluronidase.

This is due to the fact that hyaluronan's lubricating activity is manifested as **hydrodynahymic lubrication**, which is the lubrication of a fluid layer moving between

jointed surfaces. The potential of such lubrication is limited, especially in joints of the lower extremities that have been exposed to heavy static load. During in vitro experiments, hyaluronan solutions do not sustain the pressure that the joints are exposed to. The maximum load that does not destroy the supramolecular organization of hyaluronan solutions, does not exceed 0.4 kg/cm^2, whereas the load on a human knee joint in an upright position is about 3 kg/cm^2. The synovia, upon losing its viscosity at such a pressure, is 'pressed' into the extracellular matrix of articular cartilages.

The fact that mobility in joints is not impaired under these conditions means that other factors/mechanisms are of more significance in joint lubrication, in comparison with hyaluronan and the hydrodynamic mechanism. These mechanisms, enabling the lubrication of joints during movement under pressure (at static load), function as **boundary lubrication**, the essence of which is to form an immovable film on adjoining moving surfaces, which can sustain pressure and reduce friction.

Synovia's main component, which forms boundary lubrication, is a protein **lubricin** (derived from Latin *lubrico* – to make slippery) (Swann et al., 1985). This glycoprotein, with a molecular mass of 151 kDa and consisting of 1404 amino-acid residues, contains a lot of N-linked and O-linked oligosaccharide residues, as well as chondroitin sulfate and keratan sulfate glycosaminoglycans, i.e. it is a proteoglycan. The recommended modern name of lubricin, **proteoglycan 4** (PG4), is also the name of a lubricin encoding gene (*PG4*) and covers all other products of this gene, homologous to lubricin. They include a megakaryocyte stimulating factor (MSF), hemangiopoietin (HAPO) and a **superficial zone protein** (SZP) of articular cartilage – the closest to lubricin – with the only difference found in their carbohydrate components. SZP expression is a peculiar function of superficial layer chondrocytes (Rhee et al., 2005).

Lubricin is expressed and secreted into the synovia by synovial fibroblasts (type B sy-noviocytes); its concentration in the synovia reaches 30 µg/ml. Adsorbed from synovia by the cartilage surfaces, lubricin moves cartilages apart, thereby improving mobility

Lubricin has a complex domain structure. Globular hydrophobic N- and C-terminal domains, whose conformational stability is maintained by disulfide bonds, facilitate lubricin adsorption on cartilage surfaces. Generally the large C-terminal domain maintains adsorption (Jones et al, 2007; Zappone et al., 2008). Adsorption is more effective on a cartilage surface than on other artificial ones, adsorption strength being the precondition which makes the lubricin smearing action boundary (Gleghorn et al., 2009).

The primary structure of a lubricin macromolecule core protein has some similary with a the vitronectin macromolecule (see section 3.2.1.1). Unlike vitronectin, the lubricin macromolecule has a large central hydrophilic elongated mucin-like domain, containing a repeated motif KEPAPTTT.P. This domain carries numerous O-bound negatively charged oligosaccharides, which give it a form comparable to a brush, and are located on a surface at adsorption. The electostatic repulsive interactions of oligosaccharides adsorbed on opposite surfaces of articular cartilages create a free space between surfaces, thereby improving mobility (Jay et al., 2001).

The mechanism of lubricin's smearing action is probably not limited by electrostatic repulsive interactions of the molecules adsorbed. In model experiments with recombinant lubricin, it was established that the simultaneous presence of lubricin that is adsorbed and lubricin that is dissolved in the synovia increases the lubrication efficacy. This leads to the assumption about the existence of other mechanisms (Gleghorn et al., 2009).

The role of lubricin in joints is not limited to its lubricating function. It not only facilitates sliding of cartilage surfaces but prevents their deterioration due to friction. Lubricin ranges among the proteins capable of being bound to hyaluronan. This binding affects the synovia supramolecular structural organization formed by hyaluronan. It provides the synovia with certain elasticity, promoting the dispersion of energy stress on joints during movement. This effect of lubricin is also chondroprotective (protecting joints), but it is also of independent significance unrelated to its lubricating function (Jay et al., 2007).

Silencing (a homozygous negative mutation) the gene *Prg4* in mice causes pathological changes of articular cartilage surfaces, which appear several months after birth. These changes, like the pannus observed in rheumatic (inflammatory) arthritis, constitute protein depositions and the colonization of cartilage surfaces by proliferating synovial fibroblasts. Thus, lubricin appears to control the proliferation of type B synoviocytes and protect cartilage surfaces (Rhee et al., 2005). People who lack the *PRG4* gene exhibit autosomal-recessive pathology, described as a CACP (camptodactyly–arthropathy–coxa vara–pericarditis) syndrome. Arthropathy manifests itself as a subintimal fibrosis of the synovial capsule and a non-inflammatory hyperplasia of synoviocytes (Faivre et al., 2000).

The expression of lubricin by synoviocytes and SZP (superficial zone protein) that is almost identical to it by chondrocytes is suppressed by pro-inflammatory cytokines and growth factors, particularly IL-1 and TNF-α, and is stimulated by TGF-β and oncostatin M (Jones and Flannery, 2007).

Even before the discovery of lubricin, when hydrodynamic hyaluronan smearing was thought to be the main lubricating factor of the synovia, it was commonly believed that the lubrication mechanism in diarthroidal joints was an exception to the general pattern. It was known that, in all cases where adjoining biological tissues are in movement (sliding) towards each other (for example, in pleural, pericardiac and peritoneal cavities), there is a functioning boundary lubrication mechanism, which implies that the adjoining surfaces are covered with the finest (oligolamellar) layer of sur-

face-active phospholipids (**SAPL**). This general mechanism corresponds to the hydrophoby (nonwettability with water) of adjoining surfaces; by the way, the articular cartilage surfaces are hydrophobic (Hills, 2000). Therefore, attempts to find a similar, lipid components-based mechanism of boundary lubrication in joints were undertaken.

It was supposed that cholesterol esters in a liquid-crystal state might play the role of a lubricant in boundary lubrication (Bely et al., 1984). Cholesterol concentration in the synovia is about 3 mM/l; polarization- microscopic examinations enabled the detection of lighting aggregates similar to cholesterol crystallites, which can reduce friction on the surface of articular cartilage (Voronovich et al., 1987).

These investigations were not further developed and the researchers' attention switched to the above surface-active phospholipids (SAPL), which are detected by electron microscopy in the form of so-called lamellar bodies on a synoviocyte B surface inside a joint cavity and on an articular cartilage surface. SAPL are synthesized by synoviocytes B; this synthesis and secretion of SAPL into the synovia are stimulated by glycocorticoids (Hills et al., 1998). SAPL form a film adsorbed on a surface of articular cartilages, which is composed of phosphatidylcholine (41%), phosphatidylethanolamine (27%), sphingomyelin (32%) (Sarma et al., 2001). The destruction of this film by a phospholipase 2 enzyme sharply enlarges the friction coefficient in a joint that confirms the role of phospholipids as a factor in boundary lubrication (Hills and Monds, 1998).

Synoviocytes B maintain their ability to produce SAPL for many years after a total endoprosthesis replacement of joints (Purbach et al., 2002). Many SAPL, including eight types of diphosphatidylcholines, are found on all carrying surfaces of artificial joints, irrespective of the nature of materials used therein (Gale et al., 2007). This fact is important evidence of the lubricating role of SAPL in joint functions.

There is data suggesting that surface-active phospholipids act as a lubricating factor in joints, not by themselves but as lubricin components. According to this data, lubricin is a lipoglycoprotein, and phospholipids compose about 11% of its molecular mass. Lubricin plays the role of a carrier for a water-insoluble (and therefore, in the synovia) active lubricant agent–SAPL (Schwarz and Hills, 1998). The proteolytic destruction of lubricin, by exposing the synovia to trypsin action, does not lead to the deterioration of its lubricating properties.

Moreover, it has been established in an in vitro experiment that for synovia that has been treated by trypsin, the coefficient of friction between articular cartilages even decreases because SAPL are easier precipitated and adsorbed on the cartilage surface upon losing their carrier (Hills and Monds, 1998). Nonetheless, the opinion exists that the lubricating efficiency of SAPL is higher when they are bound to lubricin rather than when they are free (Jay & Cha, 1999).

Determining the role of SAPL in joint lubrication brings this lubricant into line with lubricating mechanisms in all other cases involving the movement of adjoining biological tissues, acting as boundary lubrication with the participation of surface-active phospholipids. However, at the same time, the mechanism of articular lubrication is thought to be more complex, and complications raise its reliability.

Firstly, lubricin's own boundary lubricating activity due to the above-mentioned peculiarities of its polypeptide core central domain structure, along with the activity of surface-active phospholipids, becomes apparent. In other words, two interconnected complementary factors of boundary lubrication affect joints.

Secondly, hyaluronan, to some extent, contributes to the boundary lubrication of articular cartilages. The method of confocal scanning laser microscopy (CSLM) has revealed that the synovia hyaluronan assumes a liquid crystal structure in those zones where the gap between opposed cartilage surfaces is especially narrow. The film with such a structure withstands intra-articular pressure and can serve as boundary lubrication. It is interesting that this film is not formed on the surface of artificial materials used in the endoprosthesis replacement of joints (Kobayashi and Oka, 2003). Hyaluronan is an effective carrier of lubricin in the synovia, it promotes lubricin adsorption on the cartilage surfaces and enhances its anti-adhesive action (Chang et al., 2008). Besides, high-molecular hyaluronan protects SAPL from degrada-

tion by the synovia endogenous phospholipase A2 (Nitzan et al., 2001).

Thirdly, it should be noted that almost all research on the synovia's lubricating function in vivo was carried out on knee and coxofemoral joints. Therefore, we cannot rule out the possibility that in joints, especially small ones in humans' upper extremities, where static load is not so great, the boundary lubrication by lubricin and SAPL is supported by the hydrodynamic lubrication of hyaluronan. Anyway, the role of hyaluronan as a component in the synovia's lubricating function should not be underestimated (Schmidt et al., 2007).

In reducing intra-articular friction, together with the synovia's lubricating activity, the viscoelasticity and the hydraulic permeability anisotropism of articular cartilage have great value as well. The capacity for viscoelastic deformation and the nonuniformity of pressed interstitial tissue fluid distribution (Ateshian, 2009) provide such a dynamic redistribution of load in cartilages during movement in a joint, as a result of which its surface appears, at any moment, almost ideally adapted for the optimization of movements. Owing to the combination of these specific properties of the material and the articular cartilage surfaces and the high efficiency of synovial lubrication, the friction coefficient in the joints of a healthy person is much less than that which h has been achieved in the most perfect technical units.

Chapter 10

MOLECULAR
BIOLOGICAL
AND BIOCHEMICAL
REGULARITIES
OF CONNECTIVE
TISSUE
STRUCTURES
ONTOGENESIS

10.1. MOLECULAR BIOLOGICAL AND BIOCHEMICAL MECHANISMS OF MESENCHYME CONDENSATION. REGULATION SYSTEMS OF CONNECTIVE TISSUE STRUCTURES MORPHOGENESIS

The formation of connective tissue structures begins with forming condensations in embryonal mesenchyme; this process is referred to as condensation (Hall & Miyake, 2000). Originating essentially from mesoderm, the middle germ layer, and comprising the basic embryo body mass until a certain period (in a human, until the end of the eighth week), embryonal mesenchyme contains pluripotent mesenchymal progenitor cells, which can serve as precursors of various connective tissue cellular differons (fibroblastic, chondroblastic, osteoblastic). Mesenchymal condensations are localized clusters of a progenitor cells, which constitute the first stage in the formation of all dense connective tissue structures, such as tendons and ligaments, aponeuroses and fascia; the derma undergoes a condensation stage in its evolution as well (Michon et al., 2007). Other mesenchymal conden-sations serve as source material for the formation of cartilaginous and bone structures.

Becoming regulating signaling systems beforehand is a necessary precondition for condensation formation, the most important stage of embryonal morphogenesis. These systems consist of signaling molecules, components (extra- and intracellular) of the signal transduction pathways, and cell (cytoplasmic) membrane receptors.

The so-called maternal effect produces the earliest regulating influence on morphogenesis. This effect is due to the presence of protein molecules in a zygote (fertilized ovum) and, possibly, related transfer RNAs, which originate in a mother's body and remain unchanged in an oocyte (Elis et al., 2008).

These molecules serve as primary signals for the expression of earliest activated genes' (genes of the maternal effect) encoding of a number of signaling molecules–morphogens, determining the onset of gastrulation and the formation of a body segmented pattern. A set, called a **morphome** (by analogy with genome) of the intrinsic genes of the zygote, including the gap, *pairrule*, bicoid and other families, has been described in detail in the drosophila (Surkova et al., 2007). A homologous mechanism for activating zygote genes by maternal effect factors functions at even significantly higher steps of phylogenesis, including in mammals (Minami et al., 2007). In vertebrates' zygote, "zinc fingers" containing

transcription factor XDFL156, functions. In inhibiting the activity of the *p53* gene, this factor controls the formation of germ layers and mesoderm differentiation (Sasai et al., 2008).

With the onset of gastrulation, a number of regulation signaling systems, establishing the bonds between the gastrula proliferating cells, join the regulation factors encoded by the zygote genes. The main families of signaling molecules among these systems operating on a genetic level are:

a) morphogenes of the Hh and Wnt families;

b) members of the transforming growth factors-β (TGF-β) superfamily, primarily bone morphogenetic proteins (BMPs);

c) members of the fibroblast growth factors (FGF) family;

d) a signaling system associated with Notch trans-membrane receptors; and e) a the retinoic acid system.

The leading role in controlling cell differentiation, proliferation and functions is transferred to these signaling systems comprising a comprehensive regulatory network. These systems control gastrula morphogenesis, particularly the formation of the primitive streak, a transient structure wherein mesoderm and endoderm differentiation begins. Later, the same systems control the detailed patterning of an organism, namely the formation of cell condensations, including those that determine segmentation (assembling an organism from uniform modules–segments) inherent to the majority of multicellular organisms.

The effectiveness of signaling molecules actions is provided by the early active expression of related transmembrane receptors by the cell. The receptors are a starting point for intracellular signal transduction pathways, eventually achieving the cell nucleus and regulating gene expression.

Signaling molecules (messengers) affect the cells by means of serpentine receptors (molecules with convoluted conformation, crossing the cytoplasmic membrane seven times, i.e. they contain seven transmembrane domains). The majority of such receptors, called GPCR, are coupled with G proteins (guanine nucleotide binding proteins), located within the cytoplasm immediately under the membrane. G proteins are latent guanosine triphosphatases (GTPases), whose enzymatic activity appears in the interaction of GPCRs with ligands (Neves et al., 2002). GTP hydrolysis, the initial link of the intracellular transduction of a signal arising from a ligand, is controlled by proteins–regulators of G-protein signaling (RGS). RGS-5, RGS-7 and RGS-10 stimulate condensation

---

[1] Many genes discovered mainly in genetic investigations were named in relation to the development defects (malformation) observed in the mutations of these genes. Thus, a gene whose mutation resulted in the malformation of wings was given the name Wingless.

Hedgehog (Hh) is a gene that, when absent, the larva exhibits spicules.
Having identified proteins encoded by these genes, the gene names were transferred to the proteins.

The functions of orthologic proteins subsequently found in mammals appeared to be more manifold in the majority than their names have implied.

(and the subsequent chondroblastic differen-tiation) of progenitor mesenchymal cells, with RGS-4 acting in the opposite direction (Appleton et al., 2006).

Among messengers, **morphogens** of the Hh and Wnt[1] families play a leading role in regulating morphogenetic processes (see section 4.2).

Hh (Hedgehog) family consist of three homologous proteins of the morphogen family, among which Shh (Sonic hedgehog, the alternative name of which is HHG-1) plays a more significant generalized role in regulating the development of mammals. The involvement of other Hh, Ihh and Dhh. in morphogenetic processes is restrained by certain localizations; thus, the role of Ihh is especially important in enchondral ossification (Varjusalo & Taipale, 2008).

Produced by cells as a preprotein consisting of 424 amino acid residues (in mice), Shh is exposed to proteolytic processing (autoproteolysis) within the endoplasmic reticulum, where is deprived of the signal peptide and the large C-terminal region. The N-terminal peptide (Shh-N), consisting of 173 amino acid residues (residues 25 to 198), possess the specific morphogenetic effect. Another peculiar effect of processing is the coupling of lipid components to Shh, the residue of a palmitic acid (palmitate) to the N-terminal, and of cholesterol molecules to the C-terminal (Nusse, 2003). Shh-N affects cells as a ligand via the Patch receptor. The Patch bound to its ligand derepresses the co-receptor, Smo, which serves as a source for signals coming into the cell that influence the processing of transcription factors with zinc fingers from the Gli protein family. Impairments in processing inhibit their function as transcription repressors (Ehlen et al., 2006). Many molecular details of this process are not clarified (Jia & Liang, 2006).

Shh, by affecting cell proliferation and differentiation, plays a key role in many aspects of patterning an organism's development, with the direction of its activity altered at various embryogenesis stages. The expression of the *Shh* gene in mouse embryos becomes distinctly apparent on the midline by the eighth day. In this early stage it controls the left-right and dorsal-ventral axis specification of an embryo. Later, the Shh expression is of critical importance in forming the limb distal parts and in the development of structures of ectodermal origin. The switching off (or deletion) of Shh results in the malformation of somites, a lack of vertebrae and ribs, limb and lung hypoplasia (Varjusalo & Taipale, 2008). Shh is also essential in an adult, where it maintains tissue homeostasis and participates in the regulation of stem cell differentiation.

According to some data (Dorus et al., 2006), molecular evolution of the Shh gene occurred in primates in an accelerated manner. Herewith, intensive accumulation of serine and threonin residues, which are potential substrates of posttranslational modification, occurred. These gene altera-tions were especially pronounced in the central nervous system of anthropoidea (prehominids)–and could be one of the factors promoting the origin of the human being.

In comparison with the Hh family, the morphogen family comprising the Wnt signaling system (the name is derived from the names of two orthologic genes of this family–*Wingless* in a drosophila and *Int* in a mouse) is more complex and numerous. It includes at least 22 secreted glycoproteins (19 are known in a mouse). The proteins' identification as part of the Wnt family is determined by the similarity of their amino acid sequences, ranging from 27% to 83%, as well as homology to the first discovered representative–a mouse Wnt1 (primarily named Int1) and a general predecessor of the Wnt genes–a Wg (Wingless) gene of the drosophila–rather than by their functions, which are diverse. A common peculiarity of the Wnt primary structure is a high content of cystein, at not less than 23–24 of cystein residues (i.e. more than 7%). Like macromolecules of the Hh family, Wnt macromolecules also contain two lipid components. As in Hh, a palmitic acid residue is attached to the N-terminal region (at Cys77), and a monounsaturated palmitoleic acid residue (palmitoleate) is attached to a Wnt molecule closer to C-terminal (at Cys209), wherein cholesterol is located in Hh (Takada et al., 2006).

The effect caused by Wnt in cells is complicated. Wnt affects cells via transmembrane multi-pass receptors of the Fzd (Frizzled) family, known in 10 isoforms, and the cytoplasmic proteins of the Dvl (Dishevelled) family related to them, with participation of Lrp5 and Lrp6 co-receptors. The interaction of Wnt with receptor proteins is regulated by a number of secreted soluble antagonists (Sfrp), some of which are Fzd analogues and act as "decoy" receptors, while others (Dkk, Dickkopf, "fatheaded") block Lrp co-receptors (Chen et al., 2008).

The binding of Wnt with related receptors involves their internalization (endocytosis), occurring in the presence of clathrin and dynamin. This results in the formation of a temporary intracellular structure–a signal endosome, serving as a connecting link between Wnt and sequential links of the intracellular signaling pathways (Blitzer & Nusse, 2006).

Fzd receptors employ several such pathways, with the choice of the pathway partially depending on which Wnt serves as a ligand. The most prevalent pathway in vertebrates is a major pathway referred to as a canonical pathway or Wnt/β-catenin. Ligands that primarily act by this pathway include nine Wnt isoforms: Wnt1, Wnt2, Wnt2b, Wnt3, Wnt3a, Wnt6, Wnt7b, Wnt8a, Wnt8b. The canonical pathway is aimed at providing stability or, in other words, interruption of the destruction of β-**catenin**, a phosphoprotein, which occurs in the absence of a ligand within the cytoplasm. The preserved β-catenin facilitates the stabilization of **cadherins**, cell adhesion molecules, and, even more important, it is transported into the nucleus and regulates the transcription of a significant number of genes controlled by Wnt (Clevers, 2006). The interaction of β-catenin and DNA takes place in the presence of the transcription factor LEF1/TCF.

Wnt-signaling pathways without β-catenin are considered "non-canonica" (Gordon & Nusse, 2006), one of these pathways being Fzd/PCP, which influences planar cell polarity (PCP) (Seifert & Mlozdik, 2007). This pathway, affecting primarily the cytoplasmic (cell) membrane and special orientation of the cytoskeleton, is of great importance in determining the correspondence of cell polarity to the body axes, as well as in regulating targeted cell motility. Fzd/PCP, where FZ, FMI, STBM membrane-bound protein factors, and DSH, DGO, PK, cytoplasmic proteins, are involved, is essential for normal gastrulation.

One more non-canonical pathway is known as Wnt/Ca2+. The main effect achieved by this pathway is increasing the calcium ion content in cells and activation of the enzyme involved in calcium metabolism, including calmodulin regulated kinase II (CamKII) and PKC kinase. Molecular mechanisms and the biological value of this signal pathway have not been studied well, but it has been found to be mainly used by three Wnt isoforms (Wnt4, Wnt5a, Wnt11), while some Fzd isoforms might be a starting point (Miller, 2001).

The action mechanism of six Wnt (Wnt5b, Wnt7a, Wnt9a, Wnt10a, Wnt10b, Wnt16) has not been characterized yet. They might employ other signaling pathways, including that where mitogen-activated JNK kinases are involved. Their characteristic is complicated by the redundancy of the Wnt isoforms: in experiments, switching off the genes of some isoforms might be compensated by others (Kemp et al., 2005).

The diversity of Wnt isoforms, their receptors and signaling pathways underly the variety of these mor-phogen effects, both in embryogenesis and in the postnatal period. The peculiarities of target cells and the entire context where various Wnt function result in diverse effects. The active expression of all 19 Wnt genes and 11 genes-antagonists is detected in a blastocyst consisting of 70–100 cells, even before its attaches to the uterine wall (implantation). The expression is of varied degrees of intensity in the inner and outer layers of the blastocyst and is ongoing in the post-implantation period (Kemp et al., 2005). The functional significance of Wnt, particularly their canonical signaling pathways in such an early stage of embryogenesis, is supported by serious impairments of gastrulation without the β-catenin expression (Haegel et al., 1995).

For the mesenchyme to be formed from embryonal pluripotent stem cells canonical Wnt signals are essential (Lindsley et al., 2006). The subsequent determining of a differentiation way (commitment) of the mesenchyme multipotent cells into chondroblasts, osteoblasts or adipocytes requires switching Wnt from the canonical signaling pathway to other ones (Davis & Nieden, 2008). Certain Wnt isoforms have apparent significance in commitment of differentiation of mesodermal cells. For example, in forming a transcriptional program of the fibroblast differon Wnt3a is involved (Klapholz-Brown et al., 2007). At the same time, the general targeting activity of the whole Wnt family on stem cells is maintenance of their non-differentiated pluripotent status or,

in other words, prevention of undue differen-tiation (Nusse, 2008).

The Wnt family morphogens' (Wnt3a and Wnt5a) effect on the condensation process manifests in regulating the coordinated migration of paraxial and lateral mesenchyme cells from the primitive streak (Sweetman et al., 2008).

Wnt are involved in embryogenesis by regulating many other processes, starting from the first days after implantation – during the formation of the germ layers and the primitive streak (Gadue et al., 2006), as well as generating the general plan of an organism's formation and axis specification, particularly the anterior-posterior axis of the embryo in organogenesis and angiogenesis, stem cell proliferation. The molecular mechanisms of these effects are not the same in different species of vertebrates (Marikawa, 2006). In adults, Wnt are essential for maintaining homeostasis in connective tissue, particularly for bone density maintenance. Wnt involvement in carcinogenesis has been recognized (Chen et al., 2008).

Morphogens of the Hh and Wnt families have a number of common characteristics; this similarity is based on the fact that macromolecules of both families are modified by linked lipid components, making macromolecules hydrophobic (Nusse, 2003). Hydrophobicity determines significant peculiarities of both morphogen functions; namely, in mutations restraining the attachment of lipid components, metabolism and the specific activity of Hh and Wnt undergo significant alterations (Gallet et al., 2003).

Hydrophobicity is a natural barrier to these molecules movements within a hydrophylic medium of the extracellular matrix; indeed, the Hh and Wnt concentration is higher in the immediate proximity to the secreting cells surface. However, part of the morphogen hydrophobic macromolecules covers a distance of 20 average cell diameters. The presence of two populations (fractions) of each morphogen macromolecules are supposed; the first fraction is short-distance and acts in accordance with the autocrine type, while the other one has more distant targets (Bartscherer & Boutros, 2008).

The similarity of Hh and Wnt is evident even at the moment of their biosythesis: in both cases, fatty acid residues (palmitate and palmeoleate) are attached in the endoplasmic reticulum in the presence of the same protein, **porcupine**, which has an enzymatic activity of acyltransferase (Bartscherer & Boutros, 2008).

Hydrophobicity determines specific regularities of intracellular post-translation processing, transport, interactions with the cell membrane, and transmembrane secretion of Hh and Wnt into the extracellular matrix. These regularities are similar for both morphogen families.

The similarity is that a great number of accompanying proteins, which can be considered as both chaperones and regulating factors, is involved in all stages of these intracellular and secretory processes. Hydrophobicity, being a natural barrier to morphogens movements, is overcome by the development of hydrophilic proteins, which are supplementary to hydrophobic morphogens, in the phylogenesis of complex specialized systems. The majority of these systems already exist in invertebrates (for example, in the drosophila), and this fact attests to the great importance of hydrophobic morphogens in embryonal development.

For example, Wnt transportation via Golgi cisternae and secretion are regulated by an Evi multipass trans-membrane protein (alias Wls or Sprinter) as a transporter. In turn, the Evi function is regulated by proteins of the Vps family, which comprise a multiprotein complex (Retromer) (Bartscherer & Boutros, 2008).

A protein known as Reggie-1 or Flotillin-2, concentrated in **caveolae** (crypts of the cell membrane) and interacting with Hh and Wnt, separates them during secretion into fractions, to be further transported long and short distances. Wnt transportation for long distances is possible due to the binding of the morphogen with lipoprotein particles, referred to as argosomes (Katanaev et al., 2008). A Disp transmembrane protein, interacting with cholesterol in Hh, is additionally involved in the analogous fractionation of Hh (Gallet et al., 2003).

The transportation of secreted Hh and Wnt macromolecules includes transcytosis, migration through cells, which enables the formation of a concentration gradient representative for morphogens. For the transcytosis of macromolecules of both morphogen families, a heparin sulphate proteoglycan, **glypican** Dlp, located on the cell membrane surface that promotes endocytosis – entering macromolecules into cells is essential (Gallet et al., 2008)

The similarity of both family morphogens is also seen in their interaction with target cells. They affect the cells by means of related seven-pass receptors – Fz and Smo, which function in the presence of related Gsk3 and Ck1-α kinases. Besides, Hh is bound to a twelve-pass Ptc receptor. To a certain extent, the intracellular pathways of these receptors signaling are similar. The differences are in the structure of membrane co-receptors, involved in binding ligands of both families, and in the composition of secreted molecules that inhibit binding (Nusse, 2003).

As for the role played by the lipid components of the Hh and Wnt macromolecules, despite the known inconsistency of the available concepts, these components might be supposed to enhance morphogen effects. This enhancement might have been due to facilitating contact of morphogen hydrophobic macromolecules with a cell membrane surface (Nusse, 2003).

Hh and Wnt function as typical morphogens in the processes of embryonal development. In the early period of embryogenesis, they generate differentiation of various types of specialized cells and affect the cells by determining their positioning in tissues and providing information on their localization. This earliest orientation of cells is manifested (immediately after implantation and even before the primitive streak formation) by the formation of the organism's anterior-posterior axis and endoderm and ectoderm patterning (Marikawa, 2006).

As it is characteristic for morphogens in general, the intensity of Hh and Wnt effects (qualitatively) are proportional to the gradients of their concentration in tissues; these gradients are due to morphogen molecules' migration from the cells producing them. The cells remote from the morphogen source react to a morphogen by expressing only those genes that are sensitive to its low concentration. The cells receiving the morphogen in a higher concentration express, in addition, less sensitive genes. In such a way, cells with various combinations of expressed genes appear; in other words, cells of various differons originate. The relation the morphogen effect – concentration gradient deter- mines the role of Hh and Wnt in control over specifying localization for the beginning of formation (initiation) and the further demarcation of condensations, including the formation of the organism segmented pattern (Kicheva & Gonzáles-Gaitán, 2008). Switching off genes encoding morphogens results in serious and, in some cases, fatal phenotype defects as exampled by Wnt (Logan & Nusse, 2004). The functions of Hh and Wnt morphogens are performed through interacting with a number of transcription factors localized within the nucleus of target cells, with other signaling molecules secreted into the extracellular matrix and the pathway components of signals generated by these molecules. These interactions include both synergism and antagonism and cross-control.

For example, the expression of **mesogenin 1**, a nuclear transcription regulator, essential for the mesoderm maturation before segmentation, is stimulated by Wnt under the condition of synergic involvement of another transcription factor – Tbx6 (Wittler et al., 2007). A zinc fingers-containing nuclear protein – Zic1 – is an activator of the Wnt expression (Merzdorf & Sive, 2006).

In regulating morphogens, as well as homeotic genes' (see below) functions in embryogenesis, interactions with the signaling systems of growth factors of the TGF-β (transforming growth factor) superfamily and the family of fibroblast growth factors (FGF) play the most important role.

In the TGF-β superfamily, members of the large combined family (sometimes also referred to as a superfamily) of bone morphogenetic proteins (BMP) and so-called growth and differentiation factors (GDF) play an especially significant role in embryogenesis.

Bone morphogenetic proteins (BMP) received their name when the first members of this large family of signaling molecules were isolated from a bone organic matrix and demonstrated their specific osteoinductive activity (the ability to induce the ectopic formation de novo of bone tissue). Their chemical nature, properties, action mechanism, and role in regulating the vital activities of bone tissue were discussed in section 8.4.2 and they will be mentioned again in discussing the molecular mechanisms of osteoblastogenesis (see section 10.2.3).

The BMP functions are characterized as **pleiotropic** (manifold) (Ripamonti, 2006): they are not restricted to their involvement in the regulation of bone tissue metabolism and skeletogenesis, but are significantly large-scaled. They demonstrate a marked morphogenetic and anabolic activity, stimulating the synthesis of many macromolecular components of the extracellular matrix, in particular, of proteoglycans and proteolytic enzyme inhibitors (Chubinskaya & Kuettner, 2003). They are involved in regulating the proliferation, differentiation and maintenance of cell vitality (Xiao et al., 2007). As regulating factors, they take part in the organogenesis of the nervous, muscular, cardiovascular and other systems. Their orthologs play an important role in regulating morphogenetic processes, not only in mammals but even in invertebrates with no bone tissue (e.g. in an urchin, rain-worm or a drosophila).

In this context, a suggestion (Reddi, 2005) seems quite reasonable to maintain BMP's historical abbreviation to understand it as "body morphogenetic proteins".

A signal role of BMPs is especially important in embryonal development, starting at an very early period of embryogenesis – passing from the stage of a blastula to gastrulation – and during gastrulation, with this role being diverse in time. BMP-2 and BMP-7 originating in an egg cell (maternal) act within the blastula, and they inhibit the formation and activity of embryonal inductors (the so-called Spemann organizer in amphibians can serve as an example of induction) secreting BMP antagonists – noggin, chordin and follistatin. This restriction of BMP activity creates the conditions for the formation of the nervous system.

With the onset of gastrulation, BMPs expressed within the zygote show activity, with the importance of individual BMPs and the targeting of individual BMP action change dependent on the process phase. BMP-2 shows activity very early, then the activity of BMP-4 increases, and a little later, that of GDF-6. These signaling molecules facilitate the normal development of the mesoderm, particularly of its dorsal regions (Marom et al., 2005). Targeting of the BMP action is determined not only by ligands (BMP themselves), but also by receptors mediating their actions. For example, an ALK2 receptor (also known as ACVRI) is essential for the normal completion of gastrulation (Komatsu et al., 2007). The same receptor is required for BMP involvement in specifying the right-left axis (Kishigami et al., 2004). The ActRIIA and ActRIIB receptors are essential in promoting the influence of GDF-11 on specifying the anterior-posterior axis and in the formation of the vertebral column (Oh et al., 2002). The BMPR IA receptor is involved in regulating limb growth and formation (Ovchinnikov et al., 2006). Thus, BMPs create conditions for forming a general organism pattern, primarily, specifying the axes (anterior-posterior, dorsal-ventral and right-left) of the three-dimensional body polarity (Kishigami & Mishina, 2005).

Even in the early stages of embryogenesis, BMPs hold a "high" leading position in relation to other local signaling factors regulating morphogenesis. In other words, the regulating activity of BMPs is subject not only to the genes responsible for the cell executive functions (e.g. the genes of various components of extracellular matrix molecules' biosynthesis), but also the genes encoding the expression of signaling molecules and components for signaling pathways.

BMPs interaction with the signaling system of retinoids, active derivatives of vitamin A, occupies a central place in the mechanism by which BMPs influences embryonal morphogenesis, particularly skeletogenesis. BMPs control this system, reducing its activity, which is targeted at inhibiting the growth of mesenchymal condensations and the chondroblastic differentiation of their cells by decreasing the expression of the Sox9 factor. The BMP target is the *Aldh1a2* gene, encoding retinal dehydrogenase 2 (RALDH2), a key enzyme for retinoid formation. This effect is most pronounced in BMP-4; BMP-2, BMP-7 and GDF-5 also possess it (Hoffman et al., 2006).

It must be taken as proved that signaling molecules of the BMP/GDF family play a central role in regulating the processes of embryonal morpho-genesis, including the morphogenesis of connective tissue structures and, in particular, of the skeleton structures (Wan & Cao, 2005). In bones that are being formed, BMPs stimulate their growth, activating the cells of both bone tissue differ-ons: osteoblastic and osteoclastic (Okamoto et al., 2006). It can be stated that the central scope of the BMP and GDF activity is the morphogenesis of connective tissue structures in the embryonal period, where they have an effect on gastrulation, mesoderm formation and the development of the left-right asymmetry, skeleton development, limb formation, organogenesis, gametogenesis and other processes (Yamaguchi et al., 2000; Zhao, 2003). How this activity is essential for normal embryogenesis can be seen in the data provided in *Table 10.1* on phenotypic defects resulting from the switching off of BMP genes and related factors.

Proteins of the SMAD family comprise the main intracellular signaling pathway from specific receptor serine-threonine kinases activated by by bone morphogenetic proteins (and other signaling molecules of the TGF-β superfamily) to the cell nucleus. They come in physical contact and interact with components of other signaling systems. For example, within the nucleus, SMADs adjoin with the LEF1/TCF transcription factor, binding to DNA along with β-catenin (this is one of the numerous examples). Due to this contact, BMPs affect the regulatory functions of the Wnt/β-catenin signaling system (Latamendia et al.,2001). SMAD also ensures BMPs influence on the expression of HOX proteins and their functions in skeletogenesis (Li & Cao, 2006).

The complexity of effects initiated by bone morphogenetic proteins within a cell is further complicated by the simultaneous employment of alternative (non-SMAD) intracellular signaling pathways by BMPs. The signaling systems of the Notch and Toll transmembrane receptors (see below), a signaling system activated by a p38 protein

Table 10.1

Switching off (knockout) effects of some BMP-ligand and BMP-receptor genes of a mouse phenotype

Gene	Phenotype
Bmp-2	Lethal (E7.5 – 10.5), defects in the development of an amnion, chorion and heart
Bmp-4	Lethal (E5.5 – 9.5), absence of mesoderm formation
Bmp-6	No visual defects of skeletogenesis
Bmp-7	Lethal, defects in the development of a(?) skull, ribs, hindlimbs
BmprIA	Lethal (E5.5 – 9.5), absence of mesoderm formation
BmprIB	Hypoplasia (shortening) of limbs
Smad1	Lethal (E10.5), defects in the development of extraembryonal ectoderm and mesoderm

E – a day of embryonal development (according to Gazzerro & Canalis, 2006).

of MAPK protein kinase, are among such pathways. Interactions between all these systems are more and more widening the scale of BMPs inf luence on the transcription process and optimize the cell response to BMP signals (Herpin & Cunningham, 2007).

It may be added that the experimentally induced local hyperexpression of **noggin**, an intense extracellular BMP antagonist, in a developing limb, completely discontinues the condensation process (the aggregation of cells into condensations); mesenchymal cells retain their non-differentiated status (Pizette & Niswander, 2000).

The total set of BMPs and their related members of the TGF-β superfamily is regulated and controlled at many levels. The most significant level of regulation is that of BMPs and their receptors' transcription; the molecular mechanisms of transcriptional regulation still cannot be considered clarified (Rosen, 2006).

There are five known levels where restraining BMP effects factors function (Gazzerro & Canalis. 2006):

The first level is restrainting BMPs interactions with their receptors by binding BMPs with antagonist-proteins within the extracellular matrix, resulting in BMPs' inability to react with their receptors. The role of antagonists is played by the above-mentioned noggin, a protein from the chordin family, a Tsg glycoprotein, the Dan family proteins (Dan, gremlin, sclerostin, Cerberus), and

follistatin. Noggin, gremlin and follistatin are expressed by osteoblasts (sclerostin is expressed by osteocytes) and are found in bone tissue (Rosen, 2006). The purposes for such multiplicity of these antagonists remain unclear. It can be supposed that BMP binding is not their only function, and this is supported by the variety of phenotypic defects, up to fatality, observed both in a knockdown of noggin, chordin, gremlin genes and in the excessive expression of these genes. An extracellular antagonist for the majority of BMPs is also, as previously mentioned, BMP-3, which is a little different than them in terms of structure and competes with them for receptors (Gamer et al., 2008).

The second level is the presence of pseudoreceptors on the cell surface, binding BMPs but not passing the signal inside the cell.

The third, fourth and fifth control levels are directed at propagating a BMP signal within a cell. The third level is an activity of the inhibitory SMAD-6 and SMAD-7, which prevents the formation of the SMAD-1 and SMAD-4 complex essential for signal propagation. Intracellular proteins that are BMP antagonists act at the fourth level. These include the protooncogene Ski and antiproliferative proteins Tob-1 and Tob-2, which bind the signal SMAD-1 and SMAD-5 (Yoshida et al., 2000). Chondrocyte-expressed calponin-3, a protein earlier known for its ability to be bound to actinin (Haag & Aigner, 2007), employs a similar mechanism for controlling BMP activity. Finally, the fifth control level involves Smurf protein factors, which prepare signaling SMAD for proteolytic degradation within proteosomes. All these control levels facilitate the coordination and balanced functioning of BMPs. Together with BMPs, other members of the TGF-β superfamily, particularly TGF-β1, whose initiating activity in the condensation process is not indirect but mediated by connective tissue growth factors (CTGF), are involved in regulating the morphogenesis of connective tissue structures (Song et al., 2007).

The condensation is also influenced by other members of the TGF-β superfamily, such as nodal and activins growth factors. The effect of those factors depends upon of their concentration and is similar to morphogen effects in this sense (Smith et al., 2008).

The expression of **nodal**, a homodimeric protein, occurs even in a blastula or in the very beginning of gastrulation; in its absence, mesoderm formation does not occur. Hereafter, nodal is essential to separate the mesoderm and endoderm and for regulating the left-right body asymmetry (Tian & Meng, 2006; Shen, 2007). In regulating the left-right asymmetry, which primarily manifests in the positioning and structure of visceral organs, nodal activity is controlled by *Tbx6*, one of genes' encoding transcription factors, containing a so-called T-box with a length of about 170 amino acid residues (Hadjantonakis et al., 2008).

The nodal function is performed by interacting with activins, pleiotropic growth factors of the activin-inhibin family that regulate cell proliferation and apoptosis (Chen et al., 2006). Nodal and activins are involved in stimulating the proliferation of embryonic stem cells (Ogawa et al., 2007).

Nodal and activins affect the cells through the same transmembrane receptors as BMPs and other members of the TGF-β superfamily, possessing the activity of serine/threonine kinases, and employ the same intracellular signaling pathway, where the Smad family proteins play a central role. The receptor ALK7 is also a nodal receptor (Reissmann et al., 2001). Moreover, the protein (glycolipoprotein) **Cripto** (also named Tdgf1), when attached onto the cell membrane surface by glycosylophosphatidylinositol, is important in terms of the effects produced by nodal and activins. Cripto promotes a stimulating effect of nodal and activins on mesoderm formation and the specification of the anterior-posterior (A–P) axis of an embryo (D'Andrea et al., 2008). In the latter case, nodal and activins are synergetic to morphogens of the Wnt family.

The system of the **fibroblast growth factors (FGF)** family is another system for regulating embryonal morphogenesis processes (Böttcher & Niehrs, 2005). FGFs affect cells through their own receptors, FGFR, which are tyrosine kinases. Four such receptors, encoded by related *Fgfr1* genes, are known to exist in mammals. These receptors serve as a starting point for signaling pathways within a cell, the components of which are a number of kinases (Laloo, Ras, Raf, MAPK, ERK), adapter (accessory) proteins FRS2/SNT-1, Nck, Grb2, and transcription factors of the AP1 and ETS families. At the same time, FGF effects are not only due to the effect on cell genetic mechanisms, but also to their chemoattractive properties (FGF-2, FGF-4, FGF-8).

In the first days of embryonal development, FGFs are involved in regulating cell migration, enabling gastrulation. Two FGF8 isoforms (FGF-8a and FGF-8b) augment each other's activity in the pre-gastrulation stage and during gastrulation. FGF-8b, in particular, induces the expression of a *Brachyury* gene, essential for mesoderm development (Guo & Li, 2007). Later on, FGFs are switched on in regulating mesoderm formation and the primitive streak buildup (at the same time, FGF-8a induces the expression of FGF-4), specifying the A-P axis of an embryo. The experimentally caused deletion of FGF-signaling results in fatal phenotype defects, mainly involving the process of gastrulation and mesoderm formation (see *Table 10.2*).

FGFs interact with Wnt morphogens in coordinating two ongoing processes in embryogenesis, such as cell proliferation and migration (growth of tissues) and the formation of multicellular structures) and the choice of cell differentiation way (commitment). In a mouse's growing limbs, such an interaction of FGF-8 and Wnt-3a coordinates growth with the simultaneous formation of cartilaginous structures and the intermediate layers of muscle connective tissue (ten Berg et al., 2008). This coordinating activity of FGF is controlled by the Ctr1 protein, also known as a copper transporter (Haremaki et al., 2007).

Besides, FGFs play an active role in regulating the later stages of embryonal morphogenesis, particularly in regulating skeletogenesis (see section 10.3.1).

One more signaling system involved in regulating embryogenesis, including its initial stages, is a system whose central component are trans-membrane (single-pass) **Notch** receptors. The Notch family consists of four large heterodimeric phosphoglycoproteins (with a molecular mass up to 2,500 kDa), which are similar in structure and encoded by four separate genes. Each macromolecule is made of two fragments, such as a large extracellular fragment and a significantly smaller one, consisting of transmembrane and cytoplasmic domains. Notch receptors interact with five ligands – three of them are known as Delta-like (Dll) and two as Jagged/Serrat. These ligands are also transmembrane proteins and, there-fore, the Notch signaling system functions in cell contacts, enabling the exchange of information between the cells (Mumm & Kopan, 2000).

In interaction between Notch and any ligands, the proteolytic cleavage of the cytoplasmic (intracellular) NCID domain occurs, whereby the domain moves into a cell nucleus. There, with the participation of various protein components, it produces an effect on gene expression (activating or inhibiting it), in particular, by affecting the expression of the HES5 transcription factor (Karlsson

Table 10.2

Switching off (knockout) effects of some FGF-ligand and FGF-receptor genes of a mouse phenotype

Gene	Phenotype
Fgfr-1	Lethal (E7.5 – 9.5), cell commitment, migration of mesoderm and endoderm cells' impairment
Fgfr-2	Lethal (E6 – 8), no endoderm formation
Fgf-4	Lethal (E4 – 5), defects in trophectoderm and visceral endoderm
Fgf-8	Lethal (E9.5), cell commitment, migration of mesoderm and endoderm cells' impairment

E – a day of embryonal development (according to Böttcher & Niehrs, 2005).

et., 2007b). This signaling pathway is considered as canonical. Non-canonical signaling pathways of signals arising from Notch are also known.

As demonstrated in an experiment with cultured in vitro cells of the embryonal mesenchyme of forming limbs, the Notch signaling system has a particular–a restraining–role in regulating the initiation, the first stage of a condensation process (Fujimaki et al., 2006). At the same time, the Notch system is involved in cell commitment (specification of the differentiation way) (Fiúza & Arias, 2007). Being of significant importance for maintaining the correct formation of organism structures, these functions are carried out by Notch, together with Wnt-morphogens (Hayward et al., 2008). The combined activity of Notch and Wnt is regulated (restrained) by the cytoplasmic protein NUMB (Katoh & Katoh, 2006), while FGFs also take part in controlling Notch and Wnt signals (Wahl et al., 2007).

The Notch signaling system, acting as a part of the so-called segmentation clock (which shall be discussed below), is also one of the leading factors for regulating the condensation and segmentation processes.

The active metabolites of **vitamin A**, retinoids, primarily retinoic acid (RA) (Niederreither & Dollé, 2008), play a pleiotropic regulating role in embryogenesis. Serious defects of embryonal development due to vitamin A deficiency during pregnancy are well known.

Along with their receptors (RAR and RAX) and enzymes that are involved in retinoid metabolism (RALDH2, CYP26), co-activators and co-repressors of retinoid signals, retinoids are deemed to be a special signaling system. Mutations of genes, encoding the protein components of this system, result in disturbances of embryogenesis that are no less severe than those caused by vitamin A deficiency. Since they are of lipid origin, retinoids

pass through cytoplasmic (cell) and nuclear membranes easily, all the main components of this system are within the nucleus.

The retinoid effect is similar to that of morphogens in that its intensity, as well as the morphogen effect, depends upon the concentration gradient. The RA concentration within embryo tissues decreases in the anterior-posterior direction and, thereafter, RA appears to be one of the factors regulating the specification of the embryo anterior-posterior axis. Retinoids are involved in regulating the choice of a differentiation way for embryonic pluripotent stem cells, as well as in the maintenance of pluripotency by a certain part of these cells. Retinoids maintain their regulating role and, in later stages of embryogenesis, they are among the factors regulating homeotic genes and, therefore, the condensation process.

Retinoic acid is involved in regulating segmentation and somitogenesis (see below), together with signaling molecules of the Wnt, FGF and Notch families. At the same time, it per-forms a specific function: it facilitates the combination of somite symmetry and the left-right asymmetry of visceral organs (Kawakami et al., 2005).

As all other regulating systems, the retinoic acid system is a component of the above-mentioned complex regulatory network in terms of embryogenesis. The interaction of the retinoic acid signaling system with that of fibroblast growth factors (FGF) is especially evident. This is due to the fact that FGF control the expression of the protein components of the RA metabolism and its signal propagation (Shiotsugu et al., 2004).

It should be emphasized that the functions of all signaling systems regulating embryogenesis cannot be addressed separately. These systems, each of which are controlled by tens of genes, are combined in an organized

gene regulatory network (GRN), otherwise referred to as a **transcriptional regulatory network** (TRN), and their action is strictly coordinated. The structure of this network has been modified and complicated during phylogenesis, but the general principles of its organization persist (Levine & Davidson, 2005; Busser et al., 2008).

Condensation starts in a homogenous embryonal mesenchyme under GRN control. Such control will continue to persist (Gridly, 2006). The process of mesenchymal condensations formation, with **segmentation** being its variant, involves five stages:

1) initiation;
2) establishing the borders of a condensation (determining its size and form);
3) proliferation of progenitor cells involved in a condensation (condensation growth);
4) cell adhesion; and
5) cell differentiation (Hall & Miyake, 2000). The final stage of condensation is also the initial stage in the morphogenesis of organism structu-res, including structural components of the locomotive system and other organs.

The central role among the factors regulating and controlling the condensation process, its two first stages, in particular–the stages of initiation and establishing condensation borders–are transferred to proteins, which are encoded by so-called **homeotic** genes.

The name of homeotic genes comes from the term "homeosis" (the Greek homoiosis, meaning similarity) implies the changing of a body part (or an organ), making it similar to the related part in relative organisms. These significant alterations, caused by mutations of homeotic genes, were first noticed in the foundational period of establishing the genetics of the fruit fly (drosophila), the main subject of classical genetic investigations, and this made the discovery of these genes possible.

The main feature of a homeotic gene structure is the presence of **homeoboxes** (HOX), from which the name for these homeotic genes was derived–homeobox genes. Homeoboxes are very similar to each other in terms of the composition of different DNA regions in various genes with at average of 180 base pairs.

Homeotic genes encode protein macromolecules (they can be referred to as homeotic proteins) of various sizes (ranging from 200 to 750 amino acid residues), many of them being phosphoproteins. Homeoboxes are responsible for encoding special domains in these proteins, called homeodomains. According to the length of homeoboxes, homeodomains contain about 60 amino acid residues, which are rich in arginyl and lysyl (N.N.Mushkambarov and S.L.Kuznetsov, 2003). Homeodomains have a helix-turn-helix conformation, which is referred to as a homeodomain fold. The first helix (from the N-terminal region of a molecule) consists of two regions separated by a small gap, which provides it with certain flexibility. The second helix, located closer to the C-terminal region, is perpendicularly oriented to the first helix. Such a conformation of homeodomains creates

especially convenient conditions for the binding and interacting of homeotic proteins with DNA. Homeodomains are especially actively bound to the nucleotide sequence of 5'-ATTA-3'.

The human genome contains 300 loci, which may be considered as homeoboxes. Among them, 235 loci are parts of functioning genes, while 65 are pseudogenes (genes that, for one reason or another, lack the protein-coding ability). Functioning genes are divided into 11 classes, subdivided into 102 families. These figures attest to the diversity of the structure and functions of homeotic genes (Holland et al., 2007).

A group of homeotic genes, the role of which is emphasized by their names, are proper **HOX**-genes in a human being and **Hox** genes in animals. These genes are of the same type in their structure: they have only two exons, separated by one intron of various length. A homeobox is invariably located in the beginning of the second exon, its encoded homeodomain being near to the carboxyl terminus of a protein molecule. Before a homeodomain, there is a domain bound to TALE family proteins,which are involved in the interaction of proteins with DNA as co-factors (Lappin et al., 2006).

HOX genes are parts of four orthologous (homologous and repeated) clusters (hoxa, hoxb, hoxc, hoxd) localized in four chromosomes (chromosome 7, 17, 12 and 2). The human genome contains a total of 39 genes (ranged from 9 to 12 in every cluster), comprising group of HOX-genes (Luisi Pollard & Earnshaw, 2002).

The structure 0f homeoboxes in other homeotic genes is more varied in comparison with *HOX* genes, with the structure of homeodomains encoded by them being more diverse. For example, in some homeotic proteins subdivided into the POU family, there is one more specific domain near to to the homeodomain. This special domain is similar to a homeodomain with approximately the same length. Such a double domain is flexible, which allows these proteins to be bound with an octamer (8-membered) nucleotide sequence of 5'-ATGCAAAT-3' in DNA (Phillips & Luisi, 2000).

Homeotic genes are very conservative. Their appearance, initially as precursors forming a primary cluster of *Proto-Hox* genes (not less than a billion years ago) coincided with origin of multicellular forms of life. The *ProtoHox* cluster is the ancestor of not only *HOX* genes, but also a number of other homeotic genes. Genes of *ParaBox* and NK clusters acting as regulators in various germ layers, are especially close to *HOX*-genes in terms of structure and functional targeting. The *ProtoHox* cluster also gave origin to families of homeotic genes, such as *Meox* (Mesenchyme homeobox), *Cdx* (Caudal-type homeobox), and a number of others (Garcia-Fernandez, 2005).

Along with homeotic genes, paired-box genes, comprising the *PAX* family, are involved in regulating the implementation of a general body pattern and cell specification in particular (Wang Q, 2008). The proteins encoded by these genes have a domain with 126 amino acid residues on average, consisting of two parts, located in the

N-terminal region. Some of the PAX proteins are homeotic at the same time–besides a paired domain, they have a somehow altered homeodomain).

The proteins encoded by homeotic genes are localized within cell nucleus and are transcription factors, affecting the genome mainly by interacting with gene promoter regions. Targeting of the controlling interaction of various homeodomain-containing proteins with DNA is manifold: homeotic proteins function as activators (or co-activators) and, on the contrary, as inhibitors (or co-inhibitors) of gene transcription. Combining all these effects results in such a modulation of cell activity, which facilitates the coordinated morphogenesis of an organism as a whole.

Homeotic proteins are not factors that directly affect cells. Since the role of homeotic proteins is only regulating and controlling, homeotic genes are sometimes referred to as selector genes (Hombria & Lovegrove, 2003). Using the concept of signaling systems, just as cascades, where a signal moves top-down, it can be said that homeotic genes are "above" numerous genes-effectors–the direct implementors of morphogenetic processes. Under the guiding influence of homeotic proteins, the function of mesenchymal cell genes, which encode the proteins determining the participation of these cells in the formation of condensations, is switched on (and off) at the right time and place. Homeotic proteins are proteins that the whole cell cycle (proliferative activity) depends upon. They are also related to the expression of adhesion factors essential to promote the stability of condensations and to establish communication–both between cells, and between cells and the extracellular matrix.

The point of application of homeotic proteins are the cis-regulatory elements (modules) of genes. These elements–enhancers and silencers–directly govern the switching on and off of genes (Pearson et al., 2005).

HOX-genes, gathered in clusters in chromosomes, as previously mentioned, are of fundamental importance in regulating the implementation of the general body pattern.

The Hox-gene expression in vertebrates starts in an early stage of gastrulation, when the specification of the main axis of an embryo occurs (Lappin et al., 2006). Hereafter, HOX-genes from every cluster, located within chromosomes in a linear sequence one after another in the direction from 5' beginning to 3' end, manifest their activity in the same sequence. This sequence coincides with the spatial (axial or, in other words, cranio-caudal) direction of an organism's formation and with the timing of the process: the expression of the first (counting from a 5' cluster beginning) genes of all clusters occurs earlier than the expression of the genes closing a cluster. The activity of gene products that are earlier in terms of the expression time is directed at controlling the development of more cranially located organism regions. Such a correlation of expression to the dynamics of an organism's development specific to Hox-genes is referred to as **colinearity** (Kmita & Duboule, 2003).

The role of Hox-genes, primarily of Hox-10 and Hox-11 from the hoxa, hoxc, hoxd clusters is especially important in controlling the patterning of the axial skeleton of vertebrates. These genes determine the initiation of condensation and, therefore, the localization of condensations by the length of the trunk and limbs (Wellik & Capecchi, 2003; Wellik, 2007). In experiments on mice, hoxa and hoxd clusters have been shown to be especially active in patterning the limb axes (Nelson et al., 1996).

Other homeotic genes, as well as HOX-genes involved in regulating condensation, have functions related to regulating the successive stages of condensation development (the size and form of a condensation, cell proliferation and differentiation, and others) rather than induction. In many cases, these genes' activity is restrained by definite condensations of certain localizations and/or certain periods of condensation development.

For example, the homeotic genes Pbx1 and Pbx2 are involved in implementing only the pattern of the skeleton structure of the limb distal regions (Capellini et al., 2006). Homeodomain-containing proteins Pitx1 and Pitx2 are essential for the morphogenesis of derivatives of the mesoderm lateral plate, for budding mouse hindlimbs specifically (Marcil et al., 2003). The homeotic gene Uncx4.1 encodes a protein (also containing a paired domain), which controls the formation of the proximal regions of ribs and vertebral transverse processes (Leitges et al., 2000). Homeobox containing the Bapx1 gene (also known as Nkx3.2) induces the initiation of chondrogenic condensation within the sclerotome; this effect of Bapx1 appears after its activation by Pax1 and Pax9 gene products, similar to homeotic ones (formed as the result of the duplication in phylogenesis) (Rodrigo et al., 2003). A homeotic gene known as Mohawk (Mkx), from the Tale/Iro family, is essential in mouse embryogenesis at the outset for forming the somite dermotomyotome, anticipating the development of skeletal muscles. Later on it is involved in the formation of condensations from which vertebra bodies and proximal ribs, as well as tendons in limbs, originate (Anderson et al., 2006). A homeodomain-containing transcription factor Barx2 regulates chondrogenesis in limb buds and participates in the development of the central nervous system as well (Meech et al., 2005).

As early as the beginning of condensation, in the initiation stage (initiation should also be implied as specifying a condensate localization), a transcription factor encoded by the homeotic gene Dlx5, acts. This factor activity continues in the succeeding stages of condensation, persisting in the chondroblastic differentiation process (Bendall et al., 2003).

Hox genes continue their regulating function in an adult organism, albeit in a somewhat changed way,. This function is required for normal hematopoiesis and, particularly, for a normal course of reproductive processes; its impairment results in endocrinopathies (Daftary & Taylor, 2006).

The activity of homeotic genes and other genes participating in patterning organism development is exhibited against the background of action in an evolving embryo of a large complex of molecular regulating mechanisms, which, as regulators, are positioned "above" the homeotic genes.

The very origin of a signaling cascade, which initiates condensation by inducing homeotic genes, are signaling molecules of the TGF-β superfamily. Bone morphogenetic proteins are especially active in this respect. For example, BMP-4 is one of the factors responsible for the initial induction of *Xvex-1* homeotic gene expression, starting at the gastrulation stage (Shapira et al., 1999). The expression of homeotic genes is influenced by a growth and differentiation factor 11 (GDF-11) from the BMP family, acting via the ALK5 receptor. This influence is important for the regionalization of an embryo on the anterior-posterior axis (Anderson et al., 2006). The fact that the expression of homeotic genes was noticed in ossification foci from the very outset in experiments where BMPs were used to induce ectopic bone formation supports the BMP position being "above" homeotic genes (Iimura et al., 1994). Regulating BMP's influence on the transcription activity of homeotic genes is made possible by a complex, sometimes antagonistic, interaction with Smad family proteins, intracellular components of BMP-signal pathways (Li et al., 2006).

The expression of homeotic genes from the *Cdx* caudal (tail) family, particularly the *Cdx1* gene, is regulated by Wnt morphogens (Pilon et al., 2007).

The expression of homeotic genes, including *Hox*-genes, is controlled by epigenetic mechanisms, where two conservative (they were found in drosophila and remain virtually unchanged in superior vertebrates and human beings) protein groups–such as **Polycomb** (PcG) and **Trithorax** (TR XG) groups–play the leading role. Proteins of these groups form composite multimeric complexes, which affect the expression of homeotic genes in opposite directions: polycomb proteins restrain expression, while trithorax proteins supporting expression are their antagonists. This action is epigenetic by nature: PcG and TRXG affect genome special elements (PRE and TRE), modulating chromatin structures of a cell nucleus rather than the genes regulating morphogenesis directly (Grimaud et al., 2006). Alterations of the histone H3 (methylation and formation of a H3.3. variant), which lead to changes in the expression of homeotic genes, are an especially important result of this influence (Ng & Gurdon, 2008). PcG has been shown, in the example of *Hoxd genes*, to be the factor that enables the sequencing (colinearity) of *Hox*-genes to switch on and switch off in accordance with morphogenesis dynamics (Mishra et al., 2007). The controlling role of polycomb proteins in regulating *Hox* gene expression in vertebrates is supported by so-called non-coding RNA (ncRNA), including microRNA (miRNA) at the posttranscription level. miRNAs are very short (21–23 nucleotides) single-stranded molecules, which are transcripts of stretches of DNA located be-

tween genes (Pearson et al., 2005). There are several hundred such non-coding transcripts (Rinn et al., 2007). Their main biological role is to control protein synthesis by restraining translation. microRNA molecules are bound to the complementary nucleotide sequences of single-stranded coding mRNA macromolecules, which transforms the molecules into double-stranded ones and resultantly blocks the translation. This phenomenon, referred to as RNA interference, reduces the intensity of Hox-protein synthesis (Lempradl & Ringrose, 2008). Coordinating the time of ncRNA synthesis and the activation of the PcG expression is of importance in maintaining the co-linearity of *Hox*-genes' function (Sessa et al., 2007). Polycomb proteins control the homeotic genes' functions in programming the general body pattern in embryogenesis, with this control starting by regulating the balanced activity of embryonic pluripotent stem cells (Sauvageau & Sauvageau, 2008). In the postnatal period, when the main functions of homeotic genes related to patterning an organism have been completed, PcG secures their "silencing" (Schwartz & Pirrotta, 2007).

Effects of endocrine factors are one more mechanism of regulating the expression of homeotic genes, including Hox-genes. Testosterone, estradiol, progesterone and vitamin D have such an effect. This is distinctly seen in the gender peculiarities of the skeleton structure and in an emerging skeleton deformity in endocrine dysregulation (Daftary & Taylor, 2006).

The main function of homeotic genes is over in embryogenesis, but their expression can frequently be reactivated when growth or tissue renewal is necessary, for example, in healing a bone fracture–a process that recapitulates the main events of the embryonal development of bone tissue (Gersch et al., 2005).

The process of **segmentation** or the formation of somites (**somitogenesis**) is one of the aspects of forming condensations preceding the structures of an axial bone-cartilaginous skeleton (vertebral column, elements of the rib cage). During their formation, segments are repetitive condensations along the anterior-posterior axis of the organism occurring in periodic intervals. These condensations are comprised by mesenchymal cells that originated in the symmetric streaks of the paraxial mesoderm, while ectodermal elements are also present. Later on, somites are formed from these condensations. Somites are repeated, unimodal, functionally equal structures that give rise to vertebrae, ribs, as well as related tendons and muscles. In condensations that are being formed, the simultaneously development of blood vessels and budding of nerves occurs. In such a way, the regularity of the general body pattern, known as **segmentation** or **metamerism**, appears, which is common for many living organisms (from arthropods to mammals).

The process of segmentation spreads along the non-organized so-called presomite mesoderm (PSM) in the anterior-posterior direction, in accordance with the direction of embryo growth. The point is that, over distinct periods of time, a group of proliferating and migrating

PSM cells loses its motility, acquires adhesive properties, and combines in a condensation, a precursor of a future somite, which has a clear-cut border with the surrounding loose mesoderm. In a chicken embryo, the period of forming one somite takes 90 minutes on average, while it takes two hours in a mouse embryo (Baker et al., 2006; Cinquin, 2007).

The segmentation process is regulated and controlled by two complementary molecular mechanisms.

The first mechanism is the so-called **"segmentation clock"**, which constitutes a coupled oscillating (pulsatile, cyclic, varying in intensity) functioning of the above-mentioned complex network, the signaling systems regulating morphogenesis. The Notch, Wnt and FGF signaling systems are the main components of this network (Dequéant et al., 2006; Goldbeter & Pourquié, 2008). Every period of increased activity of comprising genes is accompanied by the formation of another condensation; the continuing growth of an embryo during the period of low activity of oscillating genes results in a gap between the segments, filled in with loose mesenchyme. According to the figural expression of Pourquié (2003), a segmentation clock converts the embryonal time into a spatial body pattern in such a manner.

The signal's molecular nature, as the starting impulse of oscillation (pacemaker) of the segmentation clock, cannot be deemed to be completely identified (Ozbudak & Pourquié, 2008). All the components of the oscillating genes' network cannot simultaneously produce such a starting impulse; the strict synchronicity of their oscillation evidently must be due to a singlestarting impulse (Cinquin, 2007; Aulehla & Pourquié, 2008). According to relevant experimental findings, the oscillating character of the expression of genes such as *Hes1* and the more active *Hes7* (encoding transcription factors), as well as the *Lfng* gene (encoding one of the glycosyltransferase), also known as Lunatic fringe and the gene Axin2, the product of which is a negative regulator of Wnt signals (an inhibitor of axial growth), may be the primary oscillation impulses (Gridley, 2006). The oscillating expression of the *Lfng* gene plays the decisive role in regula-ting the segmentation of the anterior skeleton regions (Shifley et al., 2008).

The Notch signaling system, the activity of which increases and decreases in the presence of the *Lfng* gene and several other factors (for example, the Hairy transcription factor), is of significant importance in the trigger mechanism of the segmentation clock (Ishimatsu et al., 2007; Kugeyama et al., 2007). Besides, the Notch system, in facilitating communication between cells, plays an important role in protecting the segmentation clock against possible interference capable of impairing the synchronicity of gene expression (Horikawa et al., 2006).

The growth of a presomite mesenchyme occurs in the anterior-posterior (rostral-caudal) direction. The formation of segments progresses in the same direction. Active oscillating gene expression is localized in the caudal region of an embryo and the intensity of this expression decreases in the opposite, caudal-rostral, direction to the growth (Gridly, 2006).

The expression of oscillating genes is of importance and not only for somite formation. Oscillating signaling also serves as a factor in forming the segmented pattern of limbs (Aulehla & Pourquié, 2008).

The second molecular mechanism is the movement of a molecule mass ("wave") of the fibroblast growth factor FGF-8 and the Wnt-3 morphogen controlled by it, as well as factors of the Notch signaling system. The signaling system of Wnt-3a/β-catenin is more actively involved in controlling the condensations' posterior border (Dunty jr. et al., 2008).

Thus, proteins of the Notch system play a dual role in segmentation; they are oscillating components of the segmentation clock and, at the same time, a component of a morphogen wave moving in the cadual-rostral direction. Its intracellular domain, called NICD (Notch intracellular Domain) and affecting the Wnt3a activity, is of significant importance in this second role of the Notch trans-membrane protein (Gridley, 2006). The Notch expression is controlled (restrained) by a transcription factor encoded by the *Mesp2* (mesoderm posterior protein) gene; the localization of the *Mesp2* expression is determined by another transcription factor, the nuclear protein Tbx6, a member of the protein family containing so-called T-box (Oginuma et al., 2008).

Notch as a morphogen and its ligand Delta 1 (Dli) interact with the segmentation clock in determining an identity (individual peculiarities of the structure) of vertebrae (Cordes et al., 2004).

The movement of morphogen molecules forms a concentration gradient; the concentrations gradually decrease as they move away from the cells expressing morphogens. A localization where the morphogen concentration becomes sufficiently low not to restrain cell sensibility to the segmentation clock's actions is considered to be the "front' of the morphogen wave. This localization determines the anterior (rostral) border of a somite. The posterior (caudal) somite's border emerges in the place where the morphogen concentration exceeds the level where the segmentation clock acts. This interaction of the signaling molecules' wave and the segmenta-tion clock, which is the main mechanism of determining the somite borders (the second stage of the condensation process), is complex. The Mesp2 transcription factor, restraining the Notch receptor activity, plays a key role at this point (Saga, 2007).

The accuracy in determining somite borders (and evidently, other condensation) is facilitated by the concentration gradient of retinoic acid, which restrains the expression of FGF-8 (Dubrulle & Pourquié, 2004; Duestor, 2007). This gradient is oriented in a rostral-caudal direction, i.e. opposite to the concentration gradient of morphogens (Gridly, 2006). The molecular mechanisms of the third stage—the growth of condensations due to the proliferation of cells comprising them—have been insufficiently studied. The roles of the Cfkh-1 and Mfa-1 transcription factors, which stimulate the proliferation of condensation cells, are supposed to increase at this stage (Hall & Miyake, 2000).

The **YKL-40** glycoprotein (a protein similar to chitinase-3, with the synonime HC-gp39), whose expression, as determined histochemically, is concentrated within condensation proliferating cells, is also involved in establishing the borders of condensations (Johansen et al., 2007).

In terms of the development and stability of condensations, establi-shing communicative contacts bet-ween cells is of key importance, as the contacts promote structural and functional interaction between cells and transform a simple cell collection into an element of the organism structure that is being formed – for instance, into a future bone. Establishing contacts between cells is the main subject of the fourth, penultimate stage of the condensation process, referred to as the adhesion stage. In an early period of condensation (in mice the entire process of condensation formation lasts about 15 hours), a provisory adhesion is ensured through the accumulation of **hyaluronan** around the cells. Then adhesion occurs due to the intensive expression of adhesion factors, which are the integral protein components of a cell membrane (Hall & Miyake, 2000). These are heparan sulfate proteoglycans, including syndecans that bind the cells with the extracellular matrix. Molecules of calcium-independent cell adhesion, which are members of the gCAM superfamily, **N-CAM** (neural cell adhesion molecules) in particular, possess such properties. The same binding properties have cadherins, whose adhesion activity requires calcium. N-CAM are supposed to promote the stability of condensations already formed, as the adhesion activity of N-cadherins is essential in the condensation growth stage that it stimulates.

Among the cadherin family, N-cadherins play the most important role in this stimulation (Derycke & Bracke, 2004). The expression of N-cadherins, molecules that facilitate calcium-dependent cell adhesion, is stimulated by BMP-2, and this stimulation is apparently critically important in exerting the whole stimulating effect of BMP-2 on the buildup of mesenchymal cell condensations (Haas & Tuan, 1999). Products of the *Hoxa-13* and *Prx-1a* genes, as well as one of guanosine triphosphate hydrolases, Rac1, are involved in this effect (Woods et al., 2007c).

In vitro studies have shown that a natriuretic peptide of C-type (CNP), a small peptide produced especially actively by endothelial cells, stimulates the formation of condensations in 3D cultures of mesenchymal cells and that this stimulation is accompanied by an active expression of N-cadherins (Woods et al., 2007a). This fact confirms the importance of cell adhesion mediated by N-cadherins, which activate a number of intracellular signaling pathways in developing condensations.

The β-cathenin-mediated N-cadherin effect on proteins of the cytoskeleton promotes cell contact by changing their form (Delise & Tuan, 2002). **Gap junctions** (contacts), enabling the direct exchange of information between cells by moving molecules with a mass of up to 1 kDa, are formed between the contacting cells of a condensation.

Cadherins' adhesive function is regulated by growth factors of the TGF-β superfamily. This is one more activity of TGF-β that is seen even at the gastrulation stage, associated with the ability of TGF-β to induce the expression of a FLRT3 trans-membrane protein and the small guanosinetriphosphatase (GTP) Rnd1. The combined action of these two factors causes the endocytosis (moving into cytoplasm) of cadherins, which results in restraining cell adhesiveness to an optimal level (Ogata et al., 2007).

Two morphogens of the Wnt family – Wnt-5A and Wnt-7A – by means of the transmembrane receptor proteins Chfz-1 and Chfz-7, encoded by *Frizzled* family genes, also affect the N-cadherin function, and there-fore, the adhesion of mesenchymal cells that start differentiation (Tuan, 2003). These and other Wnt factors play a role in the later stages of differentiation.

In progenitor cells aggregating in a condensation, the expression of a number of **protein kinases**, often called kinases (ERK, p38 MAPK, PKC and others), is enhanced and corres-pondingly, their enzymatic activity increases (Lee et al., 2004).

Protein kinases are enzymes involved in the majority of intracellular signaling pathways, which activate proteins by attaching phosphate residues (phosphorylation) to them. As a rule, protein kinases are bound to the cellular membrane receptors or they are themselves transmembrane proteins, combining the receptor and enzymatic functions. The activation of receptor or receptor-linked protein kinases through interaction between receptors and their ligands serve as a primary signal, which is then propa-gated along related intracellular signaling pathways. Other protein kinases become consequentially involved in signal propagation, eventually providing a signal entry into the nucleus and triggering an adequate cell response. The role of kinases from the family of mitogen-activated protein kinases (MAP) is especially important in these signaling pathways' functioning (Stanton et al., 2003).

Phosphorylation enhances the motility and metabolic activity of protein molecules, which results in increasing the cell's general functional activity. One manifestation of this enhancement is the increased content of cyclic adenosine monophosphate (cAMP), associated with the activation of cAMP-dependent proteinkinase A (PKA), which phosphorylates a CREB protein responding to cAMP.

Protein kinase-mediated changes, affecting the propagation of stimulating and inhibiting signals, indicate that a cell is preparing for the onset of the next stage of condensation evolution – chondogenic differentiation. The activation of protein kinases is able to not only stimulate, but also inhibit a condensation's evolution. For example, kinases of the Src family (Lyn, Frk, Hck), in phosphorylating a tyrosine residue in proteins, produce an inhibiting effect. The pharmacologic inhibition of these kinases promotes chondroblastic differentiation (Bursell et al., 2007).

In accumulating multipotent mesenchymal cells into condensations, the content and functions of an extracellular matrix they produce change. The main peculiarity of the non-differentiated mesenchyme matrix is a high concentration of hyaluronan and fibronectines. Due to the peculiarities of its macromolecular structure), hyaluronan widens the interstitial space of the mesenchyme, creating the conditions for cell proliferation and their migration into condensations. Within the condensations, the same activity of hyaluronan makes the contact and adhesion of cells difficult; thus, the expression of hyaluronan synthase Has2 and the production of hyaluro-nan decrease (Li et al., 2007a).

Fibronectins form a microfibrillar network, where cells are attached by integrin trans-membrane receptors. This network controls proliferation, affecting the cell cycle (cell growth and division). The influence is preferably targeted to the phase of cell growth (phase G1), which is prolonged as a result of the inhibition of cyclin-dependent kinase and intracellular pathways of mitogen signals (Danen & Yamada, 2001). At the same time, the fibronectin network regulates cell location within a condensation. Cell motility gains a directed character (this phenomenon is referred to as **haptotaxis**) and this event exerts a decisive effect on the condensation form; this form anticipates the form of the future permanent structure, such as a bone, for instance (Newman & Bhat, 2007).

The integrin-mediated adhesion of condensation cells to the extracellular matrix is also promoted by a protein containing a "sticky" RGD-sequence, called a **collagenassociated protein** (RGD-CAP), or a protein induced by a growth factor TGF-β (β-**ig-h3** for short), or keratoepithelin. It contains 660 amino acid residues, including 25 residues of a γ-carboxyglutamic acid. This protein, expressed by cells of a condensation, enhances its growth (Ohno et al., 2002).

Along with quantitatively prevailing fibronectins, there are numerous members of families of other large multidomain glycoproteins, such as tenascins and thrombospodins, within the condensation matrix (Mackie & Murphy, 1998). Various glycoproteins have different effects on condensation evolution and the role these components play is diverse in different stages of the process. For example, some fibronectin isoforms, having a positive effect on the formation of a mesenchymal condensation, further prevent the onset of chondroblastic differentiation thrombospondin-4 has a positive affection on progress in the early stage of condensation development (Tucker et al., 1995), and thrombospodin-2 stimulates the osteoblastic differentiation of mesenchymal cells to the detriment of chondroblastic differentiation (Taylor et al., 2009). In constrast, tenascin C promotes the induction of chondroblastic differentiation, with a globular fibrino-

gen-like carboxyterminal domain of a tenascin macromolecule being essential for such an effect (Murphy et al., 2000).

Tenascin C is also involved (from the side of mesenchyme) in the interaction of mesenchymal and epithelial cells, which is required for the condensation process. This essential interaction is provided by proteins (transcription factors) that encode the homeotic (including paired-boxes genes) Pax-1 and Pax-9, Prrx1 and Prrx2, as well as Alx-3 and Alx-4 genes, expressed by basal epithelial cells (Hall & Miyake, 2000).

There are heparan sulfate and chondroitin sulfate proteoglycans within the condensation matrix. The main member of large proteoglycans is the chondroitin sulfate-containing proteoglycan, **versican**, also know as PG-M (see section 3.2.1.2.), intensively expressed in embryogenesis. It is expressed within a condensation and stabilizes it, with the deficiency of versican caused by appropriate mutation results in decreasing the condensation size (Shepard et al., 2008). Versican also has a significant effect on the subsequent condensation stage – the fifth and final one – in the differentiation of condensation cells. In its absence, in particular, the chondroblastic differentiation of mesenchymal cells is discontinued (Williams et al., 2005).

Within the context of the extracellular matrix's development, the adhesive contacts between condensation cells mediated with CAM and cadherins are supported by cell adhesion to the condensation matrix. Keratoepithelin containing RGD-sequences, binds the cells to the collagen (Ferguson et al., 2003).

Heparan sulfate proteoglycans, particularly syndecan-3, a transmembrane proteoglycan, intensively expressed by mesenchymal cells around a condensation and tenascin C, a glycoprotein, are involved in establishing the borders and a final form of a condensation. The expression of these glycoconjugates, which is essential for preventing the premature onset of chondroblastic cell differentiation, is under the control of the Hoxa-2 gene; its expression is stimulated by BMP-2. Moreover, the Notch receptor signaling system and a Pax-2 transcription factor, whose expression is controlled by BMP-7, are involved in limiting the condensation size (Hall & Miyake, 2000).

In the extracellular matrix of a mesenchymal condensation, as well as in the primary mesenchyme matrix, collagenous proteins are presented by large fiber-forming type I collagen and by type III collagen, which is, in general, specific for embryonal tissues. The final condensation stage is, at the same time, the initial stage of the next phase of morphogenesis. This stage principally involves the transformation of mesenchymal condensations into connective tissue structures. This transformation follows one of three possible ways that give rise to either tendons, ligaments or other fibrous structures, or else permanent cartilages, or else bones.

10.2. DIFFERENTIATION OF CONNECTIVE TISSUE CELLS

10.2.1. Molecular biological and biochemical mechanisms of fibroblast differentiation and formation of fibrous (dense) connective tissue structures

In the first differentiation way, multipotent cells of condensations differentiate into fibroblasts, joining the fibroblast differon during the process of fibrous structures' formation. Such differentiation is selectively promoted by the connective tissue growth factor, CTGF (see section 4.2) (Lee C.H. et al., 2006). The cells start to express fibroblast differon specific markers (see section 2.2.2) and the molecular components intrinsic to a fibrous tissue extracellular matrix (see section 3.5.3).

Within condensations, which are transformed into tendons and ligaments, the cells initially develop a significantly plastic phenotype, similar to that of the fibroblasts of other fibrous tissues–for example, to a phenotype of dermis fibroblasts (Oldfield & Evans, 2003). Hereafter, the final differentiation of these cells into tenoblasts/ tenocytes, which are very similar to other fibroblasts in terms of phenotypic characteristics, occurs. The main indicator of such differentiation is the intensive expression of the *Scleraxis (Scx)* gene and the *TNDM* gene, encoding a transmembrane glycoprotein tenomodulin (tendin) (Schweitzer et al., 2001; Brent et al., 2003). The Scx expression is stimulated by BMP-12 (Wang Q.W. et al., 2005).

The mesenchymal condensations preceding fibrous structures have several peculiarities that distinguish them from condensations that give rise to other elements of the skeleton. For example, OB-cadherin (osteoblastic), also known as cadherin-11, is said to play a prevailing role in cell adhesion in comparison with other condensations (Richardson et al., 2007). The cadherin-11-mediated adhesion of condensation cells predetermines a cell shape specific to tenoblasts and the organization of longitudinal cell rows, which enables matching the orientation of cell-produced collagen fibers to the tendon biomechanical function.

The active early expression of FGF8 and BMP-4 signal molecules is another peculiarity of condensations preceding fibrous structures.

The third significant peculiarity of differentiation stage of condensations preceding tendons is the dependency on the parallel skeletal muscle formation (in the nearest proximity). The morphogenesis of tendons is subject to signals expressed by differentiating muscular cells, such as proteins encoded by the *Myf6* and *Fgf4* genes (Edom-Vovard & Duprez, 2004).

As tendon formation in embryogenesis is coordinated time-wise to occur with cartilage and bone development, the expression of *Scleraxis*, a the central gene for tendon differentiation, is coordinated with the expression of *Sox9*, a gene responsible for chondroblast differentiation (Asou et al., 2002).

Differentiating fibroblasts of tendons and ligaments (tenoblasts) assume a molecular mechanism that prevents mineralization. This mechanism is related to the activity of the *Msx2* homeotic gene (Yoshizawa et al., 2004).

Within a condensation, from which the dermis fibrous layer is formed, the migration of differentiating fibroblasts requires the involvement of the integrin β1-subunit. Condensation stabilization is associated with the interactions of integrins with a Notch transmembrane protein (Michon et al., 2007).

10.2.2. Molecular biological and biochemical mechanisms of chondroblastic differentiation

Condensations whose transformation occurs according to the second and third ways, as precursors of future segments of a bone-cartilage skeleton, take on the shape of these segments as a result of demarcation. A system built up from these segments is formed, which some authors call a **membranous skeleton** (Hall, 1988).

The membranous skeleton segments are actually aggregations of mesenchymal progenitor cells, bound by adhesive factors and surrounded by specific extracellular matrix. The majority of these segments are transformed into cartilage structures as a result of chondroblastic (chondrogenic) differentiation. A chondroblastic differon is formed and the cells gain specific phenotypic characteristics of a chondroblast/ chondrocyte (see section 7.2.1.1).

Chondroblastic differentiation (the formation and development of the chondroblastic/chondrocytic differon), which starts in the final stage of the evolution of mesenchymal cell **condensations** (see section 10.1), initially occurs in the way common for all the future chondroblasts/chondrocytes, but ends by separating them into two various populations (Lefebvre & Smith, 2005; Goldring et al., 2006; Zuscik et al., 2008).

On this common way, pluripotent mesenchymal progenitor cells undergoing the prechondroblastic stage are transformed into chondroblasts. Later on, a part of the chondroblasts forms a numerically smaller population of **permanent chondrocytes** that have a phenotype particular to them. These permanent chondrocytes then persist in cartilage skeletal elements that do not undergo ossification (i.e. joint and rib cartilages, the nasal septum cartilage, the auricular cartilage, etc.).

Differentiation does not discontinue here for the larger population of chondroblasts forming the cartilage models of future bones. They are chondrocytes of temporary, **transitory** cartilages (also referred to as replaceable as they are replaced by bone tissue). They enter the further, final stage of the life cycle, the purpose of which is to prepare for endrochondral ossification. This stage, including hypertrophy, is referred to as one of **maturation** and it ends in apoptosis.

The main molecular and biochemical mechanisms of **condensation** (a process of forming condensations), described in details in section 10.1, proceed to function af-

Table 10.3

The main factors of molecular dynamics of chondroblastic differentiation

Chondrogenesis stages	Functional signal and transduction molecules	Functional transcription factors including homeotic gene products	Cell-secreted matrix components
1. Formation of mesen-chymal condensa-tions, proliferation and differentiation of chondroprogenitor cells (prechondrobasts)	TGF-β1, activines, BMP-2, BMP-4, BMP-7, FGF-2, FGF-4, FGF-8, FGF-10, Wnt-3A, Wnt-5A, Wnt-7A, Shh N-cadherin, β-catenin	Dlx5 HoxA, HoxD, Sox9, Gli3, Pax1, Pax9, Nkx3.1, Nkx3.2, Barx2	Fibronectins, hyaluronan, versican, type I collagen, tenascin C, thrombospodin-4, syndecan-3, COMP
2. Proliferation and differentiation of chondroblasts, production of cartilage extracellular matrix	BMP-2, BMP-4, BMP-5, BMP-7, BMP-14, CDMP-1, CDMP-2, FGF-2/FGFR2, IGF-1	Sox9, Sox5, Sox6, Cart1	Type II, IX, XI collagens, hyaluronan, aggrecan, xylosyltransferases, COMP, perlecan
3. Transformation of chondroblasts into chondrocytes and commitment of their further life cycle	BMP-2, BMP-7, FGF-18/FGFR- 3 Ihh/Ptc, Wnt-5B, Wnt-11	Sox9 Stat1, Gli3, Gli2, Runx2, Fra2/JunD	Hyaluronan, aggrecan, COMP, type II, IX, XI collagens

ter the condensations have been formed, exerting a regulating effect on the various stages of chondroblast differentiation. In particular, the signaling systems of bone morphogenetic proteins (BMP) and other members of the TGF-β growth factor superfamily, fibroblast growth factors (FGF), Hh and Wnt morphogen families, the Notch receptor system and others, are active during this process. The continuous active expression of homeotic genes is also of great importance.

For example, Hox-genes of the D cluster *(HoxD10–HoxD13)* are essential not only in the condensation stage, but during the subsequent chondroblastic differentiation of cultured *in vitro* mesenchymal cells of chicken limb buds (Jung & Tsonis, 1998).

The process of chondroblastic differentiation is divided into three stages (see *table 10.3*) (Hall & Miyake, 2000). The first stage is understood as all the steps in the formation of mesenchymal condensations.

The first stage is over with the origin of pre-chondroblasts, cells that have some specific markers of a chondroblastic phenotype.

The second stage is one when the cells gain a true chondroblastic phenotype and exhibit an intensive expression of the cartilage extracellular matrix components.

The third stage is one of completing chondroblast differentiation and determining (choosing) the possibility of their transformation into permanent chondrocytes of cartilage structures or transitory chondrocytes, facilitating the growth of bones and creating the conditions for endochondral ossification. The action end-point of molecular factors comprising the mechanism of a condroblastic differon formation is that pluripotent embryonal mesenchymal cells take on the specific phenotypic characteristics of a chondocyte by the end of the third stage. The differentiation of permanent cartilage cells discontinues here. They lose their capacity for mitotic division and, therefore, for proliferation, thereby transforming into chondrocytes. At the same time, their secretory activity decreases. This is particularly the outcome of cartilage chondrocytes

Most cells that have undergone chondroblastic differentiation persist in the transitory cartilage models of future bones, where the cells are surrounded by an extracellular matrix similar to that of hyaline cartilage in composition (it contains type II collagen and aggrecan). These chondrocytes enter the next and final stage of their life cycle, which is associated with endochondral ossification and ends with apoptosis.

The **Sox9** protein plays the central regulating role in the transition from the development of a mesenchymal cellular condensation to the differentiation of progenitor cells into chondroblasts (Crombrugghe et al., 2000).

This protein is a member of the transcription factor family, binding to a minor groove in a DNA macromolecule and belong to the superfamily (group) **of high mobility proteins** (HMG). These proteins contain amino acid sequences that are homologous and, at the same time, manifold–a so-called HMG-box, which is responsible for DNA-binding. *SOX*-genes (20 of which a re known in humans and mice) encode proteins, which contain a HMG-box specific for a Sry protein; this protein is present in a male Y-chromosome. Thus, SOX stands for Sry-related HMG-box. The functions of SOX proteins are varied, but all of them are involved in differentiation and development processes.

SOX-9, a protein localized within the cell nucleus, with a molecular mass of about 56 kDa, consists of 509 amino acid residues.

In humans, it is encoded by the *SOX-9* gene, whose mutations result in the severe malformation of the skeleton, known as **campomelic dysplasia**, one symptom of which is dwarfism. The *Sox9* gene expression regulated by the HoxA13 gene, together with other factors (Akiyama et al., 2007), is found in mice as of the eighth embryonal day; *Sox-9* gene switching off in mice causes phenotypic impairments similar to the campomelic dysplasia syndrome in humans. The artificially-caused excessive expression of one of the RAR-α receptor (retinoic acid receptor) isoforms by condensation cells has the same effect (Hoffman et al., 2003); this active metabolite of vitamin A (see 4.1) inhibits the expression of the Sox9 protein.

The expression of the *Sox9* gene begins before a condensation has finally been formed; it is essential in all forming elements of the bone-cartilage skeleton for committing progenitor mesenchymal cells into the chondroblastic differentiation way (Crombrugghe et al., 2000). No other genes can replace the *Sox9* gene in this respect. The early expression of the *Sox9* gene occurs in many other progenitor cells, but only in chondroblastic differentiation it is an essential condition (Akiyama et al., 2005).

The beginning expression of the Sox9 protein is accompanied by switching off (or restraining) the expression of extracellular matrix components, specific to mesenchymal condensations (see 10.1) and by starting the expression of genes specific to chondroblasts, in particular, the *Col2a1* gene, which encodes type II collagen, and other chondroblast markers. On this basis, some authors classify the condensation cells in the final step of the first stage of chondroblastic differentiation as **prechondroblasts** (Lefebvre & Smits, 2005).

Sox9 is a transcription factor that, upon binding to gene enhancer elements, switches on the expression of genes determining the chondroblast/chondrocyte phenotype as a secretory cell. These genes, whose main controller is Sox9, encode a whole set of specific components of the cartilaginous tissue extracellular matrix, such as type II, IX, XI collagens, aggrecan, and COMP (a cartilage oligomeric matrix protein).

If (in experiments in mice) the *Sox9* gene in a limb bud starting formation is switched off locally before the onset of mesenchymal condensation, the condensation is broken; therefore the defects are seen even in the first stage of chondrogenesis (see *Table 10.3*). This means that Sox9 is essential not only for the expression of cartilage extracellular matrix specific components, but also for other functions of condensation progenitor cells. For example, it is necessary for the expression of adhesion proteins, securing condensation integrity, and/or for changes in cytoskeleton proteins molecular conformation, upon which the contact of cells diffused along the embryonal mesenchyme depends. Moreover, Sox9 has an antiapoptotic effect: it maintains the viability of mesenchymal cells starting condensation. The absence of condensations results in the complete blockage of chondroblastic differentiation whereby the expression of phenotypic markers of chondroblasts/chondrocytes does not begin. In other words, the process stops until the initial step of the first chondrogenesis stage is completed; both the second and third stages are made infeasible. Cartilaginous tissue is not formed, which, in turn, implicates the impairment of endochondral ossification.

If the *Sox9* gene is switched off after condensation formation, chondrogenesis is delayed in the middle of the first stage, and, despite the onset of a mild expression of signal molecules, involved in regulating the second and the third stages, severe generalized chondrodysplasia develops in animals. Such a phenotype is specific to mice with a double null mutation (double switching off) of the genes that encode two other proteins of the Sox-family: Sox5 (long isoform L-Sox5) and Sox6 (Akiyama et al., 2002). These interchangeable macromolecules are similar to Sox9 in a macromolecule structure, and are involved as transcription co-factors, together with it, in regulating the expression of specific components of the cartilaginous tissue extracellular matrix by differentiating cells (Smits et al., 2001).

These results led us to conclude that Sox9 itself is not enough for adequate chondroblastic differentiation, which is infeasible during the second and third stages (see Table 10.3) without the participation of Sox5 and Sox6. For the histogenesis of permanent cartilaginous tissue, a combination of three Sox proteins–Sox9, Sox5 and Sox6, called "Sox-trio" (Ikeda et al., 2004)–is essential, while also being sufficient. Within this trio, Sox9 plays the leading role as the main controlling factor, and Sox9 not only directly affects the molecular mechanisms of a chondroblast/chondrocyte phenotype formation at all stages, but also controls the expression of the two other Sox proteins (Akiyama et al., 2002).

A transcription co-activator, the Tip60 enzyme (formally named histone acetyltransferase KAT5), is involved in the interaction of Sox9 and Sox5, forming a complex with them that is bound to DNA within the region of the *Col2a1* gene promoter. Damage to this complex formation delays chondroblastic differentiation (Hattori et al., 2008).

During chondroblastic differentiation in distal regions of a limb embryonal mesenchyme (in finger buds), the *Sox9* gene functions in cooperation with other genes of the Sox family, such as *Sox8* and *Sox10* (Chimal-Monroy et al., 2003).

Sox9 is involved in regulating chondroblastic differentiation since the first stage of this process, and its activity discontinues only at the very end of the chondroblast life cycle, in the hypertrophy stage (Akiyama et al., 2002).

The action mechanism of Sox9 within cells undergoing chondrogenic differentiation includes its stimulating effect on the expression of **furin**, an enzyme cleaving the signal peptide from the molecules of many proproteins; this cleavage provides mature proteins, particularly chromosome proteins, with the activity they need in chondrogenesis. In this function of Sox9, Sox5 and Sox6 are its antagonists (Guimont et al., 2007).

It should be noted that the Sox9 expression occurs not only in mesenchymal cells differentiating into chondroblasts, but also in other cellular differons. The special, leading role played by Sox9 in chondrogenesis is determined by the fact that, together with Sox5 and Sox6, a number of other factors specific to that very differon interact in Sox9 activity within the process of chondroblastic differentiation.

One of these factors is the specific **cytokine-like protein 1** (CYTL1), secreted by chondroblasts, or the C17 protein, which affect chondroblasts according to an autocrine type and stimulate the activity of Sox9 (Kim et al., 2007). Another co-activator of Sox9, which promotes its specific activity as a transcription factor in chondrogenic cells, is the **PGC-1**α protein, interacting directly with Sox9 and serving to enhance type II collagen expression (Kawakami et al., 2005b).

The same effect of Sox9 is enhanced by the **p300/CBP** core protein, which has the enzymatic activity of histone acetyltransferase. Histone acetylation causes conformation changes of the surrounding DNA chromatin, owing to which the effect of Sox9 on the *Col2a1* gene enhancer is selectively increased (Furumatsu et al., 2005).

The expression of the Sox9 gene is activated by the TRPV4 protein. This is a seven-pass transmembrane receptor, which functions as a calcium channel. Under its influence, the accelerated production of chondroblast-specific markers occurs (Muramatsu et al., 2007).

The stimulating effect of Sox9 on the expression of genes encoding the components specific to cartilage matrix, type II collagen in particular, is enhanced by the nucleus-localized deacetylating enzyme SirT1 (the sirtuin family) (Dvir-Ginzberg et al., 2008). This effect is also increased by **latexin**, a carboxypeptidase A inhibitor that is present in cytoplasm and whose promoter in condensation cells is activated by Sox9 (Kadouchi et al., 2009).

As a chondroblast/ chondrocyte phenotype is adapted to hypoxia, a prerequisite for the optimal functioning of

Sox9 during chondroblastic differentiation is the regulating effect of a hypoxia-induced HIF1α factor. HIF1α exerts such an effect on Sox9 expression by binding with the promoter zone of the Sox9 gene (Amarillo et al., 2007).

The action mechanism of *Sox9* during chondroblastic differentiation involves one more aspect. Sox9 acts as an antagonist with respect to Wnt morphogen inhibiting effects on this process. Sox9 comes into physical and functional interaction with β-catenin, a central component of the canonical Wnt signaling pathway within a cell (see section 10.1) (Akiyama et al., 2004). This interaction promotes phosphorylation and the destruction of β-catenin within the nucleus and, therefore, the disruption of the canonical Wnt-signaling pathway (Topol et al., 2008).

In various stages of Sox9 activity, starting with the condensation stage, a large number of factors act together with Sox9, including homeotic proteins of the Nkx family (Nkx3.1, Nkx3.2), as well as Msx1, Msx2, Barx2, homeotic proteins with paired domains of the Pax family (Pax1, Pax9), Fox family proteins, and Gli2 and Gli3 proteins with "zinc fingers". Known for its antiapoptotic activity, the Bcl-2 protein enhances the stimulating effect of Sox9 on the expression of its controlled chondrocyte genes (Yagi et al., 2005). The timing and localization of these genes' expression largely coincide and they may duplicate each other. The combined activity of the genes encoding these proteins provides mesenchymal condensations with the required shape, fitting with the form of further skeletal elements. Therefore, these genes' function is referred to as shape-generating. At the same time, they do not duplicate the central regulating role of *Sox9* in chondroblastic differon development (Lefebvre & Smits, 2005).

As stated above, pluripotent osteochondroprogenitor mesenchymal cells of condensations are capable to differentiate into three different ways:
1) chondroblasts of permanent cartilages;
2) chondroblasts of displaceable cartilages; and
3) osteoblasts. The choice of the way (commitment) is determined by the simultaneous activity of several regulating factors and mechanisms.

One of these factors is a balance between the expression activities of *Sox9* and *Runx2/Cbfa1*, the main gene determining the osteoblast phenotype. In forming this balance, the hierarchy of the genes is of importance, whereby Sox9 dominates in the case of their simultaneous expression (Eames et al., 2004). The ability of the Sox9 protein to stimulate the expression of the homeotic protein Bapx1 (known also as Nkx-3.2) is exhibited in this domination. This transcription factor represses *Runx2/ Cbfa1* expression by chondrocytes, especially in the final stage of their differentiation (Yamashita et al., 2009).

Another mechanism involved in the beginning of chondroblastic differentiation is the prevalence of the transcription factor Runx1 (known as Cbfa2 or AML1) expression over that of the above-mentioned Runx2 (Cbfa1) (Wang Y. et al., 2005).

Sox9, as the main regulation factor, specifying the development of the chondroblastic phenotype, and all the other signal molecules acting simultaneously with it in the same direction, essentially "manage" the genes that the main cell metabolic functions depend on, especially biosynthetic functions and those functions involving cell proliferation (cell cycle). At the same time, the genes encoding Sox9 and other regulation factors are under the complex control of other interacting signaling factors that are functionally "above" (or "over") them.

The signaling systems of the Hh and Wnt morphogen families (see section 10.1) and growth factors of the FGF (fibroblast growth factors) and BMP (bone morphogenetic proteins) families are among these factors. Their action, even the action of the factors comprising the same family, is divergent in direction–initiation and stimulation, or inhibition of differentiation. In some cases, the direction depends upon the process stage. In any case, all of these numerous factors regulate not the differentiation itself, but only the conditions of differentiation process. Some of them affect *Sox-9* expression, but only *Sox-9* determines the specificity of chondroblastic differentiation.

For example, Wnt-2a and Wnt-2c induce the expression of FGF-8 and FGF-10; these FGFs enable the initiation of chondroblastic differentiation within limb buds. *Hox*-genes of the *HoxA* and *HoxD* clusters are also involved in regulating differentiation in this initial stage, and are essential for the expression of FGF-8 and Shh. Shh, whose expression is maintained by the Wnt7a morphogen, acts by means of transmembrane proteins Ptc1 and Smo and involves proteins with "zinc fingers"–Gli2 and Gli3–in the transcription regulation (Tickle, 2003; Kmita et al., 2005; Goldring et al., 2005).

Wnt-3a stimulates the beginning of chondroblastic differentiation, employing the canonical pathway of its signal propagation to activate *Sox9* expression (Yano et al., 2005). Other Wnt, particularly Wnt-7a, demonstrate the opposite activity (Tuan, 2003). The equilibration and rate of differentiation are regulated in such a manner.

The leading factors, initiating and activating Sox9 expression are, collectively speaking, all bone morphogenetic proteins–BMP-2, BMP-4, BMP-5, BMP-7–and possibly some others. The well-known manifestation of this BMP function is their ability, for which they are named, to induce bone ectopic development, a process which starts with the chondroblastic differentiation of mesenchymal stem cells within surrounding tissues, and continues by the way of endochondral ossification.

Bone morphogenetic proteins stimulate cell differentiation at various stages of chondrogenesis since the earliest steps; the knockout of genes encoding BMP receptors results in a serious impairment of chondrogenesis (Kobayashi et al., 2005). But switching in the *Sox9* gene expression is of crucial importance in BMP actions. The main role of this switching in, whereby chondroblastic differentiation starts, is played by BMP-2 (BMP-4 acts simultaneously with it), which is also of utmost impor-

tance in initiating condensation. As other BMPs, BMP-2 employs the intracellular signaling pathway via the Smad protein system. An introducing of BMP-2 into a cell culture of mice embryonal fibroblasts activates the *Sox9* gene expression and transforms the cells into completely formed chondroblasts. This effect involves a CCAAT nucleotide sequence in the gene proximal promoter (Pan et al., 2008).

The role of BMP-5 and BMP-7 is manifested a little later, in the second stage of the process. BMP-5 enables chondroblast proliferation and maintains the stimulating effect of Sox9 with respect to the expression the chondroblastic differon specific markers (Mailhot, 2008). BMP-7 (Op-1) acts in the same direction; it enhances the expression of components of the cartilage extracellular matrix, aggrecan and hyaluronan, as well as enzymes of hyaluronan synthesis (hyaluronan synthases), and the transmembrane receptor CD44 essential for its catabolism (Nishida et al., 2004). Bone morphogenetic protein-related morphogenetic proteins of a cartilage origin (CDMP-1, CDMP-2), whose activity in chondroblastic differentiation is comparable to that of BMP-7, stimulate the beginning of the aggrecan expression (Bai et al., 2004).

The effect of bone morphogenetic proteins on chondrogenesis is opposed by the influence of noggin and other antagonists. In the absence of noggin condensations, the cartilage structures that are being formed of them become excessively large. Such a cartilage hyperplasia impairs the formation of joints (Rosen, 2006).

As was previously mentioned in the example of the Wnt-7 morphogen inhibiting effect on chondroblastic differentiation, a complex system of regulating this process involves negative factors, restraining or delaying differentiation, together with positive stimulating factors. Such a combination of factors promotes the optimal progress of differentiation.

One of central negative factors is **retinoic acid** and other **retinoids** that are actively involved in the mesenchymal condensation and somitogenesis processes. Retinoids retain the condensation cells in a pre-chondrogenic status, preventing premature chondrogenesis. This function of retinoids, easily penetrating the cell membrane, is enabled by their nuclear receptors RAR and RXR, which are, at the same time, the transcription factors. In switching off genes' encoding, these receptor proteins remove retinoids' inhibiting effect on chondrogenesis (Hoffman et al., 2003).

GAS6 (growth arrest specific protein 6), a γ-carboxyglutamic acid residue containing glycoprotein, whose formation depends upon vitamin K, is also a negative regulator. This secreted protein (in humans it consists of 721 amino acid residues) acts even at the very beginning of the first chondroblastic differentiation stage, blocking the chondrogenesis-initiating effect of bone morphogenetic proteins on mesenchymal condensation cells. The negative role of GAS6 persists even later, when it inhibits the expression of type II collagen and aggrecan by chondroblasts (and even by the chondrocytes of articular cartilages) (Motomura et al., 2007). GAS6 exerts its effect on chondroblast differentiation via a signaling pathway of one of the mitogen-activated protein kinases family, **p38 MAPK**.

At the same time, the signaling pathway of p38 MAPK protein kinases is involved in a BMP-2 stimulating effect on chondrogenesis. This involvement consists in decreasing ("down-regulating") the above-mentioned Wnt-7a inhibiting effect (acting via the canonical pathway with β-catenin involvement). Due to this decrease, Sox9 expression increases (Jin et al., 2006).

Besides the p38 MAPK pathway, the signaling pathways of two other members of the MAPK family–the extracellular signal-regulated kinase (**ERK1/2**) and c-jun N-terminal kinase (**JNK**)–are involved in regulating chondroblastic differentiation (Bobick & Kulyk, 2008). These signal transduction pathways are essential at various stages of chondrogenesis in order to provide the effect of positive and negative regulating signals.

Mitogen-activated protein kinases (MAPK), and protein kinases of the C, Erk-1/2 and p38 families are significant in another link of chondroblastic differentiation. As already stated, the establishment of adhesive contacts between cells is a prerequisite for the successful formation of a mesenchymal condensation. These contacts are provided by the intense expression of adhesion molecules, especially N-cadherins. However, since the onset of the formation of a chondroblast phenotype in cells, for which the deposition of massive extracellular matrix is specific, adhesion contacts become an impediment for the matrix components' secretion. Therefore, there emerges a necessity for decreasing cell adhesiveness. N-cadherin expression is inhibited by means of the MAPK signaling pathway. At the same time, MAPK reduce the expression of the α5β1 integrin and its main ligand, fibronectin. In such a way, the conditions essential for cell secretion of specific macromolecular components of the cartilage matrix are formed (Oh et al., 2000; Yoon et al., 2000).

The effects of protein kinases supplement the anti-adhesive activity of Wnt-5a and Wnt-7a morphogens, which, by employing the transmembrane receptors Chfz-1 and Chfz-7, also inhibit the N-cadherin function and expression, but in the earlier stage of chondroblastic differentiation (Tuan, 2003). This anti-adhesive action of some Wnt occurs with the participation of β-catenins–components of the canonical Wnt signaling pathway that interact with cytoskeleton proteins (Ryu et al., 2002).

The beginning of changes in the composition and supramolecular organization of the extracellular matrix coincides with the beginning of chondroblastic differentiation of mesenchymal condensations. The replacement starts of a condensation matrix, which only slightly differs from the matrix of embryonal non-differentiated mesenchyme, by a matrix inherent to cartilaginous tissue.

The key early sign of this replacement that indicates the appearance of primary representatives of a chondroblas-

tic differon, prechondroblasts, is a shift from the biosynthesis of type I collagen to the biosynthesis of the large collagen of the cartilage matrix–type II collagen. In this switch, its two isoforms–IIA and IIB–are exchanged (McAlinden et al., 2005). Polypeptide α-chains of these isoforms are encoded by the same gene, which is the *COL2A1* gene in humans. Before switching, α-chains of collagen IIA are expressed, which retain a fragment of a non-spiralized (globular) amino terminal peptide, which consists of 69 amino acid residues and is rich in cysteine. This fragment, encoded by exon 2, persists in the triple-helical macromolecules of type IIA collagen, which is deposited in the condensation matrix for some time.

Owing to the presence of a retained propeptide fragment, type II collagen is capable of binding signal molecules of the TGF-β1 growth factor superfamily, including BMP-2 and thus, able to influence the intensity of its impact on the differentiation process. It is supposed that namely this is the function of type IIA collagen (Zhu et al., 1999). Recently-discovered IIC and IID isoforms (McAlinden et al., 2008) differ only slightly (by the presence of some additional amino acid residues) from IIA isoforms and may have a similar function.

A little later in the step of prechondroblastic differentiation, the activation of intracellular N-proteinases occurs, causing the cleavage of an amino propeptide fragment of IIA collagen even before procollagen polypeptides have secreted into the matrix and accumulation of this fragment within the cell (McAlinden et al., 2002).

In passing into the second stage of the process, the stage of active chondroblastic differentiation, IIA collagen expression is completely discontinued and chondroblasts switch to expressing the IIB collagen isoform, which is the main component of the large collagen fibrils of cartilaginous tissue and serves as the main marker of a chondroblast/chondrocyte phenotype. Switching is caused by an alternative splicing of type II procollagen mRNA. Splicing results in the removal of exon 2, encoding an extension of the amino propeptide of the IIA isoform. The mechanism of this splicing is complex. It is regulated by so-called cis-acting elements of introns of the RNA itself, involving the core protein **TASR-1**, also known as FUSIP1, a special splicing factor rich in arginine and serine. This protein is also related to the splicing regulation of another cartilage collagen–type XI collagen (Matsushita et al., 2007).

The expression of type VI collagen starts very early. This collagen might be important for matrix self-assembling and later persists only in matrix pericellular zones (Ofek et al., 2008). A little later, the expression of other "cartilage" collagens–type IX and XI collagens–commences.

In passing into the second stage of chondrogenesis, significant alterations also occur in the glycoprotein composition of the extracellular matrix of a forming cartilage model of a skeleton element. The expression of the second main marker of the chondroblastic phenotype starts. It is aggrecan, large proteoglycan, which displaces versican specific to the embryonal mesenchyme. The ongoing expression of hyaluronan ensures the conditions for the formation of aggrecan aggregations essential for cartilage's biomechanical function. The expression of a cartilage oligomeric matrix protein (COMP) starts.

The intensive expression of a heparan sulfate proteoglycan, **perlecan** (see section 3.3.2), following the type II collagen deposition, is characteristic for the second stage of chondrogenesis. At first, perlecan is diffusely distributed throughout the condensation's entire matrix, but later, as chondroblastic differentiation proceeds, its content decreases and it is only found in the pericellular zone near to the cell membrane. In such localization, perlecan is present in cartilaginous tissue in the postnatal period.

Perlecan is known as one of the main components of basement membranes, and its role in forming cartilage structures and in formed cartilages is not quite clear as there are no basement membranes as fully-formed morphologic structures within the cartilaginous tissue. Culturing embryonal fibroblasts in a perlecan-bearing medium enables the induction of their chondroblastic differentiation. This effect of perlecan is considered to be a manifestation of its chondrogenic activity, which is related to the amino terminal domain of the core protein carrying glycosaminoglycan chains. However, the activity mechanism has yet to be revealed (Gomes et al., 2004). It is interesting that perlecan accumulation occurs only in condensations whose evolution ends in enchondral ossification. The evolution of condensations, undergoing ossification by a membranous type, occurs without the involvement of perlecan (French et al., 1999).

In vitro investigations of chondroblastic differentiation of the mesenchyme stem cells (Djouad et al., 2007) indicate that expression changes of extracellular matrix components in the stage corresponding to the second stage of *in vivo* chondrogenesis involve a wide range of matrix molecules. It is not only the expression of structural components that is altered. Along with collagens, large glycoproteins and proteoglycans, the expression of a number of enzymes (MMP-7 and MMP-28 metalloproteases, the ADAM and ADAMTS families) and signal molecules (connective tissue growth factor, CTGF, and chemokines) is changed.

On the one hand, these matrix changes indicate profound alterations of the functional status of differentiating cells. On the other hand, they exert the strongest effect on cells that is manifested by expression changes of the intracellular molecules, for example, of gelsolin (a factor of actin depolymerization) and numerous cell membrane receptor molecules (i.e. syndecans, glypicans, chemokine receptors), cadherins and some subunits of integrins ($\alpha 4$, $\alpha 7$, $\beta 5$) (Djouad et al., 2007).

The modification of an acting set of integrins and the activation of integrin-linked kinases (ILK) indicate changes in interactions between cells and the extracellular matrix and affect the chondrogenesis progress (Goessler et al., 2008). For example, the exchange of the isoform of a laminin-bound $\alpha 6\beta 1$ integrin is of function-

al importance. An $\alpha 6\beta$ subunit-containing isoform enhances the manifestations of chondroblastic differentiation, such as switching the expression of type I collagen to type II, inhibiting fibronectin expression, and inhibiting the growth rate. Appearing later, an isoform of the same integrin containing an $\alpha 6A$ subunit does not exhibit such activity, but enables the stabilization of the chondroblastic phenotype under in vitro cell culturing conditions (Segat et al., 2002).

In the second stage of chondroblastic differentiation, the activity of other regulating factors directly responsible for chondrocyte phenotype formation comes into the foreground. A cartilage homeoprotein 1 (CART1), a transcription factor localized within the cell nucleus, starts to act. This protein, encoded by the *Cart1* gene mentioned above, is one of the most specific chondroblast/chondrocyte markers, and is similar to the Pax and Alx family proteins that have a paired homeodomain. Another nuclear protein – P300/CBP – is its activating co-factor (Iioka et al., 2003). A HoxD11 homeotic protein from the Hox-family, whose expression is controlled by bone morphogenetic proteins, functions in the same direction. The insulin-like growth factor-1 (IGF-1) also exerts a stimulating effect at this stage.

As the results of comparative *in vivo* investigations of **transcriptome** demonstrate, the transition from the first stage of chondroblastic differentiation to the second one is associated with radical changes in a global **profile of gene expression**. These changes involve the expression of a total of 931 genes, among which 380 are decreasing, while 551 demonstrate intensification (Cameron et al., 2009).

There is no such clear-cut boundary between the second and third stages as exists between the first and second ones. In the third stage, the cells finally reach the status of chondrocytes of permanent cartilages, BMP-2 retains its regulating influence, and the role of BMP-7 (OP-1) increases. BMP-7 continues to stimulate the expression of hyaluronan synthases, hyaluronan and aggrecan. Insulin and ascorbic acid enable maintaining the irreversibility of the chondroblastic differentiation of mesenchymal cells caused by bone morphogenetic proteins in *in vitro* experiments (Nieden et al., 2005).

Among the members of the fibroblast growth factor family, FGF-18 plays a leading role, acting via the FGFR-3 receptor. FGF-4 and FGF-8 are involved in regulating the formation of cartilage models of future bones along the proximal-distal axes of limb buds (Yu & Ornitz, 2008).

One of proteins binding insulin-like growth factors – IGFBP-3 – begins to have a stimulating influence on differentiation. This effect, independent of IGF itself, is aimed at **STAT-1** (signal transducer and activator of transcription-1), a molecule that circulates between the nucleus and cytoplasm (Spagnoli et al., 2002).

The Notch system of transmembrane receptors functioning as a restrictor of condensation at its onset becomes important again. According to some data, this system is engaged in the development of a phenotypic functional heterogeneity of chondrocytes in various layers of articular cartilage during the third stage of chondrogenesis (Hayes et al., 2003).

A significant part of the information on the molecular mechanisms of chondroblastic differentiation is obtained through experimental investigations of mesenchymal cells cultured *in vitro*. The regularities revealed might be only partially characterizing a real *in vivo* setting, which is much more complex. The peculiarities of condensation and further chondroblastic differentiation in different regions of a developing skeleton are the main complicating aspects. These peculiarities are due to the involvement of other protein molecules in the process (transcription co-activators and repressors), which have not been mentioned earlier; these molecules are encoded by homeotic genes. It has been shown that homeotic proteins, such as Msx-1 and Msx-2, Cfkh-1, Mfh-1, Dkk-1 and some others, are involved in chondrogenesis in various localizations (Hall & Miyake, 2000).

In the process of forming an axial and paraxial (including somites) skeleton, the expression of *Hox*-genes essential for chondrogenesis is also controlled by other homeotic genes–those of the *Cdx*-family (Deschamps & Nes, 2005). As in all other localizations, Sox9 stimulation of chondrogenesis in somites requires the activity of one more factor, the Nkx3.2 transcription repressor, the induction of which involves Shh and BMP (Zeng et al., 2002). Non-identical impairments in chondrogenesis occur in the spine and rib cage in mutations of the *Nell1* gene, which encodes the protein kinase PKC β-1-binding protein Nell1 (Desai et al., 2006). Some peculiarities of molecular regulation are of significance in chondrogenesis in the appendicular skeleton: Pax9 and Jagged1 are essential for the proper formation of limb distal regions. Pax9 and Jagged1 are regulated by a Gli3 transcription repressor that, in turn, is under the control of the Shh morphogen (McGlinn et al., 2005).

The differentiation of permanent cartilage cells is discontinued after the third stage is over. They lose the capacity for mitotic division and therefore, for proliferation, thus transforming from chondroblasts into chondrocytes. At the same time, their secretory activity decreases significantly. This is particularly the outcome of cartilage chondrocytes.

It should be added that, in *in vitro* experiments, the chondrogenic differentiation of stem cells derived from adult organisms' tissues has proven to be feasible (Karlsson et al., 2007a). The application of this possibility is of great importance for the medical practice. The molecular mechanisms revealed upon studying stem cell differentiation are, in general, similar to the known details about the natural development of the cartilage cell differon in embryogenesis. However, it is premature to consider these processes as identical due to the significant differences in regulating effects, especially systematic ones, within embryos and adult organisms.

The majority of condensation mesenchymal cells that have undergone chondroblastic differentiation remain as chondroblasts in condensations that have been transformed into a transitory (temporal) hyaline cartilage. Such condensations, whose main extracellular matrix components are type II collagen and aggrecan, become "patterns" or "models" for future bones. Chondroblasts of transitory cartilages that retain their ability to proliferate come to the next differentiation stage, referred to as maturation. Chondrocyte maturation and further apoptosis create the conditions for their displacement by osteoblasts, and endochondral ossification takes place.

10.2.3. Molecular biological and biochemical mechanisms of osteoblastic differentiation

In osteoblastic differentiation, pluripotent cells of mesenchymal condensations acquire an osteoblast phenotype, characterized by the expression of a specific gene set. The genes that encode the proteins essential for building up a bone tissue extracellular matrix and its mineralization hold a central place in this set.

Switching in the expression of these genes occurs in embryogenesis under the control of a complex network of regulating factors employing various signaling pathways. The expression activity of 41 transcription factors is changed under their influence, indicating the participation of these factors in osteoblastic differentiation (Qi et al., 2003).

Runx2 plays a leading role among all these transcription factors (Komori, 2008; Franceshi et al., 2009). It is called as "the main organizer in gene transcription in osteoblasts" and its gene called a "master-gene" (Schroeder et al., 2005). Its significance in osteoblast differentiation is similar to that of the Sox9 factor in chondroblast differentiation (Karsenty, 2008).

By the way, a Sox8 transcription factor, which is close to Sox9, is one of regulators of osteoblastic differentiation, where it plays a negative role. Switching off a gene encoding this factor results in premature and accelerated mineralization (Schmidt et al., 2005).

Runx2, a phosphoprotein, one of the three members of the Runx family, encoded by the *Runx2* gene (in humans it is RUNX2), is a transcription factor. Its full officially recommended name, "a runt-related transcription factor 2", is based on gene similarity to a *Runt* ("shorty") gene in drosophila, which controls the expression of the factors responsible for the formation of paired structures of body segments. It also has a number of other names, such as AML-3, PEBP2a1, Osf-2 (osteoblast specific factor-2). The name Cbfa1 (core-binding factor alpha 1) is more often used, along with the name Runx2.

There are 12 known isoforms of Runx2. These isoforms arise as a result of alternative splicing and provide a certain specialization of functions dependent on the character and differentiation stage of the cells expressing them. The main isoforms–Runx2-I and Runx2-II–differ from each other in humans by the primary structure of the amino terminal region: the type II isoform (also called Osf2) has a sequence of 19 amino acid residues (MASNSLFSAVTPCQQSFFW), encoded by exon 1, which is absent in the type II isoform. The isoform expression is associated with employing different promoters (Xiao Z.S. et al., 2004).

The Runx2 primary structure differs by the presence of clusters of glutamine and alanine residues within the N-terminal region; these clusters distinguish Runx2 from Runx1 and Runx3.

The Runx2 macromolecule has a domain structure. A highly conservative (almost the same domain in a drosophila) Runt domain responsible for DNA binding occupies a central position (from the 105th to 233rd amino acid residues). Other domains perform binding with a number of transcription factors. Binding is accompanied by activation or repression of these factors, and by assembling active intranuclear complexes (Stein et al., 2003). At the same time, factors interacting with Runx2 affect its functions, proving themselves to be its co-partners (co-activators or co-repressors). These partners (c-Fos, c-Jun, C/EBPs, Dlx5, Hes1, Oct-1 and some others) facilitate the necessary specificity and efficacy of Runx2 action in osteoblastogenesis (Schroeder et al., 2005).

A Cbfβ factor, encoded by *Cbf*β, is involved in Runx2 functions. This phosphoprotein, containing 182 amino acid residues, forms a heterodimer with Runx1, another member of the Runx family. This heterodimer is essential for embryonal hematopoiesis occurring in the liver. Its absence causes embryo death, but if hematopoiesis is successfully maintained by genetic methods, animals are born with marked defects in ossification, characteristic for switching off the *Runx2* gene. This indicates a crucial role for Cbfβ in bone tissue development (Kundu et al., 2002).

The Runx2 position in a cell nucleus matrix, where it is concentrated in approximately 300 discrete loci, is of great importance for its functions. Localization accuracy is facilitated by special signal amino acid sequences (NLS, nuclear localization signal, and NMTS, nuclear matrix targeting signal) within its macromolecule.

The specificity of Runx2 activity in relation to osteoblasts is associated with the intragenic (cis-) regulation of its gene. In the gene P 1 promoter region, there are special elements, rich in purine (Y-repeats), which are stimulated by SP1 and ETS transcription factors and selectively act as enhancers only in osteoblast mesenchymal progenitors (Zhang Y. et al., 2009).

Runx2 functions in an activated state, which is achieved by post-transcriptional modification, i.e. phosphorylation. Phosphorylation is carried out by an ERK1/2 kinase signaling pathway. The role of this signaling pathway in osteoblastogenesis, especially in skull bones and the clavicle, is considered to be critical (Ge et al., 2007; Franceschi et al., 2009). At the same time, the phosphorylation of Runx2 is activated by signals propagated by other pathways (via the Smad system components and AP-1 factors, along pathways activated by PKA and PKC kinases). It assigns Runx2 the role of a center, coordinating a variety of signals involved in osteoblastic differentiation (Franceschi et al., 2003). In osteoblast progenitors, Runx2 employs one more signaling pathway, originating in a G protein bound to the cell membrane and receptors associated with this protein. These signals activate the expression of cyclic adenosine monophosphate (cAMP), which increases cell sensitivity to mitogen actions and accelerates proliferation (Teplyuk et al., 2008).

The expression of Runx2 in mesenchymal condensation cells begins even before the onset of osteoblast differentiation and occurs for some time in cells, starting both chondroblastic and osteoblastic differentiation. Then the Runx2 expression in chondroblasts weakens and is activated again in the final stages of chondrocyte maturation. With a Runx2 deficiency, chondrocyte maturation is delayed, indicating the involvement of this factor in chondrogenesis (Franceschi et al., 2009).

Mesenchymal cells achieving the preosteoblast stage restrain the expression of Runx2-I, primarily switching to the Runx2-II expression. The Runx2-II isoform essential for completing osteoblastic differentiation assumes importance as an osteogenesis early marker. Although the expression of the Runx2-I isoform continues, it is the Runx2-II isoform that distinguishes the cells of an osteoblastic differon from the total population of mesenchymal progenitor cells. Later on, it stimulates the proliferation and differentiation of preosteoblasts up to the formation of a mature osteoblast phenotype (Li & Xiao, 2007; Zhang S. et al., 2009).

The *Runx2* gene also performs another interesting function. Being inside a chromosome in the nearest vicinity of the genes encoding ribosomal RNA (rRNA) during mitosis, it controls rRNA expression involving transcription factors affecting the synthesis of RNA polymerase I. Created by this control on growth confinement, the proliferation and total biosynthetic activity of cells ensure the maintenance of commitment stability (a differentiation way) of cells undergoing subsequent mitoses (Young et al., 2007a; Ali et al., 2008). This effect is achieved owing to the stability of Runx2 binding with DNA within promoter zones of its controlled genes (Young, 2007b). Thus, Runx2/Cbfa1 acquires the role of a "factor, determining the cell fate" and serves as a center for coordinating the expression of genes specifying the osteoblastic differon (Lian et al., 2006).

Knocking out (nil mutation) the *Runx2* gene causes animals to die immediately after birth. Their skeleton is built up of only cartilaginous tissue without any signs of osteoblastic differentiation or the beginning of ossification. This proves the absolute relevance of Runx2 in terms of osteoblastogenesis (Komori, 2008).

The regulating and controlling action of Runx2 manifests itself as switching in the active expression of genes specific to the osteoblastic differon. Among these genes, the ones that prevail are those encoding proteins secreted into the bone tissue extracellular matrix and that create the conditions for matrix mineralization. It is these secreted proteins (or their mRNA, indicating their transcription) that are considered as markers of the osteoblastic phenotype. These markers are type I collagen, alkaline phosphatase, bone sialoprotein (BSP), osteocalcin, lumican, and osteocrin. Fibril-forming type XXIV collagen might be a highly specific marker of osteoblastic differentiation. This collagen has not been studied sufficiently yet. The increasing concentration of this collagen mRNA coincides in time with a period of intensive expression of osteocalcin (Matsuo et al., 2008).

The effect of Runx2 on the osteoblast expression of genes encoding components of the bone tissue extracellular matrix is due to the presence of an osteoblast specific element (OSE) within the promoter zone of these genes. Runx2 interacts with this element (Karsenty, 2001). The stimulating effect of Runx2 on osteoblast proliferation is related to the carboxyterminal domain of its macromolecule (Pratap et al., 2003).

Runx2 involvement in osteogenesis is not limited to its leading role in osteoblastic differentiation. Its stimulating effect on blood vessel invasion into avascular cartilage models of future bones is of importance for endochondral ossification (Komori, 2006).

The Runx2 function in osteoblastogenesis is closely related to another regulating factor–the **transcription factor Sp7** (a specificity protein 7; it is its official name in humans). Its alternative name **Osterix**, proposed for this factor in mice prevails (Nakashima et al., 2002).

In humans, this nuclear protein is encoded by the *OSX* gene (Gao et al., 2004). It is one of the "specificity proteins" and is a member of the large transcription factor family with "zinc fingers" of the C2H2 type. Osterix consists of 431 amino acid residues and contains three "fingers" in the macromolecule C-terminal region. "Fingers" are specific domains of a polypeptide chain, in which two cysteine residues and two hystidine residues retain one atom of zinc oriented in a certain position. "Zinc fingers" are responsible for binding and interacting with DNA.

Without the Sp7 expression as in a nil mutation of *Runx2*, osteoblastic differentiation is impossible; given the complete absence of osteoblasts in animals, neither membranous nor endochondral ossification occurs. But unlike the Runx2 deficiency, the deficiency of Osterix does not affect chondrocyte maturation, and cartilage models of bones develop normally. An excess of Osterix inhibits chondrocytes' maturation (Kaback et al., 2007). From this we know that, firstly, Osterix is not of significant importance for the differentiation of chondroblasts/chondrocytes *in vivo*, but is only essential for osteoblastic differentiation (Komori, 2008). Secondly, Osterix expression starts later, after osteoblastic commitment of mesenchymal cells in the preosteoblast stage. Osterix is necessary *in vitro* for the osteoblastic commitment of mesenchymal progenitor cells in BMP-induced differentiation (Tominaga et al., 2009).

The main factor stimulating Osterix expression is Runx2. Without Runx2, Osterix expression is inhibited. The *OSX*

gene promoter contains a specific element that perceives the influence of Runx2 (Nishio et al., 2006). Runx2 expression, on the contrary, is not afflicted in the absence of Osterix, i.e. while Osterix is no less important for osteoblastic differentiation than Runx2 (and can also serve as an osteoblast marker), it is under its control, being "downstream" in the regulation factor cascade (Deng et al., 2008).

However, the Runx2-dependent way of controlling Osterix expression is not the only one. Osteoblastic differentiation, stimulated by BMP2 and coordinated by Osterix, might occur even given a deficiency of Runx2. In this case, the mechanism of stimulating Osterix expression involves the Msx2 homeotic protein (Matsubara et al., 2008).

One of molecular mechanisms of Osterix action is its involvement in chromatin remodeling within a cell nucleus (Hatta et al., 2006).

Runx2/Cbfa1 and Sp7/Osterix are crucial transcription factors in osteoblastic differentiation. But they function involving a number of other transcription factors that they partially control, whose action is coordinated by localization in tissue and in terms of the time of the activity manifested. In particular, factors such as TAZ, Twist, ATF4, Dlx5 (and other Dlx), and Msx2 are of importance (Deng et al., 2008).

For example, the transcription co-activator **TAZ** (tafazzin/G4.5) enhances the stimulating effect of Runx2 on the expression of its activated genes and, simultaneously, inhibits the expression of genes stimulated by adipogenesis PPARγ activator. Such a double effect of TAZ promotes the commitment of mesenchymal progenitor cells into the osteoblastic differentiation way (Hong et al., 2005).

The transcription factors **Twist-1** and **Twist-2**, encoded by *Twsg1* and *Twsg2* genes–homologs of the drosophila gene *Twisted gastrulation*–are especially actively expressed in the first days after Runx2 expression starts. These proteins contain a special domain capable of occupying a DNA locus, which binds Runx2. Owing to this, Twist factors interfere with Runx2 binding and, thus, prevent premature beginning of osteoblastic differentiation (Bialek et al., 2004). Moreover, Twist-1 restrains the stimulating effect of bone morphogenetic proteins (BMP) on osteoblastogenesis; this Twist-1 activity is, in turn, controlled by the Id1 transcription factor ("an inhibitor of DNA binding") (Hayashi et al., 2007).

The Twist and Id factors belong to a large group of transcription factors, whose second structure contains a motif "helix-loop-helix", rich in essential amino acid residues (bHLH, basic helix-loop-helix). The bHLH factors are bound to a so-called E-box (enhancer box) of the gene promoter zone. These factors play a large role in regulating osteoblastic differentiation, with their effect on this process not being related to Runx2 in a number of cases. A general mechanism of activity allows us to consider them as a uniform complex regulating network (Zhang Y. et al., 2008). While the Twist and Id factors inhibit differentiation, factors of the Myc family having a bHLH motif as well and some others stimulate osteoblastogenesis. Another name of the Myc family is USF1, "upstream" stimulating factors, which is its recommended name.

ATF4 (activating transcription factor 4) is a protein with one bZIP-domain (leucine "zipper") binding to DNA as a dimer, a RSK2 kinase substrate. This factor, whose activity is controlled by another factor, FIAT/ γ-taxilin, is involved in the initiation and completion of osteoblastic differentiation, as well as in regulating the expression of type I collagen, osteocalcin and RANKL, i.e. the functions of a mature osteoblast (Komori, 2006). Moreover, it is involved in regulating amino acid inflow into a cell.

Dlx are homeotic (homeobox-containing) transcription factors similar to the Dll (distal-less) factor in a drosophila, which is essential for the development of appendicular osteogenesis. They are stimulators of osteoblastic differentiation. This effect is most pronounced in the Dlx5 factor, but it can be compensated largely by other isoforms (Dlx2, Dlx3, Dlx6) in the absence of Dlx5 (Samee et al., 2008; Li H. et al., 2008). Their interaction with the DNA regulating the Runx2 expression occurs in complexes with a HOXA10 protein and the homeotic protein Msx2, a member of the Msx family, with the complex composition changing upon passing from one osteoblast differentiation stage to the next one. Such switchings are accompanied by alterations in the phenotype of differentiating cells (Hassan et al., 2009). Homeotic proteins of the Msx family are of special significance in the osteoblastogenesis of cranio-facial skeleton bones and some mutations of the genes encoding these proteins are fatal (Alapatt et al., 2003). Dlx5 stimulates the Runx2 expression within the cells of the mesenchyme, which is found in sutures forming between skull bones, and promotes the osteogenic differentiation of these cells (Holleville et al., 2007).

Furthermore, together with Runx2, Dlx and Msx proteins cause the rearrangement of chromatin structures of a nucleus, which, in turn, affects the expression of genes specifying an osteoblastic phenotype (Hassan et al., 2009). The intensity of these effects (as well as the same effect of Osterix) has an inverse relationship to the degree of methylation (attaching methyl groups to nucleotides) of their gene promoters (Lee J.Y. et al., 2006).

Runx2 transcription activity is enhanced by transcription factors, such as the enhancer-bound C/EBPβ and C/EBPδ proteins, the ETS1 factor, Grg5/ESP1 co-activators, the interferon-induced p204 protein, the antigen FOSL1/FRA-1 of the Fos-family, and proteins with "zinc fingers" Krox-20 and SP3. The signal transducer and activator Stat1, the tyrosine-proteinkinase Yes, and TLE proteins similar to transducers (signal transmitters from transmembrane receptors) act, inhibiting its activity in distinct periods of differentiation (Komori, 2006).

The growth factor and mitogen pleiotrophin (Osf1, osteoblast specific factor 1) plays the role of a transcription factor. It contributes to the activating effect of Runx2 on osteocalcin expression and is involved in bone tissue's anabolic response to mechanical shock (Kesavan & Mohan, 2008). Cthrc1 (a protein containing a collagen-like triple-helical repeat) has a positive (anabolic) effect on osteoblastic differentiation. This protein is one of BMP-2 targets. Cthrc-1 increases the osteoblast count and bone tissue mass (Kimura et al., 2008).

Proteins, whose secondary structure is characterized by the presence of "zinc fingers", secure a large place among the transcription factors that control the different stages of osteoblastogenesis, including the subsequent mineralization of the osteoblast-produced matrix. Osterix, whose functions are supplemented by a number of other factors with a similar structure, is of primary significance among them. The SNA11 protein controlling cadherin expression should also be named together with this. The AJ18 protein (also called 354C), containing 11 "zinc fingers", restrains the Runx2/Cbfa1 activity (Ganss & Jheon, 2004). The PLZF protein (otherwise known as ZFP145), encoded by a *ZBTB16* gene, which is otherwise a Runx2 activator, induces the osteoblastic differentiation of mesenchymal stem cells of the spine longitudinal ligament, resulting in its pathologic ossification (Ikeda et al., 2005).

A protein called "four-and-half Lim 2" (**FHL2**) is an active stimulator of osteoblastic differentiation and the subsequent mineralization of the matrix. This protein, comprised of 279 amino acid residues, is built up of 4 ½ Lim domains. Every entire LIM-domain contains two "zinc fingers" that are closely located to each other. These "zinc fingers" provide FHL2 with marked activity in terms of "protein-protein" interactions. Within the cytoplasm, FHL2 facilitates the propagation of signals coming from integrins, and acts as a co-activator of many transcription factors within the nucleus. In particular, FHL2 is bound to β-catenin and, thus, activates the expression of Runx2, induced by Wnt family morphogens (Hamidouche et al., 2008). A deficiency of FHL2 decreases the total mass of bone tissue (causes osteopenia) and its degree of mineralization (Günther et al., 2005; Lai et al., 2006).

The protein (phosphoprotein) LMP-1 (LIM Mineralization Protein-1), containing 3 LIM-domains, exerts a stimulating effect on osteoblastic differentiation and osteogenesis. Of the 457 amino acid residues of LMP-1 that are encoded by the *PDLIM7* gene, 178 are in three LIM-domains. LMP-1 mediates the BMP-6 osteogenic effect, maintains the mineralization of differentiated *in vitro* osteoblast cultures, and is involved *in vivo* in endochondral ossification (Boden et al., 1999; Yoon & Boden, 2002).

Another protein that also contains 3 LIM-domains and is also a phosphoprotein, **LIMD1**, in acting as a signaling system component and as a transcription factor, appeared, to the contrary, to be a negative regulator (restrictor) of the differentiation and osteoblast functions. Its gene switching off increases the number of mesenchymal cells involved in the osteogenic differon (Luderer et al., 2008). The **TBX3** protein (a T-box-3 protein), which restrains the expression of Runx2 and Osterix, exerts its effect in the same direction. As a result of this action, the proliferation of progenitor cells is enhanced, but their osteoblastic differentiation is inhibited (Govoni et al., 2009).

The growth and differentiation of osteoblasts are, in addition, regulated by ionized calcium (Ca²⁺), whose effect on the transcription processes is determined by calcium binding with phosphoprotein **calmodulin**. This complex activates diverse intracellular factors, including those that affect osteoclastogenesis (see section 10.2.4) (Zayzafoon, 2005).

One of the conditions for completing the differentiation and final formation of a mature osteoblast phenotype is the release of an osteoblast from the cell cycle, i.e. a loss of the capability to proliferate. The achievement of this condition is a function of the **pRb** protein in osteoblastogenesis. This **protein, bound to retinoblastoma**, controls and inhibits the activity of an important inducer of the cell cycle, the E2f1 transcription factor (Berman et al., 2008).

Among the factors determining an osteoblastic way of differentiation of multipotent mesenchymal cells is **menin**, a nuclear protein consisting of 510 amino acid residues, which encodes the gene of multiple endocrine neoplasia type I (*Men1*) (Sowa et al., 2003). Menin macromolecule has a multidomain structure, enabling it to interact with many proteins, including those that are involved in regulating osteoblast differentiation (members of the TGF-β superfamily, including BMP, and IGFBP), as well as osteoclasts (NFkB) (Balogh et al., 2006). The switching off of the *Men1* gene prevents the appearance of osteoblast phenotypic features in mesenchymal cells; herein, a process of intramembranous ossification is greatly affected (Hendy et al., 2005). The menin effect is specific: its deficiency does not affect the chondrogenic and adipogenic differentiation of mesenchymal cells. On the contrary, menin inhibits the differentiation of osteoblasts that has already begun, interrupting the BMP influence on the Runx2/Cbfa1 transcription factor. This inhibition occurs due to the blockage of one of the AP-1 activating complex components encoded by the *JunD* proto-oncogene (Naito et al., 2005).

A number of enzymes are involved in the molecular mechanisms of osteoblastic differentiation. These are primarily numerous protein kinases, particularly the ERK family kinases mentioned above (kinases regulated by extracellular signals or, in other words, MAP, mitogen-activated kinases). ERK are involved in the processes of osteoblast growth and differentiation, and they are essential for integrin expression, for mineralization, and for other osteoblast functions (Lai et al., 2001). JNK (N-terminal c-Jun kinases, phosphorylating the c-Jun transcription factor) are significant; JNK are essential for activating the Atf4 transcription factor and important in the latest stage of differentiation (Matsuguchi et al., 2009).

Switching off the *Eif2ak3* gene encoding the **PERK** kinase (the full name is eukaryotic translation initiation factor kinase-3) results in a very serious impairment of osteo-

blastogenesis. In the absence of this enzyme, localized in an endoplasmic reticulum membrane, osteoblast proliferation slows down in relation to disturbances in the cell cycle due to the inhibition of cyclin and Cdc2 protein expression. Osteopenia develops due to a decrease in the number of mature osteoblasts and the osteoblast secretion of type I collagen, whose macromolecules are delayed in the endoplasmic reticulum. All these impairments are based on inhibiting the expression of Runx2 and Osterix (Wei et al., 2008).

Besides kinases, during a certain step of osteoblastogenesis *in vitro*, the expression of matrix 14 metalloprotease (MT1-MMP) by differentiating progenitor cells is of importance. In the absence of this enzyme, which is fixed on the cytoplasmatic membrane and catalyzes the proteolysis of collagens and aggrecan, the osteoblast expression of integrins and alkaline phosphatase is impaired and the matrix's mineralization is delayed (Manduca et al., 2009). In mice embryos, the intensive expression of MT1-MMP occurs within ossification foci between 14.5–17.5 days of embryogenesis, and switching off the encoding gene results in osteopenia and dwarfism.

The expression and functions of Runx2 and Osterix, which are the leading factors in controlling osteoblast differentiation at the transcription level, are object to control by a number of systems determining the general regularities of embryogenesis (see section 10.1) and associated with the higher levels of osteoblastogenesis regulation. These systems include:

1) signaling pathways of the transforming growth factor β superfamily (TGF-β), including the family of bone morphogenetic proteins (BMP);
2) signaling systems of fibroblast growth factors (FGF);
3) the Notch transmembrane signaling system;
4) the Hedgehog-morphogen signaling system;
5) the Wnt morphogen signaling system (Schroeder et al., 2005). Endocrine signals (parathyroid hormone, vitamin D, estrogens) are "upstream" in the signals cascade regulating Runx2 and Osterix (Komori, 2008). In addition, the influence of the extracellular matrix is included in this complex network of control.

The effect of regulating signaling systems on the "master-genes" of osteoblastogenesis is manifold. Some stimuli affect gene promoter zones, regulating their expression in such a way. Others activate enzymes involved in post-translation modifications of Runx2 or mobilize the co-factors listed above, interacting with Runx2 and affecting its binding with DNA. Herein the immediate interaction of various factors, resulting in the formation of active components, is of great functional importance in many cases (McCarthy et al., 2000).

Bone morphogenetic proteins (BMP), BMP-2, BMP-7 and BMP-9 in particular, are known as initiators and stimulators of osteoblastic differentiation of the mesenchyme progenitor cells; BMP-2 is especially active in this respect (Luu et al., 2007). During *in vitro* experiments in C2C12 strain cells differentiating into osteoblasts, it was stated that not less than 1,800 genes are susceptible to

BMP-2 action in the differentiation process for 24 hours after it was introduced into a culture. In approximately 100 of these genes, the expression intensity showed statistically significant changes, by 3–14 times. Nonspecific genes responsible for cell proliferation and growth were activated in the first few hours. This was followed by the activation of the genes, encoding a number of homeotic proteins and osteoblast-specific transcription factors, including Runx2. Finally the expression of genes encoding components of the bone tissue extracellular matrix (type I collagen, proteoglycans of the PRELP family) was stimulated (Balint et al., 2003).

This multivercity of BMP-2 action is largely due to its interaction with Runx2, which is bound with components of the Smad intracellular signaling system employed by all BMP. For this interaction, Runx2 has a special domain in the macromolecule carboxyterminal region (Afzal et al., 2005). As a result of the structural coupling of Runx2 with Smad in the nucleus, a complex is formed; this complex transmits an osteogenic BMP-2 signal, controlled by Runx2, to effector genes, executing differentiation directly (Javed et al., 2008).

BMP osteoinductive activity is extremely important in regulating the initial steps of embryonal skeletogenesis. For example, in the targeted (conditional) double inactivation (knock-out) of Bmp2 and Bmp4 genes in mice, bones' cartilage patterns were normally built up in forming limbs, but instead of osteoblasts, these patterns were homed by cells similar to fibroblasts, lacking some characteristic markers of the osteoblastic phenotype, of an Osterix protein for instance. The formation of full-fledged limbs did not take place (Bandyopadhyay et al., 2006).

BMP-2 stimulates the expression of Osterix. This stimulation is, in large part, secondary to BMP influence on Runx2 and Smad, but the BMP effect on Osterix can be partially mediated by Runx2 independent signaling pathways. One such pathway is associated with signals of the insulin-like growth factor-1 (IGF-1), whose effect on Osterix is synergetic to BMP action (Celli et al., 2005). Another pathway is the BMP-2-caused induction of the homeotic protein Dlx5, which activates Osterix expression after it has been phosphorylated by p38 kinases (Ulsamer et al., 2008). This BMP-2 stimulating effect on osteoblastic differentiation, very significant in embryogenesis, continues in the postnatal period (Bais et al., 2009).

Moreover, BMPs induce the expression of other proteins, which act as additional stimulators of osteoblastic differentiation, employing signaling pathways different from those employed by BMP. One of these proteins is the BMP-2 induced **osteoactivin** (see section 8.2.1.2).

Another protein induced by BMP-2 in osteoblasts is **WDR5**, whose gene is called BIG-3 (bmp-2-induced gene 3 kb; 3 kilobyte is the gene length). WDR5 is a member of a numerous family of so-called WD-40 proteins. They are proteins with WD repeats, varied in domain structure with a length of 40–42 amino acid residues, very often beginning with GH (glycine-histidine) residues and ending in WD residues (tryptophan–aspartic acid). WD re-

peats have a secondary structure that is compared to a propeller and makes WD-40 proteins highly active in intracellular interactions with other proteins. Wdr5, a phosphoprotein consisting of 334 amino acid residues, has 7 WD repeats. It radically accelerates the differentiation of osteoblasts in vitro when introduced into a culture: the expression of alkaline phosphatase begins earlier and is more than 10 times more active than that in the control group. Cell sensitivity to the parathyreotropic hormone increases so much significantly (Gori et al., 2001). Wdr5 has no less activity in accelerating osteoblastogenesis in vivo, enhancing the expression of type I collagen in embryo forming bones. This effect in vivo is mediated by activating the canonical Wnt signaling pathway (Gori et al., 2006). A deficiency of Wdr5 results in this pathway disruption (Zhu et al., 2008).

Together with all the effects of BMP-2, which are associated with the influence on Runx2 expression, this bone morphogenetic protein is capable of stimulating the early stages of osteoblastic and chondroblastic differentiation (let's recall that Runx2 is involved in regulating not only osteobalstogenesis, but also chondroblastogenesis) without Runx2. The BMP-2 stimulating effect is manifested by enhancing the expression of 66 genes, including 13 genes that are related to transcription regulation and are, at the same time, independent of Runx2. This action is enough to induce the expression by the progenitor cells of a number of specific chondroblast and osteoblast markers, but is not sufficient to complete the differentiation of mature chondrocytes and bone tissue producing osteoblasts (Liu et al., 2007).

The role of BMP-2 in osteogenesis regulation has one more aspect related to its effect on the formation of so-called microRNA (miRNA) (see 10.1). The buildup of 22 of the 25 variants of miRNA studied is reduced under the influence of BMP-2. Thus, BMP-2 diminishes the inhibition of protein synthesis caused by miRNA, stimulates the expression of Runx2, and increases its activity. This enables the osteoblastic commitment of mesenchymal progenitor cells (Li Z., 2008).

Unlike other BMP, BMP-9, which has yet not been adequately studied, has a strong osteogenic activity associated with its stimulating expression of the transcription factor **Hey1**. This protein, which contains one "helix-loop-helix" (bHLH) domain, in turn, increases Runx2/Cbfa1 expression, enabling osteoblastic differentiation and mineralization (Scharff et al., 2009).

The members of the TGF-β superfamily that are not assigned to the BMP family might affect the leading genes of osteoblastic differentiation in ways similar to the BMP pathways, i.e. preferably via the Smad system. Unlike BMP interacting with Smad1, Smad-5 and Smad-8, other TGF-βs work via Smad-2 and Smad-3 (Schroeder et al., 2005). Smad-3, in particular, stimulates the expression of genes related to mineralization (Kaji et al., 2006). In addition, TGF-β activity is controlled by their interaction with the proteins binding latent TGF-β (**LTBP**). Among the four members of the LTBP family, only two of them are of importance in osteoblastogenesis: LTBP-3 serves as a source of active TGF-β during osteoblast differentiation and deposition of the extracellular matrix and, as the matrix matures, TGF-β are bound to LTBP-1 and are deposited in the matrix in such a bound form (Koli et al., 2008). There are several known serious defects of osteogenesis, caused by TGF-β-ligand mutations and their receptors (Deng et al., 2008).

Among **fibroblast growth factors (FGF)** related to bone tissue, a few of them (FGF-1, -2, -9, -18, -22) are expressed throughout the entire life, including the embryonal period while the other FGF (FGF-3, -4, -8, -15, -17, -19) function only occurs in embryogenesis and is not found in the postnatal period. This fact permits supposing the prevailing involvement of the majority of FGF and their receptors in regulating osteoblastic differentiation in embryogenesis.

Acting via FGFP2 and FGFR3 receptors, FGF-2 promotes targeting the activity of the Runx2/Cbfa1 factor in a previously unknown signaling pathway, whose end-point is the expression of heparan sulfate proteoglycans (syndecans and glypicans), as well as a large proteoglycan versican. Activating the expression of the enzymes involved in this process–specific acetyltransferases and sulfotransferases–enables the enhancement of proteoglycan synthesis (Teplyuk et al., 2009). One of the FGF-2 isoforms has a marked stimulating effect on osteoblastogenesis. It is a small, secreted molecule with a molecular mass of 18 kDa, which, unlike other FGF, acts by the paracrine but not by the intracrine way (Xiao et al., 2009). FGF action is mainly manifested in terms of enhancing the expression of the extracellular matrix components involved in mineralization (Deng Z.L. et al., 2008). The main mechanism of the FGF action consists of activating MAP kinases (ERK, p38); the role that protein kinases play in regulating transcription factors, including Runx2, has been discussed above. FGFR2, one of the FGF-receptors involved in stimulating osteoblastic differentiation in the early stage, employs the same mechanism (Miraoui, 2009). The role of another receptor, FGFR1, changes depending on the stage of osteoblast differentiation. In an early stage, the deficiency of this receptor enhances the proliferation and delays the mineralization of the matrix; later on, switching off the *Fgfr1* gene, on the contrary, accelerates the completion of differentiation and accelerates mineralization (Jacob et al., 2006).

FGF-1 employs a peculiar mechanism of action, mainly stimulating preosteoblast proliferation and therefore, in- creasing the bone tissue mass. FGF-1 inhibits the expres- sion of "a fidgetin-like protein 1" possessing the activity of an adenosine triphosphatases, which is encoded by the *FIGNL1* gene. This enzyme delays cell proliferation in the early step of osteoblastic differentiation, although it stimulates their differentiation later; the stimulation is seen as the increased expression of alkaline phosphatase and osteopontin (Park et al., 2007).

Insulin-like growth factor IGF-1 affects bone tissue, mainly as a component of the pituitary growth hormone IGF (GH/IGF) "axis" (see section 8.5.2). Besides two ligands–IGF-1 and IGF-2–this "axis" includes two receptors (IGF1R and IGF2R) and 6 binding proteins (IGFBP1–IGFBP6). In this axis, IGF-1 mediates the stimulating effect of the growth hormone on bone growth and the anabolizing effect on osteoblast activity.

In the embryonal period, IGF-1 is essential for normal skeletogenesis; dwarfism, a delay in mineralization and bone deformities develop in the case of IGF-1 deficiency, caused by the encoding gene knockout (Wang Y. et al., 2006b). IGF-1 expresses osteoblasts, together with other cells. In osteoporosis, its content in compact bone tissue (within the cortical layer) is decreased. The osteoinductive effect of BMP-6, which has been used in an experiment to cure osteoporosis, is associated with the stimulation of IGF-1 expression by osteoblasts (Grasser et al., 2007).

The connective tissue growth factor (**CTGF**) is also involved in regulating osteoblastic differentiation. In the differentiation of cells *in vitro*, the concentration of CTGF mRNA increases in cells twice: in the period of intensive proliferation and during mineralization. Accordingly, the introduction of CTGF in a culture in the early differentiation stage enhances proliferation and increases the activity of alkaline phosphatase and the deposition of calcium salts in the later stage (Safadi et al., 2003). The Wnt-3 morphogen and BMP-9 growth factor are involved in regulating CTGF expression (Luo et al., 2004).

At the macro level, the **Notch** transmembrane receptor signaling system is one of central regulators in skeleton formation during the embryonal period due to its participation in somitogenesis in the condensation stage (see 10.1). The role of the Notch system in osteoblastic differentiation has a dimorphous (two-way direction) character. Notch hyperexpression results in osteosclerosis, which is associated with the excessive reproduction of immature osteoblasts; this reproduction is due to the activation of genes encoding cyclins (Engin et al., 2008). In cells differentiating into osteoblasts *in vitro*, alkaline phosphatase expression is enhanced and mineralization accelerated along with the activation of the Notch1 receptor by its ligands Delta1 и Jagged1 (Nobta et al., 2005). On the other hand, the excessive expression of Notch *in vivo* remarkably inhibited osteoblastogenesis and resulted in the development of osteopenia, which manifested itself as a reduction in bone volume and the number of trabecule (Zanotti et al., 2008). Switching off the Notch signaling is supposed to underlie osteoblastogenesis stimulation, caused *in vitro* by the connective tissue growth factor (CTGF) (Smerdel-Ramoya et al., 2008).

The mechanism of the inhibiting action of Notch signaling on osteoblastic differentiation probably lies in the Notch intracellular domain (NCID) diminishing the trans-activat- ing (stimulating gene expression) influence of the canoni- cal signaling pathway components of the Wnt morphogen family (Wnt/β-catenin system). To achieve this effect of NCID, so-called ankyrin amino acid repeats in its molecule are essential (Deregowski et al., 2006).

Morphogens of the **Wnt**-family, which play an important role in the formation of mesenchymal condensations and in chondroblast differentiation are also actively involved in the development of the osteoblastic differon and the further development of a bone skeleton. It is interesting that this participation was discovered not by studying Wnt-ligands, but when one of the causes of human osteoporosis was claimed to be the inactivating mutation of the *LRP5* gene (it encodes the transmembrane protein 5 similar to the low density lipoprotein receptor). LRP5 is an essential co-receptor, without which Frizzled (FZD), the main receptor of Wnt signals, does not function. This fact was confirmed in an experiment with nil mutation of *Lrp5* and *Lrp6* gene: in mice, the mass and bone tissue mineral density (BMD) sharply decreased, while the frequency of bone fractures increased. Thus, a disruption in Wnt signaling pathways results in osteoblastogenesis impairment (Bodine & Komm, 2006).

On the other hand, a mutation discontinuing the expression of a **Wnt antagonist (decoy receptor) of secreted frizzled-related** protein 1 (sFRP1)—a mutation that improves the conditions for Wnt interaction with a cell—resulted in an increase of BMD, indicating the intensification of osteoblastogenesis under Wnt-signal influence. At the same time, the buildup of trabecular bone tissue increases, while the apoptosis of osteoblasts and osteocytes, including adult organisms, is largely prevented (Bodine, 2008).

The question of exactly which members of the Wnt family are involved in osteoblastogenesis regulation has not been sufficiently studied. It is known that Wnt-10b is involved: switching off the expression of this morphogen in mice is accompanied by defects in the development of the trabecular bone tissue and a decline in the concentration of an osteoblast specific marker, osteocalcin, in blood. On the contrary, Wnt-10b hyperexpression in transgenic mice results in an abrupt bone mass increase with the simultaneous inhibition of adipocytogenesis, while preventing the development of osteoporosis caused by estrogen deficiency (Bennett et al., 2003).

The stimulating effect on osteoblastic differentiation and bone growth was revealed *in vitro* in Wnt-3a and Wnt-7b morphogens. This influence is accomplished by one of the non-canonical Wnt signaling pathways by means of a C delta type (PKCδ) protein kinase bound to receptors by a G protein (Tu et al., 2007).

The Wnt 11 morphogen also stimulates osteoblastic differentiation, but this stimulation affects later stages of the process—the maturation of cells building an extracellular matrix and the development of mineralization cellular mechanisms. In this case, a complicated canonical signaling pathway is employed with participation of a secreted glycoprotein R-spondin2 (another name is cristin). This glycoprotein, working via Fzd8 and LRP6 receptors, is an additional activator of the β-catenin signaling cascade (Friedman et al., 2009).

Returning to the main, canonical pathway and describing it from the point of view of Wnt mechanisms of ac-

tion on osteoblastogenesis, the special role of β-catenin—this pathway's central intracellular component—should be emphasized. β-catenin accumulating within a cell under the influence of Wnt stimulates the expression of a *Runx2* gene, the "master-gene' of osetoblastic differentiation. The stimulation results from a 2-5-fold activation of the *Runx2* promoter, to which β-catenin is bound (Gaur et al., 2005). Besides this direct action on the expression of *Runx2*, β-catenin exerts synergism to BMP-2, enhancing the stimulating effect of the latter on *Runx2* transcription and promoting osteoblastic differentiation and bone growth (Mbalaviele et al., 2005). β-catenin is also involved in the commitment of the osteoblastic way of mesenchymal progenitor cell differentiation, simultaneously inhibiting chondroblastic differentiation. In switching off Wnt /β-catenin signals, osteoblastic differentiation, on the contrary, is blocked and chondrogenesis is stimulated (Day et al., 2005; Hill et al., 2005). The production of Wnt-7b and Wnt-10b by mature osteoblasts is important in terms of the commitment of mesenchymal progenitor cells. A paracrine signaling of these ligands switches in the canonical intracellular signaling pathway within progenitor cells and β-catenin directs cell differentiation into osteogenesis, inhibiting chondrogenesis and adipogenesis (Zhou et al., 2008).

Thus, Wnt morphogens (at least some members of this family), in general, play a positive role in osteoblastogenesis and in the functioning of the osteoblastic differon, starting with progenitor cell commitment and ending in apoptosis (Cohen, 2006; Yavropoulou & Yovos, 2007). Herein, the main Wnt action is targeted at stimulating osteoblast proliferation and, therefore, increasing bone tissue mass. This is evidenced by the acceleration and slowdown of osteoblast proliferation and bone growth under the influence of various factors that affect the canonical Wnt signaling pathway by means of changes in the inflow of β-catenin into the cell nucleus. This pathway is employed by a Wnt antagonist (soluble decoy receptor)—Dickkopf1—encoded by the *Dkk1* gene (Pinzone et al., 2009), and the above-mentioned BMP-2-induced Wdr5 protein (Zhu et al., 2008), as well as Osterix, which stimulates differentiation but restrains proliferation (Zhang C. et al., 2009). The increase in bone tissue mass is also facilitated by a Wnt signaling-induced enhancement of osteoprotegerin expression by osteoblasts, which results in an increasing OPG/RANKL ratio (see section 8.5.2) and therefore, in delaying osteoclastogenesis (Kubota et al., 2009). However, this positive role of Wnt in osteoblastogenesis is limited by a certain timetable. Protracted active Wnt signaling, which can be induced in an experiment by lithium chloride, impairs the differentiation of osteoblasts. Under normal conditions, osteoblasts have a mechanism to prevent such an adverse effect: they respond to Wnt signaling according to the feed-back principle by expressing Wnt antagonists, in particular, a secreted frizzled-related protein-2 (Sfrp2) and a Wnt inhibiting factor 1 (Wif-1) (Vaes et al., 2005). The inactivation of **Wif-1** stimulates all stages of osteoblastic differentiation, beginning with mesenchymal progenitor cells (Cho et al., 2009). Iin addition, the fibroblast growth factor FGF1 also possesses a controlling (inhibiting) effect on transcription-stimulating Wnt-3a activity (Ambrosetti et al., 2008).

Two members of the **Hedgehog (Hh)** morphogen family – Sonic Hedgehog (SHh) and Indian Hedgehog (IHh) – are carriers of position information and are essential in this capacity for specifying the correct localization of beginning osteoblastogenesis. They also serve as inductors of the Wnt expression and, therefore, are positioned "above" Wnt in the cascade of regulating factors of osteoblastic differentiation. These Hh functions (IHh is actively involved in endochondral ossification, are short-term; they are over with the beginning of Osterix expression, and protracted Hh expression causes a delay in osteogenesis (Rodda & McMahon, 2006; Day & Yang, 2008).

The effects of **systemic regulation factors**, hormones and vitamins on osteoblasts, including the main aspects of osteoblastic differentiation, have been described in section 8.4.1. Some details in relation to the actions of these coordinating factors, which are "the upper" level of regulation in terms of factors directly involved in osteoblastogenesis, should also be noted.

The osteoblastogenesis stimulating effect (osteogenic and anabolic at the same time) of intermittent doses of the parathyroid hormone (PTH) is due to the increased expression and transactivation of Runx2/Cbfa1. The transactivation is explained by the phosphorylation of one of the serin residues by protein kinase A (Fujita et al., 2001). Moreover, the anabolic effect of the intermittent introduction of PTH is associated with activating the Wnt signaling pathway (Kousteni & Bilezikian, 2008). The continuous introduction of PTH causes the opposite effect despite Runx2 activation. It is related to enhancing the osteoblast expression of an osteoclast differentiation factor (ODF), also known as RANKL/TRANCE or Tnfsf11 (see section 8.2.1.2). The intensification of osteoclastogenesis and osteoclastic resorption in the formation of bone tissue prevents osteoblast maturation (Komori, 2008).

PTH affects osteogenesis not only directly but also given the participation of vitamin D derivatives having a hormonal activity (see 8.4.1). PTH stimulates the synthesis of the most active D-hormone – D3. The latter induces the osteoblast expression of semaphorine-3B, a trans-membrane receptor of a glycoprotein nature. This stimulates osteoclastogenesis and thereby regulates homeostasis maintenance of the bone tissue, preventing its excessive growth, and this can even cause osteopenia (Sutton et al., 2008). At the same time, D3 stimulates the expression of Runx2/Cbfa1 and Osterix genes, i.c. it promotes osteoblastic differentiation (Maehata et al., 2006). Another direct effect of D3 on osteoblasts – the inhibition of RANKL expression – also enables maintaining the balance between resorption and bone tissue formation (St-Arnaud, 2008).

The most important role of **estrogens** in regulating osteoblastogenesis is indicated by the development of osteoporosis after menopause: estrogen deficiency causes a lack of active osteoblasts and, as a consequence, a negative balance in bone tissue remodeling. Runx2/Cbfa1 is the target of an estrogen effect. Estrogens increase the activity of the *Runx2* gene promoter and induce the formation of this protein mRNA. This estrogen effect is partly due to their inhibition of interleukin IL-7 expression, which suppresses the activity of the *Runx2* promoter. For its part, Runx2 activates the estrogen receptor, ERα, which increases cell sensitivity to estrogens. Switching off *Runx2* makes osteoblast progenitors insensitive to the effects of estrogen (Komori, 2008).

The effect of **leptin**, a hormone produced by adipocytes, which functionally unites the bone system and fat depositions in an organism, on osteoblastogenesis has been discussed in section 8.4.1. It should be stressed once again, that this effect, which is significantly important in the postnatal period, is ambiguous. On the one hand, it stimulates osteoblastic differentiation of periostal progenitor cells, which enhances growth of cortical bone substance and improves bone mechanical properties (a bearing capacity in particular); this effect is due to the direct contact of leptin with cell receptors. On the other hand, leptin affects cells indirectly, via the nervous sympathetic system and its neuropeptides, resulting in the inhibition of osteoblastogenesis in trabecular bone tissue (Hamrick & Ferrari, 2008).

Apart from the transcription factors and signal molecules of local and systemic action, some other factors and mechanisms are involved in regulating osteoblastic differentiation.

One of these mechanisms constitutes the influence on the chromatin status of the cell nucleus and, more exactly, on the degree of acetylation (the number of attached acetyl groups) to histones, proteins that are part of chromatin. In differentiating osteoblasts, the enzymatic activity of the histone deacetylase 1 (**HDAC1**) decreases. This reduction especially diminishes the acetylation degree of histones localized in the promoter zones of essential genes for osteoblastogenesis genes, such as those encoding Osterix and osteocalcin. The inhibition of HDAC1 activity in an experiment accelerates differentiation, indicated by an earlier expression of alkaline phosphatase and osteopontin. Thus, HDAC1 is a regulator of influencing transcription factors on genes involved in osteoblastogenesis (Lee et al., 2006). Even more important is the fact that histone deacetylases form multiprotein complexes in the nucleus, which control the entire process of osteoblastic differentiation, functioning as a Runx2 co-repressor (Jensen et al., 2007).

Another mechanism is associated with protein's function of the tumor suppressor phosphoprotein **p53**, also known as a tumor cellular antigen p53, whose expression is controlled by the *Mdm2* gene active in embryogenesis. The p53 is a negative regulator of osteoblastic differentiation and bone growth. Nil mutations of the *Tp53* gene, encoding p53, accelerate osteoblastogenesis and increase bone tissue mass. The p53 action is related to, firstly, cell cycle (cell proliferation) impairments and, secondly, to its suppressing effect on the expression of the osteoblastogenesis "master" genes, *Runx2* and Osx (Langner et al., 2006; Wang X. et al., 2006).

Another factor influencing osteoblastic differentiation is a cell's microenvironment, determined by the extracellular matrix composition. Matrix accumulation in cell cultures increases Runx2's binding activity with DNA. The presence of type I collagen in the matrix is a prerequisite for osteoblastogenesis; type I collagen's activity is directed at Runx2 activation. Integrins and a signaling cascade of MAP kinases mediate the matrix-activating effect; MEK/ERK kinases phosphorylate a serin residue within the Runx2 activating domain (Schroeder et al., 2005).

Tenascin W, a glycoprotein component of the matrix, exerts its controlling influence on osteoblastogenesis, delaying the proliferation of preosteoblasts and their differentiation into mature osteoblasts. This influence is possible by suppressing canonical Wnt signaling pathways (Kimura et al., 2007).

The data given on the main mechanisms of genetic control and major regulation factors of osteoblastic differentiation, as well as the activity dynamics of the genes responsible for cell vitality should be supplemented by investigations results of **transcriptome** (a **transcription profile**) of differentiating cells.

Cultured *in vitro* cell were the subject for the most part of such investigations. A number of cultured osteoprogenitor cell lines, which can go through the entire osteoblastic differentiation way in the presence of ascorbic acid and β-glycerophosphate, are known. This way is subdivided into three steps, the duration of which naturally varies for different cell lines. The first step, which lasts for 9–10 days, involves the active proliferation of the original cells; during the second step (from the 11th till 25th days) differentiation proper takes place. In the third and final step (25th–35th days), a mature osteoblast actively forms an extracellular matrix intrinsic for bone tissue and carries out its mineralization. The regularities of gene expression at every step are of the same type and common in all the cell lines studied.

The intense expression of protooncogenes of the *c-fos, c-jun, c-myc* families has been observed at the very beginning of the first step, during the especially intensive proliferation of mesenchymal progenitor cells. The active expression of protooncogenes is peculiar to all cases of intensive cell reproduction. Other factors activating transcription and promoting proliferation, such as TACC3, Pr22/stathmin, Ets1 and Ets2, Tcf7, are accumulated (Raouf & Seth, 2002; Jong et al., 2004).

At the same time, the concentration of proteins regulating the cell cycle (and consequently the rate of cell mitotic division) and fulfilling it increases. They are **cyclins** (regulatory subunits of cyclin-dependent kinases). Antiapoptotic (improving vitality) factors of the Bcl2 protein family and telomerases, which inhibit cell ageing, simultaneously promote the accumulation of proliferating cells. However, closer to the end of the first (early) step of osteoblastic differentiation, the transcription profile is altered. The cells lose their ability to proliferate. Cyclin expression is abruptly inhibited and, on the contrary, the expression of cell cycle regulators (antiproliferative factors) of the Tob family, TIS21 and BTG2 factors is activated (Beck et al., 2001; Raouf & Seth, 2002).

At the end of the first step and during the second step, the expression of osteoblast-specific regulating transcription factors, such as Runx2/Cbfa1 and Osterix, and the homeotic proteins activating these factors come into the foreground (Hassan et al., 2006). In accordance with the most important role that bone morphogenetic proteins play in osteogenesis, the expression of genes related to the extra- and intracellular components of the BMP signaling pathways (including to BMP antagonists), as well as other BMP-targeted factors is activated. Factors encoded by some of these genes are transcription repressors, such as, for example, HEY1 (HESR1), whose active expression distinguishes osteoblasts from fibroblasts, or mediators of cell damage and apoptosis (DRP-1, ZIP-kinase/DAP3, dactylin/FBXW4 and others). They affix the osteoblastic commitment of cells by inhibiting myoblastic differentiation (Beck et al., 2001; Korchynskyi et al., 2003). The expression of components (including receptors and antagonists) of other signaling pathways–the Wnt morphogen signaling pathways and insulin-like growth factors (IGF)–simultaneously changes (Kolajzic et al., 2005).

The main scope of the second step is the expression of proteins specifying the cell morphology, especially of cytoskeleton, and extracellular matrix proteins, including those engaged in mineralization, such as osteocalcin, osteopontin, and bone sialoprotein (Jong et al., 2004).

The expression of secreted proteins, especially proteins engaged in mineralization, occupies the biggest place in the third step transcription profile of osteoblastic differentiation. In differentiation *in vitro*, this step is observed, on average, one month since the beginning of cultivation (Raouf & Seth, 2002). In passing from the second to the third differentiation step, a certain role is played by type B natriuretic (**BNP**) and especially by type C peptides (**CNP**) (Potter et al., 2006). They work as autocrine/paracrine regulators, restraining the proliferation of osteoblasts and simultaneously accelerating their differentiation. The high biologic activity of these small peptides (for example, CNP contains only 22 amino acid residues) is mainly determined by their connection with a signaling system, which involves specific guanylate cyclases catalyzing a buildup of guanosine monophosphate (Suda et al., 1996; Kaneki et al., 2008). Moreover, CNP employs a signaling pathway by which bone morphogenetic proteins stimulate differentiation; it enhances the phosphorylation of the Smad5 protein (Yeh et al., 2006). Signaling systems related to natriuretic peptides mediate the regulating effect on osteoblastic differentiation and bone growth of a factor secreted by osteoblasts, **osteocrin**. Similar to peptide hormones, osteocrin is a ligand of the CNP receptor (NPR-C) (Moffatt et al., 2007; Moffatt & Thomas, 2009).

As a result of investigations of the transcription profile, it was revealed that cells undergo significantly more complex changes during osteoblastogenesis than was previously supposed. A number of proteins that are not specific markers of osteoblastic differentiation, but are actually involved in differentiation according to the extent of their expression alterations (both increasing and decreasing), have been detected. The particular role these proteins play has not been determined yet. Also a number of previously unknown genes involved in differentiation have been discovered.

In the final stage of osteoblastic differentiation, before the beginning of the transformation of a mature osteoblast, into an osteoyte, the leading role is passed from the Runx2/Cbfa1 factor to an another transcription factor (activator) known by the abbreviation OASIS (which stands for old astrocyte specifically induced substance). OASIS, a protein with a molecular mass of 57 kDa, is a member of the CREB/ATF activating factors family, binding with a gene element sensitive to cyclic adenosine monophosphate (cAMP). Histochemical findings indicate a preferable accumulation of OASIS within cortical bone tissue, and its most intensive expression coincides in time with the active expression of osteocalcin and osteopontin. This permits considering OASIS as one of specific markers of the late stage of osteoblastogenesis, although the particular function of this factor has not yet been clarified (Nikaido et al., 2001).

In the third step, differentiating cells assume all the phenotype characteristics of a functionally mature osteoblast. However, for a part of the osteoblast population – according to Noble's (2003) approximate estimation that every 12th cell is in this part – differentiation does not discontinue here. These osteoblasts enter a process of further differentiation as a result of which they transform into long-living **osteocytes**, surrounded on all sides ("embedded/ immured") by the mineralized extracellular matrix. The matrix producers can be both osteoblasts differentiating into osteocytes (this is the most common variant) and osteoblasts replacing each other, ending their life cycle with apoptosis. This means that the osteoblast population is heterogenous on the molecular level in relation to their predetermined fate. Possible molecular factors of such heterogeneity include unequal sensitivity to leptin, delaying osteoblast apoptosis, and to members of the TGF-β superfamily, enhancing osteoblast biosynthetic activity due to a delay in their differentiation (Franz-Odendaal et al., 2006). Another possible molecular mechanism of choosing a way for osteoblasts is associated with the transcription factor Sox2, whose expression is induced by fibroblast growth factors by means of a FGFR2 receptor. An excess of Sox2 interrupts Wnt signaling pathways and, thus, delays postosteoblastic differentiation (Mansukhani et al., 2005).

The differentiation of osteocytes whose final "maturation" is enabled by the mineralization of the surrounding matrix (Irie et al., 2008) lasts from 2–10 days and is characterized by some peculiarities in molecular mechanisms, depending on the ossification type. It does not happen in the same way in various vertebrate species, in various bones and even in various regions of the same bone. However, ongoing changes in the transcription profile, no less pronounced than those in the previous stages of osteoblastic differentiation have the same type character.

No doubt, one of the most significant changes is the cessation of the expression of the "master" factor of osteoblastic differentiation – Runx2/Cbfa1. The expression of the second most important transcription factor for osteoblasts, Osterix, discontinues a little later. The absence of these factors results in the inhibition and complete cessation of the transcription of those genes they directly control. These are genes encoding proteins specific to the bone tissue extracellular matrix and osteoblast cytoplasmic membrane, such as type I collagen (and the enzymes involved in its synthesis and processing), bone sialoprotein, osteocalcin, alkaline phosphotase, IGF-receptors, and periostin (Osf2). The transcription of a number of other matrix and cell membrane components, such as osteonectin, fibronectin, tenascin C, vitronectin, thrombospodin, integrins, BMPR1 receptors, PTH/PTHrP-R, vitamin D3 receptor, CD44 protein, and signal molecules (BMP-2) is maintained or even activated.

At the same time, the intensive transcription of inactive or low-active genes in osteoblasts begins. Encoded by these genes, proteins are not osteocyte-specific, but the fact that their transcription becomes active in osteocytic differentiation gives evidence as to their necessity in the formation of an osteocyte functional phenotype.

Mineralization-related extracellular matrix glycoproteins **MEPE** (matrix extracellular phosphoglycoprotein or OF45, osteoblastic/osteocytic factor 45) and **DMP-1** (acid dentin matrix phosphoprotein 1) are among these proteins essential for osteocyte functioning; due to their enhanced expression, the transcription profile of osteoblasts differentiating into osteocytes changes. The expression of a cytoskeleton-related transmembrane glycoprotein – **E11 antigen**, a **XBPA** transcription factor (a X box-binding protein), and factors regulating phosphate metabolism – a **PHEX** enzyme (phosphate regulating neutral endopeptidase) and fibroblast growth factor 23 (**FGF-23**) – increases (Franz-Odendaal et al., 2006). Upon entering the blood and affecting the liver functions, FGF-23 assumes a central role in regulating the homeostasis of phosphates in the organism (Fukumoto, 2009). Phosphate homeostasis maintenance is, in turn, essential in bone tissue mineralization (Goebel et al., 2009). At the same time, independent of its systemic function, FGF-23 is essential as a local regulator in the final stage of bone tissue formation (Sitara et al., 2008).

For osteoblasts to be transformed into osteocytes, the matrix metalloproteases (matrixins) (see section 3.7.1) must be sufficiently present in the transcription profile. Osteocytic differentiation is delayed in the insignificant expression of genes that encode metalloproteases MMP-1 (interstitial collagenase), MMP-3 (stromelysin), MMP-8 (collagenase-2), MMP-14 (MT1-MMP) (Karsdal et al., 2004; Holmbeck et al., 2005). These metalloproteases actively break down the bone tissue extracellular matrix, particularly its main component, type I collagen, and are essential for forming lacunes, where osteocytes are located, and canals, where osteocyte dendrites ingrow. Especially important in this aspect is MMP-2 (gelatinase A), ensuring the passability of canals and a connection (signal propagation) between osteocytes and both osteoblasts and osteoclasts (Inoue et al., 2006).

Along with the genes whose role in osteocyte functioning has been studied well, the genes whose role in osteocyte biology remains unknown are involved in altering the transcription profile in the differentiation of osteoblasts into osteocytes. Examples of this include the significant enhancement of the expression of a nuclear receptor of DAX1 unknown ligands (such receptors are referred to as "orphans") and the expression of small guanosine triphosphatase, associated with the development of diabetes and the inhibition of the Sox4 transcription factor. The regular character of these changes in osteocyte differentiation has yet to be explained (Billiard et al., 2003).

10.2.4. Molecular biological mechanisms of osteoclastogenesis and its regulation

The osteoclast differon originates in hematopoietic line cells located within the bone marrow. These cells are precursors of monocytes/macrophages, and the molecular mechanisms of osteo-clastic differentiation differ from those involved in the differentiation of osteoblasts originating in mesenchymal progenitors.

The first molecular factor, which functions in the beginning of osteoclast differon formation, is the transcription factor **PU.1** (SPI1), containing a large (84 of 270 amino acid residues) Ets-domain of a helix-loop-helix type binding to a DNA sequence that is rich in purine. The function of this factor is committing a myeloid progenitor cell to differentiation into a macrophage. In its absence, not only is osteoclastogenesis discontinued, but also no macrophages are detected, although the ability to produce immature monocytes is retained (Boyle et al., 2003; Kobayashi & Kronenberg, 2005).

Monocytes/ macrophages committed into future osteoclasts in the presence of PU-1 become sensitive to a growth factor, known as a macrophage-colony stimulating factor (**M-CSF**), produced by bone marrow stromal cells and osteoblasts. It can be substituted by a granulocyte monocyte-colony stimulating factor (GM-CSF). The main function of both factors simulating the formation of cell colonies is to enable contact of cells prior to their fusion and the appearance of multinucleacity, the main phenotypic peculiarity of osteoclasts. Organisms in which both of these factors work via a **c-Fms** receptor (otherwise known as CSF1R or CD115) are switched off produce macrophages, but they lack osteoclasts.

A number of proteins of the cytoplasmic membrane, referred to as fusion proteins and including a macrophage fusion receptor (**MFR**) belonging to the signal regulating protein (SIRP) family and some other proteins, are involved in the fusion of cells-precursors aggregated into colonies (Vignery, 2005; Sims & Gooi, 2008). **DC-STAMP** (dendritic cell specific transmembrane protein) plays the leading role in the fusion process (Yagi et al., 2006). This protein received its name when it was originally discovered in dendritic cells related to the immune system, which originate from the same progenitors as osteoclasts. A DC-STAMP molecule contains 470 amino acid residues and 7 transmembrane segments. Mononuclear osteoclasts, formed in switching off the *DC-STAMP* gene, possess a significantly lower osteoclastic activity than normal multinuclear ones. Thus, DC-STAMP becomes of crucial significance in controlling the bone tissue mass (Iwasaki et al., 2008).

As early as the stage of multinuclearity formation, the **RANKL** factor becomes involved. This factor has a similar structure as proteins of the tumor necrosis factor (TNF) family and its name stands for a receptor activator of the nuclear factor κ (kappa) B ligand (RANK ligand). RANKL is also known by other names, such as TRANCE (TNF-related activation-induced cytokine), ODF (osteoclast differentiation factor), OPGL (osteoprotegerin ligand), the antigen CD254, and the tumor necrosis factor TNF11. RANKL is a transmembrane glycoprotein, whose molecule contains 317 amino acid residues, wherein the residues starting with the 69th one compose an extracellular domain, and the fragment beginning with the 140th residue (C-terminal) is able to cleave in the form of a soluble isoform, **sRANKL**. The soluble isoform enters the blood, which is why the RANKL effect not only has a local (contact) character, but also a systemic one (Dovio et al., 2006). An amino acid sequence 70 residues in length, found in s RANKL, is located within the molecule extracellular domain and determines RANKL activity.

The interaction of RANKL and RANK on the surface of osteoclast precursors or mature osteoclasts is accompanied by attracting one of the TRAF (TNF receptor-associated factors) family molecules – namely TRAF6 – to the cytoplasmic domain. TRAF6 provides switching in intracellular pathways to further propagate signals coming from RANK (Kobayashi et al., 2001). This function allows considering TRAF as the final link in the canonical pathway of osteoclastogenesis regulation; from this point of view, its initial one is M-CSF (Kim et al., 2005; Knowles & Athanasou, 2009).

Many cells express RANKL, particularly the cells of lymphatic glands; it is involved in the activation of immunocompetent cells. In bone tissue, osteoblasts are the main producers of RANKL as of M-CSF. This function of osteoblasts is stimulated by the insulin-like growth factor-1

(IGF-1). Its absence inhibits the osteoclastic resorption of bones (Wang Y. et al., 2006a).

Along with RANK activation, during osteoclastogenesis, RANKL induces the expression of more than 100 genes (Ishida et al., 2002), including the above transmembrane receptor CD-STAMP. Thus, it is a crucial stimulating regulator in the formation of osteoclast multinuclearity. Genes whose expression is induced by RANKL include genes that encode nuclear factors of the NFAT family, which is discussed below.

RANK, which is activated by RANKL, is a member of the tumor necrosis factor receptor (TNFR)-11A superfamily. Its alternative names are ODFR (osteoblast differentiation factor receptor) and antigen CD265. RANK is a phosphoglycoprotein, one-pass receptor with 587 amino acid residues, after the cleavage of a signal peptide.

The function of RANK is to activate nuclear factors of the κ (kappa) B family and it is for this that RANK received its name—receptor activator of nuclear factors-κB, **NF-κB**. The κB factor family consists of five proteins, which are pleiotropic (regulating the expression of many genes) transcription factors involved in immune and inflammatory response, cell differentiation and apoptosis. Two of these proteins—p50 and p52—form homo- and heterodimeric complexes and they are essential for osteoclast differentiation. NF-κB exerts its effect through the successive activation of a c-fos protooncogen (a component of an activating complex of the AP-1 transcription factor) and an activated T cell nuclear factor (NFATc1) (Yamashita et al., 2007). The binding of NF-κB with the Notch2 factor accelerates osteoclastogenesis caused by RANKL (Fukushima et al., 2008).

Signal propagation along the RANKL−RANK−NF-κB axis is the main (also called "classical" or "canonical") regulation pathway of osteoclast differentiation. (Kobayashi & Karsenty, 2005).

The action of the main osteoclastogenesis regulating factors is accompanied by the participation of a great number of molecules (about 100). A deficiency or excess of these molecules causes serious distortions in various stages of the osteoclastic differentiation process (Roodman, 2006; Yavropoulou & Yovos, 2008).

In the first stage, the stage of commitment (choice of a macrophage differentiation way), a leucine "zipper" containing transcription factor C/EBPα (α protein binding to the CCA-AT enhancer) functions, along with the PU.1 factor. The action of both these factors is controlled (restrained) by the repressor transcription factors Egr-1,2/Nab-2, Gfi-1, as well as a microphthalmia-associated transcription factor (MITF).

In the stage of aggregating macrophages into colonies, the intracellular propagation of M-CFS-originated and c-fsm receptor-mediated signals is associated with the activity of a large number of kinases, particularly P13K, p42/44ERK and phospholipase PLCγ, in addition to the protooncogen c-Cb1. In this stage, MITF retains its influence, stimulating the expression of cathepsin K, acid phosphatase 5 and an osteoclast-associated receptor (**OS-CAR**), which is essential for macrophage and osteoclast functions. The factors regulating the entry of cells into the cell cycle (i.e. intensifying proliferation and enlarging cell colonies) are also switched on. At the same time, factors repressing the cell cycle (Eos) also function.

Hereafter, when the central role in osteoclast differentiation passes to RANKL and RANK, involving transcription nuclear factors of the HF-κB family into the process, **AP-1** (activator protein-1) becomes critically important. AP-1 is a heterodimeric transcription factor, whose most prevailing components are members of the c-fos and c-Jun protooncogen families. HF-κB works via the successive activation of these components, which stimulate the expression of one of the nuclear factors–the activated T cell nuclear factor 1 (NFATc1) (Yamashita et al., 2007). This signaling pathway involves a RANKL-induced protein Slfn2 (Schlafen2), the absence of which interferes with the activation of c-Jun and the expression of NFATc1, which, in turn, inhibits osteoclastogenesis (Lee et al., 2008).

In the case of a c-Fos deficiency, differentiation is delayed in the macrophage stage, when the ways of further differentiation are determined–into an osteoclast or dendritic cell, accordingly, after the effect of the PU.1 factor. The significance of c-Jun is seen a little later, and its deficiency also interferes with NF-κB stimulated formation of the above-mentioned nuclear factors **NFAT**, which are essential for final formation of the osteoclastic phenotype (Ikeda et al., 2004). The emerging delay of osteoclastogenesis results in the development of osteopetrosis (Boyce et al., 2005; Yavropoulou & Yovos, 2008).

Osteoactivin, a protein expressed by osteoblasts and osteoclasts, has a stimulating effect, in cooperation with integrin subunits β1 and β3 and RANK, in the stage of the fusion of osteoclast-precursors cells as well as in the spreading of osteoclasts on a bone surface (Sheng et al., 2008).

Tyrosine kinase c-Src, bound to intracellular domains of c-Fms and RANK receptors, is an essential positive participant of the process at all stages of osteoclastogenesis. In particular, it is required in cell polarization prior to the beginning of osteoclast resorption activity. Another kinase (Lyn), a member of the same Src-kinase (SFK) family, inhibits c-Src activity (Kim et al., 2009).

In terms of the intracellular consequences of RANK activation, calcium ions (Ca^{2+}) play a significant role and their concentration increases manifold in cells that are in a state of intense activity. Ca^{2+} affects the cell function not only by itself, but also mainly by involving a small phosphoprotein, **calmodulin** (calcium modulated protein). It contains 148 amino acid residues. A calmodulin molecule, present in all eukaryotic cells, contains four domains to bind calcium ions. The formation of a Ca^{2+}-calmodulin complex activates calmodulin, which comes into interaction with many proteins, activating their functions and switching in various signaling pathways. An increased concentration of Ca^{2+} occurs in osteoclasts after binding RANKL to RANK, and the pharmacological antagonists of calmodulin inhibit osteoclastogenesis. The Ca^{2+} calmodulin complex induces, in particular, **calcineurin**, which exhibits the enzymatic activity of protein serine/threonin phosphatase. Calcineurin dephosphorylazes NFAT factors, which move to the nucleus and cause the expression of genes required for completing osteoclast differentiation. Thus, the signaling pathway RANK–$Ca2^+$–calmodulin–calcineurin–NFAT works in osteoclastogenesis (Zhang et al., 2005). The Ca^{2+} calmodulin complex switches in another signaling pathway, in which calmodulin-activated kinase (CaMK) and cyclic adenosine monophosphate (cAMP) act and which is also involved in osteoclastogenesis (Shinohara & Takayanagi, 2007). It should be recalled that the same signaling pathway is engaged in osteoblastic differentiation.

Moreover, the Ca2+ calmodulin complex activates a multifunctional enzyme type II serine/threonin protein kinase, which is dependent upon calcium/calmodulin (**CaMKII**). One of the effects of this enzyme is the activation of the transcription factors comprising the AP-1 complex, which stimulates osteoclast differentiation. The inhibition of CaMKII slows down osteoclastogenesis (Seales et al., 2006).

The known molecular factors acting in the canonical pathway of osteoclastic differentiation, through not an exhaustive list, include the above-mentioned signaling molecules, receptors, components of intracellular signaling pathways, and transcription factors. The regulation of osteoclastogenesis is more complicated by the existence of non-canonical pathways of osteoclast formation, along with canonical ones (Knowles & Athanasou, 2009). In non-canonical pathways, any component of two main factors inducing osteoclastogenesis (inducers) and subsequently affecting the canonical pathway–M-CSF or RANKL–may be substituted by other growth factors/cytokines. However, RANK plays the same role as within the canonical signaling pathway, i.e. the activation of NF-κB. The switching off of both inducers or their substitution by other ligands makes the formation of osteoclast impossible.

As substitutes for M-CSF *in vitro*, a vascular endothelial growth factor (VEGF), a placenta growth factor (PlGF), a hepatocyte growth factor (HGF), and a FLt3 receptor ligand (FLt3L) act. VEGF expression is stimulated by local hypoxia-induced factors HIF. RANKL can be substituted by the tumor necrosis factor TNF-α and by another member of the TNF superfamily (LIGHT), which is expressed by lymphocytes, as well as by the interleukins IL-6, IL-8, IL-11. Osteoclasts differentiated under the influence of non-canonical factors are of smaller size and contain fewer nuclei. Their destructive activity in relation to bone tissue is less effective than that of osteoclasts developed via the canonical pathway. The participation of non-canonical signaling pathways in physiologic osteoclastogenesis has not been finally determined. At the same time, the non-canonical signaling pathways of osteoclastogenesis are undoubtedly involved in the destruction of bone tissue in the pathological processes of an inflammatory and neoplastic nature (Knowles & Athanasou, 2009).

As previously mentioned, both the canonical and non-canonical signaling systems involved in osteoclast differentiation are related to the receptor-activator RANK. RANK is a starting point for most intracellular signaling pathways. But the majority of pathways originating in other receptors function in an interaction (cross-talk) with signaling systems switched on by RANK. These are receptors of the interferons IFN-β and IFN-γ, which inhibit osteoclastogenesis, from the PPAR-γ receptor and from the α6β2 integrin, also known as ITAM, which are engaged in stimulating osteoclast differentiation. The activity of the nuclear (contained in chromosomes) proteins **HMGB** depends on RANKL's influence on RANK. HMGF stimulate the expression of the TNF family factors essential for osteoclastogenesis (Yamoah et al., 2008). Therefore, we can agree with the statement, according to which all osteoclast signaling systems are "ranked" (Feng, 2005b).

Along with the effect that the many local and systemic osteoclastogenesis regulating factors have on oseoclastogenesis, a number of other paracrine and autocrine factors produced by osteoclasts themselves exert both a positive and negative influence on the differentiation and functional activity of osteoclasts. These factors, which were detected when analyzing the osteoclast genome, are annexin II (see section 8.1.2.2); one of enzymes of the disintegrin-metalloprotease family ADAM8 (see section 3.7.1); the eosinophil chemotactic factor; the C3 component of the complement; the macrophage inflammatory factor VIP-1α; and several others (Roodman, 2006).

Vitamin B_{12} is among the systemic factors affecting osteoclastogenesis. Its deficiency, the occurrence of which is not uncommon in old age, enhances the osteoblast production of an amino acid **homocysteine** (methylated derivative of cysteine) and a dicarboxylic methylmalonic acid. Both of these molecules stimulate osteoclastogenesis, which promotes the development of osteoporosis (Vaes et al., 2009).

10.3. MOLECULAR BIOLOGICAL AND BIOCHEMICAL REGULARITIES OF SKELETON FORMATION AND GROWTH

10.3.1. Molecular biological and biochemical regularities of bone formation

10.3.1.1. Ossification types. Endochondral ossification

Bone formation and growth occurs in two ways. The first way that the majority of bones are developed (these are bones originating from the paraxial mesoderm and mesoderm of a lateral plate)–the formation of bone tissue inside mesenchymal condensations transformed into a transitory (temporary) cartilage–is referred to as **endo-**

chondral ossification. This process entails that cartilage 'patterns" (or "models') of future bones are formed as a result of the chondroblast differentiation of mesenchymal condensation cells. During formation, their **segmentation** (division into various segments) occurs; thus, the localization of future joints is specified. In such a way, the primary skeleton of trunk and limbs, built up from hyaline cartilage 'models" of future bones, is formed.

The chondroblasts/ condrocytes of transitory cartilages continue their differentiation and their "maturation' occurs, altering their phenotype and ending in apoptosis, which leads to the erosion of cartilaginous tissue. Lacunae emerge, where the osteoblasts forming bone tissue enter. Resorbing cartilaginous tissue is gradually replaced by newly formed bone tissue. A cartilage "pattern" or "model" becomes a bone.

The second way to form bones, originating mainly from the neural crest and only partially from paraxial mesoderm, such as skull flat bones, is intramembraneous ossification. Intramembraneous ossification is when mesenchymal condensations gaining forms of membranes or films are directly transformed into bones, omitting the chondrogenesis stage.

General regularities of endochondral ossification can be formulated as follows (Kronenberg, 2003).

At first a cartilage model of bone increases in its size owing to the proliferation of chondroblasts retaining their proliferative potential and due to the deposition of the cartilage extracellular matrix they have produced. Chondroblast differentiation is still ongoing. They enter the stage of maturation, lose their capacity for mitotic division (exit the cell cycle) and become chondrocytes. The final step of chondrocyte maturation is **hypertrophy**. In this case, hypertrophy is not only an increase in cell sizes, but also alterations in their biosynthetic activity. Significant changes in a transcription profile take place, followed by alterations in the produced extracellular matrix. Among these alterations, the switching from the expression of the main cartilaginous tissue collagen, type II collagen, to that of type I collagen intrinsic for bone tissue and the beginning of the expression of alkaline phosphatase, are especially important. Such a changed matrix is accommodated for mineralization, and mineralization does occur (Blair et al., 2002). Hypertrophied chondrocytes also intensely express metalloproteases that degrade the matrix.

Chondrocytes' maturation and hypertrophy are completed by their apoptosis. Cell apoptosis, in combination with matrix degradation, results in the erosion of provisory cartilaginous tissue. Progenitor cells of an osteoblastic differon invade from the periphery, namely from the perichondrium covering the cartilage model of bone. Upon completing their differentiation, these cells are transformed into actively functioning osteoblasts, which produce a new extracellular matrix intrinsic for bone tissue. Mineralized remnants of the former matrix of a provisory cartilage serve as a framework for a new matrix.

In such a way, ossification centers appear, the first of which (primary) is formed in an aggregation of hypertrophied chondrocytes in the middle region of a future bone diaphysis. The primary center sprouts in two directions towards both future epiphyses, changing into spongy (trabecular) bone tissue. At nearly the same time, an addition in a ring or a "cup' form develops on the surface at the same level of the future diaphysis. The "cup' also sprouts along the diaphysis length, transforming into compact matter of the bone cortical layer.

Soon afterwards, secondary centers, appearing in both future epiphyses, are jointed to the primary ones. Upon sprouting out, they fill in the entire epiphysis volume with spongy bone tissue covered with a fine compact cortical layer, but do not expand to epiphysis surfaces inwards to the joint cavities, which remain covered by permanent articular cartilages.

Between the ossified (transformed into bone regions) diaphysis and epiphyses intermediate layers of cartilaginous tissue, referred to as metaepiphyseal or epiphyseal cartilages or physes remain in the postnatal period for a long time, up to sexual development has been completed. In these cartilages, chondroblasts are orderly arranged in columns oriented parallel to the bone longitudinal axis. Chondroblast division within columns continues, the columns are elongated and owing to this, longitudinal bone growth occurs; this gives origin to another common name of metaepiphyseal cartilages – growth plates (Ornitz & Marie, 2002).

After growth ceases, the cartilage of growth plates is ossified. It is replaced by the interlayers of compact bone tissue, referred to as epiphyseal lines.

10.3.1.2. Molecular biological and biochemical regularities of metaepiphyseal cartilage functions

In every bone that is formed according to the endochodral pathway, there are two **metaepiphyseal cartilages** (growth plates). A bone grows in length practically simultaneously from its opposite ends (epiphyses) towards its middle (median) part (diaphysis). The growth plate is subdivided into zones (layers), which are generally considered in a succession specific to such a growth direction (Burdan et al., 2009).

The **first zone** is referred to as a superficial reserve zone or a zone of resting cartilage. As it separates two metabolically different tissues – an oxybiotic (employing aerobic metabolism) bone tissue of an epiphysis and a cartilaginous tissue supplied in an anaerobic way – Pavlova (1980) has suggested the term "barrier zone" designating the interaction of two tissues that are different in nature. Blood vessels enter the growth plate via the barrier zone from an epiphysis; they supplement its blood supply primarily provided from the diaphysis to a certain degree. Cells of the first zone are chondroblasts that actively secrete the cartilage extracellular matrix and exhibit great proliferative potential.

Chondroblasts actively proliferate in the next (second) **zone of proliferation**, where cells are arranged in columns. The proliferation is maintained by the chondroblast expression of the parathyroid hormone-related protein (PTHrP); this peptide is the most important component in the local regulation of metaepiphyseal cartilage functions (see below). To arrange cell location in columns, transcription factors encoded by *Sox5* and *Sox6* genes are absolutely necessary. In the absence of these factors, which are relative to Sox9, the leading factor of chondroblast differentiation, and given the total switching off of both genes, the columns are not formed.

Proliferation is more active in the upper zone "rows" of chondroblasts in columns, adjusting to the barrier (reserve) zone; within these chondroblasts, mitotic figures can often be observed. The greater distance it is from the reserve zone, the greater the frequency of mitosis is decreased. A bone's longitudinal growth occurs due to cell division in the cross (versus the bone's longitudinal axis) direction, resulting in column elongation.

As the columns grow, the expression of genes encoding cartilage matrix structural components (type II collagen and minor IX and XI type collagens (that, together with it, comprise collagen fibrils), aggrecan, COMP, and others and the genes of regulation factors (homeotic protein Nkx3.2, Fgfr3 receptor, activating transcription factor Atf2 and many others) becomes more intensified within chondroblasts. The expression of the Runx2/Cbfa1 and Runx3 transcription factors increases later, in the transition of a chondroblast losing its proliferation ability into a prehypertrophic state (Lefebvre & Smits, 2005).

Within the zone of proliferating chondroblasts, the expression of heparane sulfate proteoglycan – one of a transmembrane syndecan, syndecan-3 – occurs (see section 3.2.1.2). It exerts an active stimulating action on chondroblast proliferation (Kirsch et al., 2002).

A small protein has been found within the matrix deposited by proliferating chondroblasts of the growth plate. After cleavage of a signal peptide and a propeptide, it contains 71 amino acid residues, having a molecular mass of 17 kDa. It is referred to as **Ucma**, (unique cartilage matrix-associated protein). Its molecule comprises 14 γ-carboxyglutamic acid residues, and 2 tyrosine residues are sulfated. In the direction from the reserve zone to the third one (the zone of hypertrophy), the Ucma concentration within the matrix decreases. Ucma is supposed to prevent the premature growth arrest of columns and delay the osteoblastic differentiation of mesenchymal progenitor cells surrounding the growth plate (Surmann-Schmitt et al., 2008; Tagariello et al., 2008).

The next, **third zone** is a zone of mature cartilage, where chondroblasts completely lose their capacity for proliferation, transforming into chondrocytes. The last and final stage of their differentiation – **hypertrophy** – begins.

The third zone, also called the zone of transformation, is subdivided into prehypertrophic (upper) and true hypertrophic (lower) zones. In the transition from proliferation to hypertrophic differentiation (within the upper zone), the role of a "switch" is played by a cGKII protein of cyclic guanidine monophosphate (cGMP) dependent type II protein kinase (Chikuda et al., 2004). This enzyme inhibits the action of the Sox9 factor that is essential for chondroblast differentiation, but delays chondrocyte hypertrophy, impairing its entry into the cell nucleus. Sox5 and Sox6 transcription factors slow down differentiation in the prehypertrophic stage, but are essential for hypertrophy to be completed. A volume of chondrocyte cytoplasm increases manifold (up to 10 times) as a result of hypertrophy.

To start chondrocyte hypertrophy (the transition to a hypertrophic state), the Runx2 factor is also essential, acting in combination with Dlx5 and Dlx6 transcription activators under the control of histone deacetylase Hdac4 (Lefeb- vre & Smits, 2005). Runx2 expression begins on the back ground of intensive hyaluronan expression. The peak of hyaluronan expression coincides with the beginning of hypertrophy, while the inhibition of hyaluronan expression results in Runx2 expression and its activity slowing down (Tanne et al., 2008).

Cystatin 10, also known as **carminerin**, facilitates chondrocyte hypertrophy. It is a member of the superfamily of cystein protease inhibitors, a small (about 150 amino acid residues) protein molecule specific to growth plate chondrocytes in the final stage of differentiation. Cystatin 10 is found in a the cytosol of prehypertrophic and hypertrophic chondrocytes; its intensive expression accelerates the beginning of type X collagen expression and of chondrocyte apoptosis (Koshizuka et al., 2003; Yamada T. et al., 2006)).

The transcription factor MEF2C, previously known for its effect on the cardiac muscle, exerts its influence in the same direction on chondrocyte differentiation. Switching off the gene encoding this factor damages chondrocyte hypertrophy, angiogenesis, mineralization and bone longitudinal growth (Arnold et al., 2007).

In the prehypertrophic stage, especially in postnatal ontogenesis, the increased expression (previously noted during the condensation stage) recommences for a TGF-β-induced, secreted adhesive protein by growth plate and perichondrium cells. This protein, containing a "sticky" RGD-sequence, abbreviated as βig-h3, is supposed to activate the hypertrophy of chondrocytes (Han et al., 2008). Hypertrophy is also activated by the transcription factor, homeotic protein Dlx5 (Magee et al., 2005), and a G-protein2 signal regulator (Rgs2) (James et al., 2005).

The radical rearrangement of the actin cytoskeleton in chondrocytes takes place in the final stage of their differentiation in the development of hypertrophy. This rearrangement occurs, influenced by one of the actin-binding proteins – **adseverin** (also known as scinderin). The expression of this phosphoprotein, containing 715 amino acid residues, sharply increases in chondrocytes; it is stimulated by protein kinases PKC and MEK. Adseverin breaks down actin filaments, resulting in the formation of a submembranous microfilamentous network that facilitates exocytosis, the release of secreted macromolecules, including type X collagen, from a cell (Nurminsky et al., 2007).

In the transition from prehypertrophy to hypertrophy, chondrocytes stop expressing components of the cartilage extracellular matrix. Hypertrophied chondrocytes begin to express **type X collagen** specific to the ossification centers of the cartilaginous tissue, type I collagen and alkaline phosphatase), as well as the vascular endothelial growth factor (VEGF) that promotes the development of blood capillaries. The expression of the receptor PPR, whose ligands are simultaneously the parathyroid hormone and the related peptide (PTHrP), begins and gradually increases. The expression of the Ihh morphogen (PTHrP and Ihh are central in regulating the functions of the metaepiphyseal cartilage, see below) also increases.

Genes of the *Snail* family (*Snail* and *Slugh*) are involved in regulating the terminal (preceding ossification) stage of maturation of growth plate chondrocytes. These genes encode transcription factors that are transcription repressors, therein regulating–restraining and then discontinuing the chondrocyte expression of the most characteristic components of the cartilage matrix–type II collagen and aggrecan (Seki et al., 2003).

Discontinuing chondrocyte proliferation is one of indicators of the completion of their differentiation. This differentiation stage is associated with the increased expression of the activating transcription factor 3 (ATF). ATF3 represses the transcription of genes that encode proteins of the cyclin family involved in the cell cycle, i.e. in cell division (James et al., 2006).

The chondrocytes of the prehypertrophic and hypertrophic zones of the growth plate express the chondrocyte protein with a poly-proline region (**CHPPR**), also known as a mitochondrium fragmentation regulator (MTFR1). In this specific region of this protein, (from the 184–197th amino acid residues) 11 of 14 residues are proline residues. This expression is so active that CHPPR, being in mitochondria, can be considered as a marker of the chondrocytes finishing the life cycle (preapoptotic) (Tonachini et al., 2004).

The extracellular matrix, deposited by chondroblasts and prehypertrophic chondrocytes, undergoes **mineralization**. Mineralization takes place in the presence of matrix vesicles. Matrix vesicles are carriers of bone morphogenetic proteins (BMP), VEGF and a number of non-collagenous proteins (BSP, SPARC, OPN, osteocalcin), specific to the bone tissue extracellular matrix. This enables supposing that matrix vesicles, besides their involvement in mineralization, play a morphogenetic role in the metaepiphyseal cartilage and promote ossification (Nahar et al., 2008).

The mineralization of the cartilage matrix is regulated by the interaction of type II and X collagens with a transmembrane glycoprotein (calcium channel)–annexin V (also known as anchorin CII). This interaction, for which the actin cytoskeleton-bound collagen receptor DDR2 is essential, enhances the Ca^{2+} influx into chondrocytes, resulting in the increased expression of alkaline phosphatase and the acceleration of mineralization (Woods et al., 2007b; Kim & Kirsch, 2008). Mineralization is promoted by the above-mentioned cystatin 10 (carminerine) (Yamada et al., 2006).

The last zone is one of cartilage **degeneration** or, in other words, the zone of **ossification**. The apoptosis of chondrocytes and resorption of the mineralized provisory cartilage matrix, which is carried out by osteoclastic type cells originating in the perichondrium of a cartilage model of bone (also referred to as chondroclasts) occurs in this zone. In this case, osteoclastogenesis is caused by hypertrophic chondrocytes, which, under the influence of BMP-2, express the main stimulator of osteoclastic differentiation–RANKL (Usui et al., 2008).

Resorption of the organic matrix within this zone is facilitated by the high activity of the matrixines (metalloproteases) MMP-2, MMP-9 and MMP-13, expressed by hypertrophic chondrocytes (Inada et al., 2004; Ortega et al., 2005).

The natural death (**apoptosis**) of hypertrophic chondrocytes, after the mineralization of the extracellular matrix produced by them has been completed, is a ubiquitous result of the final stage of chondrocyte differentiation during endochondral ossification (in the entire model of a future bone and, in particular, in the growth plate). Proteins of the Bc12 family play a central role in regulating chondrocyte apoptosis. Members of the subfamilies Bax and BH3, comprising this family, exhibit proapoptotic activity (stimulating apoptosis) while proteins of the subfamily, Bc12 in particular, demonstrate anti-apoptotic (maintaining cell viability) properties (Oshima et al., 2008).

Dying chondrocytes are replaced by migrating from the perichordium progenitor cells, gaining the osteoblast phenotype as a result of differentiation. Osteoblasts produce another–bone–extracellular matrix, its mineralization occurs, and trabeculae of the spongy bone tissue are formed.

The evolution of the metaepiphyseal cartilage, involving chondrocyte differentiation and resulting in bone growth and formation, is controlled by a complex of signaling pathways, which integrates the activity of numerous regulating factors of local (short-distance) action (Adams et al., 2007; Mackie et al., 2008).

The main elements of the central executive mechanism in this complex are three signaling molecules:
1) Ihh (Indian hedgehog) morphogen;
2) parathyroid hormone-related protein (PTHrP) and
3) fibroblast growth factor 18 (FGF-18) (Kronenberg, 2003).

Indian hedgehog (alternative name is HHG-2) is one of the three members of the Hh- morphogen family, similar to HHG-1 ("Sonic hedgehog", Shh) in terms of molecule structure and its post-translation processing (see section 10.1). As in Shh, the Ihh morphogenetic activity is concentrated in the molecule N-terminal region, also called N-product, and containing from the 28–202nd amino acid residues (in humans).

In the metaepiphyseal plate, Ihh is expressed by chondroblasts, located on the border between the second (proliferative) and third (hypertrophic) zones; these chondroblasts are referred to as prehypertrophic or early hypertrophic. Ihh is bound to its receptor Patched (Ptc-1), which is expressed by chondroblasts of the first and second zones. Ptc-1 activates the co-receptor (transmembrane protein) Smo. The latter activates intracellular processes, affecting the function of a cell genetic apparatus. This action stimulates chondroblasts' cell cycle and their proliferation within columns. In the case of a deficiency of Ihh or switching off the gene encoding Smo, chondroblast proliferation ceases and bones do not grow longer. It is significant that even a short-term 2-day break in this signaling pathway, upon switching on Smo, in growing mice causes irreversible damage to the bone structure due to the insufficiency of chondroblast proliferation and excessive widening of the hypertropic zone (Kimura et al., 2008).

At the same time, Ihh stimulates the expression of a **parathyroid hormone-related protein** (PTHrP) by chondroblasts and perichondral (surrounding a cartilage model of bone) cells starting proliferation. **PTHrP** acts as **intracrine** (entering a cell nucleus directly) factor (Fiaschi-Taesch & Stewart, 2003) and employs, as previously mentioned, the same PPR receptors as the parathyroid hormone. This protein retains the chondroblasts of the proliferation and prehypertrophic zones in the proliferation state and prevents their premature transformation into chondrocytes (cell cycle switching off), i.e. before completing metaepiphyseal cartilage growth in the direction of the bone's longitudinal axis, and the beginning of chondrocyte hypertrophy. The PTHrP effect is largely, but not exclusively, associated with its inhibiting influence on Runx2 transcription factor expression, facilitating hypertrophy (Guo et al., 2006). Chondroblasts retained in the proliferation state do not undergo hypertrophy and continue expressing Ihh. At the same time, PTHrP inhibits the expression of type X collagen by already hypertrophied chondrocytes.

Thus, both these local regulators (Ihh and PTHrP) control the process of endochondral ossification according to the principle of a "loop" or feedback (Kronenberg, 2003). Apart from involvement in the Ihh regulation "loop", independent of expression, PTHrP exerts a direct influence on chondrocytes of the hypertrophic zone, stimulating their hypertrophy (Mak et al., 2008). Another aspect of Ihh participation in endochondral ossification is that it is involved in coupling formation and growth of the metaepiphyseal cartilage with its replacement by bone tissue. This involvement is associated with its stimulating effect (mediated by the Smo co-receptor) on osteoblastic differentiation. In Smo hyperexpression, this stimulation is manifested as the accelerated growth of a cortical bone cup (Long et al., 2004). Moreover, Ihh syn-

chronizes the development of the growth plate with angiogenesis and maturation of the perichondrium (Colnot et al., 2005).

Ihh and PTHrP molecules from the metaepiphyseal cartilage, penetrating the epiphysis, enter the permanent articular cartilage where they are also involved in regulating chondrocyte proliferation and differentiation according to the same principle (Cheng X. et al., 2008).

The third component of the mechanism – **FGF-18** – arrests this mechanism of stimulating chondroblast proliferation within the growth plate columns ("disrupts the loop"), delays proliferation, facilitates chondroblasts' transformation into chondrocytes and the completion of their differentiation (hypertrophy). This fibroblast growth factor employs, in particular, the FGFR3 receptor expressed by prehypertrophic chondrocytes. This receptor, exhibiting tyrosine kinase activity, is of critical importance in controlling the bone growth (Provot & Schipani, 2005). Switching off the gene encoding this receptor, such as switching off the gene encoding FGF-18, induces prolongation of proliferation, excessive longitudinal growth of a bone cartilage model, and causes a delay in ossification. The role of FGF-18 is not restrained herein by having a direct inhibiting effect on proliferation; FGF-18 also inhibits Ihh expression (Cormier et al., 2002).

The action of three main signaling molecules regulating the evolution of the metaepiphyseal plate and transformation of cartilaginous tissue into bone tissue (Ihh, PTHrP and FGF-18) is supported by the activity of and is under the control of other factors, which are both local and systemic.

Within the complex of regulating processes ongoing within the growth plate, Wnt family morphogens, which are similar to Hh-family morphogens in terms of their chemical nature, are switched on. Many members of the Wnt family control different stages of skeletal development, employing the canonical (β-catenin-mediated) and non-canonical (mediated by calcium-dependent linase C) signaling pathways (see section 10.1) (Hartmann, 2007).

The expression of several Wnt in the growth plate occurs not only in embryogenesis, but also in the postnatal period. It is most active in chondroblasts of the proliferative and hypertrophic zones. The Wnt-2b, -4, -10b signals, propagating along the canonical pathway, and Wnt-5a, -5b, -11 signals, going along the non-canonical pathway, are important for maintaining the viability, proliferation and hypertrophy of chondroblasts/chondrocytes, with the effects of some Wnt being backed up by others (Andrade et al., 2007).

Wnt-ligands, as well as their receptors, co-receptors and the components of signaling pathways they employ exert a multidirectional influence on processes ongoing within the growth plate. For example, Wnt-4, 8-c, 9a and β-catenin stimulate chondrocyte differentiation and maturation, whereas Wnt-5a, -5b, Fzd1, Fzd7 receptors, their competitive receptor Frzb-1 and a secreted Fzd-receptor-related protein sFRP1 delay maturation (Chun et al., 2008). Such a complex of regulating exposure facilitates the optimal coordination of the processes ongoing within the metaepiphyseal cartilage. In the case of Wnt deficiency, there is interference in the assembly of the growth plate, its structural organization suffers and thus, so does endochondral ossification (Tamamura et al., 2005).

The targeting of the regulating effects of some Wnt-morphogens involving β-catenin in the growth plate is radically changed in terms of development dynamics: they delay the hypertrophy of proliferating chondroblasts but stimulate the terminal differentiation and hypertrophy of maturated chondrocytes. This variability explains the contradictory data on the role of Wnt.

Among local regulators, an important role in regulating growth plate functions is played by the superfamily of transforming factors TGF-β, and primarily by bone morphogenetic proteins (BMPs) comprising this superfamily, which can be carried from cell to cell by matrix vesicles in the mineralization stage of the provisory extracellular matrix (Nahar et al., 2008). Under the autocrine control of BMP-2 and BMP-6, expressed by prehypertrophic and hypertrophic chondrocytes, is the expression by the same cells of the Ihh morphogen, the main stimulator of chondroblast proliferation. Moreover, BMP-2 directly stimulates the proliferation of chondroblasts. The proliferating chondroblasts themselves express BMP-7. The lack of local expression of BMP or the receptor BMPRIB they employ, which chondroblasts possess, leads to restraining the longitudinal growth of limb bones (Kugimiya et al., 2006). The same growth defects were also seen in axial skeleton and maxillofacial bones in terms of restricting the local expression of BMP-2, BMP-4 and BMP-7 in metaepiphyseal cartilages (Wan & Cao, 2005).

Hypertrophic chondrocytes continue the active expression of BMP-2 and BMP-6. The selective knockout of genes encoding these proteins causes a deficiency of chondroblasts, which are replaced by chondrocytes of the resorbing metaepiphyseal cartilage. This indicates the involvement of BMP in coupling apoptosis of hypertrophied chondrocytes with osteoblast differentiation (Kugimiya et al., 2006).

The effects of bone morphogenetic proteins on metaepiphyseal cartilage are mediated in many cases by other regulating factors. For example, BMP-2 stimulates the expression of the initial link in the "regulation loop", Ihh morphogen, by chondroblasts approaching the completion of proliferation by inducing the expression of the homeotic protein MSX2 rather than doing so directly. MSX2 stimulates Ihh expression (Amano et al., 2008).

As a "conductor" (vehicle) or mediator (intermediate) of BMP-2 effects on the proliferation and differentiation of the growth plate cartilage cells, the connective tissue growth factor (CTGF/CCN2) acts by forming a complex with BMP-2 (Maeda et al., 2009).

On the other hand, in some cases, bone morphogenetic proteins' effect on processes ongoing within the growth plate is induced, controlled and modulated by "upstream" or parallel acting regulating factors.

For example, a member of the nuclear transcription factor NFκB family, namely p65 or REL-A (in humans), stimulates the proliferation of growth plate chondroblasts and bone longitudinal growth. This effect is achieved by inducing BMP-2 (Wu et al., 2007). The stimulating effect of BMP-4 on the expression of type II collagen by chondroblasts and type X collagen by hypertrophic chondrocytes is restrained by a protein encoded by a *TSWG1* ("twisted gastrulation 1") gene and forms a triple complex with BMP-4 and one of the BMP extracellular antagonists, **chordin** (see section 10.1); this complex prevents BMP-4 binding to its receptors (Schmidl et al., 2006).

The action mechanism of the TGF-β factor superfamily on chondrocytes of the growth plate is similar to that of Wnt morphogens in that both mechanisms employ β-catenin induction in chondroblasts and the TSWG1 transcription factor (see section 10.2.3) in chondrocytes. TGF-β induces the expression of Twist1 in mature chondrocytes, while, at the same time, inhibiting the expression of Runx2; the excessive expression of Twist1 arrests chondrocyte hypertrophy. Wnt-3a affects mature chondrocytes in the opposite direction. These findings indicate the involvement of TSWG1 in the control over the terminal stage of chondrocyte maturation (Dong et al., 2007).

Together with FGF-18, which, as shown above, is part of the "triad" of regulators of differentiation and the activity of the metaepiphyseal cartilage cells (Ihh – PTHrP – FGF-18), other fibroblast growth factors are also involved in control over the endochondral formation of bones. The concept of this involvement was primarily made on the basis of clinical observations, which found that the cause of many chondrodysplasia forms, manifesting as defects in skeletogenesis, are mutations of FGF receptors (**FGFR**). The FGFR3 receptor is of utmost importance, whose expression in embryogenesis begins later than that of FGFR1 and FGFR2. It is via the FGFR3 receptor that FGF-18 works, but it is necessary to note that a FGF-19 deficiency causes more serious impairments of skeletogenesis than a deficiency of FGFR3; it means that FGF-18 can employ other FGFR (Ornitz & Marie, 2002; Ornitz, 2005).

The excessive expression of FGF-2 and FGF-9, which also works via the FGFR3 receptor by chondrocytes of the growth plate, causes the inhibition of chondrocyte proliferation. It results in the shortening of long bones and dwarfism. The deficiency of these factors does not cause serious impairment to the phenotype.

FGF-7, -8, and -17 are mainly expressed around a cartilage model of future bone by condensation cells, which do not start chondrogenic differentiation and from which the perichondrium is formed (Chen & Deng, 2005). In the same cells, the expression of the Notch1 trans-membrane receptor is more intensive and prolonged (Watanabe et al., 2003).

The entire integrated complex of local regulation mechanisms of metaepiphyseal cartilage functions is controlled by systemic regulation factors, namely hormones and vitamins (Eerden et al., 2003).

The pituitary **growth hormone** (GH) is the most important among other factors for the growth plate and therefore, for the longitudinal growth of bones. The GH deficiency or the lack of receptors essential for its functioning in the signaling pathway causes growth defects. The main way of GH action is associated with the stimulation of insulin-like growth factor-1 (IGF-1) production by the liver and partly with the stimulation of the local production of this factor by cells of the growth plate proliferative and prehypertrophic zones. IFG-1 exerts an independent stimulating effect on chondrocytes, which express IGF binding proteins (IGFBP). This effect is targeted, however, to chondrocytes' hypertrophy rather than to the proliferation of chondrocytes (Nilsson et al., 2005). Along with this, GH directly affects chondrocytes, outside the signaling "axis" of GH-IGF-1, thereby stimulating their proliferation. The direct effect of GH, where the special receptor GHR and a hormone-binding protein GHBP are involved, is more pronounced in the postnatal period (Giustina et al., 2009).

The second place among hormone factors in terms of regulating the metaepiphyseal cartilage belongs to thyroid hormones – **thyroxine** (T4) and more active **triiodothyronine** (T3). Hypothyroidism slows down growth abruptly. To the contrary, hyperthyroidism accelerates the rate of bone growth, but also causes the premature ossification of growth plates and lessened growth as a result.

The mechanism of thyroid hormones' effect involves TRα and TRβ receptor-mediated interaction with the GH-IGF-1 "axis" (stimulation of the IGF-1 expression). However, the central role is played by the interaction of hormones with Wnt morphogens. The introduction of T3 into a culture of growth plate chondrocytes causes the intense expression of Wnt-4, the intracellular accumulation of β-catenin followed by the stimulation of the expression of the Runx2/Cbfa1 factor, which accelerates the terminal stage of chondrocyte maturation and stimulates ossification (L. Wang et al., 2007). Carboxypeptidase Z is involved in the interaction of the T3 signaling pathway and the canonical Wnt-morphogen signaling pathway. T3 induces this enzyme expression, which deletes the C-terminal arginine residue and, in such a way, stimulates a positive morphogen effect on chondrocyte maturation (L. Wang et al., 2009).

Glucocorticoids negatively affect the chondroblasts/chondrocytes of the growth plate. Glucocorticoids, especially active synthetic analogues of natural hormones in pharmacological doses, inhibit the proliferation of chondroblasts and deposition of the extracellular matrix. At the same time, they accelerate the apoptosis of hypertrophied chondrocytes. These effects result in the thinning of the growth plate and defects in bone longitudinal growth.

In the mechanism of action of glucocorticoids, their interference in various links of the GH-IGF-1 signaling pathway ("axis") is of significance, reducing the expression of IGF-1, GHR and IGF-1R receptors, as well as the IGFBP-5 binding protein (Nilsson et al, 2005).

Sex-steroids are of great importance in controlling bone's longitudinal growth, especially in the period of sexual development, when growth can be up to 20% (Perry et al., 2008). In both girls and boys (males and females in animals), estrogen hormones directly affect bone growth; they employ preferably one of two estrogen receptors, the ERα receptor to stimulate growth. In boys, estrogen buildup from androgens (testosterone) is catalyzed by the enzyme aromatase p450. Switching off the CYP19 gene encoding this enzyme causes the same delay in growth, as does the absence of the ERα receptor. However, the possibility of androgens' direct influence on the growth plate and developing bone tissue cannot be excluded. On the one hand, such an effect is suggested by bone growth defects in switching off the gene encoding the androgen receptor (AR), and the well-known phenomenon of skeleton masculinization influenced by androgens on the other hand (Nilsson et al., 2005). The estrogen deficiency caused by ovariectomy reduces the number of chondrocytes in the growth plate, which is a consequence of the delayed proliferation and acceleration of apoptosis (Takano et al., 2007). In the period of sexual development, the stimulation of the GH-IGF-1 signaling pathway (the "axis") becomes more important in terms of the effect of sex-steroids on bone longitudinal growth along with the direct action on growth plate chondrocytes (Perry et al., 2008).

As for the role of vitamins, the growth plate functions determining the bone longitudinal growth in the postnatal period are seriously affected in the absence of the regulating effects of the most active vitamin A metabolite, **retinoic acid**. For this effect to occur, retinoic acid nuclear receptors, especially the RARγ receptor, are essential. Defects seen in switching off the gene encoding this receptor include the reduction of aggrecan expression and deposition, which the volume of a forming matrix of growth plate cartilaginous tissue depends upon (Williams et al., 2009).

Vitamin D3 delays the terminal stage of chondrocyte differentiation, acting via the membrane-associated receptor MARRS. This effect is removed through the proteolytic deletion of the receptor; the removal stimulates insulin-like factor 1 (IGF-1) (Dreier et al., 2008a).

The extreme complexity of the entire process of endochondral ossification and especially of the final stage of chondrocyte differentiation should be noted, including the prehypertrophic and hypertrophic stages and the further ossification stage, where chondrocyte apoptosis, resorption of the provisory mineralized extracellular cartilage matrix, osteoblastogenesis and formation of a bone mineralized extracellular matrix occur. A complicated complex of interacting factors and regulation and control mechanisms corresponds to such complexity. The investigations of this complex have yet to be completed. The data provided above is illustrative of the role of the most thoroughly studied and most significant factors. The data on some other factors and mechanisms of controlling and regulating endochondral ossification are provided in *Table 10.4*.

Provisory metaepiphyseal cartilage is a **hyaline** type cartilage whose cells (chondroblasts/ chondrocytes) are surrounded by an extracellular matrix specific for this type. The cell mass in the growth plate prevails quantitatively over the matrix mass, whereas the inverse ratio is in permanent cartilages, especially in articular cartilage.

Herein, the qualitative macromolecular composition of the matrix of "upper" (from epiphysis to diaphysis corresponding to the dynamics of ongoing processes) zones of the growth plate does not principally differ from the matrix of other hyaline cartilages. The main components determining the matrix properties of these zones are type II collagen, which forms large heterotypical fibrils with the participation of type IX and X collagens and proteoglycan aggrecan aggregates that are united by hyaluronan.

Given such a principle similarity with permanent hyaline cartilages, a growth plate cartilage has some peculiarities in terms of its macromolecular composition. These peculiarities somehow differ in different zones.

They are particular in assortment, macromolecules structure and the quantitative content of proteoglycans. Aggrecan macromolecules differ from the reserve zone to the zone of mature cartilage. The character of sulfation of aggrecan chondroitin sulfates changes: the amount of chondroitin-6- sulfate increases from 32% to 53%, while the content of chondroitin-4- sulfate decreases respectively (from 53% to 35%). These alterations in the ratio of chondroitin sulfate isoforms in aggrecan macromolecules, as well as the enlargement of a macromolecule's total size due to the elongation of glycosaminoglycan chains is supposed to be one of the conditions essential for chondrocyte hypertrophy (Byers et al., 1997).

As for small proteoglycans, a peculiarity of a metaepiphyseal cartilage (as with the epiphyseal regions of a bone cartilage model) is the presence of significant amounts of **epiphycan**. Epiphycan encoded by the *EPYC* gene, also called dermatan sulfate proteoglycan 3 or PG-Lb, as the related osteoinductive factor osteoglycin, is part of the family of small leucine-rich repeat proteoglycans–it contains seven such repeating amino acid sequences (LRR). After cleavage of a signal peptide, 19 residues in length, an epiphycan core protein contains 303 amino acid residues, its molecular mass being 46 kDa. An epiphycan's total molecular mass is about 133 kDa. The only glycosaminoglycan chain that range in size from 23 to 34 kDa is supposedly attached to a Ser64 residue. In addition, epiphycan contains two O-bound (to Thr60 and Ser96) oligosaccharides. Epiphycan expression and its depositions in the extracellular matrix of the growth plate decreases from an epiphysis towards a diaphysis, and there is no epiphycan in the "lower" region of the hypertrophied chondrocyte zone. There is no distinct data on epiphycan's functions; it is supposed to be involved in the formation of the matrix supramolecular structural organization (Johnson et al., 1999).

Another small proteoglycan from the family of small leucine-rich repeat proteoglycans–**decorin**–is widely spread in the matrix of many types of connective tissue. It is just as spread out in zones of the growth plate almost as epiphycan. There is a lot of decorin in the barrier (resting) and proliferative zones. Its content progressively decreases from the prehypertrophic zone towards the ossification zone. The distribution of other members of the same family, such as biglycan and fibromodulin, is more homogeneous along the entire plate thickness (Alini & Roughley, 2001).

Like an extracellular matrix of permanent cartilages, the metaepiphyseal cartilage matrix contains a significant number of the basement membrane-specific heparan sulfate proteoglycan (PGBM), also known as **perlecan**. It is a large proteoglycan, one of the main components of basement membranes. After cleavage of a signal peptide, its core protein has 4,370 amino acid residues. Despite the absence of a basement membrane in the growth plate, gigantic molecules of perlecan are essential for every zone of the plate as a multifunctional extracellular framework, organizing and maintaining the matrix structure (Farach-Carson & Carson, 2007). Perlecan is also essential as a regulator of all stages of chondroblast/chondrocyte differentiation up to the mineralization of the hypertrophic zone matrix. This function of perlecan is related to its ability to react with many signaling molecules; this ability is provided by the presence of 48 diverse domains within the perlecan macromolecule (Rodgers et al., 2008).

The composition of collagen components changes radically in the hypertrophic zone, where type II collagen is gradually replaced by type I collagen specific to bone tissue in the extracellular matrix and where type X collagen appears, which is definitely present at the mineralization of cartilaginous tissue.

Matrix metalloproteases (matrixins) MMP-1 (interstitial collagenase), MMP-9 (gelatinase B), MMP-13 (gelatinase-3), and MMP-14 (MT1-MMP) are accumulated and demonstrate high activity in the extracellular matrix of the hypertrophic zone (see section 3.7.1). These enzymes carry out the proteolytic degradation of cartilage matrix, which makes it possible to form a new–bone matrix and creates conditions for the vascularization of developing bone tissue. The deficiency of these MMP impairs bone growth (Malemud, 2006; Mackie et al., 2009).

The high activity of alkaline phosphatase, involved in mineralization, is specific to the hypertrophic zone and especially to that of ossification.

A bone cartilage model is not a passive framework to form a true mineralized bone. Its extracellular matrix (not only enzymes but also structural components) take an active part in endochondral ossification in general and particularly in processes ongoing within the growth plate.

The main fibrillar collagen of cartilage matrix, type II collagen, is absolutely essential. There is no cartilage without type II collagen, and endochondral ossification

Table 10.4

Some factors and mechanisms of regulating and controlling enchondral ossification

Factors and Mechanisms	Authors
Oxygen reactive forms	Morita et al., 2007
Signaling pathway of epidermis growth factor receptor ErbB2	Fisher et al., 2007
Signaling pathway of receptor 48 coupled with G-protein	Luo et al., 2009
Secretion of a protein with box-1 of high mobility	Taniguch et al., 2007
Runx3/AML2/Cbfa1	Song et al., 2007
Signaling pathway of protein kinase B (RKB/Akt)	Rokutanda etal.,2007
Signaling pathway of phosphoinositide-3-kinase (P13K)	Kita et al., 2008; Ulici et al., 2008
Transcription factor Dlx5 (Distal-less homeobox 5)	Chin et al., 2007
Transcription factor Trps1 (Trichorhinophalangeal syndrome 1) interacting with transcription factor Gli3	Suemoto et al., 2007; Wuelling et al., 2009
Homeotic gene of dwarfism Shox2,action via natriuretic peptide B	Yu et al., 2007; Mar-chini et al., 2007
Activating transcription factor 2 (Akt-2), action via retinoblastoma protein pRb	Vale-Cruz et al., 2008
Natriuretic peptide C	Teixeira et al., 2008
Cyclic guanosine monophosphate (cGMP)	Teixeira et al., 2008
Interferon-induced protein p202	Kong & Liu, 2008
CCN3/NOV factor	Lafont et al., 2005
Protease Site-1 (S1P/MBTP1)	Patra et al., 2007
Signaling pathway of the Tgfbr2 receptor	Seo & Serra, 2007
Hypoxia, transcription factor HIF-1α, protein VHL	Schipani, 2006
Endoribonuclease Dicer and its formed miRNA	Kobayashi et al., 2008

is unfeasible without a cartilage model. In the knockout of a *Col2a1* gene encoding type II collagen, a mice skeleton has only bones of membranous origin, while bones formed by endochondral ossification are completely lacking (Li et al., 1995).

In metaepiphyseal cartilage, type II collagen, which interacts with cells by its triple-helical domain by means of integrins and a DD2 receptor, which is more specific to collagens, is essential for maintaining chondroblast/chondrocyte viability (Mackie et al., 2008). A cryptic amino acid sequence opening in the proteolysis of type II collagen induces the hypertrophy of chondrocytes with the expression of type X collagen and matrix metalloprotease-13 (MMP-13) specific to this stage of differentiation (Tchetina et al., 2007). The mutation of the gene encoding type II collagen, which causes internal deletion (loss of nucleotides), results in the impairment of endochondral ossification in the postnatal period; the defects are manifested as delay in bone formation, an abrupt reduction (up to 40%) in bone mass and increased resorption (Nieminen et al., 2008).

Defects in the growth plate structure in mice develop in the absence of type IX collagen that stabilizes the surface of cartilage matrix fibrils heterotypic in composition. The orderliness of columns is impaired, with preferably chondroblasts/ chondrocytes of the prehypertrophic and hypertrophic zones suffering; the total number of cells and the expression of the integrin β1 subunit is reduced. This results in the shortening and thickening of long bones (Dreier et al., 2008b).

For growth plate ossification, what is essential is the main proteoglycan of cartilage matrix, aggrecan to be precise, the proper structure of aggrecans' chondroitin sulfate. Upon switching off the gene *C4st1*, which encodes chondroitin-4-sulfotransferase 1 catalyzing sulfation of chondroitin sulfate in the fourth position, causes acceleration of proliferation and maturation and the premature apoptosis of chondrocytes. This defect might be related to the generation of an excess TGF-β growth factor (Klüppel et al., 2005).

An important event in the ossification process is the above-mentioned development of blood capillaries within ossification centers; capillaries are absent in cartilaginous tissue. Capillaries' growth is stimulated by VEGF-A, a member of the vascular endothelial growth factor (VEGF) family. VEGF-A is secreted by hypertrophied chondrocytes and acts simultaneously on the osteoblast and osteoclast signaling pathways (Dai & Rabie, 2007). The VEGF expression by chondrocytes is induced by FGF-18, which is involved in all stages of growth plate evolution (Mackie et al., 2008).

The hypoxia-induced factor α (**HIF-1α**) is also involved in activating VEGF expression and coupling angiogenesis with starting osteogenesis (Wang Y., Wan C. et al., 2007). The role this factor plays in ossification is specified by the circumstance that hypoxia (oxygen deficiency), intrinsic for the growth plate in the embryonal period (Schipani et al., 2006), stabilizes the chondrocyte phenotype but delays osteoblast differentiation, which is es-

sential for the replacement of provisory cartilaginous tissue with bone tissue (Hirao et al., 2006). The activation of VEGF expression by HIF-1α facilitates the ability to overcoming this impediment.

The growth of capillaries within ossification centers is controlled by the small (molecular mass 20 kDa) antiangiogenic peptide **endostatin**, which is a C-terminal fragment of a macromolecule of non-fibrillar **type XVIII collagen** (see section 3.1.1.1). Endostatin inhibits endochondral ossification, delaying the process at the stage of the bone cartilage model. This effect is based upon an endostatin inhibiting action on VEGF expression (Sipola et al., 2007).

Besides VEGF, angiogenesis is stimulated by the **connective tissue growth factor** (CTGF). This cysteine-rich protein, containing 323 amino acid residues, a member of the CCN family, is also known as HCS24 (**hypertrophic chondrocyte specific protein 24**) or ECOGENIN (endochondral ossification genetic factor) (Takigawa et al, 2003). The CTGF action promotes the coordination of angiogenesis with chondrogenesis (Ivkovic et al., 2003).

The role of capillaries developing in the ossification process is not restrained by promoting the aerobic metabolism of osteoblasts. The cells of capillary endothelium produce active peptide factors, **endothelins**. These small peptides, particularly endothelin-1, working via the specific osteoblast transmembrane receptor EDNRA (otherwise ETRA), stimulate osteoblast proliferation and activate their differentiation (Kasperk et al., 1997).

The combined effects of matrix metalloproteases and chondroclasts/ osteoclasts facilitate the resorption of provisory cartilage and clear a space for the invasion of blood vessels and for preosteoblasts and osteoblasts migrating from the bone marrow cavity. Osteoblasts completing differentiation produce and deposit a bone extracellular matrix. The conditions for promoting an **ossification front** are created in such a way, gradually displacing the cartilaginous tissue (Mackie at al., 2008). Ultimately in this process, a cartilage model is transformed into a bone, which retains residues of the cartilaginous tissue as specialized articular cartilages on the joints surfaces of epiphyses.

10.3.1.3. Intramembranous ossification

Intramembranous (membranous, endesmal) ossification, as it has already been noted, differs from endochondral ossification in that a bone is formed by the direct transformation of embryonal mesenchyme condensations into bone tissue without the intermediate stage of a provisory cartilage model. Condensations located on sites of future flat bones, mainly subcutaneously, change into double-layer lamellae or membranes for which this process is named. Sometimes the process is referred to as dermal ossification.

The mesenchymal cells of such condensations differentiate at first into osteochondral progenitor cells, after which their further osteoblastic differentiation occurs.

Differentiated osteoblasts produce the bone extracellular matrix, which undergoes mineralization. Surrounded by the mineralized matrix, osteoblasts complete their differentiation, changing into osteocytes. The trabeculae of spongy bone tissue are formed between ossified membranes; the space between trabeculae is filled with red bone marrow. The membranes take on the character of compact bone tissue. Their thickening occurs due to the activity of adjacent mesenchyme cells, part of which forms the periost, while the other part differentiates into osteoblasts. These osteoblasts deposit a compact bone cortical layer.

Even this schematic description of a morphological picture of intramembranous ossification allows suggesting the presence, first of all, of certain functional peculiarities in the cells involved in this ossification and, secondly, of certain qualitative peculiarities of macromolecular components of extracellular matrix and metabolic processes within forming bone tissue. Moreover, significant differences in the processes of endochondral and intramembranous ossification cannot be based on less significant differences in molecular mechanisms of regulation working in these processes.

The data on these peculiarities are fragmentary due to the suboptimal state of knowledge on intramembranous ossification compared with that concerning endochondral ossification. This evidence is based on statistical data. There have been 2,005 publications on endochondral ossification in the archive collected by the PubMed service of the U.S. National Library of Medicine from 1958 (the beginning of the modern information system) through 2009, while there were only 506 publications on intramembranous ossification in the same period.

It has been determined that the phenotypic characteristics of osteoblasts involved in intramembranous ossification depend on the sources of their origin. Osteoblasts of the parietal bone, the main source of which is the paraxial mesoderm, express alkaline phosphatase, osteopontin, type I collagen and the Wnt5a morphogen more intensively than do osteoblasts of the frontal bone originating from the neural crest. The frontal bone osteoblasts express FGF-2, cadherins and the bone morphogenetic proteins receptor BMPRIB more intensively, which can be considered as an indicator of a lower differentiation degree and capability for accelerated proliferation (Xu et al., 2007). The frontal bone, furthermore, differs from the parietal one due to the more active expression of fibroblast growth factors FGF-2, FGF-9, FGF-18 and all three known receptors of these factors–FGFR-1, -2 and -3 (Quarto et al., 2009).

Differences in the response of an osteoblast genome of skull bones, on the one hand, and that of mice fore and hind limb bones, on the other hand, on switching off the Runx2 gene have been determined. This switching off changed the expression of 1,277 genes in skull bones forming by the intramembranous way, whereas it affected the expression of 492–606 genes in long bones of endochondral genesis (Vaes et al., 2006).

Differences in the extracellular matrix composition have also been found. Skull flat bones contain eight times more collagen soluble fractions, three times more of the pigment epithelium-derived factor (PEDF or Serpin-f1, a member of the serine protease inhibitors family), and four times more osteoglycin. On the contrary, the long bones of limbs contain three times more chondrocalcin and secreted phosphoprotein (Spp-24 or phosphoprotein 2), four times more thrombospondin-1 and fetuin, and seven times more thrombin. Type I collagen of long bones contains three times more hydroxylysylpyridinoline bonds, and this can account for its lesser solubility and greater resistance to the effects of matrix metalloproteases (van den Bos et al., 2008).

The mineralization of the extracellular matrix of skull flat bones is associated with the expression of tenascin-W by osteoblasts and its presence in the matrix (Mikura et al., 2009).

The role of the bone acid glycoprotein-75 (BAG-75), which is very rich in an aspartic acid, is of more importance in the mineralization of bones formed by the intramembranous pathway than in endochondral ossification. The expression of BAG-75 begins very early, even during the stage of flat mesenchymal condensations' formation, and its presence determines the localization, size and shape of further mineralization centers. Later the expression of bone sialoprotein (BSP), considered as an immediate participant in mineralization, begins in the borders of these centers (Gorski et al., 2004).

The glycoprotein **periostin** (PN, alternative name is OSF-2), secreted into the matrix by osteoblasts in intramembranous ossification, is involved in mineralization. PN expression takes place in many tissues, but within bone tissue, it is pronounced selectively only in bones formed by the intramembranous pathway (Kashima et al., 2009).

Intramembranous ossification differs from endochondral ossification in the mechanisms of regulation–by acting factors and signaling pathways.

Ihh (Indian hedgehog) is one of the essential factors involved in endochondral ossification; it is expressed by hypertrophic chondrocytes and induces the beginning of chondrocyte proliferation of the growth plate upper (reserve, barrier) zone. The role of this morphogen in the intramembranous ossification ongoing in the absence of chondrocytes is negligible (Chung et al., 2004).

The transcription factor Runx2 plays the central role in osteoblast differentiation in the process of intramembranous ossification, just as in endochondral ossification (see section 10.3.1.1). Intramembranous ossification differs in that another transcription factor –**Runx1** (also called Cbfa2 and AML-1), a member of the same Runx family (proteins with a Runt-domain)–is actively expressed, along with Runx2, in ossification centers from their very formation; its expression continues till ossification completion. This allows us to state that Runx1 is involved in the initiation of intramembranous ossification (Yamashiro et al., 2004).

In intramembranous ossification, a somewhat different row of bone morphogenetic proteins (**BMP**) acts than is the case of endochondral ossification. In intramembranously forming bones, the expression of BMP-3, -4 and -8 is more pronounced, and there is also an expression of BMP-9 and -15. The expression of BMP-2 and -5 is more specific to bones of endochondral genesis. These differences are associated with the peculiarities of mechanisms to maintain homeostasis in bones of various types (Suttapreyasri et al., 2006).

A peculiar set of BMP begins to manifest even in the formation of the cranial region of the neural crest ongoing under the control of interacting BMP, FGF and the Wnt family morphogens, whereas the formative signal comes from BMP. BMP-4 activates the expression of the homeotic genes *Msx1* and *Msx2* and the transcription factor *Slug* gene; these genes directly affect the development of the neural crest. The homeotic protein Msx2 and the Alx4 protein (a member of the protein family with pared genes *PAX*) are essential for the proper development of mesenchymal condensations preceding skull flat bones. BMP (BMP-4 together with BMP-2 and -7), inducing the expression of these proteins and involving a transcription factor Foxc1, are intensively expressed by mesenchyme cells in the early stage of maxillofacial skeleton development (Rice et al., 2003).

The crucial role in the further genesis of skull bones is played by BMP-4, -3, -5, as well as BMP-7; BMP-2 is equally essential for the ossification of both types (Nie et al., 2006).

Both in endochondral ossification and in intramembranous ossification, the controlling role of fibroblast growth factors (**FGF**) has primarily been revealed in clinical observations. In particular, the etiology of a number of syndromes involving craniosynostosis defects (the formation of skull flat bones ongoing in the participation of FGF-2, -4, and -9) is associated with mutations affecting the expression of FGFR receptors (Ornitz & Marie, 2002). The most important is FGF-2, working via the FGFR-2 receptor and signaling pathways comprising protein kinase C (PKC) and protein tyrosine kinase Src (Marie, 2003).

The participation of individual FGF and the targeting of their action in intramembranous ossification do not, in all cases, coincide with their activity in endochondral ossification. The differences are particularly marked in targeting FGF-18 activity. It should be recalled that, in endochondral ossification, FGF-18 inhibits the proliferation of growth plate chondrocytes, restraining the longitudinal growth of bones. Thus, the factor exerts a negative effect on chondrogenesis. On the contrary, in intramembranous ossification, FGF-18, along with FGF-20 by means of FGFR1 and FGFR2 receptors, stimulates osteogenesis. Switching off the genes encoding these proteins impairs the development of skull flat bones (Ohbayashi et al., 2002).

The effect of FGFs, in particular of FGF-18, on the proliferation of osteoblast progenitors and the further differentiation of osteoblasts in intramembranous ossification is controlled by the homeotic protein **En-1** (Engrailed). This control is achieved by En-1 acting on the expression of FGFR2 receptor and a Spry-2 protein acting in the pathway of signals coming from FGFR. Nil mutation of an *En1* gene impairs the development of skull flat bones in mice (Deckelbaum et al., 2006).

The connective tissue growth factor **CCN2**, whose action in endochondral ossification is targeted predominantly at chondrogenesis, is essential for osteoblast differentiation in intramembranous ossification (Kawaki et al., 2008b).

Annexin A1 (lipocortin I), a small phospholipids-binding protein (an inhibitor of cellular phospholipase) is also essential for the differentiation of osteoblasts of skull intramembranous bones. Switching off the *Anxa1* gene, encoding annexin A1, abruptly impairs the development of skull bones in mice (Damazo et al., 2007).

Such serious defects as dysplasia (the maldevelopment) of intramembranous bones of the skull cup and maxillofacial skeleton result from switching off the oncogene (meningioma gene) *Mn1*, which functions as a transcription co-regulator of a variety of genes. Defects take place not only in homozygous but in heterozygous mice, in which the gene is only partly switched off (Meester-Smoor, 2005).

Ghrelin is of special interest among the number of regulation system factors in bone intramembranous formation. This peptide stimulates the secretion of the growth hormone (GH) and simultaneously directly stimulates bones' formation. Its ossification stimulating activity is especially high in accelerating the healing of skull bone defects; this acceleration is associated with the enhanced expression of alkaline phosphatase, osteocalcin and type I collagen (Deng et al., 2008).

Bones formed by the intramembranous pathway are connected to each other by bone sutures–**synostoses** as a rule. Bone fusion occurs. All the factors discussed, which regulate intramembranous ossification, are simultaneously regulators of synostosis formation and mineralization. Optimal synostosis formation (in terms of sutures' quality and the dynamics of their development) is feasible only given normal properties and contact of bone ends. Impairment in regulating ossification interferes with these conditions. At the same time, synostosis development is controlled by a number of special factors and mechanisms, interacting with the factors that regulate ossification.

For example, BMP-4 action, which stimulates intramembranous ossification and the fusion of skull cup bones, is controlled by one of the bone morphogenetic proteins antagonists, **noggin**, whose source is cells of the mesenchyme of uncompleted formation sutures and cells of the dura matter. Noggin expression is restrained by FGF-2, and a re- lease from this restriction by switching off the gene encod- ing the FGFR1 receptor causes the development of a clinical syndrome, which includes the symptom of premature craniosynostosis (cases of such a re- lease are known in spontaneous mutations in humans)

(Warren et al., 2003). A number of similar syndromes (and non-syndrome craniosynostosis) are known to be caused by mutations of genes encoding FGFR2, FGFR3, the homeotic protein MSX2, the transcription factor TWIST1, and the transmembrane protein EFNB1 (Morris-Kay & Wilkie, 2005).

Premature craniosynostosis develops given the deficiency of phosphoprotein **axin2** (conductin, axil), which is a negative regulator of the Wnt-morphogen canonical signaling pathway. Axin2 promotes the degradation of β-catenin, a central component of this pathway (see 10.1). A decrease in β-catenin concentration, under the influence of axin2, inhibits the proliferation and differentiation of osteoblast progenitors. On the contrary, in the absence of axin2 and therefore, given the increased concentration of β-catenin, these processes are accelerated and premature, shortly after birth, ossification of sutures occurs and craniosynostosis develops. The selectiveness of the axin2 effect on synostosis formation between skull bones is due to a special phenotype of the cells of this skeleton region originating from the neural crest (Yu et al., 2005).

A transmembrane (one-pass) receptor protein – the large chondroitin sulfate proteoglycan 4 (**CSPG4**), known as NG2 – is involved in synostosis development between intramembranous skull bones. The intense expression of CSPG4 is noted in forming bone sutures along the ossification front and in the matrix; after ossification is completed, this expression abruptly subsides. The same dynamics of CSPG4 expression takes place in the growth plate hypertrophic zone in endochondral ossification (Fukushi et al., 2003).

In forming bone sutures in direct contact with edges of intramembranous skull bones, islands of cartilaginous tissue are found; they are referred to as a **secondary cartilage** since they are formed not before but after bone tissue formation. The occurrence of secondary cartilage attests to the chondrogenic potential of mesenchymal condensations cells preceding intramembranous bones (Cohen, 2006).

The matter is that, even given marked differences, especially in terms of morphology, between endochondral ossification, which has been studied in detail in appendicular skeletogenesis, and intramembranous ossification specific to skull skeletogenesis, both of these processes, as well as that of permanent cartilage development, are governed by a common conservative program. The conservatism of this program becomes evident upon analyzing the processes from the point of view of molecular ontogenesis (Eames et al., 2003).

One of the elements of the common program of skeleton development is the exclusion of angiogenesis from all skeletogenic (prechondrogenic and preosteogenic) condensations in their early development. Although bone vascularization later takes place, the majority of permanent cartilages remains avascular (Eames & Helms, 2004). In the embryonal period in condensations preceding intramembranous skull bones in the early osteogenesis stage, the expression of structural molecules regarded as chondrogenesis markers – IIA, IX and XI type collagens and aggrecan – occurs, with this expression carried out by cells that also express alkaline phosphatase specific to bone tissue. In the later stage of condensation evolution, some cells also express markers of mature chondrocytes – IIB and X type collagens. This data suggests that the intramembranous pathway of ossification undergoes a transitory chondrogenic phase and proves the chondrogenic potential of the skull mesenchyme (Nah et al., 2000; Åberg et al., 2005).

The expression in forming endesmal (intramembranous) skull bones of signaling molecules and transcription factors, which specify the progress of endochondral ossification of axial and appendicular skeleton bones, indicates a combination of the molecular peculiarities of chondrogenesis and osteogenesis during intramembranous ossification. In mesenchymal condensations, from which skull bones are formed, the main signaling molecules act, regulating the longitudinal growth of endochondral bones – the Ihh morphogen and the parathyroid hormone-related protein (PTHrP). Herein, their function appears to vary as they regulate the differentiation of preosteoblasts into osteoblasts. Within the same condensations, the expression of transcription factors encoded by the "master"-genes of osteoblastic differentiation – *Runx2* and Ost – is combined with the expression of Sox9, a central transcription factor in chondroblastogenesis, which is essential for growth plate chondroblast proliferation (Eames & Helms, 2004; Abzhanov et al., 2007).

The differentiation program of cranial mesenchyme cells preceding parietal and frontal bones is switched from intramembranous into endochondral ossification in transgenic mice, in which these cells cause the expression of fibroblast growth factor FGF-9. The effect of this factor, working via the Fgfr2 receptor, is sufficient to induce endochondral ossification with chondroblastic differentiation, the proliferation and hypertrophy of chondrocytes, and the expression of type X collagen (Govindarajan & Overbeek, 2006). This is additional evidence of the chondrogenic potential of the cranial mesenchyme.

An analysis of the dynamics of gene expression shows that, in intramembranous skull bones involving the differentiation of mesenchymal progenitor cells into osteoblasts, a part of the cell undergoes a short-term status for which a **CLO** (chondrocyte-like osteoblast) term is proposed. For the transformation into CLO, the combined action of BMP-2, BMP-4 and BMP-7 is essential. CLO simultaneously express some chondrocyte markers – type II and IX collagens (but do not express aggrecan and Sox9) – and the osteoblast marker osteopontin. CLOs also express PTHrP and Ihh. Already in the next stage, the cell ceases expressing cartilage collagens and adds an expression of a mature osteoblast marker – the bone sialoprotein BspII – to osteopontin expression. Another part of the progenitor cells differentiates directly into osteoblasts and this differentiation occurs without the participation of BMP-7 (Abzhanov et al., 2007).

10.3.1.4. Type X collagen

Nonfibrillar **type X collagen**, essential for endochondral ossification, along with type VIII collagen, which is very close to it in terms of its primary structure and gene organization, comprise a group of so called short-chain network-forming collagens (Sutmuller et al., 1997) (see Table 3.1).

A molecule formula of type X collagen is $_3$ [α1(X)], its macromolecule with a length of about 150 nm, is made up by three short, α1(X) –identical polypeptide chains, each of which has a molecular mass of 59 kDa. The α1(X) chain contains one central continuous collagen domain (COL1), consisting of 460 amino acid residues, which are arranged into collagen protein-specific repeated triplet sequences (-Gly-Xxx-Yyy-). COL-domains form a collagen-typical triple helix.

Multiple non-reducible intermolecular cross-links – hydroxylysylpyridinoline (HP) and lysylpyridinoline (LP) – are located within the triple helix ("collagen") domain. These links can connect the macromolecules of type X collagen with adjacent macromolecules of the same collagen or with macromolecules of type II collagen. Herein the concentration of LP, a cross-link specific to type I collagen of mineralized tissues such as bone and dentin, is especially high. Collagen fibrils containing this link are noted for an increased mechanical strength (Orth et al., 1996).

Both terminal domains, NC1 and NC2, have a noncollagen- ous primary structure and are not spiralized. The C-terminal domain NC1 consists of 162 amino acid residues; the N-terminal domain (NC1) is shorter, containing 52 amino acid residues, including a signal peptide.

Type X collagen macromolecules form (possibly by means of disulfide bonds) supramolecular aggregates, like a net or a mesh with hexagonal (six-sided) cells (Bruckner & Rest, 1994). Such strong meshed structures are seen in electron microscopy in the pericellular matrix of hypertrophied chondrocytes.

The function of type X collagen is not entirely understood. The hypothesis that type X collagen function is related to mineralization has not been exactly proved. The knockout of the *Col10a1* gene causes only insignificant defects in skeletogenesis and hematopoiesis in bone marrow. More profound pathological alterations in bone growth appear in mutations, which lead to the truncation of the type X collage macromolecule. In such mutations, the disorganization of the meshed hexagonal structure of type X collagen supramolecular aggregates has been noted in the pericellular zone of the extracellular matrix, as well as the more diffuse distribution of proteoglycans throughout the matrix; severe bone deformities develop. The role of type X collagen, appearing as meshed aggregates in the hypertrophic stage, is most likely confined to strengthening hypertrophic chondrocytes' fixation within the matrix (Jacenko et al., 2001). This fixation takes place with the involvement of proteoglycans and the α2β1integrin. The type X collagen macro-

molecule binds to this integrin via its C-terminal non-collagen and the entire collagenous domains (Fukai et al., 1994).

A gene of type X collagen in humans is localized in chromosome 6. The gene's intron-exon structure is unusual. Unlike the majority of collagen protein genes, whose encoding nucleotide sequences exhibit a multiexon structure (divided into a lot of short exons), the type X collagen gene contains only three exons, with one large third exon encoding the entire C-terminal non-collagen and entire collagen domains (Fukai et al., 1994).

The expression of type X collagen is associated with the distinctly specified differentiation stage of growth plate chondrocytes. Type X collagen is expressed by **hypertrophic chondrocytes** only in the initial period of matrix mineralization almost simultaneously to the appearance of molecules that are specific to bone tissue, such as alkaline phosphatase, osteocalcin, and bone sialoprotein II. The bone morphogenetic proteins BMP-2 and BMP-6 stimulate type X collage expression, along with the expression of alkaline phosphatase (Grimaud et al., 1999). This stimulation is mediated by the effect on expression of the *CBfa1/Runx2* gene (Zheng et al., 2003).

The expression of type X collagen is regulated by transcription factors, and the so-called specificity proteins (SP) SP1 and SP3, which are members of the same family as Osterix (SP7), to be more precise, by the increase of the SP3/SP1 ratio in chondrocyte hypertrophy. This increase occurs due to a decrease in the content of SP1 (Magee et al., 2005). PTHrP is also involved in regulation; it inhibits the expression of type X collagen in an interaction with a transcription factor Gli3 (a protein with 5 "zinc fingers"), which is activated by the Ihh morphogen (Mau et al., 2007).

In beginning hypertrophy, the expression of a C-type natriuretic peptide (CNP) (see section 10.2.3) and its receptor NPR-B is increased. The introduction of CNP into a chondrocyte culture in the differentiation stage enhances the expression of type X collagen, together with the expression of N-cadherin (Alan & Tufan, 2008).

The rapidly disappearing type X collagen is more sensitive to the action of proteolytic enzymes than other collagen proteins, especially fibrillar collagens. It is broken down not only by collagenase 3 but also by other, not so specific metalloproteases, whereas there can be a disrupture of peptide bonds in the central triple helix domain of the macromolecule. This increased sensitivity to protease effects is due to the presence of several distortions of the typical triplet sequences of amino acid residues in the central domain.

The expression of type X collagen is considered as a marker of the hypertrophy of the metaepiphyseal cartilage chondrocytes of forming bones. Numerous data suggests that this collagen expression is occurring in other ossification centers of cartilaginous tissue as well. On the contrary, type X collagen is not found in cartilage, which does not undergo ossification, such as menisci of knee joints (Naumann et al., 2002).

Some data obtained through immunohistochemical methods indicates the presence of small amounts of type X collagen in centers of intramembranous ossification. However, there is no convincing confirmation of these data or an evaluation of their importance.

The expression of recently discovered small fibrillar **type XXVII collagen** coincides with type X collagen synthesis in time and location in the metaepiphyseal cartilage of forming bones (see section 3.1.1.1). This coincidence suggests a hypothesis on the similarity of these collagens' functions in ossification (Hjorten et al., 2007).

10.4 MOLECULAR BIOLOGICAL AND BIOCHEMICAL MECHANISMS OF JOINT FORMATION

10.4.1. Mechanisms of joint formation

Condensations of mesenchymal cells that are to become cartilage "patterns" (models) of future limb bones as a result of chondroblastic differentiation are initially whole continuous formations starting from a shoulder or a thigh and ending in branches in the region of the fingers or toes. Cartilage models formed from these condensations by chondroblastic differentiation are the same whole formations; these models are made up of chondroblasts/chondrocytes, which express specific components of the cartilage extracellular matrix–type II collagen and aggrecan.

The formation of a diarthrodial (synovial) joint, leading to the separation of a future skeleton into movable segments (bones), starts as early as the stage of mesenchymal condensations. A selection of cells committed (irreversibly designated) to be included into joint structures takes place. The great majority of non-differentiated condensation mesenchymal cells enter chondroblastic differentiation, transforming into provisory chondrocytes. This pathway results in the maturation, hypertrophy and apoptosis of provisory (primary) chondrocytes, changed by osteoblasts, and the formation of bone tissue. At the same time, a small part of condensation cells localized within a future joint zone is selected to build up a joint (Khan et al., 2007).

In selection, cell specialization is determined very early. Some of them, which contrasted to other condensation cells, do not start the expression of a *Matn1* gene encoding glycoprotein **matrilin-1** (a protein of cartilage matrix CMP, Table 7.4). The absence of matrilin-1 expression appeared to be a marker making it possible to further trace the differentiation of these cells into the permanent chondrocytes of articular cartilages. They soon start expressing such components specific to the articular cartilage extracellular matrix as lubricin (a surface layer protein) and glycoprotein tenascin C. The cells expressing matrilin-1 follow another pathway–they differentiate into the provisory chondrocytes of epiphyses (Hyde et al., 2007).

Other cells within the selection zone are flattened and become similar to fibroblasts. These fibroblast-like cells form a joint capsule and joint synovial membrane, intra- and periarticular ligaments. Herein, the cells from the condensation surrounding mesenchyme join selected condensation cells. Some of them might change the pathway of differentiation and gain a phenotype of permanent articular cartilage chondrocytes (Pacifici et al., 2006).

Cell selection provides **specification**, a determination of a future joint location. A triple-layer structure is formed on this site; it crosses a bone across its longitudinal axis and is referred to as an **interzone**. The latter consists of an intermediate non-chondrogenic plate (many authors prefer to call only this intermediate plate an interzone) and chondrogenic zones, bounding it on both sides. Thus, a cell population of the interzone is not homogenous and, during interzone formation, it is subdivided into subpopulations originating various joint structures. Herein, the preliminary stage of joint formation is over. During the next stage, called joint **cavitation**, the interzone intermediate plate, a fine layer of densely packed flattened cells which, unlike chondroblasts, express type I collagen, is transformed into a space referred to as a joint cavity, filled in with the synovia (synovial fluid). Proximal and distal chondrogenic layers of the interzone maintain contact with a cartilage model perichondrium and are finally transformed into bone articular cartilage (Edwards & Francis-West, 2001).

If all three layers of the interzone containing selected cells are removed before the transition from the first to the second stage, a joint does not develop, and a single fused bone appears instead of two future ones. On the contrary, joint development is not impaired in keeping the interzone and removing the chondrogenic layers it borders.

Two main mechanisms are involved in the formation of a joint cavity or a gap (cavitation). The first of them engaged in many other morphogenetic processes is **apoptosis**, which a certain part of the interzone cell population undergoes (Mariani & Martin, 2003). Apoptosis (from the Greek "dropping off petals or leaves (from plants or trees)" is a phenomenon of programmed cell death (PCD). This phenomenon is of universe importance in the development and vital activities of multicellular organisms involving practically all tissues. Apoptosis enforces the regularities of organism development and its balanced state throughout life (Salvesen, 2002).

Unlike **necrosis**, a process where a cell is a **passive object** in relation to the destructive factors affecting it, a cell in apoptosis is an **active subject**, it itself ends its life by means of own energy-consuming molecular mechanisms.

The differences between the morphologic, physiologic and biochemical characteristics of necrosis and apoptosis are listed in *Table 10.5*.

The family of proteolytic enzymes–cysteine proteases (not less than 13) (see section 1.8.1) acting intracellularly plays the main role in apoptosis. They are known as **caspases**; the name is explained by the fact that they break

Table 10.5
Distinctive patterns of necrosis and apoptosis

Necrosis	Apoptosis
Morphologic peculiarities	
Swelling of cytoplasm and mitochondria	Shrinkage of cytoplasm, chromatin condensation
Chaotic karyolysis	Fragmentation of the nucleus
Total destruction of a cell without formation of a vesicle	Formation of a structure (vesicle, apoptotic body) packed in a membrane
Physiologic and biochemical characteristics	
It is caused by non-physiologic (pathogenic) stimuli	It is caused by physiologic stimuli
Early destruction of the cytoplasmic membrane	Maintenance of signal perception mechanisms
It does not require energy	It depends on energy supply
Chaotic breakdown of DNA	Organized (arranged) DNA fragmentation in chromosomes
DNA degradation begins after permeability of toplasmic membrane abruptly inased	Caspases activation. Delayed discontinuity of cytoplasmic membrane. Alterations in cytoplasmic membrane facilitated by enzymatic mechanisms Annexin V binding
Consequences	
It affects cell groups	It affects individual cells
It causes an inflammatory response	It does not cause an inflammatory response as a rule
Necrotized cells are phagocytosed by neutrophils	Dead cells are phagocytosed by adjacent cells and macrophages

According to Kühn et al. (2004) with amendments

down peptide bonds at aspartic acid residues. Caspases are expressed as non-active zymogens and are activated by means of partial proteolysis like many other enzymes (Donepudi & Grutter, 2002).

Caspases are activated by two ways. When a cell is induced to apoptosis by outward signals coming from other cells or the extracellular matrix, we can speak of an **external** apoptosis pathway. External signals can be "negative" – a negative signal is understood as the ceasing of any signaling. In the disappearance of a "regular" signal from outside, some cell membrane receptors having an intracellular domain called addiction/dependence domains (ADD) become active; such receptors are referred to as dependence receptors (Bredesen et al., 2004). Alterations in the conformation of ADD or their proteolysis occur, resulting in proapoptotic signals appearing in a cell.

External signals (in relation to the cell), called "death activators", can be some members of the tumor necrosis factor superfamily TNF-α (Apo-3-L, TRAIL), one of the TNF-β family members, i.e. lymphotoxin and Fas-ligand (FasL), whose molecule is bound to the cell surface receptor Fas (CD95).

To percept these signals, a cell has a receptor TNF-R1 family, which includes the above Fas-receptor, the TNF-R1 receptor and special "death receptors" DR3, DR4, DR5, DR6 (Rossi & Gaidano, 2003). By involving special intracellular adaptor proteins, these transmembrane receptors activate caspase-8, transforming it from a proenzyme into an active enzyme. Caspase-8 activates other caspases, called effector caspases, as they directly accomplish apoptosis.

The external signal is propagated to the family of cytoplasmic proteins, known as signal transducers and activators of transcription (STAT) (Stephanou & Latchman, 2003). The phosphorylation of one of the serine residues in the C-terminal domain activates STAT-factors. STAT-1 comes into interaction of a "protein-protein" type with transcription factors, which directly affect the expression of the molecules determining the beginning and course of apoptosis.

Protein factors of the Bcl-2 family play the central role in the apoptosis **internal pathway** (Schinzel et al., 2004). The Bcl-2 family includes factors stimulating (proapoptotic) apoptosis, such as Bax, Bad, Bid, and those that prevent apoptosis (antiapoptotic), such as Bcl-2, Bcl-LX. Under normal conditions, Bcl-2 is present on the external membrane of mitochondria in a bound with an Apaf-1 (apoptotic protease activating factor-1) protein. When apoptosis internal signals (for example, active oxygen radicals) appear in the cell, Bcl-2 releases Apaf-1 and promotes the Bax factor in the destruction of the mitochondria external membrane. Soluble proteins, activating caspases in a complex with Apaf-1, are released into the cytosol from the mitochondrium intermembraneous space. Cytochrome C is one such protein. A heat shock protein (Hsp10) and proteins of the Smac and HtrA2 families exhibit a similar action. Influenced by internal

stimuli, the process of apoptosis starts with the activation of caspase-3 and caspase-9, whose function is to activate effector caspases, just as caspase-8 does. In turn, effector caspases activate enzymes performing DNA fragmentation – the central stage of apoptosis. They are caspase–activated deoxyribonuclease (CAD) and DNA fragmentation factors such as DFF40 and DFF45. Caspase-mediated internal and external ways of apoptosis interweave with each other, contacting when affecting the mitochondria membrane (Sprick & Walczak, 2004).

There are known caspases-independent apoptosis pathways that also come via mitochondria. One of the proteins released from the mitochondrium intermembraneous space and called AIF (apoptosis inducing factor) (Candé et al., 2002) is an evolutionally very old flavoprotein, which enters the nucleus from the cytosol and is electrostatically bound to DNA, causing a number of alterations in its function, which is manifested as chromatin condensation in particular. Other mitochondria proteins exhibiting the same activity are also known (Saelens et al., 2004). Under their influence apoptosis occurs without the involvement of caspases.

The phosphoprotein **p53**, also known as the cell tumor antigen p53 or the tumor suppressor p53, controls the induction and progress of apoptosis. The main targeting of this factor with manifold effects, encoded by a *TP53* gene, is apoptosis induction, which is achieved by stimulating the expression of proapoptotic genes (*Bax, Fas*) and repressing the expression of antiapoptotic (Bcl-2) genes (Nakamura, 2004). Thus, the "decision" of a cell to start apoptosis depends on P53 (Slee et al., 2004).

Besides apoptosis of a part of the interzone cell populationm, accumulation of extracellular macromolecular components, which then comprise the synovial fluid (synovia), are is of significant importance in the formation of a joint cavity (Pitsillides & Ashhurst, 2008). This accumulation is predetermined by changes in a phenotype of cells forming joint structuresm, in particular, the synovial membrane.

The activity of enzymatic systems involved in **hyaluronan** synthesis, the main component of synovia, is increased in the interzone cells. The increased activity of uridine diphosphoglucose dehydrogenase (UDPGD) is especially evident. This characteristic differentiates the interzone cells from chondrocytes not comprising the interzone. Kinases of the MAP/ERK superfamily (mitogen-activated kinases kinases), regulated by the extracellular signaling essential for intensifying anabolic processes, are also activated (Pitsillides, 2003).

At the same time in interzone cells, there is increased expression of various hyaladherins (hyaluronic acid binding proteins, HABP) of cell membranes (CD44, RHAMM, IVd4) and intracellular proteins of a so-called ERM (ezrin, radixin, moesin) complex, which unite HABP transmembrane receptors with actin cytoskeleton (Dowthwaite et al., 1998).

Despite the activation of the HABP-receptors' expression, an increased hyaluronan synthesis results in their satura- tion. Free, non-hyaladherin-bound hyaluronan, which begins to be accumulated in large amounts within the interzone, moves apart from the surrounding cells. It occurs by two ways: by pressure of water, fixed by hyaluronan due to its high hydrophilic property, and by the blocking of cell adhesion proteins by hyaluronan. This is the second main cavitation mechanism resulting in the appearance of a groove-like space between future bones ends filled in with the synovia.

Alterations in the typological characterisctics of fibrillar collagens in the dynamics of joint development processes have been well studied in rabbit knee and thigh joints starting with a 17-day embryo up to an adult (2 year old) animal (Bland & Ashhurst, 1996; 2001). On the 17th day of embryogenesis, the interzone has already separated the cartilage models of the femoral bone and tibia. A member of bone morphogenetic proteins Cdf5/Bmp14 family (Cdf5, Bmp14), phosphoprotein Erg and tenascin C are considered as its markers (Koyama et al., 2007). As an arthrogenesis marker, tenascin C (see 3.2.1.1) is given special importance in relation to the hypothesis on its role in the development of a specialized permanent phenotype of articular cartilage chondrocytes differing from that of epiphysis provisory chondrocytes undergoing hypertrophy and apoptosis. Moreover, tenascin C is present in the formatting of intraarticular ligaments and the synovial membrane (Mackie & Ramsky, 1996). In the interzone matrix, type I, III and V collagens are detected on the 17th day, but type IIB collagen specific to mature cartilaginous tissue is still absent. It is also absent on the 25th day when cavitation occurs, although the expression of type IIA procollagen mRNA is already revealed; this indicates the chondroblastic differentiation of some cells of the interzone. Type II collagen starts to be detected histochemically only when cavitation is over and its appearance indicates the formation of articular cartilages. At the moment of birth, a complete joint already exists and further development occurs only due to the continuing formation of the extracellular matrix. The ossification of epiphyses is completed by the sixth week after birth. By this time, chondrocytes of articular cartilages take on the spatial arrangement typical to them, type II collagen appears and spreads along the entire thickness of articular cartilages, and type I collagen specific to the mesechyme disappears. The latter, together with type III and V collagens, are retained in the joint capsule, tendons and ligaments.

As for the involvement of proteoglycans in joint morphogenesis, the fibroblast-like cell of the interzone intermediate layer continues to actively express versican, which is intrinsic for embryonal mesenchyme cells. This large chondroitin sulfate-containing proteoglycan, which forms aggregates with hyaluronan participation, might maintain the homeostasis of the interzone prior to the start of cavitation, facilitates cavitation and the formation of the surface of articular cartilage. The expression of another proteoglycan, aggrecan, a specific extracellular matrix component of cartilaginous tissue, is prevalent in the chondrogenic layers of the interzone (Shepard et al., 2007).

Dynamics of proteoglycans (aggrecan and fibromodulin) and glycoproteins (cartilage oligomeric matrix protein, COMP, and cartilage matrix protein, CMP) have been studied in an example of development of a shoulder joint in mice (from the 12th day of embryogenesis until the 37th day after birth) using imminohistochemical methods. The most pronounced expression of aggrecan took place in epiphyseal cartilages. Mesenchymal cells of the interzone are intensively stained for fibromodulin even before the be- ginning of cavitation. This response became more intensive in the matrix around differentiating chondrocytes. There was no CMP within these regions, while COMP accumulation around chondrocytes began after the 18th day, when the first movements appeared in a joint. This data gave rise to the conclusion that fibromodulin is essential in the early stage of joint chondrogenesis, and that the COMP function is related to the perception of mechanical stress on the matrix of a developing articular cartilage (Murphy et al., 1999).

Small proteoglycans (biglycan and decorin), which are absent in the interzone prior to this, and glycoprotein matrilin-1, in the deeper layers of the epiphyseal cartilage, appear in a forming articular cartilage only after cavitation. Matrilin-1 disappears after the ossification of epiphysis has been completed (Kavanagh & Ashhurst, 1999).

10.4.2. Molecular factors of regulation of joint formation

The formation of synovial joints is regulated and coordinated by a perplexed complex of molecular mechanisms, about which investigations have not yet been completed. A large number of signaling molecules comprising this complex is known, but there is no explanation why various molecular factors (as will later be shown) are essential for the development of some or other joints that are similar in function and structure. It has still not been determined which of the manifold factors working in the interzone play a decisive role in the selection of cells, committed to be involved in the interzone and, the further buildup of joints among the total number of chondrogenic condensation cells.

Factors encoded by homeotic *Hox*-genes (see section 10.1), which are considered responsible for implementation the general body pattern, are undoubted candidates for this role. It was supposed that joint specification is determined by a combination of the expression of genes of *HoxA* and *HoxD* clusters (the expression of cluster A genes occurs throughout condensations in the proximal-distal direction, while that of cluster D occurs in the anterior-posterior one). Herein, it was noted that the combination of the most intensive expression of both clusters genes often coincides with a condensation bifurcation (splitting into two parts) site (Yokouchi et al., 1991). For example, the knocking out of mutations of *Hoxa-10, -11* and

Hoxd-10, -11 or *–13* cause the fusion of bones in the radio-carpal joint, while mutations of *Hoxa-11, -13* and *Hoxd-11* or *–13* impair the segmentation of fingers' or toes' phalanges. However, these mutations did not affect the specification (of localization) of knee and elbow joints though the topography of these joints coincides with the bifurcation of condensations (it is one of the examples of the regulation peculiarities of individual joints' development) (Francis-West et al., 1999).

Other homeotic genes, *Dlx5* and *Dlx6* in particular, are involved in the commitment of condensation cells and specification of elbow joint localization. The expression of these genes, encoding transcription factors, performed by a limited group of cells, significantly outruns the onset of the interzone formation and which, of particular interest, is accompanied with a short-time delay in beginning the expression by the same cells of a cartilage morphogenetic protein CDF-5/BMP-14, known as one of the positive regulation factors in joint formation (Ferrari & Kosher, 2006).

The Wnt-9a morphogen (in the nomenclature used until recently, it was called Wnt-14) plays a central role in inducing joint formation, namely in selecting the cells essential for it and the specification of their localization. Its intense expression is found in a mesenchymal condensation in the zone of a future joint before other signs of joint genesis appear. Within the cells of this zone beginning, chondroblastic differentiation ceases and molecular factors (CDF5, CD44, chordin) appear, the expression of which is intrinsic for the interzone cells and precedes joint formation. Mutations that switch off the *Wnt9a* gene affect this process. Due to the absence of *Wnt9a* antichondrogenic activity, there is excessive growth of articular cartilages and, instead of two bones separated by a joint; a single united bone might be formed.

The negative effect that the absence of Wnt-9a signaling has on joint formation is increased if the expression of Ihh (a morphogen of the Hedgehog (Hh) family working via the trans-membrane 7-pass receptor Ptch1) is simultaneously increased (Mak et al., 2006). On the contrary, under normal conditions, Ihh (Indian Hedgehog), one of leading regulation factors of endochondral osteogenesis and the growth of long bones, is a positive regulator of joint formation mainly due to its chondrogenic activity. Switching off the *Ihh* gene results in the lack of limb distal (interphalangeal) joints, and the development of more proximal joints, such as for the elbow and knee, is also impaired, albeit to a lesser extent (Koyama et al., 2007). Ihh, whose action is mediated by "zinc finger"-containing factors (activators) of transcription Gli1, Gli2 and Gli3, is also necessary for the proper formation of a temporomandibular joint. At the same time, it is engaged in the morphogenesis of an intraarticular disk (Purcell et al., 2009). Excessive Ihh signaling creates a predisposition to synovial chondromatosis, and the growth of metaplastic cartilage nodes in the synovial membrane (Hopyan et al., 2005).

One important aspect of the Wnt-morphogens should be noted. The introduction of an exogenous Wnt-9a into a mesenchymal condensation might cause ectopic (in an unusual place) joint development; this phenomenon seems to be especially important. It is of interest that in this case, a distally nearby endogenous (located in a proper place, orthotopic) joint discontinues its development completely (Hartmann & Tabin, 2001).

Two other Wnt-family morphogens, Wnt-4 and Wnt-16, which back up the activity of Wnt-9a/14, are capable of inducing joint formation (Guo et al., 2004). The molecular mechanism of the Wnt-morphogen's influence on joint development has not been conclusively revealed. According to some data, working via transmembrane receptors of the Frizzled family, they employ the so-called canonical intracellular Wnt-signaling pathway, whose main element is a phosphoprotein β-catenin (see 10.1). Switching off the *Ctnnb* gene encoding β-catenin causes the same defects in joint development due to the disruption of the signaling pathway, as does a deficiency of Wnt-9a. The introduction of endogenous β-catenin results in the same effect as does that of the morphogen itself (Guo et al., 2004).

Contrary to the cogency of these data, the other findings indicate that the canonical Wnt-signaling pathway is essential for creating the conditions for the joint formation by means of repressing the chondrogenic potential of condensation mesenchymal cells rather than for inducing it (in the literal sense). The antichondrogenic activity of the Wnt-morphogens, including Wnt-9a, manifests itself in this repression (Später et al., 2006a). Under this influence, some cells of the interzone gain a phenotype of synovial fibroblasts and fibroblasts of the joint capsule fibrous layer, which are essential for the formation of a full-grown joint (Später et al., 2006b).

On the other hand, in forming a full-grown joint, should be involved factors that stimulate chondroblastic differentiation and are essential for building up the articular cartilages comprising a joint structure. In other words, the regulation of a joint formation requires the involvement of factors of an oppositely directed action – antichondrogenic and chondrogenic – that are balanced and coordinated in time.

The growth and differentiation factor **GDF-5**, which has already been mentioned several times (otherwise known as CDMP-1) and is a morphogenetic protein originating from a cartilage, is the main chondrogenic factor in joint development engaged in this complex system. At present, it is included in the bone morphogenetic proteins family under the name of BMP-14.

GDF-5 involvement in joint morphogenesis is of an ambiguous nature. It practically does not affect the genesis of joint soft tissue components and is, in general, targeted at regulating chondrogenesis of the epiphyseal region of a cartilage model of the future bone (Merino et al., 1999). In a mesenchymal condensation (in mice), a wide zone of GDF-5 intensive expression at first appears within the zone of a future joint; GDF-5 stimulates chondroblastic differentiation, inducing the expression of *Sox-9*, a chondroblast "master" gene (see section 10.2.2). A cell population of this forming interzone (in a general sense of the term) forming all the joint structures, at first expresses *Wnt9a, Collagen IIA* and *Erg* genes. Then selection (subpopulation generation) occurs, which is associated with the originating of selective resistance to the GDF-5 chondrogenic activity in cells of the interzone central plate (Storm & Kingsley, 1999). This cell subpopulation, falling under the antichondrogenic influence of Wnt-9a (and some other Wnt), builds up joint soft tissue structures and the most superficial, lubricin-producing layer of articular cartilages (Koyama et al., 2008). The cells of the interzone proximal and distal plates retain their sensitivity to GDF-5 chondrogenic activity and comprise the second subpopulation, which forms the remaining layers of articular cartilages, beginning the synthesis of such components of the extracellular matrix as aggrecan and type IIB collagen. This chondrogenic activity of GDF-5 is promoted by the transcription regulating factor Erg, a member of the same TGF-β superfamily, to which all GDFs belong. The hyperexpression of Wnt-9a and the BMP antagonist noggin inhibit this activity. The intensity of GDF-5 expression in a joint decreases after cavitation; if it remains at the same level, the excessive development of articular cartilages occurs, leading to the fusion of bone ends.

Considering the significance of GDF-5 in joint morphogenesis, it should be kept in mind that the same activity is intrinsic for both other GDFs (GDF-6 and GDF-7), which are expressed by the cells of various structures forming a joint. The targeting of their activity (chondrogenic effect) is synergetic to that of GDF-5, and the combination of switching off the genes encoding these factors increases the number of joints suffering in their absence on account of the elbow and radiocarpal joints (Settle et al., 2003).

A GDF-5 chondrogenic effect is specially targeted at stimulating the forming articular cartilages exactly (rather than the mineralization-undergoing cartilages of the epiphysis) owing to the involvement of the "downstream" transcription factor of phosphoprotein Erg in the propagation of these factors' signaling. The transcription regulator (transforming protein) **Erg** is a member of the protein ETS-family, united by the presence of an ETS-domain, which is responsible for binding to DNA. Erg (in humans, it is an isoform called C-1-1) affects transcription by activating one of histone methyltransferases, and this influence inhibits the expression of factors associated with the hypertrophy of chondrocytes and mineralization (Ihh, type X collagen, alkaline phosphatase, and metalloprotease MMP-13) and activates the expression of articular cartilage markers, particularly of tenascin C (Iwamoto et al., 2007).

Some BMP are also involved in joint formation, as indicated by the presence of relevant mRNAs and the proteins themselves in the interzone. This involvement is reflected in positive effects in terms of the formation of articular cartilages. BMP-4 exhibits such chondrogenic activity, which enhances chondroblastic differentiation and stimulates the growth of articular cartilages, provided that, unlike GDF-5, the late expression of BMP-4 does not affect joint formation (Tsumaki et al., 2002).

GDF-5 expression occurs in the cells of a forming interzone of future limb joints. At the same time, the participation of other members of the BMP/GDF family in regulating joint formation is characterized by a high specificity, which manifests itself in spatial and timing aspects. For example, GDF-6 is selectively present in the sites of future carpometacarpal and tarsometatarsal joints, while GDF-7 appears more selectively in the site of the future shoulder joint (Wolfman et al., 1997).

BMP-2 and BMP-7 (OP-1) are engaged in joint formation as inductors of an apoptosis onset of the interzone cells in cavitation (Macias et al., 1997). The selectiveness of individual BMP action is controlled by the expression of their receptors. A BMPR-1A receptor is essential for BMP's stimulating effects on chondroblastic differentiation; it is also necessary for preventing the early wear-out of articular cartilages (Rountree et al., 2004). Another receptor, similar to BMPR-1A in structure – BMPR-1B – maintains the influence of BMP on apoptosis. The type II TGF-β receptor function is of importance: switching off the gene (*Tgfbr2*) encoding this receptor results in the absence of interphalangeal joints. Joints' specification and interzone formation proceed normally, but then fibroblast-like cells of the interzone are displaced by proliferating chondroblasts (Seo & Serra, 2007). This *Tgfbr2* action is associated with the involvement of the TGF-β superfamily in controlling Wnt9a, GDF-5 and noggin expression (Spagnoli et al., 2007).

The selectiveness and specificity of the influence of BMP and other regulating factors of the TGF-β superfamily on joint formation is determined by their interaction with their antagonistic extracellular factors (action modulators) such as noggin, chordin, ghremlin and others. Excessive BMP chondrogenic activity is also prevented by a "special" BMP, BMP-3, which exhibits activity that is antagonistic to other BMP. BMP-3 expression is especially evident in the perichondrium surrounding a forming joint. Its switching off enhances the proliferation of articular cartilage chondroblasts and results in a joint closure (Gamer et al., 2008).

Some other growth factors and cytokines have been determined to participate in joint morphogenesis, along with factors of the TGF-β superfamily, although their exact roles have not been disclosed in every case.

Fibroblast growth factors FGF-2, FGF-4 and FGF-10 are expressed in the interzone of a forming joint. FGF are supposed to facilitate the proliferation of interzone mesenchymal cells and this effect is positive in the early stage of arthrogenesis. But the introduction of exogenous FGF-10 into the interphalangeal joints region causes defects in their formation and ends in the fusion of phalanges. This means that the FGF influence should not be excessive (Lovinescu et al., 2003).

The tumor necrosis factor TNF-α and interleukins of the IL-1 and IL-17 families exert catabolic effects on articular cartilages during their formation. Chondroblasts express particularly interleukin IL-17B, and it is therefore called a chondroleukin. This cytokine functioning is supposed to be essential, along with that of other BMP antagonists, in controlling the chondrogenic (anabolic) activity of BMP/GDF factors; it retains its importance in maintaining the postnatal homeostasis of articular cartilages (Reddi, 2003).

Moreover, the selection of goals (cell-targets) and the degree of activity of signals carried by molecules of various cytokines and growth factors, including the TGF-β superfamily growth factors and BMP/GDF, are controlled by the fibrillin microfibrils adsorbing these molecules, dosing and targeting their movement within the extracellular matrix (Ramirez & Rifkin, 2009).

An α5β1 integrin (see section 3.6.3) is also involved in choosing a way for the chondroblastic differentiation of mesenchymal condensation cells in bone buds–towards the permanent chondrocytes of articular cartilages or towards the provisory undergoing of hypertrophying and apoptosis by chondrocytes. The blocking of this integrin by specific antibodies introduced into a condensation inhibits chondrocyte hypertrophy, arrests type II collagen expression and causes the formation of ectopic joints on the border between the zones of proliferating chondroblasts and hypertrophic chondrocytes. This effect of the α5β1 integrin is not overcome by the simultaneous introduction of BMP7 (Garciadiego-Cázares et al., 2004).

Chondroblastic differentiation in condensations occurs in the background of hypoxia. This fact is confirmed by the expression of the main factor of tissue adaption to hypoxia, the **hypoxia-induced factor Hif-1**α, acting as a transcription factor by all the condensation cells in limb buds. Stimulating expression of a vascular endothelial growth factor (VEGF) is considered to be a specific sign of its activation. Switching off the gene encoding Hif-1α (*Hif1a*) impairs chondroblastic differentiation, thereby delaying hypertrophy of chondrocytes. Hif-1α expression is more intensely pronounced in the zones of forthcoming joint formation, with this local increase in expression detected even before the beginning of GDF-5 mRNA expression and before the appearance of the interzone. Such a succession of events allows supposing that the *Hif-1*α gene is epistatic (modifying expression) to the *Gdf5* gene and that it is related to specification of joints. In "conditional" (programmed) switching off, the *Hif-1*α, formation of distal joints in a limb is more impaired–interphalangeal joints are not formed at all and the formation of elbow and even scapular-humeral joints is delayed (Provot et al., 2007).

A biomechanical factor is important for the normal development of joints. Its role starts at the stage of the chondrogenic differentiation of mesenchymal condensation cells. When condensation cells from a mouse embryo's limb buds cultured *in vitro* are exposed to compression, they begin the early expression of the Sox9 transcription factor, type II collagen and aggrecan. At the same time, the expression of interleukin IL-1β decreases, its one aspect of antichondrogenic effects (as other members of the IL-1 family) being the inhibition of type II collagen transcription (Takahashi et al., 1998).

The origination and morphogenesis of joints are directly related to the generation of a limb motor function. Without movements in the embryonic period (in the pharmacological blocking of the muscle contracting function), i.e. in the absence of mechanic stress, a beginning joint formation ceases in the interzone stage. The fibroblast-like cells of the interzone become similar to chondroblasts and diminish and then completely discontinue the expression of type XII collagen and tenascin C. The deficiency of type XII collagen (a member of the FACIT family), which is of significant importance in the structural organization of dense, formatted types of connective tissue impairs the morphogenesis of joint soft tissue components. The deficiency of tenascin C spreads over epiphyseal regions of a cartilage model of the future bone and is accompanied by a malformation of articular cartilage deep layers (Mikic et al., 2000).

The aforementioned main experimental data related to the regulation of joint formation is obtained mainly when studying the small distal joints of limbs. Almost nothing is known about the regulation of joint formation of the axial skeleton and the largest synovial joints–coxofemoral and shoulder joints.

REFERENCES

Abdelmagid S.M., Barbe M.F., Arango-Hisijara I. et al. Osteoactivin acts as downstream mediator of BMP-2 effects on osteoblast function. // J.Cell.Physiol. – 2007. – vol. 210, N 1. – P. 26–37.

Abdelmagid S.M., Barbe M.F., Rico M.C. et al. Osteoactivin, an anabolic factor that regulates osteoblast differentiation and function. //. Exp.Cell Res. – 2008. – vol. 314, N 13. – P. 2334–2351.

Abe E. Function of BMPs and BMP antagonists in adult bone. // Ann.N.Y.Acad.Sci. – 2006. – vol. 1068. – P. 41–53.

Abe H., Matsubara T., Ichara N. et al. Type IV collagen is transcriptionally regulated by Smad1 under advanced glycation end product (AGE) stimulation. // J.Biol.Chem. – 2004. – vol. 279, N 14. – P. 14201–14206.

Abe.R, Donnelly S.C., Peng T. et al. Peripheral blood fibrocytes: differentiation pathway and migration to wound sites. // J. Immunol. – 2001. – vol. 166, N 12. – P. 7556–7562

Abercrombie M. Fibroblasts. // J.Clin.Pathol. – 1978. – vol. 31, Suppl. 12. – P. 1–6.

Aberdam D., Virolle T., Simon-Assman P. Transcriptional regulation of laminin gene expression. // Microsc.Res.Tech. – 2000. – vol. 51, N 3. – P. 228–237.

Åberg T., Rice R., Rice D. et al. Chondrogenic potential of mouse calvarial mesenchyme. // J.Histochem.Cytochem. – 2005. – vol. 53, N 5. – P. 653–663

Abramov M.G. and A.I. Vorobiev. Bone marrow, cell types. [in Russian] // In: A textbook of hematology, edited by A.I.Vorobiev. vol.1, Moscow: Newdiamed, 2002. P. 47–53.

Abu-Lail N.I., Ohashi T., Clark R.L. et al. Understanding the elasticity of fibronectin fibrils: unfolding strengths of FN-III and GFP domains measured by single molecule force spectroscopy. // – Matrix Biol 2006. – vol. 25, N 1. – P. 175–184.

Abzhanov A., Rodda S.J., McMahon A.P., Tabin C.J. Regulation of skeletogenic differentiation in cranial dermal bone. // Development. – 2007. – vol. 134. – P. 3133–3144.

Adams C.S., Shapiro I.M. Mechanisms by which extracellular matrix components induce osteoblast apoptosis. // Connect.Tissue Res. – 2003. – vol. 44, Suppl.1. – P. 230–239.

Adams J.C., Lawler J. The thrombospondins. // Int.J.Biochem.Cell Biol. – 2004. – vol. 36, N 6. – P. 961–968

Adams S.L., Cohen A.J., Lassova L. Integration of signaling pathways regulating chondrocyte differentiation during endochondral bone formation. // J.Cell.Physiol. – 2007. – vol. 213, N 3. – P. 635–641.

Addison W.N., Nakano Y., Loisel T. et al. MEPE-ASARM peptides control extracellular matrix mineralization by binding to hydroxyapatite: an inhibition regulated be PHEX cleavage of ASARM. // J.Bone Miner.Res. – 2008. – vol. 23, N 10. – P. 1638–1649.

Adewumi O., Aflatoonian B., Ahrlunf-Richter L. et al. Characterization of human embryonic stem cell lines by the International Stem Cell Initiative. // Nat.Biotechnol. – 2007. – vol. 25, N 7. – P. 803.

Afanasiev Yu.I. and E.D.Kolodeznikova. Brown adipose tissue. – Irkutsk: Irkutsk University Publishing, 1995. 184 pages [in Russian].

Afanasiev Yu.I. and N.P.Omelyanenko. Connective tissues. [in Russian] // In: A textbook of histology, vol.1., edited by R.K. Danilov and V.L. Bykov. St. Petersburg: SpecLit Publishing, 2001. P. 249–284.

Afzal F., Pratap J., Ito K. et al. Smad function and intranuclear targeting share a Runx2 motif required for osteogenic lineage induction and BMP2 responsive transcription. // J.Cell.Physiol. – 2005. – vol. 204. – P. 65–72.

Agarwal S.K., Lee D.M., Kiener H.P., Brenner M.B. Coexpression of two mesenchymal cadherins, cadheriN 11 and N-cadherin, on muribe fibroblast-like synoviocytes. // Arthritis Rheum. – 2008. – vol. 58, N 4. – P. 10444–10454.

Aigner T., Soeder S., Haag J. IL-1β and BMPs – interactive players of cartilage matrix degradation and regeneration. // Eur.Cells Mater. – 2006. – vol. 12, N 1. – P. 49–56.

Akiyama H., Chaboissier M.C., Martin J.F. et al. The transcription factor Sox9 has essential roles in successive steps of the chondrocyte differentiation pathway and is required for expression of Sox5 and Sox6. // Genes Dev. – 2002. – vol. 16, N 21. – P. 2813–2828.

Akiyama H., Kim J.E., Nakashima K. et al. Osteo-chondroprogenitor cells are derived from Sox9 expressing precursors. // Proc.Natl. Acad.Sci.USA. – 2005. – vol. 102, N 41. – P. 14556–14570.

Akiyama H., Lyons J.P., Mori-Akiyama Y. et al. Interaction between Sox9 and β-catenin control chondrocyte differentiation. // Genes Dev. – 2004. – vol. 19. – P. 1072–1087

Akiyama H., Stadler H.S., Martin J.F. et al. Misexpression of Sox9 in mouse limb bud mesenchyme induces polydactily and rescues hypodactily mice. // Matrix Biol. – 2007. – vol. 26, N 4. – P. 224–233.

Akmal M., Singh A., Anand A. et al. The effects of hyaluronic acid on articular chondrocytes. // J.Bone Joint Surg. – 2005. – vol. 98-B, N 8. – P. 1143–1149.

Akter R., Rivas D., Geneau G. et al. Effect of lamin A/C knockdown on osteoblast differentiation and function. // J.Bone Miner.Res. – 2008. – Epub. Oct. 10.

Akune T., Ohba S., Kamekura S. et al. PPARγ insufficiency enhances osteogenesis through osteoblast formation formation from bone marrow progenitors. // J.Clin.Invest. – 2004. – vol. 113. – P. 846–855.

Akutsu N., Milbury C. M., Burgeson R. E., Nishiyama T. Effect of type XII or XIV collagen NC-3 domain on the human dermal fibroblast migration into reconstituted collagen gel. // Exp. Dermatol. – 1999. – vol. 8, N 1. – P. 17–21.

Alan T., Tufan A.C. C-type natriuretic peptide regulation of limb mesenchymal chondrogenesis is accompanied by altered N-cadherin and collagen type X-related functions. // J.Cell.Biochem. – 2008. – vol. 105. – P. 227–235.

Alappat S., Zhang Z.Y., Chen Y.P. Msx homeobox gene family and craniofacial development. // Cell Res. – 2003. – vol. 13, N 6. – P. 429–442.

Alford A.I., Hankenson K.G. Matricellular proteins: extracellular modulators of bone development, remodeling, and regeneration. // Bone. – 2006. – vol. 38. – P. 749–757.

Ali S.A., Zaidi S.K., Dacwag C.S. et al. Phenotypic transcription factors epigenetically mediate cell growth control. // Proc.Natl.Acad.Sci. USA. – 2008. – vol. 105, N 18. – P. 6632–6637

Alini M., Roughley P.J. Changes in leucine-rich repeat proteoiglycans during maturation of the bovine growth plate. // Matrix Biol. – 2001. – vol. 19, N 8. – P. 805–813.

Allen J.M., Bateman J.F., Hansen U. et al. WARP is a novel multimeric component of the hondrocyte pericellular matrix that interacts with perlecan. // J.Biol.Chem. – 2006. – vol. 281, N 11. – P. 7341–7349.

Allison S.J., Baldock P.A., Herzog H. The control of bone remodeling by neuropeptide Y receptors. // Peptides. – 2007. – vol. 28. – P. 320–325.

Amano K., Ichida F., Sugita A. et al. MSX2 stimulates chondrocyte maturation by controlling Ihh expression. // J.Biol.Chem. – 2008. – vol. 283, N 43. –P. 29513–29521.

Amarillo R., Viukov S.V., Sharir A. et al. HIF1α regulation of Sox9 is necessary to maintain differentiation of hypoxic prechondrogenic cells during early skeletogenesis. // Development. – 2007. – vol. 134. – P. 3917–3928.

Amatangelo M.D., Bassi D.E., Klein-Szanto A.J.P., Cukierman E. Stroma-derived three-dimensional matrices are necessary and sufficient to promote desmoplastic differentiation of normal fibroblasts. // Am.J.Pathol. – 2005. – vol. 167, N 2. – P. 475–488.

Ambrosetti D., Holmes G., Mansukhani A., Basilico C. Fibroblast growth factor signaling uses multiple mechanisms to inhibit Wnt-induced transcription in osteoblasts. // Mol.Cell.Biochem. – 2008. – vol. 28, N 15. – P. 4759–4791.

Ameye L., Young M.E. Mice deficient in small leucine-rich proteoglycans: novel in vivo models for osteoporosis, osteoarthrosis, Ehlers-Danlos syndrome, muscular dystrophy, and corneal diseases // Glycobiology. – 2002. – vol. 12. – P. 107R–116R.

Anderson D.M., Arredondo J., Hahn K. et al. Mohawk is a novel homeobox gene expressed in the developing mouse embryo. // Dev.Dyn. – 2006. – vol. 235. – P. 792–801.

Anderson H.C., Garimella R., Tague S.E. The role of matrix vesicles in growth plate development and biomineralization. // Front.Biosci. – 2005. – vol. 10. – P. 822–837.

Anderson O., Reissmann E., Ibáñez C.F. Growth differentiation factor 11 signals through the transforming growth factor-β receptor ALK5 to regionalize the anterior-posterior axis. // EMBO Reports. – 2006. – vol. 7, N 5. – P. 831–837.

Anderson P.H., Atkins G.J. The skeleton as an intracrine organ for vitamin D metabolism. // Mol.Aspects Med. – 2008. – vol. 29, N 6. – P. 397–406.

Andrade A.C., Nilsson O., Barnes K.M., Baron M. Wnt gene expression in the post-natal growth plate: regulation with chondrocyte differentiation. // Bonr. – 2007. – vol. 40, N 5. – P. 1361–1369.

Anilkumar N., Annis D., Mosher D.F., Adams J.C. Trimeric assembly of the C-terminal region of thrombospondin-1 or thrombospondin-2 is necessary for cell spreading and fascin spike organisation. // J. Cell Sci. – 2002. – vol. 115. – P. 2357–2366.

Anokhin P.K. Sketches on physiology of functional systems. [in Russian] –Moscow: Medicine, 1975. 448 pages.

Antonicelli F., Bellon G., Debelle L., Hornebeck W. Elastin-elastase and inflamm-aging. // Curr.Top.Dev.Biol. – 2007. – vol. 79. – P. 99–155.

Aouacheria A., Cluzel C., Lethias C. Invertebrate data predict an early emergence of vertebrate fibrillar collagen clades and an anti-incest model. // J.Biol.Chem. – 2004. – vol. 279, N 46. – P. 47711–47719.

Appleton C.T.G., James C.G., Beier F. Regulator of G-protein signaling (RGS) proteins differentially control chondrocyte differentiation. // J.Cell.Physiol.– 2006. – vol. 207, N 3. – P. 735–745.

Archer C.W., Francis-West P. The chondrocyte. // Int.J.Biochem.Cell. Biol. – 2003. – vol. 35, N 4. – P. 401–404.

Argraves W.S. Greene L.M., Cooley M.A., Gallagher W.M. Fibulins: physiological and disease perspectives. // EMBO Rep. – 2003. – vol. 4, N 12. – P. 1127–1131.

Ariyan S., Enriquez R., Krizek T.J. Wound contraction and fibrocontractive disorders. // Arch. Surg. – 1978. – vol. 113. – P. 1034–1046.

Arlein W.J., Shearer J.D., Caldwel MD. Continuity between wound macrophage and fibroblast phenotype: analysis of wound fibroblast phagocytosis. // Am. J. Physiol. – 1998. – vol. 275, N 4, pt.2. – P. R1041–R1048.

Armstrong P.B., Armstrong M.T. Intercellular invasion and the organizational stability of tissues: a role for fibronectin. // Biochim.biophys.Acta.– 2000. – vol. 1470, N 2. – P. 9–20.

Arnesen S.M., Lawson M.A. Age-related changes in focal adhesions lead to altered cell behavior in tendon fibroblasts. // Mech.Aging Dev. – 2006. – vol. 127, N 9. – P. 726–732.

Arnold M.A., Kim Y., Czubryt M.P. et al. MEF2C transcription factor controls chondrocyte hypertrophy and bone development. // Dev.Cell. – 2007. – vol. 12. – P. 377–389.

Arnott J.A., Nuglozeh E., Rico M.C. et al. Connective tissue growth factor (CTGF/CCN2) is a downstream mediator for TGF-beta-induced extracellular matrix production in osteoblasts. // J.Cell.Physiol. – 2007. – vol. 210, N 3. – P. 843–852.

Asanbaeva A., Masuda K., Thonar E.J. et al. Regulation of immature cartilage growth by IGF-1, TGF-beta1, BMP-7, and pdgf-AB: role of metabp;oc balance between fixed charge and collagen network. // Biomech.Model.Mechanobiol. – 2007. – Epub Aug. 28.

Asano Y., Ihn H., Yamane K. et al. Increased expression of integrin αvβ5 induces the myofibroblastic differentiation of dermal fibroblasts. // Am.J.Pathol. – 2006. – vol. 168, N 2. P. 499–510.

Ashworth J.L., Murphy G., Rock M. et al. Fibrillin degradation by matrix metalloproteinases: implications for connective tissue remodeling. // Biochem.J. – 1999. – vol. 340. – P. 171–181.

Asou Y., Nifuji A., Tsuji K. et al. Coordinated expression of scleraxis and Sox9 genes during embryonic development of tendon and cartilage. // J.Orthop.Res. – 2002. – vol. 20, N 4. – P. 827–833.

Aszódi A., Bateman J.E., Gustafson E. et al. Mammalian skeletogenesis and extracellular matrix: what can we learn from kockout mice? // Cells Structure Function. – 2000. –vol.25.

Aszodi A., Hunziker E.B., Brakebusch C., Fässler R. β1 integrins regulate chondrocyte rotation, G1 progression, and cytokinesis. // Genes Dev. – 2003. – vol. 17. – P. 2465–2479.

Ateshian G.A. The role of interstitial fluid pressurization in articular cartilage lubrication. // J.Biomech. – 2009. – vol. 42, N 9. – P. 1163–1170.

Aulehla A., Pourquié O. Oscillating signaling pathways during embryonic development. // Curr.Opin.Cell Biol. – 2008. – vol. 20. – P. 1–6.

Ayad M., Marriott A., Morgan K., Grant M. Bovine cartilage types VI and Ix collagens. Characterization of their forms in vivo. // Biochem.J. – 1989. – vol. 262. – P. 753–761.

Azizan A., Gaw J.U., Govindra P. et al. Chondromodulin I and pleiotrophin gene expression in bovine cartilage and epiphysis. // Matrix Biol. – 2000. – vol. 19, N 6. – P. 521–531.

Babaie Y., Herwig R., Greber B. et al. Analysis of Oct4-dependent transcriptional network regulating self-renewal and pluripotency in human embryonic stem cells. // Stem Cells. – 2007. – vol. 25, N 2. – P. 500–510.

Bachelet I, Levi-Schaffer F, Mekori YA. Mast cells: not only in allergy. // Immunol Allergy Clin North Am. – 2006. Vol. 26, N 3. – P. 407–425.

Baek M.Y., Lee M.A., Jung J.W. et al. Positive regulation of adult bone formation by osteoblast-specific transcription factor Osteric. // J.Bone Miner.Res. – 2009. – vol. 24, N 6. – P. 1055–1065

Bahamonde M.E., Lyons K.M. BMP3: to be or not to be a BMP. // J.Bone Joint Surg. – 2001. – vol. 83-A, Suppl. 1, part 1. – P. S56–S62.

Bai P., Houton S.M., Huber A. et al. Peroxisome proliferators activated receptor (PPAR)-2 controls adipocyte differentiation and adipose tissue function through the regulation of the activity of the retinoid X receptor/PPARγ heterodimer. // J.Biol.Chem. – 2007. – vol. 282, N 52. – P. 37738–37746

Bai X., Xiao Z., Pan Y. et al. Cartilage-derived morphogenetic protein-1 promotes the differentiation of mesenchymal stem cells into chondrocytes. // Biochem.Biophys.Res.Commun. – 2004. – vol. 325. – P. 453–460

Bailey A.J., Knott L. Molecular changes in bone collagen in osteoporosis and osteoarthritis in the elderly. // Exp.Gerontol. – 1999. – vol. 34, N 3. – P. 337–351.

Bais M.V., Wigner N., Young M. et al. BMP2 is essential for post natal osteogenesis but not for recruitment of osteogenic stem cells. // Bone. – 2009. – vol. 45, N 2. – P. 254–266.

Baker A.H., Edwards D.R., Murphy G. Metalloproteinase inhibitors: biological actions and therapeutic opportunities. // J.Cell Sci. – 2002. – vol. 115. – P. 3719–3727.

Baker R.E., Schnell S., Maini P.K. A clock and wavefront mechanism for somite formation. // Dev.Biol. – 2006. – vol. 293. – P. 116–126.

Baldock C., Koster A.J., Ziese U. et al. The supramolecular organization of fibrillin-rich microfibrils. // Micron. – 2001. – vol. 152, N 5. – P. 1045–1056.

Balint E., Lapointe D., Drissi H. et al. Phenotype discovery by gene expression profiling: mapping of biological processes linked to BMP02-mediated osteoblast differentiation. // J.Cell.Biochem. – 2003. – vol. 89, N 2. – P. 401–426.

Balogh K., Rácz K., Patócs A., Hunyady L. Menin and its interacting proteins: elucidation of menin function. // Trends Endocr.Metab. – 2006. – vol. 17, N 9. – P. 357–364.

Bandyopadhyay A., Tsuji K., Cox K. et al. Genetic analysis of the roles of BMP2, BMP4, and BMP7 in limb patterning and skeletogenesis. // PLoS Genet – 2006. – vol. 2, N 12. – P. e216.

Baneyx G., Baugh L., Vogel V. Fubronectin extending and unfolding within cell matrix fibrils controlled by cytoskeletal tension. // Proc. Natl.Acad.Sci.USA. – 2002. Vol. 99, N 8. – P. 5139–5143.

Barbero A., Ploegert S., Heberer M., Martin I. Plasticity of clonal populations of dedifferentiated adult human articular chondrocytes. // Arthritis Rheumat. – 2003. – vol. 48, N 5. – P. 1315–1325.

Barker T.H., Framson P., Puolakkainen P.A. et al. Hevin suppresses inflammation, but hevin and SPARC together diminish angiogenesis. // Amer. J.Pathol. – 2005. – vol. 166, N 3. – P. 923–933.

Barnard J.C., Williams A.J., Rabier B. et al. Thyroid hormone regulate fibroblast growth factor receptor signaling during chondrogenesis. // Endocrinolgy. – 2006. – vol. 146, N 12. – P. 5568–5580.

Baron R., Rawadi G., Roman-Roman S. Wnt signaling: a key regulator of bone mass. // Curr.Top.Devel.Biol. – 2006. – vol. 76. – P. 103–127.

Bartschere K., Boutros M. Regulation of Wnt protein secretion and its role in gradient formation. // EMBO Rep. – 2008. – Epub. Sept.12.

Basbaum C.B., Werb Z. Focalized proteolysis: spatial and temporal regulation of extracellular matrix degradation at the cell surface. // Curr.Opin.Cell Biol. – 1996. – vol. 8, N 5. – P. 731–738.

Bastiaansen-Jenniskens Y.M., Koevoet W., Jansen K.M. et al. Inhibition of glycosaminoglycan incorporation influenced collagen network formation during cartilage matrix production. // Biochem.Biophys.Res.Commun. – 2009. – vol. 379. N 2. – P. 222–225.

Bastow E.R., Byers S., Golub S.B. et al. Hyaluronan synthesis and degradation in cartilage and bone. // Cell.Mol.life Sci. – 2007. – Epub.

Bauman V.K. Biochemistry and physiology of vitamin D. [in Russian] Riga: Zinante, 1989. 480 pages.

Beck G.R.jr., Zerler B., Moran E. Gene arrow analysis of osteoblast differentiation. // Cell Growth Differ. – 2001. – vol. 12. – P. 61–83.

Behnam K., Murray S.S., Brochmann B.J. BMP stimulation of alkaline phosphatase activity in pluripotent mouse C2C12 cells is inhibited by dermatopontin, one of the most abundant low molecular weight protein in deminrtalized bone matrix. // Conn.Tissue Res. – 2006. – vol. 47, N 5. – P. 271–277.

Belkin A.M., Stepp M.A. Integrins as receptor for laminin. // Microsc. Res.Tech. – 2000. – vol. 51, N 3. – P. 280–301.

Bellini A., Mattoli S. The role of the fibrocyte, a bone marrow-derived mesenchymal progenitor, in reactive and reparative diseases. // Lab.Invest. – 2007. – vol. 67, N 9. – P. 858–870.

Belousov Yu.B., Shishkin A.V. and E.P. Panchenko. Fibronectin and its clinical significance. [in Russian] // Cardiology. 1987. vol. 27, no. 1. – P. 100–104.

Bely V.A., Kupchinov B.I., Rodionov V.G. et al. Investigation of the synovial fluid's lubricating ability. [in Russian] // Friction and Wear, 1984, N 6. P. 983–987.

Bendall A.J., Hu G., Levi G., Abate-Shen C. Dlx5 regulate differentiation at multiple stages. // Int.J.Dev.Biol. – 2003. –vol. 47. – P. 335–344.

Bengtsson E., Mörgelin M., Sasaki T. et al. The leucine-rich repeat protein PRELP binds perlecan and collagens and may function as a basement membrane anchor. // J.Biol.Chem. – 2002. – vol. 277, N 17. – P. 15061–15068.

Benjamin M., Kaiser E., Milz S. Structure-function relationship in tendons: a review. // J.Anat. – 2008. – vol. 212, N 3. – P. 211–228.

Bennett C.N., Longo K.A., Wright W.S. et al. Regulation of osteoblastogenesis and bone mass by Wnt10b. // Proc.Natl.Acad.Sci.USA. – 2005. – vol. 102, N 9. – P. 3324–3329.

Berg D.ten, Brugmann S.A., Helms J.A., Nusse R. Wnt and FGF signals interact to coordinate growth with cell fate specification during limb development. // Development. – 2008. – vol. 135. – P. 3247–3257.

Berman A.E., Kozlova N.I. and Morozevich P.E. Integrins: structure and signals. [in Russian] // Biochemistry, 2003, vol. 68, N 12. P. 1284–1289.

Berman S.D., Tuan T.L., Miller E.S. et al. The retinoblastoma protein tumor suppressor is important for appropriate osteoblast differentiation and bone development. // Mol.Cancer Res. – 2008. – vol. 6, N 9. – P. 1440–1451.

Bernstein A.M., Twining S.S., Warejcka D.J. et al. Urokinase receptor cleavage: a critical step in fibroblast-to-myofibroblast differentiation. // Mol.Biol.Cell. – 2007. – vol. 18. – P. 2718–2727,

Berrier A.L., Yamada K.M. Cell-matrix adhesion. // J.Cell.Physiol. – 2007. – vol. 213. – P. 565–573

Bessa P.C., Casal M., Reis R.L. Bone morphogenetic proteins in tissue engineering: the road from the laboratory to the clinic, part I (basic concepts). // J.Tissue Eng.Regen.Med. – 2008. – vol. 2. – P. 1–13.

Betekhtin A.G. A course in mineralogy: A study guide. [in Russian] / Scientific editing by B.I. Pirogov and B.B. Shakursky. Moscow: KDU, 2008. 736 pages.

Betrand S., Godoy M., Semal P., van Gansen P. Transdifferentiation of macrophges into fibroblasts as a result of Schistosoma mansoni infection. // Int. J. Dev. Biol. – 1992. – vol. 36. – P. 179–184.

Beurden H.E.van, von den Hoff J.W., Torensma R et al. Myofibroblasts in palatal wound healing: prospects for reduction of wound contraction after cleft palate repair. // J.Dent.Res. – 2005. – vol. 84, N 10. – P. 871–879.

Beurden HE, Snoek PA, Von den Hoff JW, Torensma R, Kuijpers-Jagtman AM. //Fibroblast subpopulations in intra-oral wound healing. Wound Repair Regen – 2003 – vol. 11 – P. 55–63.

Bevilacqua M.A., Iovino B., Zambrano N. et al. Fibromodulin gene transcription is induced by ultraviolet irradiation and its regulation is impaired in senescent fibroblasts. // J.Biol.Chem. – 2005. – vol. 280, N 36. – P. 31809–31817.

Bezooijen R.L.van, Roelen B.A.J., Visser A. et al. Sclerostin is an osteocyte-expressed negative regulator of bone formation, but not a classical BMP antagonist. // J.Exp.Med. – 2004. – vol. 199, N 6. – P. 805–814.

Bezooijen R.L.van, Svensson J.P., Eefting D. et al. Wnt but not BMP signaling is involved in the inhibitory action of sclerostin on BMP-stimulated bone formation. // J.Bone Miner.Res. – 2007. – vol. 22, N 1. – P. 19–28.

Bhowmick N.A., Chytil A., Plieth D. et al. TGF-beta signaling in fibroblasts modulates the oncogenic potential of adjacent epithelia. // Science. – 2004. – vol. 303. – P. 848–851.

Bialek P., Kern B., Yang X. et al. A twist code determines the onset of osteoblast differentiation. // Dev.Cell. – 2004. – vol. 6. – P. 423–435.

Bidwell J.P., Yang J., Robling A.G. Is HMGB1 an osteocyte alarmin? // J.Cell.Biochem. – 2008. – vol. 103, N 6. – P. 1671–1680.

Billiard J., Moran R.A., Whitley M.Z. et al. Transcriptional profiling of human osteoblast differentiation. // J.Cell.Biochem. – 2003. – vol. 89, N 2. – P. 389–400.

Birk D.E. Type V collagen: heterotypic I/V collagen interactions in the regulation of fibril assembly. // Micron. – 2001. – vol. 32, N 3. – P. 223–237.

Bischoff S.C. Role of mast cells in allergic and non-allergic immune responses: comparison of human and murine data. // Nat.Rev.Immunol. – 2007. – vol. 7, N 2. – P. 93–104.

Bjarnason R., Andersson B., Kim H.S. et al. Cartilage oligomeric matrix protein increases in serum after the start of growth hormone treatment in prepubertal children. // J.Clin.Endocrinol.Metab. – 2004. – vol. 89. – P. 5156–5160.

Blain E.J., Gilber S.J., Hayes A.J., Duance V.C. Disassembly of the vimentin cytoskeleton disrupts articular cartilage chondrocyte homeostasis. // Matrix Biol. – 2996. – vol. 25, N 7. – P. 398–408.

Blair H.C., Zaidi M., Schlesinger P.H. Mechanisms balancing skeletal matrix synthesis and degradation. // Biochem.J. – 2002. – vol. 364, N 2. – P. 329–341.

Blanchette-Mackie E.J., Scow R.O. Movement of lipolytic products to mitochondria in brown adipose tissue of young rats: An electron microscope study // J. Lipid Res. – 1983. – vol. 24. – P. 229.

Bland Y.S., Ashhurst D.E. Development and ageing of the rabbit knee joint: distribution of the fibrillar collagens. // Anat.Embryol. (Berl.). – 1996. – B.194, N 6. – S.507–619.

Bland Y.S., Ashhurst D.E. The hip joint: the fibrillar collagens associated with development and ageing in the rabbit. // J.Anat. – 2001. – vol. 198, N 1. – P. 17–27.

Blaney-Davidson E.N., Scharstuhl A., Vitters P.M. et al. Reduced transforming growth factor-beta signaling in cartilage of old mive: role in impaired repair capacity. // Arthritis Res.Ther. – 2005. – vol. R1338–R1347.

Blewis M.E., Schumacher B.L.S., Klein T.J. et al. Microenvironment regulation of PRG4 phenotype of chondrocytes. // J.Orthop.Res. – 2007. – vol. 25. – P. 685–695.

Blitzer J.T., Nusse R. A critical role for endocytosis in Wnt signaling. // BMC Cell Biol. – 2006. – vol. 7. – P. 28.

Blonder J., Xiao Z., Veenstra T.D. Protemic profiling of differentiating osteoblasts. // Expert Rev.Proteomics. – 2006. – vol. 3, N 5. – P. 483–496.

Bobick B.E., Kulyk W.M. Regulation of cartilage formation and maturation by mitogen-activated protein kinase signaling. // Birth Defects Res. C. Embryo Today. – 2008. – vol. 84, N 2. – P. 131–154.

Bobick B.K., Thornhill T.M., Kulyk W.M. Fibroblast growth factors 2, 4, and 8 exert both positive and negative effects on limb, frontonasal, and nasal chondrogenesis via MEK-ERK activation. // J.Cell. Physiol. – 2007. – vol. 211, N 1. – P. 233–243.

Boden S.D., Liu Y., Hair G.A. et al. LMP-1, a LIM-domain protein, mediates BMP-6 effects on bone formation. // Endocrinology. – 1999. – vol. 139. – P. 5125–5134.

Bodine P.V.N. Wnt signaling control bone apoptosis. // Cell Res. – 2008. – vol. 18. – P. 248–253.

Bodine P.V.N., Komm B.S. Wnt signaling and osteoblastogenesis. // Rev.Endocr.Metab.Disord. – 2006. vol.7. – P. 733–739.

Boeuf S., Steck E., Pelttari K. et al. Subtractive gene exession profiling of articular cartilage and mesenchymal stem cells: serpins as cartilage-relevant differentiation markers. // Osteoarthritis cartilage. – 2008. – vol. 16, N 1. – P. 41–60.

Bogonatov B.N. and N.G. Gonchar-Zaikina. A system of bone canals as a base for bone angioarchitectonics. [in Russian] // AHE Archives, 1976, vol. 70, N 4. P. 53–60.

Bookkoff D. Adipocyte developmet and the loss of erythropoietic capacity in the bone marrow of mice after sustaine hypertransfusion. // Blood. 1982. N 60. P. 1337–1344.

Bökel C., Brown N.H. Integrins in development: moving on, responding to, and sticking to the extracellular matrix. // Dev.Cell – 2002. – vol. 3. – P. 311–321.

Bondos S. Variations on a theme: Hox and Wnt combinatorial regulation during animal development. // Science STKE. – 2006. – 355. – pe38.

Bondos S.E., Tan X.X., Matthews C.S. Physical and genetic interactions link Hox function with diverse transcription factors and cell signaling proteins. // Mol.Cell.Proteomics. – 2006. – vol. 5. – P. 824–834.

Bonewald L.F. Mechanosensation and transduction in osteocytes. // Bonekey Osteovision. – 2006. – vol. 3, N 10. – P. 7–15.

Bonnelye E., Aubin J.E. Estrogen receptor-related receptor α: a mediator of estrogen response in bone. // J.Clin.Endocrinol.Metab. – 2005. – vol. 90, N 5. – P. 3115–3121.

Boot-Handford R.P., Tuckwell D.S., Plumb D.A. et al. A novel and highly conserved collagen (proα1(XXVII)) with a unique expression pattern and unusual molecular characteristics establishes a new clade within the vertebrate fibrillar collagen family: // J.Biol. Chem. – 2003. – vol. 278, N 33. – P. 31067–31077.

Borasky R. Amino acids distribution profiles of collagen fibrils. // J. Amer. Leather chem. Ass., 1967. – vol. 62. – P. 768–780.

Bord S., Ireland D.C., Moffatt P. et al. Characterization of osteocrin expression in human bone. // J.Histochem.Cytochem. – 2005. – vol. 53, N 10. – P. 1181–1187.

Boregowda R., Paul E., White J., Ritty T.M. Bone and soft connective tissue alterations result from loss of fibrillin-2 expression. // Matrix Biol. – 2008. – vol. 27, N 8. – P. 661–666.

Bornstein P. The NH2-terminal propeptides of fibrillar collagens: highly conserved domains with poorly understood functions. // Matrix Biol. – 2002. – vol. 19. N 7. – P. 247–258.

Bornstein P., Sage E.H. Matricellular proteins: extracellular modulators of cell function. // Curr.Opin.Cell Biol. – 2002. – vol. 14, N 5. – P. 608–616

Bornstein P., Sage E.H. Thrombospondins. // In: Methods in Enzymology. Vol. 245. Academic Press Inc. – 1994. – P. 62–85.

Borradori L., Sonnenberg A. Structure and function of hemidesmosomes: more than simple adhesion complexes. // J.Invest. Dermatol. – 1999. – vol. 112, N 3. – P. 411–418.

Borsi L., Castellani P., Risso A.M. et al. Transforming growth factor-beta regulates the splicing pattern of fibronectin messenger RNA precursor. // FEBS Lett. – 1990. – vol. 261. – P. 175–178.

Bos K.J., Holmes D.F., Kadler K.E. et al. Axial structures of the heterotypic collagen fibrils of vitreous humour and cartilage. // J.Mol.Biol. – 2001. – vol. 306, N 5. – P. 1011–1022.

Bos T.van den, Speijer D., Bank R.A. et al. Differences in matrix composition between calvaria and long bone in mice suggest differences in biomechanical properties and resorption. Special emphasis on collagen. // Bone. – 2008. – vol. 43, N 3. – P. 459–468.

Boskey A.L. Amorphous calcium phosphate: the contention of bone. // J.Dental Res. – 1997. – vol. 76, N 8. – P. 1433–1436.

Boskey A.L. Mineral-matrix interactions in bone and cartilage. // Clin.Orthop. – 1992. – vol. 281. – P. 244–274.

Boskey A.L., Raggio C.L., Bullough P.G., Kinnett J.G. Changes in the bone tissue lipids in persons with steroid and alcohol-induced osteonecrosis. // Clin.Orthop. Rel.Res. – 1983. – vol. 172. – P. 289–295.

Boskey A.L., Young M.F., Kilts T., Verdelis K. Variations in mineral properties in normal and mutant bones and teeth. // Cells Tissues Organs. – 2005. – vol. 181. – P. 144–163.

Böttcher R.E., Niehrs C. Fibroblast growth factor signalling during early vertebrate development. // Endocrin.Rev. – 2005. – vol. 26, N 1. – P. 63–77.

Boyan B.D., Dean D.D., Sylvia V.L., Schwartz Z. Steroid hormone action in musculoskeletal cells involves membrane receptor and nuclear receptor mechanism. // Connect.Tissue Res. – 2003. – vol. 44, Suppl. 1. – P. 30–35.

Boyce B.F., Hughes D.E., Wright K.B. et al. Recent advances in bone biology provide insight into the pathogenesis of bone diseases. // Lab.Invest. – 1999. – vol. 79, N 2. – P. 83–94.

Boyce B.F., Xing L. Functions of RANK/RANKL/OPG in bone modeling and remodeling. // Arch.Biochem.Biophys. – 2008. – vol. 473, N 2. – P. 139–146.

Boyce B.F., Yamashita T., Yao Z. et al. Roles of NF-κB and c-Fos in osteoclasts. // J.Bone Miner.Metab. – 2005. – vol. 23, Suppl. – P. 11–15.

Boyle W.J., Simonet W.S., Lacey D.R. Osteoclast differentiation and regulation. // Nature. – 2003. – vol. 423. – P. 337–442.

Bradley E.W., Ruan M.M., Ourales M. PAK1 is a novel MEK-independent raf target controlling expression of the IAP survivin in M-CSF-mediated osteoclast survival. // J.Cell.Physiol. – 2008. – vol. 217, N 3. – P. 752–758.

Bradshaw A.D., Puolakkainen P., Dasgupta J. et al. SPARC-null mice display abnormalities in the dermis characterized by decreased collagen fibril diameter and reduced tensile strength. // J.Invest. Dermatol. – 2003. – vol. 120, N 6. – P. 949–955.

Brakebusch C., Fässler R. The integrin-actin connection, an eternal love affair. // EMBO J. – 2003. – vol. 22, N 10. – P. 2224–2233.

Brasaemle D.L. The perilipin family of structural lipid droplet proteins: stabilization of lipid droplets and control of lipolysis. // J.Lipid Res. – 2007. – vol. 48. – P. 2547–2559.

Brasaemle D.L., Dolios G., Shapiro L., Wang H. Proteomic analysis of proteins associated with lipid droplets of basal and lipolytically stimulated 3T3-L1 adipocytes. // J.Biol.Chem. – 2004. – vol. 279. N 45. – P. 46835–46842.

Braun-Falco O., Rupec M. Some observation on dermal collagen fibrils in ultra-thin section. // J. Invest. Derm. – 1964. – vol. 42. – № 1.– P. 15–19.

Brazier H., Pawlak G., Vivas V., Blangy A. The Rho GTPase Wrch1 regulates osteoclast precursor adhesion and migration. // Int.J.Biochem.Cell.Biol. – 2009. – vol. 41, N 6. – P. 1391–1401.

Bredesen D.E., Mehlen P., Rabizadeh S. Apoptosis and dependence receptors: a molecular basis for cellular addiction. // Physiol.Rev. – 2004. – vol. 84, N 2. – P. 411–430.

Brekken R.A., Puolakkainen P., Graves D.C. et al. Enhanced growth of tumors in SPARC-null mice is associated with changes in the ECM. // J.Clin. Invest. – 2003. – vol. 111, N 4. – P. 487–495.

Brekken R.A., Sage E.H. SPARC, a matricellular protein at the crossroads of cell-matrix. // Matrix Biol. – 2000. – vol. 19, N 7. – P. 569–580.

Brenner S., Horne R.W. A negative staining method for high resolution electron microscopy of viruses // Biochim. Biophys. Acta.– 1959. – vol. 34. – P. 103–110.

Brent A.E., Schweitzer R., Tabin C.J. A somatic compartment of tendon progenitors. // Cell. – 2003. – vol. 113, N 2. – P. 235–248.

Bronsky J., Prusa R., Nevoral J. The role of amylin and related peptides in osteoporosis. // Clin.Chim.Acta. – 2006. – vol. 373, N 1–2. – P. 9–16.

Bronson R.E., Argenta J.G., Siebert E.P., Bertolami C.N. (1988). Distinctive fibroblastic subpopulations in skin and oral mucosa demonstrated by differences in glycosaminoglycan content. // In Vitro Cell Dev. Biol. – 1988. – V 24. – P. 1121–1126.

Bruckner P., Rest M.van der. Structure and function of cartilage collagens. // Microsc.Res.Technic. – 1994. – vol. 28, N 3. – P. 378–384.

Bubnoff A.von, Cho K.W.Y. Intracellular BMP signalling regulation in vertebrates: pathway or network. // Devel.Biol. – 2001. – vol. 239, N 1. – P. 1–14.

Bucala R., Spiegel L.A., Chesney J. et al. Circulating fibrocytes define a new leukocyte subpopulation that mediates tissue repair. // Mol. Med. – 1994. – vol. 1. – P. 71–81

Buckwalter J.A., Glimcher M.J., Cooper R.B., Recker R. Bone biology. Part I: Structure, blood supply, cells, matrix, and mineralization. // J.Bone Joint Surg. – 1995. – vol. 77-A. – P. 1256–1289.

Budde B., Blumbach K., Ylöstalo J. et al. Altered integration of matrilin-3 into cartilage extracellular matrix in the absence ofcollagen IX. // Mol.Cell.Biol. – 2005. – vol. 25, N 23. – P. 10465–10478.

Burdan F., Szumilo J., Korobowicz A. et al. Morphology and physiology of the epiphysial growth plate. // Folia Histochem.Cytobiol. – 2009. – vol. 47, N 1. – P. 5–16.

Burgeson R.E. Type VII collagen. // Structure and function of collagen types (Mayne R, Burgeson R.E., eds.) Orlando e.a.: Academic Press. – 1987. – P. 145–172.

Burgeson R.E., Nimni M.E. Collagen types. Molecular structure and tissue distribution. // Clin.Orthop. – 1992. – vol. 282. – P. 250–272.

Burridge K., Chrzanowska-Wodnicka M. Focal adhesions, contractility, and signaling. Annu. Rev. Cell Dev. Biol. – 1996. – vol. 12. – P. 463–518.

Bursell L., Woods A., James C.G. et al. Src kinase inhibition promotes the chondrocyte phenotype. // Arthritis Res.Ther. – 2007. – vol. 9. – P. R105.

Busser B.W., Bulyk M.L., Michelson A.M. Toward a systems level understanding of developmental regulating networks. // Curr.Opin. Genet.Dev. – 2008. – Epub. Oct. 8.

Byers P.H. Collagens: building blocks at the end of the developmental line. // Clin.Genet. – 2000. – vol. 58, N 2. – P. 270–278.

Byers s., Rooden J.C.van, Foster B.K. Structural changes in the large proteoglycan, aggrecan, in different zones of the ovine growth plate. // Calcif.Tiisue Int. – 1997. – vol. 60, N 1. – P. 71–78.

Calderwood D.A. Integrin activation. // J.Cell Sci. – 2004. – vol. 117, N 5. – P. 657–686.

Cameron T.L., Belluccio D., Farlie P.C. et al. Global comparative transcriptome analysis of cartilage formation in vivo. // BMC Dev. Biol. – 2009. – vol. 9. – P. 20.

Caminos J.E., Gualillo O., Lago F. et al. The endogenous growth hormone secretagogue (Ghrelin) is synthesized and secreted by chondrocytes. // Endocrinology. – 2005. – vol. 146. – P. 1285–1292.

Canalis E. Mechanism of glucocorticoid action in bone. // Curr.Osteoporosis Rep. – 2005. – vol. 3, N 3. – P. 98–102.

Canalis E., Deregowski V., Pereira R.C., Gazzerro E. Signals that determine the fate of osteoblastic cells. // J.Endocrinol.Invest. – 2005. – vol. 28, Suppl. – P. 3–78.

Canalis E., Economides A., Gazzerro E. Bone morphogenetic proteins, their antagonists, and the skeleton. // Endocrin.Rev. – 2003. – vol. 24. – №2. – P. 218–235.

Candé C., Cecconi F., Dessen P., Kroemer G. Apoptosis-inducing factor (AIF): key to the conserved caspase-independent pathway of cell death. // J.Cell Sci. – 2002. – vol. 115. – P. 4727–4734.

Cannon B., Nedelgaard J. Brown adipose tissue: function and physiological significance. // Physiol.Rev. – 2004. – vol. 84. – P. 277–359.

Canty E.G., Kadler K.E. Procollagen trafficking, processing and fibrillogenesis. // J.Cell.Sci. – 2005. – vol. 118. – P. 1341–1353.

Capellini T.D., Di Giacomo G., Salsi V. et al. Pbx1/Pbx2 requirement for distal limb patterning is mediated by the hierarchical control of Hox gene spatial distribution and Shh expression. // Development. – 2006. – vol. 133. – P. 2263–2273.

Caplan A.I. Mesenchymal stem cells: cell-based reconstructive therapy in orthopedics. // Tissue Eng. – 2005. – vol. 11, N 7–8. – P. 1198–1211.

Caplan A.I., Dennis J.E. Mesenchymal stem cells as trophic mediators. // J Cell Biochem. – 2006. – vol. 98, N 5. – P. 1076–1084.

Cardoso L., Herman B.C., Verborgt O. et al. Osteocyte apoptosis controls activation of intracortical resorption in response to bone fatigue. // J.Bone Miner.Res. 2009. Vol. 24, P. 597–605.

Carmichael G.G., Fullmer H.M. The fine structure of the oxytalan fiber // J. Cell Biol. – 1966. Vol. 28. – P. 33–36.

Cartwright M.J., Tchkonia T., Kirkland J.L. Aging in adipocytes: potential impact of inherent, depot-specific mechanisms. // Exp.Gerontol. – 2007. – vol. 42, N 6. – P. 463–471.

Carvalho H.F., Felisbino S.L., Keene D.R., Vogel K.G. Identification, content, and distribution of type VI collagen in bovine tendons. // Cell Tissue Res. – 2006. – vol. 325, N 2. – P. 315–324.

Case N., Ma M., Sen B. et al. Beta-catenin levels influence rapid mechanical response in osteoblasts. // J.Biol.Chem. – 2008. – vol. 283, N 43. – P. 29196–29205.

Castells M.C., Friend D.S., Bunnell C.A et al. The presence of mmembrane-bound stem cell factor on highly immature nonmetachromatic mast cells in the systemic mastocytoma. // J.Allergy Clin. Immunol. – 1996. – vol. 98, N 4. – P. 831–840.

Castor C.W., Prince R.K., Dorstewitz E.L. (1962). Characteristics of human "fibroblasts" cultivated in vitro from different anatomical sites. // Lab Invest. – 1962. – vol. 11. – P. 703–713.

Cattaruzza S., Perris B. Approaching the proteoglycome: molecular interactions of proteoglycans and their functional output. // Macromol.Biosci. – 2006. – vol. 6, N 8. – P. 667–680.

Celli A.B., Hollinger J.O., Campbell P.G. Osx transcriptional regulation is mediated by additional pathways to BMP2/Smad signals. // J.Cell.Biochem. – 2005. – vol. 95, N 3. – P. 518–528.

Chabot B., Stephenson D.A., Chapman V.M. et al. The protooncogene c-kit encoding a transmembrane tyrosine kinase receptor maps to the mouse W locus. // Nature. – 1988. Vol. 335, N 6185. – P. 88–9.

Chadjichristos C., Chayor C., Kypriotou M. et al. Sp1 and Sp3 transcription factors mediate interleukin-1β down-regulation of human type II collagen gene expression in articular chondrocytes. // J.Biol.Chem. – 2003. – vol. 278, N 41. – P. 39762–39772.

Chaffer C.L., Thompson E.W., Williams E.D. Mesenchymal to epithelial transition in development and disease. // Cells Tissues Organs. – 2007. – vol. 185, N 1. – P. 7–19.

Chang D.P., Abu-Lail N.I., Guilak F. et al. Conformational mechanics, adsorption, and normal force interactions of lubricin and hyaluronic acid on model surfaces. // Lsngmuir. – 2008. – vol. 24, N 4. – P. 1183–1193.

Chang H.Y., Chi J.-T., Dudoit S. et al. Diversity, topographic differentiation, and positional memory in human fibroblasts. // Proc.Natl. Acad.Sci. USA. – 2002. – vol. 99. N 20. – P. 12877–12882.

Chang W., Shoback D. Extracellular Ca2+ -sensing molecules. // Cell Calcium. – 2004. – vol. 35, N 3. – 183–196.

Chapman J.A., Kellgarn J.H., Steven F.S. Assembly of collagen fibrils. // Fed. Proc. 1966. – vol. 25. – P. 1811–1812.

Charbonneau N.L., Dzamba B.J., Ono R.N. et al. Fibrillin can co-assemble in fibrils, but fibrillin fibril composition displays cell-specific differences. // J.Biol.Chem. – 2003. – vol. 278, N 4. – P. 2740–2749.

Chellaiah M.A., Kizer N., Biswas R. Osteopontin deficiency produces osteoclast dysfunction due to reduced CD44 surface expression. // Mol.Biol.Cell. – 2003. – vol. 14, N 1. – P. 173–189.

Chen F.H., Herndon M.E., Patel N. et al. Interaction of cartilage oligomeric matrix protein/thrombospondiN 5 with aggrecan. // J.Biol. Chem. – 2007. – vol. 282, N 34. – P. 24591–24598.

Chen F.H., Thomas A.O., Hecht J.T. et al. Cartilage oligomeric matrix protein/thrombospondi N 5 supports chondrocyte attachment through interaction with integrin. // J.Biol.Chem. – 2005. – vol. 280., N 38. – P. 32655–32660

Chen L., Deng C.X. Roles of FGF signaling in skeletal development and human genetic diseases. // Front.Biosci. – 2005. – vol. 10. – P. 1961–1976.

Chen S.S., Falcovitz Y.H., Schneiderman R. et al. Depth-dependent compressive properties of normal aged human femoral head articular cartilage: relationship to fixed charged density. // Osteoarthritis Cartilage. – 2001. – vol. 9, N 6. – P. 561–569.

Chen X., Macica C.M., Nasiri A., Broadus A.E. Regulation of articular chondrocyte proliferation and differentiation by Indian hedgehog and parathyroid hormone-related protein in mice. // Arthritis Rheum. – 2008. – vol. 58, N 12. – P. 3778–3797.

Chen X., Yang J., Evans P.M., Liu C. Wnt signaling: the good and the bad. // Acta Biochim.Biophys.Sin. – 2008. Vol.40, N 7. – P. 577–594.

Chen X.D., Dusevich V., Feng J.Q. et al. Extracellular matrix made by bone marrow cells facilitate expansion of marrow-derived mesenchymal progenitor cells and prevents their differentiation into osteoblasts. // J.Bone Miner.Res. – 2007. – vol. 22, N 12. – P. 943–956.

Chen Y., Alman B.A. Wnt pathway: an essential role in bone regeneration. // J.Cell.Biochem. – 2009. – vol. 106, N 2. – P. 353–362.

Chen Y., Zardi L., Peters D.M. High-resolution cryo-scanning electron microscopy study of the macromolecular structure of fibronectin fibrils. // Scanning. – 1997. – vol. 19, N 5. – P. 349–355.

Chen Y.G., Wang Q., Lin S.L. et al. Activin signaling and its role in regulation of cell proliferation, apoptosis, and carcinogenesis. // Exp.Biol.Med. – 2006. – vol. 231. – P. 534–544.

Cheney C.M., Lash J. W. Diversification within chick somites: Differential response to notochord. // Dev. Biol. – 1981. – vol. 81. – P. 288–298.

Cheng H., Jiang W., Phillips F.M. et al. Osteogenic activity of the fourteen types of human bone morphogenetic proteins. // J.Bone Joint Surg. – 2003. – vol. 85-A. N 8. – P. 1544–1552.

Cheng S.L., Lecanda F., Davidson M.K. et al. Human osteoblasts express a repertoire of cadherins, which are critical for BMP-2-induced osteogenic differentiation. // J.Bone Miner.Res. – 1998. – vol. 13, N 4. – P. 633–644.

Chertkov I.L. and A.Ya. Friedenstein. Cellular fundamentals of hematopoiesis (hematopoietic progenitor cells). [in Russian] Moscow: Medicine, 1977. 290 pages.

Chertkov I.L. and O.A. Gurevich. Stem hematopoietic cell and its microenvironment. [in Russian] Moscow: Medicine, 1984. 240 pages.

Chesney J., Bacher M., Bender A., Bucala R. The peripheral blood fibrocyte is a potent antigen-presenting cell capable of priming naive T cells in situ. // Proc. Natl. Acad. Sci. USA. – 1997. – vol. 94. – P. 6307–6312.

Chesney J., Bucala, R. Peripheral blood fibrocytes: mesenchymal precursor cells and the pathogenesis of fibrosis. // Curr. Rheumatol. Rep. – 2000. – vol. 2. – P. 501–505.

Chesney J., Metz C., Stavitsky A. B. et al. (1998) Regulated production of type I collagen and inflammatory cytokines by peripheral blood fibrocytes. // J.Immunol. – 1998. – vol. 160. – P. 419–425.

Chevrier A., Nelea M., Hurtig M.B. et al. Meniscus structure in human, sheep, and rabbit for animal models of meniscur repair. // J.Orthop.Res. – 2009. – vol. 27, N 9. – P. 1197–1103.

Chihara Y., Rakugi H., Ishikawa K. et al. Klotho protein promotes adipocyte differentiation. // Endocrinology. – 2006. – vol. 147. – P. 3835–3842.

Chikuda H., Kugimiya F., Hoshi K. et al. Cyclic GMP-dependent protein kinase II is a molecular switch from proliferation to hypertrophic differentiation of chondrocytes. // Genes Devel. – 2004. – vol. 18. – P. 2418–2429.

Chimal-Monroy J., Rodrigez-Leon J., Montero J.A. et al. Analysis of the molecular cascade responsible for mesodermal limb chondrogenesis: Sox genes and BMP signaling. // Dev.Biol. – 2003. – vol. 257. – P. 292–301.

Chin H.J., Fischer M.C., Li Y. et al. Studies on the role of Dlx5 in regulation of chondrocyte differentiation during endochondral ossification in the developing mouse limb. // Dev.Growth Differ. – 2007. – vol. 49, N 6. – P. 515–521.

Chipev C.C., Simon M. Phenotypic differences between dermal fibroblasts from different body sites determine their responses to tension and TGFbeta1. // BMC Dermatol. – 2002. – Vol. 2. P. 13.

Chiquet M. Regulation of extracellular matrix gene expression by mechanical stress. // Matrix Biol. – 1999. – vol. 18, N 5. – P. 417–426.

Chiquet-Erisman R. Tenascins. // Int.J.Biochem.Cell Biol. – 2004. – vol. 36, N 6. – P. 986–990.

Cho S.H., Oh C.D., Kim S.J. et al. Retinoic acid inhibits chondrogenesis of mesenchymal cells by sustaining expression of N-cadherin and its associated proteins. // J.Cell.Biochem. – 2003. – vol. 89, N 4. – P. 837–847.

Cho S.W., Yang J.Y., Sun H.J. et al. Wnt inhibitory factor (WIF)-1 inhibits osteoblastic differentiation in mouse embryonic mesenchymal cells. // Bone. – 2009. – vol. 44, N 6. – P. 1069–1077.

Chou M.Y., Li H.C. Genomic organization and characterization of the human type XXI collagen (COL21A1). // Genomics. – 2002. – vol. 79, N 3. – P. 395–401.

Chu M.L., Tsuda T. Fibulins in development and heritable disease. // Birth Defects Res. C. Embryo Today. // – 2004. – vol. 72, N 1. – P. 25–36.

Chubinskaya S., Hakamiya A., Pacione C. et al. Synergistic effect of IGF-1 and OP-1 on matrix formation by normal and OA chondrocytes cultured in alginate beads. // Osteiarthritis Cartilage. – 2007a. – vol. 15, N 4. – P. 421–430.

Chubinskaya S., Kawakami M., Rappoport L. et al. Anti-catabolic effect of OP-1 in chronically compressed intervertebral discs. // J.Orthop.Res. – 2007b. – vol. 25, N 4. – P. 517–530.

Chubinskaya S., Kuettner K.E. Regulations of osteogenic proteins by chondrocytes. // Int.J.Biochem.Cell Biol. – 2003. – vol. 35. – P. 1323–1340.

Chubinskaya S., Segalite D., Pikovsky D. et al. Effects induced by BMPs in cultures of human articular chondrocytes: comparative assay. // Growth Factors. – 2008. – vol. 26, N 5. – P. 275–283.

Chun J.S., Oh H., Yang S., Park M. Wnt signaling in cartilage development and degeneration. // BMB Rep. – 2008. – vol. 81, N 7. – P. 485–498.

Chung U.I., Kawaguchi H., Takato T., Nakamura K. Distinct osteogenic mechanisms of bones of distinct origin. // J.Orthop.Sci. – 2004. – vol. 9. – P. 410–414.

Cinquin O. Understanding the somitogenesis clock: What's missing? // Mech.Dev. – 2007. – vol. 124. – P. 501–517.

Civitelli R. Cell-cell communication in the osteoblast/osteocyte lineage. // Arch.Biochem.Biophys. – 2008. – vol. 473. – P. 188–193.

Claassen H., Cellarius C., Scholz-Ahrens K.E. et al. Extracellular matrix changes in knee joint cartilage following bone-active drug treatment. // Cell Tissue Res. – 2006. – vol. 324. – P. 279–289.

Claassen H., Schlüter M., Schunke M., Kurz B. Influence of 17β-estradiol and insulin on type II collagen and protein synthesis of articular chondrocytes. // Bone. – 2006. – vol. 39, N 2. – P. 310–317.

Clark A.G., Korbaugh A.L., Otterness T., Kraus V.G. The effects of ascorbic acid on cartilage metabolism in guinea pig articular cartilage explants. // Matrix Biol. – 2002. – vol. 21, N 2. – 175–184.

Clevers H. Wnt/βcatenin signaling in development and disease. // Cell. – 2006. – vol. 127. – P. 469–480

Coetzee M., Kruger M.C. Osteoprotegerin – receptor activator of nuclear factor-kappaB ligand ratio: a new approach to osteoporosis treatment. // Southern Med.J. – 2004. – vol. 97, N 5. – P. 506–511.

Cohen M., Kam Z., Addadi L., Geiger B. Dynamic study of the transition from hyaluronan- to integrin mediated adhesion in chondrocytes. // EMBO J. – 2006. – vol. 25, N 2. – P. 302–311.

Cohen M.M.jr. The new bone biology. Pathologic, molecular, and clinicall correlates. // Am.J.Med.Genet Part A. – 2006. – vol. 140 A. – P. 2646–2706.

Coleman P.J., Scott D., Mason R.M. et al. The proteoglycans and glycosaminoglycan chains of rabbit synovium. // Histochem.J. – 1998. – vol. 30, N 7. – P. 519–524.

Colnot C., Fuente L.de la, Huang S. Indian hedgehog synchronize skeletal angiogenesis and perichondrial maturation with cartilage development. // Development. – 2005. – vol. 132. – P. 1057–1067.

Colognato H., Yurchenko P.D. Form and function: the laminin family of heterotrimer. // Dev.Dyn. – 2000. – vol. 218, N 2. – P. 243–248.

Comerford E.J., Tarlton J.F., Innes J.F. et al. Metabolism and composition of the canine anterior cruciate ligament relate to differences in knee joint mechanics and predisposition to ligament rupture. // J.Orthop.Res. – 2005. – vol. 23, N 1. – P. 61–66.

Contard P., Bartel R. L., Jacobs L. et al. Culturing keratinocytes and fibroblasts in a three-dimensional mesh results in epidermal differentiation and formation of a basal lamina-anchoring zone. // J. Invest. Dermatol. – 1993. – vol. 100. – P. 35–39.

Coordinated expression of scleraxis and Sox9 genes during embryonic development of tendon and cartilage. // J.Orthop.Res. – 2002. – vol. 20. – P. 827–833.

Copeland N.G., Gilbert D.J., Cho B.C., et al. Mast cell growth factor maps near the steel locus on mouse chromosome 10 and is deleted in a number of steel alleles. // Cell – 1990. – vol. 63, N 1. P 175–183.

Cordes R., Schuster-Gossler K., Serth K., Gossler A. Specification of vertebral identity is coupled by Notch signaling and the segmentation clock. // Development. – 2004. – vol. 131. – P. 1221–1233.

Cormier S., Delezoide A.L., Benoist-Lasselin C. et al. Parathyroid hormone receptor type I/Indian hedgehog expression is preserved in the growth plate of human fetuses affected with fibroblast growth factor type 3 activating mutation. // Amer.J.Pathol. – 2002. – vol. 163, N 4. – P. 1325–1335.

Cornelissen A.M., Stoop R., Von den Hoff H.W. et al. (2000). Myofibroblasts and matrix components in healing palatal wounds in the rat. // J.Oral Pathol. Med. – vol. 29. – P. 1–7.

Cornish J., Grey A., Callon K.N. et al. Shared pathways of osteoblast mitogenesis induced by amylin, adrenomedullin, and IGF-1. // Biochim.Biophys.Res.Commun. – 2004. – vol. 318, N 1. – P. 240–246.

Corson G.M., Charbonneau N.L., Keene D.R., Sakay L.Y. Differential expression of fibrillin-3 adds to microfibril variety in human and avian, but not rodents, connective tissues. // Genomics. – 2004. – vol. 83, N 3. – P. 461–472.

Costell M., Gustafson E., Aszodi A. et al. Perlecan maintains the integrity of cartilage and some basement membranes. // J.Cell Biol. – 1999. – vol. 147, N 5. – P. 1109–1122.

Couchman J.R., Chen L., Woods A. Syndecans and cell adhesions. // Int.Rev.Cytol. – 2001. – vol. 207. – P. 113–150.

Cowin S.C. Mechanosensation and fluid transport in living bone. // J.Musculoskelet. Neuron Interact. – 2002. – vol. 2, N 3. – P. 256–260.

Cox R.W., Dell B.L. High resolution electron microscope observation on normal and pathological elastin // J. roy. microscop. Soc. 1966. – vol. 85. – P. 401–409

Crickmore M.A., Mann R.S. Hox control of morphogen mobility and organ development through regulation of glypican expression. // Development. – 2007. – vol. 134. – P. 327–334.

Crockett R., Grubelnik A., Roos S. et al. Biochemical composition of the superficial layer of articular cartilage. // J.Biomed.Mater.Re. – 2007. – vol.82A. – P. 958–964.

Crombrugghe B.de, Lefebvre V., Behringer R.R. et al. Transcriptional mechanis, of chondrocyte differentiation. // Matrix Biol. – 2000. – vol. 19, N 5. – p. 389–394.

Csiszar K. Lysyl oxidases: a novel multifunctional amine oxidase family. // Prog.Nucleic Acid Res. – 2001. – vol. 70. – P. 1–32.

Cullinane D.M. The role of osteocytes in bone regulation: mineral homeostasis versus mechanoreception. // J.Musculoskelet. Neuronal Interact, – 2002. – vol. 2, N 3. – 242–244.

D'Andrea D., Liguori G.L., Le Good J.A. Cripto promotes A-P axis specification independently of its stimulatory effect on Nodal autoinduction. // J.Cell Biol. – 2008. – vol. 180, N 3. – P. 597–605.

Daftary G.S., Taylor H.S. Endocrine regulation of HOX genes. // Endocrine Rev. – 2006. – vol. 27, N 4. – P. 331–355.

Dahl C., Hoffmann H.J., Saito H., Schiøtz P.O. Human mast cells express receptors for IL-3, IL-5 and GM-CSF; a partial map of receptors on human mast cells cultured in vitro. // Allergy. – 2004. Vol. 59, N 10. – P. 1087–1096.

Dai J., Rabie A.B.M. VEGF: an essential mediator of both angiogenesis and endochondral pssification. // J.Dent.Res. – 2007. – vol. 86, N 10. – P. 937–950.

Dallas S.L., Chen Q., Sivakumar F. Dynamics of assembly and reorganization of extracellular matrix proteins. // Curr.Top.Dev.Biol. – 2006. – vol. 75. – P. 1–24.

Damazo A.S., Moradi-Bidhendi N., Oliani S.M., Flower R.J. Role of annexiN 1 gene expression in mouse craniofacial bone development. // Birth Defects Res.A. Clin.Mol.Teratol. – 2007. – vol. 79, N 7. – P. 1524–1532.

Danen E.H., Yamada K.M. Fibronectin, integrins, and growth control. // J.Cell Physiol. – 2001. – vol. 189, N.1. – P. 1–13.

Danfelter M., Innerfjord P., Heinegård D. Fragmentation of proteins in cartilage treated with IL-1. Specific cleavage of type IX collagen by MMP-13 releases the NC4 domain. // J.Biol.Chem. – Epub. October 19, 2007.

Danilov R.K. General principles of the cell structure, development and classification of tissues. [in Russian] // In: A textbook of his-

tology (iN 2 volumes). Vol. 1. St. Petersburg: SpecLit, 2001. P. 95–105.

Darby I., Skalli O., Gabbiani G. Alpha-smooth muscle actin is transiently expressed by myofibroblasts during experimental wound healing. // Lab.Invest – 1990. – vol. 63. – P. 21–29.

Darnel J., Lodish H., Baltimore D. (eds). Molecular cell biology. // N.Y.: Scientific American Books. – 1990

Davey R.A., Turner A.G., McManus J.F. et al. Calcitonin receptor plays a physiological role to protect against hypercalcemia in rats. // J.Bone Miner.Res. – 2008. – vol. 23, N 8. – P. 1182–1193.

Davidson L.A., Keller R., DeSimone D.W. Assembly and remodeling of the fibrillar fibronectin extracellular matrix during gastrulation and neurulation in Xenopus laevis. // Dev.Dyn. – 2004. – vol. 231, N 4. – P. 888–895.

Davis L.A., Nieden N.I.zur Mesodermal fate decision of a stem cell: the Wnt switch. // Cel.Mol.Life Sci. – 2008. – vol. 65, N 17. – P. 2658–2674.

Day A.J., Prestwich G.D. Hyaluronan-binding proteins: tying up the giant. // J.Biol.Chem. – 2002. – vol. 277, N 7. – P. 4385–4388

Day T.F., Guo X., Garrett-Beal L., Yang Y. Wnt/ β-catenin signaling in mesenchymal progenitors control osteoblast and chondrocyte differentiation during vertebrate skeletogenesis. // Dev.Cell. – 2005. – vol. 8. – P. 739–750.

Day T.F., Yang Y. Wnt and hedgehog signaling pathways in bone development. // J.Bone Joint.Surg.Am. – 2008. – vol. 90, Suppl.1. – P. 19–24.

De Luca F., Barnes K.M., Uyeda A. et al. Regulation of growth plate chondrogenesis by bone morphogenetic protein-2. // Endocrinology. – 2001. – vol. 142, N 1. – P. 430–436.

DeAngelo P.I. Hyaluronan synthases: fascinating glycosyltransferases from vertebrates, bacterial pathogens, and algal viruses. // Cell.Mol.Life. – 1999. – vol. 56. – P. 670–682

Debelle L., Tamburro A.M. Elastin: molecular description and function. // Int.J.Biochem. Cell Biol. – 1999. – vol. 31, N 3. – P. 261–272.

Deckelbaum R.A., Majithia A., Booker T. et al. The homeoprotein engrailed 1 has pleotropic function in calvarial intramembranos formation and remodeling. // Development. – 2006. – vol. 133, N 1. – P. 63–74.

Dedukh N.V., E.Ya. Pankov. Skeletal tissues. [in Russian] // In: A textbook of histology. vol. 1, edited by R.K.Danilov and V.L.Bykov. St. Petersburg: SpecLit, 2001. P. 284–336.

Delany A.M., Kalajzic I., Bradshaw A.D. et al. Osteonectin-null mutation compromises osteoblast formation, maturation, and survival. // Endocrinology. – 2003. – vol. 144, N 6. – P. 2588–2596.

Delise A.M., Tuan R.S. Analysis of N-cadherin function in limb mesenchymal chondrogenesis in vitro. // Dev.Dyn. – 2002. – vol. 235. – P. 195–204.

Dell'Accio F., De Bar C., El Tawl N.M.F. et al. Activation of WNT and BMP signaling in adult human articular cartilage following mechanical injury. // Arthritis Res.Ther. – 2006. – vol. 8. – P. R139.

Délot E., King L.M., Briggs M.D. et al. Trinucleotide expansion mutations in the cartilage oligomeric matrix protein (COMP) gene. // Hum.Mol.Gen. – 1999. – vol. 8, N 1. – P. 123–128.

Deng F., Ling J., Ma J. et al. Stimulation of intramembranous bone repair in rats by ghrelin. // Exp.Physiol. – 2008. – vol. 93, N 7. – P. 872–879.

Deng Z.L., Sharff K.A., Tang N. et al. Regulation of osteogenic differentiation during skeletal development. // Front.Biosci. – 2008. – Epub. Jan.1.Dermatol. – 1999. – vol. 112, N 3. – P. 411–418.

Denisov-Nikolsky Yu.I. Morphofunctional characteristics of bone as an organ. [in Russian] // In: Current issues of theoretical and clinical osteoarthrology, written by Denisov-Nikolsky Yu.I., Mironov S.P., Omelyanenko N.P., I.V. Matveichuk, 2005. P. 15–35.

Denisov-Nikolsky Yu.I., Zhilkin B.A., Doktorov A.A., I.V. Matveichuk. Ultrastructural organization of a lamellar bone tissue mineral component in adult and old persons. [in Russian]// Morphology, 2002, vol. 122, no. 5. P. 79–83.

Dequéant M., Glynn E., Gaudenz K. et al. A complex oscillating network of signaling genes underlies the mouse segmentation clock. // Science. – 2006. – vol. 314, N 5805. – P. 1595–1598.

Deregowski V., Gazzerro E., Priest L. et al. Notch 1 overesxpression inhibits osteoblastogenesis by suppression Wnt/β-catenin but not bone morphogenetic protein signaling. // J.Biol.Chem. – 2006. – vol. 281, N 10. – P. 6203–6210.

Derfoul A., Perkins G.L., Hall D.J., Tuan R.S. Glucocorticoids promote chondrogenic differentiation of adult mesenchymal stem cells by enhancing expression of cartilage extracellular matrix genes. // Stem Cells. – 2006. – vol. 24. – P. 1487–1495.

Derycke L.D.M., Bracke M.E. N-cadherins in the spotlight of cell-cell adhesion, differentiation, embryogenesis, invasion and signaling. // Int.J.Dev.Biol. – 2004. – vol. 48. – P. 463–476.

Desai J., Shannon M.E., Johnson M.D. et al. Nell1-deficient mice have reduced expression of extracellular matrix proteins causing cranial and vertebral defects. // Hum.Mol.Genet. – 2006. – vol. 15, N 8. – P. 1329–1341.

Deschamps J., Nes J.van. Developmental regulation of the Hox genes during axial morphogenesis in the mouse. // Development. – 2005. – vol. 132. – P. 2931–2942.

Desmouliere A, Gabbiani G. The role of the myofibroblast in wound healing and fibrocontractive diseases. In: The molecular and cellular biology of wound repair (Clark R.A.F., edit.). New York: Plenum Press. – 1996. P. 391–413.

Desmouliere A. Factors influencing myofibroblast differentiation during wound healing and fibrosis. // Cell Biol.Int. – 1995. – Vol. 19. – P. 471–476.

Desmouliere A., Geinoz A., Gabbiani F., Gabbiani G. Transforming growth factor-beta 1 induces alpha-smooth muscle actin expression in granulation tissue myofibroblasts and in quiescent and growing cultured fibroblasts. // J. Cell Biol. – 1993. – vol. 122. – P. 103–111.

Desmouliere A., Rubbia-Brandt L., Abdiu A. et al. Alpha-smooth muscle actin is expressed in a subpopulation of cultured and cloned fibroblasts and is modulated by gamma-interferon. // Exp.Cell. Res. – 1992. – vol. 201. – P. 64–73.

Destaing O., Sanjay A., Itzstein C. et al. The tyrosine kinase activity of c-Src regulates actin dynamics and organization of podosomes in osteoclasts. // Mol.Biol.Cell. – 2008. – vol. 19. – P. 394–404.

Diab M. The role of type IX collagen in osteoarthritis and rheumatoid arthritis. // Orthop.Rev. – 1993. – vol. 22, N 2. – P. 165–170.

Dietz U.H., Sandell L.J. Cloning of a retinoic acid-sensitive mRNA expressed in cartilage and during chondrogenesis. // J.Biol.Chem. – 1996. – vol. 271, N 6. – P. 3311–3316.

Dieudonne M.N., Pecquery B., Leneveu M.C., Guidicelli Y. Opposite effects of androgens and estrogens on adipogenesis in rat preadipocytes: Evidence for sex and site-related specificities and possible involvement of insulin-like growth factor 1 receptot and peroxisome proliferator-acivated receptor γ2. // Endocrinology. – 2000. – vol. 141, N 2. – P. 649–656.

Dijke P.ten, Krause C., Gorter D.J.de et al. Osteocyte-derived sclerostin inhibits bone formation: its roile in bone morphogenetic protein and Wnt signaling. // J.Bone Joint Surg,Am. – 2008. – vol. 90, Suppl.1 – P. 31–35.

Dijkstra C. D., Damoiseaux J. G. Endocytosis. // Physiol. Rev. – 1997. – vol. 77. – P. 759–803,

Dijkstra C. D., Damoiseaux J. G. Macrophage heterogeneity established by immunocyto-chemistry. // Prog. Histochem. Cytochem. – 1993. – vol. 27. – P. 1–65,.

Djouad F., Delome B., Maurice M. et al. Microenvironmental changes during differentiation of mesenchymal stem cells towards chondrocytes. // Arthritis Res.Ther. – 2007. – vol. 9. – P.R33.

Docheva D., Hunziker E.B., Fässler R., Brandau O. Tenomodulin is necessary for tenocyte proliferation and tendon maturation. // Mol.Cell.Biol. – 2005. – vol. 25, N 2. – P. 669–705.

Dodson R.E., Shapiro D. Regulation of pathways of mRNA destabilization and stabilization. // Progr.Nucleic Acid Res. – 2002. – vol. 72. – P. 129–164.

Doege K.J., Coulter S.N., Meek L.M. et al. A human specific polymorphism in the coding region of the aggrecan gene. // J.Biol.Chem. – 1997. – vol. 272, N 21. – P. 13974–13979.

Doljanski F. The sculpture role of fibroblast-like cells in morphogenesis. // Persp.Biol.Med. – 2004. – vol. 47, N 3. – P. 339–356.

Domaratskaya E.I. Stem cells – bone marrow residents. [in Russian] Izvestiya RAN. Seriya Biologicheskaya, 2011, no. 3. P. 1–12.

Donepudi M., Grutter M. Structure and zymogen activation of caspases. // Biophys.Chem. – 2002. – vol. 101–102. – P. 145–153.

Dong Y.F., Soung do Y., Chang Y. et al. Transforming growth factor-beta and Wnt signals regulate chondrocyte differentiation through Twist1 in a stage-specific manner. // Mol.Endocrinol. – 2007. – vol. 21, N 11. – P. 2805–2820.

Dorus S., Anderson J.R., Vallender E.J. et al. Sonic hedgehog, a key developmental gene, experienced intensified molecular evolution in primates. //Hum.Mol.Genet. – 2006. – vol. 15, N 13. – P. 2031–2037

Douglas T., Heinemann S., Bierbaum S. et al. Fibrillogenesis of collagen types I, II, and III with small leucine-rich proteoglycans decorin and biglycan. // Biomacromolecules. – 2006. – vol. 7, N 8. – P. 2388–2393.

Dovio A., Data V., Angeli A. Circulating osteoprotegerin and soluble RANKL: do they have future in clinical practice. // J.Endocrinol. Invest. – 2005. – vol. 24, Suppl. 10 – P. 14–22.

Dowthwaite G.P., Edwards J.C.W., Pitsillides A.A. An essential role for hyaluronan and hyaluronan binding proteins during joint development. // J.Histochem.Cytochem. – 1998. – vol. 46, N 5. – P. 641–652.

Dreier R., Günther B.K., Mainz T. et al. Terminal differentiation of chick embryo chondrocytes requires shedding of a cell surface protein that binds 1,25-dihydroxyvitamin D3. // J.Biol.Chem. – 2008a. – vol. 283, N 2. – P. 1104–1112.

Dreier R., Opolka A., Grifka J. et al. Collagen IX deficiency seriously compromises growth cartilage development in mice. // Matrix Biol. – 2008b. – vol. 27, N 4. – P. 319–329.

Dubrulle J., Pourquié O. Coupling segmentation to axis formation. // Development. – 2004. – vol. 131. – P. 5783–5793

Ducy P., Schinke T., Karsenty G. The osteoblast: a sophisticated fibroblast. // Science. – 2000. – vol. 289, N 5484. – P. 1501–1504.

Dudas J., Mansuroglu T., Batusic D. et al. Thy-1 is an in vivo and in vitro marker of liver myofibroblasts. // Cell Tissue Res. – 2007. – Vol. 329. – P. 503–514.

Dudhia J. Aggrecan, aging and assembly in articular cartilage. // Cell.Mol.Life Sci. – 2005. – vol. 62. – P. 2241–2256.

Duester G. Retinoic acid regulation of somitogenesis clock. // Birth Defects Res.C.Embryo Today. – 2007. – vol. 81. P. 84–92

Dugina V., Fontao L., Chaponnier C. et al. Focal adhesion features during myofibroblastic differentiation are controlled by intracellu-

lar and extracellular factors. // J.Cell Sci. – 2001. – vol. 114. –
P. 3285–3296.

Dunty W.C.jr., Biris K.K., Chalamalasetty R.B. et al. Wnt3a/β-catenin
signaling controls posterior body development by coordinating
mesoderm formation and segmentation. // Development. –
2008. – vol. 135. – P. 85–94.

Dusso A.S., Brown A.J., Slatopolsky E. Vitamin D. // Am.J.Physiol.Renal
Physiol. – 2005. – vol. 289. – P.F8–F28.

Dvir-Ginzberg M., Gagarina V., Lee E.J., Ha; D.J. Regulation of cartilage-
specific gene expression in human chondrocytes by SirT1 and
NAMPT. // J.Biol.Chem. – Epub 2008. Oct.28

Dvorak M.M., Riccardi D. Ca2+ as an extracellular signal in bone. //
Cell Calcium. – 2004. – vol. 35, N 3. – P. 249–255.

Eames B.F., Helms J.A. Conserved molecular program regulating cranial and appendicular skeletogenesis. // Dev.Dyn. – 2004. –
vol. 231, N 1. – P. 4–13.

Eames B.F., La Fuente L., Helms J.A. Molecular ontogeny of the skeleton. // Birth Defects Res. C. Embryo Today. – 2003. – vol. 69, N 2. –
P. 93–103.

Eames B.F., Sharpe P.T., Helms J.A. Hierarchy revealed in the specification of three skeletal fates by Sox9 and Runx2. // Dev.Biol. –
2004. – vol. 274, N 1. – P. 188–200.

Eble J.A. Collagen-binding integrins as pharmacological targets. //
Curr.Pharmacol.Des. – 2005. – vol. 11. – P. 867–880.

Eckes B., Dogic D., Colucci-Guyon E. et al. Impaired mechanical
stability, migration and contractile capacity in vimentin-defi-
cient fibroblast. // J.Cell Sci. – 1998. – vol. 111. – P. 1897–1907.

Edom-Vovard F., Duprez D. Signals regulating tendon formation during chick embryonic development. // Dev.Dyn. – 2004. – vol. 229. –
P. 449–457

Edom-Vovard F., Schuler B., Bonnin M.A. et al. Fgf4 positively regulates
scleraxis and tenascin expression in chick limb tendons. //
Dev.Biol. – 2002. – vol. 247. – P. 351–366.

Edwards C.J., Francis-West P.H. Bone morphogenetic proteins in the
development and healing of synovial joints. // Semin.Arthrit.
Rheum. – 2001. – vol. 31, N 1. – P. 33–42.

Edwards C.M., Mundy G.R. Eph receptors and ephrin signaling pathways: a role in bone homeostasis. // Int.J.Med.Sci. – 2008. –
vol. 5, N 5. – P. 263–272.

Edwards J.C.W. Fibroblast biology. Development and differentiation
of synovial fibroblasts in arthritis. // Arthritis Res. – 2000. –
vol. 2. – P. 344–347.

Eerden B.C.J.van der, Karperien M., Wit J.M. Systemic and local regulation of the growth plate. // Endocrine Rev. – 2003. – vol. 24, N 6. –
P. 782–801.

Effect of type XII or XIV collagen NC-3 domain on the human dermal fibroblast migration into reconstituted collagen gel. //
Exp.Dermatol. – 1999. – vol. 8, N 1. – P. 17–21.

Eger W., Schumacher B.L., Mollenhauer J. et al. Human knee and ankle
cartilage explants: catabolic differences. // J.Orthop.Res. – 2002. –
vol. 20, N 3. – P. 526–534.

Egging D.F., van Vlijmen I., Starcher B. Dermal connective tissue development in mice: an essential role for tenascin X. // Cell Tissue
Res. – 2006. – vol. 323, N 3. – P. 463–474.

Ehlen H.W., Buelens L.A., Vortkamp A. Hedgehog signaling in skeletal
development. // Birth Defects Res.C,Embryo Today. – 2006. –
vol. 78, N 3. – P. 267–279.

Ehnis T., Dieterich W., Bauer M. et al. Localization of a binding site for
the proteoglycan decorin on collagen XIV (undulin). //
J.Biol.Chem. – 1997. – vol. 272, N.33. – P. 20414–20419.

Ekblom P., Ionai P., Talts J.F. Expression and biological role
of laminin-1. // Matrix Biol. – 2003. – vol. 22, N 1. – P. 35–47.

El-Amin S.F., Lu H.H., Khan Y. et al. Extracellular matrix production
by human osteoblasts cultured in biodegradable polymers applicable for tissue engineering. // Biomaterials. – 2003. – vol. 24,
N 7. – P. 1213–1221.

Elefteriou F. Regukation of bone remodeling by the central and peripheral nervous system. // Arch.Biochem.Biophys. – 2008. –
vol. 473, N 2. – P. 231–236.

Elefteriou F., Esposito J.Y., Garrone R., Lethias C. Binding of tenascin-C
to decorin. // FEBS Lett. – 2001. – vol. 495, N 1–2. – P. 44–47

Elenius K., Jalkanen M. Functions of syndecans – a family of cell surface proteoglycans. // J.Cell Sci. – 1994. – vol. 107, N 11. –
P. 2975–2982.

Elis S., Batellier F., Couty I. et al. Search for the genes involved in oocyte maturation and early embryo development in the hen. //
BMC Genomics. – 2008. – vol. 9. – P. 110.

Eliseev V.G. Connective tissue. [in Russian] Moscow: Medgiz, 1961.
416 pages.

Ellman M.B., An H.S., Muddasani P., Im H.J. Biological impact of the
fibroblast growth factor family on articular cartilage and intervertebral disc homeostasis. // Gene. – 2008. – vol. 420,
N 1. – P. 82–89.

Engel J. Role of oligomerization domains in thrombospondins and
other extracellular matrix proteins. // Int.J.Biochem.Cell Biol. –
2004. – vol. 36, N 6. – P. 997–1004.

Engin F., Yan Z., Yang T. et al. Dimorphic effects of Notch signaling in
bone homeostasis. // Nat.Med. – 2008. – vol. 14, N 3. – P. 299–305.

Enomoto-Iwamoto M., Nakamura T., Aikawa T. et al. Hedgehog proteins
stimulate chondrogenic cell differentiation and cartilage formation. // J.Bone Miner.Res. – 2000. – vol. 15, N 9. – P. 1659–1668.

Erickson A.C., Couchman J.R. Still more complexity in mammalian
basement membranes. // J.Histochem.Cytochem. – 2000. –
vol. 48, N 10. – P. 1291–1306.

Eriksen T.A., Wright D.M., Parslow P.P. Duance V.C. Role of Ca2+ for the
mechanical properties of fibrillin. // Proteins: Struct.Funct.Gen-
et. – 2001. – vol. 45. – P. 90–95.

Everts V., Korper W., Hoeben R.A. et al. Osteoblastic bone degradation
and the role of different cysteine proteinases and matrix metalloproteinases: differences between calvaria and long bone. //
J.Bone Miner.Res. – 2006. – vol. 21, N 9. – P. 1399–1408.

Evistar T., Kauffman H., Maroudas A. Synthesis of insulin-like growth
factor binding proteiN 3 in vitro in human articular cartilage
cultures. // Arthritis Rheum. – 2003. – vol. 48, N 2. – P. 410–417.

Eyden B.P. Brief review of the fibronexus and its significance for myofibroblastic differentiation and tumor diagnosis. // Ultrastruct.
Pathol. – 1993. – vol. 17. – P. 611–622.

Eyre D.R., Pietka T., Weis M.A., Wu J.J. Covalent cross-linking of the
NC1 domain of collagen type IX to collagen type II in cartilage. //
J.Biol.Chem. – 2004. – vol. 279, N 23. – P. 2568–2574.

Eyre D.R., Weis M.A., Wu J.J. Articular cartilage cikkagen: an irre-
placeable framework. // Eur.Cells Mater. – 2006. – vol. 12. –
P. 57–63.

Eyre D.R., Wu J.-J. Collagen cross links. // Topics in Current Chemistry. – 2005. – vol. 247. – P. 207–229.

Faccio R., Novack D.V., Zallone A. et al. Dynamic changes in the osteoclast cytoskeleton in response to growth factors and cell attachment are controlled by β3 integrin. // J.Cell Biol. – 2003. – vol. 162,
N 3. – P. 499–509.

Faivre L., Prieur A.M., Le Merrer M. et al. Clinical variability and genetic homogeneity of the camptodactyly-arhropathy-coxa vara-peri-

carditis syndrome. // Am.J.Med.Genet. – 2000. – vol. 95, N 3. – P. 213–216.

Faivre L., l Prieur A.M., Le Merrer M. et al. Clinical variability and genetic homogeneity of the campodactily-arthropathy-coxa vara-pericarditis syndrome. // Am.J.Med.Genet. 2000. vol. 95. №3. – P. 213–216.

Falahati-Nini A., Riggs B.L., Atkinson E.J. et al. Relative contributions of testosterone and estrogen in regulating bone resorption and formation in normal elderly men. // J.Clin.Invest. – 2000. – vol. 106, N 12. – P. 1553–1560.

Fallahi A., Kroll B., Warner L.R. et al. Structural model of the amino propeptide of collagen XI α1 chain with similarity to the LNS domain. // Protein Sci. – 2005. – vol. 14. – P. 1526–1537.

Fam H., Bryant J.T., Kontopoulou M. Rheological properties of synovial fluid. // Biorheology. – 2007. – vol. 44, N 2. – P. 59–74.

Fan D., Chen Z., Wang D. Osterix is a key target for mechanical signals in human thoracic ligament flavum cells. // J.Cell.Physiol. – 2007. – vol. 211. – P. 577–584.

Fan L., Sebe A., Péterfi Z. et al. Cell contact-dependent regulation of epithelial-mesenchymal transition via the Rho-Rho kinase-phospho-myosin pathway. // Mol.Biol.Cell. – 2007. – vol. 18. – P. 1083–1097.

Farach-Carson M.C., Carson D.D. Perlecan – a multifunctional extracellular proteoglycan scaffold. // Glycobiology. – 2007. – vol. 17, N 9. – P. 897–905.

Farach-Carson M.C., Carson D.D. Perlecan – a multifunctional extracellular proteoglycan scaffold. // Glycobiology. – 2007. – vol. 17, N 9. – P. 895–903.

Feng J.Q., Ward L.M., Liu S. et al. Loss of DMP1 causes rickets and osteomalacia and identifies a role for osteocytes in mineral metabolism. // Nat.Gen. – 2006. – vol. 38, N 11. – P. 1230–1231

Feng X. RANKing intracellular signaling in osteoclasts. // IUBMB Life. – 2005b. – vol. 57, N 6. – P. 389–395.

Feng X. Regulatory roles and molecular signaling of TNF family members in osteoclasts. // Gene. – 2005a. – vol. 350. – P. 1–13.

Ferguson J.W., Mikesh M.F., Wheeler E.F., LeBaron R.G. Development expression pattern of Beta-ig (βIG-H3) and its function as a cell adhesion protein. // Mech.Dev. – 2003. – vol. 120. – P. 851–864.

Ferland G. The vitamin K-dependent proteins: an update. // Nutrit. Rev. – 1998. 0 vol. 56, N 8. – P. 223–230.

Fernandez E.J., Lolis E. Structure, function, and inhibition of chemokines. // Annu.Rev. Pharmacol.Toxicol. – 2002. – vol. 42. – P. 469–499.

Fernandez R., Schmid T.M., Eyre D.R. Assembly of collagen II, IX and XI into nascent hetero-fibrils by a rat chondrocyte linr. // Eur.J.Biochem. – 2003. – vol. 270. – P. 3243–3250.

Fernandez R., Weis M., Scott M.A. et al. Collagen XI chain assembly in cartilage of the chondrodysplasi (cho) mice. // Matrix Biol. – 2007. – vol. 26, N 9. – P. 597–603.

Ferrara N. Vascular endothelial growth factor: basic science and clinical progress. // Endocr.Rev. –2004. – vol. 25, N 4. – P. 581–611.

Ferrari D., Kosher R.A. Expression of Dlx5 and Dlx6 during specification of the elbow joint. // Int.J.Dev.Biol. – 2006. – vol. 50. – P. 709–713.

Fertala A., Sieron A.L., Hojima Y. et al. Self-assembly of collagen II by enzymic cleavage of recombinant procollagen II. // J.Biol.Chem. – 1994. – vol. 269, N 15. – P. 11584–11589.

Fetter M.L., Leddy H.A., Guilak F., Nunley J.A. Composition and transport properties of human ankle and knee cartilage. // J.Orthop.Res. – 2006. – vol. 24, N 2. – P. 211–219.

Feugate J.E, Li Q, Wong L, Martins-Green M. The cxc chemokine cCAF stimulates differentiation of fibroblasts into myofibroblasts and accelerates wound closure. // J.Cell Biol. 2002. – vol. 156. – P. 161–172.

Ffander D., Rahmansadeh R., Scheller E.E. Presence and distribution of collagen II, collagen I, fibronectin, and tenascin in adult normal and osteoarthritic rabbit cartilage. // J.Rheumatol. – 1999. – vol. 26, N 2. – P. 386–394.

Fiashi-Taesch N.M., Stewart A.F. Parathyroid hormone-related protein is an intracrine factor – trafficking, mechanisms and functional consequences. // Endocrinology. – 2003. – vol. 144, N 2. – P. 407–411.

Fichard A., Kleman J.P., Ruggiero F. Another look at collagen V and XI molecules. // Matrix Biol. – 1995. – vol. 14, N 7. – P. 515–531.

Filmus J. Glypicans in growth control and cancer. // Glycobiology. – 2001. – vol. 11, N 3. – P. 19R 23R

Filmus J., Capurro M., Rat J. Glypicans. // Genome Biology. – 2008. – vol. 9. – P. 224.

Filmus J., Selleck S.B. Glypicans: proteoglycans with a surprise. // J.Clin.Invest. – 2001. – vol. 108, N 5. – P. 497–500.

Findlay D.M., Sexton P.M. Calcitonin. // Growth factors. – 2004. – vol. 22, N 4. – P. 217–224.

Fisher G.J. The pathophysiology of photoaging of the skin. // Cutis. – 2005. – vol. 75, 2 Suppl. – P. 5–8

Fisher L.W., Fedarko N.S. Six genes expressed in bone and teeth encode the current members of the SIBLING family of proteins. // Connect.Tissue Res. – 2003. – vol. 44, Suppl.1. – P. 33–40.

Fisher M.C., Clinton G.M., Maihle M.J., Dealy C.M. Requirement for ErbB2/ErbB signaling in defeloping cartilage and bone. // Dev.Growth Differ. – 2007. – vol. 49, N 6. – P. 503–513.

Fitzgerald J., Bateman J.F. A new FACIT of the collagen family: COL21A1. // FEBS Lett. – 2001. – vol. 505, N 2. – P. 275–280.

Fiúza U.M., Arias A.M. Cell and molecular biology of Notch. // J.Endocrinol. – 2007. – vol. 194. – P. 459–474.

Flannery C.R. MMPs and ADAMTSs: functional studies. // Front.Biosci. – 2006. – vol. 11. – P. 544–569.

Fleisch H. Development of bisphophonates. // Breast Cancer Res. – 2002. – vol. 4. – P. 30–34.

Fleischmajer R., MacDonald E. D.II, Contard P, Perlish J.S. Immunochemistry of a keratinocyte-fibroblast co-culture model for reconstruction of human skin. J. Histochem. Cytochem – 1993 – V. 41. – P. 1359–1366.

Fleischmajer R., Schechter A., Bruns M. Skin fibroblasts are the only source of nidogen during early basal lamina formation in vitro. // J. Invest. Dermatol. – 1995. – vol. 105. – P. 597–601.

Flier A. van der, Sonnenberg A. Function and interactions of integrins. // Cell Tissue Res – 2001. – vol. 305. – P. 285–298.

Flint M.H., Merrilless M.J. Relationship between the axial periodicity and staining of collagen by the Masson trichrome procedure. // Histochem. J. – 1977. – vol. 9. – P. 1–13.

Forsberg E., Kjellén L. Heparan sulfate: lessons from knockout mice. // J.Clin.Invest. – 2001. – vol. 108, N 2. – P. 175–180

Fosang A., Last K., Knäuper V. et al. Degradation of cartilage aggrecan by collagenase-3. // FEBS Lett. – 1996. – vol. 380, N 1–2. – P. 17–20.

Franceschi R.T. Functional cooperativity between osteoblast transcription factors: evidence for the importance of cubnuclear macromolecular complexes? // Calcir.Tissue Int. – 2003. – vol. 72. – P. 638–642.

Franceschi R.T., Ge C., Xiao G. et al. Transcriptional regulation of osteoblasts. // Cells, Tissues, Organs. – 2009. – vol. 189, N 1–4. – P. 144–152.

Franceschi R.T., Xiao G., Jiang D. et al. Multiple signaling pathways converge on the Cbfa1/Runx2 transcription factor to regulate osteoblast differentiation. // Connect.Tissue Res. – 2003. – vol. 43, Suppl.1. – P. 109–116.

Franchi M., Trirè A., Quarante M. et al. Collagen structure of tendon relates to function. // The Scientific World J. – 2007. – vol. 7. – P. 404–420.

Franchimont N., Wertz S., Malaise M. Interleukin-6: an osteotropic factor influencing bone formation? // Bone. – 2005. – vol. 37, N 5. – P. 601–605l.

Francis-West P.H., Parish J., Lee K., Archer C.W. BMP/GDF-signaling interactions during synovial joint development. // Cell Tissue Res. – 1999. – vol. 296. – P. 111–119.

Frank S., Schulthess T., Landwehr R. et al. Characterization of the matrilin coiled-coil domains reveal seven novel isoforms. // J.Biol.Chem. – 2002. – vol. 277, N 21. – P. 19071–19079.

Fransson L.A., Belting M., Cheng F. et al. Novel aspects of glypican glycobiology. // Cell.Mol.Life Sci. – 2004. – vol. 61, N 9. – P. 1016–1024.

Franzén A., Hultenby K., Reinholt F.P. et al. Altered osteoclast development and function in osteopontin deficient mice. // J.Orthop.Res. – 2008. – vol. 26, N 5. – P. 721–728.

Franzke C.-W., Bruckner P., Bruckner-Tuderman l. Collagenous transmembrane proteins. Recent insights into biology and pathology. // J.Biol.Chem. – 2005. – vol. 280, N 6. – P. 4005–4008.

Franz-Odendaal T.A., Hall B.K., Witten P.E. Buried aliwe: how osteoblasts become osteocytes. // Dev.Biol. – 2006. – vol. 235. – P. 176–190.

Fraser J.R.E., Laurent T.C., Laurent U.B.G. Hyaluronan: its nature, distribution, functions and turnover. // J.Intern.Med. – 1997. – vol. 242. – P. 27–33.

Freemont A.J., Hoyland J.A. Morphology, mechanisms and pathology of musculoskeletal ageing. // J.Pathol. – 2007. – vol. 211. – P. 252–259.

French M.M., Rose S., Canneco J., Athanasiou K.A. Chondrogenic differentiation of adult dermal fibroblasts. // Ann.Biomed.Engin. – 2004. – vol. 32, N 1. – P. 50–56.

French M.M., Smith S.E., Akanbi K. et al. Expression of the heparin sulfate proteoglycan perlecan during mouse embryogenesis and perlecan chondrogenic activity in vitro. // J.Cell Biol. – 1999. – vol. 145, N 5. – P. 1103–1115.

Friedenstein A.Ya. and K.S. Lalykina. Induction of bone tissue and osteogenic progenitor cells. [in Russian] Moscow: Medicine, 1973. 224 pages.

Friedman M.S., Oyserman S.M., Hankenson K.D. Wnt11 promotes osteoblast maturation and mineralization through R-spondiN 2. // J.Biol.Chem. – 2009. – vol. 284, N 21. – P. 14117–14125.

Frübeck G. Intracellular signaling pathways activated by leptin. // Biochem.J. – 2006. – vol. 393. – P. 7–20.

Frutos C.A.de, Dacquin R., Vega S. et al. Snail1 controls bone mass by regulating Runx2 and VDR expression during osteoblast differentiation. // EMBO J. – 2009. – vol. 28, N 6. – P. 686–696.

Fubini S.L., Todhunter R.J., Burton-Wurster N. et al. Corticosteroids alter the differentiation phenotype of articular chondrocytes. // J.Orthop.Res. – 2001. – vol. 19. – P. 688–695.

Fuchs S., Rolauffs B., Amdt S. et al. CD44 and the isoforms CD44v5 and CD44v6 in the synovial fluid of the osteoarthritic human knee joint. // Osteoarthritis Cartilage. – 2003. – vol. 11, N 6. – P. 839–844.

Fujimaki R., Toyama Y., Hozumi N., Tezuka K. Involvement of Notch signaling in initiation of prechondrogenic condensation and nodule formation in micromass culture. // J.Bone Miner.Metab. – 2006. – vol. 24. – P. 191–198.

Fujimura T., Moriwaki S., Imokawa G., Takema Y. Crucial role of fibroblast integrins alpha2 and beta1 in maintaining structure and mechanical properties of the skin. // J.Dermatol.Sci. – 2007. – vol. 45, N 1. – P. 45–53.

Fujisawa T., Hattori T., Ono M. et al. CCN family 2/connective tissue growth factor (CCN2/CTGF) stimulates proliferation and differentiation of auricular chondrocytes. // Osteoarthritis Cartilage. – 2008. – vol. 16, N 7. – P. 782–795.

Fujita T., Fukuyama R., Izumo N. et al. Transactivation of core binding factor α1 as a basic mechanism to trigger parathyroid hormone-induced osteogenesis. // Jpn.J.Pharmacol. – 2001. – vol. 86. – P. 405–416

Fukai N., Apte S.S., Olsen B.R. Nonfibrillar collagen. // Methods in Enzymology. – 1994. – vol. 245. Extracellular matrix components (Ruoslahti E., Engvall E., edit.). – P. 3–28.

Fukumoto S. The role of bone in phosphate metabolism. // Mol.Cell. Endocrinol. – 2009. – vol. 310, N 1–2. – P. 63–70.

Fukumoto S., Iwamoto T., Sakai E. et al. Current topics in pharmacological research on bone metabolism: osteoclast differentiation regulated by glycosphingolipids. // J.Pharmacol.Sci. – 2006. – vol. 100. – P. 195–200.

Fukushi J., Inatani M., Yamaguchi Y., Stallcup W.B. Expression of NG2 proteoglycan during endochondral and intramembranous ossification. // Dev.Dyn. – 2003. – vol. 228, N 1. – P. 143–148.

Fukushima H., Nakao A., Okamoto F. et al. The association of Notch2 and NF-kB accelerates RANKL-induced osteoclastogenesis. // Mol.Cell.Biol. – 2008. – vol. 28, N 20. – P. 6402–6412.

Fukushima N., Hanada R., Teranishi H. et al. Ghrelin directly regulates bone formation. // J.Bone Miner.Res. – 2005. – vol. 20, N 5. – P. 790–798.

Fuller G.M., Shield D. Molecular Basis of Medical Cell Biology. Stamford, Connecticut, Appleton & Lange, 1998

Fullmer H.M. Differential staining of connective tissue fibers in areas of stress // Science 1960. – vol. 127. – P. 240.

Fullmer H.M., Lillie R.D. The oxytalan fiber: a previously undescribed connective tissue fiber // J. Histochem. Cytochem. – 1958. – vol. 6. – P. 425.

Funari V.A., Day A., Krakow D. et al. Cartilage-selective genes identified in genome-scale analysis of non-cartilage and cartilage gene expression. // BMC Genomics. – 2007. – vol. 8. – P. 165.

Funato N, Moriyama K, Shimokawa H, Kuroda T. Basic fibroblast growth factor induces apoptosis in myofibroblastic cells isolated from rat palatal mucosa. // Biochem Biophys Res Commun. – 1997. – V. 240. – P. 21–26.

Furlan S., La Penna G., Perico A., Cesaro A. Hyaluronan chain conformation and dynamics. // Carbohydr.Res. – 2005. – vol. 340, N 5. – P. 959–970.

Furumatsu T., Tsuda M., Yoshida K. et al. Sox 9 and p300 cooperatively regulate chromatin-mediated transcription. // J.Biol.Chem. – 2005. – vol. 280, N 42. – P. 35203–35208.

Furuya K., Nifuji A., Rosen V., Noda M. Effects of GDF7/BMP12 on proliferation and alkaline phosphatase expression in rat osteoblastic osteosarcoma ROS 17/2.8 cells. // J.Cell.Biochem. – 1999. – vol. 72, N 2. – P. 177–180.

Gabbiani G. Evolution and clinical implications of the myofibroblast concept. // Cardiovasc. Res. 1998. vol. 38 – P. 545–548

Gabbiani G. Modulation of fibroblastic cytoskeletal features during wound healing and fibrosis. // Pathol.Res. Pract. – 1994. – V. 190. – P.: 851–853.

Gabbiani G. The biology of the myofibroblast. // Kidney Int. – 1992. – vol. 41. – P. 530–532.

Gabbiani G. The myofibroblast in wound healing and fibrocontractive diseases. // J. Pathol. – 2003. – vol. 200. – P. 500–503.

Gabbiani G., Badonnel M.C. Contractile events during inflammation. // Agents Actions. – 1976. – vol. 6. – P.:277–280.

Gabbiani G., Ryan G.B., Majne G. Presence of modified fibroblasts in granulation tissue and their possible role in wound contraction. // Experientia. – 1971. – vol. 27. – P. 549–550.

Gadue P., Huber T.L., Paddison P.J., Keller G.M. Wnt and TGF-β signaling are required for the induction of an in vitro model of primitive streak formation using embryonic stem cells. // Proc.Natl.Acad. Sci.USA. – 2006. – vol. 103, N 45. – P. 16806–16811.

Gale L.R., Chen W., Hills B.A., Crawford R. Boundary lubrication of joints. Characterization of surface active phospholipids found on retrived implants. // Acta Orthopaed. – 2007. – vol. 78. – № 3. P. 309–314.

Galera P., Park R.W., Ducy P. et al. c-Krox binds to several sites in the promoter of both mouse type I collagen genes. // J.Biol.Chem. – 1996. – vol. 271, N 35. – P. 21331–21339.

Gallet A., Rodriguez R., Ruel L., Therond P.P. Cholesterol modification of Hedgehog is required for trafficking and movement, revealing an asymmetric cellular response to Hedgehog. // Development. – 2003. – vol. 4. – P. 191–204.

Gallet A., Staccini-Lavenant L., Therond P.P. Cellular trafficking of the glypican Dally-like is required for full-strength hedgehog signaling and wingless transcytosis. // Dev.Cell. – 2008. – vol. 14, N 5. – P. 712–725

Galli S.J. New concepts about the mast cell. // N.Engl.J. Med. – 1993. – vol. 328. – P. 257–265.

Galli S.J., Maurer M., Lantz C.S. Mast cells as sentinels of innate immunity. // Curr.Opin. Immunol. – 1999. – vol. 11, N 1. P. 53–59.

Galli S.J., Nakae S., Tsai M. Mast cells in the development of adaptive immune responses. // Nat. Immunol. – 2005. vol. 6, N 2. – P. 135–42.

Galliford T.M., Murphy E., Williams A.J. et al. Effects of thyroid status on bone metabolism: a primary role for thyroid stimulating hormone or thyroid hormone // Minerva Endocrinol. – 2005. – vol. 30, N 4. – P. 237–246.

Gamer L.W., Ho V., Cox K., Rosen V. Expression and function by BMP-3 during chick limb development. // Dev.Dyn. – 2008. – vol. 237, N 6. – P1691–1698.

Gan O.,Yoshida T., Li J., Owens G.K. Smooth muscle cells and myofibroblasts use distinct transcriptional mechanisms for smooth muscle alpha-actin expression. // Circ.Res. – 2007. – vol. 101, N 9. – P. 883–892.

Gañan Y., Macias D., Basco R.D. et al. Morphological diversity of the avian foot is related with the pattern of msx gene expression in the developing autopod. // Dev.Biol. – 1998. – vol. 196, N 1. – P. 33–41

Ganss B., Jheon A. Zinc finger transcription factors in skeletal development. // Crit.Rev.Oral Biol. – 2004. – vol. 15 – № 5. – P. 282–297.

Gao G., Westling J., Thompson V.P. et al. Activation of proteolytic activity of ADAMTS4 (aggrecanase-1) by C-terminal truncation. // J.Biol.Chem. – 2002. – vol. 277, N 13. – P. 11034–11041.

Gao Y., Grassi F., Ryan M.R. et al. IFN-γ stimulates osteoclast formation and bone loss in vivo via antigen-driven T cell activation. // J.Clin.Invest. – 2007. – vol. 117, N 1. – P. 122–132.

Gao Y., Jheon A., Nourkeyhani H. et al. Molecular cloning, structure, expression, and chromosomal localization of the human Osterix (SP7) gene. // Gene. – 2004. – vol. 341. – P. 101–110.

Garciadiego-Cázares D., Rosales C., Katoh M., Chimal-Monroy J. Coordination of chondrocyte differentiation and joint formation be α5β1 integrin in the developing appendicular skeletpn. // Development. – 2004. – vol. 131. – P. 4735–4742.

Garcia-Fernandez J. The genesis and evolution of homeobox gene clusters. // Nat.Rev.Genet. – 2005. – vol. 6. – P. 881–892.

Garimella R., Tague S.E., Zhang J. et al. Expression and synthesis of bone morphogenetic proteins by osteoclasts: a possible path to anabolic bone remodeling. // J.Histochem.Cytochem. – 2008. – vol. 56, N 6. – 569–577.

Garnero P., Piperno M., Gineyts E. et al. Cross sectional evaluation of biochemical markers of bone, cartilage, and synovial tissue metabolism in patients with knee osteoarthritis: relation with disease activity and joint damage. /. Ann.Rheum.Dis. – 2001. – vol. 40, N 6. – P. 619–626.

Gaur T., Lengner C.J., Hovhannisyan H. et al. Canonical WNT signaling promotes osteogenesis by directly stimulating Runx2 gene expression. // J.Biol.Chem. – 2005. – vol. 280, N 39. – P. 33132–33140.

Gay S., Miller E.J. Collagen in the physiology and pathology of connective tissue, //Stuttgart-New York. Gustav Fischer Verl. 1978.

Gazzerro E., Canalis E. Bone morphogenetic proteins and their antagonists. // Rev.Endocr.Metab.Disord. – 2006. – vol. 7. – P. 51–65.

Ge C., Xiao G., Jiang D., Franceschi R.T. Critical role of the the extracellular signal-regulated rinase – MAPK pathway in osteoblast differentiation and skeletal development. // J.Cell Biol. – 2007. – vol. 176, N 5. – P. 709–718.

Geiger B., Bershadsky A., Pankov R., Yamada K.M. Transmembrane extracellular matrix-cytoskeleton crosstalk. // Nat.Rev.Mol.Cell Biol. – 2001. – vol. 2. – P. 793–805.

Geng H., Carlsen S., Nandakumar K.S. et al. Cartilage oligomeric matrix protein deficiency promotes early onset and the chronic development of collagen-induced arthritis. // Arthritis Res.Ther. – 2008. – vol. 10. – P. R134.

Geng Y., McQuillan D., Roughley P.J. SLRP interaction can protect collagen fibrils from cleavage by collagenases. // Matrix Biol. – 2006. – vol. 25, N 8. – P. 484–491.

Gennari L., Nuti R., Bilezikian J.P. Aromatase activity and bone homeostasis in men. // J.Clin.Endocrinol. – 2004. – vol. 89, N 12. – P. 5898–5907.

George A., Hao J. Role of phosphophoryn in dentin mineralization. // Cells Tissues Organs. – 2005. – vol. 181. – P. 232–240.

Gerecke D.R., Foley J.W., Castagnola P. et al. Type XIV collagen is encoded by alternative transcripts with distinct 5' regions and is a multidomain protein with homologies to von Willebrand's factor, fibronectin, and other matrix proteins. // J.Biol.Chem. – 1993. – vol. 268, N 16. – P. 12177–12184.

Gerke V., Creutz C.E., Moss S.E. Annexins: linking Ca2+ signalling to membrane dynamics. // Nat.Rev.Mol.Cell Biol. – 2005. – vol. 6. – P. 449–461.

Gersch R.P., Lombardo F., McGovern S.C., Hadjiargyrou M. Reactivation of Hox gene expression during bone regeneration. // J.Orthop. Res. – 2005. – vol. 24, N 4. – P. 882–890.

Gersdorff N., Müller M., Otto S. et al. Basement membrane composition in the early mouse embryo day 7. // Dev.Dyn. – vol. 233, N 3. – P. 1140–1148.

Gersdorff N., Müller M., Schall A., Miosge N. Secreted modular calcium-binding protein-1 localization during mouse embryogenesis. // Histochem.Cell Biol. – 2006. – vol. 126, N 6. – P. 705–712.

Ghadially F.N., Lalonde J.M.A., Long M.K. Ultrastructure of amianthoid fibers in os¬teoarthritic cartilage. // Virchow Arch. Cell Path. 1979. vol. 31. P. 81–86.

Ghosh A.K. Factors involved in the regulation of type I collagen gene expression: Implication in fibrosis. // Exp.Biol.Med. – 2002. – vol. 227, N 5. – P. 301–314.

Gibson P.G., Allen C.J., Yang J.P. et al. Intraepithelial mast cells in allergic and nonallergic asthma. Assessment using bronchial brushings. // Am.Rev. Respir.Dis. – 1993. – vol. 148, N 1. – P. 80–86.

Gieseking R. Elektronenmikrospischen Benbachtungen zur Anordnung der Kollagen-Elementarfibrillen in der Sehnenfaser. // Z. Zellforsch. – 1962. – Bd. 58. – S.160.

Gill M.R., Oldberg A., Reinholt F.P. Fibromodulin-null murine knee jointdisplay increased incidence of osteoarthritis and alterations in tissue biochemistry. // Osteoarthritis Cartilage. – 2002. – vol. 10, N 10. – P. 751–757.

Gimble J.M., Zvonic S., Floyd Z.E. et al. Playing with bone and fat. // J.Cell.Biochem. – 2006. – vol. 98. N 2. – P. 251–286.

Gingery A., Bradley E.W., Pederson L. et al. TGF-beta coordinately activates TAK1/MEK/AKT/NFkB and SMAD pathways to promote osteoclast survival. // Exp.Cell Res. – 2008. – vol. 314, N 15. – P. 725–738.

Giudici C., Raynal N., Wiedemann H, et al. Mapping of SPARC/BM-40/osteonectin binding sites on fibrillar collagens. // J.Biol.Chem. – 2008. – vol. 283, N 28. – P. 19551–19560.

Giustina A., Mazziotti G., Canalis E. Growth hormone, insulin-like growth factors, and the skeleton. // Endocrine Rev. – 2009. – vol.29, N 5. – P. 535–559.

Glade M.J., Kanwar Y.S., Stern P.H. Insulin and thyroid hormone stimulate matrix metabolism in primary cultures of articular chondrocytes from young rabbit independently and in combination. // Connect.Tissue Res. – 1994. – vol. 11, N 1. – P. 37–44.

Glass D.A. II, Bialek P., Aho J.D. Canonical Wnt signaling in differentiated osteoblasts controls osteoclast differentiation. // Dev.Cell. – 2005. – vol. 6., P. 751–764.

Gleghorn J.P., Jones A.R.C., Hannen C.R., Bonassar L.J. Boundary mode lubrication of articular cartilage by recombinant human lubricin. // J.Orthop.Res. – 2009. – vol. 27, N 6. – P. 771–777.

Glimcher M.J. Bone: nature of the calcium phosphate crystals and cellular, structural, and physical chemical mechanisms in their formation. // Rev.Mineral.Geochem. – 2006. – vol. 64. – P. 223–283.

Globus R.K., Doty S.B., Lull J.C. et al. Fibronectin is a survival factor for differentiated osteoblasts. // J.Cell Sci. – 1998. – vol. 111. – P. 1385–1393.

Gobezie R., Kho A., Krastins B. et al. High abundance synovial fluid proteome: distinct profiles in health and osteoarthritis. // Arthritis Res.Ther. – 2007. – vol. 9. – P.R36.

Goebel S., Lienau J., Rammoser U. et al. FGF23 is a putative marker for bone healing and regeneration. // J.Orthop.Res. – 2009. – Epub. Feb.12.

Goessler U.R., Bugert P., Bieback K. et al. Expression of collagen and fiber-associated proteins in human septal cartilage during in vitro dedifferentiation. // Int.J.Mol.Med. – 2004. – vol. 14, N 6. – P. 1015–1022.

Goessler U.R., Bugert P., Bieback K. et al. In-vitro analysis of the expression of TGFβ-superfamily-members during chondrogenic differentiation of mesenchymal stem cells and chondrocytes during dedifferentiation in cell culture. // Cell.Mol.Biol.Lett. – 2005. – vol. 10. – P. 343–362.

Goessler U.R., Bugert P., Bieback K. et al. Invitro-analysis of integrinexpression in stem-cells from bone marrow and cord blood during chondrogenic differentiation. // J.Cell.Mol.Med. – 2008. – Epub Aug.4.

Gokel J.M., Hubner G. Occurrence of myofibroblasts in the different phases of morbus Dupuytren (Dupuytren's contracture). // Beitr.Pathol. – 1977. – Bd.161. – S.166–175.

Goldbeter A., Pourquié O. Modeling the segmentation clock as a network of coupled oscillations in the Notch, Wnt and FGF signaling pathways. // J.Theor.Biol. – 2008. – vol. 252. – P. 574–585.

Goldring M.B., Berenbaum F. The regulation of chondrocyte function by proinflammatory mediators. Prostaglandins and nitric oxide. // Clin.Orthop. – 2004. – 427 Suppl. – P.S37–S46.

Goldring M.B., Tsuchimochi K., Ijiri K. The control of chondrogenesis. // J.Cell.Biochem. – 2006. – vol. 97. – P. 33–44.

Gomes jr.R.R., Farachi-Carson M.C., Carson D.D. Perlecan functions in chondrogenesis: insights from in vitro and in vivo models. // Cells Tissues Organs. – 2004. – vol. 176, N 1/3. – P. 79–86.

Gomperts B.N., Strieter R.M. Fibrocytes in lung diseases. // J.Leukoc. Biol. – 2007. – vol. 82, N 3. – P. 449–456.

Goodison S., Urquidi V., Tarin D. CD44 cell adhesion molecules. // J.Clin.Pathol.Med.Pathol. – 1999. – vol. 52. – P. 189–199

Gordeladze J.O., Drevon C.A., Syversen U., Reseland J.R. Leptin stimulates human osteoblastic cell proliferation, de novo collagen synthesis, and mineralization: impact on differentiation markers, apoptosis, and osteoclastic signaling. // J.Cell.Biochem. – 2002. – vol. 85, N 4. – P. 825–836.

Gordeladze J.O., Reseland J.E., Drevon C.A. Pharmacological interference with transcriptional control of osteoblasts: a possible role for leptin and fatty acids in maintaining bone strength and body lean mass. // Curr.Pharmacol.Design. – 2001. – vol. 7. – P. 275–291.

Gordon J.S., Lash J.W. In vitro chondrogenesis and cell viability. // Dev.Biol. – 1974. – vol. 36. P. 88–104.

Gordon M.D., Nusse R. Wnt signaling: Multiple pathways, multiple receptors, and multiple transcription factors. // J.Biol.Chem. – 2006. – vol. 281, N 32. – P. 22429–22433.

Gori F., Divieti P., Demay M.B. Cloning and characterization of a novel WD-40 repeat protein that dramatically accelerates osteoblast differentiation. // J.Biol.Chem. – 2001. – vol. 276, N 49. – P. 46515–46522.

Gori F., Friedman L.G., Demay M.B. Wdr5, a WD-40 protein, regulates osteoblast differentiation during embryonic bone development. // Dev.Biol. – 2006. – vol. 295, N 2. – P. 498–506.

Gori F., Schipani E., Demay M.B. Fibromodulin is expressed by both chondrocytes and osteoblasts during fetal bone osteogenesis. // J.Cell.Biochem. – 2001. – vol. 82, N 1. – P. 46–57.

Gorski J.P. Acidic phosphoproteins from bone matrix: a structural rationalization of their role in biomineralization. // Calc.Tissue Int. – 1992. – vol. 50, N 4. – P. 391–396.

Gorski J.P., Wang A., Lovitch D. et al. Extracellular bone acidic glycoprotein-75 defines condensed mesenchyme regions to be niberalized and localizes withbone sialoprotein during intramembranous bone formation. // J.Biol.Chem. – 2004. – vol. 279, N 24. – P. 25455–25463.

Gosline J. The physical properties of elastic tissue // Int. Rev. connect. Tissue Res. New York. – 1976. – vol. 7. – P. 211–249.

Goto T., Yamaza T., Tanaka T. Cathepsins in the osteoclast. // J.Electron Microscopy. – 2003. – vol. 52, N 6. – P.551–558.

Gotte L., Volpin D. The ultrastructural organization of elastin. // Proc. 22nd colloq. Brugge 1974 (II. Peeter, edit). New York, Pergamon Press, Oxford, 1974.

Govoni K.E., Baylink D.J., Chen J., Mohan S. Dosruption of Four-and-a half LIM2 decreases bone mineral content and bone mineral density in femur and tibia bones of female mice. // Calcif.Tissue Int. – 2006. – vol. 79, N 1. – P. 112–117.

Govoni K.E., Linares G.R., Chen S.T. et al. T-box 3 negatively regulates osteoblast differentiation by inhibiting expression of osterix and runx2. // J.Cell.Biochem. – 2009. – vol. 106, N 3. – P. 482–490.

Gowen L.C., Petersen D.N., Mansolf A.L. et al. Targeted disruption of the osteoblast/osteocyte factor 45 gene (OF45) results in increased bone formation and bone mass. // J.Biol.Chem. – 2003. – vol. 278, N 3. – P. 1998–2003.

Granemann J.H., Moore H.P.H. Location, location: protein trafficking and lipolysis in adipocytes. // Trends Endocrin.Metab. – 2008. – vol. 19, N 1. – P. 3–9.

Grasser W.A., Orlic I., Borovecki F. BMP-6 exerts its osteoinductive effect through activation of IGF-1 and EGF pathways. // Int.Orthop. – Epub. 19 Jul. 2007.

Green K.J., Jones J.C.R. Desmosomes and hemidesmosomes: structure and function molecular components. // FASEB J. – 1996. – V. 10. – P. 871.

Gregg S.J., Sing K.S.W. Adsorption, Surface Area and Porosity. 2nd ed., ACADEMIC PRESS, 1982. – 304 p.

Gregoire F.M. Adipocyte differentiation: from fibroblast to endocrine cell. // Exp.Biol.Med. – 2001. – vol. 226, N 11. – P. 997–1002.

Gregoire F.M., Smas C.M., Sul H.S. Understanding adipocyte differentiation. // Physiol.Rev. – 1998. – vol. 78, N 3. – P. 783–809.

Gregory J.D. Structure and aggregation of proteoglycans of cartilage // Proteides of biological fluids (Peetrs H., edit.). New York, Pergamon Press. Oxford. – 1974. – P. 321–328.

Gren B., Stoltze K., Anderson A., Dabelsteen E. Oral fibroblasts produce more HGF and KGF than skin fibroblasts in response to co-culture with keratocytes. // APMIS. – 2002. – vol. 110, N 12. – P. 292–298.

Gridley T. The long and short of it: somite formation in mice. // Dev.Dyn. – 2006. – vol. 235. – P. 2330–2336.

Grigolo B., Lisignoli G., Piacentini A. et al. Evidence for redifferentiation of human chondrocytes grown on a hyaluronan-based biomaterial (HYAff11): molecular, immunohistochemical and ultrastructural analysis. // Biomaterails. – 2001. – vol. 23, N 4. – P. 1187–1195.

Grimaud C., Nègre N., Cavalli G. From genetics to epigenetics: the tale of Polycomb group and trithorax group genes. // Chromosome Res. – 2006. – vol. 14. – P. 363–375.

Grimaud C.D., Romano P.K., D'Souza M. et al. BMP-6 is an autocrine stimulator of chondrocyte differentiation. // J.Bone Miner.Res. – 1999. – vol. 14, N 4. – P. 475–482.

Grinnell F. Fibroblasts, myofibroblasts, and wound contraction. // J Cell Biol. – 1994. – V. 124: – P. 401–404.

Gross J. Electron microscope studies of sodium hyaluronate // J.Biol. Chem. – 1948. – vol. 172. – P. 511.

Grossmann J. Molecular mechanism of "detachment-induced apoptosis – anoikis". // Apoptosis. – 2002. – vol. 7, N 2. – P. 247–260.

Gu G., Mulari M., Peng Z. et al. Death of osteocytes turns off the inhibition of osteoclasts and triggers local bone resorption. // Biochem. Biophys.Res.Commun. – 2005. – vol. 335, N 4. – P. 1095–1101.

Gu J., Taniguchi N. Regulation of integrin functions by N-glycans. // Glycocoj.J. – 2004. – vol. 21, N 1–2. – P. 9–15

Guerreiro P.M., Renfro J.L., Power D.M., Canario A.V. The parathyroid hormone family of peptides: structure, tissue distribution, regulation, and potential functional roles in calcium and phosphate metabolism in fish. // Am.J.Physiol.Integr.Comp.Physiol. – 2007. – vol 292, N 2. – P.R679–R696.

Guilak F., Alexopoulos L.G., Upton M. et al. The pericellular matrix as a transducer of bio¬mechanical and biochemical signals. // Ann. N.Y. Acad. Sci. 2006. vol. 1068. P. 498–512.

Guilmette R.A., Hakimi R., Durbin P.W. et al. Competitive binding of Pu and Am with bone mineral and novel chelating agents. // Radiat.Prot.Dosimetry. – 2003. – vol. 105, # 1–4. – P. 527–534.

Guimont P., Grondin F., Dubois C.M. Sox9-dependent transcriptional trgulation of the proprotein convertase furin. // Am.J.Physiol. Cell Physiol. – 2007. –vol.293, N 1. – P.C172–C173.

Günther T., Poli C., Müller J.M. et al. Fhl2 deficiency results in osteopenia due to decreased activity of osteoblasts. // EMBO J. – 2005. – vol. 24. – P. 3049–3056.

Guo J., Chung U.I., Yang D. PTH/PTHrP receptor delays chondrocyte hypertrophy via both Runx2-dependent and –independent pathways. // Dev.Biol. – 2006. – vol. 292, N 1. – P. 116–128.

Guo Q., Li J.Y.H. Distinct functions of the major Fgf8 spliceform, Fgf8b, before and during mouse gastrulation. // Development. – 2007. – vol. 134. – P. 2251–2260.

Guo X., Day T.F., Jiang X. et al. Wnt/β-catenin signaling is sufficient and necessary for synovial joint formation. // Genes Dev. – 2004. – vol. 18. – P. 2404–2417.

Gurlek A., Pittelkow M.R., Kumar R. Modulation of growth factor/cytokine synthesis and signaling by 1α,25(OH)2-dihydroxyvitamin D3: implications in cell growth and differentiation. // Endocrin. Rev. – 2002. – vol. 23, N 6. – P. 763–796.

Guschina Yu.Yu., Plokhov P.A. and A.V. Zeveke. Investigation of effects of proteoglycan hydration, pH and modulators on the morphology of collagen fibrils and subfibers. [in Russian] //Vestnik of Lobachevsky State University of Nizhny Novgorod, 2007, no. 1. P. 114–119.

Gustafsson E., Fässler R. Insights into extracellular matrix functions from mutant mouse model. // Exp.Cell.Res. – 2000. – vol. 261, N 1. – P. 52–68.

Haag J., Aigner T. Identification of calponiN 3 as a novel Smad-binding modulator of BMP signaling expressed in cartilage. // Exp.Cell Res. – 2007. – vol. 313. – P.P. 3386–3394.

Haas A.R., Tuan R.S. Chondrogenic differentiation of murine C3H10T1/2 multipotential mesenchymal cells. II. Stimulation by bone morphogenetic protein-2 requires modulation of N-cadherin expression and function. // Differentiation. – 1999. – vol. 64, N 2. – P. 77–89.

Habuchi H., Habuchi O., Kimata K. Sulfation pattern in glycosaminoglycans: does it have a code? // Glycoconj.J. – 2004. vol. 21, N 1–2. – P. 47–52.

Hadjantonakis A.K., Pisano E., Papaioannu V.E. Tbx6 regulates left/right patterning in mouse embryos through effects on nodal cilia and prinodal signaling// PLoS ONE. – 2008. – vol. 3, N 6. – P.e2511.

Haegel H., Larue L., Ohaugi M. et al. Lack of β-catenin affects mouse development at gastrulation. // Development. – 1995. – vol. 121. – P. 3429–3537.

Hafizi S., Dahlbäck B. Gas6 and protein S. Vitamin K-dependent ligfands for the Axl receptor tyrosine kinase subfamily. // FEBS J. – 2006. – vol. 273. – P. 5231–5244.

Halbrooks P.J., Ding R., Wozney Y.M., Rain G. Role of RGM coreceptors in bone morphogenetic protein signaling. // J.Mol.Signal. – 2007. – P. 2–4.

Hall B.K. Earliest evidence of cartilage and vone development in embryonic life. // Clin.Orthop. – 1088. – N 225. – P. 255–272.

Hall B.K., Miyake T. All for one and one for all: cell condensations and the initiation of skeletal development. // Bioessays. – 2000. – vol. 22, N 2. – P. 138–147.

Hall, S. E., J. S. Pavill, P. M. Henson, C. Haslett. Apoptotic neutrophils are phagocytosed by fibroblast with participation of fibroblast vitronectin receptor and involvement of

Halleen J.M., Tiitinen S.L., Ylipahkala H. et al. Tartrate-resistant acid phosphatase 5b (TRACP5b) as a marker of bone resorption. // Clin.Lab. – 2006. – vol.52, N 9–10. – P.499–509.

Hallmans R., Horn N., Selg M. et al. Expression and function of laminins in the embryonic and mature vasculature. // Physiol. Rev. – 2005. – vol. 85, N 3. – P. 979–1000.

Hallösz K., Kassner A., Mörgelin M. et al. COMP acts as a catalyst in collagen fibrillogenesis. // J.Biol.Chem. – 2007, Aug.22. M705735200.

Hamidouche Z., Hay E., Vaudin P. et al. FHL2 mediates dexamethasone-induced mesenchymal cell differentiation into osteoblasts by activated Wnt/Beta-catenin signaling-dependent Runx2 expression. // FASEB J. – 2008. – vol. 22, N 11. – P. 3813–3822.

Hamrick M.W., Ferrari S.L. Leptin and the sympathetic connection of fat to bone. // Osteoporosis Int. – 2008. – vol. 19, N 7. – P. 905–912

Han M.S., Kim J.E., Shin H.I., Kim I.S. Expression patterns of βig-h3 in chondrocyte differentiation during endochondral ossificxation. // Exp.Mol.Med. – 2008. – vol.40, N 4. – 453–460.

Han X., Amar S. Identification of genes differentially expressed in cultured human periodontal ligament fibroblasts vs. gingival fibroblasts by DNA microarray analysis. // J.Dent.Res. – 2002. – vol. 81, N 6. – P.399–405.

Han X., Bolcato A.L., Amar.S. Identification of genes differentially expressed in cultured human osteoblasts versus human fibroblasts by DNA microarray analysis. // Connect.Tissue Res. – 2002. – vol.43, N 1. – P.63–75.

Handford P.A. Fibrillin-1: a calcium binding protein of extracellular matrix. // Biochim. Biophys. Acta. – 2000. – vol. 1498, N 2/3. – P.84–90.

Hankenson K.D., Ausk B.J., Bain S.D. et al. Mice lacking thrombospondoN 2 show an atypical pattern of endocortical and periosteal bone formation in response to mechanical loading. // Bone. – 2006. – vol.38. – P.310–316.

Hansen J.B., Jørgensen C., Petersen R.K. et al. Retinoblastoma protein functions as a molecular switch determining white versus brown adipocyte differentiation. // Proc.Natl.Acad.Sci.USA. – 2004. – vol. 101, N 12. – P.6172–6174.

Hansen U., Bruckner P. Macromolecular specificity of collagen fibrillogenesis. Fibrils of collagens I and XI contain a heterotypic alloyed core and a collagen I sheath. // J.Biol.Chem. – 2003. – vol. 278, N 39. – P.37352–37359.

Hansen U., Bruckner P. Macromolecular specificity of collagen fibrillogenesis: fibrils of collagen I and XI contain a heterotypic alloyed core and a collagen I sheath. // J.Biol.Chem. – 2003. – vol. 279, N 39. – P.37352–37359.

Hansson GK, Hellstrand M, Rymo L et al. – Interferon gamma inhibits both proliferation and expression of differentiation-specific alpha-smooth muscle actin in arterial smooth muscle cells. // J Exp.M.ed. – 1989. – vol. 170. – P. 1595–1608.

Harada S.I., Rodan G.A. Control of osteoblast function and regulation of bone mass. // Nature. – 2003. – vol.423, N 6937. – P. 349–355.

Hardingham T.E., Fosang A. The structure of aggrecan and its turnover in cartilage. // J.Rheumatol – 1995. – voil.23, Suppl.1. – P.86–90.

Haremaki T., Fraser S.T., Kuo Y.M. et al. Vertebrate Ctr1 coordinates morphogenesis and progenitor cell fate and regulates embryonic stem cell differentiation. // Proc.Natl.Acad.Sci.USA. – 2007. – vol.104, N 29. – P. 12029–12034.

Harnett M. Antigen receptor signalling: from the membrane to the nucleus // Immunology Today. – 1994.– vol. 15. – P. 15.

Harney D., Hessle L., Narisawa S. et al. Concerted regulation of of inorganic pyrophosphate and osteopontin by Akp2, Enpp1. and Ank. // Am.J.Pathol. – 2004. – vol. 164, N 4. – P. 1199–1209.

Harst M.R.van der, Brama P.A.J., Lest C.H.A.van der et al. An integral biochemical analysis of the main constituents of articular cartilage, subchondral and trabecular bone. // Osteoarthritis Cartilage. – 2004. – vol. 12. – P. 752–761.

Hartmann C. Skeletal development – Wnts are in cintrol. // Mol.Cell. – 2007. – vol. 24, N 2. – P. 177–184.

Hartmann C., Tabin C.J. Wnt-14 plays a pivotal role in inducing synovial joint formation in the developing appendicular skeleton. // Cell. – 2001. – vol. 104. – P. 341–351.

Hartung A., Bitton-Worms K., Rechtman M.M. et al. Different routes of bone morphogenetic protein (BMP) receptor endocytosis influence BMP signaling. //Mol.Cell.Biol. – 2006. – vol. 26, N 20. – P. 7791–7805.

Hascall V.C., Laurent T.C. Hyaluronan structure and physical properties. //1998. – http:/www.glycoforum.gr.jp

Hasegawa K., Yoneda M., Kuwabara H. et al. Versican, a major hyaluronan-binding component of the dermis, loses its hyaluronan-binding activity in solar elastosis. // J.Invest.Dermatol. – 2007. – vol. 127, N 7. – P. 1657–1663.

Hashimoto K., Di Bella R.J. Electron microscopic studies of normal and abnormal elastic fibers of the skin // J. Invest. Derm. – 1967. – vol. 48, N 5. – P. 405–423

Hashimoto M., Nakasa T., Hikata T., Asabara H. Molecular network of cartilage homeostasis and osteoarthritis. // Med.Res.Rev. – 2007. – Epub. SeP. 19

Hassan M., Tare R.S., Lee S.H. et al. BMP2 commitment to the osteogenic lineage involves activation of Runx2 by DLX3 and a homeodomain transcriptional network. // J.Biol.Chem. – 2006. – vol. 281, N 52. – P. 40515–40526.

Hassan M.Q., Saini S., Gordon J.A. et al. Molecular switches including homeodomain proteins, Hoxa10 and Runx2 domain proteins regulate osteoblastogenesis. // Cells, Tissues, Organs. – 2009. – vol. 189, N 1–4. – P. 122–125.

Hatta M., Yoshimura Y., Deyama Y. et al. Molecular characterization of the zinc finger transcription factor Osterix. // Int.J.Mol.Med. – 2006. – vol. 17. – P. 425–430.

Hattori T., Coustry F., Stephens S. et al. Transcriptional regulation of chondrogenesis by coactivator Tip60 via chromatin association with Sox9 and Sox5. // Nucleic Acid Res – 2008. – vol. 16, N 9. – P. 3011–3024.

Haudenschild D.R., Mcpherson J.M., Turo R., Binette F. Differential expression of multiple genes during articular chondrocyte redifferentiation. // Anat.Rec. – 2001. – vol. 263. – P. 91–98.

Hauser H.J., Ruegg M.A., Brenner R.E., Ksiazek I. Agrin is highly expressed by chondrocytes and is required for normal growth. // Histochem.Cell.Biol. – 2007. – vol. 127. – P. 363–374.

Hayashi M., Nimura K., Kashiwagi K. et al. Comparative roles of Twist-1 and Id1 in transcriptional regulation by BMP signaling. // J.Cell Sci. – 2007. – vol. 120. – P. 1350–1357.

Hayer B., Fagerlie S.R., Ramakrishnan A. et al. Derivation, characterization, and in vitro differentiation of canine embryonic stem cells // Stem Cells. – 2008. – vol. 26, N 2. – P. 465–473.

Hayes A.J., Dowthwaite G.P., Webster S.V., Archer C.W. The distribution of Notch receptors and their ligands during articular cartilage development. // J.Anat. – 2003. – vol. 202. – P. 495–502.

Haylock D.M., Nilsson S.K. Osteopontin: a bridge between bone and blood. // Br.J.Haematol. – 2006. – vol. 134, N5. – P. 467–474.

Hayward P., Kalmar T., Arias A.M. Wnt/Notch signaling and information processing during development. // Development. – 2008. – vol. 125. – P. 411–424.

Heaton J.M. The distribution of brown adipose tissue in the human // J. Anat. – 1972. – vol. 112, N1. – P. 105–108.

Hedlund H., Hedbom E., Heinegård D. et al. Association of the aggrecan keratin sulfate-rich region with collagen in bovine articular cartilage. // J.Biol.Chem. – 1999. – vol. 274, N9. – P. 5777–5781.

Heino T.J., Hentunen T.A., Väänänen H.K. Osteocytes inhibit osteoclastic bone resorption through transforming growth factor beta enhancement by estrogen. // J.Cell.Biochem. – 2002. – vol. 85, N1. – P. 185–197.

Henderson M., Polewski R., Fanning J.C., Gibson M.A. Microfibril-associated glycoprotein-1 (MAGP-1) is specifically located on the beads of the beaded-filament structure for fibrillin-containing microfibrils as visualized by the rotary shadowing technique. // J.Histochem.Cytochem. – 1996. – vol. 44, N12. – P. 1389–1397

Hendy G.N., Kaji H., Sowa H. et al. Menin and TGF-beta superfamily member signaling via the Smad pathway in pituitary, parathyroid and osteoblast. // Horm.Metab.Res. – 2005. – vol37, N6. – P. 375–379.

Henriksen K., Leeming D.J., Berjalsen I. et al. Osteoclasts prefer aged bone. // Osteoporosis Int. – 2007. – vol. 18. – P. 751–759.

Henrotin Y.E., Zheng S.X., Labasse A.M. et al. Modulation of human chondrocyte metabolism by recombinant human interferon. // Osteoarthritis Cartilage. – 2000. – vol. 8, N6. – P. 74–82.

Henry G., Garren W.L. Inflammatory mediators in wound healing. // Surg.Clin.N.Am. – 2003. – vol. 83, N3. – P. 483–485.

Henry L.R., Lee H.O., Lee J.S. et al. Clinical implications of fibroblast activation protein in patients with colon cancer. // Clin.Cancer Res. – 2007. – vol. 13, N6. – P. 1736

Herpin A., Cunningham C. Cross-talk between the bone morphogenetic protein pathway and other major signaling pathways results in tightly regulated cell-specific outcomes. // FEBS J. – 2007. – vol. 274. – P. 2977–2985.

Herpin A., Lelong C., Favrel P. Transforming growth factor-beta-related proteins: and ancestral and widespread superfamily of cytokines in metazoans. // Dev.Comp.Immunol. – 2004. – vol. 28, N5. – P. 1461–1485.

Hill T.P., Später D., Taketo M.M. et al. Canonical Wnt/ β-catenin signaling prevents osteoblast differentiation into chondrocytes. // Dev.Cell. – 2005. – vol. 8. – P. 727–738.

Hillman R.A., Ault K.A. Hematology in Clinical Practice. New York: McGraw-Hill, 1995, P. 304.

Hills B.A. Boundary lubrication in vivo. // Proc.Inst.Mech.Eng part H. – 2000. – vol. 214, N1. – P. 83–94.

Hills B.A., Ethell M.T., Hodgson D.B. Release of lubricating synovial surfactant by intra-articular steroid. // Br.J.Rheum. – 1998. – vol. 37. – P. 649–652.

Hills B.A., Monds M.K. Enzymatic identification of the load-bearing lubricant in the joint. // Br.J.Rheum. – 1998. – vol. 37, N3. – P. 137–142.

Hinz B., Gabbiani G. Mechanisms of force generation and transmission by myofibroblasts. // Curr.Opin.Biotechnol. – 2003. – V. 14. – P. 538–546.

Hinz B., Mastrangelo D., Iselin C.E. et al. Mechanical tension controls granulation tissue contractile activity and myofibroblast differentiation. // Am.J.Pathol. 2001. – vol. 159. – P. 1009–1020.

Hinz B., Phan S.H., Thannickal V.J. et al. The myofibroblast. One function, multiple origin. // Am.J.Pathol. – 2007. – vol. 170, N6. – P. 1807–1816.

Hirao M., Tamai N., Tsumaki N. et al. Oxygen tension regulates chondrocyte differentiation and function during endochondral ossification. // J.Biol.Chem. – 2006. – vol. 281, N41. – P. 31079–31092.

Hirao M.,, Hashimoto J., Yamasaki N. et al. Oxygen tension i san important mediator of the transformation of osteoblasts in osteocytes. // J.Bone Miner.Metab. – 2007. – vol. 25. – P. 266–276.

Hirose J., Masuda I., Ryan L.M. Expression of cartilage intermediate layer protein/nucleotide pyrophosphohydrolase parallels the production of extracellular inorganic pyrophosphate in response to growth factors and with aging. // Arthritis Rheum. – 2000. – vol. 43, N12. – 2703–2711.

Hiscock D.R., Caterson B., Flannery C.R. Expression of hyaluronan synthases in articular cartilage. // Osteoarthritis Cartilage. – 2000. – vol. 8, N2. – P. 120–126.

Hishida T., Naito K., Osada S. et al. Peg10, an imprinted gene plays a crucial role in adipocyte differentiation. // FEBS Letters. – 2007. – vol. 581, – P. 4272–4278.

Hitchcock A.M., Yates K.E., Costello C.E., Zaia J. Comparative glycomics of connective tissue glycosaminoglycans. // Proteomics. – 2008. – vol. 8, N7. – P. 1384–1397.

Hjorten R., Hansen U., Underwood R.A. et al. Type XXVII collagen at the transition of cartilage to bone during skeletogenesis. // Bone. – 2007. – vol. 41, N4. – P. 335–342.

Hock J.M., Krishnan V., Onyia J.E. et al. Osteoblast apoptosis and bone turnover. // J.Bone Miner.Res. – 2001. – vol. 16, N6. – P. 975–984.

Hodge A.J., Scmitt F.O. The charge profile of the tropocollagen macromolecule and the packing arrangement in native-type collagen fibrills. // Proc. Nat. Acad. Sci. USA. – 1960. – vol. 46. – P. 186–197.

Hoffman L.M., Garcha K., Karamboulas K. et al. BMP action in skeletogenesis involves attenuation of retinoid signalin. // J.Cell Biol. – 2006. – vol. 176, N1. – P. 101–113.

Hoffman L.M., Weston A.D., Underhill T.M. Molecular mechanisms regulating chondroblast differentiation. // J.Bone Joint Surg. – 2003. – vol. 85-A, Suppl.2. – P. 124–123.

Hoffmann A., Pelled G., Turgeman G. et al. Neotendon formation induced by manipulation of the Smad8 signaling pathway in mesenchymal stem cells. // J.Clin.Invest. – 2006. – vol. 116, N4. – P. 940–952.

Holland P.W.H., Booth H.A.F., Bruford E.A. Classification and nomenclature of all human homeobox genes. // BMC Biology. – 2007. – vol. 5. – P. 47.

Holleville N., Mateos S., Bontoux M. et al. Dlx5 drives Runx2 expression and osteogenic differentiation in developing cranial sutures. // Dev.Biol. – 2007. – vol. 394, N2. – P. 860–874.

Holmbeck K., Bianco P., Pidou I. et al. The metalloproteinase MT1-MMP is required for normal development and maintenance of osteocyte processes in bone. // J.Cell Sci. – 2005. – vol. 118, N1. – P. 147–156.

Holmen S.L., Zylatra C.R., Mukherjee A. et al. Essential role of β-catenin in postnatal bone acquisition. // J.Biol.Chem. – 2005. – vol. 280, N22. – P. 21162–21168.

Hombria J.C.G., Lovegrove B. Beyond homeosis –HOX function in morphogenesis and organogenesis. // Differentiation. – 2003. – vol. 71. – P. 461–476

Hong J.H., Hwang E.S., McManus M.T. et al. TAZ, a transcriptional modulator of mesenchymal stem cell differentiation. // Science. – 2005. – vol. 309, N.5737. – P. 1074–1078.

Hong K.M., Belperlo J.A., Keane M.P. Differentiation of human circulating fibrocytes as mediated by transforming growth factor-β and peroxisome proliferators-activated receptot γ. // J.Biol.Chem. – 2007. – vol. 282, N 31. – P. 22910–22920.

Hong Y.H., Hishikawa D., Miyahara H. et al. Up-regulation of adipogenin, an adipocyte plasma transmembrane protein, during adipogenesis,// Mol.Cell. Biochem. – 2005. – vol. 276. – P. 133–141.

Hoogendam J., Parlevliet E., Miclea R. et al. Novel early target genes of parathyroid hormone-related peptide in chondrocytes. // Endocrinology. – 2006. – vol. 147. – P. 1141–1152.

Hooper N.M. Proteases: a primer. // Essays Biochem. – 2002. – V. 38. – P. 1–8.

Hopkins D.R., Keles S., Greenspan D.S. The bone morphogenetic proteiN 1/Tolloid-like metalloproteinases. // Matrix Biol. – E-pub. 2007. May 18.

Hopyan S., Nadesan P., Yu C. et al. Dysregulation of hedhehog signaling predisposes to synovial chondromatosis. // J.Pathol. – 2005. – vol. 206, N 2. – P. 143–150.

Horikawa K., Ishimatsu K., Yoshimoto E. et al. Noise-resistant and synchronized oscilklation of the segmentation clock. // Nature. – 2006. – vol. 441, N 7094. – P. 719–723.

Horikawa O., Nakajima H., Kikuchi T. et al. Distribution of type VI collagen in chondrocyte microenvironment: study of chondron isolated from human normal and degenerative articular cartilage and cultured chondrocytes. // J.Orthop.Sci. – 2004. – vol. 9, N 1. – P. 29–36

Horiuchi K., Amizuka N., Takeshita S. et al. Identification and characterization of a novel protein, periostin, with restricted expression to periosteum and periodontal ligament and increased expression by transforming growth factor beta. // J.Bone Miner. Res. – 1999. – vol. 14, N 7. – P. 1239–1249.

Hou W.S., Li Z., Gordon R.E. et al. Cathepsin K is a critical protease in synovial fibroblast-mediated collagen degradation. // Am.J.Pathol. – 2001. – vol. 159, N 6. – P. 2167–2177.

Houston B., Stewart A.J., Farquharson C. PHOSPHO1 – a novel phosphatase specifically expressed at sites of mineralization in bone and cartilage. // Bone. – 2004. – vol. 34. – P. 629–637.

Hsia H.C., Schwarzbauer J.E. Meet the tenascins: multifunctional and mysterious. // J.Biol.Chem. – 2005. – vol. 280, N 29. – P. 26641–26644.

Hsu S.H., Noamani B., Abernethy D.E. et al. Dlx5- and Dlx6-mediated chondrogenesis: differential domain requirements for a conserved function. // Mech. Dev. – 2006. – vol. 129, N 11. P. 819–830.

Hu J.C., Athanasiou K.A. Chondrocytes from different zones exhibit characteristic differences in high density culture. // Connect.Tissue Res. – 2006. – vol. 47, N 3. – P. 133–140.

Huang G., Zhang Y., Kim B. et al. Fibronectin binds and enhances the activity of bone morphogenetic proteiN 1. // J.Biol.Chem. – 2009, Epub. – July 18.

Huang L.E., Bunn H.F. Hypoxia-inducible factor and its biomedical relevance. // J.Biol.Chem. – 2003. – vol. 279, N 22. – P. 19575–19578.

Hubmacher D., Tiedemann K., Reinhardt D.P. Fibrillins: from biogenesis of microfibrils to signaling function. // Curr.Top.Dev.Biol. – 2006. – vol. 75. – P. 93–123.

Hudson B.G., Reeders S.T., Tryggvason K. Type IV collagen: Structure, gene organization, and role in human diseases. Molecular basis of Goodpasture and Alport syndromes and diffuse leiomyomatosis. // J.Biol.Chem. – 1993. – vol. 268, N 35. – P. 28033–28038.

Hugo H., Ackland M.L., Blick T. et al. Epithelial-mesenchymal and mesenchymal epithelial transition in carcinoma progression. // J.Cell.Physiol. – 2007. – vol. 213, N 2. – P. 374–383.

Huh Y.H., Ryu J.H., Chun J.S. Regulation of type II collagen expression by histone deacetylase in articular chondrocytes. // J.Biol.Chem. – 2007. – vol. 282, N 23. – P. 17123–17131.

Huiskes R. If bone is the answer, then what is the question?// J.Anat. – 2003. – vol. 197, N 2. – P. 145–156.

Hulmes D.J.S. Building collagen molecules, fibrils, and suprafibrillar structures. // J.Struct.Biol. – 2002. – vol. 137, N 1–2. – P. 2–10.

Humphries M.J. Insight into integrin-ligand binding and activation from the first crystal structure. // Arthritis Res. – 2004. – V. 4, Suppl. 3. – P. S69–S78.

Hurle J.M., Corson G., Daniels K. et al. Elastin exhibits a distinctive temporal and spatial pattern of distribution in the developing chick limb in association with the establishment of the cartilaginous skeleton. // J.Cell Sci. – 1994. – vol. 107. – P. 2623–2634.

Hutter H., Vogel B.E., Plenefisch J.D. et al. Conservation and novelty in the evolution of cell adhesion and extracellular matrix genes. // Science. – 2000. – vol. 287, N 5455. – p. 989–994.

Hyc A., Osiecka-Iwan A., Niederla-Bielinska J., et al. Pro- and anti-inflammatory cytokines increase hyaluronan production by rat synovial membrane in vitro. // Int.J.Mol. Med. 2009. vol. 24, № 4. P. 579–585.

Hyde G., Dover S., Aszodi A. et al. Lineage tracing using matrilin-1 gene expression reveals that articular chondrocytes exist as the joint interzone forms. // Dev.Biol. – 2007. – vol. 304. – P. 825–833.

Hynes R.O. Integrins: bidirectional allosteric signaling machines. // Cell. – 2002. – vol. 110, N 6. – P. 673–687.

Hynes R.O., Zhao Q. The evolution of cell adhesion. // J.Cell Biol. – 2000. – vol. 150, N 2. – P. F89–F95.

Iimura T., Oida S., Takeda K. et al. Changes in homeobox-containing gene expression during ectopic bone formation induced by bone morphogenetic protein. // Biochem.Biophys.Res.Commun. – 1994. – vol. 201, N 2. – P. 980–987.

Iioka T., Furukawa K., Yamaguchi A. et al. P300/CBP acts as a coactivator to cartilage homeoprotein-1 (Cart1), paired-like homeoprotein, through acetylation of the conserved lysine residue adjacent to the homeodomain. // Matrix Biol. – 2003. – vol/18, N 8. – P. 1419–1429.

Ikeda F., Nishimura F., Matsubara T. et al. Critical roles of c-Jun signaling in regulation of NFAT family and RANKL-regulated osteoclast differentiation. // J.Clin.Invest. – 2004. – vol. 114, N 4. – P. 475–484.

Ikeda R., Yoshida K., Tsukahara S. The promyelotic leukemia zinc finger promotes osteoblastic differentiation of human mesenchymal stem cells as an upstream regulator of CBFA1. // J.Biol.Chem. – 2005. – vol. 280, N 9. – P. 8523–8530

Ikeda T., Kamekura S., Mabuchi A. et al. The combination of SOX5, SOX6, and SOX9 (the SOX trio) provides signals sufficient for induction of permaneny cartilage. // Arthritis Rheum. – 2004. – vol. 50, N 11. – P. 3561–3573

Imai S., Heino T.G., Hienola A. et al. Osteoclast-derived HB-GAM (pleiotrophon) is associated with bone formation and mechanical loading. // Bone. – 2009. – vol. 44, N 5. – P. 785–794.

Inada M., Wang Y., Byrne M.H. et al. Critical roles for collagenase-3 (Mmp13) in development of growth plate cartilage and in endochondral ossification. // Proc.Natl.Acad.Sci.USA. – 2004. – vol. 101, N 49. – P. 17193–17197.

Ingham P.W., McMahon A.P. Hedgehog signalling. // Genes.Devel. – 2001. – vol. 15. – P. 3058–3087.

Inoue K., Mikuni-Takagaki Y.M., Oikawa K. et al. A crucial role for matrix metalloproteinase 2 in osteocytic canalicular formation and bone metabolism. // J.Biol.Chem. – 2006. – vol. 281, N 44. – P. 33814–33824.

Iozzo R.V. Basement membrane proteoglycans: from cellar to ceiling. // Nat.Rev.Mol.Cell Biol. – 2005. – vol. 6, N 8. – P. 646–656.

Iozzo R.V. Heparan sulfate proteoglycans: intricate molecules with intriguing functions. // J.Clin.Invest. – 2001. – vol. 108, N 2. – P. 165–167.

Iozzo R.V. Matrix proteoglycans: from: from molecular design to cellular function. // Annu.Rev.Biochem. – 1998. – vol. 67. – P. 609–652.

Irie K., Ejiri S., Sakakura Y. et al. Matrix mineralzation as a trigger for osteocyte maturation. // J.Histochem.Cytochem. – 2008. – vol. 56, N 6. – P. 561–567.

Irie N., Takeda Y., Watanabe Y. et al. Bidirectional signaling through ephrinA2-EphA2 enhances osteoclastogenesis and suppresses osteoblastogenesis. // J.Biol.Chem. – 2009. – vol. 284, N 21. – P. 14637–14644.

Iruela-Araspe M.L., Liska D.J., Sage E.H., Bornstein P. Differential expression of thrombospondiN 1, 2, and 3 during murine development. // Dev.Dyn. – 2005. – vol. 197, P. 40–56.

Ishida N., Hayashi K., Hoshijima M. et al. Large scale gene expression analysis of osteoclastogenesis in vitro and elucidation of NFAT2 as a key regulator. // J.Biol.Chem. – 2002. – vol. 277, N 43. – P. 41147–41156.

Ishii M., Egen J.G., Klauschen F. et al. Sphingosine-1-phosphate mobilizes osteoclast precursors and regulates bone homeostasis. // Nature. – 2009. – vol. 458, N 7237. – P. 524–528.

Ishimatsu K., Horikawa K., Takeda H. Coupling cellular oscillators: a mechanism that maintains synchrony against developmental noise in the segmentation clock. // Dev.Dyn. – 2007. – vol. 236. – P. 1416–1421.

Isogai Z., Aspberg A., Keene D.R. et al. Versican interacts with fibrillin-1 and links extracellular microfibrils to other connective tissue network. // J.Biol.Chem. – 2002. – vol. 277, N 6. – P. 4565–4572.

Issack P.S., Helfet D.L., Lane J.M. Role of Wnr signaling in bone remodeling and repair. // HSS J. – 2008. – vol. 4. – P. 66–70.

Ivkovic S., Yoon B.S., Popoff S.N. et al. Connective tissue growth factor coordinates chondrogenesis and angiogenesis during skeletal development. // Development. – 2003. – vol. 130. – P. 2779–2791.

Iwamoto J., Takeda T., Sato Y. Effects of vitamin K2 in osteoporosis. // Curr.Pharmaceut.Des. – 2004. – vol. 10. – P. 2557–2576.

Iwamoto M., Tamamura Y., Koyama E. et al. Transcription factor ERG and joint cartilage formation during mice limb and spine skeletogenesis. // Dev.Biol. – 2007. – vol. 305, N 1. – P. 40–51.

Iwanaga T., Shikuchi M., Kitamura H. et al. Morphology and functional role of synoviocytes in the joint. // Arch.Histol.Cytol. – 2000. – vol. 63, N 1. – P. 17–31.

Iwaniec U.T., Boghossian S., Lapke P.D. et al. Central leptin gene therapy corrects skeletal abnormalities in leptin deficient ob/ob mice. // Peptides. – 2007. – vol. 28. – P. 1012–1019.

Iwano M., Plieth D., Danoff T.M. et al. Evidence that fibroblasts derive from epithelium during tissue fibrosis. // J.Clin.Invest. – 2002. – vol. 119, N 3. – P. 341–350.

Iwasaki R., Ninomiya K., Miyamoto K. et al. Cell fusion in osteoclasts plays a critical role in controlling bone mass and osteoblast activity. // Biochem.Biophys.Res.Commun. – 2008. – vol. 377, N 3. – P. 899–904.

Jacenko O., Chan D., Franklin A. et al. A dominant interference collagen X mutation disrupts hypertrophic chondrocyte pericellular matrix and glycosamine and proteoglycan distribution in transgenic mice. // Amer.J.Pathop. – 2001. – vol. 159, N 6. – P. 2257–2269.

Jacob A.L., Smith C., Partanen J., Ornitz D.M. Fibroblast growth factor receptor 1 signaling in osteo-chondrogenic cell lineage regulates sequential steps of osteoblast maturation. // Dev.Biol. – 2006. – vol. 296. – P. 315–328.

Jacob M.P., Sauvage M., Osborne-Pellegrin M. Regulation of elastin synthesis. // J.Soc. Biol. – 2001. – vol. 195, N 2. – P. 131–141.

Jacques C., Recklies A.D., Levy A., Berenbaum F. HC-gp39 contributes to chondrocyte differentiation by inducing SOX9 and type II collagen expression. // Osteoarthritis Cartilage. – 2007. – vol. 15, N 2. – P. 138–146.

Jäger I., Fratzl P. Mineralized collagen fibrils: a mechanical model with a staggered arrangement of mineral particles. // Biophys.J. – 2005. – vol. 79, N 10. – P. 1737–1746.

James C.G., Appleton C.T.G., Ulici V. et al. Microarray analysis of gene expression during chondrocyte differentiation identifies novel regulators of hypertrophy. // Mol.Biol.Cell. – 2005. – vol. 16. – P. 5316–5333.

James C.G., Ulici V., Tuckerman J. et al. Expression profiling of dexamethasone-treated primary choncrocytes identifies targets of glucocorticoid signaling in endochondral bone development. // BMC Genomics. – 2007. – vol. 8. – P. 205.

James C.G., Woods A., Underhill T.M., Beier F. The transcription factor ATF3 is upregulated during chondrocyte differentiation and represses cyclin D1 and A gene transcription. // BMC Mol.Biol. – 2006. – vol. 7. – P. 30.

Jang J,C., Tsonis P.A. Role of 5'HoxD genes in chondrogenesis in vitro. // Int.J.Dev.Dyn. – 1998. – vol. 42. – P. 609–615.

Janig E., Haslbeck M., Aigelsreiter A. et al. Clusterin associates with altered elastic fibers in human photoaged skun and prevents elastin from ultraviolet-induced aggregation in vitro. // Am.J.Pathol. – 2007. – vol. 171. – N 5. – P. 1474–1482.

Jans D.A., Thomas R.J., Gillespie M.T. Parathyroid hormone-related protein (PTHrP): a nucleocytopkasmic shuttling protein with distinct paracrine and intracrine roles. // Viotam.Horm. – 2003. – vol. 66. – P. 345–384.

Janssens K., Dijke P.van, Janssens S., Hul W.V. Transforming growth factor-β1 to the bone. // Endocrin.Rev. – 2005. – vol. 26. – P. 743–774.

Javed A., Bae J.S., Afzal F. et al. Structural coupling of Smad and Runx2 for execution of the BMP2 jsteogenic signal. // J.Biol.Chem. – 2008. – vol. 283, N 13. – P. 8412–8422.

Jay G.D., Cha C.J. The effect of phospholipase digestion upon the lubricating ability of synovial fluid. // J.Rheumatol. – 1999. – vol. 26, N 11. – P. 2454–2457.

Jay G.D., Harris D.A., Cha C.J. Boundary lubrication by lubricin is mediated by O-linked β(1-3)Gal-GaINAc oligosaccharides. // Glycoconj.J. – 2001. – vol. 18. – P. 807–815.

Jay G.D., Tantravahi U., Britt D.E. et al. Homology of lubricin and superficial zone protein (SZP): products of megakarycyte stimulating factor (MSF) gene expression by human synovial fibroblasts and articular chondrocytes localized to chromosome 1q25. // J.Orthop.Res. – 2001. – vol. 19. – P. 677–687.

Jay G.D., Torres J.R., Warman M.L. et al. The role of lubricin in the mechanical behavior of synovial fluid. // Proc.Natl.Acad.Sci.YSA. – 2007. – vol. 104, N 15. – P. 6194–6199.

Jenkins C.L., Bretscher L.E., Guzel I.A., Raines R.T. Effect of 3-hydroxyproline on collagen stability. // J.Am.Chem.Soc. – 2003. – vol. 123, N 21. – P. 6422–6427.

Jensen E.D., Nair A.K., Westendorf J.J. Histone deacetylase co-repressor complex control of Runx2 and bone formation. // Crit.Rev.Eukaryot. Gene Expr. – 2007. – vol. 17, N 3. – P. 187–196.

Jia D., O'Brien C.A., Stewart S.A. et al. Glucocorticoids act directly on osteoclasts to increase their life span and reduce bone density. // Endocrinology. – 2006. – vol. 147, N 12. – P. 5592–5599.

Jia J., Jiang J. Decoding the Hedgehog signal in animal development. // Cell.Mol.Life Sci. – 2006. – vol. 63. – P. 1246–1265.

Jiang J., Leong M.L., Mung J.C. et al. Interaction between zonal populations of articular chondrocytes suppresses chondrocyte mineralization and this process is mediated by PTHrP. // Osteoarthritis Cartilage. – 2007. – Epub Jul. 20.

Jiang J.K., Siller-Jackson A.J., Burra S. Roles of gap junctions and hemichannels in bone cell functions and in signal transmission of mechanical stresses. // Front.Biosci. – 2007. – vol. 12. – P. 1450–1462.

Jin E.J., Lee S.Y., Choi Y.A. et al. BMP-2-enhanced chondrogenesis involves p38 MAPK-mediated down-regulation of Wnt7a pathway. // Mol.Cells. – 2006. – vol. 22, N 3. – P. 353–359.

Jinguji Y. Developmental stage dependent expression of the endothelial stress fibers and organization of fibronectin fibrils in the aorta of chick embryos. // Zool.Sci. – 2003. – vol. 20. – P. 1359–1366

Johansen J.S., Heyer P.E., Larsen L.A. et al. YKL-40 protein expression in the early developing human musculoskeletal system. // J.Histochem.Cytochem. – 2007. – vol. 55, N 12. – P. 1213–1228.

John T., Kohl B., Mobasheri A. et al. Interleukin-18 induces apoptosis in human articular chondrocytes. // Histol.Histopathol. – 2007. – vol. 22, N 5. – P. 469–482.

Johnson J., Shinomura T., Eberspaecher H. et al. Expression and localization of PG-Lb/Epiphycan during mouse development. // Dev.Dyn. – 1999. – vol. 219. – P. 419–510.

Johnson K., Farley D., Hu S.I., Terkeltaub R. One of two chondrocyte-expressed isoforms of cartilage intermediate-layer protein functions as an insulin-like growth factor 1 antagonist. // Arthritis Rheum. – 2003. – N 5. – P. 1302–1314.

Johnson R.G., Poole A.R. The early response of articular cartilage to ACL transsection in a canine model. // Exp.Pathol. – 1990. – vol. 38. – P. 37–52.

Jones A.R., Gleghorn J.P., Hughes C.E. et al. Binding and localization of recombinant lubricin to articular cartilage surfaces. // J.Orthop. Res. – 2007. – vol. 25, N 3. – P. 283–292.

Jones A.R.C., Flannery C.R. Bioregulation of lubricin expression by growth factors and cytokines. // Eur.Cells Materials. – 2007. – vol. 13. – P. 40–45.

Jones D.C., Wein M.M., Glimcher L.H. Schnurri-3: a key regulator of postnatal skeletal remodeling. // Adv.Exp.Med.Biol. – 2007. – vol. 602. – P. 1–13.

Jones G.C., Kiley G.P., Buttle D.J. The role of proteases in pathologies of the synovial joint. // Int.J.Biochem.Cell Biol. – 2008. – vol. 40, N 6–7. – P. 1199–1218.

Jones G.C., Riley G.R. ADAMTS proteinases: a multi-domain, multi-functional family with roles in extracellular matrix turnover and arthritis. // Arthritis Res.Ther. – 2005. – vol. 7, N 5. – P. 160–169.

Jong D.S.de, Vaes B.L.T., Dechering K.J. et al. Identification of novel regulators associated with early phase osteoblast differentiation. // J.Bone Miner.Res. – 2004. – vol. 19, N 6. – P. 947–958.

Jordan C.D., Charbonneau N.L., Sakai L.Y. Fibrillin microfibrils: connective tissue pathways that regulate shape and signaling. // J.Musculoskelet.Neuronal Interact. – 2006. – vol. 6, N 4. – P. 366–367.

Jorgensen N.R. Short-range calcium signaling in bone. // APMIS Suppl. – 2005. – N 118. – P. 5–36.

Josephson K., Praetorius J., Frische S. et al. Targeted disruption of the Cl-/HCO3- exchanger Ae2 results in osteopetrosis in mice. // Proc.Natl.Acad.Sci. USA. – 2009. – vol. 106, N 5. – P. 1638–1641.

Jung J.C., Tsonis P.A. Role of 5' HoxD genes in chondrogenesis in vitro. // – Int.J.Dev.Biol. – 1998. – vol. 42. – P. 609–615.

Kaback L.A., Soung D.Y., Naik A. et al. Osterix/Sp7 regulates mesenchymal stem cell mediated endochondral ossification. // J.Cell.Physiol – 2007. – vol. 214. – P. 173–182.

Kadar A. The elastic fiber normal and pathological condition in the arteries. Jena, VEB, Gustav Fischer Verlag. – 1979. – P. 311.

Kadereit B., Kumar P., Wang W.J. et al. Evolutionary conserved gene family important for fat storage. // Proc.Natl.Acad.Sci.USA. – 2008. – vol. 105, N 1. – P. 94–99.

Kadler K. Extracellular matrix 1: Fibril-forming collagens. // Protein Profile. – 1995. – vol. 2, N 5. – P. 491–619.

Kadler K. Matrix loading: assembly of extracellular matrix collagen fibrils during embryogenesis. // Birth Defects Res. C. – 2004. – vol. 72, N 1. – P. 1–11.

Kadler K.E. Holmes D.F., Trotter J.A., Chapman J.A. Collagen fibril formation. // Biochem.J. – 1996. – vol. 316, N 1. – P. 1–11.

Kadouchi I., Sakamoto K., Tangjiao L. et al. Latexin is involved in bone morphogenetic protein-2-induced chondrocyte differentiation. // Biochem.Biophys.Res.Commun. – 2009. – vol. 378, N 3. – P. 600–604.

Kadoya K., Sasaki T., Kostka G. et al. Fibulin-5 deposition in human skin: decrease with aging and ultraviolet B exposure and increase in solar elastosis. // Br.J.Dermatol. – 2005. – vol. 153, N 3. – P. 607–612.

Kagan H.M., Li W. Lysyl oxidases: Properties, specificity, and biological roles inside and outside of the cell. // J.Cell Biochem. – 2003. – vol. 88, N 4. – P. 660–672.

Kaji H., Naito J., Sowa H. et al. Smad3 differently affects osteoblast differentiation dependent upon the differentiation stage. // Horm.Metab.Res. – 2006. – vol. 38, N 11. – P. 740–745.

Kalajzic I., Staal A., Yang W-P. et al. Expression profile of osteoblast lineage at defined stages of differentiation. // J.Biol.Chem. – 2005. – vol. 280, N 26. – P. 24618–24626.

Kalluri R., Neilson E.G. Epithelial-mesenchymal transition and its implications for fibrosis. // J.Clin.Invest. – 2002. – vol. 112, N 12. – P. 1776–1784.

Kamioka H., Sugawara Y., Honjo T. et al. Terminal differentiation of osteoblasts to osteocytes is accompanied by dramatic changes in the distribution of actin-binding proteins. // J.Bone Miner.Res. – 2004. – vol. 18, N 3. – P. 471–478.

Kamiya N., Watanabe H., Habuchi H. et al. Versican/PG-M regulates chondrogenesis as an extracellular matrix molecule crucial for mesenchymal condensation. // J.Biol.Chem. – 2006. – vol. 281, N 4. – P. 2390–2400.

Kamphorst J.J., van der Heijden K., DeGroot J. et al. Profiling of endogenous peptides in human synovial fluid by NanoLC-VS: method validation and protein identification. // J.Proteome Res. 2007. – vol. 6. № 11. P. 4388–4396.

Kanaan R.A., Kanaan L.A. Transforming growth factor β1, bone connection. // Med.Sci.Monit. – 2006. – vol. 12, N 9. – P.RA164–RA169.

Kanda T., Funato N., Baba Y., Kuroda T. Evidence for fibroblast growth factor receptors in myofibroblasts during palatal mucoperiosteal repair. // Arch.Oral.Biol. – 2003. – vol. 48. – P. 213–221.

Kaneki H., Kurokawa M., Ide H. The receptor attributable to C-type natriuretic peptide-induced differentiation of osteoblasts is switched from type B- to type C-natriuretic peptide receptor with aging. // J.Cell.Biochem. – 2008. – vol. 103, N 3. – P. 753–764.

Kang Q., Sun M.H., Cheng H. et al. Characterization of the distinct orthtotopic bone-forming activity of 14 BMPs using recombinant adenovirus-mediated gene delivery. // Gene Therapy. – 2004. – vol. 11. – P. 1312–1320.

Kania M., Reichenberger E., Baur S.T. et al. Structure variation of type XII collagen at its carboxyl-terminal NC1 domain generated by tissue-specific alternative splicing//. – J.Biol.Chem. – 1999. – vol. 274, N 31. – P. 22053–22059.

Käpylä I., Jäälinoja J., Tulla M. et al. The fibril associated collagen IX provides a novel mechanism for cell adhesion to cartilaginous matrix. // J.Biol. Chem. – 2004. – vol. 279, N 49. – P. 51677–51687.

Karlsson C., Brantsing C., Svensson T. et al. Differentiation of human mesenchymal stem cells and articular chondrocytes: analysis of chondrogenic potential and expression pattern of differentiation-related transcription factors. // J.Orthop.Res. – 2007a. – vol. 25, N 2. – P. 152–163.

Karlsson C., Jonsson M., Asp J. Notch and HES5 are regulated during human cartilage differentiation. // Cell Tisse Res. – 2007b. – vol. 327. – P. 539–551.

Karousou E., Ronga M., Vigetti D. et al. Collagen, proteoglycans, MMP-2, MMP-9 and TIMPs in human Achilles tendon rupture. // Clin.Orthop. Rel.Res. – 2008. – Epub. Apr.19.

Karp G. Cell and molecular biology. – N.Y.e.a.: John Wiley & Sons. – 1999.

Karperien M., van der Eerden B.C.J., Wu J.M. Genomic and non-genomic actions of sex steroids in the growth plate. // Pediatr.Nephrol. – 2005. – vol. 20. – P. 323–329.

Karsdal M.A., Andersen T.A., Bonewald L., Christiansen C. Matrix metalloproteases (MMPs) safeguard from apoptosis during transdifferentiation into osteocytes: MT1-MMP maintains osteocyte viability. // DNA Cell Biol. – 2004. – vol. 23, N 3. – P. 155–165.

Karsdal M.A., Martin T.J., Bollerslev J. et al. Are nonresorbing osteoclasts sources of bone anabolic activity? // J.Bone Miner.Res. – 2007. vol. 22, N 4. – P. 487–494.

Karsdal M.A., Tanko L.B., Riis B.E. et al. Calcitonin is involved in cartilage homeostasis: is calcitonin a treatment for OA? // Osteoarthritis Cartilage. – 2006. – vol. 14, N 7. – P. 617–624.

Karsenty G. Convergence between bone and energy homeostasis: leptin regulation of bone mass. // Cell Metabolism. – 2006. – vol. 4. – P. 341–348.

Karsenty G. Transcriptional control of osteoblast differentiation. // Endocrinology. – 2001. – vol. 142, N 7. – P. 2731–2733.

Karsenty G. Transcriptional control of skeletogenesis. // Annu.Rev. Genomics Hum.Gen. – 2008. – vol. 9. – P. 183–196.

Kashima T.G., Nishiyama T., Shimazu K. et al. Periostin, a novel marker of intramembranous ossification, is expressed in fibrous dysplasia and in c-Fos-overexpressing bone lesions. // Hum.Pathol. – 2009. – vol. 40, N 2. – P. 226–237.

Kashiwagi M., Tortorella M., Nagase H., Brew K. TIMP-3 is a potent inhibitor of aggrecanase 1 (ADAM-TS4) and aggrecanase 2 (ADAM-TS5). // J.Biol.Chem. – 2001. – vol. 276, N 16. – P. 12501–12504.

Kasperk C.H., Borcsok I., Schreier H.U. et al. Endothelin-1 is a potent regulator of human bone cell metabolism in vitro. // Calcif.Tissue Int. – 1997. – vol. 60, N 4. – P. 368–374.

Kassner A., Hansen U., Miosge N. et al. Discrete integration of collagen XVI into tissue-specific collagen fibrils or beaded microfibrils. // Matrix Biol. – 2003. – vol. 22, N 2. – P. 131–143.

Katanaev V.L., Solis G.P., Hausmann G. et al. Reggie-1/flotillin-2 promotes secretion of the long-range signaling forms of Wingless and Hedgehog in Drosophila. // EMBO J. – 2008. – Epub.Jan.24

Kato M., Patel M.S., Levasseur R. et al. Cbfa1-independent decrease in osteoblast proliferation, osteopenia, and persistent embryonic eye vascularization in mice deficient in Prp5, a Wnt coreceptor. // J.Cell Biol. – 2002. – vol. 157, N 2. – P. 305–314.

Katoh M., Kato M. NUMB is a break of Wnt-Notch signaling cycle. // Int.J.Mol.Med. – 2006. – vol. 18. – P. 517–521.

Katoh.Y., Katoh M. Comparative integromics on BMP/GDF family. // Int.J.Mol.Med. – 2006. – vol. 17, N 5. – P. 951–955.

Katsumi A., Ort A.W., Tzima E., Schwartz M.A. Integrins in mechanotransduction. // J.Biol.Chem. – 2004. – vol. 279, N 13. – P. 12001–12004

Kaunitz J.D., Yamaguchi D.T. TNAP, TrAP, ecto-puringeric signaling, and bone remodeling. // J.Cell.Biochem. – 2008. – vol. 105, N 3. – P. 655–662.

Kavanagh E., Ashhurst D. Development and ageing of the articular cartilage of the rabbit knee joint: distribution of biglycan, decorin, and matrilin-1. // J.Histochem.Cytochem. – 1999. – vol. 47. – P. 1603–1616.

Kawakami Y., Raya A., Raya R.M. et al. Retinoic acid signaling links left-right asymmetric patterning and bilaterally symmetric somitogenesis in the zebrafish embryo. // Nature. – 2005. – vol. 415. – P. 165–172.

Kawakami Y., Tsuda M., Takahash., et al. Transcriptional coactivator PGC-1α regulates chondrogenesis via association with Sox9. // Proc.Natl.Acad.Sci. USA. – 2005. – vol. 102, N 7. – P. 2414–2419.

Kawaki H., Kubota S., Suzuki A. et al. Cooperative regulation of chondrocyte differentiation by CCN2 and CCN3 shown by a comprehensive analysis of the CCN family proteins in cartilage. // J.Bone Miner.Res. – 2008a. – vol. 23, N 11. – P. 1751–1764.

Kawaki H., Kubota S., Suzuki A. et al. Functional requirement of CCN2 for intramembranous bone formation in embryonic mice. // Biochem.Biophys.Res.Commun. – 2008b. – vol. 366, N 2. – P. 450–456.

Kawamura N., Kugimiya F., Oshima Y. et al. Akt1 in osteoblasts and osteoclasts control bone remodeling. // PLoS ONE. – 2007. – vol. 2, N 10. – P. 1058.

Ke H.Z., Qi H., Crawford D.T. et al. A new vitamin D analog, 2MD, restores trabecular and cortical collagen bone mass and strength in ovariectomized rats with extablished osteopenia. // J.Bone Miner.Res. – 2005. – vol. 20, N 10. – P. 1742–1755.

Kearns A.E., Khosla S., Kostenuik P.J. Receptor activator of nuclear factor κB ligand and osteoprotegerin regulation of bone remodeling in health and disease. // Endocrine Rev. – 2008. – vol. 29, N 2. – P. 156–192.

Keeley F.W., Bellingham C.M., Woodhouse K.A. Elastin as a self-organizing biomaterial: use of recombinantly expressed human elastin polypeptides as a model for investigations of structure and self-assembly of elastin. // Philos.Trans.R.Soc.Lond.B.Biol.Sci. – 2002. – vol. 357, N 1418. – P. 185–189.

Keene D.R., Jordan C.D., Reinhardt D.P. et al. Fibrillin-1 in human cartilage: developmental expression and formation of special banded fibrils. // J.Histochem. Cytochem. – 1997. – vol. 45, N 8. – P. 1069–1082.

Keene D.R., Sakai L.Y., Burgeson R.E. et al. Human bone contains type III collagen, type VI collagen, and fibrillin: type III is present on specific fibers that mediate attachment of tendons, ligaments and periosteum on calcified bone cortex. // J.Histochem Cytochem. – 1991. – vol. 39, N 1. – P. 59–69.

Kemp C., Wilems E., Abdo S. et al. Expression of all Wnt genes and their secreted antagonists during mouse blastocyst and postimplantation development. // Dev.Dyn. – 2005. – vol. 233. – P. 1064–1075.

Kempuraj D., Saito H., Kaneko A. et al. Characterization of mast cell-committed progenitors present in human umbilical cord blood. // Blood. – 1999. – vol. 93, N 10. – P. 3338–3346.

Kennedy L., Liu S., Shi-wen X. et al. CCN2 is necessary for the function of mouse embryonic fibroblasts. // Exp.Cell Res. – 2007. – vol. 313. – P. 952–964.

Kershaw E.E., Schupp M., Guan H.P. et al. PPAR(gamma) regulates adipose triglyceride lipase in adipocytes in vitro and in vivo. // Am.J.Physiol. Endocrinol.Metab. // 2007. – vol. 293, N 6. – P. E1736–1745.

Kesavan C., Mohan S. Lack of anabolic response to skeletal loading in mice with targeted disruption of the pleiotrophin gene. // BMC Res.Notes. – 2008. – vol. 1. – P. 124.

Kewley M.A., Steven F.S., Williams G. The presence of fine elastin fibrils within the elasting fibre observed by scanning electron microscopy // J. Anat. 1977. – vol. 123, N 1. – P. 129–134.

Khalafi A., Schmidt T.M., Neu C., Reddi A.H. Increased accumulation of superficial zone protein (SZP) in articular cartilage in response to bone morphogenetic protein-7 and growth factors. // J.Orthop.Res. – 2007. – vol. 25, N 3. – P. 293–303

Khan I.M., Redman S.N., Williams R. et al. The development of synovial joints. // Curr.Top.Dev.Biol. – 2007. – vol 79. – P. 1–36.

Khan I.M., Salter D.M., Bayliss M.T. et al. Expression of clusterin in the superficial zone of bovine articular cartilage. // Arthritis Rheum. – 2001. – vol. 44, N 8. – P. 1795–1799.

Khasigov P.Z., Khasanbaeva G.Sh., Rubachev P.G. et al. Proteins of basement membranes. [in Russian]//Biochemistry, 1996, vol. 61, N 7. P. 1152–1168.

Khilkin A.M., Shekhter A.B. and L.P. Istranov. Collagen and its medical application. [in Russian] Moscow: Medicine, 1976. 320 pages.

Khosla S. Leptin – central or peripheral to the regulation of bone metabolism. // Endocrinology. – 2002. – vol. 143, N 11. – P. 4161–4164.

Khruschev N.G. Histogenesis of connective tissue. [in Russian] Moscow: Science, 1976. 116 pages.

Kiani C., Chen L., Wu Y.J. et al. Structure and function of aggrecan. // Cell Res. – 2002. – vol. 12, N 1. – P. 19–32.

Kicheva A., Gonzáles-Gaitán M. The Decapentaplegic morphogen gradient: a precise definition. // Curr.Opin.Cell Biol. – 2008. – vol. 20, N 2. – P. 137–143.

Kielty C.M., Baldock C., Lee D. et al. Fibrillin: from microfibril assembly to biomechanical function. // Philos.Trans.R.Soc.London. B. Biol.Sci. – 2002a. – vol. 357, N 1418. – P. 207–217.

Kielty C.M., Sherrat M.J., Shuttleworth C.A. Elastic fibres. // J.Cell.Sci. – 2002b. – vol. 115, N 14. – P. 2817–2828.

Kielty C.M., Sherratt M.J., Marson A., Baldock C. Fibrillin microfibrils. // – Adv.Protein Chem. – 2005. – vol. 70. – P. 405–436.

Kim C.W., Cho E.H, Lee Y.J. et al. Disease-specific proteins from rheumatoid arthritis patients. // J.Korean Med.Sci. – 2006. – vol. 21. P. 476–484.

Kim H., Choi H.K., Shin J.H. Selective inhibition of RANK blocks osteoclast maturation and function and prevents bone loss in mice. // J.Clin.Invest. – 2009. – vol. 119, N 4. – P. 613–625

Kim H.J., Kirsch T. Collagen/annexin V interactions regulate chondrocyte mineralization. // J.Biol.Chem. – 2008. – vol. 283, N 16. – P. 10310–10317.

Kim H.J., Zhang K., Zhang L. et al. The Src family kinase, Lyn, suppresses osteoclastogenesis in vitro an in vivo. // Proc.Natl.Acad. Sci.USA. – 2009. – vol. 106, N 7. – P. 2325–2330.

Kim H.J., Zhao H., Kitaura S. et al. Glucocorticoids suppress bone formation via the osteoclast. // J.Clin.Invest. – 2006. – vol. 116, N 8. – P. 2152–2160.

Kim J.S., Ryoo Z.Y., Chun J.S. Cytokine-like 1 (CYTl1) regulates the chondrogenesis of mesenchymal cells. // J.Biol.Chem. – 2007. – vol. 282, N 40. – P. 28359–28367.

Kim J.Y., Wu Y., Smas C.M. Characterization of ScAP-23, a new cell line from murine cutaneous adipose tissue, identifies genes for the molecular definition of preadipocytes. // Physiol.Genomics. – 2007. – vol. 31, N 2. – P. 328–342.

Kim N., Kadono Y., Takani M. et al. Osteoclast differentiation independent of the TRANCE-RANK-TRAF6 axis. // J.Exp.Med. 2005. – vol. 202, N 5. – P. 589–595.

Kim S., Koga T., Isobe M. et al. Stat1 functions as a cytoplasmic attenuator of Runx2 in the transcriptional program of osteoblast differentiation. // Genes Dev. – 2003. – vol. 17. – P. 1979–1991.

Kim S.J., Kim E.J., Kim E.J. et al. The modulation of integrin expression by the extracellular matrix in articular chondrocytes. // Yonsei Med.J. – 2003. – vol. 44, N 3. – P. 493–501.

Kimura H., Akiyama H., Nakamura T., Crombrugge B.de. Tenascin =W inhibits proliferation and differentiation of preosteoblasts during endochondral bone formation. // Biochem. Biophys. Res. Commun. – 2007. – vol. 356. – P. 935–941.

Kimura H., Kwan K.M., Zhang Z. et al. Cthrc1 is a positive regulator of osteoblastic bone formation. // PLoS ONE. – 2008. – vol. 3, N 9. – e 3174.

Kimura H., Ng J.M.Y., Curran T. Transient inhibition of the Hedgehog pathway in young mice causes permanent defects in bone structure. // Cancer Cell. – 2008. – vol. 13. – P. 249–260.

Kinloch A., Lundberg K., Wait R. et al. Synovial fluid is a site of citrullination of autoantigens in inflammatory arthritis. // Arthritis Rheum. – 2008. – vol. 58, N 8. – P. 2287–2295.

Kirimoto A., Takagi Y., Chya K., Shimokawa H. Effects of retinoic acid on the differentiation of chondrogenic progenitor cells ATDC5. // J.Med.Dent.Sci. – 2005. – vol. 52, N 3. – P. 153–162.

Kirsch T., Ishikawa Y., Mwale F., Wuthier R.E. Roles of nucleational core complex and collagens (types II and X) in calcification of growth plate cartilage matrix vesicles. // J.Biol.Chem. – 2004. – vol. 269, N 31. – P. 20103–20109.

Kirsch T., Kin H.J., Winkles J.A. Progressive ankylosis gene (Ank) regulates osteoblast differentiation. // Cells Tissues Organs. – 2009. – vol. 189. – P. 158–163.

Kirsch T., Pfafle M. Selective binding of anchorin CII (annexin V) to type II and X collagen to chondrocalcin (C-propeptide of type II collagen). Implication for anchoring function between matrix vesicles and matrix proteins. // FEBS Lett. – 1992. – vol. 28, N 2. – P. 143–147.

KirschT., Koyama E., Liu M. et al. Syndecan-3 is a selective regulator of chondrocyte proliferation. // J.Biol.Chem. – 2002. – vol. 277, N 44. – P. 42171–42177.

Kirshenbaum A.S., Goff J.P., Semere T. et al. Demonstration that human mast cells arise from a progenitor cell population that is CD34(+), c-kit(+), and expresses aminopeptidase N (CD13). // Blood. – 1999. –Vol. – 94, N 7. – P. 2333–42.

Kishigami S., Mishina Y. BMP signaling in early embryonic development. // Cytokine Growth Factors Rev. – 2005. – vol. 16, N 3. – P. 265–278.

Kishigami S., Yoshikawa S.I., Castranio I. et al. BMP signaling through ACVRI is required for left-right patterning in the early mouse embryo. // Dev.Bio. – 2004. – vol. 276. – P. 185–293.

Kita K., Kimura T., Nakamura N. et al. PI3/Akt signaling as a key regulatory pathway for chondrocyte terminal differentiation. // Genes to Cells. – 2008. – vol. 13. – P. 839–850.

Kitahama S., Gibson M.A., Hatzinikolas G. et al. Expression of fibrillin and other microfibril-associated proteins in human bone and osteoblast-like cell. // Bone. – 2000. – vol. 7, N 1. – P. 61–67.

Kitahara H., Hayami T., Tokunagi K. et al. Chondromodulin expression in rat articular cartilage. // Arch.Histol.Cytol. – 2003. – vol. 66, N 3. – P. 221–228.

Kitamura Y., Yokoyama M., Matsuda H. et al. Spleen colony-forming cell as common precursor for tissue mast cells and granulocytes. // Nature. – 1981. – vol. 291, N 5811. P. 159–60.

Kitisin K., Saha T., Blake T. et al. TGF–β signaling in development. // Sci. STKE. – 2007. – N 399. – cm1.

Kizawa H., Kou I., Iida A. et al. An aspartic acid repeat polymorphism in asporin inhibits chondrogenesis and increases susceptibility to osteoarthritis. // Nat.Genet. – 2005. – vol. 37, N 2. – P. 138–145.

Kjaer M. Role of extracellular matrix in adaptation of tendon and skeletal muscle to mechanical loading. // Physiol.Rev. – 2004. – vol. 84, N 2. – P. 649–696.

Kjaer M., Magnusson P., Krogsgaard M. et al. Extracellular matrix adaptation of tendon and skeletal muscle to exercise. // J.Anat, – 2006. – vol. 208. – P. 445–450.

Kjellén L., Lindahl U. Proteoglycans: structures and interactions. // Ann.Rev.Biochem. – 1991. – vol. 60. – P. 443–475.

Klapholz-Brown Z., Walmsley G.G., Nusse Y.M. et al. Transcriptional program induced by Wnt protein in human fibroblasts suggests mechanisms for cell cooperatiuvity in defining tissue microenvironment. // PLoS ONE. – 2007. – vol. 2, N 9. – P. e945.

Klatt A.B., Nitsche D.P., Kobbe B. et al. Molecular structure and tissue distribution of matrilin-3, a filament-forming extracellular matrix protein expressed during skeletal development. // J.Biol.Chem. – 2000. – vol. 275, N 6. – P. 3099–4006.

Klein-Nulend J., Nijweide P.J., Burger E.H. Osteocyte and bone structure. // Curr.Osteoporosis Rep. – 2003. – vol. 1, N 1. – P. 5–10.

Klishov A.A. Histogenesis and tissue regeneration. [in Russian] – Leningrad: Medicine, 1984.

Klüppel M., Wight T.N., Chan C. et al. Maintenance of chondroitin sulfation balance by chondroitin-4-sulfotransferase 1 is required for chondrocyte development and growth factor signaling during cartilage morphogenesis. // Development. – 2005. – vol. 132. – P. 3989–4003.

Kmita M., Duboule D. Organizing axes in time and space; 25 years of collinear tinkering. // Science. – 2003. – vol. 301, N 5631. – P. 331–333.

Kmita M., Tarchini B., Zakány J. et al. Early developmental arrest of mammalian limbs lacking HoxA/HoxD gene function. // Nature. – 2005.– vol. 435, N 7035. – P. 1113–1116.

Knorr T., Obermayr F., Bartnik E. et al. YKL-39 (chitinase 3-like proteiN 2), but not YKL-40 (chitinase 3-like proteiN 1) is up regulated in osteoarthritic chondrocytes. // Ann.Rheum.Dis. – 2003. – vol. 62. – P. 995–998.

Knorre A.G. Embryonal histogenesis. Leningrad, Medicine, 1971. 432 pages.

Knott L., Bailey A.J. Collagen cross-links in muneralizing tissues: a review of their chemistry, function, and clinical relevance. // Bone. – 1998. – vol. 22, N 3. – P. 181–187.

Knowles H.J., Athanasou N.A. Canonical and non-canonical pathways of osteoclast formation. // Histol.Histopathol. – 2009. – vol. 24. – P. 337–346.

Knox S.M., Whitelock J.M. Perlecan: how does one molecule do so many things? // Cell.Mol.Life Sci. – 2006. – vol. 63. – P. 2435–2445.

Knudson C.B., Knudson W. Hyaluronan and CD44. Modulators of chondrocyte metabolism. // Clin.Orthop. – 2004. – vol. 472S. – P. S152–S162.

Knudson C.B., Knudson W. Cartilage proteoglycans. // Semin.Cell.Dev. Biol. – 2001. – vol. 12, N 2. – P. 69–78.

Knudson C.B., Knudson W. Hyaluronan-binding proteins in development, tissue homeostasis, and disease. // FASEB J. – 1993. – vol. 7, N 13. – P. 1233–1241.

Knudson W., Chow G., Knudson C.B. CD44-mediated uptake and degradation of hyaluronan. // Matrix Biol. – 2002. – vol. 21, N 1. – P. 15-23.

Knupp C., Pinall C., Munro P.M. et al. Structural correlation between collagen VI microfibrils and collagen VI banded aggregates. // J.Struct.Biol. – 2006. – vol. 154, N 3. – P. 312–326.

Ko A.R., Huh Y.H., Lee H.C. et al. Identification and characterization of arginase II as a chondrocyte phenotype-specific gene. // IUBMB Life. – 2006. –vol.58, N 10. – P. 597–605.

Kobata A. Glycobiology in the field of aging research – introduction to glycogerontology. // Biochimie. – 2003. – vol. 85, N 1–2. – P. 13–24.

Kobayashi M., Oka M. The lubricative function of artificial joint material surfaces by confocal laser electron microscopy. Comparison of natural synovial joint surfaces. // Biomed.Mater.Eng. – 2003. – vol. 13, N 4. – P. 429–437

Kobayashi N., Kadono Y., Naito et al. Segregation of TRAF6-mediated signaling pathways clarifies its role in osteoclastogenesis. // EMBO J. – 2001. – vol. 20, N 6. – P. 1271–1280.

Kobayashi T., Kronenberg H. Minireview: Transcriptional regulation in development of bone. // Endocrinology. – 2005. – vol. 146, N 3. – P. 1012–1017.

Kobayashi T., Lu J., Cobb B.S. et al. Dicer-dependent pathways regulate chondrocyte proliferation and differentiation. // Proc.Natl.Aca. Sci.USA. – 2008. – vol. 105, N 6. – P. 1949–1954.

Kobayashi T., Lyons K.M., McMahon A.P., Kronenberg H.M. BMP signaling stimulates cellular differentiation at multiple steps during cartilage development. // Proc.Natl.Acad.Sci.USA. – 2005. – vol. 102. N 50. – P. 18023–18027.

Kobayashi T., Udagawa N., Takahashi N. Action of RANKL and OPG for osteoclastogenesis. // Crit.Rev.Eukaryot.Gene Expr. – 2009. – vol. 19. N 1. – P. 61–72.

Koch M., Foley J.E., Hahn R. et al. α1(XX) collagen a new member of the collagen subfamily, fibril associated collagens with interrupted triple helices. // J.Biol.Chem. – 2001. –V. 276, N 25. – P. 23120–23126

Koch M., Laub F., Zhou P. et al. Collagen XXIV, a vertebrate collagen with structural features of invertebrate collagen. Selective expression in developing cornea and bone. // – J.Biol.Chem. – 2003. – vol. 278, N 44. – P. 43236–43244.

Koch M., Murrell J.R., Hunter D.D. et al. A novel member of the netrin family, β-netrin, chares homology with β-chain of laminin. // J.Cell Biol. – 2000. – vol. 151, N 2. – P. 221–234.

Koellig S., Clauditz T.S., Kaste M., Miosge N. Cartilage oligomeric matrix protein is involved in human limb development and in the pathogenesis of osteoarthritis. // Arthritis Res.Ther. – 2006. – vol. 8. – P.R56.

Koga T., Matsui Y., Asagiri M. et al. NFAT and Osterix cooperatively regulate bone formation. // Nat.Med. – 2005. – vol. 11, N 8. – P. 880–885.

Kohfeldt E., Sasaki T., Yasuda T. et al. Nidogen-2: a new basement membrane protein with diverse binding properties. // J.Mol.Biol. – 1998. – vol. 282, N 1. – P. 99–109.

Kokkinos M.I., Wafai R., Wong M.K. et al. Vimentin and epithelial-mesenchymal transition in human breast cancer – observations in vitro and in vivo. // – Cells Tissues Organs. – 2007. – vol. 185. – P. 191–203.

Kolajzic I., Staal A., Yang W.P. et al. Expression profile of osteoblast lineage ar different stages of differentiation. // J.Biol.Chem. – 2005. – vol. 289, N 26. – P. 24618–24626.

Koli K., Ryynänen M.J., keski-Oja J. Latentb TGF-beta binding proteins (LTBPs)-1 and -3 coordinate proliferation and osteogenic differentiation of human mesenchymal stem cells. // Bone. – 2008. – vol. 41, N 4. – P. 679–688.

Kolodeznikova E.D. Responsive changes of the skin and brown adipose tissue in long-term exposure to cold. [in Russian] // PhD thesis abstract. Moscow, 1971.

Kolodsick J.E., Peters-Golden M., Larios J. et al. Prostaglandin E2 inhibits fibroblast to myofibroblast transition via E. prostanoid receptor 2 signaling and cyclic adenosine monophosphate elevation. // Am.J.Respir.Cell.Mol.Biol. – 2003. Vol.29. – P. 537–544.

Komatsu Y., Scott G., Nagy A. et al. BMP type I receptor ALK2 is essential for proper patterning at late gastrulation during mouse embryogenesis. // Dev.Biol. – 2007. – vol. 236. – P. 512–517.

Komori T. Regulation of bone development by Runx2. // Front.Biosci. – 2008. – vol. 13. – P. 898–903.

Komori T. Regulation of osteoblast differentiation by transcription factors. // J.Cell.Biochem. – 2006. – vol. 99. – P. 1233–1239.

Kong L., Liu C.J. Mediation of chondrogenuc and osteogenic differentiation by an interferon-inducible p202 protein. // Cell.Mol.Life Sci. – 2008. – vol. 65. – P. 3494–3506.

König A., Bruckner-Tuderman L. Epithelial-mesenchymal interactions enhance expression of collagen VII in vitro. // J.Invest.Dermatol. – 1991. – vol. 96. – P. 803–808.

König A., Bruckner-Tuderman L. Transforming growth factor-β promotes deposition of collagen VII in a modified organotypic skin model. // Lab. Invest. 1994 – vol. 70. – P. 203–209.

Korchynskyi O., Dechering K.J., Sijbers A.M. et al. Gene array analysis of bone morphogenetic protein type I receptor-induced osteoblast differentiation. // J.Bone Miner.Res. – 2003. – vol. 18, N 7. – P. 177–185.

Kortesidis A., Zannettino A., Isenmann S. et al. Stromal-derived factor-1 promotes growth, survival, and development of human bone marrow stromal stem cells. // Blood. – 2005. – vol. 105, N 10. – P. 3793–3801.

Kosher, R.A., Lash J.W. Notochordal stimulation of in vitro somite chondrogenesis before and after enzymatic removal of perinotochordal materials. // Dev. Biol. – 1975. – vol. 42: – P. 362–378.

Koshizuka Y., Yamada T., Hoshi K. et al. CystatiN 10, a novel chondrocyte-specific protein, may promote the last steps of the chondrocyte differentiation pathway. // J.Biol.Chem. – 2003. – vol. 278, N 48. – P. 48259–48266.

Kotadiya P., McMichael B.K., Lee B.S. High molecular weight tropomyosine reegulates osteoclast cytoskeletal morphology. // Bone. – 2008. – vol 43. N 5. – P. 951–960.

Kou I., Ikegawa S. SOX9-dependent and –independent transcriptional regulation of human cartilage link protein. // J.Biol.Chem. – 2004. – vol. 279, N 49. – P. 50942–50948.

Kousteni S., Bilezikian J.P. The cell biology of parathyroid hormone in osteoblasts. // Curr.Osteoporos.Rep. – 2008. – vol. 6, N 2. – P. 72–76.

Koyama E., Ochiai T., Rountree R.B. et al. Synovial joint formation during mouse limb skeletogenesis. Role of Indian hedgehog signaling. // Ann.N.Y.Acad.Sci. – 2007. – vol. 1116. – P. 100–112.

Koyama E., Shibukawa Y., Nagayama M. et al. A distinct cohort of progenitor cells participates in synovial joint and articular cartilage formation during mouse limb development. // Dev.Biol. – 2008. – vol. 316. – P. 62–73.

Kozel B.A., Wachi H., Davis E.C., Mecham R.P. Domains in tropoelastin that mediated elastin deposition in vitro and in vivo. // J.Biol.Chem. – 2003. – vol. 278, N 20. – P. 18491–18498

Krebs D.L., Hilton D.J. SOCS proteins: negative regulators of cytokine signaling. // Stem Cells. – 2001. – vol. 19. – P. 378–387.

Kreici P., Krakow D., Mekikian P.B., Wilcox W.R. Fibroblast growth factors 1, 2, 17, and 19 are the predominant FGF ligans expressed in human fetal growth plate cartilage. // Pediatr.Res. – 2007. – vol. 61, N 3. – P. 267–272.

Kresse H., Schönherr E. Proteoglycans of extracellular matrix and growth control. // J.Cell.Physiol. – 2001. – vol. 189, N 3. – P. 266–274.

Krishnan V., Bryant H.U., MacDougald D.A. Regulation of bone mass by Wnt signaling. // J.Clin.Invest. – 2006. – vol. 116, N 5. – P. 1202–1209.

Kronenberg H.M. Developmental regulation of the growth plate. // Nature. – 2003. – vol. 423, N 6937. – P. 332–336,

Krtolica A., Parrinello S., Lockett S. et al. Senescent fibroblasts promote epithelial cell growth and tumorigenesis: a link between cancer and aging. // Proc.Natl.Acad.Sci.U S A. – 2001. – vol. 98. – P. 12072–12077.

Kruse M.N., Becker C., Lottaz D. et al. Human meprin α and β homo-oligomers: cleavage of basement membrane proteins and sensitivity to metalloprotease inhibitors. // Biochem.J. – 2004. – vol. 378. – P. 383–389.

Kubota S., Takigawa M. Role of CCN2/CTGF/Hcs24 in bone growth. // Int.Rev.Cytol. – 2007. – vol. 257. – P. 1–41.

Kubota T., Michigami T., Ozono K. Wnt signaling in bone metabolism. // J.Bone Miner.Metab. – 2009. – vol. 27. – P. 265–271.

Kucia M., Wysoczynski M., Baskiewicz'Masiuk M. et al. Morphological and molecular characterization of novel population of CXCR4+SSEA-4+Oct-4+ very small embryonic-like cells purified from human cord blood: preliminary report // Leukemia, 2007, vol. 21, no. 2. P. 297–303.

Kucia M., Wysoczynski M., Wu W. et al. Evidence that very small embryonic-like stem cells are mobilized into peripheral blood // Stem Cells. 2008, vol. 26. P. 2083–2092.

Kugeyama R., Masamizu Y., Niwa Y. Oscillator mechanism of Notch pathway in the segmentation clock. // Dev.Dyn. – 2007. – vol. 236. – P. 1403–1409.

Kugimiya F., Ohba S., Nakamura K. Kokubo T. et al. Physiological role of bone morphogenetic proteins in osteogenesis. // J.Bone Miner. Metab. – 2006. – vol. 24. – P. 95–99.

Kühn K. The classical collagens: types I, II, and III. // In: Structure and function of collagen types (Mayne R, Burgeson R.E., eds.) Orlando e.a.: Academic Press. – 1987. – P. 1–42.

Kühn K., D'Lima D.D., Hashimoto S., Lotz M. Cell death in cartilage. // Osteoarthritis Cartilage. – 2004. – vol. 12, N 1. – P. 1–16.

Kume S., Kato S., Yamaguchi S. et al. Advanced glycation end-products attenuate human mesenchymal stem cells and prevent cognate differentiation into adipose tissue, cartilage, and bone. // J.Bone Miner.Res. – 2005. –V. 20, N 9. – P. 1647–1658.

Kundu M., Javed A., Jeon J.P. et al. Cbfβ interacts with Runx2 and has a critical role in bone development. // Nat.Genet. – 2002. – vol. 32. – P. 547–552

Kupriyanov V.V., Karaganov Ya.L. and V.N. Kozlov. Microcirculatory bloodstream. [in Russian] Moscow: Medicine, 1975. 213 pages.

Kuroda K., Tajima S. Proliferation of HSP47-positive skin fibroblasts in dermatofibroma. // J.Cutan.Pathol. – 2008. – vol. 35, N 1. – P. 21–26.

Kuznetsova N., Leikin S. Does the triple helical domain of type I collagen encode molecular recognition and fiber assembly while telopeptides serve as catalytic domains. // J.Biol.Chem. – 1999. – vol. 274, N 51. – P. 36083–36089.

Kvist A.J., Johnson A.E., Mörgelin M. et al. Chondroitin sulfate perlecan enhances collagen fibril formation. Implications for chondrodysplasias. // J.Biol. Chem. – 2006. – vol. 281, N 28. – P. 33127–33139.

Kvist A.J., Nyström A., Hultenby K. et al. The major basement membrane components localize in the chondrocyte pericellular matrix – a cartilage basement membrane equivalent. // Matrix Biol. – 2008. – vol. 27, N 1. – P. 22–33.

Labat M. L., Bringuier A. F., Arys-Philippart C. et al. Monocytic origin of fibrosis. In vitro transformation of HLA-DR monocytes into neo-fibroblasts: inhibitory effect of all-trans retinoic acid on this process. // Biomed. Pharmacother. – 1994. – vol. 48. – P. 103–111

Labat-Robert J. Age-dependent remodelling of connective tissue: role of fibronectin and laminin. // Pathol.Biol. – 2003. – vol. 51, N 10. – 563–568.

Lafont J.E., Jacques C., Le Dreau G. et al. New target genes for NOV/CCN3 in chondrocytes: TGF-β2 and type X collagen. // J.Bone Miner.Res. – 2005. – vol. 20, N 12. – P. 2213–2223.

Lafont J.E., Talma S., Murphy C.L. Hipoxia-inducible factor HIF-2α is essential for the hypoxic induction of the human articular chondrocyte phenotype. // Arthritis Rheum. – 2007. – vol. 56, N 10. – P. 3297–3306.

Lai C.F., Bai S., Uthgenanni B.A. et al. Four and Half Lim proteiN 2 (FHL2) stimulates osteoblast differentiation. // J.Bone Miner. Res. – 2006. – vol. 21, N 1. – P. 17–28.

Lai C.F., Chaudhary L., Fausto A. et al. Erk is essential for growth, differentiation, integrin expression, and cell functions in human osteoblastic cells. // J.Biol.Chem. – 2001. – vol. 276, N 17. – P. 14443–14450.

Lai C.F., Cheng S.L. αvβ integrins play an essential role in BMP-2 induction of osteoblast differentiation. // J.Bone Miner.Res. – 2005, – vol. 20, N 2. – P. 330–340.

Lai S.F., Wu S., Li L.M. et al. An in vivo genome-wide gene expression study of circulating monocytes suggested GBP1, STAT1 and CXCL10 as novel risk genes for the differentiation of peak bone mass. // Bone. – 2009. – vol. 44, N 5. – P. 1010–1014.

Lake A.C., Sun Y., Li J.L. et al. Expression, regulation, and triglyceride hydrolase activity of Adiponitrin family members. // J.Lipid Res. – 2005. – vol. 46. – P. 2477–2487.

Lam M.H.C, Thomas R.J., Martin T.J. et al. Nuclear and nucleolar localization of parathyroid hormone-related protein. // Immunol.Cell Biol. – 2000. – vol. 78. – P. 395–402.

Landis W.J., Silver F.H. Mineral deposition in theextracellular matrices of vertebral tissues: identification of possible apatite nucleation sites on type I collagen. // Cells, Tissues, Organs. – 2009. – vol. 189, N 1–4. – P. 20–24.

Lane N.E., Yao W., Nakamura M.C. et al. Mice lacking the integrin beta5 subunit have accelerated osteoclast maturation and increased activity in the estrogen-deficient state. // J.Bone Miner. Res. – 2005. – vol. 20, N 1. – P. 58–66.

Lange M.A. Radioautographic investigation of the origin of fibroblast-like elements of a connective tissue neoplasm site. [in Russian] // PhD thesis abstract. Moscow, 1975.

Langner C., Steinman H.A., Gagnon J. et al. Osteoblast differentiation and skeletal development are regulated by Mdm2-p53 signaling. // J.Cell Biol. – 2006. – vol. 172, N 6. – P. 909–921.

Lanzardo S., Curcio C., Forni G., Antón I.M. A role for WASP interacting protein, WIP, in fibroblast adhesion, spreading and migration. // Int.J.Biochem.Cell Biol. – 2007. – 2007. – vol. 39, N 1. – P. 262–274.

Lappin T.R.J., Grier D.G., Thompson A., Halliday H.L. HOX genes: seductive science, mysterious mechanisms. // Ulster Med.J. – 2006. – vol. 75, N 1. – P. 23–31.

Latvanlehto A., Snellman A., Tu H., Pihlajaniemi T. Type XIII collagen and some other transmembrane collagens contain two separate coiled-coil motifs, which may function as independent oligomerization domains. // J.Biol.Chem. – 2003. – vol. 278, N 39. – P. 37590–37599.

Lauer-Fields J.I., Juska D., Fields G.B. Matrux metalloproteinases and collagen metabolism. // Biopolymers. – 2002. – vol. 66, N 1. – P. 19–32.

Laurent T.C., Laurent U.B.G., Fraser J.R.E. Functions of hyaluronan. // Ann.Rheum.Dis. – 1995. – vol. 54, N 5. – P. 429–432.

Lavietes B.B., Carsons S., Diamond H.S., Laskin R.S. Synthesis, secretion, and deposition of fibronectin in cultured human synovium. // Arthritis Rheum. – 1985. – vol. 28, N 9. – P. 1016–1026.

Lawson W.E., Polosukhin V.V., Zoia O. et al. Characterization of fibroblast-specific proteiN 1 in pulmonary fibrosis. // Am.J.Respir.Crit. Care Med. – 2005. – vol. 171, – N 8. – P. 899–907.

Le Goff C., Somerville R.F., Kesteloot F. et al. Regulation of procollagen amino-propeptide processing during mouse embryogenesis by specializtion of homologous ADAMTS proteases: insight on collagen biosynthesis and dermatosparaxis. // Development. – 2006. – vol. 133, N 8. – P. 1587–1596.

Leask A., Abraham D.J. All in the CCN family: essential matricellular signaling modulators emerge from the bunker. // J.Cell Sci. – 2006. – vol. 119. – P. 4803–4810.

Leask A., Abraham D.J. The role of connective growth factor, a multifunctional matricellular protein, in fibroblast biology. // Biochem.Cell Biol. – 2003. – vol. 81, N 6. – P. 355–363.

Leckband D., Prakasam A. Mechanism and dynamics of cadherin adhesion. //Annu.Rev.Biomed. Eng. – 2006. – vol. 8. – P. 259–287.

Lee C.H., Moioll E.K., Mao J.J. Fibroblast differentiation of human mesenchymal stem cells using connective tissue growth factor. // Conf.Proc.IEEE Eng.Med.Biol.Soc. – 2006. – vol. 1. – P. 775–778.

Lee C.R., Sakai D., Nakai T. et al. A [henoptypic comparison of intervertebral disc and articular cartilage cells in the rat. // Eur.Spine J. – 2007. – vol. 16. – P. 2174–2185.

Lee D.H., Kim T.S., Choi Y., Lorenzo J. Osteoimmunology: cytokines and the skeletal system. // BMB Rep. – 2008. – vol. 41, N 7. – P. 495–510.

Lee D.Y., Yeh C.R., Chang S.F. et al. Integrin-mediated expression of bone formation-related genes in osteoblast-like cells in response to fluid shear stress: roles of extracellular matrix, Shc, and mitogen-activated protein kinase. // J.Bone Miner.Res. – 2008. – vol. 23, N 7. – P. 1140–1149.

Lee H.G., Eun H.C. Differences between fibroblasts cultured from oral mucosa and normal skin: implication to wound healing. // J.Dermatol. Sci. – 1999. – vol. 2. – P. 176–182.

Lee H.W., Suh J.H., Kim A.Y. et al. Histone deacetylase 1-mediated histone modification regulates osteoblst differentiation. // Mol. Endocrinol. – 2006. – vol. 20, N 10. – P. 2432–2443

Lee J.Y., Lee Y.M., Kim M.J. et al. Methylation of the mouse Dlx5 and Osx gene promoters regulate cell-type specific gene expression. // Mol.Cells. – 2006. – vol. 22, N 2. – P. 182–188.

Lee J.Y., Spicer A.P. Hyaluronan: a multifunctional megaDalton, stealth molecule. // Curr.Opin.Cell Biol. – 2000. – vol. 12. – P.581–586.

Lee M.H., Murphy G. Matrix metalloproteinases at a glance. // J.Cell Sci. – 2004. – vol. 117. – P.4015–4016.

Lee N.K., Choi H.K., Yoo H.J. RANKL-induced schlafen2 is a positive regulator of osteoclastogenesis. // Cell.Signal. – 2008. – vol.20, N 12. – P.2302–2309.

Lee S.J., Jeon H.B., Lee J.H. et al. Identification of proteins differentially expressed during chondrogenesis of mesenchymal cells. // FEBS Lett. – 2004. – vol.563, N 1. – P.35–40.

Lee Y.J., Lee F.B., Kwon Y.E. et al. Effect of estrogen on the expression of matrix metalloproteinase (MMP)-1, MMP-3, and MMP-13 and tissue inhibitor of metalloproteinase-1 in osteoarthritic chondrocytes. // Rheumatol.Int. – 2003. – vol.23. – P.282–288.

Lee Y.S., Chuong C.M. Activation of protein kinase A is a pivotal step involved in both BMP-2- and cyclic AMP-induced chondrogenesis. // J.Cell.Physiol. – 1997. – vol.170, N 2. – P.153–165.

Lefebvre V., Smits P. Transcriptional control of chondrocyte fate and differentiation. // Birth Defects Res.C. – 2005. – vol.75. – P.200–212.

Leimeister C., Steidl C., Schunacher N. et al. Developmental expression and biochemical characterization of Emu family members. // Dev.Biol. – 2002. –V. 249, N 2. – P.204–218.

Leites M., Neidhardt L., Haenig B. et al. The paired homeobox gene Uncx4.1 specified pedicles, transverse processes and proximal ribs of the vertebral column. // Development. – 2000. – vol.127. – P.2259–2267.

Leitinger B. Molecular analysis of collagen binding by the human discoidin domain receptors, DDR1 and DDR2. // J.Biol.Chem. – 2003. – vol. 278, N 19. – P. 16761–16769.

Léjard V., Brideau G., Blais F. et al. Scleraxis and NFATc regulate the expression of the Pro-α1(I) collagen gene in tendon fibroblasts. // J.Biol.Chem. – 2007. vol.282, N 24. – P. 17665–17675.

Lely A.J.van der, Tschop M., Heiman M.I., Ghigo E. Biological, physiological, pathophysiological, and pharmacological aspects of ghrelin. // Endocrine Rev. – 2004. – vol.25, N 3. – P.426–457.

Lemann J.jr., Bushinsky D.A., Hamm L.L. Bone buffering of acid and base in humans. // Am.J.Physiol.Renal Physiol. – 2003. – vol.285. – P.F811–F832.

Lenga Y., Koh A., Perera A.S. et al. Osteopontin expression is required for myofibroblast differentiation. // Circ.Res. – 2008. – vol. 102, N 3. – P. 319–327.

Lengner C.J., Hassan M.Q., Serra R.W. et al. Nkx3.2 –mediated repression of Runx2 promotes chondrogenic differentiation. // J.Biol.Chem. – 2005. – vol. 280, N 16. – P. 15872–15879.

Lensch M.W., Daheron L., Schlaeger T.M. Pluripotent stem cells and their niches. // Stem Cell Dev. – 2006. – vol. 2, N 3. – P. 185–201.

Lepekhin E., Gron B., Berezin V. et al. Differences in motility pattern between human buccal fibroblasts and periodontal and skin fibroblasts. // Eur J Oral Sci – 2002. – vol. 110. – P. 13–20.

Lerner U.H. Deletions of genes encoding calcitonin/α-CGRP, amylin and calcitonin receptor have given new and unexpected insights into the function of calcitonin receptors and calcitonin receptor-like receptors in bone. // J.Musculoskelet.Neuronal Interact. – 2006. – vol.6, N 1. – P.87–95.

Letamendia A., Labbé E., Artisano L. Transcriptional regulation by Smads: crosstalk between the TGF-β and Wnt pathways. // J.Bone Joint Surg. – 2001. – vol.83-A, Suppl.1. – P.S31–S39

Lethias C., Carney A., Comte J. et al. A model of tenascin X integration within the collagenous network. // FEBS Lett. – 2006. – vol. 580. – P.6281–6285.

Levick J.R., McDonald J.N. Microfibrillar meshwork of the synovial lining and associated broad banded collagen: a clue to identity. // Ann.Rheum.Dis. – 1990. – vol.49, N 1. – P.31–36.

Levine M., Davidson E.H. Gene regulatory networks for development. // Proc.Natl.Acad.Sci.USA. – 2005. – vol. 102, N 14. – P.4936–4942.

Levine S.J. Mechanisms of soluble cytokine receptor generation. // J.Immunol. – 2004. –V. 173, N 9. – P.5343–5348.

Li S.S., Liu Y.H., Tseng C.N. Characterization and gene expression profiling of five new human embryonic stem cell lines derived in Taiwan. // Stem Cells Dev. – 2006. – vol. 25, N 4. – P.532–555.

Li H., Marjanovic I., Kronenberg M.S. et al. Expression and function of Dlx genes in the osteoblast lineage. // Dev.Biol. – 2008. – vol.316, N 2. – P.458–470.

Li S.W., Prockop D.J., Helminen H. et al. Transgenic mice with targeted inactivation of the Col2a1 gene for collagen II develop a skeleton with membranous and periosteal bone but no endochondral bone. – // Genes.Dev. – 1995. – vol.9. – P.2821–2830.

Li S.-W., Sieron A.L., Fertala A. et al. The C-proteinase that processes procollagens to fibrillar collagens is identical to protein previously identified as bone morphogenetic protein-1. // Proc.Natl. Acad.Sci.USA. – 1996. – vol. 93. – P.5127–5130.

Li T.F., Warris V., Ma J. et al. Distribution of tenascin-X in different synovial samples and synovial membrane-like interface tissue from aseptic loosening of total hip replacement. // Rheumatol. Int. – 2000. – vol. 19, N 5. – P. 177–183.

Li X., Cao X. BMP signaling and skeletogenesis. // Ann.N.Y.Acad.Sci. – 2006. – vol. 1068. – P. 26–40.

Li X.,Nie S., Chang C. et al. Smads oppose Hox transcriptional activities. // Exp.Cell Res. – 2006. – vol. 312, N 6. – P. 854–864.

Li Y., Toole B.P., Dealy C.N., Kosher R.A. Hyaluronan in limb morphogenesis. // Dev.Biol. – 2007. – vol.305, N 2. – P.411–420.

Li Y.L.,Xiao Z.S. Advances in Runx2 regulation and its isoforms. // Med.Hypotheses. – 2007. – vol.68, N 1. – P. 169–175.

Li Z., Hassan M.Q., Volinia S. et al. A microRNA signature for a BMP2-induced osteoblast lineage commitment program. // Proc. Natl. Acad.Sci.USA. – 2008. – vol. 105, N 37. – P. 13906–13911).

Li Z., Kong K., Qi W. Osteoclasts and its roles in calcium metabolism and bone development and remodeling. // Biochem.Biophys.Res. Comm. – 2006. – vol. 343. – P. 345–50.

Lian J.B., Stein G.S., Javed A. et al. Networks and hubs for transcriptional control of osteoblastogenesis. // Rev.Endocr.Metab.Disord. – 2006. – vol. 7. – P. 1–16.

Liao J., McCauley L.K. Skeletal metastasis: established and emerging roles of parathyroid hormone related protein. // Cancer Metastasis Rev. – 2006. – vol.25. – P.559–571.

Liao Y.F., Gotwals P.J., Koteliansky V.E. The EIIIA segment of fibronectin is a ligand for integrins alpha 9beta 1 and alpha 4beta 1 providing a novel mechanism for regulating cell adhesion by alternative splicing. // J. Biol. Chem. – 2002. – vol. 277. – P. 14467–14474.

Lieder A., Kaspar D., Blakytny R. et al. Signal transduction pathways involved in mechanotransduction in bone cells. // Biochem.Biophys. Res.Comm. – 2006. – vol.349, N 1. – P. 1–5.

Lillie M.A., Gosline J.M. The viscoelastic basis for the tensile strength of elastin. // Int.J.Biol.Macromol. – 2002. – vol. 30, N 2. – P. 119–127.

Lin G., Tiedemann K., Vollbrandt T. et al. Homo- and heterotypic fibrillin-1 and –2 interactions constitute the basis for the assembly of microfibrils. // J.Biol.Chem. – 2002. – vol. 277, N 52. – P.50795–50804.

Lin X. Functions of heparan sulfate proteoglycans in cell signaling during developing. // Development. – 2004. – vol. 131. – P. 6009–6021.

Linck G., Stocker S., Grimaud J.A., Porte A. Distribution of immunoreactive fibronectin and collagen (type I, III, IV) in mouse joints. // Histochemistry. – 1983. – vol. 77, N 3. – P. 323–328.

Lindsley R.C., Gill J.G., Kyba M. et al. Canonical Wnt signaling is required for development of embryonic stem cell-derived mesoderm. // Development. – 2006. – vol. 133, N 19. – P. 3787–3796.

Lisignoli G., Codeluppi K., Todoerti K. et al. Gene array profile identifies collagen type XV as a novel human osteoblast-secreted matrix protein. // J.Cell.Physiol. – 2009. – Epub. Apr.13.

Litjens S.H., de Pereda J.M., Sonnenberg A. Current insights into the formation and breakdown of hemidesmosomes. // Trends Cell Biol. – 2006. – vol. 16, N 7. – P. 376–383.

Little C.B., Ghosh P. Variation in proteoglycan metabolism by articular chondrocytes in different joint regions is determined by postnatal mechanical loading. // Osteoarthritis Cartilage. – 1997. – vol. 5, N 1. – P. 49–62.

Little C.B., Mecker C.T., Golub S.B. et al. Blocking aggrecanase cleavage in the aggrecan interglobular domain abrogates cartilage erosion and promotes cartilage repair. // J.Clin.Invest. – 2007. – vol. 117, N 6. – P. 1627–1636.

Litvin J., Selim A.H., Montgomery M.O. et al. Expression and function of periostin isoforms in bone. // J.Cell Biochem. – 2004. – vol. 92, N 5. – P. 1044–1061.

Liu T., Gao Y., Sakamoto K. et al. BMP-2 promotes differentiation of osteoblasts and chondroblasts in Runx2-deficient cell lines. // J.Cell. Physiol. – 2007. – vol. 211, N 3. – P. 728–735.

Liu X.S., Luo H.J., Yang H. et al. Palladin regulates cell and extracellular matrix interaction through maintaining normal actin cytoskeleton architecture and stabilizing beta integrin. // J.Cell.Biochem. – 2007. – vol. 100, N 5. – P. 1288–1300.

Liu Y., Porta A., Peng X. et al. Prevention of glucocorticoid-induced apoptosis in osteocytes and osteoblasts by calbindin-D28k. // J.Bone Miner.Res. – 2004. – vol. 19, N 4. – P. 479–490.

Lo S.H. Focal adhesions: what's new inside. // Dev.Biol. – 2006. – vol. 294. – P., 280–291.

Locksley R.M., Killeen N., Lenardo M.J. The TNF and TNF receptor superfamilies: integrating mammalian biology. // Cell. – 2001. – V. 104. – P. 487–501

Loeser R. Integrins and cell signaling in chondrocytes, // Biorheology. – 2002. – vol. 32. – P. 119–124.

Logan C.Y., Nusse R. The Wnt signaling pathway in development and disease. // Annu.Rev.Cell Dev.Biol. – 2004. – vol. 20. P. 781–810.

Lohwasser C., Neureiter D., Weigle B. et al. The receptor for advanced glycation end products is highly expressed in the skin and upregulated by advanced glycation end products and tumor necrosis factor alpha. // J.Invest.Dermatol. – 2006. – vol. 126. – P. 291–299.

Long F., Chung U.-i., Ohba S. et al. Ihh signaling is directly required for the osteoblast lineage in the endochondral skeleton. // Development. – 2004. – vol. 131. – P. 1309–1318.

Lopes C.C., Dietrich C.P., Nader H.B. Specific structural features of syndecans and heparan sulfate chains are needed for cell signaling. // Braz. J.Med.Biol.Res. – 2006. – vol. 39. – P. 157–167.

Lorena D., Uchio K., Alto Costa A.M., Desmouliere A. Normal scarring: importance of myofibroblasts // Wound Repair Regen. – 2002. – vol. 10. – P. 86–92.

Lorenzo J., Horowitz M., Choi Y. Osteoimmunology: interaction of the bone and immune system. // Endocrine Rev. – 2008. – vol. 29, N 4. – P. 403–440.

Lovinescu I., Koyama E., Pacifici M. Roles of FGF-10 on the development of development diarthrodial limb joints. // Penn.Dent.J. – 2003. – vol. 103, N 5. – P. 9.

Lu J., Lian G., Lekinski R. et al. Filamin B mutations cause chondrocyte defects in skeletal development. // Hum.Mol.Genet. – 2007. – vol. 16, N 14. – P. 1661–1675.

Lu X., Gilbert L., He X. et al. Transcriptional regulation of the Osterix (Osx, Sp7) promoter by tumor necrosis factor identifies disparate effects of mitogen-activated protein kinase and NFκB pathways. // J.Biol.Chem. – 2006. – vol. 281, N 10 – P. 6297–6306.

Lu Y., Holmes D.F., Baldock C. Evidence for the intramolecular pleating model of fibrillin microfibril organization from single particle image analysis. // J.Mol.Biol. – 2005. – vol. 349. – P. 73–85.

Lucic D., Mollenhauer J., Kilpatrick K.E., Cole A.A. N-telopeptide of type II collagen interacts with annexin V on human chondrocytes. // Connect.Tissue Res. – 2003. – vol. 44. – P. 225–239.

Luckman S.P., Rees E., Kwan A.P. Partial characterization of cell – type X collagen interactions. // Biochem.J. – 2003. – vol 372, N 2. – P. 485–493.

Luderer H.F., Bai S., Longmore G.D. The LIM protein LIMD1 influence osteoblast differentiation and function. // Exp.Cell.Res. – 2008. – vol. 314, N 15. – P. 2884–2894.

Luft J.H. Ruthenium red and violet. I. Chemistry, purification, methods of use for electron microscopy and mechanism of action // Anat. Rec. – 1971a. – vol. 171, N 3. – P. 347–368.

Luft J.H. Ruthenium red and violet. II. Fine structural localization in animal tissues // Anat. Rec. 1971b. – vol. 171, N 3. – P. 369–416.

Luft J.H. The fine structure of hyaline cartilage matrix following ruthenium red fixative and staining // J.Cell Biol. – 1965. – vol. 27. N 2. – P. 61A.

Luo J., Wan Y. Tightly regulated distribution of family members of proteins is related to social properties in the open body system. // Intern.J.Mol.Med. – 2006. – vol. 17. – P. 411–418.

Luo J., Zhou W., Zhou X. et al. Regulation of bone formation and bone remodeling by G-protein-coupled receptor 48. // Development. – 2009. – vol. 136, N 16. – P. 2747–2756.

Luo Q., Kang Q., Si W. et al. Connective tissue growth factor (CTGF) is regulated by Wnt and bone morphogenetic proteins signaling in osteoblast differentiation of mesenchymal stem cells. // J.Biol.Chem. – 2004. – vol. 279, N 51. – P. 55958–55968.

Luo W., Guo W., Zheng J. et al. Aggrecan from start to finish. // J.Bone Miner.Metab. – 2000. – vol. 18, N 1. – P. 51–56.

Luu H.H., Song W.X., Luo X. et al. Distinct roles of bone morphogenetic proteins in osteogenic differentiation of mesenchymal stem cell. // J.Orthop.Res. – 2007. – vol. 25, N 5. – P. 665–677.

Lygoe K.A., Wall I., Stephens P., Lewis M.P. Role of vitronectin and fibronectin receptors in oral mucosal and dermal myofibroblast differentiation. // Biol.Cell. – 2007. – vol. 99, N 11. – P. 601–614.

Lysy P.A., Smets F., Sibile C. et al. Human skin fibroblasts: from mesodermal to hepatocyte-like differentiation. // Hepatology. – 2007. – vol. 46, N 3. – P. 1574–1585.

Macias D., Cahan Y., Sampath T.K. et al. Role of BMP-2 and OP-1 (BMP-7) in programmed cell death and skeletogenesis during chick limb development. // Development. – 1997. – vol. 124, – P. 1109–1117.

Mackie E.J. Osteoblasts: novel roles in orchestration of skeletal architecture. // Int.J.Biochem.Cell Biol. – 2003. – vol. 15, N 9. – P. 102–110.

Mackie E.J., Ahmed Y.A., Tatarczuch L. et al. Endochondral ossification: how cartilage is converted into bone in the developing skeleton. // Int.J.Biochem.Cell.Biol. – 2008. – vol. 40, N 1. – P. 46–62.

Mackie E.J., Ramsky S. Expression of tenascin in joint-associated tissues during development and postnatal growth. // J.Anat. – 1996. – vol. 188. – P. 157–165.

Mackley J.R., Ando J., Herzyk P., Winder S.J. Phenotypic responses to mechanical stress in fibroblasts from tendon, cornea and skin. // Biochem.J. – 2006. – vol. 396. – P. 307–316.

Maden M. The role of retinoic acid in embryonic and post-embryonic development. // Proc.Nutrit.Soc. – 2000. – vol. 59. – P. 65–73.

Maden M., Hind M. Retinoic acid, a regeneration-inducing molecule. // Dev.Dyn. – 2003. – vol. 226, N 2. – P. 237–244.

Maeda A., Nishida T., Aoyama K. et al. CCN family 2/connective tissue growth factor modulates BMP-2 signaling as as a signal conductor, which action regulates the proliferation and differentiation of chondrocytes. // J.Biochem. – 209. – vol. 145, N 2. – P. 207–216.

Maeda T., Jikko A., Abe M. et al. Cartducin, a paralog of Acrp30/adiponectin, is induced during chondrogenic differentiation and promotes proliferation of chondrogenic precursors and chondrocytes. // J.Cell.Physiol. – 2006. – vol. 206, N 2. – P. 537–544.

Maehata Y., Takamizawa S., Ozawa S. et al. Both direct and collagen-mediated signals are required for active vitamin D3-elicited differentiation of human osteoblastic cells: Roles of osterix, an osteoblast related transcription factor. // Matrix Biol. – 2006. – vol. 25, N 1. – P. 47–59\8.

Magee C/. Nurminskaya M., Faverman L. et al. SP3/SP1 transcription activity regulates specific expression of collagen type X in hypertrophic chondrocytes. // J.Biol.Chem. – 2005. – vol. 280, N 27. – P. 25331–25338.

Mailhot G., Yang M., Mason-Savas A. et al. BMP-5 expression increased during chondrocyte differentiation in vivo and in vitro and promotes proliferation and cartilage matrix synthesis in primary chondrocyte culture. // J.Cell.Physiol. – 2008. – vol. 214, N 1. – P. 156–164.

Mak K.K., Chen M.H., Day T.F. et al. Wnt/β-catenin signaling interacts differentially with Ihh signaling in controlling endochondral bone and synovial joint formation. // Development. – 2006. – vol. 133. – P. 3695–3707.

Mak K.K., Kronenberg H.M., Chuang P.T. et al. Indian hedgehog signals independently of PTHrP to promote chondrocyte hypertrophy. // Development. – 2008. – vol. 135. – P. 1947–1956.

Malavia L., Wade-Guéye, Boudiffa M. et al. Bone sialoprotein plays a functional role in bone formation and osteoclastogenesis. // J.Exp.Med. – 2008. – vol. 205, N 5. – P. 1145–1143.

Male D., Brostoff J., Roit I. Immunology. Saunder, 2012, P. 482

Malemud C.J. Matrix metalloprotcases (MMPs) in health and disease: an overview. // Front.Biosci. – 2006. – vol. 11. – P. 1696–1701.

Malemud C.J. Matrix metalloproteinases: role in skeletal development and growth plate disorders. // Front.Biosci. – 2006. – vol. 11. – P. 1702–1715.

Malone J.P., Alvares K., Veis A. Structure and assembly of the heterotrimeric and homotrimeric C-propeptide of type I collagen: significance of the alpha2(I) chain. // Biochemistry. – 2005. – vol. 44, N 46. – P. 15269–15279.

Malta J., Blitterwijk C.A.van, Geffen M.van et al. Low oxygen tension stimulates the redifferentiation of dedifferentiated adult human nasal chondrocytes. // Osteoarthritis cartilage. – 2004. – vol. 12, N 4. – P. 306–313.

Mandrup S., Lane M.D. Regulating adipogenesis. // J.Biol.Chem. – 1997. – vol. 272, N 9. – P. 5367–5370.

Manduca P., Castagnino A., Lombardini D. et al. Role of MT1-MMP in the osteogenic differentiation. // Bone. 0 2009. – vol. 44, N 2. – P. 251–265.

Manfroid I., Caubit X., Marcelle C., Fasano L. Teashirt 3 expression in the chick embryo reveals a remarkable association with tendon development. // Gene Expr.Patterns. – 2006. – vol. 6, N 8. – P. 908–912.

Mann H.H., Özbek S., Engel J. et al. Interactions between the cartilage oligomeric matrix protein and matrilins. Implications for matrix assembly and pathogenesis of chondroplasias. // J. Biol. Chem. – 2004. – vol. 279, N 24. – P. 25294–25298.

Mann H.H., Sengle G., GebauerJ.M. et al. Matrilins mediate weak cell attachment without formation focal adhesion formation. // Matrix Biol. – 2007. – vol. 26, N 3. – P. 167–174.

Manolagas S.C., Kousteni S., Jilka R.L. Sex steroids and bone. // Rec.Progr.Bone Horm.Res. – 2002. – vol. 57. – P. 385–409.

Månsson B., Wenglén C., Mörgelin M. et al. Association of chondroadherin with collagen type II. // J.Biol.Chem. – 2001. – vol. 276, N 35. – P. 32883–32888.

Mansukhani A., Ambrosetti D., Holmes G. et al. Sox2 induction by FGF and FGRF2 activating mutations inhibits Wnt signaling and osteoblast differentiation. // J.Cell Biol. – 2005. – vol. 168, N 7 – P. 1065–1076.

Mao Y., Schwarzbauer J.E. Fibronectin fibrillogenesis, a cell-mediated matrix assembly process. // Matrix Biol. – 2005. – vol. 24, N 6. – P. 389–399.

Maquart F.X., Bellon G., Pasco S., Monboisse J.C. Matrikines in the regulation of extracellular matrix degradation. // Biochimie. – 2005. – vol. 87, N 2–3. – P. 353–360.

Marchini A., Hacker B., Marttila T et al. BNP is a transcriptional target of the short stature homeobox gene SHOX. // Hun.Mol.Genet. – 2007. – vol. 16, N 24. – P. 3081–3087

Marcil A., Dumontier E., Chamberland M. et al. Pitx1 and Pitx2 are trquired for development of hindlimb buds. // Development. – 2003. – vol. 130. – P. 45–55.

Mariani F.V., Martin D.R. Deciphering skeletal patterning: clues from the limb. // Nature. – 2003. – vol. 423, N 6937. – P. 319–325.

Marie P.J. Fibroblast growth factor signaling sontrolling osteoblast differentiation. // Gene. – 2003. – vol. 316. – P. 23–32.

Marikawa Y. Wnt/beta-catenin signaling and body plan formation in mouse embryo. // Semin.Cell Dev.Biol. – 1996. – vol. 17, N 2. – P. 175–184.

Marill J., Idres N., Capron C.C. et al. Retinoic acid metabolism and mechanism of action: a review. // Curr.Drug Metabolism. – 2003. – vol. 4. – P. 1–10.

Marinkovich M. P., Keene D. R., Rimberg C. S., Burgeson R. E. Cellular origin of the dermal-epidermal basement membrane. // Dev. Dyn. – 1993. – vol. 197. – P. 255–267.

Mark K.von der,, Wandt P., Roxrodt F., Kühn K. Direct evidence for a correlation between amino acid sequence and cross striation pattern of collagen // FEBS Letters 1970. – vol. 11, № 2. – P. 105–108.

Marom K., Levy V., Pillemer G., Fainsod A. Temporal analysis of the early BMP d\functions identifies distinct anti-organizer and mesoderm patterning phases. // Dev.Biol. – 2005. – vol. 282. – P. 442–454.

Maroudas A., Bayliss M.T., Uchitel-Kaushansky N. Aggrekan turnover in human articular cartilage: use of aspartic acid racemization as marker of molecular age. // Arch.Biochem.Biophys. – 1998. – vol. 350, N 1. – P. 61–71.

Martin J.A., Miller B.A., Scherb M.B. et al. Co-localization of insulin-like growth factor binding protein-3 and fibronectin in human articular cartilage. // Osteoarthritis Cartilage. – 2002. – vol. 10, N 7. – P. 556–563.

Martin R.B. Porosity and specific surface of bone // CRC Critical reviews in biomedical engineering – 1986. – vol. 10. – N 3. – P. 179–222.

Martin S., Parton R.C. Lipid droplets: a unified view of a dynamic organelle. // Nat.Rev.Mol.Cell Biol. – 2006. – vol. 7. – P. 373–378.

Martin T.J., Sims N.A. Osteoclast-derived activity in the coupling of bone formation to resorption. // Trends Mol.Med. – 2005. – vol. 11, N 2. – P. 76–81.

Martinovic S., Borovecki F., Mijavac V. et al. Requirement of a bone morphogenetic protein for the maintenance and stimulation of osteoblast differentiation. // Acta Histol.Cytol. – 2006. – vol. 69, N 1. – P. 23–36.

Masur S.K., Conors R.J.J., Cheung J.K., Antohi S. Matrix adhesion characteristics of corneal myofibroblasts. // Invest.Ophthalmol.Vis.Sci. – 1999. –V. 40. – P. 904–910.

Masur S.K., Dewal H.S., Dinh T.T. et al. Myofibroblasts differentiate from fibroblasts when plated at low density. // Proc.Natl.Acad.Sci. USA. – 1996. – vol. 93. – P. 4219–4223.

Matheson S., Larjava B., Hakkinen L. Distinctive localization and function for lumican, fibromodulin and decorin to regulate collagen fibril organization in periodontal tissues. // J.Periodontol.Res. – 2005. – vol. 40, N 4. – P. 312–324.

Matsubara T., Kida K., Tamaguchi A. et al. BMP2 regulates osterix through Msx2 and Runx2 during osteoblast differentiation. // J.Biol.Chem. – 2008. – vol. 283, N 43. – P. 29119–29125.

Matsuguchi T., Chiba N., Bandow K. et al. JNK activity is essential for Atf4 expression and late-stage osteoblast differentiation. // J.Bone Miner.Res. – 2009. – vol. 24, N 3. – 398–410.

Matsumoto K., Kamiya N., Suwan K. et al. Identification and characterization of versican/PG-M aggregates in cartilage. // J.Biol.Chem. – 2006. – vol. 281, N 26. – P. 18257–18263.

Matsuo K., Ray N. Osteoclasts, mononuclear phagocytes, and c-Fos: new insights in osteoimmunology. // Keio J.Med. – 2005. – vol. 53, N 2. – P. 78–84.

Matsuo N., Tanaka S., Gordon M.K., Koch M. et al. CREB-AP1 protein complexes regulate transcription of the collagen XXIV gene (Col24a1) in osteoblasts. // J.Biol.Chem. – 2006. – vol. 281, N 9. – P. 5445–5452.

Matsuo N., Tanaka S., Yoshioka H. et al. Collagen XXIV (Col24a1) gene expression is a specific marker of osteoblast differentiation and bone formation. // Connect.Tissue Res. – 2008. – vol. 49, N 2. – P. 68–75.

Matsushita H., Blackburn M.L., Klineberg E. et al. TASR-1 regulates alternative splicing of collagen genes in chondrogenic cells. // Biochem.Biophys.Res.Commun. – 2007. – vol. 356, N 2. – P. 411–417.

Mau E., Whertstone H., Yu C. et al. PTHrP regulates growth plate chondrocyte differentiation and proliferation in a Gli3 dependen manner utilizing hedgehog ligand dependen and independent mechanisms. // Dev.Biol. – 2007. – vol. 305, N 1. – P. 28–39.

Maximov A.A. Fundamentals of histology: Part II. A theory of tissues. [in Russian] – Leningrad: B.M.I., 1925. 316 pages.

Maximow A.A. Bin de gewebe und blutbildende Gewebe. [in German] // In: Möllendorfs Handbuch der microskopischen Anatomie des Menschen. Berlin: Springer, 1927. Bd. 21. P. 232–560.

Mayer U., Kohfeldt E., Timpl R. Structural and genetic analysis of laminin-nidogen interaction. // Ann.NY Acad.Sco. – 1998. vol. 857. – P. 30–42.

Mayne R., Mark K.von der. Collagens of cartilage. // In: Cartilage (Hall B.K., ed.). Vol.1. N.Y.: Acad.Press. – 1983. – P. 181–214.

Mazerbourg S., Sangkuhl K., Lui C.W. et al. Identification of receptors and signaling pathways for orphan bone morphogenetic protein/ growth differentiation factor ligands based on genomic analyses. – 2005. – vol. 280, N.37. – P. 32122–32132.

Mbalaviele G., Sheikh S., Stains G.P. et al. Beta-catenin and BMP-2 synergize to promote osteoblast differentiation and new bone formation. // J.Cell.Biochem. – 2005. – vol. 94, N 2. – P. 403–418.

Mbuyi-Muamba J.M., Dequecker J., Gevers G. Collagen and non-collagenous proteins in different mineralization stages of human femur. // Acta Anat. – 1989. – vol. 134, N 4. – P. 265–268.

McAlinden A., Havlioglu N., Liang L et al. Alternative splicing of type II procollagen exoN2 is regulated by the combination of weak 5' splice site and adjacent introne stem-loop cis element. // J.Biol. Chem. – 2005. – 280, N 38. – P. 32700–32711.

McAlinden A., Johnstone B., Kollar J. et al. Expression of two novel alternatively spliced COL2A1 isoforms during chondrocyte differentiation. // Matrix Biol. – 2008. – vol. 27, N 3. – P. 254–266.

McAlinden A., Smith T.A., Sandell L.J. et al. α-Helical coiled-coil oligomerization domains are almost ubiquitous in the collagen superfamily. // J.Biol.Chem. – 2003. – vol. 278, N 43. – P. 43200–43207.

McAlinden A., Zhu Y., Sandell L.J. Expression of type II procollagens during development of the human intervertebral disc. // Biochem.Soc.Trans. – 2002. – vol. 30, N 6. – P. 831–838.

McAnulty R.J. Fibroblasts and myofibroblasts: their source, function and role in disease. // Int.J.Biochem.Cell Biol. – 2007. – vol. 39, N 4. – P. 666–671.

McCarthy T.L., Ji C., Centrella M. Links among growth factors, hormones, and nuclear factors with essential roles in bone formation. // Crit.Rev.Oral Biol.Med. – 2000. – vol. 11, N 4. – P. 409–422

McDevitt C.A. Biochemistry of articular cartilage. // Ann. Rheum. Dis. – 1973. – vol. 32. – P. 364–373.

McDonald J.A., Camenish T.D. Hyaluronan: genetic insight into the complex biology of a simple polysaccharide. // Glycoconj.J. – 2002. – vol. 19, N 4–5. – P. 331–339.

McGlinn E., Beuren K.L.van, Fiorenza S. et al. Pax9 and Jagged1 act downstream of Gli3 in vertebrate limb development. // Mech.Dev. 2005. – vol122., N 11. – P. 1218–1233.

McKee M.D., Farach-Carson M.C., Butler W.T et al. Ultrastructural immunolocalization of noncollagenous (osteopontin and osteocalcin) and plasma (albumin and alpha2HS-glycoprotein) proteins in rat bone. // J.Bone Miner.Res. – 1993. – vol. 8, N 4. – P. 485–496.

McLean R.M., Podell D.N. Bone and joint manifestations of hypothyroidism. // Semin.Arthritis Rheum. – 1995. – vol. 24, N 4. – P. 282–290

McNamara L.M., Majeska R.J., Weinbaum S, et al. Attachment of osteocyte cell processes to the bone matrix. // Anat.Rec. – 2009. – vol. 292, N 3. – P. 355–363.

McNulty A.L., Vail T.P., Kraus V.B. Chondrocyte transport and concentration of ascorbic acid is mediated by SVCT2. // Biochim.Biophys. Acta. – 2005. – vol. 1712, N 2. – P. 212–221.

Mecham R.R., Whitehouse L., Hay M. et al. Ligand affinity of the 67-kDa elastin/laminin binding protein is modulated by the protein's lectin domain. // J.Cell Biol. – 1991. – vol. 113, N 1. – P. 187–194.

Meech R., Edelman D.B., Jones F.S., Makarenkova H.R. The homeobox transcription factor Barx2 regulates chondrogenesis during limb development. // Development. – 2005. – vol. 132. – P. 2135–2146.

Meester-Smoor M.A., Vermeij M., Helmond M.J.L.van et al. Targeted disruption of the Mn1 oncogene results in severe defects in development of membranous bones of the cranial skeleton. // Mol.Ce.Biol. – 2005. – vol. 25, N 10. – P. 4229–4236.

Meirelles L.da S., Chagastelles P.C., Nardi N.B. Mesenchymal stem cells reside in virtually all post-natal organs and tissues. // J.Cell Sci. – 2006. – vol. 119. – P. 2204–2213.

Melrose J., Roughley P., Knox S. et al. The structure, location, and function of perlecan, a prominent pericellular proteoglycan of fetal, postnatal, and mature hyaline cartilage. // J.Biol.Chem. – 2006. – vol. 281., N 48. – P. 36905–36914.

Meng Q.G., Long X. A hypothetical biological synovial fluid for treatment of temporomandibular joint disease. // Med. Hypotheses. – 2008. – vol. 70, N 4. – P. 835–837.

Meran S., Thomas D., Stephens P. et al. Involvement of hyaluronan in regulation of fibroblast phenotype. // J.Biol.Chem. – 2007. – vol. 282, N 35. – P. 25687–25697.

Mercer D.K., Nicol P.P.,Kimbembe C., Robins S.P. Identification, expression, and tissue distribution of the three rat lysyl hydroxylase isoforms. // Biochem.Biophys.Res.Commun. – 2003. – vol. 307, N 4. – P. 803–809.

Meredith D., Gehl K.A., Seymour J. et al. Characterization of sulphate transporters in isolated bovine articular chondrocytes. // J.Orthop.Res. – 2007. – vol. 25, N 9. – P. 1145–1153

Merino R.,Macias D., Gañan Y. et al. Expression and function of GDF-5 during skeletogenesis in the embryonic chick limb bud. // Dev.Biol. – 1999. – vol. 206, N 1. – P. 33–45.

Merzdorf C.S., Sive H.L. The zic1 gene is an activator of Wnt signaling. // Int.J.Dev.Biol. – 2006. – vol. 50. – P. 611–617.

Metz C. N. Fibrocytes: a unique cell population implicated in wound healing. // Cell.Mol. Life Sci. – 2003. – vol. 60. – P. 1342–1350.

Metz M, Siebenhaar F, Maurer M. Mast cell functions in the innate skin immune system. // Immunobiology. – 2008. – vol. 213, N 3–4. – P. 251–60.

Miao D., He B., Jiang Y. et al. Osteoblast-derived PTHrP is a potent endogenous bone anabolic agent that modifies the therapeutic efficacy of administered PTH 1-34. // J.Clin.Invest. – 2005. – vol. 115, N 9. – P. 2402–2411.

Michon F., Charveron M., Dhoually D. Dermal condensation formation in the chick embryo: Requirement for integrin engagement and subsequent stabilization by a possible Notch/integrin interaction. // Dev.Dyn. – 2007. – vol. 236. – P. 755–768.

Midura R.J., Wang A., Lovitch D. et al. Bone acidic glycoprotein-75 delineates the extracellular sites of future bone sialoprotein accumulation and apatite nucleation in osteoblast cultures. // J.Biol.Chem. – 2004. – vol 279, N 24. – P. 25464–25473.

Mihai C., Iscru D.F., Druhan L.J. et al. Discoidin domain receptor 2 inhibits fibrillogenesis of collagen type I. // J.Mol.Biol. – 2006. – vol. 361, N 5. – P. 364–376.

Mikhailov A.N. Integumentary collagen and principles of its processing. [in Russian] Moscow: "Light industry", 1971. 528 pages.

Mikhailov A.N. Physics and chemistry of integumentary collagen. [in Russian] Moscow: "Leg. prom.", 1981. 232 pages.

Mikic B., Wong M., Chiquet M., Hunziker E.B. Mechanical modulation of tenascin-C and collagen-XII expression during avian joint formation. // J.Orthop.Res. – 2000. – vol. 18, N 3. – P. 406–415.

Mikura A., Okuhara S., Saito M. Association of tenascin-W expression with mineralization in mouse calvarial development. // Congenit. Anom. (Kyoto). – 2009. – vol. 49, N 2. – P. 77–84.

Miller E.J. Chemistry of the collagens and their distribution. // In: Extracellular matrix biochemistry (K.A.Piez, A.H.Reddi, eds.). – N.Y.a.o.: Elsevier. – 1984. – P. 41–81

Miller J.R. The Wnts. // Genome Biol. – 2001. – vol. 3, N 1: reviews. – P. 3001.1–3001.15.

Miller J.S., Schwartz L.B. Human mast cell proteases and mast cell heterogeneity. // Curr Opin Immunol – 1989. – vol. 1. – P. 637–642.

Milner J.M., Kevorkian L., Young D.A. et al. Fibroblast activation protein alpha is expressed by chondrocytes following a pro-inflammatory stimulus and is elevated in osteoarthritis. // Arthritis Res. Ther. – 2005. – vol. 8. – P. R23.

Milz S., Benjamin M., Puyz R. Molecular parameters indicating adaptation to mechanical stress in fibrous connective tissues. // Adv.Anat.Embryol.Cell Biol. – 2005. – vol. 178. – P. 1–71.

Milz S., Tischer T., Buettner A. et al. Molecular composition and pathology of enthuses on the medial and lateral epicondyles of the humans: a structural basis for epicondylitis. // Ann.Rheum.Dis. – 2004. – vol. 63. – P. 1015–1021.

Minami N., Suzuki T., Tsukamoto S. Zygotic gene activation and maternal factors in mammals. // J.Reprod.Dev. – 2007. – vol. 53, N 4. – P. 707–715.

Minamitani T., Ariga H., Matsumoto K. Deficiency of tenascin-X causes a decrease in the level of expression of type VI collagen. // Exp. Cell Res. – 2004. – vol. 297, N 1. – P. 49–60.

Minamitanii T., Ikuta T., Saito Y. et al. Modulation of collagen fibrillogenesis by tenascin-X and type VI collagen. // Exp.Cell Res. – 2004. – vol. 298, N 1. – P. 305–315.

Minamizato T., Sakamoto K., Liu T. et al. CCN/NOV inhibits BMP-2 inhibit osteoblast differentiation by interacting with BMP and Notch signaling pathways. // Biochem.Biophys.Res.Commun. – 2007. – vol. 354. – P. 567–573.

Minguell J.J., Erices A., Conget P. Mesenchymal stem cells. // Exp.Biol. Med. – 2001. – vol. 226, N 6. – P. 507–520.

Miraoui H., Oudina K., Petite K. et al. Fibroblast growth factor receptor 2 promotes osteogenic differentiation in mesenchymal cells via extracellular-related kinase and protein kinase C signaling. // J.Biol.Chem. – 2009. – vol. 284, N 8. – P. 4897–4904.

Mironov S.P., Omelyanenko N.P., Kozhevnikov O.V., Il'yna V.K., and A.V. Ivanov. Usage of autologous stromal bone marrow cells in the surgical treatment of shin bones' congenital pseudarthrosis in children. [in Russian] Annals of Traumatology & Orthopedics (named in honour of N.N. Priorov), 2011, no.2. P. 46–52.

Mironov S.P., Omelyanenko N.P., Kozhevnikov O.V., Il'yna V.K., Ivanov A.V., Karpov I.N., and Lazarev V.A. Usage of cell-based technology in the surgical correction of congenital leg length discrepancy in children. [in Russian]. Annals of Traumatology & Orthopedics (named in honor of N.N. Priorov), 2011, no.1. P. 3–9.

Mironov S.P., Omelyanenko N.P., Kozhevnikov O.V., Il'yna V.K., Ivanov A.V., and I.N. Karpov. Effects of cultured autologous connective tissue (stromal) cells of bone marrow on slowly forming distraction regenerates in children. [in Russian] Cell Transplantation and Tissue Engineering, 2011, vol. VI, no. 2. P. 104–112.

Mishra R.K., Yamaguchi T., Vasanthi D. et al. Involvement of Polycomb-Group genes in establishing HoxD temporal colinearity. // Genesis. – 2007. – vol. 45. – P. 570–576.

Misra A., Lim R.P.Z., Wu Z., Thanabalu T. N-WASP plays a crucial role in fibroblast adhesion and spreading. // Biochem.Biophys.Res. Comm. – 2007. – vol. 374, N 4. – P. 908–912.

Mithieux S.M., Weiss A.S. Elastin. // Adv.Protein Chem. – 2005. – V. 70. – 437–461.

Mo R., Freer A.M., Zinyk D.L et al. Specific and redundant functions of Gli2 and Gli3 zinc finger genes in skeletal patterning and development. // Development. – 1997. – vol. 124. – P. 113–123.

Mochida Y., Parisuthiman D., Pornprasertsuk-Damrongsri S. et al. Decorin modulates collagen matrix assembly and mineralization. // Matrix Biol. – 2009. – vol. 28, N 1. – P. 44–52.

Moffatt P., Thmas G. Osteocrin beyond just another bone protein. // Cell.Mol.Life Sci. – 2009. – Epub.Feb.24.

Moffatt P., Thomas G., Sellin K. et al. Osteocrin is a specific ligand of the natriuretic peptide clearance receptor that modulates bone growth. // J.Biol.Chem. – 2007. – vol. 282, N 50. – P. 36454–36462.

Mohan S., Kapoor A., Singgih A. et al. Spontaneous fractures in the mouse mutant sfx are caused by deletion of Gulonolactone Oxidase gene, causing viyamin C deficiency. // J.Bone Miner.Res. – 2005. – vol. 20, N 9. – P. 1597–1610/

Monical, P. L., Kefalides, N. A. Coculture modulates laminin synthesis and mRNA levels in epidermal keratinocytes and dermal fibroblasts. // Exp. Cell. Res. – 1994. – vol. 210. – P. 154–159.

Montagna W., Parakkal P.F. The structure and function of skin. – New York – London, Acad. Press. – 1974.

Moreno M., Munoz R., Aroca F. et al. Biglycan is a new extracellular component of the chordin-BMP4 signaling pathway. // EMBO J. – 2005. – vol. 24. – P. 1397–1405.

Mori M., Nakajima M., Mikami Y. et al. Transcriptional regulation of the cartilage intermediate layer protein. // Biochem.Biophys.Res. Commun. – 2006. – vol. 341, N 1. – P. 121–127.

Morita K., Miyamoto T., Fujita N. et al. Reactive oxygen species induce chondrocyte hypertrophy in endochondral ossification. // J.Exp.Med. – 2007. – vol. 204, N 7. – P. 1613–1627.

Morris-Kay G.M., Wilkie A.O.M. Growth of the normal skull vault and its alterations in craniosynostosis: insights from human genetics and experimental studies. // J.Anat. – 2005. – vol. 207. – P. 637–653.

Mort J.S., Billington C.J. Articular cartilage and changes in arthritis. Matrix degradation. // Arthritis Res. – 2001. – vol. 3. – P. 337–341

Mosher D.E., Fogerty E.J., Chernousov M.A., Barry E.L.R. Assembly of fibronectin into extracellular matrix. // Ann.N.Y.Acad.Sci. – 1991. – vol. 614. – P. 167–180

Moss J.M., Van Damme M.P., Murphy W.H. et al. Purification, characterization, and biosynthesis of bovine cartilage lysozyme isoforms. // Arch.Biochem.Biophys. – 1997. – vol. 339. – P. 172–182.

Motomura H., Niimi H., Sugimori K. et al. Gas6, a new regulator of chondrogenic differentiation from mesenchymal cells. // Biochem.Biophys.Res. Commun. – 2007. – vol. 357. – P. 997–1003.

Moulin K., Truel N., André M. et al. Emergence during development of white-adipocyte cell phenotype is independent of the brown-adipocyte cell phenotypr. // Biochem.J. – 2001. – vol. 356. – P. 659–664.

Moulin V, Auger FA, Garrel D, Germain L. Role of wound healing myofibroblasts on re-epithelialization of human skin. // Burns. – 2000. – vol. 26, N 1. – P. 3–12.

Moulin V., Castilloux G., Auger F.A. et al. Modulated response to cytokines of human wound healing myofibroblasts compared to dermal fibroblasts. // Exp.Cell.Res. – 1998. – vol. 238. – P. 283–293.

Moulin V., Tam B., Castilloux G. et al. Fetal and adult human skin fibroblasts display intrinsic differences in contractile capacity. // J.Cell.Physiol. – 2000. – vol. 188. – P. 211–222.

Muir H. The chondrocyte, architect of cartilage. Biomechanics, structure, function and molecular biology of cartilage matrix macromolecules. // Bioessays. – 1995. – vol. 17, N 12. – P. 1039–1049.

Mukai Y., Otsuka F., Otani H. et al. TNF-α inhibits BMP-induced osteoblast differentiation through activating SAPK/JNK signaling. // Biochem.Biophys.Res.Commun. – 2007. – vol. 356. – P. 1004–1010.

Mukherjee A., Rotwein P. Insulin-like growth factor binding protein-5 in osteogenesis: facilitator or inhibitor? // Growth Horm. – 2007. – vol. 17, N 3. – P. 179–185.

Mukudai Y., Kubota S., Kawaki H. et al. Posttranslational regulation of chicken ccn2 gene expression by nucleophosmin/B23 during chondrocyte differentiation. // Mol.Cell.Biol. – 2008. – vol. 28, N 19. – P. 6134–6147.

Mumm J.S., Kopan R. Notch signaling: from the outside in. // Dev.Biol. – 2000. – vol. 228. – P. 151–165.

Mummert M.E. Immunologic roles of hyaluronan. // Immunol.Res. – 2005. – vol 31, N 3. – P. 189–206.

Muramatsu S., Wakabayashi M., Ohno T. et al. Functional gene screening system identified TRPV4 as a regulator of chondrogenic differentiation. // J.Biol.Chem. – 2007. – vol. 282, N 44. – P. 32158–32162.

Murchison N.D., Price B.A., Conner D.A. et al. Regulation of tendon differentiation by scleraxis distinguishes force-transmitting tendons from muscle anchoring tendons. // Development. – 2007. – vol. 134. – P. 2697–2708.

Muro A.F., Chauhan A.K., Gajovic S. et al. Regulated splicing of the fibronectin EDA exon is essential for proper skin wound healing and normal lifespan. // J.Cell Biol. – 2003. – vol. 162. – P. 149–160.

Murphy E., Williams G.H. The thyroid and the skeleton. // Clin.Endocrinol. – 2004. – vol. 61. – P. 285–298.

Murphy J.M., Heinegård R., McIntosh A. et al. Distribution of cartilage molecules in the developing mouse joint. // Matrix Biol. – 1999. – vol. 18, N 5. – P. 487–497.

MurphyL.I., Fischer D., Chiquet-Ehrismann R., Mackie J. Tenascin-C induced stimulation of chondrogenesis is dependent on the presence of the C-terminal fibrinogen-like globular domain. // FEBS Lett. – 2000. – vol. 480. – P. 189–192

Murphy-Ulrich J.E. The de-adhesive activity of matricellular proteins: is intermediate cell adhesion an adaptive state? // J.Clin.Invest. – 2001. – vol. 107, N 7. – P. 785–790.

Murray T.M., Rao L.G., Divieti P., Bringhurst F.R. Parathyroid hormone secretion and action: evidence for discrete receptors for the carboxyl-terminal region and related biological actions of carboxyl-terminal ligand. // Endocrine Rev. – 2005. – vol 26, N 1. – P. 78–113.

Murshed M., Harmey D., Millán et al. Unique coexpression in osteoblasts of broadly expressed genes accounts for the spatial restriction of the ECM mineralization to bone. // Genes Dev. – 2005. – vol. 19. – P. 1093–1194.

Mushkambarov N.N. and S.L. Kuznetsov. Molecular biology. [in Russian] Moscow: Med. Inform. Agency, 2003, 544 pages.

Musri M.M., Gomis R., Párrizas M. Chromatin and chromatin-modifying proteins in adipogenesis. // Biochem.Cell Biol. – 2007. – V. 85. – P. 397–410.

Muto J., Kuroda K., Wachi H. et al. Accumulation of elafin in actinic elastosis of sun-damaged skin: elafin binds to elastin and prevents elastolytic degradation. // J.Invest.Dermatol. – 2007. – V. 127. – P. 1358–1366.

Myllyharju J. Prolyl 4-hydroxylases, the key enzymes of collagen biosynthesis. // Matrix Biol. – 2003. – vol. 22, N 1. – P. 15–24.

Myllyharju J., Kivirikko K.I. Collagens, modifying enzymes and their mutations in humans, flies and worms. // Trends Genet. – 2004. – vol. 20, N 1. – P. 33–43.

Nadra R., Menuelle P., Chevallier S., Berdal A. Regulation by glucocorticoiud of cell differentiation and insulin-like growth factor binding protein production in cultured fetal rat nasal chondrocytes. // J.Cell.Biochem. – 2003. – vol. 88, N 5. – P. 911–922.

Nagase H., Brew K. Designing TIMP (tissue inhibitors of metalloproteinases) variants that are selective metalloproteinase inhibitors. // Biochem.Soc. Symp. – 2003. – vol. 70. – P. 201–212.

Nagata K.H. SP47 as a collagen-specific molecular chaperone: function and expression in normal mouse development. // Semin.Cell Dev.Biol. – 2003. – vol. 14, N 5. – P. 275–282.

Nah H.D., Pacifici M., Gerstenfeld L.C. et al. Transient chondrogenic phase in the intramembranous pathway during dermal skeleton development. // J.Bone Miner.Res. – 2000. – vol. 15, N 3. – P. 522–533.

Nahar N.N., Nissana L.R., Garimella R. et al. Matrix vesicles are carriers of bone morphogenetic proteins (BMPs), vascular endothelial growth factor (VEGF), and noncollagenous matrix proteins. // J.Bone Miner.Metab. – 2008. – vol. 26, N 5. – P. 514–519.

Nair R.R., Preete R., Smitha G., Adiga I. Variation in mitogenic response of cardiac and pulmonary fibroblasts to cerium. // Biol.Trace Elem.Res. – 2003. – vol. 94, N 3. – P. 237–246.

Naito J., Kaji H., Sowa H. et al. Menin suppresses osteoblast differentiation by antagonizing the AP-1 factor, JunD. // J.Biol.Chem. – 2005. – vol. 280, N 6. – P. 4785–4791.

Naito Z. The role of small leucine-rich proteoglycan (SLRP family) in pathological lesions and cancer cell growth. // J.Nippon Med. Sch. – 2005. – vol. 72, N 3. – P. 137–145.

Nakahata T., Kobayashi T., Ishiguro A. et al. Extensive proliferation of mature connective-tissue type mast cells in vitro. // Nature. – 1986. – vol. 324, N 6092. P. 65–7

Nakajima M., Kizawa H., Saitoh M. et al. Mechanisms for asporin function and regulation in articular cartilage. // J.Biol.Chem. – 2007. – vol. 282, N 44. – P. 32185–32192.

Nakamura I., Duong L.T., Rodan S.R., Rodan G.A. Involvement of of αVβ3 integrins in osteoclast function. // J.Bone Miner.Metab. – 2007. – vol. 25. P. 337–344.

Nakamura M., Udagawa N., Matsuura S. et al. Osteoprotegerin regulates bone formation through a coupling mechanism with bone resorption. // Endocrinology. – 2003. – vol. 144, N 12. – P. 5441–5449.

Nakamura T., Lozano P.R., Ikeda Y. et al. Fibulin-5/DANCE is essential for elastogenesis in vivo. // Nature. – 2002. – vol. 415, N 6868. – P. 171–175.

Nakamura Y. Isolation of p53-target genes and their functional analysis. // Cancer Sci. – 2004. – vol. 95, N 1. – P. 7–11.

Nakase T., Yoshikawa H. Potential role of bone morphogenetic proteins (BMPs) in skeletal repair and regeneration. // J.Bone Miner.Metab. – 2006. – vol. 24. – P. 425–433.

Nakashima K., Zhou X., Kunkel G. et al. The novel zinc finger-containing transcription factor Osterix is required for osteoblast differentiation and bone formation. // Cell. – 2002. – vol. 106, N 1. – P. 17–29.

Nakashima Y., Kariya Y., Yasuda C., Miyasaki K. Regulation of cell adhesion and type VII collagen binding by the beta3 chain short arm of laminin-5: effect of its proteolytic cleavage. // J.Biochem. (Tokyo). – 2005. – vol. 138, N 5. – P. 539–552.

Nakatani T., Honda E., Hayakawa S. et al. Effects of decorin on the expression of α-smooth muscle actin in a human myofibroblast cell line. // Mol.Cell.Biochem. – 2008. – vol. 308, N 1–2. – P. 201–207.

Nakayama Y., Shirai Y., Yoshikara K., Uesaka S. Evaluation of glycosaminoglycan levels in normal joint fluid of the knee. // J.Nippon Med. Sci. – 2000, – vol. 67, N 2. – P. 92–95.

Nampei A., Hashimoto J., Hayashida K. et al. Matrix extracellular phosphoglycoprotein (MEPE) is highly expressed in osteocytes in human bone. // J.Bone Miner.Metab. – 2004. – vol. 22, N 3. – P. 176–184.

Naot D., Cornish J. The role of peptides and receptors of thecalcitonin family in the regulation of bone metabolism. // Bone. – 2008. – vol. 43, N 5. – P. 813–818.

Naot D., Grey A., Reid I.R., Cornish J. Lactoferrin – a novel bone growth factor. // Clin.Med.Res. – 2005. – vol. 3, N 2. – P. 93–101.

Naumann A., Dennis J.E., Awadallah A. et al. Immunochemical and mechanical characterization of cartilage subtypes in rabbit. // J.Histochem.Cytochem. – 2002. – vol. 50. – P. 1049–1058.

Neame P.J., Tapp H., Azizan A. Noncollagenous, nonproteoglycan macromolecules of cartilage. // Cell.Mol.Life Sci. – 1999. –vol.55, N 10. – P. 1327–1340.

Need A.G. Bone resorption markers in vitamin D insufficiency. // Clin.Chim.Acta. – 2006. – vol. 368, N 1–2. – P. 48–52.

Neiva K., Sun Y.-X., Taichman K.S. The role of osteoblasts in regulating hematopoietic stem cell activity and tumor metastasis. // Braz.J.Med. Biol.Res. – 2005. – vol. 38. – P. 1449–1454.

Nelson C.E., Morgan B.A., Burke A.C. et al. Analysis of Hox gene expression in the chick limb bud. // Development. – 1996. – vol. 122. – P. 1449–1466.

Neves S.R., Ram P.T., Iyengar R. et al. G protein pathways. // Science. – 2002. – vol. 296, N 5573. – P. 1636–1639.

Newman B., Gigout L.I., Sudre L. et al. Coordinated expression of matrix Gla protein is required during endochondral ossification for chondrocyte survival. // J.Cell Biol. – 2001. – vol. 154, N 3. – P. 659–666.

Newman S.A., Bhat R. Activator-inhibitor dynamics of vertebrate limb pattern formation. // Birth Defects Res. C. Embryo Today. – 2007. – vol. 81, N 4. – P. 305–319.

Ng R.K., Gurdon J.B. Epigenetic inheritance of cell differentiation status. // Cell Cycle. – 2008. – vol. 7, N 9. – P. 1173–1177.

Nicolae C., Ko Y.P., Miosge N. et al. Abnormal collagen fibrils in cartilage of matrilin-1/matrilin-3 deficient mice. // J.Biol.Chem. – 2007. – vol. 282, N 30. – P. 22163–22175.

Nie X., Luukko K., Kettunen P. BMP signaling in craniofacial development. // Int.J.Dev.Biol. – 2006. – vol. 50. – P. 511–521.

Nie X., Luukko K., Kettunen P. FGF signalling in craniofacial development and developmental disorders. // Oral Dis. – 1996. – vol. 12, N 2. – P. 102–111.

Nieden N.I zur, Kempka G., Rancourt D.E., Ahr H. Induction of chondro-, osteo- and adipogenesis in embryonic stem cells by bone morphogenetic protein-2: effect of cofactors on differentiating lineages. // BMC Dev.Biol. – 2005. – vol. 5. – P. 1–15.

Niederreithe K., Dollé P. Retinoic acid in development: towards an integrated view. // Nat.Rev.Gen. – 2008. – vol. 9. – P. 541–553.

Niemeier A., Kassem M., Toedter K. et al. Expression of LRP1 by human osteoblasts: a mechanism for the delivery of lipoproteins and vitamin K1 to bone. // J.Bone Miner.Res. – 2005. – vol. 20, N 2. – P. 283–293.

Nieminen J., Sahlmab J., Hirvonen T. et al. Disturbed synthesis of type II collagen interfers with rate of bone formation and growth and increases bone resorption in transgenic mice. – Calcif.Tissue Int. – 2008. – vol. 82. – P. 229–237.

Niikura T., Reddi A.H. Differential regulation of lubricin/superficial zone protein by transforming growth factor beta/bone morphogenetic protein superfamily members in articular chondrocytes and synoviocytes. // Arthritis Rheum. – 2007. – vol. 56, N 7. – P. 2312–2321.

Nikaido T., Yokoya S., Mori T. et al. Expression of the novel transcription factor OASIS, which belongs to the CREB/ATF family, in mouse embryo with special embryo with special reference to bone development. // Histochem.Cell Biol. – 2001. – vol. 116. – P. 141–148.

Nilsson O., Marino R., De Luca F. et al. Endocrine regulation of the growth plate. // 2005. vol. 64, P. 157–165.

Ninomiya K., Miyamoto T., Imai J. et al. Osteoclastic activity induces osteomodulin expression in osteoblasts. // Biochem.Biophys.Res. Commun. – 2007. – vol. 362, N 2. – P. 460–466.

Nishida T., Kawaki H., Baxter R.M. et al. CCN2 (connective tissue growth factor) is essebtial for extracellular matrix production and integrin signaling in chondrocytes. // J. Cell. Commun. Signal. – 2007. – vol. 1. – P. 45–58.

Nishida Y., Knudson C.B., Knudson W. Osteogenic protein-1 inhibits matrix depletion in a hyaluronan-induced model of osteoarthritis. // Osteoarthritis Cartilage. – 2004. – vol. 12, N 5. – P. 374–382.

Nishio Y., Dong Y., Paris M. et al. Runx2-mediated regulation of the zinc finger Osterix/Sp7 gene. // Gene. – 2006. – vol. 372. – P. 62–70.

Nitzan D.W., Nitzan L., Dan P., Yedgar S. The role of hyaluronic acid in protecting surface-active phospholipids from lysis by exogenous phospholipase A2. // Rheumatol. – 2001. – vol. 40. – P. 336–340.

Noble B.S. Bone microdamage and cell apoptosis. // Eur.Cells Materials. – 2003. – vol. 6, N 1. – P. 46–56

Noble B.S. The osteocyte lineage. // Arch.Biochem.Biophys. – 2008. – vol. 473, N 2. – P. 106–111.

Noble B.S., Reeve J. Osteocyte function, osteocyte death and bone fracture resistance. // Mol.Cell.Endocrinol. – 2000. – vol. 159, N 1–2. – P. 7–13.

Nobta M., Tsukazaki T., Shibata Y. et al. Critical regulation of bone morphogenetic protein-induced osteoblastic differentiation by Delta1/Jagged1-activated Notch1 signaling. // J.Biol.Chem. – 2005. – vol. 280, N 16. – P. 15842–15848.

Nochi H., Sung J.H., Lou J. et al. Adenovirus mediated BMP-13 gene transfer induces chondrogenic differentiation of murine mesenchymal progenitor cells. – J.Bone Miner.Res. – 2004. – vol. 19, N 1. – P. 111–122.

Nohe A., Keating E., Knaus P., Petersen N.O. Signal transduction of bone morphogenetic protein receptors. // Cell.Signaling. – 2004. – vol. 16. – P. 291–299.

Nolte S.V., Xu W., Renekampff H.O., Rodemann H.P. Diversity of fibroblasts – a review on implications for skin tissue engineering. // Cells Tissue Organs. – 2007. – Epub. NoV. 28.

Nomura S., Takano-Yamamoto T. Molecular events caused by mechanical stress in bone. // Matrix Biol. – 2000. – vol. 19, N 2. – P. 91–96.

Nomura Y. Structural change in decorin with skin aging. // Connect. Tissue Res. – 2006. – vol. 47, N 5. – P. 249–255.

Norman A.W. Vitamin D receptor: new assignments for already busy receptor. // Endocrinology. – 2006. – vol. 147, N 12. – P. 5542–5548.

Noyori K., Takagi T., Jasin H.A. Characterization of the macromolecular components of the articular cartilage surface. // Rheumatol. Int. – 1998. – vol. 18, N 2. – P. 71–77.

Nugent G.E., Aneloski N.M., Schmidt T. et al. Dynamic shear stimulation of bovine cartilage biosynthesis of proteoglycaN 4. // Arthritis Rheum. – 2006. – vol. 54, N 6. – P. 1888–1896

Nurminskaya M., Kaartinen M.T. Transglutaminases in mineralized tissues. // Front.Biosci. – 2006. – vol. 11. – P. 1591–1606.

Nurminsky D., Magee C., Faverman L., Nurminskaya M. Regulation of chondrocyte differentiation by actin-severing protein adseverin. // Dev.Biol. – 2007. – vol. 302. – P. 427–437.

Nusgens B., Humbert P., Rougier A. et al. Topically applied vitamin C enhances the mRNA level of collagens I and III, their processing enzymes and tissue inhibitor of matrix metalloproteinase 1 in the human dermis. // J.Invest.Dermatol. – 2001. – vol. 116. – P. 853–859.

Nusse R. Wnt signaling and stem cell control. // Cell Research. – 2008. – vol. 18. – P. 523–527

Nusse R. Wnts and Hedgehogs: lipid-modified proteins and similarities in signaling mechanisms at the cell surface. // Development. – 2003. – vol. 130. – P. 5297–5305.

O'Brien C.A., Jia D., Plotkin L.I. et al. Glucocorticoids act directly on osteoblasts and osteocytes to induce their apoptosis and reduce bone formation and strength. // Endocrinology. – 2004. – vol. 145, N 4. – P. 1835–1841.

O'Shea P.J., Narvey C.B., Suzuki H. et al. A thyrotoxic skeletal phenotype of advanced bone formation in mice with resistance to thyroid hormone. // Cell. – 2003. – vol. 17, N 7. – P. 1410–1424.

Obregon M.J. Thyroid hormone and adipocyte differentiation. // Thyroid. – 2008. – vol. 18, N 2. – P. 185–195.

Ochi H., Hirani W.M., Yuan Q. et al. T helper cell type 2 cytokine-mediated comitogenic responses and CCR3 expression during differentiation of human mast cells in vitro. // J.Exp. Med. – 1999. – vol. 190, N 2 – P. 267–80.

Oestergaard S., Sondergaard B.C., Andersen P.H. et al. Effect of overiectomy and estrogen therapy on type II collagen degradation and structural integrity of articular cartilage in rats. // Arthritis.Rhemat. – 2006. – vol. 54, N 8. – P. 2441–2451

Ofek G., Revell C.M., Hu J.C. et al. Matrix development in self-assembly of articular cartilage. // PloS ONE. – 2008. – vol/3, N 7. – P. e2795.

Ofek O., Karsak M., Leclerc N. et al. Peripheral cannabinoid receptor, CB2, regulates bone mass. // Proc.Natl.Acad.Sci.USA. – 2006. – vol. 103, N 3. – P. 696–701.

Ogata S., Morokuma J., Hayata T. et al. TGF-β signaling-mediated morphogenesis: modulation of cell adhesion via cadherin endocytosis. // Gened Dev. – 2007. – vol. 21. – P. 1817–1831.

Ogawa K., Saito A., Matsui H. et al. Activin-Nodal signaling is involved in propagation of mouse embryonic stem cells. // J.Cell Sci. – 2007. – vol. 120, N 1. – P. 55–65.

Ogawa M., LaRue A., Drake C.J. Hematopoietic origin of fibroblasts/myofibroblasts: pathophysiologic implications. // Blood. – 2006.– vol. 106, N 9. – P. 2893–2986.

Oginuma M., Niwa Y., Chapman D.L., Saga Y. Mesp2 and Tbx6 cooperatively create periodic patterns coupled with the cloick machinery during mouse somitogenesis. // Development. – 2008. – vol. 135. – P. 2555–2562.

Ogita H., Takai Y. Nectins and nectin-like molecules: roles in cell adhesions, polarization, movement, and proliferation. // IUBMB Life. – 2006. – vol. 58, N 5–6. – P. 334–343.

Oh C.D., Chang S.H., Yoon Y.M. et al. Opposing role of mitogen-activated protein kinase subtypes, Erk-1/2 and p38, in the regulation of chondrogenesis of mesenchymes. // J.Biol.Chem. – 2000. – vol. 275, N 5. – 5613–5619.

Oh E.S., Couchman J.R. Syndecans-2 and -4: close cousins, but not identical twins. // Mol.Cells. – 2004. – vol. 17, N 2. – P. 181–187.

Oh S.P., YeoC.Y., Lee Y. et al. Activin type IIA and IIB receptors mediate Gdf11 signaling in axial vertebral patterning. // Genes Dev. – 2002. – vol. 16. – P. 2749–2754.

Ohbayashi N., Shibayama M., Kurotaki Y. et al. FGF18 is required for normal cell proliferation and differentiation during osteogenesis and chondrogenesis. // Genes Dev. – 2002. – vol. 16. – P. 870–879.

Ohlsson C., Bengtsson B.Å, Isaksson O.G.P. et al. Growth hormone and bone. // Endocrine Rev. – 1998. – vol. 19, N 1. – P. 55–79.

Ohnishi Y., Tajima S., Akiyama M. et al. Expression of elastin-related proteins and matrix metalloproteases in actinic elastosis of sun-damaged skin. // Arch.Dermatol. – 2000. – vol. 292, N 1. – P. 127–131.

Ohno S., Doi T., Tsutami S. et al. RGD-CAP (beta)ig-h3) is expressed in precartilage condensations and in prehypertrophic chondrocytes during cartilage development. // Biochim.Biophys.Acta. – 2002. – vol. 1572, N 1. – P. 114–122.

Okamoto M., Murai J., Yoshikawa H., Tsumaki N. Bone morphogenetic proteins stimulate osteoclasts and osteoblasts during bone development. // J.Bone Miner.Res. – 2006. – vol. 21, N 7. – P. 1022–1033.

Okayama Y, Kawakami T. Development, migration, and survival of mast cells. // Immunol Res. 2006. – vol. 34, N 2. – P. 97–115.

Okitsu Y., Takahashi S., Minegishi N. et al. Regulation of adipocyte differentiation of bone marrow stromal cells by transcription factor GATA-2. // Biochem.Biophys.Res.Comm. – 2007. – vol. 364. – P. 383–387.

Oklu R., Hesketh R. The latent transforming growth factor-beta binding protein family. // Biochem.J. – 2000. – vol. 352, N 3. – P. 601–610.

Okumuro-Nakanishi S., Saito M., Niwa H., Ishikawa F. Oct-3/4 and Sox2 regulate Oct-3/4 gene in embryonic stem cells. // J.Biol.Chem. – 2005. – vol. 280, N 7. – P. 5307–5317.

Oldfield S.F., Evans D.J.R. Tendon morphogenesis in the developing avisn limb. // J.Anat. – 2003. – vol. 202, P. 153–164.

Olin A.I., Mörgelin M., Sasaki T. The proteoglycans aggrecan and versican form networks with fibulin-2 through their lectin domain binding. // J.Biol.Chem. – 2001. – vol. 276, N 2. – P. 1253–1261.

Olsen A.K., Sondergaard B.C., Byrjalsen I. et al. Anabolic and catabolic function of chondrocytes ex vivo is reflected by the metabolic processing of type II collagen. // Osteoarthritis Cartilage. – 2007. – vol. 15, N 3. – P. 335–342.

Olsen B.R. Life without perlecan has its problems. // J.Cell Biol. – 1999. – vol. 147, N 5. – P. 909–911.

Olsen S.K., Garbi M., Zampieri N. et al. Fibroblast growth factor (FGF) homologous factors share structural but not functional homology with FGFs // J.Biol.Chem. – 2003. – vol. 278, N 36. – P. 34226–34236.

Omelyanenko N.P., Slutsky L.I. Connective tissues. vol.I. Ed. Mironov S.P. [in Russian] – Moscow: Izvestiy, 2009. 380 pages.

Omelyanenko N.P., Slutsky L.I. Connective tissues. vol.II. Ed. Mironov S.P. [in Russian] – Moscow: Izvestiy, 2009. 600 pages.

Omelyanenko N.P. Regularities of the structural organization of fibrous stroma in some human organs. Abstract print. 2nd Pan-Pacific Connective Tissue Societies Symposium, Indonesia, Poster Abstracts. 1993. – XI.

Omelyanenko N.P., Zherebtsov L. D., I.N. Mikhailov. Ultrastructure of collagen fibers and ground substance of the human dermis. [in Russian] // AHE Archives. 1977. vol. 72, N 4. P. 69–76.

Omelyanenko N.P, Zherebtsov L.D, Yu.A. Khoroshkov. Peculiarities of the special organization of human Achilles tendon collagen fibers. [in Russian] // AHE Archives, 1981. vol. 84, N 8. P. 77–82.

Omelyanenko N.P, Zherebtsov L.D., L.A. Deev. Ultrastructural relationships of fibrous components in human connective tissue. [in Russian]// AHE Archives, 1979. vol. 74, N 5. P. 65–70.

Omelyanenko N.P., G.M. Butyrin. A quantitative assay of the interstructural space of a human bone compact substance. [in Russian] // Annals of Traumatology & Orthopedics, 1994. N 1. P. 51–54.

Omelyanenko N.P., P.M. Itskov. Morphologic peculiarities of articular cartilage boundary structures. [in Russian] // Morphology. 2002. 121, N 2–3. P. 117.

Omelyanenko N.P. Articular cartilage. [in Russian] // In: Current issues of theoretical and clinical osteoarthrology, written by Denisov-Nikolsky Yu.I., Mironov S.P., Omelyanenko N.P. and I.V. Matveichuk, Moscow: Novosti, 2005. P. 184–205.

Omelyanenko N.P. Bone tissue. Structural functional characteristics of its basic components. [in Russian] //In: Current issues of theoretical and clinical osteoarthrology, written by Denisov-Nikolsky Yu.I., Mironov S.P., Omelyanenko N.P. and I.V. Matveichuk. Moscow: Novosti, 2005. P. 37–81.

Omelyanenko N.P. Connective tissues. [in Russian] // In: Atlas of scanning electron microscopy of cells, tissues and organs, edited by O.V. Volkova, V.A.Shakhlamov and A.A.Mironov. Moscow: Medicine, 1987. P. 463.

Omelyanenko N.P. Orientation analysis of ultrastructural architectonics of a human articular cartilage fibrous framework. [in Russian] // AHE Archives. 1989. Vol. 97, N 7. P. 39–47.

Omelyanenko N.P. Regularities of the organization of connective tissue fibrous elements and ground substance of a human locomotive apparatus. [in Russian] // Doctoral dissertation abstract. Moscow, 1991. 58 pages.

Omelyanenko N.P. Regularities of the structural organization of fibrous stroma of some human organs. [in Russian] // AHE Archives, 1984. vol. 79, N 8. P. 65–75.

Omelyanenko N.P. Structural-functional organization of a human Achilles tendon fibrous framework. [in Russian]// AHE Archives, 1983. N 2. P. 69–77.

Omelyanenko N.P. Ultrastructural organization of a fibrous framework and interstitial canals of human compact bone. [in Russian]// Collected papers of the N.N. Priorov Central Research Institute of Traumatology and Orthopedics. – Moscow, 1990. P. 10–16.

Omelyanenko N.P. Ultrastructural organization of the human dermis ground substance. [in Russian] // AHE Archives, 1978, vol. 74, N 4. P. 101–108.

Omelyanenko N.P. Ultrastructure of the human articular cartilage interstitial space and ground substance. [in Russian] // AHE Archives, 1990, vol. 98, N 6. P. 77–83.

Omelyanenko N.P., Il'yna V.K., and I.N. Karpov. Bone Marrow. [in Russian] // In: Current issues of theoretical and clinical osteoarthrology, written by Denisov-Nikolsky Yu.I., Mironov S.P., Omelyanenko N.P. and I.V. Matveichuk, 2005. P. 164–181.

Omelyanenko N.P., Ilizarov G.A. and V.N. Stetsula. Bone tissue regeneration. [in Russian] // In: Traumatology and Orthopedics/ A textbook. 1997, vol. 1. P. 393–481.

Omelyanenko N.P., Mironov S.P., Denisov-Nikolsky Yu.I., Matveichuk I.V., and I.N. Karpov. Reparative bone regeneration. [in Russian] // In: Current issues of theoretical and clinical osteoarthrology, written by Denisov-Nikolsky Yu.I., Mironov S.P., Omel'yanenko N.P., and I.V. Matveichuk, 2005. P. 239–271.

Omelyanenko N.P., Sokolov V.N., Yurkovets D.I. and O.V. Razgulina. Investigative techniques of quantitative morphologic parameters of a biologic object surface relief. [in Russian] // Biomedical technologies. Collection of scientific papers of the Research Center of Biomedical Engineering. Moscow, 2000, issue 14. P. 102–110.

Omelyanenko N.P., Zherebtsov L.D. Skin and its derivatives. [in Russian] // In: Atlas of scanning electron microscopy of cells, tissues and organs, edited by O.V. Volkova, V.A.Shakhlamov and A.A.Mironov. Moscow: Medicine, 1987. P. 463.

Onoprienko G.A. Bone vascularization in fractures and defects. [in Russian] – Moscow: Medicine, 1993. 224 pages.

Opolka A., Ratzinger S., Schubert T. et al. Collagen IX is indispensable for timely maturation of cartilage during fracture repair In mice. // Matrix Biol. – 2007. – vol. 26, N 2. – P. 85–95.

Orend G. Potential oncogenic action of tenascin-C in tumorigenesis. // Int.J.Biochem.Cell Biol. – 2005. – vol. 37, N 5. – P. 1066–1083.

Ornitz D.M. FGF signaling in the developing endochondral skeleton. // Cytokine Growth Factor Rev. – 2005. –vol.16, N 2. – P. 205–213.

Ornitz D.M., Itoh N. Fibroblast growth factors. // Genome Biol. – 2001. – vol. 2, N 3. – P. 1–12.

Ornitz D.M., Marie P.J. FGF signaling pathways in endochondral and intramembranous bone development and human genetic disease. // Genes.Dev. – 2002. – vol. 16, N 12. – P. 1446–1465.

Ortega N., Behonick D.J., Colnot C. et al. Galectin-3 is a downstream regulator of matrix metalloproteinase-9 function during endochondral bone formation. // Mol.Biol.Cell – 2005. – vol. 16. – P. 3028–3039.

Ortega T. Collagen fibers, reticular fibers and elastic fibers. A comprehensive understanding from a morphological viewpoint. // Arch.Histol.Cytol. – 2002. – vol. 65, N 2. – P.109–126.

Orth M.W., Luchene L.D., Schmid T.M. Type X collagen from the hypertrophic cartilage of the embryo chick tibiae contains both hydroxylysyl – and lysylpiridinoline cross-links. // Biochem.Biophys.Res.Commun. – 1996. – vol. 219, N 2. – P. 301–303.

Osakabe T., Hayashi M., Hasegawa K. et al. Age- and gender-related changes in ligament components. // Ann.Clin.Biochem. – 2001. – vol. 38. – P. 527–532.

Oshima Y., Akiyama T., Hikita A. et al. Pivotal role of Bcl-2 family proteins in the regulation of chondrocyte apoptosis. // J.Biol.Chem. – 2008. – vol. 283, N 39. – P. 26499–26508.

Otterness I.C., Bliven M.L., Eskra J.D. et al. Cartilage damage after intraarticular exposure to collagenase 3. // Osteoarthritis Cartilage. – 2000. – vol. 8, N 5. – P. 366–373.

Ovchinnikov D.A., Selever J., Wang Y. et al. BMP receptor IA in limb bud mesenchyme regulates distal outgrowth and patterning. // Dev.Biol. – 2006. – vol. 295. – P. 103–115.

Ozaki K., Leonard W.J. Cytokine and cytokine receptor pleiotropy and redundancy. // J.Biol.Chem. – 2002. – vol. 277, N 33. – P. 29355–29358.

Özbek S., Engel J., Stetefeld J. Storage function of cartilage oligomeric matrix protein: the crystal structure of the coiled-coil domain in complex with vitamin D3. // The EMBO J. – 2002. – vol. 21, N 22. – P. 5960–5968.

Ozbudak E.M., Pourquié O. The vertebrate segmentation clock: the tip of the icebrtg. // Curr.Opin.Genet.Dev. – 2008. – Epub. Aug.14.

Pace J.M., Corrado M., Missero C., Byers P.H. Identification, characterization and expression analysis of a new fibrillar collagen gene, COL27A1. // Matrix Biol. – 2003. – vol. 22, N 1. – P. 3–14.

Pacifici M., Koyama E., Shibukawa Y. et al. Cellular and molecular mechanisms of synovial joint and articular cartilage formation. // Ann.N.Y.Acad.Sci. – 2006. – vol. 1068. – P. 74–86.

Palacios C. The role of nutrients in bone health, from A to Z. // Curr. Rev.Food Sci.Nutrit. – 2006. – vol. 46, N 8. – P. 621–628.

Palaiologou A.A., Yukna R.A., Moses R., Lallier T.E. Gingival, dermal, and periodontal ligament fibroblasts express different extracellular matrix receptors. // J.Periodontol. – 2001. – vol. 72. – P. 798–807.

Pan Q., Yu Y., Chen Q., Li C. et al. Sox9, a kley transcriptional factor of bone morphogenetic protein-2-induced chondrogenesis, is activated through BMP pathway and CCAAT box in the proximal promoter. // J.Cell.Physiol. – 2008. – vol. 217, N 1. – P. 228–241

Pankov R., Yamada K.M. Fibronectin at a glance. // J.Cell Sci. – 2002. – vol. 115, N 20. – P. 3861–3863.

Parisi M.S., Gazzerro E., Rydziel S., Canalis E. Expression and regulation of CCN genes in murine osteoblasts. // Bone. – 2006. – vol. 38, N 5. – P. 671–677.

Park P.W., Reizes O., Bernfield M. Cell surface heparan sulfate proteoglycans: selective regulators of ligand receptor encounters. // J.Biol.Chem. – 2000. – vol. 275, N 39. – P. 29923–29926.

Park S.J., Kim S.J., Rhee Y. et al. Fidgetin-like gene inhibited by basic fibroblast growth factor regulates the proliferation and differentiation of osteoblasts. // J.Bone Miner.Res. – 2007. – vol. 22, N 6. – P. 889–896.

Parker A.E., Boutell J., Carr A., Maciewicz R.A. Novel cartilage-specific variants of fibronectin. // Osteoarthritis Cartilage. – 2002. – vol. 10, N 7. – P. 528–534.

Parker E.A., Hegde A., Buckley M. et al. Spatial and temporal regulation of GF-IGF-related gene expression in growth plate cartilage. // J.Endocrinol. – 2007. – vol. 194, N 1. – 31–40.

Parsons K.K., Maeda N., Yamauchi M. et al. Ascorbic acid-independent synthesis of collagen in mice. // Am.J.Physiol.Endocrinol.Metab. – 2006. – vol. 290. – P. E1131–E1139.

Pasquali-Ronchetti I., Baccarini-Contri M. Elastic fiber during development and aging. // Microsc.Res.Tech. – 1997. – vol. 38, N 4. – P. 428–435.

Patel M.S., Elefteriou F. The new field of neuroskeletal biology. // Calcif.Tissue Int. – 2007. vol.80, N 5. – P. 337–347.

Patra D., Xing X., Davies S. et al. Site-1 protease is essential for endochondral bone formation in mice. // J.Cell Biol. – 2007. – vol. 179, N 4. – P. 687–700.

Pavalko F.M., Norvell S.M., Burr D.B. et al. A model for mechanotransduction in bone cells: the load bearing mechanosomes. // J.Cell.Biochem. – 2003. – vol. 88, N 1. – P. 104–112.

Pavlova V.N. Synovial medium of joints. [in Russian] – Moscow: Medicine, 1980.

Pavlova V.N., Kopieva T.N., Slutsky L.I. and G.G. Pavlov. Cartilage. [in Russian] Moscow: Medicine, 1988. 320 pages.

Pearson J.C., Lemons D., McGinnis W. Modulating Hox gene functions during animal body patterning. // Nat.Rev.Genet. – 2005. – vol. 6. – P. 893–904.

Pease D., Bouteille M. The tridimensional ultrastructure of native collagenous fibrils: cytochemical evidence for a carbohydrate matrix // J. Ultrastruct. Res. 1971. – vol. 35. N°3–4. – P. 339–358.

Pederson L., Ruan M., Westendorf J.J. et al. Regulation of bone formation by osteoclasts involves Wnt/BMP signaling and the chemokine sphingosine-1-phosphate. // Proc.Natl.Acad.Sci.USA. – 2008. – vol. 105< N 52. – P. 20764–20769.

Penner A.S., Rock M.J., Kielty C.M., Shipley J.M. Microfibril-associated glycoprotein-2 interacts with fibrillin-1 and fibrillin-2 suggesting a role of MAGP-2 in elastic fiber assembly. // J.Biol.Chem. – 2002. – vol. 277, N 38. – P. 35044–35049.

Perret S., Merle C., Bernocco S. et al. Unhydroxylated triple helical collagen I produced in transgenic plants provides new clues on the role of hydroxyproline in collagen folding and fibril formation. // J.Biol.Chem. – 2001. – vol. 276, N 47. – P. 43693–43698.

Perry R.J., Farquharson C., Ahmed S.F. The role of sex steroids in controlling pubertal growth. // Clin.Endocrinol. – 2008. – vol. 68. – P. 4–15.

Pfander D., Cramer T., Schipani E, Johnson R.S. HIF-1α control extracellular matrix synthesis by epiphyseal chondrocytes. // J.Cell.Sci. – 2003. – vol. 116. – P. 1819–1826

Pfister B.E., Aydelotte M.B., Burkhardt W. et al. Del1: a new protein in the superficial layer of articular cartilage. // Biochem.Biophys. Res.Commun. – 2001. – vol. 286. – P. 268–273.

Phan S.H. Fibroblast phenotypes in pulmonary fibrosis. // Am.J.Respir.Cell Mol.Biol. – 2003. – vol. 29, 3 Suppl. – P.S87–S92.

Phillips K., Luisi B. The virtuoso of versatility: POU proteins that flex to fit. // J.Mol.Biol. – 2000. – vol. 302, N 5. – P. 1023–1039.

Phillips R. J., Burdick M. D, Hong K. et al. Circulating fibrocytes traffic to the lungs in response to CXCL12 and mediate fibrosis. // J. Clin. Invest. 2004. – vol 114. – P. 438–446.

Phornphutkul C., Wu K.Y., Gruppuso P.A. The role of insulin in chon-drogenesis. // Mol.Cell.Endocrinol. – 2006. – vol. 249, N 1–2. – P. 107–115.

Picard F., Géhin M., Annicotte J.S. et al. SRC-1 and TIF-2 control energy balance between white and brown adipose tissues. // Cell. – 2002. – vol. 111. – P. 931–941.

Piecha D., Wiberg C., Mörgelin M. et al. Matrin-2 interacts with itself and with other extracellular matrix proteins. // Biochem.J. – 2002. – vol. 367. – P. 715–721.

Pihlajamaa T., Peräla M., Vuoristo M.M. et al. Characterization of re-combinant human type IX collagen. Association of alpha chains into homotrimeric and heterotrimeric moleculs. // J.Biol.Chem. – 1999. – vol. 274, N 32. – P. 22464–22468.

Pilon N., Oh K., Sylvestre J.R. et al. Wnt signaling is a key mediator of Cdx1 expression. // Development. – 2007. – vol. 134. – P. 2315–2323.

Pinheiro S.W., Micheletti A.M., Crema V.O. et al. The different concen-trations of mast cells in the musculature of the esophagus and the colon. // Hum Pathol. – 2007. – vol. 38, N 8. – P. 1256–1264.

Pinzone J.J., Hall B.M., Thudi N.K. et al. The role of Dickkopf-1 in bone development, homeostasis, and disease. // Blood. – 2009. – vol. 113, N 3. – P. 317–325.

Pirok E.W 3rd, Henry J., Schwartz N. Cis-elements that control the ex-pression of chick aggrecan. // J.Biol.Chem. – 2001. – vol. 276, N 20. – P. 16894–16903.

Pitsillides A.A. Identifying and characterizing the joint cavity form-ing cells. // Cell Biochem Function. – 2003. – vol. 21. – P. 235–240.

Pitsillides A.A., Ashhurst D.K. A critical evaluation of specific aspects of joint development. // Dev.Dyn. – 2008. – vol. 237. – P. 2284–2294.

Pittet B., Rubbia-Brandt L., Desmouliere A., et al. Effect of gamma-inter-feron on the clinical and biologic evolution of hypertrophic scars and Dupuytren's disease: an open pilot study. // Plast.Reconstr. Surg. – 1994. – vol. 93. – P. 1224–1235.

Pizette S., Niswander L. BMPs are required at two steps of limb chond-srogenesis: formation of prechondrogenic condensations and their differentiation into chondrocytes. // Dev.Biol. – 2000. – vol. 219. – P. 237–249.

Planque N. Nuclear trafficking of secreted factors and cell-surface receptors: new pathways to regulate cell proliferation and differ-entiation, and involvement in cancers. // Cell Commun. Signal. – 2006. – vol. 4. – P. 7.

Plantin P., Durigon M., Boileau C., Le Parc J. Mise en evidence d'un re-seau de fibrilline dans le tissue osseux normal. // Ann.Pathol. – 2000. – vol. 20, N 2. – P. 115–118.

Plisov S.Y., Ivanov S.V., Yoshino K. et al. Mesenchymal-epithelial transi-tion in the developing metanphric kidney: gene expression study by differential display. // Genesis. – 2000. – vol. 27, N 1. – P. 22–31.

Plotkin L.I., Manolagas S.C., Bellido T. Transduction of cell survival sig-nals by connexin-43 hemichannels. // J.Biol.Chem. – 2002. – vol. 277, N 10. – P. 8648–8657.

Plotkin L.I., Mathov I., Aguirre J.I. et al. Mechanical stimulation pre-vents osteocyte apoptosis: requirement of integrins. Src kinases, and ERKs. // Am.J.Physiol.Cell Physiol. – 2005. – vol. 289. – P. 633–643.

Plumb M.S., Aspden R.M. High levels of fat and (n-6) fatty acids in can-cellous bone in osteoarthritis. // Lipids in health and disease. – 2004. – vol. 3. – P. 12.

Poduval P., Sillat T., Beklen A. et al. Type IV collagen α-chain composi-tion in synovial lining from tgrauma patients and patients with rheumatoid arthritis. // Arthritis Rheum. – 2007. – vol. 56, N 12. – P. 3959–3967.

Pogue R., Sebald E., King L. et al. A transcriptional profile of human bone cartilage. // Matrix Biol. – 2004. – vol. 23, N 5. – P. 299–307.

Pol A., Martin S., Fernandez M.A. et al. Dynamic and regulated associa-tion of caveolin with lipid bodies: Modulation of lipid body mo-tility and function by a dominant negative mutant. // Mol.Biol. Cell. – 2004. – vol. 15. – P. 99–110.

Pollard T.D., Earnshaw W.C. Cell Biology. Phil.e.a.: Saunders Elsevier Sci. – 2002.

Pompe T., Renner L., Werner C. Nanoscale features of fibronectin fibrillogenesis depend on protein-substrate interaction and cytoskeleton feature. // Biophys.J. – 2006. – vol. 88. – P. 527–534.

Ponta H., Sherman L., Herrlich P.A. CD44: from adhesion molecules to signaling trgulators. // Nat.Rev.Mo.Cell Biol. – 2003. – vol. 4, N 1. – P. 33–45.

Poole A.R., Kojima T., Yasuda T. et al. Composition and structure of ar-ticular cartilage. // Clin.Orthop.Rel.Res. – 2001. – vol. 391S. – P.S26–S33.

Poole C.A. Articular cartilage chondrons: form, function and fail-ure. // J.Anat. – 1997. – vol. 191, N 1. – P. 1–13

Poole K.E.S., Reeve J. Parathyroid hormone – a bkne anabolic and cata-bolic agent. // Curr.Opin.Pharmacol. – 2005. – vol. 5. – P. 612–617.

Porter S., Clark I.M., Kevorkian L., Edwards D.R. The ADAMTS metallo-proteinases. // Biochem.J. – 2005. – vol. 386, N 1. – P. 15–27.

Pöschl E., Schlötzer-Schrehardt U., Brachvogel I. et al. Collagen IV is es-sential for basement membrane stability but dispensable for initiation of its assembly during early development. // Develop-ment. – 2004. – vol. 131, N 7. – P. 619–628.

Posey K.L., Hankenson K., Veerisetty A.C. et al. Skeletal abnormalities in mice lacking extracellular matrix proteins, thrombospondin-1, thrombospondin3, thrombospondin-5, and type IX collagen. // Amer.J.Pathol. – 2008. – vol. 172, N 6. – P. 1664–1674.

Posner A.S. The mineral of bone. // Clin.Orthop. – 1985. – vol. 200. – P. 87–99.

Potter L.R., Abbey-Hosch S., Dickey D.M. Natriuretic peptides, their re-ceptors. and cyclic guanosin monophosphate-dependent signal-ing function. // Endocrin.Rev. – 2006. – vol. 27, N 1. – P. 47–72.

Potts J.T. Parathyroid hormone: past and present. // J.Endocrinol. – 2005. – vol. 187. – P. 311–325.

Pourquié O. The segmentation clock: converting embryonic time into spatial pattern. // Science. – 2003. – vol. 301. – P. 328–330.

Powell D.W., Mifflin R.C., Valentich J.D. et al. Myofibroblasts. I. Parac-rine cells important in health and disease. // Am.J.Physiol. 1999. – vol. 277, N 1, pt1. – P.:C1–C9.

Pratap J., Galindo M., Saidi S.K. et al. Cell growth regulatory role of Runx2 during proliferative expansion of preosteoblasts. // Cancer Res. – 2003. – vol. 63, N 17. – P. 5357–5362

Pratta M.A., Yao W., Decicco C. et al. Aggrecan protects cartilage colla-gen from proteolytic cleavage. // J.Biol.Chem. – 2003. – vol. 278, N 46. – P. 45539–45545.

Prêle C.M., Horton M.A., Caterina P., Stenbeck G. Identification of the molecular mechanisms contributing to polarized trafficking in osteoblasts. // Exp.Cell Res. – 2003. – vol. 282, N 1. – 24–34.

Prestvich T.C., MacDougald O.A. Wnt/β-catenin signaling in adipogen-esis and metabolism. // Curr.Opin.Cell.Biol. – 2007. – vol. 19. – P. 612–617.

Price P.A., Toroian D., Lim J.E. Mineralization by inhibitory exclusion: the calcification of collagen with fetuin. // J.Biol.Chem. – 2009. – vol. 284, N 25. – P. 17092–17101.

Primakoff P., Myles D.G. The ADAM gene family: surface proteins with adhesion and protease activity. // Trends Genet. – 2000. – V 16, N 2. – P. 83–87.

Provot S., Schipani E. Molecular machanisms of endochondral bone development. // Biochem.Biophys.Res.Commun. – 2005. – vol.328. – P.658–665.

Provot S., Zinyk D., Gunes Y. et al. Hif-1α regulates differentiation of limb bud mesenchyme and joint development. // J.Cell Biol. – 2007. – vol.177, N3. – P.451–464.

Pufe T., Groth G., Goldring M.B et al. Effect of pleiotrophin, a heparin-binding growth factor, on human primary and immortalized chondrocytes. // Osteoarthritis Cartilage. – 2007. – vol.15, N2. – P.155–162.

Pullig G., Weseloh G., Klatt A.R. et al. Matrilin-3 in human articular cartilage: increased expression in osteoarthritis. // Osteoarthritis Cartilage. – 2002. – vol.10, N4. – P.253–263.

Punzi L., Calò L., Plebani M. Clinical significance of cytokine determination in synovial fluid. // Crit.Rev.Clin.Lab.Sci. – 2002. – vol.39, N1. – P.61–88.

Puolakkainen P., Bradshaw A.D., Kyriakides T.R. et al. Compromised production of extracellular matrix in mice lacking secreted protein, acidic and and rich in cysteine (SPARC) leads to a reduced foreign body reaction to implanted biomaterials. // Amer.J.Pathol. – 2003. – vol. 162, N2. – P.627–635.

Purbach B., Hills B.A., Wroblewski B.M. Seum-active phospholipids in total hip arthroplasty. // Clin.Orthop. – 2002. – vol.396. – P.115–118.

Purcell P., Joo B.W., Hu J.K. Temporomandibular joint formation requires two distinct hedgehog-dependent steps. // Proc. Natl.Acad.Sci.USA. – 2009. – vol. 106, N42. – P.18297–18302.

Puri V., Kondo S., Ranjit S. et al. Fat-specific proteiN 27, a novel lipid droplet protein that enhancesd triglyceride storage. // J.Biol.Chem. – 2007. – vol. 282, N47. – P.34213–34218.

Purroy J., Spurr N.K. Molecular genetics of calcium sensing in bone cells. // Hum.Mol.Genetics. – 2002. – vol. 11, N20. – P.2377–2384.

Qi H., Agular D.J., Williams S.M. et al. Identification of genes responsible for osteoblast differentiation from human mesodermal progenitor cells. // Proc.Natl.Acad.Sci.USA. – 2003. – vol. 100, N6. – P.3305–3310.

Qi W., Scully S.P. Type II collagen modulates the composition of extracellular matrix synthesized by articular chondrocytes. // J.Orthop.Res. – 2003. – vol.21. – P.282–289.

Qiao B., Padilla S.R., Benya P.D. Transformin growth factor (TGF)-β-activated kinase 1 mimics and modulate TGF-β-induced stimulation of type II co;;agen synthesis in chondrocytes independent of Col2a1 transcription and Smad3 signaling. // J.Biol.Chem. – 2005. – vol.280, N17. – P.17562–17571.

Qin C., D'Souza R., Feng J.Q. Dentin matrix proteiN1 (DMP1). // J.Dent.Res. – 2007. – vol.86. – P.1134–1141.

Qin J., Vinogradova O., Plow E.F. Integrin bidirectional signaling: a molecular view. // PLoS Biology. – 2004. – vol. 2, N6. – P. Q726–Q729.

Quarles L.D. Endocrine function of bone in mineral metabolism regulation. // J.Clin.Invest. – 2008. vol. 118. – P 3820–3828.

Quarto N., Behr B., Li S., Longaker M.T. Differential FGF ligands and FGF receptor expression pattern in frontal and parietal calvarial bone. // Cells Tissues Organs. – 2009. – vol.190, N3. – P.158–169.

Quian R.Q., Glanville R.W. Alignment of fibrillin molecules in elastic microfibrils is defined by transglutaminase-derived crosslinks. // Biochemistry. – 1997. – vol. 36. – P.15841–15847.

Quondamatteo F., Reinhardt D.P., Charbonneau N.L. et al. Fibrillin-1 and fibrillin-2 in human embryonic and fetal development. // Matrix Biol. – 2002. – vol. 21, N2. – P.637–646.

Raabe H.M., Molsen H., Mlinaric S.M. et al. Biochemical alterations in collagen IV induced by in vitro glycation. // Biochem.J. – 1996. – vol. 319. – P.699–704.

Rabier B., Williams A.J., Mallein-Gerin F. et al. Thyroid hormone-stimulated differentiation of primary rib chondrocytes in vitro requires thyroid hormone receptor β. // J.Endocrinol. – 2006. – vol. 191. – P.221–228.

Rabinovitch M. Professional and non-professional phagocytes: an introduction. // Trends Cell Biol. – 1995. – vol. 5. – P. 85–88.

Rachfal A.W., Brigstock D.R. Structural and functional properties of CCN proteins. // Vitamins Horm. – 2005. – vol. 70. – P.69–103.

Raducanu A., Hunziker E.B., Drosse I., Aszódi A. β1 integrin deficiency results in multiple abnormalities of the knee joint. // J. Biol. Chem. – 2009. – vol. 284. – P. 23780–23792.

Rahmani M., Wong B.A., Ang L. Versican signaling to transcriptional control pathways. // Can.J.Physiol.Pharmacol. – 2006. – vol. 84, N1. – P.77–92

Rajpurohit R., Koch C.J., Tao E. et al. Adaptation of chondrocytes to low oxygen tension: relationship between hypoxia and cellular metabolism. // J.Cell.Physiol. – 1996. – vol. 168, N2. – P.424–432.

Ramachandran G.N., Reddi A.H. Biochemistry of collagen. – New York and London, Plenum press. – 1976.

Ramirez F., Carta L., Lee-Arteaga S. et al. Fibrillin-rich microfibrils – structural and instructive determinants of mammalian development and physiology. // Connect.Tissue Res. – 2008. – vol. 49, N1. – P. 1–6.

Ramirez F., Dietz H.C. Fibrillin-rich microfibrils: structural determinants of morphogenetic and homeostatic events. // J.Cell.Physiol. – 2007. – vol. 213. – P.326–330.

Ramirez F., Rifkin D.B. Extracellular microfibrils: contextual platforms for TGF-β and BMP signals. // Curr.Opin.Cell.Biol. – 2009. – vol. 21, N5. – P.616–622.

Ramirez F., Sakai L.Y. Biogenesis and function of fibrillin assemblies. // Cell Tissue Res. – 2009. – Epub. Jine 10

Ramirez F., Sakai L.Y., Dietz H.C., Rifkin D.B. Fibrillin microfibrils: multipurpose extracellular network in organismal physiology. // Physiol.Genomics. – 2004. – vol. 19, N2. – P.151–154.

Rao H., Lu G., Kajiya H. et al. Alpha9beta1: a novel osteoclast integrin that regulates osteoclast formation and function. // J.Bone Miner.Res. – 2006. – vol. 21, N10. – P.1657–1665.

Raouf A., Ganss B., McMahon C. et al. Lumican is a major proteoglycan component of the bone matrix. // Matrix Biol. – 2002. – vol. 21, N21. – P.361–367.

Raouf A., Seth A. Discovery of osteoblast-associated genes using cDNA microarrays. // Bone. – 2002. – vol. 30, N3. – 463–471

Rappolee D.A., Mark D., Banda M.J., Werb Z. Wound macrophages express TGF-α and other growth factors in vivo. Analysis by mRNA phenotyping. // Science. – 1988. – vol. 241. – P. 708–712.

Rapraeger A.C. Syndecan-regulated receptor signaling. // J.Cell Biol. – 2000/ – vol. 149, N5. – P.995–997.

Rasmussen H., Barrett PQ. Calcium mes¬senger system: an integrated view. // Physiol Rev. 1984. 64 (3). P. 408–419.

Rauner M., Sipos W., Pietschmann P. Age-dependent Wnt gene expression in bone and during the course of osteoblast differentiation. // Age (Dordr.). – 2008. – vol. 30. – P. 273–282.

Ray D., Osmundson E.C., Kiyokawa N. Constitutive and UV-induced fibronectin degradation is a ubiquitination-dependent process controlled by beta-TrCP. // J.Biol.Chem. – 2006. – vol. 281, N32. – P. 23060–23065.

Raymond L., Esk S., Hays E. et al. RelA is required for IL-1β stimulation of matrix metalloproteinase-1 expression in chondrocytes. // Osteoarthritis Cartilage. – 2007. – vol. 15, N4. – P. 431–441.

Reddi A.H. BMPs: from bone morphogenetic proteins to body morphogenetic proteins. // Cytokine growth Factor Rev. – 2005. – vol. 16, N3. – P. 1249–1250.

Reddi A.H. Bone morphogenetic proteins: from basic science to clinical applications. // J.Bone Joint Surg. – 2001. – vol. 83–A, Suppl.1., part 1. – P. S1–S6.

Reddi A.H. Cartilage morphogenetic proteins: role in joint development, homeostasis, and regeneration. // Ann.Rheum.Dis. – 2003. – vol. 62, Suppl.II. – P. II73–II78

Redselli A., Vesentini S., Soncini M. et al. Possible role of decorin glycosaminoglycans in fibril to fibril force transfer in relative mature tendons. // J.Biochem. – 2003. – vol. 36, N10. – P. 1555–1569.

Rehn A.P., Cerny R., Sugars R.V. et al. Osteoadherin is upregulated by mature osteoblasts and enhances their in vitro differentiation and mineralization. // Calcif.Tissue Int. – 2008. – vol. 82. – P. 454–464.

Reichrath J., Lehmann B., Carlsberg C. et al. Vitamins as hormones. // Horm.Metab.Res. – 2007. – vol. 39, N2. – P. 71–84

Reigle K.L., Di Lullo G., Turner K.R. et al. Non-enzymatic glycation of type I collagen diminishes collagen-proteoglycan binding and weakens cell adhesion. // J.Cell.Biochem. – 2008. – vol. 104, N5. – P. 1684–1698.

Reijnders C.M.A., Bravenboer N. Holzmann P.J. et al. In vivo mechanical loading modulates insulin-like growth factor binding protein-2 gene expression in rat osteocytes. // Calcif.Tissue Int. – 2007. – vol. 60. – P. 137–143.

Reinboth B., Hanssen E., Cleary E.G., Gibson M.A. Molecular interactions of biglycan and decorin with elastic fiber components: biglycan forms a ternary complex with tropoelastin and microfibril-associated glycoproteiN 1. // J.Biol.Chem. – 2002. – vol. 277, N6. – P. 3950–3957.

Reingold A., Ringrose L. How does noncoding transcription regulate Hox genes? // Bioessays. – 2008. Vol.30. – P. 110–121.

Reinhardt D.P., Gambee J.E., Ono R.N. et al. Initial steps in assembly of microfibrils. Formation of disulfide-cross-linked multimers containing fibrillin-1. // J.Biol.Chem. – 2000. – vol. 275, N3. – P. 2205–2210.

Reiser K.M., Hennessy S.M., Last J.A. Analysis of age-associated changes in collagen crosslinks in the skin and lung of monkey and rats. // Biochim.Biophys.Acta. – 1987. – vol. 926, N3. – P. 339–348.

Reissmann E., Jörnvall H., Blokzijl A. et al. The orphan receptor ALK7 and the activin receptor ALK4 mediate signaling by Nodal proteins during vertebrate development. // Genes Dev. – 2001. – vol. 15. – P. 2010–2022.

Retta S.F., Balzac F., Avolio M. Rap1: a turnabout for the crosstalk between cadherins and integrins. // Eur.J.Cell Biol. – 2006. – V. 85, N3–4. – P. 283–293.

Revel J.P., Karnovsky M.J. Hexagonal array of subuita in intercellular junctions of the mouse heart and liver // J. Cell Biol. 1967. – V. 33. – P. 67.

Revell P. A , Al-Saffar N., Fish Ş., Qsei D. Extracellular matrix in the synovial intimal cell layer. // Ann.Rheum.Dis. – 1995. – vol. 54, N5. – P. 404–407.

Rhee D.K., Marcelino J., Baker M. et al. The secreted glycoprotein lubricin protects cartilage surfaces and inhibits synovial cell overgrowth. // J.Clin. Invest. – 2005. – vol. 115, N.3. – P. 422–432.

Rice R., Rice D.P.C., Olsen B.R.,Thesleff I. Progression of calvarial bone development requires Foxc1 regulation of Msx2 and Alx4. // Development. – 2003. – vol. 262. – P. 75–87.

Richardson D.W., Dodge G.R. Dose-dependent effects of corticosteroids on the expression of matrix-related genes in normal and cytokine-treated articular chonbdrocytes. // Inflamm.Res. – 2003. – vol. 32, N1. – P. 39–49.

Richardson S.H., Starborg T., Lu Y. et al. Tendon development require regulation of cell condensation and cell shape via cadherin-11-mediated cell-cell adhesion. // Mol.Cell.Biol. – 2007. – vol. 27, N17. – P. 6218–6228.

Rifkin D.B. Latent transforming growth factor-β (TGF-)β binding proteins: orchestration of TGF-β availability. // J.Biol.Chem. – 2004. – vol. 280, N9. – P. 7409–7412.

Riggs B.L., Khosla S., Melton L.J.III. Sex steroids and the construction and the conservation of the adult skeleton. // Endocrine Rev. – 2002, vol. 23, N3. – P. 279–302.

Riggs B.L., Parfitt A.M. Drugs used to treat osteoporosis: the critical need for a uniform nomenclature based on their action on bone remodeling. // J.Bone Miner.Res. – 2005. – vol. 20. – P. 177–184.

Rinn J.L., Bondre C., Gladstone H.B. et al. Anatomic demarcation by positional variation in fibroblast gene expression programs. // PLoS genetics. – 2006. – vol. 2, N7. – P. 1084.

Rinn J.L., Kortesz M., Wang J.K. et al. Functional demarcation of active and silent chromatin domains in human HOX loci by non-coding RNAs. // Cell. – 2007. – vol. 129, N7. – P. 1311–1323.

Ripamonti U. Soluble osteogenic molecular signals and the induction of bone formation. // Biomaterials. – 2006. – vol. 27. – P. 507–522.

Risteli M., Niemitalo O., Lankinen H. et al. Characterization of collagenous peptides bound to lysyl hydroxylase isoforms. // J.Biol.Chem. – 2004. – vol. 279, N36. – P. 37535–37543.

Ritty T.M., Ditsios K., Starcher B.C. Distribution of the elastic fiber and associated proteins in flexor tendon reflects function. // Anat. Rec. – 2002. – vol. 268, N4. – P. 230–240.

RittyT.M., Roth R., Heuser J.E. Tendon cell array isolation reveals a previously unknown fibrillin-2-containing macromolecular assembly. // Structure. – 2003. – vol. 11. – P. 1179–1188.

Robenek H., Hofnagel O., Buers L. et al. Adipophilin-enriched domains in the ER membrane are sites of lipid droplet biogenesis. // J.Cell Sci. – 2006. – vol. 119. – P. 4215–4224.

Robenek H., Robenek M.J., Troyer D. PAT family proteins pervade lipid droplet cores. // J.Lipid Res. – 2005. – vol. 46. – P. 1331–1338.

Robert L. [The fibroblast, definition of its "programme" of biosynthesis of the extracellular matrix]. // Pathol.Biol. (Paris). – 1995. – T.40, N9. – P. 851–858.

Robert L., Robert A.M., Fülöp T. Rapid increase in human life expectance: will it soon be limited by the aging of elastin. // Biogerontology. – 2008. – vol. 9, N2. – P. 119–133.

Robertson J.A., Chatterjee-Kishore M., Yaworski P.J. et al. WNT/β-catenin signaling is a normal physiological response to mechanical loading in bone. // J.Biol.Chem. – 2006. – vol. 281, N42. – P. 31720–31728.

Robins S.P. Biochemistry and functional significance of collagen cross-linking. // Biochem.Soc.Trans. – 2007. – vol. 35, N5. – P. 849–852.

Roche S., Provansal M., Tiers L. et al. Proteomics of primary mesenchymal stem cells. // Regenerative Med. – 2006. – vol. 1, N4. – P. 511–517.

Rodda S.J., McMahon A.F. Distinct roles for Hedgehog and canonical Wnt signaling in specification, differentiation, maturation and maintenance of osteoblast progenitors. // Development. – 2006. – vol. 133, N 6. – P. 3231–3244.

Rodgers K.D., San Antonio J.D., Jacenko O. Heparan sulfate proteogly-cans: a GAGgle of skeletal-hematopoietic regulators. // Dev.Dyn. – 2008. – vol. 237, N 10. – P. 2622–2642.

Rodionova N.V. Functional morphology of cells in osteogenesis. [in Russian] Kiev: Naukova-Dumka, 1989. 192 pages.

Rodrigo I., Hill R.E., Balling R. et al. Pax1 and Pax9 activate Bapx1 to in-duce chondrogenic differentiation in the sclerotome. // Develop-ment. – 2003. – vol. 130. – P. 473–482.

Rodriguez R.R., Seegmiller R.E., Stark M.R., Bridgewater L.C. A type XI collagen mutation leads to increased degradation of type II colla-gen in articular cartilage. // Osteoarthritis Cartilage. – 2004. – vol. 12, N 4. – P. 314–320.

Rogers B.A., Murphy C.L., Cannon S.R., Briggs T.W.R. Topographical vari-ation in glycosaminoglycan content in human articular carti-lage. // J.Bone Joint Surg. – 2006. – vol. 88–B, N 12. – P. 1670–1674.

Roh S., Song S.H., Choi K.C. et al. Chemerin – a new adipokine that modulates adipogenesis via its own receptoe. // Biochem.Biophys. Res. Comm. – 2007. – vol. 362. – P. 1013–1018.

Rokutanda S., Fujita T., Kanatani N. et al. Akt regulates skeletal devel-opment through GSK3, mTOR, and FoxOs. // Dev.Biol. – 2009. – vol. 328, N 1. – P. 78–94.

Ronnov-Jessen L., Petersen O.W. Induction of alpha-smooth muscle ac-tin by transforming growth factor-beta 1 in quiescent human breast gland fibroblasts. Implications for myofibroblast genera-tion in breast neoplasia. // Lab.Invest. 1993. – vol. 68. – P. 696–707.

Roodman G.D. Regulation of osteoclast differentiation. // Ann.N.Y.Acad.Sci. – 2006. – vol. 1068. – P. 100–109

Rosen E.D., Spiegelman B.M. Molecular regulation of adipogenesis. // Annu.Rev.Cell.Dev.Biol. – 2000. – vol. 16. P. 145–171.

Rosen E.D., Spiegelman B.M. PPARγ: a nuclear regulator of metabo-lism, differentiation, and cell growth. // J.Biol.Chem. – 2001. – vol. 278, N 41. – P. 37731–37734.

Rosen V. BMP and BMP inhibitors in bone. // Ann.N.Y.Acad.Sci. – 2006. – vol. 1068. – P. 19–25.

Rosenbloom J., Abrams W.R., Mecham R. Extracellular matrix 4: The elastic fiber. // FASEB J. – 1993. – vol. 7, N 13. – P. 1208–1218.

Roseti L., Suda R., Cavallo C. et al. Ligament repair: a molecular and immunohistological characterization. // J.Biomed.Mater.Res.A. – 2008. – vol. 34, N 1. – P. 17–27.

Ross A.S., Tsang R., Shewmake K., McGehee R.E.jr. Expression of p107 and p130 during human adipose-derived stem cell adipogenesis. // Biochem.Biophys. Res.Comm. – 2008. – vol. 366, N 4. – 927–931.

Ross F.R., Teitelbaum S.L. Alphavbeta3 and macrophage-colony-stimu-lating factor: partners in osteoclasr biology. // Immunol.Rev. – 2005. – vol. 208. – P. 88–105.

Ross R., Fialkov R.J., Altman L.K. The morphogenesis of elastic fibers // Adv.Exp.Med.Biol.– 1977. – P. 7–17.

Rossi D., Gaidano G. Messengers of cell death: apoptosis signaling in health and disease. // Haematologica. – 2003. – vol. 88, N 2. – P. 212–218.

Rottem M., Okada T., Goff J.P., Metcalfe D.D. Mast cells cultured from the peripheral blood of normal donors and patients with masto-cytosis originate from a CD34+/FcεRI. cell population. // Blood. – 1994. –V. 84, N 8. – P. 2489–2496.

Roughley P.J. Articular cartilage and changes in arthritis. Noncolla-genous proteins and proteoglycans in the extracellular matrix of the cartilage. // Arthritis Res. – 2001. – vol. 3, N 6. – P. 342–347.

Roughley P.J. The structure and function of cartilage proteogly-cans. // Eur.Cells Materials. – 2006. – vol. 12. – P. 92–101.

Rountree R.B., Schoor M., Chen H. et al. BMP receptor signaling is re-quired for postnatal maintenance of articular cartilage. // PLoS Biol. – 2004. – vol. 2, N 11. – P. 355.

Rubbia-Brandt L., Sappino A.P., Gabbiani G. Locally applied GM-CSF in-duces the accumulation of alpha-smooth muscle actin contain-ing myofibroblasts. // Virchows Arch.B.Cell Pathol.Incl.Mol. Pathol. – 1991. – vol. 60. – P. 73–82.

Rubin J., Rubin C., Jacobs C.R. Molecular pathways mediated mechani-cal signaling in bone. // Gene. – 2006. – vol. 367. – P. 1–16.

Ruiz-Romero C., López-Armada M.J., Blanco P.J. Proteomic characteriza-tion of human normal articular chondrocytes a novel tool for the study of osteoarthritis and other rheumatic diseases. // Proteomics. – 2005. – vol. 5, N 12. – P. 3048–3059.

Ryoo H.M., Lee M.H., Kim Y.J. Critical molecular switches involved in BMP-2-induced osteogenic differentiation of mesenchymal cells. // Gene. – 2006. – vol. 366, N 1. – P. 51–57.

Ryu J.H., Kim S.J., Kim S.H. et al. Regulation of the chondrocyte pheno-type by beta-catenin. // Development. – 2002. – vol. 129, N 23. – P. 5541–5550.

Saar G., Shinar H., Navon G. Comparison of the effects of mechanical and osmotic pressures on the collagen fiber architecture of in-tact and proteoglycan-depleted articular cartilage. // Eur.Biophys.J. – 2007. – vol. 36. – P. 529–538.

Saas J., Haag J., Rueger D. et al. IL-1beta, but not BMP-7 leads to a dra-matic change in the gene expression pattern of human adult articular chondrocytes – portraying the gene expression pattern in two donors. // Cytokine. – 2006. – vol. 36, N 1–2. – P. 190–199.

Sado Y., Kagawa M., Naito I. et al. Organization and expression of basement membrane collagen IV genes and their role in human disorders. // J.Biochem. (Tokyo). – 1998. – vol. 123, N 5. – P. 767–776.

Saelens X., Festjens N., Walls V. et al. Toxic proteins released from mi-tochondria in cell death. // Oncogene. – 2004. – vol. 23, N 16. – P. 2861–2874.

Sáez J.C., Berthoud V.M., Brañes M.C. et al. Plama membrane channels formed by connexins: their regulation and functions. // Physiol. Rev. – 2003. – vol. 83, N 4. – P. 1359–1400.

Safadi F.F., Xu J., Smock S.L. et al. Cloning and characterization of oste-oactivin, a novel cDNA expressed in osteoblasts. // J.Cell.Biochem. – 2001. – vol. 84, N 1. – P. 12–26.

Safadi F.F., Xu J., Smock S.L. Expression of connective tissue growth factor in bone: its role in osteoblast proliferation and differentia-tion in vitro and bone formation in vivo. // J.Cell.Physiol. – 2003. – vol. 196. – P. 51–62.

Saga Y. Segmental border is defined by the key transcription factor Mesp2, by means of suppression of Notch activity. // Dev.Dyn. – 2007. – vol. 236. – P. 1450–1455.

Sage E.H. Regulation of interactions between cells and extracellular matrix: a command performance on several stages. // J.Clin.Invest. – 2001. – vol. 107, N 7. – P. 781–783.

Saha S., Ghosh P., Mitra D. et al. Localization and thyroid hormone in-fluenced expression of collagen II in ovarian tissue. // Cell. Physiol.Biochem. – 2007. – vol. 19. – P. 67–76.

Saito M., Fujii K., Marumo K. Degree of mineralization-related colla-gen crosslinking in the femoral neck cancellous bone in cases of hip fracture and controls. // Calcif.Tissue Int. – 2006. – vol. 79, N 3. – P. 160–168.

Sakai E., Miyamoto H., Okamoto K. et al. Characterization of phagoso-mal subpopulations along endocytic routes in osteoclasts and macrophages. // J.Biochem. – 2001. – vol. 130, N 6. – P. 823–831.

Sakakura T., Kusano I. Tenascin in tissue perturbation repair. // Acta Pathol.Japon. – 1991. – vol. 41, N 4. – P. 247–258.

Salingcarnboriboon R., Tauji K., Komori T. et al. Runx2 is a target of mechanical unloading to alter osteoblasts activity and bone formation in vivo. // Endocrinology. – 2006. – vol. 147, N 5. – P. 2296–2305.

Salvesen G.S. Caspases and apoptosis. // Essays Biochem. – 2002. – vol. 38, N 1. – P. 9–19.

Samee N., Geoffroy V., Marty C. et al. Dlx5, a positive regulator of osteoblastogenesis. is essential for osteoblast-osteoclast coupling. // Am.J.Pathol. – 2008. – vol. 173, N 3. – P. 173–180.

Sarma A.V., Powell G.L., LaBerge M. Phospholipid composition of articular cartilage boundary lubricant. // J.Orthop.Res. – 2001. – vol. 19, N 4. – P. 671–676.

Sasai N., Yakura R., Kamiya D. et al. Ectodermal factor restricts mesoderm differentiation by inhibiting p53. // Cell. – 2008. – vol. 133. – P. 878–890.

Sasaki T., Fässler R., Hohenester E. Laminin: the crux of basement membrane assembly. // J.Cell Biol. – 2004. – vol. 164, N 7. – P. 959–963.

Sasaki T., Göhring W., Miosge N. et al. Tropoelastin binding to fibulins, nidogen-2 and other extracellular matrix proteins. // FEBS Lett. – 1999. – vol. 460, N 2. – P. 280–284.

Satdykova G. P. Fibroblast-like cells of an aseptic inflammation focus (radioautographic, electron microscopic and electron-histochemical examination). [in Russian] // PhD thesis abstract. Moscow, 1974.

Sato K., Yomogida K., Wada T. et al. Type XXVI collagen, a new member of the collagen family, is specifically expressed in the testis and ovary. // J.Biol.Chem. – 2002. – vol. 277, N 40. – P. 37678–37684.

Saulgozis Yu.Zh., Slutsky L.I., Knets I.V. and Kh.A. Janson. Investigations of dependencies between different mechanical properties and the human bone tissue biochemical composition. [in Russian] // Mechanics of polymers, 1973, no. 1. P. 138–145.

Saunders KB, D'Amore PA. An in vitro model for cell-cell interactions. // In Vitro Cell Dev Biol – 1992 – vol. 28A – P. 521–528.

Sauvageau M., Sauvageau G. Polycomb group genes: keeping stem cell activity in balance. // PLoS Biology. – 2008. – vol. 6, N 4. – P. e113.

Savarese J.J., Erickson H., Scully S.P. Articular chondrocyte tenascin-C production and assembly into de novo extracellular matrix. // J.Orthop.Res. – 1996. – vol. 14. – P. 273–281.

Savini I., Rossi A., Pierro C. et al. SVCT1 and SVCT2: key proteins for vitamin C uptake. // Amino Acids. – 2007. – vol. 34, N 3. – P. 347–355.

Sawaguchi N., Najima T., Iwasaki N. et al. Extracellular matrix modulates expression of cell-surface proteoglycan genes in fibroblasts. // Connect.Tissue Res. – 2006. – vol. 47, N 3. – P. 141–148.

Sawai N., Koike K., Mwamtemi H.H. et al. Thrombopoietin augments stem cell factor-dependent growth of human mast cells from bone marrow multipotential hematopoietic progenitors. // Blood. – 1999. – vol. 93, N 11 – P. 3703–3712.

Scaffidi A.K., Moodley Y.P., Weichselbaum M. et al. Regulation of human lung fibroblast phenotype and function by vitronectin and vitronectin integrins. // J.Cell.Sci. – 2001. – vol. 114. – P. 3507–3516.

Schaller M.D. FAK and paxillin: regulators of N-cadherin adhesion and inhibitors of cell migration. // J.Cell Biol. – 2004. – vol. 166, N 2. – P. 157–159.

Scharff K.A., Song W.X., Luo X. et al. Hey1 basic helix-loop-helix protein plays an important role in mediating BMP-9-induced osteogenic differentiation of mesenchymal progenitor cells. // J.Biol.Chem. – 2009. – vol. 284, N 1. – P. 649–659.

Schinzel A., Kaufmann T., Borner C. Bcl-2 family members intracellular targeting, membrane insertion, and changes in subcellular localization. // Biochim.Biophys.Acta. – 2004. – vol. 1644, N 2–3. – P. 95–105.

Schipani E. Hypoxia and HIF-1α in chondrogenesis. // Ann.N.Y.Acad. Sci. – 2006. – vol. 1068. – P. 66–73

Schmid F.X. Prolyl isomerases join the fold. // Curr.Biol. – 1995. –V. 5, N 9. – P. 993–994.

Schmidl M., Adam N., Surmann-Schmitt C. et al. Twisted gastrulation modulates bone morphogenetic protein-induced collagen II and X expression in chondrocytes in vitro and in vivo. // J. Biol. Chem. – 2006. – vol. 281, N 42. – P. 31790–31800.

Schmidt K., Schinke T., Haberland M. et el. The high mobility group transcription factor Sox8 is a negative regulator of osteoblast differentiation. – J.Cell Biol. – 2005. – vol. 168, N 6. – P. 899–910

Schmidt T.A., Gastelum N.S., Hguyen Q.T. et al. Boundary lubrication of articular cartilage. // Arthritis Rheum. 2007. vol. 56. № 3. P. 682–691.

Schmidt T.A., Gastelum N.S., Nguyen Q.T. et al. Boundary lubrication of articular cartilage. Role of synovial fluid constituents. // Arthritis Rheum. – 2007. – vol. 56, N 3. – P. 882–891.

Schmidt T.A., Plaas A.H., Sandy J.D. Disulfide-bonded multimers of proteoglycaN4 PRG4 are present in normal synovial fluids. // Biochim.Biophys.Acta. – 2009. – vol. 1790, N 5. – P. 375–384.

Schmitt F.O., Gross J. Further progress in the electron microscopy of collagen. //J. Amer. Leather Chem. Ass. – 1948. – vol. 43. – P. 658–675.

Schmitt-Graff A., Desmouliere A., Gabbiani G. Heterogeneity of myofibroblast phenotypic features: an example of fibroblastic cell plasticity. // Virchows Arch. – 1994. – vol. 425. – P. 3–24.

Schneider G.B., Zaharias R., Stanford C. Osteoblast integrin adhesion and signaling regulate mineralization. // J.Dent.Res. – 2001. – vol. 80, N 6. – P. 1540–1544.

Schneider H., Můhle C., Pacho F. Biological function of laminin-5 and pathogenic impact of its deficiency. // Eur.J.Cell Biol. – 2007. – vol. 86, N 11–12. – P. 701–717.

Schofield J.D., Weightman B. New knowledge of connective tissue ageing. // J.Clin.Pathol. – 1978. – vol. 31, Suppl.(Roy.Coll.Path.) 12. – P. 174–190.

Schoppet M., Chavakis T., Al-Fakri N. et al. Molecular interactions and functional interference between vitronectin and transforming growth factor-β. // Lab.Invest. – 2002. – vol. 82, N 1. – P. 37–46,

Schroeder T.M., Jensen E.D., Westendorf J.J. Runx2: a master organizer of gene transcription in developing and maturing osteoblasts. // Birth Defects Res. (Part C). – 2005. – vol. 75. – P. 213–225.

Schvartz I., Seger D., Shaltfiel S. Vitronectin:// Int.J.Biochem.Cell Biol. – 1999. – vol. 31, N 5. – P. 539–544.

Schwartz N.B., Pirok 3rd E.W., Mensch jr. J.B., Domowicz M.S. Domain organization, structure, evolution, and regulation of aggrecan gene family. // Progr. Nucleic Acid Res.Mol.Biol. – 1999. – vol. 62. – P. 177–225.

Schwartz Y,B., Pirrottaa V. Polycomb silencing mechanisms and the management of genomic programmes. // Nat.Rev.Genet. – 2007. – vol. 8, N 1. – P. 9–22.

Schwartz Z., Brooks B., Swain L. et al. Production of 1,25-dihydroxyvitamin D3 and 24,25-dihydrocyvitamin D3 by growth zone and resting zone chondrocytes is dependent on cell maturation and is regulated by hormones and growth factors. // Endocrinology. – 1992. – vol. 130, N 5. – P. 2495–2504.

Schwarz L.M., Hills B.A. Surface-active phospholipids as a lubricating component of Lubricin. // Brit.J.Rheum. – 1998. – vol. 37, N 1. – P. 21–26.

Schweitzer R., Chyung J.H., Murtaugh L.C. et al. Analysis of the tendon cell fate using Scleraxis, a specific marker for tendons and ligaments. // Development. – 2001. – vol. 128. – P. 3855–3866.

Scott J.E. Elasticity in extracellular matrix 'shape modules' of tendon, cartilage, etc. A sliding proteoglycan filament model. // J.Physiol. – 2003. – vol. 553, N 2. – P. 335–343.

Scott J.E. Extracellular matrix, supramolecular organization and shape. // J.Anat. – 1995. – vol. 187, N 3. – P. 259–269.

Scott J.E. Structure and function in extracellular matrices depend on interactions between ionic glycosaminoglycans. // Pathol.Biol. (Paris). – 2001. – vol. 49, N 4. – P. 284–289.

Scott J.E. The first and second 'laws' of chemical morphology, exemplified in mammalian extracellular matrix. // Eur.J.Histochem. – 2002. – vol. 46, N 2. – P. 111–124.

Scott J.E., Heatley F. Hyaluronan forms specific stable tertiary structures in aqueous solutions: a 13C NMR study. // Proc.Natl.Acad. Sci.USA. – 1999. – vol. 96, N 9. – P. 4850–4855.

Scully S.P., Lee J.W., Chert P.M.A., Qi W. The role of the extracellular matrix in articular chondrocytes regulation. // Clin.Orthop. – vol. 391, Suppl.1. – P. S72–S89.

Scults F.M., Johnston J.M. The synthesis of higher glycerides via the monoglyceride pathway in hamster adipose tissue. // J. Lipid Res. – 1971. – vol. 12. – P. 132.

Seales E.C., Micoll K.J., McDonald J.M. Calmodulin is a critical regulator of osteoclastic diofferentiation, function, and survival. // J.Cell.Biochem. – 2006. – vol. 97, N 1. – 45–55.

Segade F., Trask B.C., Broedelman T.J. et al. Identification of a matrix-binding domain in the microfibril associated glycoproteins 1 and 2 (MAGP1 and 2) and intracellular localization of alternative splice forms// J.Biol.Chem. – 2002. – vol. 277, N 13. – P. 11050–11057.

Segat D., Comai B., Di Marco E. et al. Integrins α6Aβ1 and α6Bβ1 promote different stages of chondrogenic cell differentiation. // J.Biol.Chem. – 2002. – vol. 277, N 35. – P. 31612–31622.

Segovia-Silvestre T., Neutzsky-Wulff A.V., Sorensen M.G. et al. Advances in osteoclast biology resulting from the study of osteopetrosis mutation. // Hum.Genet. – 2009. – vol. 134. – P. 561–577.

Seifert J.R.K., Mlozdik M. Frizzled/PCP signaling: a conserved mechanism regulating cell polarity and directed motility. // Nat.Rev. Genet. – 2007. – vol. 8. – P. 126–138.

Seki K., Fujimori T., Savagner P. et al. Mouse Snail family transcription repressors regulate chondrocyte, extracellular matrix, type II collagen, and aggrecan. // J.Biol.Chem. – 2003. – vol/278, N 43. – P. 41862–41870.

Sekiya I., Koopman P., Tsuji K. et al. Dexamethasone enhances SOX9 expression in chondrocytes. // J.Endocrinol. – 2001b. – vol. 169. – P. 573–579.

Sekiya I., Koopman P., Tsuji K. et al. Transcriptional suppression of Sox9 expression in chondrocytes by retinoic acid. // – J.Cell.Biochem.Suppl. – 2001a. – Suppl.1. – P. 71–78.

Selim A.A. Osteoactivin bioinformatic analysis: prediction of novel functions, structural features, and modes of action. // Med.Sci. Monit. – 2009. – vol. 15, N 2. – P. 19–33.

Seo H.S., Serra R. Deletion of Tgfbr2 in Prx1-cre expressing mesenchyme results in defects in development of long bones and joints. // Dev.Biol. – 2007. – vol. 310, N 21. – P. 304–316.

Sepulveda J.L., Wu C. The parvins. // Cell mol.Life Sci. – 2006. – vol. 63, N 1. – P. 25–35.

Serini G., Bochaton-Piallat M.L., Ropraz P. et al. The fibronectin domain ED-A is crucial for myofibroblastic phenotype induction by transforming growth factor-beta1 // J. Cell Biol. – 1998. – vol. 142. – P. 873–881.

Serov V.V. and A.B. Shekhter. Connective tissue (Functional morphology and general pathology). [in Russian] Moscow: Medicine, 1981. 312 pages.

Sessa L., Breiling A., Lavorgna et al. Noncoding RNA synthesis and loss of Polycomb group repression accompanies the collinear activation of the human HOXA cluster. // RNA. – 2007. – vol. 13. – P. 223–239.

Seta N., Kuwana M. Human circulating monocytes as multipotential progenitors. // Keio J.Med. – 2007. – vol. 56, N 2. – P. 41–47.

Settle S.H.jr., Rountree R.B., Sinha A. et al. Multiple joint and skeletal patterning defects caused by single and double mutations in the mouse GDF6 and GDF5 genes. // Dev.Biol. – 2003. – vol. 254,N 1. – P. 116–130.

Shapira E., Marom K., Yelin R. et al. A role for the homeobox gene Xvex-1 as part of the BMP-4 signaling pathway. // Mech.Dev. – 1999. – vol. 86. – P. 99–111.

Shekhter A.B., Nikolaev A.V., and Berchenko G.N. Macrophage-fibroblast interaction and its potential role in regulating collagen metabolism in wound healing. [in Russian] Bulletin of Experimental Biology and Medicine, 1977, no. 5. P. 627–630.

Shen B., Bhargav D., Wei A. et al. BMP-13 emerges as a potential inhibitor of bone formation. // Int.J.Biol.Sci. – 2009. – vol. 5, N 2. – P. 192–200.

Shen M.M. Nodal signaling: developmental roles and regulation. // Development. – 2007. – vol. 134. – P. 1023–1034.

Sheng M.H.C., Lau K.H.W. Role of protein-tyrosine phosphatases in regulation of osteoclastic activity. // Cell.Mol.Life Sci. – 2009. – vol. 66, N 11–12. – P. 1946–1961.

Sheng M.H.C., Wergedal J.E., Mohan S., Lau K.H.W. Osteoactivin is a novel osteoclastic protein and plays a key role in osteoclast differentiation and activity. // FEBS Lett. – 2008. – vol. 582. – P. 1451–1458.

Sheng W., Wang G., LaPierre D.P. et al. Versican mediates mesenchymalepithelial transition. // Mol.Biol.Cell. – 2006. – vol. 17. – P. 2009–2020.

Shepard J.B., Gliga D.A., Morrow A.P. et al. Versican knock-down compromises chondrogenesis in the embryonic chick limb. // Anat. Rec. – 2008. – vol. 291, N 1. – P. 19–27.

Shepard J.B., King H.A., LaFoon B.A. et al. Versican expression during synovial joint morphogenesis. // Int.J.Biol.Sci. – 2007. – vol. 3, N 6. – P. 380–384.

Sher L.B., Harrison J.R., Adams D.J., Kream B.E. Impaired cortical bone acquisition and osteoblast differentiation in mice with osteoblast-targeted disruption of glucocorticoid signalin. // Calcif.Tissue Int. – 2006. – vol. 79, N 2. – P. 118–125.

Shi J., Son M.Y., Yamada S. et al. Membrane-type MMPs enable extracellular matrix permissiveness and mesenchymal cell proliferation during embryogenesis. // Dev.Biol. – 2008. – vol. 313, N 1. – P. 196–209.

Shierinsky V.P. and Vorotnikov A.V. Cell motility in the cardiovascular system. [in Russian] Nature, 2005, no. 12. P. 39–44.

Shifley E.T., VanHorn K.M., Perez-Balaguer A. et al. Oscillatory lunatic fringe activity is crucial for segmentation of the anterior but not posterior skeleton. // Development. – 2008. – vol. 135. – P. 899–908.

Shigematsu M., Watanabe H., Sugihara H. Proliferation and differentiation of unilocular fat cells in the bone marrow. // Cell structure and function. 1999. N 24. P. 89–100.

Shikhman A.R., Brinson D.C., Lota M. Profile of glycosaminoglycan-degrading glycosidases and glycoside sulfatases secreted by human articular chondrocytes in homeostasis and inflammation. // Arthritis Rheum. – 2000. – vol. 43, N 6. – P. 1307–1314.

Shikumani C., Takimoto A., Ono M., Hiraki Y. Scleraxis positively regulates the expression of tenomodulin, a differentiation marker of tenocytes. // Dev.Biol. – 2006. – vol. 298. – P. 234–247.

Shinohara M., Takayanagi H. Novel osteoclast signaling mechanism. // Curr.Osteopor.Rep. – 2007. – vol. 5, N 2. – P. 67–72.

Shiotsugu J., Katsuyama Y., Arima K. et al. Multiple points of interaction between retinoic acid and FGF signaling during embryonic axis formation. // Development. – 2004. – vol. 131. – P. 2653–2667.

Shukunami C., Kondo J., Wakai H. et al. Molecular cloning of mouse and bovine chondromodulin II cDNA and the growth-promoting actions of bovine recombinant protein. // J.Biochem. (Tokyo). – 1999. – vol. 125, N 3. – P. 436–442.

Sidman R.L., Perkins M., Weiner N. Noradrenaline and adrenaline content of adipose tissue. // Nature. – 1962. – vol. 193. – P. 36–37.

Siebers M.C., Brugge P.J. der, Walboomers X.F., Jansen J.A. Integrins as linker protein between osteoblast and bone replacing material. // Biomaterials. – 2005. – vol. 26. – P. 137–146.

Siljander P.R.M., Hamaia S., Peachy A.R. Integrin activation state determines selectivity for novel recognition sites in fibrillar collagens. // J.Biol. Chem. – 2004. – V 279, N 46. – P. 67763–47772.

Silver F.H., DeVore D., Siperko L.M. Role of mechanophysiology in aging of ECM: effects in mechanochemical transduction. // J.Appl.Physiol. – 2003. – vol. 95. – P. 2134–2141.

Silver F.H., Horvath I., Foran D.J. Mechanical implications of the domain structure of fiber-forming collagens: comparison of the molecular and fibrillar flexibilities. // J.Theor.Biol. – 2002. – vol. 216, N 2. – P. 243–254.

Silver F.H., Siperko L.M. Membranosensing and mechanochemical transduction: how is mechanical energy sensed and converted into chemical energy in an extracellular matrix? // Crit.Rev.Biomed.Eng. – 2003. – vol. 31, N 4. – P. 255–331.

Sim A.T., Ludowyke R.I., Verrills N.M. Mast cell function: regulation of degranulation by serine/threonine phosphatases. // Pharmacol. Ther. – 2006. – vol. 112, N 2. – P. 425–439.

Simkin P.A. Synovial perfusion and synovial fluid solutes. // Ann.Rheum.Dis. – 1995. – vol. 54, N 5. – P. 424–428.

Simons K., Toomre D. Lipid rafts and signal transduction. // Nat.Rev. Mol.Biol. – 2000. – vol. 1, N 1. – P. 31–39.

Simons M., Horowitz A. Syndecan-4-mediated signaling. // Cell.Signal. – 2001. – vol. 13, N 12. – P. 855–862.

Simpson D.M., Ross R. The neutrophilic leukocyte in situ cell death detection kit, again as directed. Control sections in wound repair—a study with antineutrophil serum. // J. Clin.Invest. – 1972. – vol. 51. – P. 2009–2023.

Simpson A.H.K.W., Mills L., Noble B. The role of growth factors and related agents in accelerating fracture healing. // J.Bone Joint Surg. – 2006. – vol. 88-B, N 6. – P. 701–705.

Sims N.A., Gooi J.H. Bone remodeling: multiple cellular interactions required for coupling of bone formation and resorption. // Semin.Cell Dev.Biol. – 2008. – vol. 19. – P. 444–451.

Sims N.A., Jenkins B.J., Nakamura A. et al. Interleukin-11 receptor signaling is required for normal bone remodeling. // J.Bone Miner. Res. – 2005. – vol. 20, N 7. – P. 1093–1102.

Sims N.A., Jenkins B.J., Quinn J.M.W. et al. GlycoproteiN 130 regulates bone turnover and bone size by distinct downstream signaling pathways. // J.Clin.Invest. – 2004. – vol. 113, N 3. – P. 379–389.

Singer I.I., Kawka D.W., Kazazis D.M., Clark R.A. In vivo codistribution of fibronectin and actin fibers in granulation tissue: immunofluorescence and electron microscope studies of the fibronexus at the myofibroblast surface. // J.Cell Biol. – 1984. – vol. 98. – P. 2091–2106.

Sipola A., Ilvesaro J., Birr E. et al. Endostatin inhibits endochondral ossification. // J.Gene Med. – 2007. – vol. 9. – P. 1057–1064.

Sitara D., Kim S., Bazzaque M.S. et al. Genetic evidence of serum phosphate independent functions of FGF23 in bone. // PLoS Genet. – 2008. – vol. 4, N 8. – P. e1000154.

Sitaru C., Mihai S., Otto C. Induction of dermal-epidermal separation in mice by passive transfer of antibodies specific to collagen type VII. // J.Clin.Invest. – 2005. – vol. 115, N 4. – P. 870–878.

Skerry T.M. The role of glutamate in the regulation of bone mass and architecture. // J.Musculoskelet.Neuronal Interact. – 2008. – vol. 8, N 2. – P. 166–173.

Skulachev V.P. (Скулачев В.П.). Uncoupling: new approaches to an old problem of bioenergetics. // Biochem. Biophys.Acta. – 1998. – vol. 1363. – P. 100–124.

Skulachev V.P. Uncoupling: new approaches to an old problem of bioenergetics. [in Russian] // Biochem. Biophys. Acta, 1998, vol. 1363. P. 100–124.

Slatter D.A., Avery N.C., Bailey A.J. Collagen in fibrillar state is protected from glycation. // Int.J.Biochem.Cell.Biol. – 2008. – Epub. Mar.16.

Slee E.A., O'Connor D.J., Lu X. To die or not to die: how does p53 decide. // Oncogene. – 2004. – vol. 23, N 16. – P. 2809–2818.

Slutsky L.I. and Pfafrod G.O. Collagen and non-collagenous proteins of human compact bone tissue in ageing. [in Russian] // Gerontology and geriatrics. Locomotive system in ageing: Annals, 1980. P. 26–29.

Slutsky L.I. Biochemistry of normal and pathologically altered connective tissue. [in Russian] – Leningrad: Medicine, 1969. 370 pages.

Slutsky L.I. Supporting tissues and the joint –biochemistry and functions. [in Latvian] Riga: Academic publishing of the Latvian University, 2006. 412 pages.

Slutsky L.I., Petukhova L.I. Supportive function of the articular cartilage and its biochemical alterations in coxarthrosis. [in Russian] // Scientific papers of Riga Research institute of traumatology and orthopedics, 1971, vol. 10. P. 235–239.

Smerdel-Ramoya A., Zanotti S., Deregowski V., Canalis E. Connective tissue growth factor enhance osteoblastogenes in vitro. // J.Biol.Chem. – 2008. – vol. 283, N 33. – P. 22690–22699.

Smith G.N jr., BrandtK.D. Hypothesis: can type IX collagen "glue" together intersecting type II fibers in articular cartilage matrix? // Rheumatol. – 1992. – vol. 19, N 1. – P. 14–17.

Smith J.C., Hagemann A., Saka Y., Williams P.H. Understanding how morphogens work. // Phil.Trans.Roy.Soc.B. – 2008. – vol. 363. – P. 387–392.

Smith J.W., Serafini-Fracassini A. The distribution of proteinpolysaccharide complex in the nucleus pulposus matrix in yong rubbits // J.Cell Sci. 1968. – vol. 3. – P. 33–40.

Smith T.J. Insights into the role of fibroblasts in human autoimmune diseases. // Clin.Exp.Immunol. – 2005. – vol. 141, N 3. – P. 388–397.

Smith-Mungo L.I., Kagan H.M. Lysyl oxidase: properties, regulation and multiple functions in biology. // Matrix Biol. – 1998. – V. 16, N 7. – P. 387–398.

Smits P., Li P., Mandel J., Zhang Z. et al. The transcription factors L-Sox5 and Sox6 are essential for cartilage formation. // Dev.Cell. – 2001. – vol. 1. – P. 277–290.

Smola H., Stark H.-J, Thiekötter G. et al. Dynamics of basement membrane formation by keratinocyte-fibroblast interactions in organotypic skin culture. // Exp. Cell Res. – 1990. – vol. 239. P. 399–410.

Sodek J., Zhu B., Huynh M.H. et al. Novel functions of the matricellular proteins osteopontin and osteonectin/SPARC. // Connect.Tiss. Res. – 2002. – vol. 43, N 2–3. – P. 308–319.

Södersen F., Ekman S., Eloranta M.L. et al. Ultrastructural immunolocalization of cartilage oligomeric matrix protein (COMP) in relation to collagen fibrils in the equine tendone. // Matrix Biol. – 2005. – vol. 24, N 5. – P. 376–385.

Sokolov V.N. Quantitative assay of the ground structure. [in Russian] // In Current Engineering Geology: concepts, practice, challenges. – Moscow: MSU publishing, 1988. P. 174–175.

Sondergaard B.C., Wulf H., Henriksen K. et al. Calcitonin directly attenuates collagen type II degradation by inhibition of matrix metalloproteinase expression and activity by articular chonfdrocytes. // Osteoarthritis Cartilage. – 2006. – vol. 14, N 8. – P. 759–768.

Song F., Wisithphrom K., Zhou J., Windsor L.J. Matrix metalloproteinase dependent and independent collagen degradation. // Front.Biosci. – 2006. – vol. 11. – P. 3100–3120.

Song J.J., Aswad R., Kanaan R.A. et al. Connective tissue growth factor (CTGF) acts a downstream mediator of TGF-β1 to induce mesenchymal cell condensation. // J.Cell.Physiol. – 2007. – vol. 210. – P. 398–410.

Song N.H., Filmus J. The role of glypicans in mammalian development. // Biochim.Biophys. Acta. – 2002. – vol. 1573, N 3. – P. 241–246.

Sorrell J.M., Caplan A.I. Fibroblast heterogeneity: more than skin deep. // J.Cell Sci. – 2004. – vol. 117. – P. 667–675

Sottile J., Chandler J. Fibronectin matrix turnover occurs through a caveolin-1-dependent process. // Mol.Biol.Cell – 2005. – vol. 16, N 2. – P. 757–768.

Sottile J., Hocking D.C. Fibronectin polymerization regulates the composition and stability of extracellular matrix fibrils and cell matrix adhesions. // Mol.Biol.Cell – 2002. – vol. 13. – P. 3546–3549.

Soulhar J., Buschmann M.D., Shirazi-Ali A. A fibril-network-reinforced biphasic model of cartilage in uncontrolled compression. // J.Biomech.Eng. – 1999. – vol. 121, N 3. – P. 340–347.

Soung D.Y., Donh Y., Wang Y. et al. Runx3/AML2/Cbfa3 regulates early and late chondrocyte differentiation. // J.Bone Miner.Res. – 2007. – vol. 22, N 8. – P. 1260–1270.

Sowa H., Kaji H., Canaff L. et al. Inactivation of menin, the product of multiple endocrine neoplasia type I gene, inhibits the commitment of multipotential mesenchymal stem cells into the osteoblast lineage. // J.Biol.Chem. – 2003. – vol. 278, N 23. – P. 21058–21069.

Soysa N.S., Alles N., Shimokawa H. et al. Inhibition of the classical NF-κB pathway prevents osteoclast bone-resorbing activity. // J.Bone Miner.Metab. – 2009. – vol. 27. – P. 131–139.

Spagnoli A., O'Rear L., Chandler R.L. TGF-β signaling is essential for joint morphogenesis. // J.Cell Viol. – 2007. – vol. 177, N 6. – P. 1105–1117

Spagnoli A., Torello M., Nagalla S.R. et al. Identification of STAT-1 as a molecular target of IGFBP-3 in the progress of chondrogenesis. // J.Biol.Chem. – 2002. – vol. 277, N 21. – P. 18860–18867

Später D., Hill T.P., Gruber M., Hartmann C. Role of canonical Wnt signaling in joint formation. // Eur.Cells Mater. – 2006a. – vol. 12. – P. 71–80.

Später D., Hill T.P., O'Sullivan R.J. et al. Wnt9a signaling is required for joint integrity and regulation of Ihh during chondrogenesis. // Development. – 2006b. – vol. 133. – P. 3039–3049.

Spencer G.J., Hitchcock I.S., Genever P.G. Emerging neuroskeletal signaling pathways. // FEBS Lett. – 2004. – vol. 559, N 1. – P. 6–12.

Spicer A.P., Tien J.Y. Hyaluronan and morphogenesis. // Birth Defects Res.C.Embryo. Today. – 2004. – vol. 72, N 1. – P. 89–108.

Sprick M.R., Walezak H. The interplay between the Bcl-2 family and death receptor mediated apoptosis. // Biochim.Biophys.Acta. – 2004. – vol. 1644, N 1–2. – P. 125–132.

Spyrou G.E., Naylor I.L. The effect of basic fibroblast growth factor on scarring. // Br.J. Plast.Surg. – 2002. – vol. 55. – P. 275–282.

Squier C.A., Kremenak C.R. Myofibroblasts in healing palatal wounds of the beagle dog. // J.Anat. – 1980. – vol. 130. – P. 585–594.

Stabler T.V., Kraus V.B. Ascorbic acid accumulates in cartilage in vivo. // Clin.Chim.Acta. – 2003. – vol. 334, N 1–2. P. 157–162.

Stains J.P., Civitelli R. Cell-to-cell interactions in bone. // Biochem.Biophys.Res.Commun. – 2005. – vol. 328. – P. 721–727.

Stanton H., Ung L., Fosang A.J. The 45 kDa collagen-binding fragment of fibronectin induces matrix metalloproteinase synthesis by chondrocytes and aggrecan degradation by aggrecanases. // Biochem.J. – 2002. – vol. 364. – P. 181–190.

Stanton L.A., Underhill T.M., Beier F. MAP kinases in chondrocyte differentiation. // Dev.Biol. – 2003. – vol. 263. – P. 165–174.30.

St-Arnaud R. The direct role of vitamin D on bone homeostasis. // Arch.Biochem.Biophys. – 2008. – vol. 473, N 2. – P. 225–230.

Steck E., Benz K., Lorenz H. et al. Chondrocyte expressed protein-68 (CEP-68), a novel human marker gene for cultured chondrocytes. // Biochem.J. – 2001. – vol. 353. – P. 169–174.

Steck E., Braun J., Peltari K. et al. Chondrocyte secreted CRTAC1: a glycosylated extracellular matrix molecule of human articular cartilage. // Matrix Biol. – 2007. – vol. 26, N 1. – P. 30–41.

Stein G.S., Lian J.B., Stein J.L et al. Intranuclear organization of RUNX transcriptional regulatory machinery in biological control of skeletogenesis and cancer. // Blood Cells Mol.Dis. – 2003. – vol. 30, N 2. – P. 170–176.

Stephanou A., Latchman D.S. STAT-1 – a novel regulator of apoptosis. // Int.J.Exp.Pathol. – 2003. – vol. 84, N 6. – P. 239–244.

Stephens P., Davies K.J., Occleston N. Skin and oral fibroblasts exhibit phenotypic differences in extracellular matrix reorganization and matrix metalloproteinase activity. // Br.J. Dermatol. – 2001. – vol. 144. – P. 229–237.

Steplewski A., Brittingham R., Jimenez S.A., Fertala A. Single amino acid substitutions in the C-terminus of collagen II alter its affinity for collagen IX. // Biochem.Biophys.Res.Commun. – 2005. – vol. 335, N 3. – P. 749–755.

Stern R. Hyaluronan catabolism: a new metabolic pathway. // Eur.J.Cell Biol. – 2004. – vol. 83, N 7. – P. 317–325.

Stern R., Asari A.A., Suguhara K.N. Hyaluronan fragments: an information-rich system. // Eut.J.Cell Biol. – 2006. – vol. 85, N 9. – P. 698–715.

Stokes D.G., Liu G., Coimbra I.B. et al. Assessment of the gene expression profile of differentiated and dedifferentiated human fetal chondrocytes by microarray analysis. // Arthritis Rheum. – 2002. – vol. 46, N 2. – P. 404–419.

Storm E.E., Kingsley D.M. GDF5 coordinates bone and joint formation during digit development. // Dev.Biol. – 1999. – vol. 209. – P. 11–27.

Stracke J.O., Fosang A.J., Ledbetter S. et al. Matrix metalloproteinases 19 and 20 cleave aggrecan and cartilage oligomeric matrix protein. // FEBS Lett. – 2000. – vol. 478, N 1–2. – P. 52–56.

Strewler G.H. The physiology of parathyroid hormone-related protein. // New Engl.J.Med. – 2000. – vol. 342, N 3. – P. 177–185.

Strutz F., Okada H., Lo C.W. et al. Identification and characterization of a fibroblast marker: FSP-1. // J.Cell Biol. – 1995. – vol. 130, N 2. – P. 393–405.

Suda N., Tanaka S., Fukushima M. et al. C-type natriuretic peptide as autocrine/paracrine regulator of osteoblast. Evidence for possible presence of bone natriuretic peptide system. // Biochem.Biophys.Res.Commun. – 1996. – vol. 223, N 1. – P. 1–6.

Suda T., Ueno Y., Fujii K., Shinki T. Vitamin D and bone. // J.Cell.Biochem. – 2003. – vol. 88, N 2. – P. 259–266.

Suemoto H., Moragaki Y., Nishioka K. et al. Trps1 regulates proliferation and apoptosis of chondrocytes through Stat3 signals. // Dev.Biol. – 2007. – vol. 312, N 2. – P. 572–581.

Sugahara K., Kitagawa H. Recent advances in the study of the biosynthesis and functions of sulfated glycosaminoglycans. // Curr.Opin.Struct.Biol. – 2000. – vol. 10, N 5. – P. 518–527.

Sullivan M.M., Barker T.H., Funk S.E. et al. Matricellular hevin regulates decorin production and collagen assembly. // J.Biol.Chem. – 2006. – vol. 281, N 37. – P. 27621–27632.

Sun J.S., Wu C.X., Tsuang Y.H. et al. The in vitro effects of dehydroepiandrosterone on chondrocyte metabolism. // Osteoarthritis Cartilage. – 2006. – vol. 14, N 3. – P. 238–249.

Surkova S. (С.Суркова), Kosman D., Kozlov K. et al. Characterization of the Drosophila segment determination morpphome. // Dev.Biol. – 2007. – vol. 313, N 2. – P. 844–862.

Surmann-Schmitt C., Dietz U., Kireva T. et al. Ucma, a novel secreted cartilage specific protein with implications in osteogenesis. // J.Biol.Chem. – 2008. – vol. 283, N 11. – P. 7082–7093.

Sutmuller M., Brujin J.A., de Heer E. Collagen types VIII AND X, ywo non-fibrillar short-chain collagens. Structure, homolgirs. functions and involvement in pathol. // Histol.Histopathol. – 1997. – vol. 12, N 2. – P. 357–366.

Suttapreyasri S., Koontongkaew S., Phongdara A., Leggat U. Expression of bone morphogenetic proteins in normal human intramembranous and endochondral bones. // Int.J.Oral Maxillofac.Surg. – 2006. – vol. 35, N 5. – P. 444–452.

Sutton A.L., Zhang X., Dowd D.R. et al. SemaphoriN 3B is a 1,25-dehydrovitamin D3-induced gene in osteoblasts that promotes osteoclastofenesis and induces osteopenia in rats. // Mol.Endocrinol. – 2008. – vol. 22, N 6. – P. 370–381.

Suzdaltseva Yu.G., Burunova V.V., Vakhrushev I.V. et al. The ability of human mesenchymal cells derived from different sources to differentiate into mesodermal tissues. [in Russian] // Bulletin of Experimental Biology and Medicine, 2007, vol. 143, N 1. – P. 114–121.

Suzuki N., Yokoyama F., Nomizu M. Functional sites in the laminin alpha chain. // Connect.Tissue Res. – 2005. – vol. 46, N 3. – P. 142–152.

Svensson L., Aszódi A., Reinholt F.P. et al. Collagen-binding proteins. // Osteoarthritis Cartilage. – 2001. – vol. 9, Suppl.A. – P. 523–528.

Swann A., Amer H., Dieppe P. The value of synovial fluid assays in the diagnosis of joint disease: a literature survey. // Ann. Rheum.Dis. – 2002. – vol. 61. – P. 493–498.

Swann D.A., Silver F.H., Slayter H.S. et al. The molecular structure and lubricating activity of lubricin isolated from human and bovine synovial fluid. // Biochem.J. – 1985. – vol. 225, N 1. – P. 195–201.

Sweetman D., Wagstaff L., Cooper O. et al. The migration of paraxial and lateral plate mesoderm cells emerging from the late primitive streak is controlled by different Wnt signals. // BMC Dev.Biol. – 2008. – vol. 8. – P. 63.

Sychenikov I.A., Aboyants R.K., Dronov A.F., Istranov L.P., Nikolaev A.V. and A.B. Shekhter. Collagen plastic reconstruction in medicine. [in Russian], edited by V.V. Kovanov and I.A. Sychenikov. Moscow: Medicine, 1978. 256 pages.

Syed F., Khosla S. Mechanisms of sex steroid effects on bone. // Biochem.Biophys.Res.Commun. – 2005. – vol. 328, N 3. – P. 688–696.

Sylvia V.L., Gay I., Hardin R. et al. Rat costochondral chondrocytes produce 17β-estradiol and regulate its production by 1α,25(OH)2D3. // Bone. – 2002. – vol. 30, N 1. – P. 57–63.

Tagariello A., Luther J., Streiter M. et al. Ucma – a novel secreted factor represents a highly specific marker for distal chondrocytes. // Matrix Biol. – 2008. – vol. 27, N 1. – P. 3–11.

Takada R., Satomi Y., Kurata T. et al. Monounsaturated fatty acid modification of Wnt protein: its role in Wnt secretion. // Dev.Cell. – 2006. – vol. 11. – P. 791–801.

Takagi J. Structural basis for ligand recognition by RGD (Arg-Gly-aAsp)-dependent integrins. // Biochem.Soc.Trans. – 2004. – V. 32, N 3. – P. 403–406.

Takahashi I., Nickolls G.H., Takahasi K. et al. Compressive force promotes Sox9, type II collagen and aggrecan and inhibits IL-1β expressing resulting in chondrogenesis in mouse embryonic limb bud mesenchymal cells. // J.Cell Sco/ – 1998. – vol. 111, N 14. – P. 2067–2076.

Takahashi T., Ogasawara T., Asawa Y., Mori Y. et al. Three-dimensional microenvironment retain chondrocyte phenotype during proliferation culture. // Tisse Eng. – 2007. – vol. 13, N 7. – P. 1583–1592.

Takano H., Aizawa T., Irie T. et al. Estrogen deficiency leads to decrease in chondrocyte numbers in the rabbit growth plate. // J.Orthop.Res. – 2007. – vol. 12, N 4. – P. 366–374.

Takayanagi H. Mechanistic insight into osteoclast differentiation in osteoimmunology. // J.Mol.Med. – 2005. – vol. 83. – P. 170–179.

Takayanagi H. Osteoimmunology: shared mechanisms and cross-talk between the immune and bone system. // Nat.Rev.Immunol. – 2007. – vol. 7, N 4. – P. 292–304.

Takayanagi H., Sato K., Takaoka A., Taniguchi T. Interplay between interferon and other cytokine systems in bone metabolism. // Immunol.Rev. – 2005. – vol. 208. – P. 181–193.

Takeuchi S., Mukai N., Tateichi T., Niyakawa S. Production of sex steroid hormones from DHEA in articular chondrocytes of rats. // Am.J.Physiol.Endocrinol.Metab. – 2007. – vol. 293, N 1. – P. 410–E415.

Takigawa M., Nakamashi T., Kubota S. et al. Role of CTGF/HCS24/ecogenin in skeletal growth control. // J.Cell,Physiol. – 2003. – vol. 194, N 3. – P. 256–266.

Tallheden T., Karlsson C., Brunner A. et al. Gene expression during redifferentiation of human articular chondrocytes. // Osteoarthritis Cartilage. – 2004. – vol. 12. – P. 525–535.

Talwar R.M., Wong B.S., Svoboda X., Harper R.P. Effects of estrogen on chondrocyte proliferation and collagen synthesis in skeletally mature articular chondrocytes. // J.Oral Maxillofac.Surg. – 2006. – vol. 64, N 4. – P. 600–609.

Tamamura Y., Otani T., Kanatani N. et al. Developmental regulation of Wnt/β-catenin signals is required for growth plate assembly, cartilage integ-. Jrity and endochondral ossification. // J.Biol.Chem. – 2005. – vol. 280, N 19. – P. 19185–19195.

Tamburro A.M., Bochicchio B., Pepe A. The dissection of human tropoelastin: from the molecular structure to self-assembly to the elasticity mechanism. // – Pathologie Biologie. – 2005. – vol. 53. – P. 383–389.

Tamma R., Colaianni G., Zhu L.L. et al. Oxytocun is an anabolic bone hormone. // Proc.Natl.Acad.Sci.USA. – 2009. – vol. 106, N 17. – P. 7149–7154.

Tammi M.I., Day A.J., Turley E.A. Hyaluronan and homeostasis: a balancing act. // J.Biol.Chem. – 2002. – vol. 277, N 7. – P. 4581–4584.

Tamura M., Ishikawa O. An increase in mature type skin collagen cross-link, histidinohydroxylysinonorleucine, in the sclerotic skin of morphea. // J.Dermatol.Sci. – 2001. – vol. 25, N 1. – P. 83–86

Tan X., Weng T., Zhang J. et al. Smad4 is required for maintaining normal murine postnatal bone homeostasis. // J.Cell Sci. – 2007. – vol. 120. – P. 2162–2170.

Taniguchi N., Yoshida K., Ito T. et al. Stage-specific secretion of HMGB1 in cartilage regulates endochondral ossification. // Mol. Cell. Biol. – 2007. – vol. 27, N 16. – P. 5650–5663.

Tanne Y., Tanimoto K., Tanaka N. et al. Expression and activity of Runx2 mediated by hyaluronan during chondrocyte differentiation. // Arch.Oral Biol. – 2008. – vol. 53, N 5. – P. 478–487.

Tasheva E.S., Klocke B., Conrad G.W. Analysis of transcriptional regulation of the small leucine-rich proteoglycans. // Mol.Vis. – 2004. – vol. 10. – P. 758–772.

Tatham A.S., Shewry P.R. Elastomeric proteins: biological roles, structures and mechanisms. // Trends Biochem.Sci. – 2000. – vol. 25, N 11. – P. 567–571.

Taylor A.F., Saunders M.M., Shigle D.I. et al. Mechanicallyu stimulated osteocyte regulate osteoblast activity via gap junction. // Am.J.Physiol.Cell Physiol. – 2007. – vol. 292. – P. C545–C552.

Taylor D.K., Meganck J.A., Terkhorn S. et al. Thrombospondin-2 influences the proportion of cartilage and bone during fracture healing. // J.Bone Miner.Res. – 2009. – Epub.Jan.5

Taylor P.R., Martinez-Pomares L., Stacey M. et al. Macrophage receptors and immune recognition. // Annu.Rev. Immunol. – 2005. – vol. 23. – P. 901–944.

Tchetina E.V., Kobayashi M., Yasuda T. et al. Chondrocyte hypertrophy can be induced by a cryptic sequence of type II collagen and is accompanied by the induction of MMP-13 and collagenase activity: implications for development and arthritis. // Matrix Biol. – 2007. – vol. 26, N 4. – P. 247–258.

Teitelbaum S.L. Bone resorption by osteoclasts. // Science. – 2000. – vol. 289, N 5484. – P. 1504–1508

Teitelbaum S.L. Osteoclasts and integrins. // Ann.N.Y.Acad.Sci. – 2006. – vol. 1068. – P. 95–99.

Teitelbaum S.L. Osteoclasts: what do they do and how do they do it. // Am.J.Pathol. – 2007. – vol. 170, N 2. – P. 427–438.

Teixeira C.C., Agoston H., Beier F. Nitric oxide, C-type natriuretic peptide and cGML as regulators of endochondral ossification. // Dev.Biol. – 2008. – vol. 319, N 2. – P. 171–178

Teng Y., Zeisberg M., Kalluri R. Transcriptional regulation of epithelial-mesenchymal transition. // J.Clin.Invest. – 2007. – vol. 117, N 2 – P. 304–306.

Teplyuk N.M., Galindo M., Teplyuk V.I. et al. Runx2 regulates G-protein coupled signaling pathways to control growth of osteoblast progenitors. // J.Biol.Chem. – 2008. – vol. 283, N 41. – P. 27585–27597.

Teplyuk N.M., Haupt L.M., Ling L. et al. The osteogenic transcription factor Runx2 regulates components of the fibroblast growth factor/proteoglycan signaling axis in osteoblasts. // J.Cell.Biochem. – 2009. – vol. 107, N 1. – P. 144–154.

Termaat M.F., Boer D., Baker E.C. et al. Bone morphogenetic proteins. // J.Bone Joint Surg. – 2005. – vol. 87-A. – P. 1367–1378.

Teti A., Zallone A. Do osteocytes contribute to bone mineral homeostasis? Osteocytic osteolysis revised. // Bone. – 2009. – vol. 44, N 1. – P. 11–16.

Tetlow L.C., Woolley D.E. Expression of vitamin D receptors and matrix metalloproteinases in osteoarthritic cartilage and human articular chondrocytes in vitro. // – Osteoarthritis Cartilage. – 2001. – vol. 9, N 5. – P. 423–431.

Tfelt-Hansen J., Brown E.M. The calcium-sensing receptor in normal physiology and pathophysiology. // Crit.Rev.Clin.Lab.Sci. – 2005. – vol. 42, N 1. – P. 35–70.

Thiale H. Histolyse und Histogenese. – Frankfurt a.M., Springer-Verlag. – 1967.

Thibault D.L., Utz P.J. Interpreting interest in interferon-α. // Arthritis Res.Ther. – 2003. – vol. 5, N 5. – P. 246–248.

Thomas G., Moffatt P., Salois P. et al. Osteocrin, a novel bone-specific secreted protein that mediates the osteoblast phenotype. // J.Biol.Chem. – 2003. – vol. 278, N 50. – P. 50563–50571.

Thomas J.T., Prakash D., Weih K., Moos M.jr. CDMP1/GDF5 has specific processing requirements that restrict its action to joint surfaces. // J.Biol.Chem. – 2006. – vol. 281, N 36. – P. 26725–26733.

Thomas T. The complex effects of leptin on bone metabolism through multiple pathways. // Curr.Opin.Pharmacol. – 2004. – vol. 4, N 5. – P. 295–300.

Thrailkill K.M., Lumpkin C.K.jr., Bunn R.C. et al. Is insulin an anabolic agent in bone? Dissecting the diabetic bone for clues. // Am.J.Physiol.Endocrinol.Metab. – 2005. – vol. 289. – P.E735–E745.

Thyberg J. Electron microscopy of cartilage proteoglycans // Histochem. J. 1977. – vol. 9. – P. 259–266.

Tian T., Meng A.M. Nodal signals pattern vertebrate embryos. // Cell. Mol.Life Sci. – 2006. – vol. 63. – P. 672–685.

Tickle C. Patterning systems – from one end of the limb to the other. // Dev.Cell. – 2003. – vol. 4. – P. 449–458.

Timpl R., Sasaki T., Kostka G., Chu M.L. Fibulin: a versatile family of extracellular matrix proteins. // Nat.Rev.Mol.Cell.Biol. – 2003. – vol. 4, N 6. – P. 479–489.

Tomasek J.J., Gabbiani G., Hinz B. et al. Myofibroblasts and mechanoregulation of connective tissue remodeling. // Nat. Rev. Mol. Biol. – 2002. – vol. 3. – P. 348–355.

Tominaga H., Maeda S., Miyoshi H. et al. Expression of osterix inhibits bone morphogenetic protein-induced chondrogenic differentiation of mesenchymal protenitor cells. // J.Bone Miner.Metab. – 2009. – vol. 27, N 1. – P. 36–45.

Tonachini L., Monticone M., Di Marco E. et al. Chondrocyte protein with a poly-proline region is a novel protein expressed by chondrocytes in vitro and in vivo. // Biochim.Biophys.Acta. – 2002. – vol. 1577, N 3. – P. 431–439.

Toole B.P. Hyaluronan in morphogenesis and tissue remodeling. // http://www.glycoforum.gr.jp/ – 1998.

Topol L., Chen W., Song H. SOX9 inhibits WNT signaling by promoting β-catenin phosphorylation in the nucleus. // J.Biol.Chem. -Epub 2008 Dec.1. M808048200

Toricelli P., Fini M., Gavarese G. et al. Effects of systemic glucocorticoid administration on tenocytes. // Biomed.Pharmacother. – 2006. – vol. 60, N 6. – P. 380–385.

Tovey N.K. A digital computer technique for orientation analysis of micrographs of soil fibric // Microsc., 1980. – vol. 120. – P. 303–317.

Trackman P.C. Diverse biological functions of extracellular collagen ptocessing enzymes. // J.Cell.Biochem. – 2005.– vol. 96, N 5. – P. 927–937.

Trayhurn P., Beattie J.H. Physiological role of adipose tissue: white adipose tissue as an endocrine and secretory organ. // Proc. Nutr. Soc. 2001. N 60. P. 329–339.

Trelstadt R.L. Matrix macromolecules: spatial relationships in two dimensions. // Ann.N.Y.Acad.Sci. – 1990. – vol. 580. – P. 391–420.

Trowbridge I.M., Gallo R.L. Dermatan sulfate: new functions for an old glycosaminoglycan. // J.Glycobiol. – 2002. – vol. 12, N 9. – P. 117R–125R.

Tsai J., Tong Q., Tan G. et al. The transcription factor GATA2 regulates differenbtiation of brown adipocytes. // EMBO reports. – 2005. – vol. 6, N 9. – P. 879

Tseng S., Reddi A.H., Di Cesare P.E. Cartilage oligometic matrix protein (COMP): a biomarker of arthritis. // Biomarker Insights. – 2009. – vol. 4. – P. 33–44.

Tsuji K., Nakahata T., Takagi M. et al. Effects of interleukin-3 and interleukin-4 on the development of "connective tissue-type" mast cells: interleukin-3 supports their survival and interleukin-4 triggers and supports their proliferation synergistically with interleukin-3. // Blood. – 1990. – vol. 75, N 2. – P. 421–427

Tsumaki N., Nakase T., Miyaji T, Kakiuchi M. et al. Bone morphogenetic protein signals are required for cartilage formation and differently regulate joint development during skeletogenesis. // J.Bone Miner,Res. – 2002. – vol. 17, N 2. – P. 898–906.

Tu Q., Pi M., Quarles L.D. Calcyclin mediates serum response element (SRE) activation by an osteoblastic extracellular cation-sensing mechanism. // J.Bone Miner.Res. – 2003. – vol. 18, N 10. – P. 1825–1833.

Tu X., Joeng K.S., Nakayama K.I. et al. Noncanonical Wnt signaling through G protein-linked PKCδ activation promotes bone formation. // Dev.Cell. – 2007. – vol. 12. – P. 113–127.

Tuan R.S. Cellular signaling in developmental chondrogenesis: N-cadherin, Wnts, and BMP-2. // J.Bone Joint Surg. – 2003. – vol. 85-A, Suppl.2. – P. 137–141.

Tucker R.P. The thrombospondin type I repeat superfamily. // – Int.J.Biochem.Cell Biol. – 2004. – vol. 36, N 6. – P. 969–974.

Tucker R.P., Adams J.C., Lawler J. Thrombospondin-4 is expressed by early osteogenic tissues in the chick embryo. // Dev.Biol. – 1995. – vol. 203, N 4. – P. 477–490.

Tucker R.P., Drabikowski K., Hess J.F. et al. Phylogenetic analysis of the tenascin gene family: evidence of origin early in the chordate lineage. // BMC Evol.Biol. – 2006. – vol. 6, N 1. – P. 60.

Tuckwell D. Identification and analysis of collagen α1(XXI), a novel member of the FACIT collagen family. // Matrix Biol. – 2002. – vol. 21, N 1. – P. 63–66.

Tufan A.C., Tuan R.S. Wnt regulation of limb mesenchymal chondrogenesis is accompanied by altered N-cadherin-related functions. // FASEB J. – 2001. – vol. 15, N 8. – P. 1436–1438.

Tulla M., Pentikainen O.T., Viitasalo T. et al. Selective binding of collagen subtypes by integrin α1I, α2I, and α10I domain. // J.Biol.Chem. 2001. – vol. 276, N 51. – P. 48206–48212.

Tupler R., Perini G., Green M.R. Expressing the human genome. // Nature. – 2001. – vol. 409. – P. 832–833.

Turker S., Keratosun Y., Gunal I. β-blockers increase bone mineral density. // Clin.Orthop. – 2006. – vol. 443. – P. 73–74.

Turley E.A., Noble P.W., Bourguignon L.Y.W. Signaling properties of hyaluronan receptors. // J.Biol.Chem. – 2002. – vol. 277, N 7. – P. 4589–4592.

Turner C.H., Robling A.C., Duncan R.I., Burr D.B. Do bone cell behave like a neuronal network? // Calcif.Tissue Int. – 2002. – vol. 70, N 6. – P. 435–442.

Turner C.H., Warden S.J., Bellido T. et al. Mechanobiology of the skeleton. // Sci.Signal. – 2009. – vol. 2 (68), pt.3.

Twai W.O., Czirok A., Hegedus B. et al. Fibulin-1 suppression of fibronectin-regulated cell adhesion and motility. // J.Cell Sci. – 2001. – vol. 114, N 24. – P. 4587–4598.

Tzortzaki E.G., Koutsopoulos A.V., Dambaki K.I. et al. Active remodeling in idiopathic interstitial pneumonias: evaluation of collagen types XII and XIV. // J.Histochem.Cytochem. – 2006. – vol. 54, N 6. – P. 693–700.

Udagawa N., Kotake S., Kamatani N. et al. The molecular mechanisms of osteoclastogenesis in rheumatoid arthritis. // Arthritis Res. – 2002. – vol. 4, N 3. – P. 281–289.

Uitto J. The role of elastin and collagen in cutaneous aging: intrinsic aging versus photoexposure. // J.Drugs Dermatol. – 2008. – vol. 7, Suppl 2. – P. s12–s16.

Ulici V., Hoenselaar K.D., Gillespie J.R., Beier F. The PI3K pathway regulates endochondral bone growth through control of hypertrophic chondrocyte differentiation. // BMC Dev.Biol. – 2008. – vol.8. P. 40.

Ulsamer A., Ortuño M.J., Ruiz S. et al. BMP-2 induces Osterix expression through upregulation of Dlx5 and its phosphorylation by p38. // J.Biol.Chem. 2008. – vol. 283, N 7. – P. 3816–3826.

Umlauf E., Csaazar E., Moertelmaier M. et al. Association of stomatin with lipid bodies. // J.Biol.Chem. – 2004. – vol. 279, N 22. – P. 23699–23709.

Ureña P., Vermejoul M.C.de. Circulating biochemical markers of bone remodeling in uremic patients. // Kidney Int. – 1999. – vol. 53. – P. 2141–2156.

Urist M.R., Behnam K., Kerendi F. et al. Lipids closely associated with bone morphogenetic protein (BMP) and induced heterotopic bone formation. // Connect.Tissue Res. – 1997. –vol.36, N 1. – P. 9–20.

Urry D.W., Hugel T., Seitz M. et al. Elastin: a representative ideal protein elastomer // Philos.Trans.R.Soc. London. B. Biol.Sci. – 2002. – vol. 357, N 1418. – P. 169–184.

Ushiki T. Collagen fibers, reticular fibers and elastic fibers. A comprehensive understanding from a morphological viewpoint. // Arch.Histol.Cytol. – 2002. – vol. 65, N 2. – P. 109–126.

Usui M., Xing L., Drissi H. et al. Murine and chicken chondrocytes regulate osteoclastogenesis by producing RANKL in response to BMP2. // J.Bone Miner.Res. – 2008. – vol. 23, N 4. – P. 314–325.

Vaage J., Harlos. J.P. Collagen production by macrophages in tumour encapsulation and dormancy. // Br. J. Cancer. – 1992 – vol. 66. – P. 220–221.

Vaage J., Lindblad W. J. Production of collagen type 1 by mouse peritoneal macrophages. // J. Leukoc. Biol – 1990. – vol.48: – P. 274–280.

Vääräniemi J., Halleen J.M., Kaarlonen K. et al. Intracellular machinery for matrix degradation in bone-resorbing osteoclasts. // J.Bone Miner.Res. – 2004. – vol. 19, N 9. – P. 1432–1449.

Vaes B.L., Dechering K.J., van Someren E.P. et al. Microarray analysis reveals expression regulation of Wnt antagonists in differentiating osteoblasts. // Bone. – 2005. – vol. 36, N 5. – P. 803–811.

Vaes B.L., Ducy P., Sijbers A.M. Microarray analysis on Runx2-deficient mouse embryos reveals novel Runx2 functions and target genes during intramembranous and endochondral boneformation. // Bone. – 2006. – vol. 39, N 4. – P. 724–738.

Vaes B.L.T., Lute C., Blom H.J. et al. Vitamin B12 deficiency stimulates osteoclastogenesis via increased homocysteine and methylmalinic acid. // Calcif.Tissue Int. – 2009. – vol. 84. – P. 413–422.

Vale-Cruz D.S., Ma Q., Syme J., LuValle P.A. Activating transcription factor-2 affects skeletal growth by modulating pRb gene expression. // Mech.Dev. – 2008. – vol. 125, N 9–10. – P. 843–858.

Valentich J.D., Popov V., Saada J.I., Powell D.W. Phenotypic characterization of an intestinal subepithelial myofibroblast cell line. // Am J Physiol. – 1997. – vol. 272. – P. C1513–1524.

Vanderschueren D., Vandenput L., Boonen S. et al. Androgens and bone. // Endocrine Rev. – 2004. – vol. 25, N 3. – P. 389–425.

Vankemmelbeke M.N., Holen L., Wilson A.L. et al. Expression and activity of ADAMTS-5 in synovium. // Eur.J.Biochem. – 2001. – vol.268, N 5. – P. 1259–1268.

Vannahme C., Gosling S., Paulsson M. et al. Characterization of SMOC-2, a modular extracellular calcium-binding protein. // Biochem.J. – 2003. – vol. 373, N 3. – P. 805–814.

Vannahme C., Smyth N., Miosge N. et al. Characterization of SMOC-1, a novel modular calcium binding protein in basement membranes. // J.Biol.Chem. – 2002. – vol. 277, N 41. – P. 3797

Varedi M., Ghahary A., Scott P.G., Tredget E.E. Cytoskeleton regulates expression of genes for transforming growth factor-beta 1 and extracellular matrix proteins in dermal fibroblasts. // J.Cell.Physiol. – 1997. – vol. 172. – P. 192–199.

Varjusalo M., Taipale J. Hedgehog: functions and mechanisms. // Genes Dev. – 2008. – vol. 22. – P. 2454–2472.

Vaughan M.B., Howard E.W., Tomasek J.J. Transforming growth factor-beta1 promotes the morphological and functional differentiation of the myofibroblast. // Exp.Cell.Res. – 2000. – vol. 257. – P. 180–189.

Veit G., Hansen U., Keene D.R. Collagen XII interacts with avian tenascin-X through its NC3 domain. // J.Biol.Chem. – 2006. – V. 281, N 37. – P. 27461–27470.

Veit G., Kobbe B., Keene D.R. et al. Collagen XXVIII, a novel VWA-domain-containing protein with many imperfections in the collagenous domain. // J.Biol.Chem. – 2006. – vol. 281, N 6. – P. 3494–3504.

Venkov C.D., Link A.J., Jennings J.L. et al. A proximal activator of transcription in epithelial-mesenchymal transition. // J.Clin.Invest. – 2007. – vol. 117, N 2. – P. 482–491.

Verborgt O., Tatton N.A., Majeska R.J., Schaffler M.B. Spatial distribution of Bax and Bcl-2 in osteocytes after bone fatigue: complementary role in bone remodeling regulation. // J.Bone Miner.Res. – 2002. – vol. 17, N 8. – P. 907–914.

Verkman A.S., Mitra A.K. Structure and function of aquaporin water channels. // Am.J.Physiol.Renal Physiol. – 2000. – vol. 278, N 1. – P. F13–F.28.

Vermeer C., Jie K.S., Knapen M.H. Role of vitamin K in bone metabolism. // Annu.Rev.Nutr. – 1995. – vol. 15. – P. 1–22.

Vermeulen K., Berneman Z.N., Van Bockstaele D.R. Cell cycle and apoptosis. // Cell Prolif. – 2003. – vol. 36. – P. 165–175.

Vestweber D., Blanks J.E. Mechanisms that regulate the function of selectins and their ligands. // Physiol.Rev. – 1999. – vol. 79, N 1. – P. 181–213.

Veverka V., Henry A.J., Slocombe P.M. et al. Characterization of the structural features and interactions of sclerostin: molecular isights into a key regulator of the Wnt-mediated bone formation. // J.Biol.Chem. – 2009. – vol. 284, N 16. – P. 10890–10900.

Viegas M., Gomez E., Brooks J., Davies R.J. Changes in nasal mast cell numbers in and out of the pollen season. // Int.Arch. Allergy. Appl.Immunol. – 1987. – vol. 82, N 34. – P. 275–276.

Vignery A. Macrophage fusion: the making of osteoclasts and giant cells. // J.Exp.Med. – 2005, vol. 202, N 3. – P. 337–340.

Vinall R.L., Reddi A.H. The effect of BMP on the expression of cytoskeletal proteins and its potential relevance. // J.Bone Joint Surg. – 2001. – vol. 83-A, Suppl.1. – P. S63–S69.

Vincent T.L., McLean C.J., Full L.V. et al. FGF-2 is bound to perlecan in the pericellular matrix of articular cartilage, where it acts as a chondrocyte mechanotransducer. // Osteoarthritis Cartilage – 2007. – vol. 15, N 7. – P. 752–763.

Vincourt J.B., Lionneton F., Kratassiouk G. et al. Establishment of a reliable method for direct proteome characterization of human articular cartilage. // Mol.Cell.Proteomics. – 2006. – vol. 5, N 10. – P. 1984–1995.

Vinogradov V.V., Akulinin G.E., Vorobieva N.F. and G.V. Pravotorov. Type differences of loose connective tissue in rodents of various ecological importance. [in Russian] // In: IX All-Soviet Union congress of anatomists, histologists and embryologists. Novosibirsk: Abstracts, 1981. p. 80.

Visse R., Nagase H. Matrix metalloproteinases and tissue inhibitors of metalloproteinases. Structure, function, and biochemistry. // Circ.Res. – 2003. – vol. 92. – P. 827–839.

Vlasov B.Ya. Bioenergetic aspect of posttraumatic regeneration of bone tissue. [in Russian] // Doctoral dissertation abstract. Moscow, 1987. P. 43.

Vogel K.G., Peters J.A. Histochemistry defines a proteoglycan-rich layer in bovine flexor tendon subjected to bending. // J.Musculoskel-et.Neuronal Interact. – 2005. – vol. 5, N 1. – P. 64–69.

Vogel W.F., Abdulhussein R., Ford C.E. Sensing extracellular matrix: an update on discoidin domain receptor function. // Cell.Signal. – 2006. – vol. 18, N 8. – P. 1108–1116.

Voronovich I.R., Kupchinov B.I., Rodionov V.G. et al. Biological mechanisms to reduce intraarticular friction. [in Russian] // Orthop., Traumatol., Prosthet. 1987, N 4. P. 71–73.

Vranka J.A., Sakai L.Y., Bächinger H.P. Prolyl 3-hydroxylase 1, enzyme characterization and identification of a novel family pf enzymes. // J.Biol.Chem. – 2004. – vol. 279, N 22/ – P. 23615–23621.

Vrotsos Y., Miller S.C., Marks S.C. Prostaglandin E – a powerful anabolic agent for generalized or site-specific bone formation. // Crit. Rev.Eukaryot.Gene Expr. – 2003. – vol. 13, N 2–4. – P. 253–263.

Vuillermoz B., Wegrowski Y., Contet-Audonneau J.L. et al. Influence of aging on glycosaminoglycans and small leucine-rich proteoglycan production by skin fibroblasts. // Mol.Cell.Biol. – 2005. – vol. 277, N 1–2. – P. 63–72.

Wachmuth L., Söder S., Fan Z. et al. Immunolocalization of matrix proteins in different human cartilage subtypes. // Histol.Histopathol. – 2006. – vol. 21, N 5. – P. 477–485.

Wacker S.A., McNulty C.L., Durston A.J. The initiation of Hox gene expression in Xenopus laevis is controlled by Brachyury and BMP-4. // Dev.Biol. – 1994. – vol. 266. – P. 123–133.

Wada H., Okuyama M., Sato N., Zhang S. Molecular evolution of fibrillar collagen in chordates, with implications for the evolution of vertebrate skeleton and chordate phylogeny. // Evol.Dev. – 2006. – vol. 8. – P. 370–377.

Waddington R.J., Roberts H.C., Sugars R.V., Schönherr E. Differential roles for small leucine-rich proteoglycans in bone formation. // Eur.Cell Mater. – 2003. – vol. 6, N 1. – P. 12–21.

Wagener R., Ehleb H.W., Ko Y.P. et al. The matrilins – adaptor proteins in the extracellular matrix. // FEBS Lett. – 2005. – vol. 579, N 15. – P. 3323–3329.

Wahl M.B., Deng C., Lewandoski M., Pourquié O. FGF signaling acts upstream of the NOTCH and WNT signaling pathways to control segmentation clock oscillations in mouse somitogenesis. // Development. – 2007. – vol. 124. – P. 4033–4041.

Wälchli C., Koch M., Chiquet M. et al. Tissue-specific expression of fibril-associated collagens XII and XIV. // J.Cell Sci. – 1994. – V. 107. – P. 669–681.

Walker E.C., McGregor N.E., Poulten I.J. et al. Cardiotrophin-1 is an osteoclast-derived stimulus of bone formation required for normal bone remodeling. // J.Bone Miner.Res. – vol. 23, N 12. – P. 2025–2032.

Wan M., Cao X. BMP signaling in skeletal development. // Biochem. Biophys.Res.Commun. – 2005. – vol. 328. – P. 651–657.

Wang H., Yoshiko Y., Yamamoto R. et al. Overexpression of fibroblast growth factor 23 suppresses osteoblast differentiation and matrix mineralization in vitro. // J.Bone Miner.Res. – 2008. – vol. 23, N 6. – P. 939–948.

Wang J., Elewaut D., Hoffman I. et al. Physiological levels of hydrocortisone maintain an optimal chondrocyte extracellular matrix metabolism. // Ann.Rheum.Dis. – 2004. – vol. 63, N 1. – P. 61–66.

Wang J.F., Jiao H., Stewart T.L. et al. Fibrocytes from burn patients regulate the activities of fibroblasts. // Wound Repair Regen. – 2007. – vol. 15, N 1. – P. 113–121.

Wang J.H., Thampatty B.F., Lin J.S., Im H.J. Mechanotransduction of gene expression in fibroblasts. // Gene. – 2007. – vol. 391, N 1–2. – P. 1–15.

Wang Q., Yang W.H., Krupinski J. et al. PAX genes in embryogenesis and oncogenesis. // J.Cell.Mol.Med. – 2008. – Epub. Jul. 4.

Wang Q.W., Chen Z.L., Piao Y.J. Mesenchymal stem cells differentiate into tenocytes by bone morphogenetic protein (BMP) 12 gene transfer. // J.Biosci.Bioeng. – 2005. – vol. 100, N 4. – P. 418–422.

Wang W., Kirsch T. Annexin V/β5 integrin interactions regulate apoptosis of growth plate chondrocytes. // J.Biol.Chem. – 2006. – vol. 281, N 41. – P. 30848–30856.

Wang X., Kua H.Y., Hu Y. et al. p53 functions as a negative regulator of osteoblastogenesis, osteoblast-dependent osteoclastogenesis, and bone remodeling. // J.Cell Biol. – 2006. – vol. 172, N 1. – P. 115–125.

Wang X.M., Yao T.W., Nadvi N.A. et al. Fibroblast activation protein and chronic liver disease. // Front.Biosci. – 2008. – vol. 13. – P. 3168–3180.

Wang Y., Beflower R.M., Dong Y.-F. et al. Runx1/AML1/Cbfa2 mediates onset of mesenchymal cell differentiation toward chondrogenesis. // J.Bone Miner.Res. – 2005. – vol. 20, N 9. – P. 1624–1636.

Wang Y., Kim K.A., Kim J.H., Sul H.S. Pref-1, a preadipocyte secreted factor that inhibit adipogenesis. // J.Nutrit. – 2006 – vol. 136. – P. 2953–2956.

Wang Y., McL.M., Schaffler M.B., Weinbaum S. A model for the role of integrins in flow induced mechanotransduction in osteocytes. // Proc.Natl.Acad. Sci.USA. – 2007. – vol. 104, N 40. – P. 15541–15546.

Wang Y., Nishida S., Elalieh H.Z. et al. Role of IGF signaling in regulating osteoclastogenesis. // J.Bone Miner.Res. – 2006a. – vol. 21, N 9. – P. 1350–1358.

Wang Y., Nishida S., Sakata T. et al. Insulin-like growth factor-1 is essential for embryonic bone development. // Endocrinolohy. – 2006b. – vol. 147, N 10. – P. 4753–4761.

Wang Y., Wan C., Deng L. et al. The hypoxia-inducible factor α pathway couples angiogenesis to osteogenecis during skeletal development. // J.Clin.Invest. – 2007. – vol. 117, N 6. – P. 1616–1626.

Warnke P.H., Springer I.N., Russo P.A.J. et al. Innate immunity in human bone. // Bone. – 2006. – vol. 38. – P. 400–408.

Warren S.M., Brunet K.L.J., Harland R.M. et al. The BMP antagonist noggin regulates cranial suture fusion. // Nature. – 2003. – vol. 422. – P. 625–629.

Watanabe H., Gao L., Sugiyama S. et al. Mouse aggrecan: a large proteoglycan proteoglycan protein sequence, gene structure and promoter sequence. // Biochem.J. – 1995. – vol. 308, N 2. – P. 433–440.

Watanabe H., Yamada Y. Mice lacking link protein develop dwarfism and craniofacial abnormality. // Nat.Genet. – 1999. – vol. 21, N 2. – P. 225–229.

Watanabe N., Tezuka Y., Matsuno K. et al. Suppression of differentiation and proliferation of early chondrogenic cells by Notch. // J.Bone Miner.Metab. – 2003. – vol. 21. – P. 344–352.

Watson P., Forster R., Palmer K.J. et al. Coupling of ER exit to microtubules through direct interaction of COPII with dynactin. // Nat.Cell Biol. – 2005. – vol. 7, N 1. – P. 48–55.

Watson R.E., Ball S.G., Craven N.M. et al. Ultrastructure and expression of type VI collagen in photoaged skin. // Br.J.Dermatol. – 2001. – vol. 144, N 4. – P. 751–759.

Webb C.M., Zaman G., Mosley J.R. et al. Expression of tenascin-C in bones responding to mechanical loads. // J.Bone Miner.Res. – 1997. – vol. 12, N 1. – P. 52–58.

Wet J., Sheng X., Feng D. et al. PERK is essential for neonatal skeletal development to regulate osteoblast proliferation and differentiation. // J.Cell.Physiol. – 2008. – vol. 217, N 3. – P. 693–707.

Weiler T., Du Q., Krokhin O. et al. The identification and characterization of a novel protein c19orf10 in the synovium. // Arthritis Res. Ther. 2007. Vol.9. R30.

Welch M.P., Odland G.F., Clark R.A. Temporal relationships of F-actin bundle formation, collagen and fibronectin matrix assembly, and fibronectin receptor expression to wound contraction. // J.Cell Biol. – 1990. – Vl.110. –P. 133–145.

Wellik D.M. Hox patterning of the vertebrate axial skeleton. // Dev.Dyn. – 2007. – vol. 236. – P. 2454–2463.

Wellik D.M., Capecchi M.R. Hox 10 and Hox11 genes are required toi globally pattern the mammalian skeleton. // Science. – 2003. – vol. 301. – P. 363–367.

Wendel M., Sommarin Y., Heinegård D. Bone matrix proteins isolation and characterization of a novel cell-binding keratin sulfate proteoglycan (osteoadherin) from bovine bone. // J.Cell Biol. – 1998. – vol. 141, N 3. – P. 839–847.

Wenstrup R.J., Florer J.B., Davidson J.M. et al. Murine model of the Ehlers-Danlos syndrome: COL5A1 haploinsufficiency disrupts collagen fibril assembly at multiple stages. // – J.Biol.Chem. – 2006. – vol. 281, N 18. – P. 1288–12895.

Werner S., Krieg T., Smola H. Keratinocyte-fibroblast interactions in wound healing. // J.Invest.Dermatol. – 2007. – vol. 127, N 5. – P. 998–1008.

Weston A.D., Chandraratna R.A.S., Torchia J., Underhill T.M. Requieremnt for RAR-mediated gene repression in skeletal progenitor differentiation. // J.Cell Biol. – 2002. – vol. 158, N 1. – P. 39–51.

Whittaker C.A., Hynes R.O. Distribution and evolution of von Willebrand/Integrin A domains: widely dispersed domains with roles in cell adhesion and elsewhere. // Mol.Biol.Cell. – 2002. – vol. 13. – P. 3369–3387.

Wiberg C., Klatt A.R., Wagener R. et al. Complexes of matrilin-1 and biglycan or decorin connect collagen VI microfibrils to both collagen II and agrecan. // J.Biol.Chem. – 2003. – vol. 278, N 30. – P. 27898–27904.

Wiesmann H.P., Meyer U., Plate U., Hohling H.J. Aspects of collagen mineralization in hard tissue formation. // Int.Rev.Cytol. – 2005. – vol. 242. – P. 121–156.

Wiezrbicka-Patinowski I., Schwarzbauer J.E. The ins and outs of fibronectin matrix assembly. // J.Cell.Sci. – 2003. – vol. 116, N 16. – P. 3269–3276

Wight T.N. Versican: a versatile extracellular matrix proteoglycan in cell biology. // Curr.Opin.Cell Biol. – 2002. –V. 14, N 5 – P. 617–623.

Williams D.R.jr., Presar A.R., Richmond A.T. et al. Limb chondrogenesis is compromised in the versican deficient hdf mouse. // Biochem.Biophys.Res.Comm. – 2005. – vol. 334. – P. 960–966.

Williams J.A., Kondo N., Okabe T. et al. Retinoic acid receptors are required for skeletal growth, matrix homeostasis and growth plate function in postnatal mouse. // Dev.Biol. – 2009. – vol. 328, N 2. – P. 315–327.

Williamson A.K., Chen A.C., Masuda K. et al. Tensile mechanical properties of bovine articular cartilage: variations with growth and relationship to collagen network components. // J.Orthop.Res. – 2003. – vol. 22, N 8. – P. 871–878.

Wilson R., Lees J.F., Bulleid N.J. Protein disulfide isomerase acts as a molecular chaperone during the assembly of procollagen. // J.Biol.Chem. – 1998. – vol. 273, N 16. – P. 9637–9643.

Wilson S.R., Peters C., Saftig P., Bromme D. Cathepsin K activity-dependent regulation of osteoclast actin ring formation and bone resorption. // J.Biol.Chem. – 2009. – vol. 284, N 4. – P. 2584–2592.

Winslow B.B., Takimoto-Kimura R., Burke A.C. Global patterning of the vertebrate mesoderm. // Dev.Dyn. – 2007. – vol. 236. – P. 2371–2381.

Winslow M.M., Pan M., Starbuck M. et al. Calcineurin/NFAT signaling in osteoblasts regulate bone mass. // Dev.Cell. – 2006. – vol. 10. – P. 771–782.

Wiren K.M., Toombs A.R., Semirale A.A., Zhang X. Osteoblast and osteocyte apoptosis associated with androgen action in bone: requirement of increased Bax/Bcl-2 ratio. // Bone. – 2006. – vol. 38. – P. 637–651.

Witowski J., Jörres A. Peritoneal cell culture: fibroblasts. // Peritoneal Dialysis Int. – 2006. – vol. 26. – P. 292–299

Wittler L., Shin E.H., Grote P. et al. Expression oif Msgn1 in the presomitic mesoderm is controlled by synergism of WNT signaling and Tbx6. // EMBO Rep. – 2007. – vol. 8, N 8. – P. 184–189.

Woessner J.F.,jr. The impish TIMP: the tissue inhibitor of metalloproteinase-3. // J.Clin.Invest. – 2001. – vol. 108, N 6. – P. 799–800.

Wolf J., Carsons S.E. Distribution of type VI collagen expression in synovial tissue and cultured synoviocytes. Relation to fibronectin expression. // Ann.Rheum.Dis. – 1991. – vol. 50, N 7. – P. 493–496.

Wolfman N.M., Hattersley C., Cox K. et al. Ectopic induction of tendon and ligament in rats by growth and differentiation factors 5, 5, and t members of the TGF-β family. // J.Clin.Invest. – 1997. – vol. 100, N 2. – P. 321–330.

Wolins N.E., Brasaemle D.L., Bickel P.E. A proposed model of fat packaging by exchangeable lipid droplet proteins. // FEBS Lett. – 2006. – vol. 580. – P. 5484–5491.

Wongdee K., Pandaranandakli J., Teerapornpuntakli J. et al. Osteoblasts express claudins and tight junction-associated proteins. // Bichem.Cell Biol. – 2008. – vol. 130. – P. 79–90.

Wood I.S., Trayburn P. Glucose transporters (GLUT and SGLT) expanded families of sugar transport proteins. // Br.J.Nutr. – 2003. – V. 89. – N 1. – P. 3–9.

Woods A., Khan S., Beier F. C-type natriuretic peptide regulates cellular condensation and glycosaminoglycan synthesis during chondrogenesis. // Endocrinology. – 2007. – vol. 148. – P. 5030–5041.

Woods A., Wang G., Beier F. Regulation of chondrocyte differentiation by the actin cytoskeleton and adhesive interactions. // J.Cell. Physiol. – 2007. vol.213, N 1. – P. 1–8.

Woods A., Wang G., Dupuis H. et al. Rac1 signaling stimulates N-cadherin expression, mesenchymal condensation, and chondrogenesis. // J.Biol.Chem. – 2007. – vol. 282, N 32. – P. 23500–23508.

Worrall J.G., Bayliss M.T., Edwards J.W. Morphological localization of hyaluronan in normal and diseased synovium. // J.Rheumatol. – 1991. – vol. 18, N 10. – P. 1466–1472.

Wu S., Flint J.K., Rezvani G., De Luca F. Nuclear factor NF-κB p65 facilitates longitudinal bone growth by inducing growth plate chondrocyte proliferation and differentiation and by preventing apoptosis. // J.Biol.Chem. – 2007. – vol. 282, N 46. – P. 33698–33706.

Wu X., Pan G., McKenna M.A. et al. RANKL regulates Fas expression and Fas-mediated apoptosis in osteoclasts. // J.Bone Miner.Res. – 2005. – vol. 20, N 1. – P. 107–116.

Wu Y., Humphry M.B., Nakamura M.C. Osteoclasts – the innate immune cells of the bone. // Autoimmunity. – 2008. – vol. 41, N 3. – P. 183–194.

Wuelling M., Kaiser F.J., Buelens L.A. et al. Trps1, a regulator of chondrocyte proliferation and differentiation, interacts with the activator form of Gli3. // Dev.Biol. – 2009. – vol. 328, N 1. – P. 40–53.

Wynn T.A. Cellular and molecular mechanisms of fibrosis. // J.Pathol. – 2008. – vol. 214. – P. 199–210.

Xia Y., Pauza M.E., Feng L., Lo D. RelB regulation of chemokine expression modulates local inflammation. // Am.J.Pathol. – 1997. – vol. 151. – P. 375–387.

Xiao L., Liu P., Li X. et al. Exported 18-kDa isoform of fibroblast growth factor-2 is a critical determinant of bone mass in mice. // J.Biol.Chem. – 2009. – vol. 284, N 5. – P. 3170–3182.

Xiao L., Naganawa T., Obugunde E. et al. Stat1 controls postnatal bone formation by regulating fibroblast growth factor signaling in osteoblasts. // J.Biol.Chem. – 2004. – vol. 279, N 26. – P. 27743–27752.

Xiao X.M., Liao E.Y., Zhou H.D. et al. Ascorbic acid inhibits osteoclastogenesis of RAW264.7 cells induced by receptor activated nuclear activated kappaB ligand (RANKL) in vitro. // J.Endocrinol.Invest. – 2005. – vol. 28, N 3. – P. 253–260.

Xiao Y.T., Xiang L.X. Shao J.Z. Bone morphogenetic proteins. // Biochem.Biophys.Res.Commun. – 2007. – vol. 362. – P. 550–553.

Xiao Z., Camalier C.E., Nagashima K. et al. Analysis of the extracellular matrix vesicle proteome in mineralizing osteoblasts. // J.Cell.Physiol. – 2007. – vol. 210. – P. 325–335.

Xiao Z.S., Hlelmeland A.B., Quarles L.D. Selective deficiency of the "bone-related" Runx2-II unexpectedly preserve osteoblast-mediated skeletogenesis. // J.Biol.Chem. – 2004. – vol. 279, N 10. – P. 20307–20313.

Xing L., Boyce B.F. Regulation of apoptosis in osteoclastic and osteoblastic cells. // Biochem.Biophys.Res.Commun. – 2005. – vol.328. – P. 709–720.

Xing W., Singgih A., Kappor A. et al. Nuclear factor-E2 trlated factor-1 mediates ascorbic acid induction of osterix acid expression. // J.Biol.Chem. – 2007, May 17. – Manuscript 702614200.

Xu S., Yu J.J. Beneath the minerals, a layer of round lipid particles was identified to mediate collagen calcification in compact bone formation. // Biophys.J. – 2006. – vol 91, N 11. – P. 4221–4229.

Xu Y., Mallach P., Zhou D., Longaker M.T. Molecular and cellular characterization of mouse calvarial osteoblasts derived from neural crest and paraxial mesoderm. // Plast.Reconstr.Surg. – 2007. – vol. 120. – P. 1783–1795.

Yagi M., Miyamoto T., Toyama Y. Suda T. Role of DC-STAMP in cellular fusion of osteoclasts and macrophage giant cells. // J.Bone Miner. Metab. – 2006. – vol. 24, N 5. – P. 355–358.

Yagi R., McBurney D., Horton W.E.jr. Bcl-2 positively regulates Sox9-dependent chondrocyte gene expression by suppressing the MEK-ERK1/2 signaling pathway. // J.Biol.Chem. – 2005. – vol. 280, N 34. – P. 30517–30525

Yagishita N., Yamasaki S., Nishioka K., Nakajima T. Synoviolin protein folding and the maintenance of joint homeostasis. // Nat.Clin/Pract/Rheumatol. – 2008. – vol. 4, N 2. – P. 91–97.

Yagishita N., Yamasaki S., Nishioka K., Nakajima T. Synovium protein folding and mauntenance of joint homeostasis. // Nat.Clin.Pract. Rheumatol. 2008. vol.4. N 2. P. 91–97.

Yamada K.M. Fibronectin peptides in cell migration and wound repair. // J.Clin.Invest. – 2000. – vol. 105, N 11. – P. 1507–1509.

Yamada T., Kawano H., Koshizuka Y. et al. Carminerin contributes to chondrocyte calcification during endochondra; ossification. // Nat.Med. – 2006. – vol. 12, N 6. – P. 665–670.

Yamagishi S, Kobayashi K, Yamamoto H. // Vascular pericytes notonly regulate growth, but also preserve prostacyclin-producing ability and protect against lipid peroxide-induced injury of co-culturedendothelial cells. Biochem Biophys Res Commun – 1991 – V. 190, – P. 418–425.

Yamaguchi M., Igarashi A., Misawa H., Tsurusaki Y. Enhancement of albumin expression in bone tissue with healing rat fractures. // J.Cell.Biochem. – 2003. – vol. 89, N 2. – P. 356–363.

Yamanaka S., Li J., Kania G., Elliott S. et al. Pluripotency of embryonic stem cells. // Cell Tissue Res. – 2008. – vol. 331, N 1. – P. 5–22.

Yamashiro T., Wang X.P., Li Z. et al. Possible roles of Runx1 and Sox9 in incipient intramembranous ossification. // J.Bone Miner.Res. – 2004. – vol. 19, N 10. – P. 1671–1677.

Yamashita S., Andoh M., Ueno-Kudoh H. et al. Sox9 directly promotes Bapx1 gene expression to repress Runx2 in chondrocytes. // Exp.Cell Res. – 2009. – vol. 315, N 13. – P. 2231–2240.

Yamashita T., Yao Z., Li F. et al. NF-kB p50 and p52 regulate receptor activatkr of NF-κB ligand (RANKL) and tumor necrosis factor induced osteoblast precursor differeb\ntiation by activating c-Fos and NFATc1. // J.Biol.Chem. – 2007. – vol. 282, N 25. – P. 18245–18263.

Yamoah K., Brebene A., Ballram R. et al. High-mobility group box proteins modulate tumor necrosis factor-α expression in osteoclastogenesis via a novel deoxyribonucleic acid sequence. // Mol.Endocrinol. – 2008. – vol. 22, N 5. – P. 1141–1153.

Yan Q., Sage E.H. SPARC, a matricellular glycoprotein with important biological functions. // J.Histochem.Cytochem. – 1999. – vol. 47, N 12. – P. 1495–1505.

Yanagisawa H., Davis E.C., Starcher B.C. et al. Fibulin-5 is an elastin-binding protein essential for elastic fibre development in vitro. // Nature. – 2002. – vol. 415, N 6868. – P. 168–171.

Yang Q., McHugh K.P., Patntirapong S. et al. VEGF enhancement of osteoclast survival and bone resorption involves VEGF receptor-2 signaling and beta3 integrin. // Matrix Biol. – 2008. – vol. 27, N 7. – P. 589–599.

Yang V.W., LaBrenz S.R. Decorin is a Zn2+ metalloprotein. // J.Biol.Chem. – 1999. – vol. 274, N 18. – P. 12454–12460.

Yang W., Kalajzic I., Lu Y. et al. In vitro and in vivo study on osteocyte-specific mechanical signaling pathways. // J.Musculoskel.Neuron Interact. – 2004. – vol. 4, N 4. – 386–387.

Yang X., Yip J., Anastassiades T. et al. The action of TNFalpha and TGF-beta include specific alterations of the glycosilation of bovine and human chondrocytes. // Biochim.Biophys.Acta. – 2007. – vol. 1773, N 2. – P. 264–272.

Yano F., Kugimiya F., Ohba S. et al. The canonical Wnt signaling pathways promotes chondrocyte differentiation in a Sox9-dependent manner. // Biochem.Biophys.Res.Commun. – 2005. – vol. 333. – P. 1300–1308.

Yao J.Q., Seedhom B.B. Mechanical conditioning of articular cartilage to prevalent stresses. // Brit. J. Rheumatol. 1993. vol. 32, N 9. P. 856–965.

Yao Z., Nakamura N., Masuko-Hongo K. et al. Characterization of cartilage intermediate layer protein (CILP)-induced arthropathy in mice. // Ann.Rheum.Dis. – 2004. – vol. 63. – P. 252–258.

Yates K.E., Shortkroff S., Reish R.G. Wnt influence on chondrocyte differentiation and cartilage function. // DNA Cell Biol. – 2005. – vol. 24. – P. 446–457.

Yavropoulou M.P., Yovos J.G. Osteoclastogenesis – current knowledge and future perspectives. // J.Musculoskelet.Neuron.Interact. – 2008. – vol. 8, N 3. – P. 204–216.

Yavropoulou M.P., Yovos J.G. The role of the Wnt signaling pathway in osteoblast commitment and differentiation. // Hormone, – 2007. – vol. 6, N 4. – P. 279–294.

Yeh L.C., Tsai A.D., Lee J.C. Cartilage-derived morphogenetic proteins induce osteogenic gene expression in the C2C12 mesenchymal cell line. // J.Cell.Biochem. – 2005. – vol. 95, N 1. P. 173 188.

Yeh L.C., Zavala M.C., Lee J.C. C-type natriuretic peptide enhances osteogenic protein-1-induced osteoblastic cell differentiation via Smad5 phosphorylation. // J.Cell.Biochem. – 2006. – vol. 97, N 3. – P. 494–500

Yin T., Li L. The stem cell niches in bone. // J.Clin.Invest. – 2006. – vol. 116, N 5. – P. 1185–1201.

Yirmiya R., Goshen I., Bajayo A. et al. Depression induces bone loss through stimulation of the sympathetic nervous system. // Proc.Natl.Acad.Sci. USA. – 2006. – vol. 103, N 45. – P. 16876–16881.

Yokouchi Y., Sasaki H., Kuroiwa A. Homeobox gene expression correlates with the bifurcation of limb cartilage development. // Nature. – 1991. – vol. 353, N 6343. – P. 443–445.

Yokozeki M., Baba Y., Shimokawa H. et al. Interferon-gamma inhibits the myofibroblastic phenotype of rat palatal fibroblasts induced by transforming growth factor-beta1 in vitro. // FEBS Lett. – 1999. – vol. 442. – P. 61–64.

Yokozeki M., Moriyama K., Shimokawa H., Kuroda T. Transforming growth factor-beta 1 modulates myofibroblastic phenotype of rat palatal fibroblasts in vitro. // Exp Cell Res – 1997. – vol. 231. – P. 328–336.

Yonekawa M., Kondo S., Sugura H. et al. Serum cartilage-derived retinoic acid-sensitive protein (CD-RAP) levels in Swarm rat chondrosarcoma. // J.Orthop.Res. – 2002. – vol. 20. – P. 382–386.

Yoon S.T., Boden S.D. Osteoinductive molecules in orthopaedics: basic science and preclinical studies. // Clin.Orthop. – 2002. – vol. 395. – P. 33–43.

Yoon Y.M., Oh C.D., Kim D.Y. et al. Epidermal growth factor negatively regulates chondrogenesis of mesenchymal cells by modulating the protein kinase C-α, Erk-1, and p38 MAPK signaling pathways. // J.Biol.Chem. – 2000. – vol. 275, N 16. – P. 12353–12359.

Yoshida Y., Tanaka S., Umemori H. et al. Negative regulation of BMP/Smad signaling by Tob in osteoblasts. // Cell. – 2000. – vol. 103. – P. 1085–1097.

Yoshikawa K., Takahashi S., Imamura Y. et al. Secretion of non-helical collagenous polypeptides of alpha1(IV) upon depletion of ascorbate by cultured human cells. // J.Biochem. (Tokyo) – 2001. – vol. 129, N 6. – P. 929–936

Yoshiko Y., Maeda N., Aubin J.E. StanniocalciN 1 stimulates osteoblast differentiation in rat calvaria cell cultures. // Endocrinology. – 2003. – vol. 144, N 9. – P. 4134–4143.

Yoshizawa T., Takizawa F., Iizawa F. et al. Homeobox protein Msx2 acts as a molecular defense mechanism for preventing ossification of ligament fibroblasts. // Mol.Cell.Biol. – 2004. – vol. 24, N 8. – P. 3460–3472.

Young B.B., Gordon M.K., Birk D.E. Expression of type XIV collagen in developing chicken tendons: association with assembly and growth of collagen fibrils. // Dev.Dyn. – 2000. – vol. 217. – P. 430–439.

Young D.W., Hassan M.Q., Pratap J. et al. Mitotic occupancy and lineage-specific transcriptional control of rRNA genes by Runx2. // Nature. – 2007a. – vol. 445. – P. 442–446.

Young D.W., Hassan M.Q., Yang X.Q. et al. Mitotic retention of gene expression pattern by the cell fate-determining transcription factor. // Proc.Natl.Acad.Sci.USA. – 2007b. – vol. 104, N 9. – P. 3189–3194.

Young M.F. Bone matrix proteins: their function, regulation, and relationship to osteoporosis. // Osteoporosis Int. – 2003. – vol. 14, Suppl. 3. – P. S35–S42.

Yu H.M.I., Jerchow B., Sheu T.J. et al. The role of Axin2 in calvarial morphogenesis and craniosynostosis. // Development. – 2005. – vol. 132, N 8. – P. 1995–2005.

Yu K., Ornitz D.M. FGF signaling regulates mesenchymal differentiation and skeletal patterning along the limb bud proximodistal axis. // Development. – 2008. – vol. 125. – P. 483–491.

Yu L., Liu H., Yan M. et al. Shox2 is required for chondrocyte proliferation and maturation in proximal limb skeleton. // Dev.Biol. – 2007. – vol. 306, N 2. – P. 549–559.

Yurchenco P.D., Schittny J.C. Molecular architecture of basement membranes. // FASEB J. – 1990. – vol. 4, N 6. – P. 1577–1590

Yurchenko P.D., Wadsworth W.G. Assembly and tissue functions of early embryonic laminins and netrins. // Curr.Opin.Cell Biol. – 2004. – vol. 16, N 5. – P. 572–579.

Zaidel-Bar R., Cohen M., Addadi L., Geiger B. Hierarchical assembly of cell-matrix adhesion complexes. // Biochem.Soc.Trans. – 2004. – vol. 32, N 3. – P. 416–420.

Zaidi M., Moonga B.S., Huang C.L. Calcium sensing and cell signaling processes in the local regulation of osteoclastic bone resorption. // Biol. Rev.Camb.Philos.Soc. – 2004. – vol. 79, N 1. – P. 79–100.

Zaman G., Jessop H.L., Muzylak M. et al. Osteocytes use estrogren receptor α to respond to strain but their ERα content is regulated by estrogen. // J.Bone Miner.Res. – 2006. – vol. 21, N 8. – P. 1297–1306.

Zambotti A., Makhluf H., Shen J., Ducy F. Characterization of an osteoblast-specific enhancer element in the CBFA1 gene. // J.Biol.Chem. – 2002. – vol. 277, N 44. – P. 41497–41506.

Zamir E., Geiger B. Molecular complexity and dynamics of cell-matrix adhesions. // J.Cell Sci. – 2001. – vol. 114. – P. 3583–3590.

Zanotti S., Smerdel-Ramoya A., Stadmeyer L. et al. Notch inhibits osteoblast differentiation and causes osteopenia. // Endocrinology. – 2008. – vol. 149, N 8. – P. 3890–3899.

Zappone B., Greene G.W., Oroudjev C. et al. Molecular aspects of boundary lubrication by human lubricin: effect of disulfide bonds and enzymatic digesion. // Langmuire. – 2008. – vol. 24, N 4. – P. 1495–1508.

Zaucke F., Dinser R., Maurer P., Paulsson M. Cartilage oligomeric matrix protein (COMP) and collagen IX are sensitive markers for the differentiation state of articular primary chondrocytes. // Biochem.J. – 2001. – vol. 358, N 1. – P. 17–24.

Zavadil J., Böttinger E.P. TGF-β and epithelial-to-mesenchymal transitions. // Oncogene. – 2005. – vol. 24. – P. 5764–5774.

Zavarzin A.A. and A.V. Rumyantsev. A course of histology. [in Russian] Moscow: Medgiz, 1946. 723 pages.

Zayzafoon A. Calcium/calmodulin signaling controls osteoblast growth and differentiation. // J.Cell.Biochem. – 2005. – vol. 97. – P. 56–70.

Zeisberg M., Yang C., Martino M. et al. Fibroblasts derive from hepatocytes in liver fibrosis via epithelial to mesenchymal transition. // J.Biol.Chem. – 2007. – vol. 282, N 32. – P. 23337–23347.

Zeng L., Kempf H., Murtaugh C.L. et al. Shh establishes an Nkx2/Sox9 autoregulatory loop that is maintained by BMP signals to induce somatic chondrogenesis // Genes Dev. – 2002. – vol. 16. – P. 1990–2005.

Zeveke A.V., Plohov J. R. A., Gushina Yu., Ashutov A. N. The investigation of water regime influence on the collagen structure by AFM. // Pys. Low-Dim. Struct. – 2004. – N ½. – P. 71–75.

Zhang C., Cho K., Huang Y. et al. Inhibition of Wnt signaling by the osteoblast-specific transcription factor Osterix. // Proc.Natl. Acad. Sci USA. – 2008. – vol. 105, N 19. – P. 5936–5941.

Zhang G., Young B.B., Birk D.E. Differential expression of type XII collagen in developing chicken metatarsal tendons. // J.Anat. – 2003. – vol. 202. – P. 411–420.

Zhang H., Marshall K.W., Tang H. et al. Profiling genes expressed in human fetal cartilage using 13,356 expressed sequence tags. // Osteoarthritis Cartilage. – 2003. – vol. 11, N 5. – P. 1309–1319.

Zhang L., McKenna M.A., Said-Al-Naief N. et al. Osteoclastogenesis: the role of calcium and calmodulin. // Crit.Rev.Eukaryot.Gene Expr. – 2005. – vol. 15, N 1. – P. 1–13.

Zhang S., Xiao Z., Luo J. rt al. Dose-dependent effects of Runx2 on bone development. // J.Bone Miner.Res. – 2009. – Epub. May 6.

Zhang Y., Hassan M.Q., Li Z.Y. et al. Intricate gene regulatory networks of helix-loop-helix (HLH) proteins support regulation of bone-tissue related genes during osteoblast differentiation. // J.Cell.Biochem. – 2008. – vol. 105, N 2. – P. 487–496.

Zhang Y., Hassan M.Q., Xie R.L. et al. Co-stimulation of the the the bone-related Runx2 P1 promoter in mesenchymal by SP1 and ETS transcription factors at polymorphic purine-rich DNA sequences (Y-repeats). // J.Biol.Chem. – 2009. – vol. 284, N 5. – P. 3125–3135.

Zhang Z., Fan J., Becker K.G. et al. Comparison of gene expression profile berween human chondrons and chondrocytes: a cDNA microarray study. // Osteoarthritis Cartilage. – 2006. – vol.14, N 5. – P.449–459.

Zhao G.Q. Consequences of knocking out BMP signaling in the mouse. // Genesis. – 2003. – vol. 35, N 11.– P. 143–156.

Zhao L., Gregoire F., Sul H.S. Transient induction of ENC-1, a Kelch-related actin-binding protein, is required for adipocyte differentiation. // J.Biol.Chem. – 2000. – vol. 275, N 22. – P. 16845–16850.

Zhao W., Byrne M.H., Wang Y., Krane S.M. Osteocyte and osteoblast apoptosis and excessive bone deposition accompany failure of collagenase cleavage of collagen. // J.Clin.Invest. – 2000. – vol.106, N 8. – P. 941–949.

Zheng Q., Itokawa T., Sridhar S. Effects of glucose-dependent insulinotropic peptide on osteoclast function. // Am.J.Physiol. Endocrinol. Metab. – 2007. – vol. 292. – P.E543–E548.

Zheng Q., Zhou G., Morello R. et al. Type X collagen gene regulation by Runx2 contributes directly to its hypertrophic chondrocyte-specific expression in vivo. // J.Cell Biol. – 2003. – vol/162, N 5. – P. 833–842.

Zherebtsov L.D. Age-related changes of facial skin elastic structures. [in Russian] // Pathology Archives, 1960, no. 7. P. 45–51.

Zhou H., Mak W., Zheng Y. et al. Osteoblast directly control lineage commitment of mesenchymal progenitor cells through Wnt signaling. // J.Biol.Chem. – 2008. – vol. 283, N 4. – P. 1936–1945.

Zhu A.J., Scott M.P. Incredible journey: how do developmental signals travel through tissue?// Genes Dev. – 2004. – vol. 18. – P. 2985–2997.

Zhu E., Demay M.B., Gori F. Wdr5 is essential for osteoblast differentiation. // J.Biol.Chem. – 2008. – vol. 283, N 12. – P. 7361–7367.

Zhu S., Barbe M.F., Liu C. et al. Periostin-like factor in osteogenesis. // J.Cell.Physiol. – 2009. – vol. 218, N 3. – P. 584–592.

Zhu Y., Oganesian A., Keene D.R., Sandell L.J. Type IIA procollagen containing the cystein-rich amino propeptide is deposited is deposited in the extracellular matrix of prechondrogenic tissue and binds to TGFβ1 and BMP-2. // J.Cell.Biol. – 1999. – vol. 144, N 5. – P. 1069–1080.

Zien A., Gebhard P.M., Fundel K., Aigner T. Phenotyping of chondrocytes in vivo and in vitro using cDNA array technology. // Clin.Orthop.Rel.Res. – 2007. – N 460. – P. 226–233.

Zimmerman D., Jin F., Leboy P. et al. Impaired bone formation in transgenic mice resulting from altered integrin function in osteoblasts. // Dev.Biol. – 2000. – vol. 220. – P. 2–15.

Zimmermann P., David G. The syndecans, tuners of transmembrane signaling. // FASEB J. – 1999. – vol. 13, Suppl. – P. S91–S100.

Ziros P.G., Rojas Gil A.-P., Georgakopoulos T. et al. The bone-specific transcriptional regulator Cbfa1 is a target of mechanical signal in osteoblastic cells. // J.Biol.Chem. – 2002. – vol. 277, N 26. – P. 23934–23941.

Zuscik M.J., Hilton M.J., Zhang X. et al. Regulation of chondrogenesis and chondrocyte differentiation by stress. // J.Clin.Invest. – 2008. – vol. 118, N 2. – P. 429–438.

Zweers M.C., Vlijmen-Williams I.M.van, Kuppevelt T.H. et al. Deficiency of tenascin-X causes abnormalities in dermal elastic fiber morphology. // J.Invest.Dermatol. – 2004. – vol. 122, N 4. – P. 885–891.

Zwijsen A., Verschueren K., Huylebroeck D. New intracellular components of bone morphogenetic protein/Smad signaling cascades. // FEBS Lett. – 2003. – vol. 546, N 1. – P. 133–139.

LIST OF ABBREVATIONS

A

11-βHSD – 11-β-hydroxysteroid dehydrogenase

5-HT – 5-hydroxytriptamine

A118 – a zinc finger protein transcription factor (syn. – Zfp34p)

Aa – amino acids

AA – amino acids

ABHD5 – an adipocyte lipase

Acrp30 – adiponectin (syn. – AdipoQ, agM1, GB-28)

ActR – activin and BMP receptors

ACVR1, ACVR2 – activin receptors

ADAM – a disintegrin and matrix metalloprotease (syn. – MDC0)

ADAM – a disintegrin and metalloproteinase domain-containing protein

ADAMTS – a disintegrin and matrix metalloprotease with thrombospondin motif

ADD – addiction/dependence domain

AdipoQ – see: Acrp30

AdipoR – adiponectin receptor

ADP – adenosine diphosphate

Adrb2 – beta-2 adrenergic receptor encoding gene

ADRP – adipose differentiation-related protein

Ae2 – anion exchanger Cl/HCO3

aFABP – FABP (see:) encoding human gene

AGE – advanced glycation endproducts

AGM1 – see: Acrp30

AIF – apoptosis-inducing factor 1, mitochondrial

AJ – adherens junctions

Akp2 – tissue-nonspecific alkaline phosphatase encoding gene (syn. Alpl)

ALCAM – activated leucocyte cell adhesion molecule

Aldh1a2 – enzyme retinal dehydrogenase (see: Raldh2) encoding gene

ALK – a TGF-β receptor –bound kinase

Alx – a family of homeodomain proteins

AMP – adenosine monophosphate

Ang-1 – angiopoietin-1

ANK –

Anxa-1 – annexin A1 encoding gene

AP-1 – activator protein-1, a family of transcription factors

aP2 – see: FABP (syn.- FABP4)

Apaf-1 – apoptotic protease activating factor 1

Ar – amino acid residues

AR – androgen receptor

ARG2 – enzyme arginase II coding human gene

ASARM – see: MEPE

ATDC5 – cultivated line of chondrogenic cells

ATF4 – activating transcription factor 4

ATGL – desnutrin encoding human gene

ATGL – desnutrin, an adiponutrin family adipocyte lipase

ATP – adenosine triphosphate

Axin2 – beta-catenin stability and Wnt signaling regulating protein Axin-2 encoding gene

B

BAD – Bcl2 antagonist of cell death, proapoptotic factor

BAG-75 – bone acidic glycoprotein-75

Bapx – a family of homeotic genes (syn. – Nkx)

Barx – an ANTP class family of homeotic genes

BAT – brown adipose tissue

Bax – a proapoptotic factor

Bax – aproapoptotic transcription factor

Bax – Bax (see) encoding gene

Bcl2 – an antiapoptotic factor

BGP – bone gla protein (syn. Osteocalcin)

BH3 – a domain of some proapoptotic proteins

bHLH – basic helix-loop-helix, protein molecular conformation structural motif rich in basic amino acid residues

Bid – proapoptotic factor

BIG3 – see: Wdr5

BM-40 – see: SPARC

BM-4o – see; SPARC

BMD – bone mineral density

BMF – biomineralization foci

BMP – bone morphogenetic proteins

BMPR – bone morphogenetic protein receptors

BMU – bone metaboli/multicellular unit

BNP – B-type natriuretic peptide

BO – bone as an organ

BP120, BP-230 – hemidesmosome proteins

BRAL1 – a hyaluronan receptor

BRC – bone remodeling compartment – see: BMU

BSP-I, BSP-II – bone sialoproteins

BTEB – transcription-activating factor, a zink finger protein, Krueppel-like subfamily member (syn. – KLF)

BUB1 – serin/threonin protein kinase, a cell cycle-activating enzyme

bZIP basic leucine zipper, structural domain of many transcription factors

C

C/EBPs – CCAAT/enhancer-binding proteins (see: CAAT)

C2C12 – cultivated cell line differentiating in osteoblasts

C4st1 – chondroitin sulfotransferase 1 encoding gene

CAAT – CAAT DNA nucleotide sequence-binding transcription factors (syn. – C/EBP)

CACP – campodactily – arthropathy – coxa vara – pericarditis

CAD – caspase –activated deoxyribonuclease (syn. – DFF40)

CAM – cell adhesion molecules

cAML – cyclic adenosine monophosphate

CART – cocaine and amphetamine regulated transcript

CART1 – cartilage homeotic protein (syn. – TRAF4)

CaSR – calcium sensing receptor (syn. – CaR)

CB2 – endogenous cannabioids receptor 2 (syn. – CNR2)

cbEGF – epidermal growth factor calcium-binding motif

CBF – an activating transcription factor

Cbfa1 – core binding factor alpha 1 (syn. Runx2, Oncogene AM, OSF2)

Cbfb – core binding factor beta

CBP – a transcription coactivator

CC – coiled coil, a secondary protein molecular structure motif

CCL – chemokins (chemotactic cytokines)

CCN2 – see: CTGF

CCN3/NOV – protein NOV homolog, nephrablostoma overexpressed protein, syn. – IGFBP9

CD – cell surface antigens (centres, clusters of differentiation)

CD44 – hyaluronan transmembrane receptor

CDC – cell division cycle proteins

CDMP – cartilage-derived morphogenetic proteins

cDNA – complementary deoxyribonucleic acid

CD-RAP – cartilage-derived retinoic acid sensitive protein

Cdx – caudal typr homeobox a family of homeotic genes

CDX2 – caudal type homeobox protein 2, a transcription factor

CEP68 – 68Da chondrocyte expresses protein

Cfkh-1 – condensate cells proliferation stimulating
    transcription factor

c-Fms – macrophage colony stimulating factor 1 receptor,
    syn. – M-CSFR, CD115

c-Fos – transcription factor, cellular protooncogene,
    a member of the AP-1 family (see)

CFU – colony forming unit – granulocyte/monocyte

cGKII – cGMP dependent type II protein kinase

cGMP – cyclic guanosine monophosphate

Chfz – transmembrane receptor proteins encoded
    by Fzd family genes (see)

CHOP – C/EBP-homologous protein

CHPPR – chondrocyte protein with a polyproline region
    (syn. – MTFR1)

CIC-7 – a chloride transporting ion exchanger

CILP – cartilage intermediate layer protein

c-Jun – transcription factor, cellular protooncogene,
    a member of the AP-1 family (see)

Ck1α – casein kinase 1α

c-Krox – activating transcription-factor, a zinc finger protein

CLO – chondrocyte-like osteoblast

CLP – cartilage link protein

CLR – a calcitonin receptor

CMP – cartilage matrix protein (syn. – matrilin-1)

c-Myc – cellular protooncogene, transcription factor

c-Myc – protooncogene-related multifunctional
    transcription factor

CNP – C-type natriuretic peptide

Col – collagen encoding animal genes

COL – collagen encoding human genes

COL – collagen macromolecules three-helical
    ("collagenous") domains

COMP – cartilage oligomeric matrix protein

COPI, COPII – coat proteins

CP191A – cytochrome P450 19A1

cPLA2 – cytosoliv phospholipase A2

CPPD – crystalline calcium pyrophosphate dehydrate

CPTHR – PTH carboxyterminal fragment specific receptor

CPZ – carboxypeptidase Z

CRE – cAMP response element of DNA

CREB – cAMP response elemen binding, a transcription factor

CRLR – calcitonin receptor-like receptor

CRTAC1 – cartilage acidic protein 1

Crtl1 – cartilage link protein encoding gene

CS – chondroitin sulfate

Csf – colony stimulating factor

CSPG1 – chondroitin sulfate proteoglycan 1, aggrecan

CSPG2 – chondroitin sulfate proteoglycan 2, versican, fibroblast
    large proteoglycan (syn. – PG-M)

CSPG4 – chondroitin sulfate proteoglycan 4,
    melanoma chondroitin sulfate proteoglycan

CT – connective tissue

CT-1 – cardiotrophin-1

CTGF – connective tissue growth factor (syn. – CCN2, HCSP24)

CTGF – connective tissue growth factor (syn.: CCN2)

CTR – calcitonin receptor

Ctr – copper transport protein 1

CUGBP1 – adipogenesis inhibiting protein

CYP19 – cytochrome P450 encoding human gene

CYP26 – cytochrome P450 26A1

CYP27B1 – cytochrom P450 subfamily XXVIIB polypeptide 1

CYR61 – a CCN family glycoprotein

CYTL1 – cytokine-like protein 1

D

DAF – decay accelerating factor, complement system protein

Dan – TGF-β superfamily signal molecules inhibitors

DANCE – fibulin-5 (syn. – EVEC)

DAP3 – death-associated protein 3 (syn. – MRP-S29)

DAPK3 – death-associated protein kinase (syn. – ZIP-kinase)

DAX1 – a nuclear receptor of unknown ligands ("orfan")

DAXX – death associated proteins

DBM – demineralized bone matrix

DCD-1 – dermicidin-1

DC-STAMP – dendritic cell specific transmembrane protein

DDR1, DDR2 – discoidin domain receptors

DDR2 – discoidin domain-containing receptor 2 (syn. – CD176b)

DEJ – dermal-epidermal junction

Del1 – developmentally regulated endothelial cell locus protein 1

DFF40 – see: CAD

DFF45 – DNA fragmentataion factor 45 kDa subunit alpha

DGO – a cytoplasmic protein

Dhh – a Hh family morphogene

Disp – a transmembrane protein, peptide transporter

Dkk – "Dickkopf", Lrp coreceptors blocker

DKK1 – Dickkopf-related protein 1, a secreted protein

Dll – Delta-like transmembrane proteins, Notch family
    ligands receptors

Dlp – a glypican, promoter of Wnt ahd Hh morphogens endocytosis

Dlx – family of homeotic proteins

DLX5 – a homeobox protein, transcription factor

DMP1 – dentin matrix protein 1

DNA – deoxyribonucleic acid

DPPA4 – protein expressed in undifferentiated embryonal
    stem cells

DR – death receptors

DRP-1 – density-regulated protein 1 (syn. – SMAP3)

DS – dermatan sulfate

DSH – a cytoplasmic protein

DS-PGI – dermatan sulfate proteoglycan I, biglycan

DS-PGII – dermatan sulfate proteoglycan II, decorin

DS-PGIII – dermatan sulfate proteoglycan III, epiphycan
    (syn. – PG-Lb)

Dvl – "disheveled", cytoplasmic proteins associated
    with Fzd receptors (see.)

E

EBAP – see: LEFTA)

E-box – DNA enhancer boxes

ED-A – a fibronectin isoform specific domain

EDNRA – endthelin 1 receptor (syn. – ETRA)

EF hand – a helix-loop-helix structural domain found in a large
    family of calcium-binding proteins

EFNB – ephrin B1 (syn. – LERK-2)

EGF – epidermal growth factor

EGF – epithelial growth factor

EGFR – epidermal growth factor receptor
Egr-1 – early growth response factor 1 (syn. NaB-2, Krox-24)
Eif2a3 – PERK (see.) encoding gene
EM – extracellular matrix
EMT – epithelial-mesenchymal transition
Emu – emilins (elastinmicrofibril interfacers)-containg
    glycoproteins
EMX – a homeotic protein
En1 – homeobox protein engrailed-1
ENC-1 – actin-bound phosphoprotein
EOMES – Eomesodemis homolog (syn. – TBR), a nuclear protein
EPAS-1 – see: HIF-2α
EPR – subtype EP prostaglandin receptors
EPYC – epyphycan encodinf human gene
ER – estrogen receptors
ErbB2 – receptor tyrosine protein kinase (syn. – EGFR, CD340)
Erg – Ers-related gene
ERK – extracellular signal-regulated protein kinases
ERM – protein family ezrin – radixin – moesin
ERRα – estrogen receptor-related receptor α (syn. – ERR1)
ESI – elastase-specific inhibitor (syn. – elafin, SKALP)
ESP1 – amino terminal enhancer of split, a nuclear protein
    (syn. – Grg5)
ETS – "E-twenty six", a transcription factor family
Eve – Golgi cisternae transmembrane protein
EVEC – see: DANCE
EYA – Eyes absent homolog, cytoplasm abd nucleus protein

F

FA – fatty acids
FA – focal adhesions (syn. – FC)
FABP – fatty acids-binding proteins
FACIT – fibril-associated collagens with interrupted triple helices
FACIT – fibril-associated collagens with interrupted triple helix
FAK – focal adhesion kinase (syn. – PTK2)
FAK – focal adhesion protein kinases
FAPα – fibroblast activation protein alpha
FAS – fatty acid synthase
FAS – TNF receptor superfamily member 6 (syn. – FASL, CD95)
FBN – fibrillins
FBN1 – fibrillin 1 encoding human gene
FBN1, FBN2, FBN3 – fibrillins
FBN1, FBN2, FBN3 – fibrillins encoding human genes
Fbn2 – fibrillin 2 encoding gene
FBXW4 – F-box WD repeat-containing protein 4
FC – focal contacts (syn. – FA, focal adhesions)
FCD – fixed charge density
Fck – tyrosine protein kinases family Src subfamily
    tyrosine protein kinase
FGF – fibroblast growth factors
FGFR – fibroblast growth factor receptors
FHL2 – "four and a half LIM domains protein 2",
    a transcription factor
FIAF – fasting-induced adiposity factor
FIAT – factor inhibiting ATF4-mediated transcription
FIT1, FIT2 – fat-inducing transcripts
FN – fibronectin
FN-f 45 – fibronectin macromolecule 45 kDa fragment
FOSL1 – see: FRA-1
Fox – RNA-binding protein family

Foxc – a transcription factor
Foxc, Foxd3 – Forkhead box proteins (syn. FKHL),
    nuclrat proteins proteins
FOXF1 – a human gene
FRA-1 – Fos-related antigen 1, a nuclear protein (syn. – FOSL1)
Fra-2 – Fos-related antigen 2, a transcription factor (syn. JunD)
FRS2 – fibroblast growth factor receptor substrate 2 (syn. – SNT)
Frzb1 – frizzled-related protein 1 (syn. – sFRP3)
FSP1 – fibroblast specific protein 1 (syn. – S100A4)
FX – focal complexes
FZ – cell-membrane associated protein
Fzd – "frizzled", Wnt receptor
Fzd – Fzd receptor encoding gene

G

G – guanine nucleotide binding proteins,
    latent guanosine triphosphatase (see: GTPases)
G1 – growth phase of the cell sycle
GABA – γ-aminobutyric acid
GADD153 – growth arrest and DNA damage-inducible protein
GAS6 – growth arrest specific protein 6
GATA1, GATA2 – GATA nucleotide sequence-binding
    multifunctional zinc finger transcription factors
Gbx2 – multifunctional transcription factor, a homeobox protein
G-CSF – granulocyte colony-stimulating factor
GDF – growth and differentiation factors (see: CDMP)
GER, GFOGER – collagens triple helical domains
    adhesive amino acid sequences
GH – growth hormone
GHBP – growth hormone binding protein
GHR – growth hormone receptor
GHS – growth hormone secretagogue
GIP – gastric inhibitory polypeptide
GIPS – GIP receptor
GJ – gap junctions
GLAST glutamate aspartate transporter
Gli – transcription factors
GLUT4 – glucose transmembrane transporter
    encoding human gene
GM-CSF – granulocyte macrophage colony-stimulating factor
GM-CSF – granulocyte monocyte colony stimulating factor
GM-CSFR – granulocyte macrophage colony-stimulating
    factor receptor
Gp130 – glycoprotein 130,, IL-6 coreceptor
GPCR – G protein-coupled seven pass transmembrane receptors
GR – glycocorticoid receptor
Grb2 – growth factor receptor-bound protein 2, an adapter protein
GRB7 – growth factor receptor-bound protein 7
Grg5 – amino terminal enhancer of split 1,
    a nuclear phosphoprotein
GRN – gene regulatory network
Gsk3 – glycogen synthase kinase 3
GTP – guanosine triphosphate
GTPase – guanosine triphosphatase
Gulo – gulonolactone oxidase encoding gene
GULO – gulonolactone oxidase encoding human gene

H

H3 – histone H3

H3K4 – a histone

HABP – hyaluronic acid binding proteins

HAPLN – hyaluronanand proteoglycan link protein

Has – hyaluronan synthase encoding animal gene

HAS – hyaluronan synthases

hBD – human beta-defensins

HB-GAM – heparin-binding growth-associated molecule
    (syn. – OSF1)

Hck – Src subfamily tyrosine protein kinase

HCS24 – hypertrophic chondrocyte specific protein 24
    (syn. – CCN2, IGFBP8)

HDAC1 – histone deacetylase 1

H-E – hematoxylin and eosin stain

Hes – Hess factors encoding genes

hESC – human embryonic stem cells

HESS – transcription factor family

HEY-1 – a transcription factor (syn. – HESR1, CHF2, Herp2)

HGF – hepatocyte growth factor

Hh – Hedgehog morphogene family

HHG – see: Ihh

HIF-1α – HIF-1α encoding human gene

HIF-1α – hypoxia-induced factor 1α

HIF-2α – hypoxia-induced factor 2α (syn. – EPAS-1)

HMG – high mobility group

HMGB1 – high mobility group protein box 1

HOX – homeobox

HOXA5 – a homeobox protein

HP – hydroxylysylpyridinolin

HRE – hypoxia response element, a DNA fragment

HSC – hemopoietic stem cell

HSL – hormone-sensitive lipase

Hsp – heat shock proteins

HSP47 – heat shock protein 47 (syn. – Serpin H1, CBP1)

Htr12 – high temperature requirement protein 12

HU-K5 – adipocyte monoglycerol lipase (syn. – MGLL)

Hyal – hyaluronan

I

ICAM – IgCAM (see) family adhesive molecule

ICAM-1 – intercellular adhesion molecule 1 (syn. – CD54)

Id – inhibitor of DNA binding

ID2 – DNA-binding protein inhibitor 2, a nuclear protein

IF1, IF2 – transcription inhibition factors

IFN – interferons

IFNR – interferon receptors

Ig – immunoglobulins

IgCAM – immunoglobulin domain-containing cell adhesion mole-
    cules

IGD – interglobular domain

IGF – insulin-like growth factors

IGFBP – insulin-like growth factors binding proteins

IGFB – IGF-binding proteins

IGFR – IGF receptors

IGFR – insulin-like growth factor s receptors

IHABP – intracellular hyaluronan-binding proteins

Ihh – Indian hedhehog, Hh family morphogen (syn. – HHJ)

IKK – inhibitor of nuclear factor kappa B (syn. IKKB)

IL – interleukins

ILK -integrin-linked kinase

IP3 – inositol triphosphate

IR – insulin receptor

ITAM – immunoreceptor tyrosine-based activation motif

J

Jag1 – "jagged", Notch signal system ligand

JNK – c-Jun terminal kinases (syn – MAP)

JNK – c-Jun transcription factors-phosphorylating protein kinases

JunD – see: Fra2

K

KAT5 – histone acetyltransferase KAT5 (syn. – Tip60)

KGF – keratinocyte growth factor

KLF – Krueppel-like factors, zinc finger-containing
    transcription factors

Krox20 – a transcription factor (syn. – Egr2)

KS – keratin sulfate

L

LAP – TGF-β transcript latency peptide

LD – lipid droplets

LECT – leukocyte cell-derived chemotaxin, a glycoprotein
    secreted by embryonal stem cells

LEF1 – lymphoid enhancer binding factor 1 (syn. – TCF)

LEFTA – Left-right determination factor 2, a secreted protein
    (syn. – EBAP

LFA-3 – lymphocyte function-associated antigen 3

Lfng – glycosyl transferase encoding gene

LG4 – laminin macromolecule globular domain

LIF – leukemia inhibiting factor, a cytokine

LIM – protein macromolecules two "zinc finger" –
    containing domains

LIM – protein structural domains, composed of two zinc fingers,
    separated by a two-amino acid residue hydrophobic linker

LIMD – 3 LIM domains containing phosphoprotein

LIMK1 – LIM domain (see) kinase, a zinc finger protein

LIV1 – a zinc transporter protein (syn. – ZIP6, SLC39A6)

LLC – large latent complex

LM – light microscopy

LMP-1 – LIM mineralization protein-1

LOX – lysyl oxidase

LP – link protein

LP – lysylpyridinoline

LPS – lipoplysaccharides

LRP – leucine-rich repeats

Lrp – Lrp coreceptors encoding genes

LRP1 – low density lipoprotein receptor-related protein 1
    (syn. – CD91)

Lrp5, Lrp6 – receptors Dvl coreceptors (see: Dvl)

LRR – leucine-rich repeat

L-Sox5 – Sox family transcription factor Sox 5 long form

LTB – lymphotoxin beta (TNF superfamily member 3)

LTBP – latent TGF-beta binding proteins

LTBP-2 – fibrillin microfibrils-associated LTBP (see)

Lyn – Src family (see) tyrosine protein kinase

LYVE-1 – a hyaluronan receptor

M

MAGP – microfibril-associated glycoprotein

MAGP-1, MAGP-2 – microfibrillar glycoproteins

MAPK – mitogen-activated protein kinases

MARRS5 (1,25D# membrane associated rapid response steroid receptor (syn. – Erp57/GRp58/Erp60)

Matn1 – matrilin-1 encoding gene

MATN3 – matrilin-3 encoding human gene

MC – melanocortin

MC3T3-E1 – a cultivated osteoblast cell line

MC4r – melanocortin receptor

MCAM – melanoma cell adhesion molecule (syn. – MUC18, CD146), a glycoprotein, IgCAM (see) family adhesive molecule

M-CSF – macrophage colony-stimulating factor

MDC – see: ADAM

MEF2C – myocyte-specific enhacer factor 2C

MEK – mitogen activated kinases kinases

Meox – Mesenchyme homeobox genes

MEPE – matrix extracellular phosphoglycoprotein (syn. – OF45, see)

Mesp2 – mesoderm posterior protein 2

MET – mesenchymal-epithelial transition

Mfa-1 – a transcription factor

MFR – macrophage fusion receptor (syn. – Sirp-α1, p84, CD172a)

MG-53 – a cultivated osteoblast cell, line

MGLL – see: HU-K5

MGP – matrix Gla protein

MIP-1α – macrophage inflammatory protein 1α (syn. – C-C motif chemokine 3)

miRNA – micro ribonucleic acid

MITF – microphthalmia-associated transcription factor

Mkx – a homeotic gene (syn. – Mohawk)

MLDP – myocardial LD protein a perilipin, lipid droplet-associated protein (syn. – Plin5, Pat1, OXPAT)

MMP – matrix metalloproteases (syn. – MP, metalloproteinases, matrixins)

MMP2 – gelatinase A

Mn1 – possible tumor suppressor Mn1

mRNA – matrix ribonucleic acid

MSC – mesenchyme stem cells

MSF – megakaryocyte-stimulating factor (syn. – PTG4, SZP, ke, hbwby)

MSF – MSF encoding human gene

Msp – major sperm proteins

Msx – ANTP class homeotic proteins

Msx – Msx encoding genes

MT/MMP – membrane-type matrix metalloproteases

MT1-MMP – matrix metalloprotease (syn. – MMP14)

MTA3 – metastasis-associated protein 3, a nuclear protein

MTFR – see: CHPPR

MUC1 – mucin 1, cell surface associated (syn. – PEM), a keratinocyte marker

MV – matrix vesicles

Myf6 – myogenic factor 6 encoding gene

N

Nab-2 – see: Egr-1

NADPH – nicotinamide adenine dinucleotide phosphate

NANOG – homeobox protein, a transcription factor

NC – non-collagenous (non-triple helical) domains in collagenous proteins molecules

NC – non-collagenous (non-triple helical) domains in collagenous proteins molecules

N-CAM – neural cell adhesion molecules

NCID – Notch intracellular domain

Nck – a cytoplasmic adapter protein

N-CoR1 – nuclear receptors 1 coreceptor

ncRNA – non-coding RNA

NFAM – NFAT activation molecule

NFATc1 – activated T cell nuclear factor

NF-kB – nuclear factor –kappa B

NFkB – nuclear factor kappa B, complex of transcription factors

NIK – serine/threonine protein kinase (syn. MAP3K14)

NK – natural killer

NK1-R – substance P receptor

Nkx – ANTP family homeotic proteins (syn. –Bapx)

Nkx – Nkx proteins encoding genes

NLS – nuclear localization signal

NMP4 – nuclear matrix transcription phosphoprotein 4

NMTS – nuclear matrix targeting signal

NOS – nitric oxide synthase

NOV – CCN family glycoprotein

NPP1 – nucleotide pyrophosphate phosphodiesterase (syn. – PC-1)

NPR-C – natriuretic peptide receptor C

NTPPase – nucleoside tripyrophosphate hydrolase (syn. – CILP)

N-WASP – neural Wiskott-Aldrich syndrome protein (syn. – WASL) involved in transduction of signals from receptors to the actin cytoskeleton

O

OASIS – old astrocyte specifically induced substance

OB-R – leptin receptor

OCIF – osteoblast inhibitory factor – see: OPG

Oct-1 – octamer 5'-ATTTGCAT-3'-binding transcription factor 1

OCT4 – octamer-binding transcription factor 4 (syn. – POU5F1), critical factor in self-renewal of embryonal undifferentiated mesenchymal stem cells

ODF – osteoclast differentiation factor – see: RANKL

OF45 – osteoblast/osteocyte factor 45 (syn. – MEPE)

OPG – osteoprotogerin (syn. – OCIF)

OPGL – osteoprotegerin ligand (see: RANKL)

OPN – osteopontin

OPN – osteopontin encoding human gene

Opn – osteopontin encoding gene

ORP150 – 150 kDa oxygen-regulated protein

OSCAR – osteoclast –associated receptor

OSE – osteoclast specific element

OSF-1 – osteoblast-specific factor 1 (syn. – pleiotrophin, HB-GAM)

OSF-2 – osteoblast specific factor 2 (syn. – periostin)

Osterix – see: SP7

Ostn – osteocrin (syn. – musclin)

OSX – Osterix encoding human gene

OT – oxytocin

OXPAT – see: MLDP

Oxtr – oxytocin receptor

P

p202 – interferon inducible protein 292

p204 – interferon inducible protein 204

P3 – prolyl 3-hydroxylase, procollagen-proline 3-dioxygenase

p300 – histone acetyltransferase p300

p38 – MAPK protein kinase activating and Dlx5 inducing protein kinase

P4 – prolyl 4-hydroxylase, procollagen-proline 4-dioxygenase

p42 – see: p44

p44ERK – extracellular signal regulated kinase 1 (syn. – MAPK1, p42)

p53 – a cell cycle suppressor, upregulated modulator of apoptosis, pro-apoptotic tumor protein 53 encoding multifunctional animal gene

p53 – tumor protein 53, a cekk cycle suppressor

p65 – see RELA

PAK1 – p21 activated kinase 1

PAPS – 3'-phosphoadenosine-5'-phosphosulfate

PARP – proline and arginin-rich protein

PARP- 2 – poly(ADP-ribose) polymerase 2

PAT – a perilipin family (syn. – PLIN, PERI)

PAX – paired box, PRD class homeobox protein family

Pax – PAX proteins encoding genes

Pbx – homeotic genes family

PC – a thrombospondin macromolecule modulus

PC1 – see: NPP1

PCD – programmed cell death, apoptosis

PcG – Polycomb-group proteins

PCM – pericellular (territorial) matrix

PCP – planar cell polarity

PDBM – partly demineralized bone matrix

PDGF – platelet-derived growth factors

PDGFR – PDGF receptors

PDLIM7 – LMP-1 encoding human gene

PEDF – pigment epithelium-derived factor, stromal cell-derived factor 3, Serpin-f, Caspin

Pem – multifunctional transcription factor

PERK – eukaryotic translation initiator factor 2-α kinase 3

PG4 – PG4 encoding human gene (see: SZP)

PG4 – proteoglycan 4 (see: MSF)

PG-40 – biglycan (syn. – PG-S1)

PGBM – basement membrane-specific heparin sulfate proteoglycan 2, perlecan (syn. – PLC, HSPG)

PGC-1α – peroxisome proliferator-activated receptor gamma coactivator 1α

PGE – prostaglandins E

PGHS-2 – prostaglandin G/H synthase 2

PG-I – proteoglycan I, biglycan

PGI2 – prostaglandin 12

PG-II – proteoglycan II, decorin (syn. – PG-40)

PG-Lb – proteoglycan Lb, epiphycan,dermatan sulfate proteoglycan 3

PG-M – versican (syn. –VCAN, CSPG2)

PG-31 – see. PG-40

PG-S2 – decorin (syn. – PG I)

PHEX – phosphate regulating neutral endopeptidase

PHOSPHO1 – phosphoethanolamine/phospholine phosphatase

PI3K – 3-phosphoinositol kinase

PINCH – a focal contact protein

PIP – focal contact protein triple complex containing PINCH, ILK (see), parvin

Pitx – homeotic genes family

PK – prickle1, a nuclear receptor

PKA – CREB phosphorylatin protein kinase A

PKC – phospholipid-dependent protein kinase C

PKCδ – delta type protein kinase C

PLCγ – phospholipase C gamma-1

PLF – periostin-like factor

PlGF – placenta growth factor

PLINA – perilipin A encoding human gene

PLOD – protein lysyl hydroxylase, procollagen-lysine 5-dioxygenase

PN – periostin (see: OSF-2)

PN-1 – serine protease inhibitor

PNPLA1 – an adipocyte lipase

POU – POU domain-containing homeotic protein family

POU5F1 – Oct-4 (see) encoding human gene

PP – inorganic pyrophosphate

PP – pyrophosphate phosphatase

PP1, PP2A – collagen type I expression regulating phosphatases

PPAR – peroxisome proliferator-activated receptors, nuclear receptor group

PPARγ – peroxisome proliferator-activated receptor γ

PPI – peptidylprolyl isomerase

PPRC1 – peroxisome proliferator-activated receptor gamma coactivator-related protein 1, cold-induced nuclear protein

PPRE – DNA peroxysome proliferator responsive element

Pr22 – growth arrest specific protein homolog

pRB – retinoblastoma protein, a tumor suppressor protein

pRb – retinoblastoma-associated protein

PRE – nuclear chromatin structure modulating genome element

pref-1 – preadipocyte secreted factor

PRELP – proline/arginine-rich and leucine-rich repeat protein

PRELP – proline-arginine-rich end leucine-rich repeat protein, SLRP protein family (seeJ member

Prrx – class PRD homeotic

PSGL-1 – P-selectin glycoprotein ligand 1

PSM – presomite mesoderm

Ptc – "patched", Hh-morphogens binding 12-pass transmembrane receptor

PTH – parathyroid hormone

PTHR – PTH and PTHrP-binding receptor

PTHrP – parathyroid hormone-related protein

PTP – proteintyrosine phosphatase

PU.1 – PU-box-binding transcription factor

Pyk2 – proteintyrosine kinase 2

R

Rac – Rho (see:) family small guanosine triphosphatases subfamily

Raf – c-Raf, a serine/threonine protein kinase

RALDH – retinaldehyde dehydrogenaqse

RALDH2 – retinalaldehyde dehydrogenase

RAMP – receptor activity modifying protein

RANK – receptor activator of nuclear factor kappa-B (syn. ODFR, TNFR 11A, CD265

RANKL – receptor activator of nuclear factor kappa-B ligand (syn. – TRANCE, Tnsf1, ODF, OPGL, CB254)

Rap1 – Rab5 GDP/GTP exchange factor, an enzyme/nucleotide exchanger involved in integrin-cadherin interaction

RAR – retinoic acid nuclear receptors

Ras – Src family protein kinases, Ras/ERK/MAPK
    signaling pathway components
Ras – superfamily of proteins involved in intracellulsr signal
    transduction
RelA – RELA transforming factor (syn. – p65)
REX1 – a zinc finger nuclear protein (syn. – ZFP42)
RGD – "adhesive" tripeptide arginineglycineasparagine
RGD-CAP – RGD containing collagen-associated protein
    (see: β-ig-h3)
RGM – repulsive guidance molecules, BMPR coreceptors
RHAMM – hyaluronan-mediated motility receptor
    (syn. – HMMR, IHABP, CD165)
rhBMP – recombinant human bone morphogenetic protein
Rho – family of GTPases (see) involved in intracellular
    signal transduction
Rho – superfamily Ras small guanosin triphosphatases family
RNA – ribonucleic acid
Rnd1 – a small guanosin triphosphatase
ROLDH a retinoic acid dehydrogenase
ROS – reactive oxygen species
rRNA – ribosomal ribonucleic acid
RSK – ribosomal protein S6 kinase 2
RTEF-1 – transcriptional enhancer factor (syn. – TEAD-4, TEF-1))
Runx1 – Runt family transcription factor (see: Cbfβ
Runx2 – see: Cbfa1
RXR – a nuclear retinoid receptor
RXR – retinoid receptors
RyR – ryanodine receptors, a class of intracellular calcium
    transmembrane channels
RyR2 – ryanodine receptor 2

S

S100A4 – see: FSP1
S1P – sphingosine-1-phosphate
SAA – serum amyloid A protein
SALL4 – sal-like protein 4, a zinc finger transcription factor
SAPK – see: MAP
SAPK – serin/threonine protein kinases
SAPL – surface-active phospholipids
SC1 – SPARC-like protein (see: SPARC)
SCD1 – stearoyl CoA desaturase-1 (an enzyme involved in fatty
    acid metabolism) encoding human gene
SCF – SCF complex (Skp-Cullin-F-box), a multiprotein ligase
    complex catalyzing the ubiquitination of proteins destined
    for proteasome degradation
SCFR – SCF receptor
SCTMC – stem connective tissue multipotency cell
Scx – Scleraxis encoding gene
SDF-1 – stromal cell-derived factor 1 (syn. – STRO-1)
SEM – scanning electron microscopy
SER – smooth endoplasmic reticulum
SF – synovial fibroblast, B type synoviocyte
sFRP1 – secreted frizzled-related protein 1
S-Gal – a transmembrane receptor interacting with elastin
    and laminins
SGLT – sodium ions and glucose transmembrane transporter
Shh – Sonic hedgehog, Hh family morphogen
Shox2 – short stature homeobox protein 2 (syn. – SHOT, Ogl2x)
Shox2 – Shox2 encoding gene
SHP-1 – a tyrosineprotein phosphatase

SIBLING – small integrin-binding ligand N-linked glycoproteins
SIP1 – survival of motor neuron protein-interacting protein 1,
    a member of intracellular signal pathways
Sir2 – a sirtuin (see: Sirt1) encoding gene
SIRP – signal regulating proteins
SirT1 – NAD-dependent deacetylase Sirtuin 1
SIRT1 – sirtuin1, a NAD-dependent protein deacetylase,
    involved in longevity regulation
Site-1 – serine-type endopeptidase 1 (syn. – S1P, Mbtps1)
Ski – Ski oncogene, BMP intracellulat antagonist
SLC – small latent complex
SLC – soluble carrier family members
SLC25A7 – solute carrier family 25 member 7, mitochondrial
    brown fat uncoupling protein (syn. – UCP1)
Slfn2 – Schlafen2, transcription factor
SLRP – small leucine-rich proteoglycans
SLS – segment long spacing, collagen crystallites
Smac – second mitochondria-derive activator of caspase
SMAD – TGF-β intracellular signal pathway component
SMADs – intracellular proteins that transducer
    extracellular TGF-β signals to the nucleus
SMAF-1 – small adipocyte factor 1, adipogenin
SMA-α – actin, alpha skeletal muscle
Smo – "smoothened", Hh and Wnt morphogens 7-pass
    transmembrane receptor
SMOC-1, SMOC-2 – SPARC-related modular calcium-binding
    proteins (see: SPARC)
Snail – a transcription factor
SOCS – suppressors of cytokine signaling
SOST – sclerostin encoding human gene
SOX2 – transcription factor essential to maintain self-renewal
    of ubdifferentiated embryonic stem cells
    (syn. – SRY[sex determining region Y]-box 2)
Sox4 – Sox family activating transcriptrion factor
Sox6 – Sox family transcription factor
Sox9 – Sox family transcription factor, main regulator
    of chondroblast differentiation
SP – SP neuropeptides
Sp – specificity proteins
SP1 – a transcription factor
Sp1, Sp2 – "specificity proteins", activating transcription factors
    involved in gene expression in early embryonic development
Sp3 – specificity protein Sp3
Sp7 – specicificity protein Sp7, osteoblast differentiation
    important regulator (syn. – Osterix)
SPARC – secreted protein acidic and rich in cystein
    (syn. – osteonectin, BM-40)
SPP – see: BSP-1
Spp-24 – secreted phosphoprotein 24, endopeptidases inhibitor
sRANKL – RANKL (seeJ soluble isoform
Src – tyrosineprotein kinases family
SRC-1 – a nuclear protein, steroid receptor coactivator 1
SSEA – cell membrane stage-specific embryonic glycolipid
    external antigens
STAT – signal transducers and activators of transcription,
    components of intracellular signal pathways
STC1 – stanniocalcin-1
Stem – stem cell markers
STRO-1 – see: SDF-1
SVCT – transmembrane sodium vitamin C and glucose
    cotransporters

SVCT2 – sodium vitamin C cotransporter 2
Syk – spleen tyrosine kinase
SZP – superficial zone protein

T

T1DM – type 1 diabetes mellitus
T2DM – type 2 diabetes mellitus
T3 – triiodothyronine
T4 – thyroxine
TACC3 – transforming acidic coiled coil containing protein 3, cytoplasmic protein (syn. – ERIC-1)
TAG – triacylglycerols (syn. – TG, triglycerides)
TAK1 – transforming growth factor-β-activated kinase (syn. – MAP3K7)
Tale – homeotic protein (syn. – Iro)
TASR – arginine and serine-rich splicing factor (syn. – SFR13A, FUSIP1)
TAZ – tafazzin, component of the Hippo signaling pathway, transcription modulator and coactivator that controls tissue growth (syn. – EFE2, G4.5)
TAZ – translin-associated zinc finger protein (syn. – RP58)
TBX – nuclear proteins, transcription factors containing a DNA-binding domain, the T-box
TCF – see: LEF1
Tcf7 – T-cell factor 7 (syn. – LAPIS, OP18
Tdgf1 – teratocarcinoma-derived growth factor 1 (syn. – Cripto)
TDGF1 – teratocarcinoma-derived growth factor 1, secreted by embryonal stem cells (syn. – Cripto-1)
TEAD-4 – see: RTEF-1
TG – see: TAG
TG – transglutaminases
Tgfbr – transforming growth factor-beta receptors
TGF-β – transforming growth factor -beta superfamily
TGFβR – TGF-β receptors
THY1 – thymocyte cell surface antigen 1 (syn. – CD90), a specific marker of mesenchyme stem cells
TIF-2 – eukaryotic translation initiation factor 2, a nuclear protein
TIMP – tissue inhibitors of matrix metalloproteases
TIP47 – a perilipin
Tip60 – see: KAT5
TIS21 – antiproliferative transcription factor (syn. – BIG2)
TJ – tight junctions
TLE – transducer-like enhancer protein
TM – transmission electron microscopy
TNAP – tissue nonspecific alkaline phosphatase
TNF – tumor necrosis factors
TNFR – TNF receptor superfamily
TNFR – TNF (see) receptors
Tnfsf1 – see: RANKL
TNMD – tenomodulin encoding gene
Tob – antiproliferative proteins
Tp53 – p53 (see:) encoding gene
TPR – tandem proteoglycan repeat unit
TR – thyroid hormone receptor
TRA-1 – stem cell surface keratin sulfate-containing antigen
TRACP5 – tartrate-resistant acid phosphatase 5 (syn. – TRAP)
TRAF – TNF receptor-associated factor, adapter protein
TRAIL – TNF-related apoptosis-inducing ligand (syn. – TNF SF10, APO-21)
TRANCE – TNF-related activation-induced cytokine

(syn. – TNF11, CD254) (see: RANKL)
TRAP – see: TRACP
TRCP – cell membrane transient receptor potential calcium ion channel
TRE – DNA thyroid-reactive element
TRE – thyroid hormone response element
Trps1 – tricho-rhino-phalangeal syndrome type 1 protein
TRPV4 – transient receptor potential cation channel subfamily V member 4
TRSP1 – trichorhinophalangeal syndrome 1, zinc finger transcription factor encoding human gene
TRXG – Trithorax proteins
TSG-6 – TNF-stimulated gene 6 protein (syn. – TNAFIP6)
TSH – thyroid-stimulating hormone, thyrotropin
TSHR – TSH-receptor
TSP – thrombospondins
TSR – thrombospondin type I repeat, a thrombospondin macromolecule modulus
Twist – twist-related proteins, transcription factors, cell differentiation negative regulators
TWSG1 – twisted gastrulation homolog 1, a BMP antagonist
TβR – TGF-β receptors

U

Ucma – unique cartilage matrix-associated protein (syn. – Gla-rich protein)
UCP1 – see: SLC25A7
UDP – uridine diphosphate
UDPGD – uridine diphosphate glucose dehydrogenase
Uncx – homeotic genes family
uPA – urokinase-type plasminogen activator
uPAR – uPA receptor
UPO – UPO receptors (syn. – Axl-oncogenes)
UTF1 – undifferentiated embryonic cell transcription factor 1, a nuclear multifunctional phosphoprotein

V

VAMP1 – vesicle-associated membrane protein 1
V-ATPase – vacuolar-type adenosine triphosphatase
VAV3 – guanine nucleotide exchange factor (GEF), member of the family
VCAM – vascular adhesion cell molecule, IgCAM (see) family adhesive molecule
VCAM-1 – vascular adhesion protein 1 (syn. – CD106)
VCAN – versican encoding human gene
VDR -vitamin D receptor
VDRP – vitamin D-binding protein
VEGF – vascular endothelial growth factor
VEGFR – vascular endothelial growth factor receptor
VGVAPG – elastin polypeptide chain characteristic hexapeptide repeat
VHL – Von Hippel-Lindau disease tumor suppressor (syn. – pVHL, protein G7)
VIP – vasoactive intestinal peptides
Vsp – Eve transporter-regulating protein family
vWA – von Willebrand factor A domain

W

WARP – von Willebrand factor A domain-related protein

WAT – white adipose tissue

WD repeat – protein molecule domain beginning
   by glycine-histidine residues and ending by triptophan
   and aspartic acid residues

Wdr5 – WD repeat-containing protein 5
   (syn. – BMP-2-induced 3 kb gene protein

Wif-1 – Wnt inhibitory factor 1

WIP – Wiscott-Aldrich syndrome protein- interacting protein
   (see: N-WASP; syn. – PPRL-2)

WISP – CCN family glycoproteins

Wnt – Wnt morphogen family, components of Wnt
   signaling pathway

Wrch – Wnt-1-responsive Cdc 42 homolog 1 (syn. – RhoU) (see: Cdc)

X

XBP-1 – X box-binding protein 1, a transcription factor

XDL156 – a zinc finger containing transcription factor

XRP – retinoid receptor

Xvex – homeotic genes family

Y

Yes – proto-oncogene tyrosineprotein kinase

YKL-39 – chitinase-3-like protein 2, gene CHI3L2 encoded
   chondrocyte protein

YKL-40 – chitinase-3-like protein 1, gene CHI3L1encoded
   chondrocyte glycoprotein

Z

ZBTB16 – ZBTB16 encoding human gene

ZBTB16 – zinc finger and BTB domain- containing protein 16

Zfx – Zinc finger protein X-linked, a multifunctional nuclear protein

Zic1 – zinc finger nuclear protein, Wnt morphogens expression activator

Zic3 – Zic family member 3 heterotaxy 1, embryonic stem cell zinc
   finger nuclear protein

ZO-1 – zona occludens 1 (tight junction protein 1), marker of epithelial cells

αCGRP – α-calcitonin gene-related peptide

β-ig-h3 – protein induced by growth factor TGF-β
   (syn. BIGH3, keratoepithelin, RGD-CAP

δEF – elongation factor delta, eukaryotic translation
   elongation factor complex member

INDEX

A

Achilles tendon, 157
Actin filaments, 21, 27, 183, 362
Activating transcription factor 4 (ATF4), 510
Actomyosin microfilaments, 24
ADAMTS (a disintegrin and metalloproteases with
    thrombospondin motifs), 187
Adenosine monophosphate (AMP), 397
Adenosine triphosphate (ATP), 84
Adhesion loci, 183
Adhesive junctions (AJs), 357
Adipocytes, 56, 211, 213. *See also* Adipose cells
    biochemical characteristics, 64
    biomolecular characteristics, 64
    differentiated, 65
    gene expression, 65
    leptin, as source of, 439
    lipases, 65
    phenotyoes, 67
Adipogenesis, 66, 206
Adiponutrin, 65
Adipose cells
    biochemical characteristics, 64
    biomolecular characteristics, 64
    brown adipose tissue (BAT); *see* Brown adipose tissue (BAT)
    description, 56
    fat accumulation, 57
    fat deposition, 57
    fat-inducing transcripts, 64
    histophysiologic characteristics, 56–57
    metabolism, 56–57
Adrenal medulla, 436
Adrenomedullin, 436
Advanced glycation end-products (AGEs), 201–202
Adventitial cells, 211
Aggrecans, 176, 298, 301, 305, 326, 478
Aging
    adipogenesis, impact on, 206
    bone tissue, 451
    characterizations of, 200
    connective tissue changes, 205–206
    epigenetic influences, 200
    genetic factors, 200
    glycosaminoglycans, changes in, 205
    light aging, 200
    process, 200
    signs of, 200
Agrin, 150
Allysine aldol, 91
Amianthoid, 327
Amino acids
    regular tripeptides, 80–81
    residues, 4
    sticky, 184
Amphiarthrosis, 479–480, 480
Amylin, 436
Androgens, 318, 436–437
Annexins, 313, 397
Aponeurosis, 169
Apotosis, 200–201, 358, 394, 451

Aquaporins, 181
Arthritis, 297
Asporin, 306
Auricle tissue, 275
Autocrine, 193

B

B-lymphocytes, 77
Bamacan, 150
Barium, 386
Basement membranes (BMs)
    appearance and description, 144
    biochemistry, 144–145
    collagens of, 145, 148
    laminins, 148–149
    overview, 144
    structure, 144
Basic metabolic units (BMUs), 434, 451, 452
BAT. *See* Brown adipose tissue (BAT)
Bcl-2 gene, 451
Beta-catenin, 487
Bisphosphonates, 400
Blastocysts, 14
BMPs. *See* Bone morphogenetic proteins (BMPs)
Bone fusion, 531
Bone marrow, 211, 213, 215. *See also* Bone tissue
    stem cells, 323
    stroma, 355
Bone mineral density (BMD), 434, 440
Bone morphogenetic proteins (BMPs), 7, 320–321, 445t, 446, 447,
    448, 489, 490, 491, 492, 512, 531
Bone tissue. *See also* Bone marrow
    aging, 451
    biomechanical properties, 410–411
    blood supply of, 244
    bone morphogenetic proteins; *see* Bone morphogenetic proteins
    bone morphogenetic proteins (BMPs); *see* Bone morphogenetic
        proteins (BMPs)
    bone organ, 209
    bone proper, 209
    canals, bone, characteristics of, 411, 419, 421
    cell distribution, 218–219, 224
    cell division, 225, 230, 231, 236
    cell types, 211, 215, 217–218, 225, 231
    chemical composition, 343, 345, 376
    collagenous proteins in, 346
    colony formation, 230–231
    constituents, 208
    cranial bones, of, 343
    demineralization, 405
    formation, 246
    functional characteristics, 209
    growth plates, 247
    heterogeneous crystallization, 394
    hormones regulating, 421, 434
    innervation, 244
    lamellae, 375, 376, 387
    lamellar, 342–343
    lipids in, 374–375
    macro-architectonics, 361

matrix vesicles (MVs), 394, 397
mature, 342, 346, 348, 355
metabolic functions, regulation factors of, 443–450
mineral, 400
morphogenesis, 421, 437
multiphasic nature of, 343
non-collagenous components, 371, 373–374
osteoblasts; *see* Osteoblasts
osteoclasts; *see* Osteoclasts
osteocytes; *see* Osteocytes
osteons; *see* Osteons
osteopontin; *see* Osteopontin
partially demineralized bone matrix (DBM, PDBM), 405
phosopholipids in, 375
preosteoblasts; *see* Preosteoblasts
prostaglandins, relationship between, 442
remodeling/rebuilding; *see* Bone tissue remodeling
reticulofibrous, 342
rough fibrous, 342
structural foundation of, 208
structure, 209, 225, 227, 342
tibia, of, 345
Bone tissue remodeling
    characteristics, 450
    classifications, 450
    complexity of, 455
    defining, 450
    mechanisms of, 450–451, 454–456
    pathological, 450
    physiological, 450
    reparative, 450
    stages, 450
Bowman's layer, 161
Brown adipose tissue (BAT), 57, 62, 64, 67
Byglycan, 136

C

C-calcitriol, 438
C-jun N-terminal kinase (JNK), 505
C-Krox factor, 88
C-peptide, 177
C-procollagen proteinase, 177
C-type natriuretic peptide receptor (NPR-C), 356
Cadherins, 181–182, 498
Calcitonin, 318, 435–436, 442
Calcium, 203, 345, 381, 386, 397, 454
Calcium pyrophosphate dihydrate (CPPD) crystals, 298
Calcium salts, 400
Calcium/calmodulin (CaMKII), 520
Calcyclin, 397
Calmodulin, 297
CAMP, 498
Cartilage, 209, 211
    articular, 249–250, 275, 284, 286, 294, 323–326
    cartilage intermediate layer protein (CILP); *see* Cartilage intermediate layer protein (CILP)
    cartilage link protein gene (CTRL1); *see* Cartilage link protein gene (CTRL1)
    cell types, 269
    characteristics, 246

chondrocytes, 250, 255–256, 262–263, 265, 269, 270, 285
connective tissue, relationship between, 247
costal, 298
cultures, tissue, 313
differons, 249–250
elastic cartilage-cartilaginous tissue, 327
epiphyseal, 298
extracellular matrix, 275, 299–300
fetal, 300–301
fibrous cartilage-cartilaginous tissue, 334, 336, 339
hyaline non-articular cartilage-cartilage tissue, 326–327
metabolism, 314–316
mutations, genetic, 269–270
polymorphism, 256
proteoglycans in, 301
regulation of metabolic functions, 317–320
tissue types, 246
Cartilage end-plate (CEP), 327
Cartilage intermediate layer protein (CILP), 249, 298
Cartilage link protein gene (CTRL1), 304
Cartilage matrix protein (CMP), 311
Cartilage oligomeric matrix protein (COMP), 176, 297, 447, 506
Cartilage-derived morphogenetic proteins (CDMP), 321–322, 444, 445t
Cathepsins, 368
Caveolae, 489
Caveolin-1, 64
CD14-positive monocytes, 68
CD44, 138, 312–313
CDMP. *See* Cartilage-derived morphogenetic proteins (CDMP)
CDNA, 110–111, 314
Cell adhesion molecules (CAM), 181
Cells
    differentiation, 14–15
    extracellular matrix surrounding, 4
    significance of, 4
CEP. *See* Cartilage end-plate (CEP)
Chaperones, 49, 89, 179
Chemerin, 66
Chemical mediators, 7
Chemokines, 194
Chondoblastic differentiation, 500–501, 503–504
Chondroadherin, 299
Chondroblasts, 250, 270, 300, 522. *See also* Chondrocytes
Chondrocalcin, 177
Chondrocyte expressed protein (CEP), 265
Chondrocytes
    cartilage, relationship between, 250, 255–256, 262–263, 265, 269, 270, 275, 285, 297
    differentiation, 322
    expression, 300
    hormonal influences, 317
    IL-4, 326
    perception of, 313
    shapes, 326
    spatial fixation, 298
Chondrodisplasias, 448
Chondromodulin-II, 300
Chorda, 12
Chromatin, 190
Clusterin, 204–205

Collagens, 9, 54
    adjacent fibers of, maximal distances between, 153
    aging, 451
    basement membranes, of; *see* Basement membranes (BM)
    biochemistry of, 80
    defining, 80
    disulfide bonds, 90
    dynamic structuring, 95
    families of, 87
    fiber-forming, 80, 95
    fibrils, 90, 92, 93, 95, 97–98, 309, 311, 312, 327, 386
    fish, in, 80
    flattened, 161
    intermolecular crosslinks, 86
    invertebrates, of, 80
    mammalian, 80
    microfibrils, 109
    non-fibrillar, 92
    proteins, 80, 81, 87, 97
    reptiles, in, 80
    segments long spacing (SLS), 85, 95
    shape, 375
    structure of, 155, 157, 410
    synovial membrane, as component of; *see under* Synovial mem-
        brane
    synthesis, 87
    transmembrane types, 184
    type I, 84, 90, 172, 271, 370, 374, 398, 434
    type II, 86, 88, 92, 271, 272, 273, 274, 275, 311, 316, 321, 398
    type III, 86, 92, 370, 371
    type IV, 145, 161, 169, 243, 306
    type IX, 272, 273, 274, 275, 311
    type V, 86, 92
    type VI, 87, 174–175, 275, 311, 370, 474
    type VII, 149, 184, 187
    type VIII, 370
    type X, 318, 394, 398, 533–534
    type XI, 86, 273, 274
    type XII, 173–174, 370
    type XIII, 184
    type XIV, 174
    type XVIII, 145, 148, 370
    type XXIV, 86, 87
    type XXVI collagen macromolecule, 81
    type XXVII, 86, 87
    type XXVIII, 87
COMP. *See* Cartilage oligomeric matrix protein (COMP)
Connective tissue. *See also* specific types and organs
    adipose, 2
    allocation of, 155
    classification, 2
    defining, 2
    density of, 155
    differentiation, 500
    distention of, 153
    elastic fibers, 107
    embryonic histogenesis, 12–13
    evaluating, 3
    extracellular matrix, 2, 8
    fibrous; *see* Fibrous connective tissue (FCT)
    fibrous, dense, regular, characteristics of, 171–177

    formation, 486
    functions of, 3–4, 157
    interstitial space of, 152, 171
    intraorgan, 2
    looseness of, 153–154
    macrophages, 68–69, 72
    mast cells (tissue basophiles) (MC), 72–73, 76
    morphogenesis, 487
    organ structure, specificity of, 2
    organ-specific progenitors, 19
    plasma cells (plasmocytes), 76–77
    skeletal, 2
    stress conditions, behavior under, 157
    structure of, 154–155, 157
    tooth; *see* Tooth connective tissue
Coral skeleton, 410
Cornea, 161, 169
Corticotrophin, 25
CRIPTO (TDGF1), 13
Crystalline hydroxyapatite, 376, 381
CTGF/CCN2, 321–322
CYIQNC-PLG, 441
Cystatin A, 478
Cysteine, 107
Cysteine knot, 446
Cytokine-like protein 1 (CYTL1), 503
Cytokines, 52, 193
    inflammatory nature of, 322
    receptors, 440
Cytoplasmic membranes, 5, 45, 54
Cytoskeletons, 21, 41, 183

D

D-hormones, 438
Decorin, 55, 136, 137, 175
    functions, 180
    rigidity, 180
Dehydromerodesmosine, 110
Delta 1, 497
Dematerialized bone matrix (DBM), 45
Demineralized bone matrix (DBM), 236
Demineralized bone matrix (DBM), 405. *See also* Bone tissue
Demosomes, 183
Dentin. *See* Tooth connective tissue
Dermatones, 11–12
Dermicidin, 478
Desmosine, 110
Desnutrin, 65
Diaphragm, 169
Diarthrosis, 474
Differons, 49
    bone cells; *see* Osteoblasts; Preosteoblasts
    cartilage, 249–250
    fibroblastic, 55, 154
Dimorphism, sexual, 437
Dura matter, 169
Dynactine, 89
Dynein, 89
Dysplasia, 531

E

Earthworm genome mapping, 144
ED-A fibronectin (ED-A FN), 30, 31
Ehlers-Danlos syndrome, 175
Elafin, 204
Elastin, 11
    aging, 115
    cDNA, 110–111
    elastic fibers, relationship between, 110, 112, 115, 121
    insolubility, 109
    overview, 109–110
    premRNA, 111
    structure, 110, 115, 118
Elastokines, 203
EMT. See Epithelial-mesenchymal transition (EMT)
En-1. See Engrailed (En-1)
Enamel, tooth. See Tooth connective tissue
Endoplasmic reticulum, 45
Endosteum, 421
Engrailed (En-1), 531
Enzymes, 4, 8
Epidermal growth factor (EGF), 136, 194
Epiligrin, 149
Epithelial-mesenchymal transition (EMT), 49, 50, 53
ERK1/2, 505
Estrogens, 318, 360, 436–437
Euchromatin, 19
EVEC/DANCE, 129
Exon 2, 502
Extracellular matrix, 2, 45
    cells, relationship between, 4, 181
    classes of, 8
    composition of, 7, 180
    connective tissue, in, 8
    differentiated cells, surrounding, 67
    domain structure, 177
    fibroblasts, relationship between, 25
    fibroblasts, relationship between, 54–55
    isoforms, 177
    macromolecular components, 177, 179
    morphogenesis, role in, 179–180
    myofibroblast differentiation, role in, 52
    polymers' construction, 177
    production of, 181
    proteins, formed by, 6–7
    self-assembly, 180
    stroma connective tissue, of, 243

F

F-actin, 21
Fascia, 169
Fatty acids binding protein (FABP4), 65
Fatty acids synthase, 65
Femural chondyles, 285
Fibrillin, 9, 107
    elastic structures, in, 121
    microfibrils, 109, 121
Fibrillin-1 (FBN-1), 107, 205, 371
Fibrillin-2 (FBN-2), 107, 371

Fibrillin-3 (FBN-3), 107
Fibrillinopathy, 109
Fibrillogenesis, 93, 95
Fibrils, 112, 115
    collagen; see under Collagen
    elastic, 327
    skeletal, 112, 115
Fibroblast growth factors (FGFs), 320, 322, 448, 449, 489
Fibroblasts
    actin filaments; see Actin filaments
    activation protein alpha, 50
    collagens, 49, 50
    culturing conditions, under, 33–34, 38, 41, 55
    dermis, 49, 50, 51
    differon functional program, 49
    epithelial cells, relationship between, 25
    extracellular matrix, relationship between, 25, 54–55
    fibroclasts; see Fibroclasts
    fibrocytes; see Fibrocytes
    growth factor; see Fibroblast growth factors (FGFs)
    heterogeneity, 45, 50
    lymphocytes, relationship between, 25
    macrophages, relationship between, 25
    mast cells, relationship between, 25
    morphology, 51
    myofibroblasts; see Myofibroblasts
    phenotypes, 26, 45, 49
    polymorphism, 21
    proliferation, 19, 25–26
    properties of, 54
    reparative, 26–27
    role of, 21
    smooth muscle cells, relationship between, 25
    specific protein 1, 49
    structural dynamics, 41, 45
    systemic regulation factors, role in, 25
    topographic differentiation, 50
Fibroclasts, 19, 31, 33
Fibrocytes, 19, 52–53
    forms of, 26
Fibromodulin, 138, 175
Fibronectins, 299, 373, 474
    blood, 128
    functions, 127, 128
    intracellular processes, influence on, 128
    microfibrils, 128
Fibrous connective tissue (FCT), 2
    cells of, 18
    collagens; see Collagens
    dermis, 157
    differon, cells of, 18, 19
    helical form of, 98
    overview, 80
    structures of, 80
    tissue level, 101
Fibrous membranes, connective tissue in, 169, 171
Fibulin-1, 111
Fibulin-2, 111
Fibulin-5, 111, 129
Fibulins, 111
    cardiac valves, in, 129

functions, 129
  isoforms, 111–112
Filamin, 183
Fimbrin, 183
Fixed-charge density, 311
Flotillin-2, 489
Focal adhesion kinases (FAK), 312
Focal adhesions, 54, 183
Focal contacts, 183
Four-and-a-half Lim 2 (FHL2), 510
Frizzled family. *See* Fzd receptors
Fzd receptors, 487, 488

G

Galactosamine, 247
Gelatinases, 187
Gene regulatory network, 494
Gene-related peptides, 435
Genomes, 5. *See also* specific genomes, genes
  earthworm, mapping of, 144
Ghrelin, 531
Glucocorticoids, 25, 317, 436
Glucosamine, 247
Glucosepane, 201
Glucosylgalactosylpyridinoline non-reducib-le cross-link
  (Glc-Gal-PYD), 475
Glycine, 109
Glycoconjugates, 9
  biochemical properties, 121, 125
  non-collagenous, 346
  overview, 121
  secretion, 121
Glycome, 205
Glycoproteins, 530. *See also* specific glycoproteins
  biochemical characteristics, 294
  functions, 125, 128, 129, 130–131, 132
  laminin-like, 149, 150
  overview, 125
  properties, 127
  proteins, differences from other, 125
  proteoglycans, relationship between, 150, 151
  structures, 125, 127, 128, 129, 130, 131, 132, 294
Glycosaminoglycans, 9, 69, 125, 132, 135, 294, 303
Glycosphingolipids, 375
Glycosyltransferase, 132
Glycotransferases, 140
Golgi apparatus, 121, 348, 358
Granular endoplasmic reticulum (GER), 21
Growth and differentiation factors (GDFs), 489
Growth arrest specific protein 6 (GAS6), 504
Growth factors. *See also* specific growth factors
  bone tissue, accumulation in, 374
  insulin-like growth factors (IGFs); *see* Insulin-like
    growth factors (IGFs)
  overview, 193
  transforming; *see* Transforming growth factors
Growth hormone binding protein (GHBP), 421
Growth hormones, 421
Growth retardation, 439
Guanosine triphosphatase (GTPase), 55

H

Hedgehog (Hh), 486, 487, 488, 489, 514
Helminthiases, 73
Hematopoietic stem cell (HSC), 243
Hematopoietic tissue, 243
Hemidemosomes, 183
Heparin, 130, 151
Hepatocyte growth factor (HGF), 50
Hepatocytes, 127
Hexabrachion, 129
Hexosamines, 247–248
Hey1, 512
Hh. *See* Hedgehog (Hh)
High mobility proteins (HMG), 502
Histones, 271
HMG. *See* High mobility proteins (HMG)
HMGB, 520
Homeoboxes (HOX). *See* HOX genes
Homocysteine, 520
Homologs, 8
Hormones, regulating through, 182, 317, 318. *See also* specific
  hormones bone tissue morphogenesis and function; *see* under
    Bone tissie
D-hormones, 438
  thyroid, 438
HOX genes, 494, 495
Human embryonic stem cells (hESC)
  cytoplasmic membrane, 13–14
  genes in, 13
Hyaladherins, 134
Hyalectans, 135, 305
Hyaline, 527
Hyaluronan, 15, 55, 132, 133, 134, 298, 303, 305, 311, 314, 476.
  See also under Synovia
Hyaluronic acid synthases (HAS), 140
Hydrodynahymic lubrication, 482
Hydroxyapatite, 375
Hydroxylapatite, 457
Hydroxylysyls, 91
Hydroxyproline, 81, 88
Hypertrophic chondrocyte-specific gene product 24 (HCS24), 321
Hypofibronectinemia, 128
Hypothyroidism, 318
Hypovitaminosis A, 319, 320
Hypoxia response element (HRE), 315–316

I

ICAM-1, 475
Ihh. *See* Indian hedgehog (Ihh)
Imino acids, 81, 84
Immunoglobulins, 15
Indian hedgehog (Ihh), 530
Insulin, 320
Insulin-like growth factors (IGFs), 449, 455
Integrins, 182, 184, 313, 360, 369, 506
Interleukins, 194, 326, 434
Intermediate filaments, 24
Intracellular HA-binding proteins (IHABP), 133
Isodesmosine, 110

J

Joint formation, mechanisms of, 534, 536–537
Joint formation, molecular factors, 537–540

K

Kalinin, 149
Keratan sulfate, 132
Keratan sulfate glycosaminoglycans, 482
Keratan sulfate136
Keratinocyte growth factor (KGF), 51
Keratinocytes, 144
Kinases, 452
Klotho, 66
Knee synovia. *See* under Synovia

L

L-ascorbate. *See* Vitamin C
Lactoferrin, 443
Lamellopodia, 24
Lamina spendens, 275
Laminins, 148–149
    basement membranes, relationship between, 151
    binding to, 182
Lapatite, 468
Larynx, 275
Latency-associated peptides (LAPs), 444
Lecticans, 135
Leptin, 67, 439, 440–441
Leucine, 357, 373
Leukocytes, 203–204
Ligamentum flavum, 357
Lipocortins, 313
Lipocytes, 56–57. *See also* Adipose cells
Lipogenesis, 66
LMP-1, 510
Lubricin, 482, 483, 484
Lumican, 306
Lumican deficiency, 175
Lysyl oxidase, 90–91
Lysyls, 89, 91, 110

M

Macromolecules, 7, 8
Maillard reaction, 201, 202, 206
Marfan's syndrome, 371
Matricellular proteins, 125
Matrilin-2, 181
Matrilins, 131, 298
Matrix extracellular phosphoglycoprotein
    (MEPE), 517
Matrix Gla protein (MGP), 300
Matrix metalloproteases (matrixins), 527
Matrix metalloproteases (MMP), 185, 187
Matrix ribonucleic acid (mRNA), 4, 6
    expression, in collagen, 131, 175
    Klotho, in, 66
Mechanotransduction, 183

Meprins, 189
Merosin, 149
Mesenchyma, 376, 500
Mesenchymalepithelial transition (MET), 55, 56
Mesenchyme, 12, 13
Mesenchyme stem cells (MSC), 14, 15
Mesochyme, 14
Mesoderm, 11
Mesogenin 1, 489
Messenger RNA, 269
Metabolism, 4
    biochemistry of, 8
Metalloproteases
    inhibitors, 189
    overview, 187, 189
Metalloproteinase-2 (MMP-2), 26
Metalloproteinases, 185
Micro-ribonucleic acids (microRNA), 13
Microfibril-associated glycoprotein-1 (MAGP-1), 107
Microfibrilopathy, 109
Microfibrils, human embryo, 371
Microfilaments, 21
Microtubules, 24
MMP-1, 527
MMP-13, 527
MMP-14, 527
MMP-9, 527
Moesin, 183
Mohawk gene, 495
Morphogenesis, 437
Morphogens, 8, 193, 194
Mucopolysaccharides. *See* Glycosaminoglycans
Multiplexins, 145
Myofibroblasts, 27
    culturing conditions, under, 55
    cytokines, role of, 31
    extracellular matrix, role of, 52
    origins, 30
    signaling activity, 51–52
Myosin filaments, 21
Myosin light chain phosphatase, 24

N

N-acetylglucosamine, 132
N-cadherin, 475
N-glycosylation, 107
N-linked oligosaccharides, 171–172
N-linked oligosaccharides, 125, 132
Nanocrystals, 400
Nectins, 182
Netrins, 149
Neural tube, 12
Neuropeptides, 194, 441
Neurotransmitters, 441
Nexilin, 183
Nicein, 149
Nidogens, 149–150
Nitric oxide, 322
Normoxia, 315
Notch receptors, 497, 513

Nuchal ligament, 157
Null mutations, 177

O

O-linked oligosaccharides, 125
OCT4, 13
OF450 protein, 355
Oligomeric, 151
Oligosaccharides, 171–172, 322
Oligosaccharides, 125
Ontogenesis, 436–437
Organelles, 64
Ossification, delayed, 439
Ossification, intramembranous, 530
Osteoactivin, 356
Osteoblastic differentiation, 507–508
Osteoblastogenesis, 455
Osteoblasts, 346, 348, 354–357, 421, 434, 440, 530
Osteocalcin, 355, 373, 434, 531
Osteoclasts, 361–363, 363–364, 368, 369, 434, 436, 437
Osteoclasts452
Osteocytes, 358–361, 451, 454–455, 455
Osteogenic cells, 211
Osteonectins, 149, 371
Osteons, 376
Osteopontin, 52, 369, 374
Osterix, 439, 441, 509
Oxytalan, 115

P

P38 MAPK, 505
Paired-box genes (PAX). *See* PAX genes
Palladin, 54
Parathyroid hormone, 444
Parenchymal organs, connective tissue in, 169
Partially demineralized bone matrix (DBM, PDBM), 405. *See also* Bone tissue
PAX proteins, 495
Paxillin, 183
Pentisidine, 201
Peptide hormone parathyroidin (PTH), 318–319
Peptides, 193
Perichondrium, 169
Pericytes, 346
Perididymis, 169
Perilipin, 64
Perilipin A, 64
Periosteum, 169
Periostin, 530
Perlecan, 150, 506
    mice experiments with nil mutation of gene, 151
Peroxisome proliferator activated receptors (PPAR), 65–66
PG-M. *See* Versicans
Phagocytosis, 68
Phenotypes, 5
Phosphotungstic acid (PTA), 85
Phospolipids, 482
Plasmocytes, 76–77
Platelet-derived growth factors (PDGF), 194

Plectins, 149
Pluripotent stem cells, 13
Plutonium, 386
Podosomes, 363
Polycomb, 496
Polypeptides, 421, 443
    assembly, 4
    defining, 4
Porograms, 152
Prefibroblasts, 19
PremRNA, 111
Premyofibroblasts, 30
Preosteoblasts, 346
Presomite mesoderm (PSM), 496
Procollagen, 89
Profilin, 21
Proline, 89, 109
Proline/arginine-rich protein (PARP), 299
Prolyl-3-hydroxylase (P3H), 88
Prolyl-4-hydroxulase (P4H), 88
Prostaglandins, 442
Protein kinase A (PKA), 64
Protein kinases, 498
Proteins, 4. *See also specific proteins*
    biosynthesis of, 4
    bone morphogenetic proteins, 7
    calcium-binding, 397
    cartilage-derived morphogenetic proteins (CDMP); *see* Cartilage-derived morphogenetic proteins (CDMP)
    collagenous, 7, 316, 346
    conservatism, 8
    families of, 6
    function of, 410
    human genome, in, 6
    number of, 6
    structural, 4
    superfamilies of, 6, 7
    vitamin D-binding protein (VDBP), 438
Proteoglycan-4 (PG-4), 249, 478, 482
Proteoglycans, 9, 121, 125. *See also specific proteoglycans*
    biochemical characteristics, 294
    biosynthesis, 132–133, 139, 303
    cartilage tissue, in, 301
    cell membranes, connected to, 138
    classes, 136–137
    description, 132
    functions, 132–133
    ground substance PGs, 141
    hyaluronan; *see* Hyaluronan
    large, 135
    properties, 133
    small leucin-rich proteoglycans (SLRP); *see Small leucin-rich proteoglycans (SLRP)*
    space-occupying, 135
    structures, 132, 133, 175
    sulfation, degree of, 132
    versicans; *see* Versicans
Proteolysis, 203
Pulp, tooth. *See* Tooth connective tissue
Pyrophosphate, 400

R

Radium, 386
RAMPs, 452
RANKL, 363, 369, 435, 437, 438, 440, 451, 459, 520
Reactive oxygen species (ROS), 200
Reggie-1, 489
Repulsive guidance molecules (RGMs), 446
Reticulocytes, 211
Retinoic acid, 493
Retinol. See Vitamin A
Reuss model, 410
Rheumatoid arthritis, 479
Ribosomes, 4, 19
Runx1, 503
Runx2, 356, 363, 439, 455, 507, 508, 509, 512
Runx2/Cbfa1, 356–357

S

SAPL. See Surface-active phospholipids (SAPL)
Sclera, 161, 169
Scleraxis, 172
Secreted modular calciumbinding proteins, 132
Secreted protein, acidic and rich in cysteine (SPARC), 131, 149, 180
Secretion, 6
Segmentation, 496–497
Segmentation clock, 497
Selectins, 182
Semaphorin 3B, 438
Sex steroids, 318
Sexual dimorphism, 437
Short distance regulators, 7
Signaling molecules, 5–6, 8
Skeletal (striated) muscles, connective tissue in, 157, 161
SLRP. See Small leucin-rich proteoglycans (SLRP)
SMAD proteins, 446, 490, 491–492
Small leucin-rich proteoglycans (SLRP), 136, 177, 306, 317, 373
Small-angle x-ray scattering (SAXS), 386
SMOC-1, 132
SMOC-2, 132
Sodium hyaluronate, 141
Somites, 496
SOX2, 13
SOX9, 502, 507
Sox9, 329
SPARC. See Secreted protein, acidic and rich in cysteine (SPARC)
Spectrin, 21
Src family, 498–499
Stem connective tissue multipotent (polypotent) cells (SCTMC), 211
Stem multipotent circulating (mobile) CT-cells, 18
Stem polypotent CT cells, 19
Stomatin, 64
Stromlysins, 187
Strontium, 386
Superficial zone protein (SZP), 305, 492, 493
Surface-active phospholipids (SAPL), 483, 484
Syndecans, 138, 184
Syndesmosis, 479
Synostoses, 531

Synovia. See also Synovial membrane
    alkiline properties, 476
    biochemistry, 477–478
    defining, 476
    distinctness, 479
    hyaluronan, 480–482
    knee, 477
    lubricating function, 482–484
    osmolality, 477
    protein, 477
Synovial membrane. See also Synovia
    collagen components, 474–475
    fibroblasts, 478
    fineness, 474
    glucosylgalactosylpyridinoline non-reducib-le cross-link (Glc-Gal-PYD), 475
    immunohistochemical findings, 474, 475
    joint formation, role in, 536
    overview, 474
    structure, 476, 478
Synoviocytes, 479. See also Synovia; Synovial membrane
SZP. See Superficial zone protein (SZP)

T

T-cells, mature, 19
Tandem proteoglycan repeat units (TPR), 301
Tartaric salts acid phosphatase 5 (TRAP), 362, 369
TASR-1, 502
Tbx6, 489
Tenascin-C, 129
Tenascin-R, 129
Tenascin-X, 129, 175, 180
Tenascins, 128
Tendogenesis, 172
Tenoblasts, 171
Tenomodulin, 171, 172
Teriparatide, 434
TGF-beta, 489
Thermogenin, 67
Thrombospondin-3, 297
Thrombospondins, 130
Thymosine, 21
Thyroid hormones, 438
Thyroid-stimulating hormone (TSH), 439
Thyroxine, 438
TIMP-1, 176
TIMP-2, 176
Tissue inhibitors of metalloproteinases (TIMPs), 26
TNF. See Tumour necrosis factor (TNF)
Tooth connective tissue
    animal, 457
    dentin, 457, 468
    enamel, 468
    human, 457
    pulp, 157
Topographic differentiation, 50
Transcription factors, 316, 509. See also specific transcription factors
Transcriptional regulatory network (TRN), 494
Transcriptosome, 4

Transcytosis, 368
Transforming growth factors
    bone tissue, in, 443–444
    isoforms, 443–444
    regulatory factors, interaction with, 444
Transmission electron microscopy (TEM), 386
Triglycerides, 65
Trithorax (TR XG) group, 496
Tropocollagen, 90
Tropoelastin, 110, 111
Tumour necrosis factor (TNF), 202, 322
Twist-1, 509
Twist-2, 509
Tyrosine, 130

U

Uridine diphosphate nucleotides, 139

V

Vacuolar adenosine triphosphatase (V-ATPase), 368
Vascular endothelial growth factor (VEGF), 194
Vascular endothelial growth factor (VEGF), 363
VCAM-1, 475
Versican, 15, 176, 304, 305
    role of, 181
Versicans, 135–136
Vimentin, 49, 52, 56
Vitamin A, 192–193, 319, 493
Vitamin C, 192, 320, 442, 443
Vitamin D, 319, 438
Vitamin D deficiency, 438
Vitamin D-binding protein (VDBP), 438
Vitamin K, 443
Vitronectin, 130
Voigt model, 410
Von Willebrand factor, 7
Von Willebrand factor A-domain-related protein
    (WARP), 299

W

White adipose tissue (WAT), 67
Wnt, 450, 486, 487–488, 488, 489, 498, 505, 513
Wolff's law, 361

X

Xylosyltransferase, 139

Y

YKL-40, 498

Z

Zinc fingers, 7, 15, 172